André Jaggy (ed.)

Small Animal Neurology

An Illustrated Text

André Jaggy (ed.)

Small Animal Neurology

An Illustrated Text

Associate editor
Simon R. Platt

English translation
Teresa J. Gatesman

schlütersche

© 2010, Schlütersche Verlagsgesellschaft mbH & Co. KG, Hans-Böckler-Allee 7, 30173 Hannover
E-mail: info@schluetersche.de

Original edition: Atlas und Lehrbuch der Kleintierneurologie, 2. überarbeitete und erweiterte Auflage, © 2007,
Schlütersche Verlagsgesellschaft mbH & Co. KG, Hans-Böckler-Allee 7, 30173 Hannover

Printed in Germany

ISBN 978-3-89993-026-9   **1006073810**

CD-ROM included

Bibliographic information published by Die Deutsche Nationalbibliothek

Die Deutsche Nationalbibliothek lists this publication in the Deutsche Nationalbibliografie; detailed bibliographic data are available in the Internet at http://dnb.ddb.de.

Frontispiece: Hand-drawn sketch, neurophysiology introductory course: part 2

To the memory of Rudolf Frankenhauser

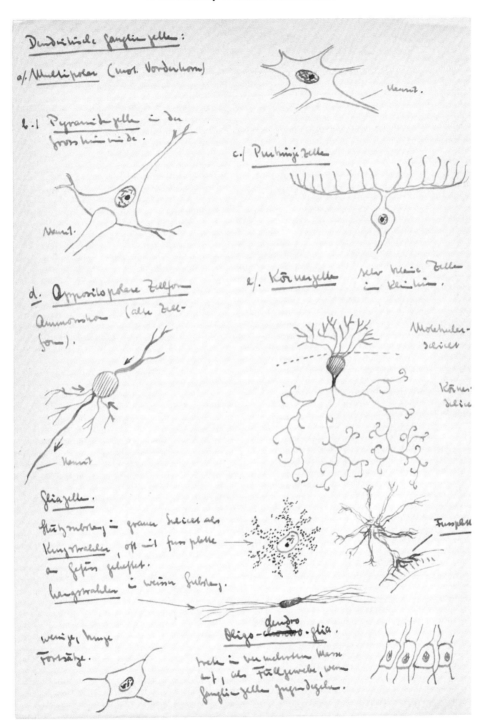

"Everything should be made to be as simple as possible, but no simpler"
ALBERT EINSTEIN

Contents

Contributors

Filippo Adamo DVM Dipl ECVN
President Bay Area VCN (Veterinary Neurology
  Neurosurgery Consulting)
208 Santa Clara Way
San Mateo, CA, 94403
USA
Chap. 13: Peripheral Nervous System and Musculature (co-author)

Gina Aeschbacher DVM Dipl ACVA and ECVA
Senior Assistant, Anaesthesiology
Veterinary Clinical Sciences
Department of Clinical Veterinary Medicine
Vetsuisse Faculty Bern
Länggassstrasse 128
3012 Bern
Switzerland
Chap. 5: Anaesthesia (author) and Chap. 9.3: Analgesics (author)

Susi Arnold DVM FVH PD
Instructor; Head of the Department of Small Animal
  Reproduction
Dept. of Small Animal Medicine / Small Animal
  Reproduction
Vetsuisse Faculty Zurich
Winterthurerstrasse 260
8057 Zurich
Switzerland
Chap. 14.2: Bladder Disturbances (author)

Massimo Baroni DVM Dipl ECVN
Practitioner, Specialist for Veterinary Neurology
Clinica Veterinaria Valdinievole
Via Mascagni 112
51015 Montecatini Terme
Pistoia
Italy
Chap. 15: Vestibular Apparatus (author)

Luciana Bergamasco DVM Prof.
Assistant professor
Via Leonardo da Vinci 44
10095 Gruliasco Torino
Italy
Chap. 7.2.1 Electroencephalography (author)

Massimo Bernardini DVM Dipl ECVN Prof.
Assistant professor
University of Padua
Via Montebello 7
40121 Bologna
Italy
Chap. 14: Spinal Cord (co-author)

Thomas Bilzer DVM Prof.
Professor for Neuropathology
Specialist for Pathology
Institute of Neuropathology of the University Clinic
  Düsseldorf
Moorenstrasse 5
40225 Düsseldorf
Germany
*Chap. 2: Neuropathology (author) and Chap. 18: Cerebrum
(co-author)*

Tim Bley DVM
Assistant Department Neurology
Department of Clinical Veterinary Medicine
Vetsuisse Faculty Bern
Länggassstrasse 128
3012 Bern
Switzerland
Chap. 7.3: Biopsy (author)

Laurent Cauzinille DVM Dipl ECVN and ACVIM
  (Neurology)
Specialist for Veterinary Neurology
Clinique Fregis
43 Avenue Aristide Briand
94110 Arcueil
France
*Chap. 13: Peripheral Nervous System and Musculature
(co-author)*

Iris Challande-Kathmann DVM Dipl ECVN
Assistant
Department of Clinical Veterinary Medicine
Department Neurology
Vetsuisse Faculty Bern
Länggassstrasse 109a
3012 Bern
Switzerland
*Chap. 8: Rehabilitation (author) and Chap. 17.6: Differential
Diagnoses for Primary and Secondary Epilepsy (co-author)*

Sigitas Cizinauskas DVM Dipl ECVN
Lecturer, Head of the Department of Neurology
Department of Clinical Studies
Faculty of Veterinary Medicine
University of Helsinki
P.O. Box 57
00014 Helsinki
Finland
Chap. 16: Cerebellum (author)

Peter Deplazes DVM FVH Dipl EVPC Prof.
Professor in Ordinary, Institute for Parasitology
Vetsuisse Faculty Zurich
Winterthurerstrasse 266a
8057 Zurich
Switzerland
Chap. 20: Parasitic Neurological Diseases in the Dog and Cat
(author)

Dominik Faissler DVM Dipl ECVN Prof.
Assistant Professor Neurology – Neurosurgery
Tufts University
200 Westboro Road
North Grafton MA 01536
USA
Chap. 13: Peripheral Nervous System and Musculature (author)

Gaby Flühmann DVM
Assistant
Institute of Animal Anatomy
Vetsuisse Faculty Bern
Länggassstrasse 128
3012 Bern
Switzerland
Chap. 7: Electrodiagnostics (co-author)

Franck Forterre DVM Dipl ECVS
Senior assistant
Department Surgery
Department of Clinical Veterinary Medicine
Vetsuisse Faculty Bern
Länggassstrasse 128
3012 Bern
Switzerland
Chap. 10: Neurosurgery (co-author)

Claude Gaillard Dipl Ing. Agr. Prof.
Retired Professor in Ordinary, Director of the Institute of
   Genetics, Nutrition and Husbandry of Domestic Animals
Vetsuisse Faculty Bern
Länggassstrasse 109a
3012 Bern
Switzerland
Chap. 3: Genetic Diseases and Breed Disposition (author)

Gualtiero Gandini DVM DECVN Prof.
Department of Veterinary Clinical Sciences
University of Bologna
Via toara di sopra 50
40064 Ozzano Emilia
Italy
Chap. 18: Cerebrum (author)

Frédéric Gaschen DVM Dipl ACVIM and
   ECVIM-CA Prof.
Associate Professor of Veterinary Medicine
Department of Veterinary Clinical Science
Louisiana State University
Baton Rouge, LA 70803
USA
Chap. 4: Laboratory Investigations (author) and Chap. 12:
Peripheral Nervous System and Musculature (co-author)

Nicole Gassner DVM
Department of Clinical Veterinary Medicine
Vetsuisse Faculty Bern
Länggassstrasse 128
3012 Bern
Switzerland
Appendix

Olivier Glardon DVM FVH
Department of Clinical Veterinary Medicine
Vetsuisse Faculty Bern
Bremgartenstrasse 109a
3012 Bern
Switzerland
Chap. 11: Acupuncture (author)

Tony Glaus DVM Dipl ACVIM (Internal Medicine) and
   ECVIM (Internal Medicine and Cardiology) PD
Instructor, Scientific Head of the Department of Cardiology
Vetsuisse Faculty Zurich
Winterthurerstrasse 260
8057 Zurich
Switzerland
Chap. 9.1: Antibiotic Therapy in Neurological Diseases (author)

Thomas Gödde DVM Dipl ECVN
Specialist for Neurology
General veterinary practise
Heurungstrasse 10
83451 Piding
Germany
Chap. 17: Brain Stem (co-author)

André Jaggy DVM Dipl ECVN PhD Prof.
Associate Professor, Departmental Head
Department of Clinical Veterinary Medicine
Department Neurology
Vetsuisse Faculty Bern
Länggassstrasse 109a
3012 Bern
Switzerland
Chap. 1: Neurological Examination of Small Animals (author),
Chap. 2.3: Investigation of the Cerebrospinal Fluid (author),
Chap. 7.2.1 Electroencephalography (co-author), Chap. 13:
Peripheral Nervous System and Musculature (co-author), Chap. 15:
Vestibular Apparatus (co-author) Chap. 16: Cerebellum (author),
Chap. 18: Cerebrum (author)

Konrad Jurina DVM Dipl ECVN
Specialist for Veterinary Neurology
Specialist Veterinary Clinic for Small Animals
Keferloher Strasse 25
85540 Haar
Germany
*Chap. 12: Peripheral Nervous System and Musculature
(co-author)*

Marion Kornberg DVM Dipl ECVN
Specialist for Veterinary Neurology
Pellingerstrasse 57
54294 Trier
Germany
Chap. 14: Spinal Cord (co-author)

Johann Lang DVM Dipl ECVDI Prof.
Associate Professor, Head of Department of Clinical
    Radiology
Department of Clinical Veterinary Medicine
Vetsuisse Faculty Bern
Länggassstrasse 128
3012 Bern
Switzerland
Chap. 6: Neuroradiology (author)

Christophe Lombard DVM Dipl ACVIM (Internal
    Medicine) and ECVIM (Internal Medicine and
    Cardiology) Prof.
Professor in Ordinary for Internal Medicine and Cardiology
Department of Clinical Veterinary Medicine
Vetsuisse Faculty Bern
Länggassstrasse 128
3012 Bern
Switzerland
Chap. 18.6.2: Syncope (author)

Massimo Mariscoli DVM Dipl ECVN Prof.
Assistant Professor
Department of Clinical Veterinary Science
Faculty of Veterinary Medicine
University of Teramo
Viale Crispi 212
64100 Teramo
Italy
Chap. 15: Vestibular apparatus (co-author)

Petra Mertens DVM FTAV CAAB DECVBM-CA
    DACVB Prof.
Assistant Professor
University of Minnesota
College of Veterinary Medicine
1352 Boyd Avenue South
St. Paul MN 55108
USA
*Chap. 19: Behavioural Problems and Disturbances in Behaviour
(author)*

Anne Muhle DVM Dipl ECVN
Specialist for Veterinary Neurology
Centro Veterinario Gregorio VII
Via Gregorio VII 518
00615 Rome
Italy
*Chap. 7: Electrodiagnostics (co-author) and Chap. 16: Brain Stem
(co-author)*

Claudia Reusch DVM Dipl ACVIM and ECVIM Prof.
Professor in Ordinary, Director of Clinic of Small Animal
    Medicine
Clinic for Small Animal Medicine
Vetsuisse Faculty Zurich
Winterthurerstrasse 260
8057 Zurich
Switzerland
Chap. 9.2: Steroid Therapy (author)

Ulrich Rytz DVM Dipl ECVS
Senior Assistant
Department of Clinical Veterinary Medicine
Small Animal Clinic, Department of Surgery
Vetsuisse Faculty Bern
Länggassstrasse 128
3012 Bern
Switzerland
Chap. 10: Neurosurgery (author)

Hugo Schmökel DVM Dipl ECVS
Senior Assistant, Specialist for Veterinary Surgery
Institute of Biotechnology of EPFL LMRP
AA B o46
1015 Lausanne
Switzerland
Chap. 10: Neurosurgery (co-author)

Gabriela Seiler DVM Dipl ECVDI
Lecturer in Radiology
School of Veterinary Medicine
University of Pennsylvania
3900 Delancey Street
Philadelphia PA 19104–6010
USA
Chap. 6: Neuroradiology (co-author)

Nadja Sigrist DVM FVH Dipl ACVECC
Senior Assistant
Department of Clinical Veterinary Medicine
Vetsuisse Faculty Bern
Länggassstrasse 128
3012 Bern
Switzerland
*Chap. 12 Stabilization of the neurological emergency patient
(author)*

Bernhard Spiess DVM Dipl ACVO and
Dipl ECVO Prof.
Full Professor, Head of Department
Department of Small Animals
Department Ophthalmology
Vetsuisse Faculty Zurich
Winterthurerstrasse 260
8057 Zurich
Switzerland
*Chap. 1.5: Ophthalmological Examination (author) and
Chap. 17.3: Neuro-ophthalmology (author)*

David Spreng DVM Dipl ECUS and ACUECC Prof.
Titular Professor
Department Surgery
Department of Clinical Veterinary Medicine
Vetsuisse Faculty Bern
Länggassstrasse 128
3012 Bern
Switzerland
*Chap. 12 Stabilization of the neurological emergency patient
(author)*

Petr Srenk DVM Dipl ECVN
Specialist for Veterinary Neurology
Referral Clinic JAGGY Brno
Komárovská 5
61700 Brno
Czech Republic
Chap. 7: Electrodiagnostics (author)

Frank Steffen DVM Dipl ECVN
Senior House Officer
Department of Small Animals / Neurology –
Neurosurgery
Vetsuisse Faculty Zurich
Winterthurerstrasse 260
8057 Zurich
Switzerland
*Chap. 17: Brain Stem (author) and Chap. 14.2 Bladder
Disturbances (co-author)*

Andrea Tipold DVM Dipl ECVN Prof.
Clinic for Small Animal Medicine in Hanover
Foundation Veterinary High School Hanover
Bischofsholer Damm 15
30173 Hanover
Germany
Chap. 14: Spinal Cord (author)

Marc Vandevelde DVM Dipl ECVN Prof.
Professor in Ordinary, Director of the Department of Clinical
Veterinary Medicine
Vetsuisse Faculty Bern
Bremgartenstrasse 109a
3012 Bern
Switzerland
*Chap. 2.2: Classification of Neurological Diseases: VITAMIN D
(author)*

Cornelius von Werthern DVM FVH Dipl ECVS
Specialist for Veterinary Surgery
Surgical Referral Practise
Centralstrasse 25
6210 Sursee
Switzerland
Chap. 10: Neurosurgry (co-author)

Associate editor

Simon R. Platt BVM&S MRCVS, Dipl. ACVIM
(Neurology) and Dipl. ECVN
Associate Professor Neurology Service
College of Veterinary Medicine
University of Georgia
501 DW Brooks Drive
Athens, GA, 30602
USA

English translation

Teresa J. Gatesman BVSc
Striet 9
37083 Göttingen
Germany

Preface to the English edition

It has been a great honour to edit the English language version of this extremely comprehensive veterinary neurology and neurosurgery text. This is a textbook which could proudly sit next to any of authoritative neurology books of our time. The attention to detail and its clarity in presentation make this a phenomenal reference for veterinary students, clinicians in general practice, neurologists in training, and board certified neurologists all around the world.

In editing this book for a wider English speaking audience, I was able to draw on my experience of clinical neurology in referral practice and academic environments in Europe and in the USA. Such experience has allowed me to understand the views and needs of students and clinicians both in learning and undertaking veterinary neurology from many walks of life. The benefit of the time I have been glad to spend sharing my views with students, interns, residents, and colleagues', learning from them as I go, has helped me undertake this editing role and it is to them that I dedicate this text.

It is a testament both to the authors of this book and the tremendous worldwide advances made in veterinary neurology that only minor additions and amendments were necessary ensuring that disease predispositions, clinician preferences and drug availabilities were geographically addressed. Diagnostic capabilities vary within small geographical areas, let alone between countries, and between the variety of practices and hospitals where we all work. However, this textbook has successfully addressed this issue without the need for any adaptation for the English speaking audience. To me, as I read through this work, it served as tremendous evidence of the globalisation of veterinary neurology and a phenomenal inspiration. We should all be proud, wherever we feel we are in this profession, of the contributions we have made to help in whatever small way to accomplish this.

It would be unfair to identify any of the chapters within this book above another. However, in identifying the unique and therefore outstanding aspects of this book, the chapters on neuroimaging, neurosurgery, neuropharmacology and electrodiagnosis deserve special attention by the reader. The inclusion of MRI based neuroanatomy and frequently used drug appendices are exceptional.

I would like to thank Dr. Andre Jaggy for his friendship and insight over the years and most of all for this excellent opportunity to be involved with this outstanding book.

Athens, October 2009
Simon R. Platt

Preface to the second German edition

»Im eigenen Auge schau mit Lust
Was Plato von Anbeginn gewusst!
Und will Dir's nicht von selbst gelingen
So wird Purkinje Dir es bringen.«[*]

JOHANN WOLFGANG VON GOETHE

The text and figures in the chapters of this second edition have been revised and amended. We have remained true to our maxim of describing the organic diseases so that their weighting, classification, or grouping caters for both the student as well as the practicing veterinarian.

In addition, two renowned specialists – Prof. Spreng and Dr. Sigrist – were won over to allow inclusion of their profound knowledge about emergency medicine into the redesigned Chapter 12. Using simple flow diagrams and clear statements, they have been able to present the complexity of neurological emergencies in a didactically precise manner. Furthermore, the interested reader will find an excellent presentation of magnetic resonance images and macrosections in Appendix 1 (under the title »Comparative sectional anatomy of the canine and feline brain«). The experts – Prof. Lang and Prof. Vandevelde in cooperation with Drs. Gassner, Rossi, and Konar – have made a solid contribution to the understanding of neur-

ological diagnostics with their work here. A clear overview of the most common sequences in MRI diagnostics is given and their implementation is explained in an understandable manner using clinical examples.

I wish to give my thanks to all the coauthors for their contributions. The revision of this book has also caused the publishers an especially large amount of work; therefore, I wish to give a big thanks to Dr. Ulrike Oslage, without whom the second edition would not have been so quickly completed. I would also like to especially thank Bettina Sodemann for her exertions and careful editing.

I wish to send heartfelt thanks also to all the readers and friends whose critical comments have led to the removal of inaccuracies or mistakes. Indeed, we would be thankful for any future critical comments.

Bern, Spring 2007
André Jaggy

---

[*] *»With your own eye show with pleasure, What Plato knew from the start! And if you cannot do it on your own, So will Purkinje teach you.«*

Preface to the first German edition

This book unites a highly motivated and predominantly internationally renowned group of neurologists, radiologists, internists, surgeons, anaesthetists, cardiologists, pathologists, geneticists, behavioural therapists and parasitologists. It was my job, as professor of neurology and neurosurgery at the Vetsuisse Faculty in Bern, to plan, organise and edit the different chapters so that the book is homogeneous – which is most evident in the clinical chapters (12–19).

Most of the neurologists come from the **Bern School of Clinical Animal Neurology**, which was set up by Prof. Marc Vandevelde and then continued by myself in the late 1980s. I am grateful to Prof. Vandevelde and my early mentor – Prof. John Oliver, University of Georgia, USA – as both of them taught me how important it is to always combine clinical experience with relevant research results. I have tried to fulfil this premise with respect to the knowledge in my area of research – epilepsy in the dog – and later in my tuition of students and the further education of veterinarians, both nationally and internationally.

This book consists of two parts. The first part includes the process of the neurological examination, an introductory chapter on neuropathology as well as a somewhat detailed discourse of adjunct examination methods such as electro-diagnosis, laboratory investigations and radiology; without which neurology could not be conceivable. Detailed information about anaesthesia, pharmacology and rehabilitation is also included. The first part is rounded off by chapters on neurosurgery, neurogenetics and acupuncture. The second part of the book is dedicated to the clinical aspects of neurology and is subdivided according to the different sections of the nervous system: from the peripheral structures such as nerves and muscles to the higher centres of the brain.

The practised reader will quickly notice that the different chapters are subdivided according to the acronym VITAMIN D and then follow the respective incidences of the diseases.

Despite its extensiveness, this book does not under any circumstances purport to be all encompassing. It is the authors' intentions that the book describes the most important aspects of neurological disease. The literature listed in the text enables the reader to easily acquire in-depth information about the individual facets. The diagnosis of neurological disease is not conceivable without the examination methods shown in great detail in the illustrations. However, the authors see in these methods primarily a means of confirming a previously formulated tentative clinical diagnosis. The latter is achieved as a rule from a careful anamnesis, a thorough clinical investigation and a precise localisation. May this book serve in the further development of this knowledge.

A CD-ROM has been produced as an accompaniment to the book to provide a better understanding of the neurological examination and so, the anatomical localisation of the lesion. Nine neurological cases for self-evaluation have been included. My thanks go to Dr. Fabrice Hamann and Dr. Sam Jaggy, who both did so much for the realisation of this project.

The authors also wish to thank Dr. Ulrike Oslage of the Schlütersche Verlagsgesellschaft for the careful design and production of this book.

Many people have helped in the acquirement of literature and pictures, in the critical appraisal of the chapters and the careful production of the appendices. Our especial thanks go to Tim Bley, Yvonne Reimer, Ales Tomek, Martin Konar and Patrick Kirchner. We also wish to particularly thank Stan Demiere for the graphics and line drawings. In addition, special thanks should go to my colleague, Johann Lang for the radiographs, CT and MRI pictures.

I feel a need to thank all those who have helped us in various ways in our work: the academic and technical co-workers at the Clinic for Small Animal Medicine; the veterinarians and specialists who referred patients to us – without these, we as a predominantly referral practise would be on a very weak footing – the students who challenge us daily, who criticize and bring us back to reality, who give meaning to our teaching and provide us with pleasure. Merci …

Bern, October 2004
André Jaggy

For Danielle
My thanks to her for her love, support and understanding
as well as for my sons, Thomas, Stefan and Samuel.

Abbreviations

5-HT	5-hydroxytryptamine (serotonin)	EMG	electromyogram / electromyography
AASL	atlanto-axial subluxation	EPA	tissue-type plasminogen activator
ACE	angiotensin converting enzyme	EPSP	excitatory postsynaptic potential
ACh	acetylcholine	ERG	electroretinogram
ACP	acupuncture	Ext	extensors
ACTH	adrenocorticotrophic hormone	FeLV	feline leukaemia virus
AEP	auditory evoked potentials	FET	functional electrical therapy
ALAT	alanine aminotransferase	FIP	feline infectious peritonitis
ALD	acral lick dermatitis	FIPs	fibrillation potentials
ALT	alanine aminotransferase	FIV	feline immunodeficiency virus
ANA	antinuclear autoantibodies	FLAIR	fluid light attenuation inversion recovery
ANS	autonomic nervous system	Flex	flexors
AP	alkaline phosphate	FLM	fasciculus longitudinalis medialis
aPPT	activated partial thromboplastin time	FR	reticular formation
AST	aspartate aminotransferase	free T_4 or fT_4	free biologically active thyroxin fraction
ATP	adenosine triphosphate	FSE	feline spongiform encephalopathy
BAEP	brain stem auditory evoked potentials	GABA	γ-aminobutyric acid
BD	Borna disease	Gd	gadolinium
BDV	Borna disease virus	Gd-DTPA	gadolinium diethylenetriaminepenta-acetic acid
BID	twice daily		
BSE	bovine spongiform encephalopathy	GFAP	glial fibre protein
cAMP	cyclic adenosine monophosphate	GGT or γ-GT	gamma glutamate transferase
CBASS	completely balanced steady state	GI	gastrointestinal
CBC	complete blood count	GLDH	glutamate dehydrogenase
CBF	cerebral blood flow	GME	granulomatous meningoencephalitis
CCSM	cervical caudal spondymyelopathy	GOBF	giant onion bulb formation
CD	cognitive dysfunction	Hct	haematocrit
cGMP	cyclic guanidine monophosphate	HE	hepatoencephalopathy
CK (= CPK)	creatine kinase (= creatine phosphokinase)	HU	Hounsfield units
CMAP	compound muscle action potential	HVSF	high voltage, slow frequency (activity)
CMO	craniomandibular osteoarthropathy	Hz	Hertz
CMO_2	cerebral oxygen consumption	ICP	intracranial pressure
CN	cranial nerve	IgA	immunoglobulin A
CNS	central nervous system	IgG	immunoglobulin G
CPP	cerebral perfusion pressure	IgM	immunoglobulin M
CRC	corrected reticulocyte count	IM	intramuscular
CRH	corticotrophin releasing hormone	IP3	inositol triphosphate
CSF	cerebrospinal fluid	IPSP	inhibitory postsynaptic potential
CT	computed tomography	IR	inversion recovery
cTSH	canine thyroid stimulating hormone	IU/kg	international units / kilogramme body weight
CVP	central venous blood pressure		
DD	differential diagnosis	IV	intravenous
DIC	disseminated intravascular coagulation	LAD	leucocyte adhesion protein deficiency
DISH	disseminated idiopathic skeletal hyperostosis	LDH	low density lipoproteins
		LMN	lower motor neuron
DLSS	degenerative lumbosacral stenosis	LMNS	lower motor neuron system
DV	dorsoventral	LSD	lysosomal storage disease
EAP	electroacupuncture	LVFA	low voltage, fast activity
ECT	emissions computer tomography	MAC	minimal alveolar concentration
ED_{50}	effective dose 50	MAO	monoamine oxidase
EEG	electroencephalogram / electroence-phalography	MAOB	monoamine oxidase B
		MAP	mean arterial blood pressure

MCE	multiple cartilaginous exostoses
MCHC	mean corpuscular haemoglobin concentration
MCV	mean corpuscular volume
MEP	miniature endplate potential
MHC	major histocompatibility complex
mNCV	motoric nerve conduction velocity
MP	myotonic potential
MPS	mucopolysaccharidosis
MPSS	methylprednisolone sodium succinate
MR	magnetic resonance
MRI	magnetic resonance imaging
mRNA	messenger RNA
NCV	nerve conduction velocity
NMDA	N-methyl-D-aspartate
NMR	nuclear magnetic resonance
NSAID	non-steroidal anti-inflammatory drug
OAAM	occipito-atlanto-axial malformation
OCD	osteochondritis dissecans
$PaCO_2$	arterial carbon dioxide partial pressure
PaO_2	arterial oxygen partial pressure
PCR	polymerase chain reaction
PET	positron emission tomography
PLR	pupillary light reflex
PMMA	polymethylmetacrylate
PMP	pseudomyotonic potentials
PNCV	peripheral nerve conduction velocity
PNS	peripheral nervous system
PO	per os, orally
PSS	portosystemic shunt
PSW	positive sharp waves
PU /PD	polyuria/polydipsia
Pw	proton weighted
QID	four times daily
REM	rapid eye movement
RMI	reticulocyte maturation index

RNA	ribonucleic acid
RNS	repetitive nerve stimulation
RPI	reticulocyte production index
RT-PCR	reverse transcriptase polymerase chain reaction
SA	stimulation artefact
SBM	submaximal stimulation
SID	once daily
SSRI	selective serotonin reuptake inhibitor
SSS	sick sinus syndrome
SPECT	single photon emission tomography
SPM	supramaximal stimulation
SRME	steroid-responsive meningoencephalo-myelitis
STIR	short T1 inversion recovery
$t_{1/2}$	elimination half-life
T1	T1 relaxation time
T1w	T1-weighted
T2	T2 relaxation times
T2w	T2-weighted
T_4	serum thyroxin
TBE	tick-borne encephalitis
TCM	traditional Chinese medicine
TENS	transcutaneous electrical nerve stimulation
TID	three times daily
tPA	tissue plasmogen activator
TPA	tissue polypeptide antigen
TRH	thyrotropin releasing hormone
TSH	thyroid stimulating hormone
UE	uraemic encephalopathy
UMN	upper motor neuron
UMNS	upper motor neuron system
V	volt
VD	ventrodorsal
VLDH	very low density lipoprotein
WHO	World Health Organisation

V
I
T
A
M
I
N

D

Instructions for the Reader

The authors have followed the acronym VITAMIN D for the clinical diagnosis of neurological diseases. Due to their colour coding, these tables can be quickly found in the respective chapters. If no clinically relevant disease has been documented, the letter for that group of diseases has been left out.

1 Neurological Examination of Small Animals

André Jaggy
Bernhard Spiess

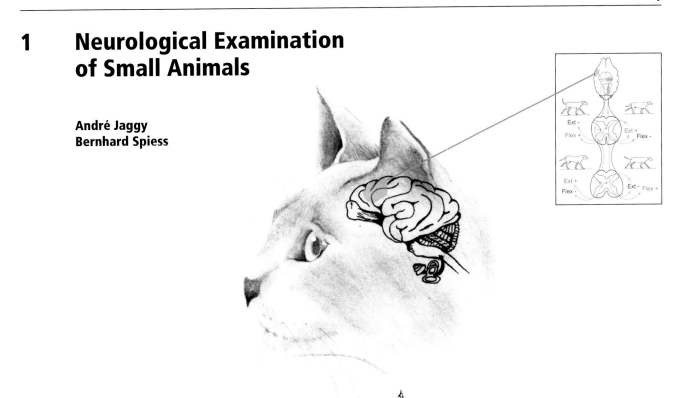

The neurological examination is the basis of clinical neurology and serves to recognize abnormal clinical signs. Identifiable pathological symptoms form the fundamental framework of neurological syndromes.

The aims of the examination are:
- Confirmation and differentiation of neurological and non-neurological abnormalities.
- Localisation of the lesion in the central (CNS) or peripheral (PNS) nervous system.
- Determination of the severity of the lesion(s).
- Development of a differential diagnosis and prognosis.

The neurological examination, therefore, forms an integral part of the clinical examination. After the determination of the localisation and the suspected diagnoses, more specific investigations can be undertaken to establish the exact cause of the disease which will help to predict a more accurate prognosis.

1.1 Signalment

Some neurological diseases are more common in specifc breeds (e.g. disc herniation in the Dachshund, epilepsy in the Golden Retriever, syringomyelia in the Cavalier King Charle's spaniel or hydrocephalus in the Chihuahua), while others are more common at certain ages (e.g. hereditary and infectious disease in puppies and young dogs, degenerative or neoplastic changes in older/geriatric animals). In some diseases, a sex predisposition has been observed (see Appendix 2). In addition, functionally related disturbances in the CNS due to hypoglycaemia can occur in dogs trained for specific purposes (e.g. police or hunting dogs) or in toy breeds on poor diets.

1.2 Anamnesis

The neurological examination always begins with a determination of the history of the case (anamnesis). This is the initial and most important element on the way to determining the differential diagnosis and in certain cases can be used to predict the diagnosis. The observations and comments of the owner or care-giver are essential for the interpretation of all further examinations, but should be judged carefully. Certain clinical signs can be better delineated/defined by well aimed questioning. The onset and course of the disease (acute, chronic, intermittent, progressive, non-progressive, relapsing) must be taken into consideration. An acute onset of clinical signs can indicate (a) toxicosis, (b) trauma, (c) vascular insult, (d) inflammatory disease, or (e) neoplasia. In comparison, a

1

chronic progression can be indicative of a degenerative, neoplastic or infectious aetiology. It is important to determine whether or not the process is progressive (as in degenerative myelopathy in the German Shepherd dog), non-progressive (as in traumatic lesions) or relapsing (often seen with disc herniations). The description of the initial clinical signs as well as of the subsequent disease development can help to determine a focal (such as vascular or neoplastic disease) vs. a multifocal process (such as inflammation).

Some diseases, such as idiopathic epilepsy in the Golden and Labrador Retrievers, occur in families. In such cases, information about the patient's origin (family tree analysis) can provide the basis for a genetic cause of the disease. Information about possible behavioural disturbances and/or changes in personality should be determined in discussion with the owner/care-giver. This information can be important in the determination of the lesion localisation and the differential diagnosis. For instance, the acute occurrence of unmotivated anxiety attacks or untargeted aggression can indicate either a functional psychomotor epilepsy (temporal lobe epilepsy) or a space-occupying lesion in the cerebrum.

Sometimes there is a relationship between the animal's nutritional status and neurological symptoms; for example, hypervitaminosis A or thiamine deficient encephalopathy, most commonly seen in the cat. The initial origin of the animal (kennel, import, stray, etc.) is important. Previous medical diseases, concurrent medications, toxin exposure as well as the animal's vaccination and worming/parasite status should all be taken into consideration.

1.3 General examination

When there is suspicion of a neurological disease, examination of the extraneural body functions is essential. Accordingly, the general clinical examination plays an integral part in the neurological investigation. Numerous clinical signs can indicate a primary organic disease outside of the CNS or PNS. Even when the patient has been presented with well-defined neurological signs, a systemic cause of the dysfunction (e.g. liver insufficiency, endocrine disease or sepsis) should be investigated.

The differentiation between a focal and a generalised disease process or a primary vs. a secondary disturbance can in some cases be achieved during a general examination. For example, infectious diseases which affect the nervous system are often associated with clinical signs occurring in other organ systems (e.g. respiratory or gastrointestinal symptoms with distemper or toxoplasmosis).

Clinical experience teaches the veterinarian to use routine laboratory investigations and more specialised tests both in a targeted and an economic manner. A useful rule is that the longer a case remains unclear, the more specialised investigations need to be implemented.

1.4 Neurological status

1.4.1 Neurological examination methods

The neurological examination must be undertaken methodically. A logical sequence should be established so that incorrect conclusions are not reached and so that the results can be easily assessed. It is important to write down all the results so that no test or result is forgotten (Table 1.1).

The examination undertaken should be as complete as possible but may be varied from case to case, depending on the size, breed and personality of the animal. Using the following sequence of tests, both the CNS and the PNS are systematically examined from the "higher" to the "lower" centres. The neurological examination can be broken down into several important subdivisions including observation (information about mental status, behaviour, posture and movement), palpation (muscle mass, muscle tone, pain), cranial nerve function, spinal reflex function, superficial sensory function and postural reaction testing.

Manipulations that cause either excitement or pain should not be undertaken at the start of the examination (e.g. the testing of flexor reflexes or deep pain). In order to gain the trust of the animal, it is sometimes advisable to undertake the examination in a playful manner. If the animal is frightened or puts up a fight, then many reflexes and reactions are difficult to interpret.

1.4.2 The sequence of the neurological examination

While questioning the owner or care-giver, the level of consciousness, behaviour, posture and movement of the animal should be carefully observed. The behaviour and movement can be examined in depth at a later time (see Chaps. 1.4.3.2 and 1.4.3.4).

1.4.3 The main aspects of the examination

1.4.3.1 Mental status

The state of consciousness, the animal's behavioural patterns and the ability of the patient to interact with its environs are assessed. Small differences in standard behaviour can be indi-

Table 1.1: Neurological Examination

1. **Consciousness:** normal / abnormal; obtunded / stupor / coma _____

2. **Behaviour:** normal / abnormal _____

3. **Posture:** normal / abnormal _____

4. **Gait:** normal / abnormal _____

5. Cranial nerves		7. Spinal reflexes	
left	right	left	right
		Forelegs	
_____ II Vision _____			
_____ Menace response (II, VII) ___			
_____ II Cotton ball test _____		_____ Ext. carpi radialis _____	
_____ II + III PLR _____		_____ Flexor _____	
_____ Stimulation left _____			
_____ Stimulation right _____		**Hindlegs**	
_____ III, IV, VI Strabismus _____			
_____ VIII + III, IV, VI Nystagmus ___		_____ Patellar _____	
_____ V Sensory _____		_____ Tibialis cranialis _____	
_____ V Chewing _____		_____ Flexor _____	
_____ VII Facial _____			
_____ V, VII Corneal _____			
_____ V, VII Palpebral _____		**Other**	
_____ IX, X Swallowing _____			
_____ X Sensory _____		_____ Perineal _____	
_____ XI Neck muscles _____		_____ Vulvourethral _____	
_____ XII Tongue _____		_____ Panniculus _____	
Muscle palpation _____			
Otoscopy _____		Comments: _____	
Ophthalmoscopy _____		_____	
_____ II Fundus _____		_____	
Comments: _____		_____	

6. Postural reactions		8. Sensation	
left	right		
_____ *Hopping*		_____ Superficial _____	
_____ Front _____		_____ Deep pain _____	
_____ Back _____		_____ Hyperaesthesia _____	
_____ *Knuckling* _____		_____ Hypaesthesia _____	
_____ Front _____		_____ Analgesic zone _____	
_____ Back _____			
_____ *Righting* _____			
_____ Extensor Postural Thrust ___		Comments: _____	
_____ *Wheelbarrow* _____		_____	
_____ *Visual placing* _____		_____	
_____ *Neck extension* _____		_____	
_____ *Placing test* _____		_____	
_____ Tactile _____		_____	
_____ Optical _____		_____	
_____ *Neck reactions* _____		_____	

Evaluation: –2 absent; –1 reduced; 0 normal; +1 increased
PLR: pupillary light reflex

vidual, breed or family specific. Labrador Retrievers, Golden Retrievers and Persian cats are in general very cooperative and sociable. In contrast, other breeds are rather exuberant and difficult to examine. The history of the animal's actions and the owner's opinion will help to classify its behaviour as being normal or not.

Anatomy and physiology
The reticular formation, an extensive nuclear area in the brain stem, extends from the medulla oblongata to the diencephalon and receives information via the majority of the sensory tracts (exteroception, interoception and proprioception), which it then diffusely projects to the cerebral cortex (Fig. 1.1). The functions of the reticular formation are as follows: maintaining consciousness, reflex and reaction readiness, maintenance of alertness and the control of sleep-related activity levels

A focal or diffuse lesion in the brain stem or a diffuse bilateral lesion in the cerebral cortex can lead to an interruption in this feedback control system; the cause of which can be primary or secondary.

Examination and assessment
The level of consciousness can be determined by observing the animal and from the answers to the following questions: Is the animal attentive? Does it react with its environment? Does it react to various stimuli (calling, touching or pain)?

The four levels of consciousness are:
- Normal.
- Obtunded: the animal is awake but disinterested. Almost every disease can be the cause of this state.
- Stuporous: the animal is unconscious and can only be aroused by the application of strong stimuli (e.g. pain). This state is mainly observed in association with an interruption between the reticular formation and the cortex.
- Comatose: the animal exhibits a deep loss of consciousness and does not react even to painful (noxious) stimuli. A coma is often observed when there is a complete interruption between the reticular formation and the cortex. A lesion of the brain stem is the cause in the majority of these cases.

1.4.3.2 Behaviour
Behaviour is the result of a very complex series of physiological processes, whose anatomic features lie in the cerebral cortex and the limbic system.

Anatomy and physiology
Behaviour is controlled by the limbic system and is the result of the interactions of stimuli from the environment and those which originate from within the body itself (Fig. 1.2). Behavioural disturbances can either be of a primary (in association with primary CNS dysfunction) or a secondary nature (e.g. subsequent to systemic disease).

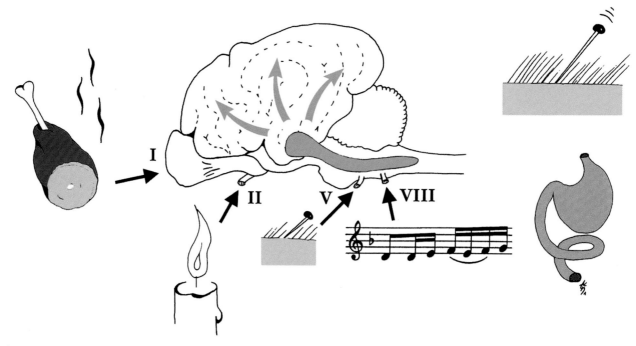

Fig. 1.1
Consciousness. The reticular formation, a fine network that extends from the upper cervical spinal cord to the thalamus, is primarily responsible for consciousness. The rostral part of the brain stem forms a key part in this relay system. It transmits stimuli directly (without an interchange) or indirectly (with an interchange) from the periphery to the cortex, which is neurophysiologically subordinate to it.

Examination and assessment

Fear, aggressiveness, shyness or disorientation are examples of abnormal behaviour. Often these are associated with chewing, licking, yawning and compulsive pacing movements. These signs can rarely be associated with the dysfunction of a single anatomical structure, as the manifestations of disease of the cortex and limbic system are very similar. An indispensable part of the examination is a discussion with the owner or care-giver targeted at elucidating any changes in behaviour as well as prolonged observation in a relaxed environment.

1.4.3.3 Posture

A healthy animal takes on a normal body posture when a standing as it counters the effects of gravity on its body weight. The limbs are in extension and a the line running through the pelvis, back, and chest is parallel to the ground, while the head is held in balance with the neck.

Anatomy and physiology

A reflex arc ensures normal posture. The afferent pathway is the sensory part and this transmits the necessary information from various receptors in the limbs and body, from the eyes, and from the vestibular system via sensory nerves to the CNS. The vestibular receptors are mainly responsible for the appreciation of movement and changes in the position of the head. Receptors in the limbs (e.g. stretch receptors) report on the tension within the muscles, tendons, and the joint capsules. Such information is sent partly via the cerebellum and the brain stem. It is interpreted in the cortex and then transmitted via the efferent (motor) tracts to the α- and γ-motor neurons that innervate the neck, body, and limb muscles. The cerebellum and the vestibular apparatus are also responsible for the maintenance of normal body posture.

Examination and evaluation

When observing the animal, the posture of the head, neck, trunk, and limbs are evaluated. In many cases, variations from the norm are first seen during movement (dynamic posture).

The characteristics of abnormal posture are:
- Head tilted (principally with vestibular lesions).
- Head turned sideways / pleurothotonus (mainly with cerebral lesions).
- Head and neck tilted sideways / torticollis (chiefly with brain stem lesions).
- Head and neck flexed downwards (especially with vestibular brain stem lesions or cervical lesions).
- Kyphosis (especially with spinal cord lesions in the thoracolumbar region; Fig. 1.3a).
- Scoliosis (lateral curvature of the spine; Fig. 1.3c) and lordosis (ventral curvature of the spine; Fig. 1.3b) in diseases of the spinal column.

Reduced muscle tone in a limb or more than one limb results in a wide-based gait or knuckling of the feet (especially with lesions affecting the lower motor neurone system [LMNS]).

Increased muscle tone in one or more limbs is conspicuous as a hyperextension of the affected limbs (stiffness, spasticity). This is seen particularly with lesions of the upper motor neurone system (UMNS).

Opisthotonus (extension of the head and neck) is observed with lesions of the rostral brain stem.

Decerebrate rigidity, an involuntary extension of all the extremities in response to external stimuli, arises with lesions in the rostral brain stem / mesencephalon / pons. In some cases, this can occur in combination with opisthotonus.

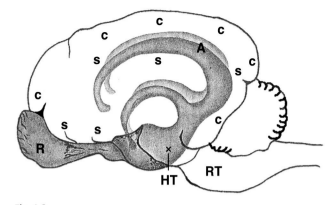

Fig. 1.2
The limbic system consists of the rhinencephalon (R), the hypothalamus (HT), the hippocampus (A), the subcortical (s) and cortical (c) centres and part of the reticular formation (RT). This system is responsible for the complex behaviour of animals.

1.4.3.4 Movement

Anatomy and physiology
Movement with displacement of the body from one place to another in principle requires the movement of the body's centre of gravity forwards, to the side or backwards. This process is regulated by the **afferent** (spinocortical) and **efferent** (corticospinal) tracts (Fig. 1.4a) as well as the **locomotion centres** (Fig. 1.4b).

Afferent nerves
The afferent sensory pathways are categorized according to their target and modality, into spinocortical and the spinocerebellar pathways (Fig. 1.4a).

Efferent nerves
In order to understand the concept of the efferent motor pathways, it is necessary to explain the concepts of the lower motor neuron (LMN) and the upper motor neuron (UMN) (Fig. 1.4a).

The LMN
The lower motor neurons originate as cell bodies in the ventral horn of the grey matter of the spinal cord and the motor centres in the brain stem. There are two types of neurons, α and γ, each of which innervate the striated muscle. Both of these types of neurons can be stimulated or even inhibited at the segmental, intersegmental and suprasegmental levels. The summation of these stimuli determines whether or not the LMN is sufficiently activated to elicit a contraction of the musculature. As the stimulation of the LMN results in muscle contraction, a lesion in the LMN causes a flaccid paresis or paralysis, with reduced or absent reflexes and neurogenic muscle atrophy. Such clinical-neurological phenomena do not occur in lesions of the UMN. Anatomically, the LMN system is composed of the ventral horn (α-motor neurons), the ventral root, spinal nerves, the peripheral nerves, the neuromuscular end-plate and the muscles (target organs).

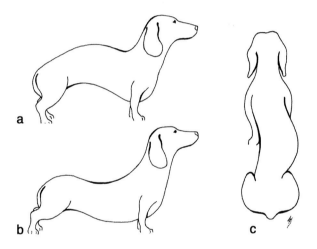

Fig. 1.3a–c
Abnormal body positions: kyphosis (a), lordosis (b) and scoliosis (c).

The UMN
The upper motor neurons (UMN) are suprasegmental neurons, which directly or indirectly influence the LMN or LMNS. In human beings, the UMN is found in the primary motor cortex and affects the LMN or LMNS via the UMNS (corticospinal tract).

The UMNS is more extensive in veterinary neurology as it includes not only **neurons in the cortex**, but also ones in the **basal nuclei**, the **brain stem** and the **cerebellum**. The UMNS influences the LMN via interneurons. The overall effect of the UMNS is an inhibition of the LMN. A lesion in the UMN or UMNS results in a loss of this inhibition (dysinhibition) of the LMN. If the segmental reflex arc remains

1

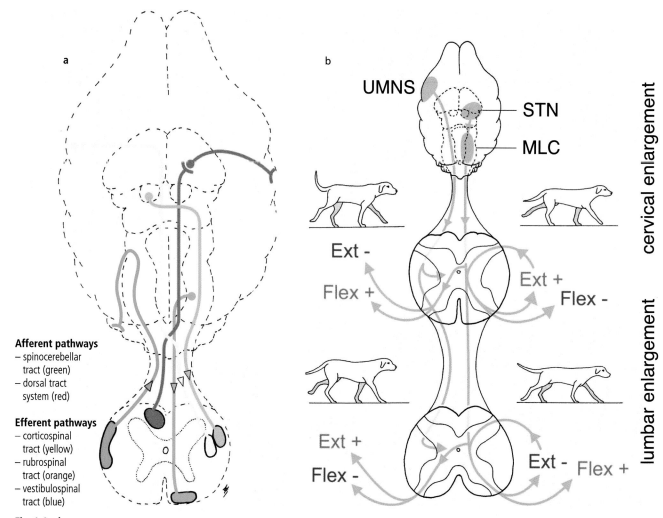

a

b

UMNS

STN

MLC

Ext -

Flex +

Ext +

Flex -

Ext +

Flex -

Ext -

Flex +

cervical enlargement

lumbar enlargement

Afferent pathways
– spinocerebellar
  tract (green)
– dorsal tract
  system (red)

Efferent pathways
– corticospinal
  tract (yellow)
– rubrospinal
  tract (orange)
– vestibulospinal
  tract (blue)

Fig. 1.4a, b
(a) Ascending and descending pathways. The ascending sensory pathways are divided into two main groups according to their target and their modality. In the first group, information reaches the consciousness via the spinocortical tracts, which end in the cerebrum. The second group which deals with the stimuli "subconsciously" end in the cerebellum via the spinocerebellar tracts. This information is very important for the feedback of reflex activation and modulation during movement. In addition to these primary endings, the ascending tracts give off collateral branches, which have synapses at the level of the spinal cord (and that enter the dorsal horn for the activation or inhibition of segmental or intersegmental reflexes) and the brain stem (via the dorsal spinocerebellar tracts to the reticular formation and which are important in the brain stem reflexes). The descending pathways are divided into an upper motor neuron system (UMNS) and a lower motor neuron system (LMNS).
(b) Physiological gait consists of an afferent and an efferent part coming from the cortex, thalamus (subthalamic nuclei, STN), brain stem (mesencephalic locomotion centre, MLC) and the spinal locomotion centres. Each limb has its own pacemaker, which is located in the cervical enlargement for the forelimbs and the lumbar enlargement for the hindlimbs. These two spinal enlargements are coordinated with each other and are influenced by a motor centre in the mesencephalon, which in turn is influenced by a higher centre in the subthalamus. Stimulation of this system results in an alternating flexion (swing phase) and extension (support phase) of the limbs. Together these two dynamic elements form a single step. The flexor and extensor reflexes are proof for the presence of the pacemaker.

intact, the reflexes can be exaggerated (hyperreflexia). The muscle tone can either be normal or increased (spastic). The degree of paresis depends on the extent of the lesion affecting the UMNS.

In addition to an understanding of the LMN and UMN systems, an understanding of the concept of the mechanisms responsible for locomotion, is important in the appreciation of the processes involved in movement.

Locomotion centres
The locomotion centre for the forelegs lies in the cervical enlargement, whilst that for the hindlegs is in the lumbar enlargement (Fig. 1.4).

Relays at the level of a single limb
The stimulation of the skin afferents of a limb results in an activation of the motor neurons of the flexors and an inhibition of the motor neurons of the extensors in the same limb. As a result, the limb is flexed.

Stimulation of the afferent muscle spindles causes an activation of the motor neurons of the extensor muscles and an inhibition of the feedback system of the antagonistic flexor muscles in the same limb. The limb is then extended (support phase).

Relays at the level of a pair of limbs (thoracic or pelvic)

If a limb is in the initial swing phase (extensors −; flexors +), for example in the left leg, then the contralateral limb influenced via an internal feedback circuit comprising segmental reflex arcs, will be in the support phase (extensors +; flexors −). In this manner, it is possible for the animal to balance out its centre of gravity. The crossed extensor reflex indicates damage to this internal feedback circuit; with lesions of the thoracolumbar spinal cord, stimulation of the skin of one pelvic limb, results in an extension of the contralateral limb, in addition to flexion of the stimulated limb. In chronic cases of paraplegia, due to lesions at the level of the thoracolumbar spinal cord, every form of external stimulus can initiate an alternating motor response in the limbs.

In an animal with paraplegia due to a thoracolumbar lesion, it is certainly possible for an incoordinated and involuntary gait (spinal walking) to arise. In spinal walking, the cervical pacemaker centre is stimulated by a displacement of the centre of gravity resulting in the thoracic limbs taking a step forwards. The concurrent displacement of the pelvic region then stimulates the pacemaker centre of the pelvic limbs, and so they then take a pace forwards, albeit in an incoordinated manner

Relays at the level of both pairs of limbs

The coordination of the thoracic limbs with the pelvic limbs is regulated through the cervical and the lumbar enlargements (pacemaker centres). For the production of such movements, both the afferent and the efferent pathways work in consortium with the propriospinal tracts.

Higher centres of locomotion

The mesencephalic locomotion centre (MLC) is responsible for the coordination of spontaneous movement and lies symmetrically and bilaterally at the level of the rostral mesencephalon. Electrical stimulation of this centre leads to both normal and spontaneous movements. Directed spontaneous movement is not possible after experimental sectioning of the rostral mesencephalon. As the subthalamic nuclei (STN) are responsible for the determination or orientation of spontaneous movement, these nuclei are superior to the MLCs.

If a lesion is in the STN itself, then the animal's gait is almost normal; what is missing in such patients is an ability to determine their movements. Often, such patients present with the urge to be always be on the move.

In conclusion, all the important relay stations responsible for the normal sequence of movements involved in gait lie in the subthalamus, the mesencephalon and the spinal cord.

Influences on the locomotion centres

The complex systems described above are physiologically inferior to the cerebral cortex, the cerebellum and the vestibular apparatus. The cerebral cortex is responsible for "will" and decision-making, the cerebellum for the fine tuning of movement and muscle tone, and the vestibular apparatus is responsible for balance and sustaining muscle tone in conjunction with the cerebellum. The influence of these structures on the locomotion centres takes place via the descending motor pathways.

Corticospinal tracts

The motor pathways are subdivided according to their course and their localisation. They are divided into the pyramidal and the extrapyramidal tracts. The **pyramidal tracts** originate in the cerebral motor cortex and extend as "pyramids" to the medulla oblongata. Some tracts leave the main "pathways" at the level of the brain stem to go directly to the brain stem nuclei (corticolbulbar tracts). The rest of the fibres cross over at the level of the medulla and then descend through the spinal cord as the corticospinal tracts (in the lateral funiculi). These tracts synapse via interneurons on α-motor neurons. A lesion of this system results in spastic paralysis. The corticospinal tracts exert their greatest influence **on the distal limb musculature** and are most highly developed in primates, but have minimal function in companion veterinary species.

Extrapyramidal tracts

These tracts have their greatest influence on the proximal limb musculature. They are made of polysynaptic circuits of differing complexities. The **basal ganglia**, **subthalamic nuclei** and the **substantia nigra** (in the mesencephalon) comprise the largest part of this system. The nuclei are connected with the cortex via polysynaptic loops. These regulatory circuits have a direct influence on the nuclei in the mesencephalon and the reticular nuclei in the pons and medulla. The descending tracts of these brain stem and vestibular nuclei have an indirect influence on the LMN.

The descending tracts can be characterised according to their functionality. There is a direct connection between the functional effects of the LMNS and its phylogenetic development. The phylogenetically oldest system is responsible for posture. It has a greater positive effect on the anti-gravity muscles (extensors) than on the gravity muscles (flexors). These tracts contain vestibulospinal and recticulospinal "transmission lines" and are found in the ventral funiculus. The phylogenetically newer motor system is responsible for the initiation and modulation of spontaneous and rhythmic motor actions (running, jumping, etc.). To achieve this, the extensor tonus must be partially reduced, which is made possible via the lateral funiculi (corticospinal, rubrospinal and lateral reticulospinal tracts).

The corticospinal tracts are far better developed in human beings than in animals. Their animal counterparts are the ru-

1

brospinal tracts. The red nucleus is directly affected by the motor cortex via the phylogenetically younger cortico-rubrospinal tracts. Older tracts influence the red nucleus indirectly via the motor cortex and the basal nuclei. The rubrospinal tracts cross caudal to the red nucleus and descend via the lateral funiculi to the segmental interneurons in the dorsal horn of the spinal cord. The vestibulospinal tract is one of the phylogenetically oldest parts of the motor system. The vestibular nuclei receive only a little information from the cortex. They are mainly stimulated by the peripheral vestibular apparatus (inner ear) and modulated by the cerebellum.

Examination and assessment

Abnormality of the gait can be seen as proprioception disturbances, paresis or paralysis, circling movements, ataxia and/or dysmetria.

Disturbances in proprioception

Proprioception is the mechanism involved in the self-regulation of posture and movement through an awareness of the position of the limbs in space. A deficit results in an abnormal placing of the feet or knuckling of the limbs, which is not necessarily seen with every step taken. It can also result in one of the three types of ataxia.

Paresis or Paralysis

Paralysis or plegia is defined as the complete inability to activate one or more muscles. Paresis is an incomplete paralysis. The affected limbs show either inadequate or no contraction of their musculature. Depending on the clinical signs, the following terms are used: **monoparesis** (paresis of one limb); **paraparesis** (paresis of both hindlimbs); **tetraparesis** (paresis of all four limbs); **hemiparesis** (paresis of an ipsilateral pair of limbs); and **claudication** (limping or lameness). The cause of paresis or paralysis lies in a failure of the motor function of a nerve or its target organ, e.g. the muscle. The lesion can lie either in the UMNS or the LMNS. One, therefore, speaks of a UMN or LMN paresis or paralysis.

Depending on the tone in the musculature, paresis or paralysis can be divided into three forms: spastic (increased tone = UMN or central lesion), flaccid (reduced tone = peripheral or myogenic [LMN unit] lesion, or a rarely a chronic central lesion resulting from disuse of the limb(s)) and intermittent paresis or paralysis.

Circling

Clinically, circling movements can be defined as a drifting to one side with either large or small diameters, or as a turning motion. The direction of the displacement is towards the side of the lesion in the majority of cases, but not all. Circling can be seen with prosencephalic or brainstem lesions. Concurrent torticollis and/or head tilt occur mainly in association with lesions in the vestibular system.

Ataxia

A disturbance in the coordination of movement or collaboration of muscle groups is called ataxia. Ataxia can, but not always, be associated with paresis or involuntary movements depending on the localisation of the causative lesion. The degree of the ataxia present may be described as slight, medium or severe ataxia, although this is qualitative, and may be focal or generalised in its distribution. Depending on the location of the responsible lesion, ataxia can be subdivided into peripheral/spinal (proprioceptive), cerebellar, or vestibular forms. The clinical picture depends on the type and form of the ataxia, though it is always important to look for incoordinated movements. A base wide stance, crossing over of the limbs, shortened or elongated stride length are all typical of the majority of the different forms of ataxia. The responsible lesion can be neuro-anatomically located utilising the additional clinical signs present in the patient, and the type of ataxia can be defined. For example, when the cerebellum is affected hypermetria, intention tremors and loss of the menace response may be seen in addition to the ataxia.

Dysmetria

Dysmetria describes stride lengths that are either too big (hypermetria) or too small (hypometria). Often "goose-stepping" strides can be observed: the stride is stopped suddenly and the patient sways. Dysmetria of the head is best seen when the patient drinks or eats and is often termed an intention tremor. The distance to the target (food bowl) is usually overestimated or even underestimated. This form of ataxia can occur with lesions of the cerebellum or the cerebellar pathways.

1.4.4   Postural reactions

Postural reactions entail complex normal regulatory processes in which motor, sensory and coordination pathways are involved. Testing of the postural reactions enables the examination of not only the afferent pathways but also the efferent ones, too. Such testing is also useful in registering subtle abnormalities or for a clearer recognition of a neurological problem. It is very important to compare all four limbs with each other because these tests often show differences between the right and left half of the body, which can assist with developing a differential diagnosis list

1.4.4.1   Hopping on one leg or a pair of legs

Peripheral nerves, the spinal cord, brain stem, cerebellum and cerebrum are all involved in hopping. The hopping test is undertaken as follows: the patient is held so that it stands on one leg or a pair of legs. The patient is then pushed to one side (Fig. 1.5).

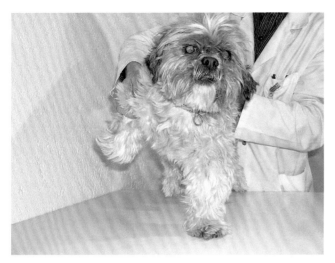

Fig. 1.5
Hopping on a foreleg.

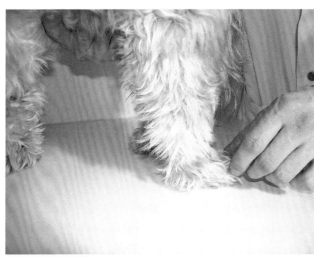

Fig. 1.6
Knuckling of the left hindleg.

An **extension of the supporting leg(s)** followed by a quick correction whilst being pushed to one side is considered as being normal. Abnormal reactions include a **reduced speed of reaction** (mainly a proprioception deficit), an **abnormal placement of the foot** (motor deficit), **hypometria** defined as a reduced correction reaction (lesion in the spinal cord [C6–T2]) and **hypermetria** (cerebellar lesion, spino-cerebellar pathways).

Patients with lesions in the cervical spinal cord cannot hop or stand normally on the ipsilateral pair of limbs.

1.4.4.2   Knuckling
With the knuckling test, both the sensory afferent pathways and the motor efferent pathways in the limb are tested. The former are responsible for the perception of the position of the limb in space, while the latter are responsible for the normal placement of the foot. The distal part of the limb is flexed, so that the dorsal surface of the metacarpus (or metatarsus) lies on the floor. The animal should put its limb back in its normal position within a second. It is remarkable that the musculoskeletal diseases which cause severe disturbances in gait are associated with little or no disturbances in this reaction (Fig. 1.6).

1.4.4.3   Righting reaction
With this test, the ability of the patient to take on a normal position in the gravitational field is assessed. Of the four systems which play a part in maintaining a balanced posture, the visual and the vestibular systems are activated first of all, followed by the proprioceptive and the motor systems (Fig. 1.7).

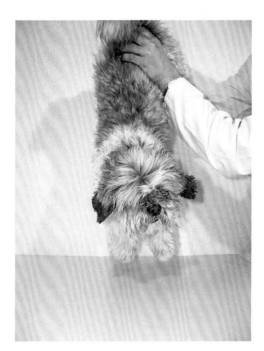

Fig. 1.7
Righting reaction.

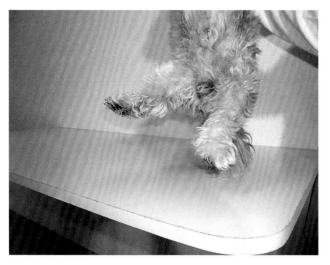

Fig. 1.8
Extensor postural thrust reaction.

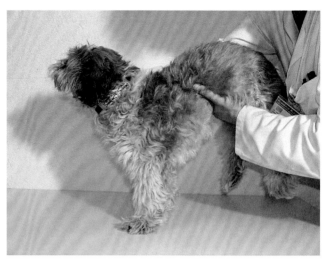

Fig. 1.9
Wheelbarrow.

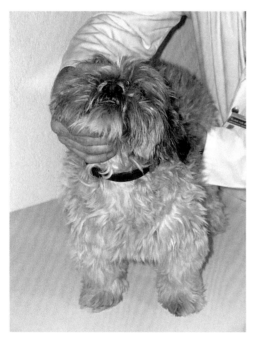

Fig. 1.10
Wheelbarrow with head held high.

There are two methods of testing the righting reaction:
1. The animal is held up by the pelvis and the placement of its head with respect to the body is observed, while the forelegs are well flexed. A body-head angle of 45° is expected in normal cases. If the vestibular system is to be tested, the patient should be blindfolded, although this is rarely necessary.

2. The animal is placed in lateral recumbency and then observed as it gets up. Healthy animals that do not have a one-sided lesion of the vestibular system should first roll onto their sternum and then get up. This is incoordinated or even impossible in an animal with a disease of its vestibular system.

1.4.4.4   Extensor postural thrust reaction

In this two-stage test, the animal is held behind the shoulder blades and lifted so that it no longer touches the floor and then it is carefully placed back on the floor again. **Hyperextension** of the limbs should be observed. In the second part of the test, the animal is pushed gently backwards, so that an **alternating flexion and extension of the hindlimbs** is elicited. Lesions in the spinocortical, corticospinal and the vestibulocerebellar pathways cause disturbances in the movement processes and such clinical signs should be interpreted as pathological (Fig. 1.8).

1.4.4.5   Wheelbarrow test or walking on the forelimbs

Lifting of the patient, whereby the abdomen is supported so that the animal's hindlegs no longer touch the floor, enables the animal's ability to walk on its forelimbs to be judged. Normally, the head is carried parallel to the floor and the animal moves its legs forwards in symmetrical, short and alternating steps (Fig. 1.9). Pathological findings are a hesitant gait, knuckling or buckling of the limbs and a slowing down of the beginning or intention phase of the movement. Severe lesions in the cervical spinal cord cause a severe flexion of the head such that the nose touches the floor. To ensure that the patient can only correct its position using proprioceptive information alone, the wheelbarrow test is done with the ani-

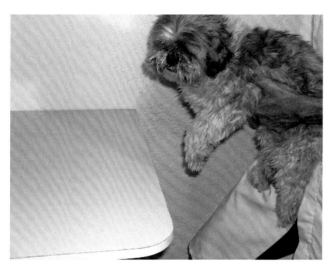

Fig. 1.11
Visual placement test.

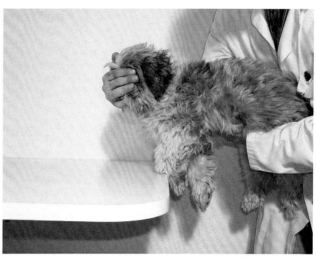

Fig. 1.12
Tactile placement test.

mal's head in extension (head held high) (Fig. 1.10). A slight increase in tone of the foreleg extensors is to be seen. This technique is particularly useful in animals with cerebral lesions as they usually exhibit a normal gait.

1.4.4.6 Placement test

This test has both a visual and a tactile component, which are undertaken one after the other. The visual placement test is very good for testing visual-assisted integration of movement. The animal is held up by its thorax and slowly pushed towards a barrier (table edge or top of a wall). The normal reaction is a coordinated stepping on the barrier without there having been any contact (Fig.1.11).

The tactile placement test is done in a similar manner though the animal is either blindfolded or has its head held in hyperextension. The thoracic limbs are then brought into contact with the edge of the table at the level of the carpus. The animal should immediately pick up its feet and lay them on the table. This test can be repeated with each limb individually, but as an adaptation (quick learning of the reaction) can take place, it is suggested that the animal should be turned around once between each test (Fig.1.12).

Knuckling, awkward or a lack of foot placement, excessive placement movements, excessively slow or a hesitant correction of movements are all to be interpreted as abnormal reactions.

1.4.4.7 Tonic neck reactions

These tests are infrequently done because they are difficult to interpret. The complex reactions to these movements are initiated by the receptors in the cervical muscles and by a fine

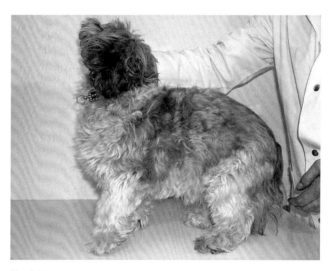

Fig. 1.13
Tonic neck reaction (hyperextension of the forelegs and hyperflexion of the hindlegs).

coordination of the vestibular apparatus with the neck musculature and the receptors in the neck.

This test assesses the normal reaction of a flexion of the pelvic limbs and an extension of the thoracic limbs associated with raising the animal's head. Abnormal reactions are asymmetrical movements, stretching or abnormal bending of one or more limbs (Fig. 1.13).

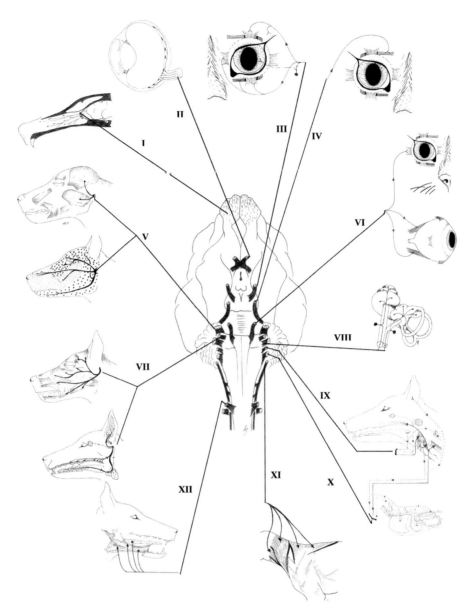

Fig. 1.14
Schematic overview of the twelve pairs of cranial nerves (I–XII). The majority of the cranial nerves originate in the midbrain, pons and medulla oblongata. The two exceptions are the olfactory nerve and the optic nerve.

If the head is bent downwards, a normal semiflexion of the thoracic limbs and an extension of the pelvic limbs occur. If the head is rotated to one side, then an extension of the limbs on the same side can be seen.

Cervical spinal lesions cause an abnormal flexion of all limbs during these tests in most cases.

1.4.5 Investigation of the cranial nerves

1.4.5.1 Cranial nerve function

The cranial nerves (CN) are conventionally numbered from I to XII. They originate either in the brain stem (III–X, XII) or outside it (I, II, XI). Simple examination methods can be used to investigate the functions of all the cranial nerves, which are comprised of motor and/or sensory fibres (Fig. 1.14). Parasympathetic fibres run within CN III (Fig. 1.15), VII, IX and X, while the sympathetic fibres lie separately (Fig. 1.16).

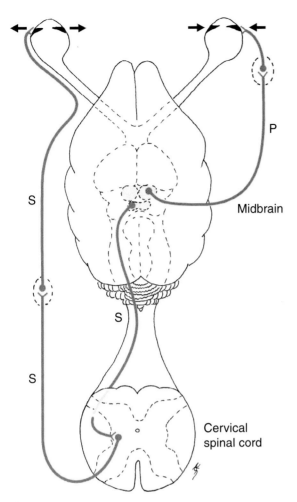

Sympathetic nervous system   Parasympathetic nervous system

1

Fig. 1.15
Parasympathetic (P) and sympathetic innervation (S) of the pupils.
(Pupil dilatation ← →; pupil constriction → ←).

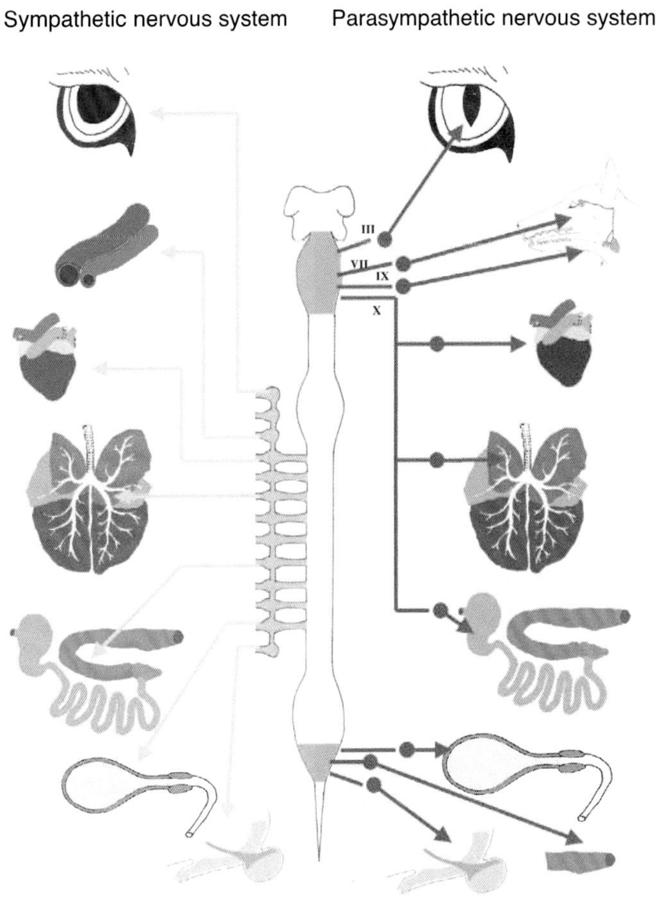

Fig. 1.16
Parasympathetic (red) and sympathetic (blue) innervation of the organs.

I.   Olfactory nerve (sense of smell)

Anatomy and physiology
The chemical stimuli are transferred via the olfactory bulb to the olfactory part of the cerebral cortex for the conscious perception of smell.

Examination and assessment
The anamnesis (the observations of the owner or care-giver) with respect to the animal's behaviour in the presence of food or scents is most informative.

The objective assessment of the sense of smell is very difficult. In the dog, repulsive or pleasant test substances can be used. It should be ensured that substances are not used that will irritate the mucous membranes (ammonia or tobacco smoke), otherwise the receptors of the trigeminal nerve (CN V) will be stimulated causing a behavioural "defence" reflex to occur. Food, alcohol fumes or cloves are well suited to test whether a total loss in the sense of smell has occurred (**anosmia**). An incomplete loss, in contrast, cannot be diagnosed with any certainty.

Tumours or infectious disease are the most common causes of anosmia. However, this clinical sign is considered to be very rarely associated with a neurological lesion and so is not frequently tested.

1

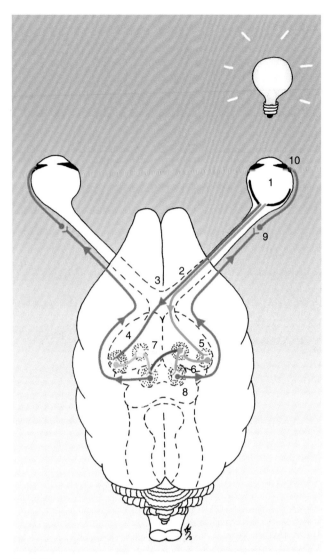

Fig. 1.17
Pupillary light reflex. The electrical impulses are transmitted in part by anatomical structures similar to those involved in the menace response. These are the temporal and nasal retina (1), the optic nerve (2), the optic chiasma (3) and the optic tract (4).The latter tract has synapses with the pretectal nuclei and further on with the parasympathetic nuclei (Edinger-Westphal nuclei, 5) of the oculomotor nerve. The majority of the optic fibres responsible for the pupillary light reflex come from the temporal side of the retina, do not cross over and run via pretectal fibres to the lateral (direct reflex arc, 6) and contralateral (indirect reflex arc, 7) Edinger-Westphal nuclei. This is the reason why the reactions of the direct pupillary light reflex are stronger than those of the indirect reflex. The preganglionic parasympathetic neurons of CN III (8) lie in the rostral part of the midbrain ventral to the mesencephalic aqueduct. These fibres go ventral to the crus cerebri, pass through the dura mater and join up with CN IV and VI. Afterwards, they then pass through the orbital fissure. The parasympathetic part of CN III has its synapses in the ciliary ganglion (9). Short postganglionic fibres go to the ciliary and the sphincter pupillae muscles (10). The sympathetic fibres innervate the dilator pupillary muscles. The reflex arc originates in the hypothalamus and has its first synapses in the midbrain. From there, it continues on to the preganglionic neurons in the spinal cord between T1–T3 (Fig. 1.15). After leaving the spinal cord, these neurons run within the vagosympathic trunk to the cervical ganglia. The postganglionic fibres travel with the internal carotid artery, then pass through the middle ear, to finally innervate the smooth muscle, glands and blood vessels in the head and neck.

II. Optic nerve (sense of sight)

Anatomy and physiology

Light stimulates the photoreceptors of the retina and subsequently, the neurons of the retina and then highly specialised ganglion cells. The axons of the latter cells form the optic nerve. The majority of fibres of CN II cross over at the optic chiasm and then run as the optic tracts to the lateral geniculate body of the thalamus. The neurons from this body project via the optic radiation to the optic cortex, where the stimulus is perceived at a conscious level.

In animals, the majority of the optic fibres cross over at the level of the optic chiasm to the contralateral side, whereas in primates only those fibres which have their origin in the nasal half of the retina cross over. In dogs, the majority of the nasal fibres and about 50% of the temporal fibres cross over to the contralateral side. In animals within the same genus, about 75% of the fibres cross over, while in cats it is roughly 65%. From a clinical point of view, the majority of animals behave as if all the fibres crossover. Therefore, the left and right fields of vision are examined separately, and a patient with a one-sided lesion of the cerebral cortex will appear clinically to be blind only on the contralateral side.

The reflex arc for the pupillary light reflex partially contains the same anatomical-physiological structures as the pathways for sight (Fig. 1.17).

Examination and assessment

The sense of sight is responsible for vision and the pupillary light reflex. A number of neurological tests are used to examine these processes: the menace response, the pupillary light reflex, the cotton ball test, the visual placement test and an ophthalmological examination (see Chap. 1.5). Observation of the patient while navigating around obstacles is a rather unreliable test as other neurological abnormalities can affect the results.

Menace response
Both eyes are investigated separately. A sudden movement with the hand is made towards one eye. The normal response is a closing of the eyelids; this is not a reflex (Fig.1.18). This response is not present in animals under 10 to 12 weeks of age and **has to be learnt**. The hand movement should not be too harsh or the tactile receptors of the cornea will be stimulated, thereby initiating the corneal reflex.

Diffuse cerebellar lesions maybe associated with a loss of the menace response. Such patients are not blind and they have a normal palpebral reflex.

Pupillary light reflex
The pupillary light reflex tests, amongst other things, the function of the peripheral visual pathways. First of all, the size and symmetry of the pupils are examined. Physiologically, the pupils are the same size in both eyes. If the pupils are of different sizes, it is called anisocoria (mydriasis = enlarged pupil; miosis = small pupil).

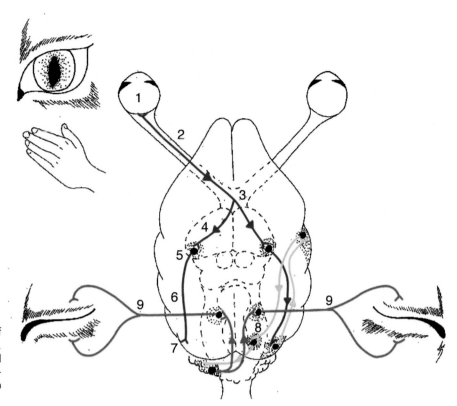

Fig. 1.18
menace response. This "reflex" arc consists of the receptors in the retina (1), the optic nerve (2), the optic chiasma (3), the optic tract (4), the lateral geniculate body (5), the optic radiation (6), the visual cortex (7), the crossed descending pathways to the brain stem (8) and the facial nerve (9).

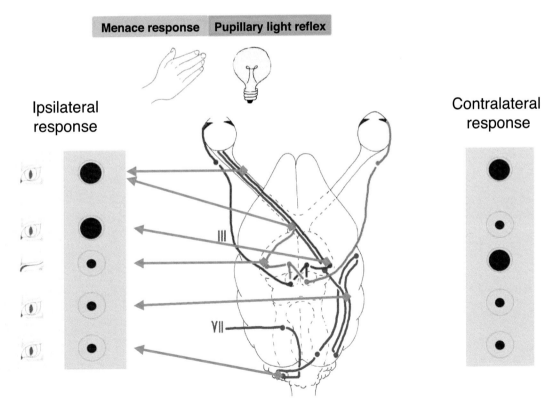

Fig. 1.19
Ipsilateral and contralateral reactions of the pupil to a light stimulus affecting the left eye. Ipsilateral response to a menace. The different lesions that are possible along the visual pathway are shown in green.

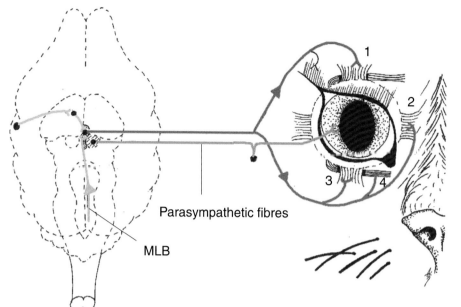

Parasympathetic fibres

MLB

Fig. 1.20
Innervation of the eyeball via the motor nuclei of the oculomotor nerve (red) to the dorsal (1), medial (2) and ventral (3) rectus muscles as well as the ventral oblique muscle (4) and levator palpebrae muscle. The medial longitudinal fasciculus (MLB) connects these three cranial nerve nuclei with the vestibular system and the motor centres of the eye muscles. Movement of the head to the side activates the vestibular system (orange) and subsequently, the nerves to the eye muscles causing a physiological nystagmus.

The examination is undertaken by shining a strong source of light into the eye. The normal reaction is a constriction of the pupil both on the side of the light stimulation (direct reflex) and on the other side (indirect reflex).

An incomplete lesion of the optic nerve is usually only associated with a partial dysfunction. A lesion of the retina, optic nerve or optic tract causes a peripheral blindness with a greatly delayed pupillary light reflex (Fig. 1.19).

A lesion affecting only the parasympathetic nucleus of CN III on one side is rather rare as this nucleus lies only a few millimetres from the rest of CN III. Clinically, an unresponsive enlarged pupil is seen.

If there is a lesion in CN III, not only is an enlarged pupil evident but there is also a ventrolateral strabismus.

Cotton ball test
A ball of cotton wool is allowed to fall within one side of the visual field. The normal reaction is a movement of the head or eye in the direction of the ball. The left and right visual fields can be tested separately. A reaction to this test necessitates an intact optic nerve and also an intact optic cortex. A lesion in the optic region of the cerebral cortex is known as a "central" blindness.

Visual placement test
With this test, subtle abnormalities in sight can be differentiated. The neurological pathway consists of the optic nerve as well as the efferent motor pathways to the limbs.

Ophthalmological examination
If there are no obvious changes in the cornea, lens, aqueous humour or vitreous body, then the ocular fundus is also examined (see Chap. 1.5). Gross abnormalities such as inadequate filling of the blood vessels, bleeding, a loss in colour of the retina or a swelling of the optic disc can be recognised.

Using the abovementioned tests, a lesion in the visual pathways can be more accurately localised.

III.	Oculomotor nerve	} (eye position
IV.	Trochlear nerve	and movement)
VI.	Abducens nerve	

The oculomotor nerve is primarily responsible for the normal movement of the eyeballs. The trochlear nerve is responsible for the movement of the eyeball upwards and the abducens nerve for its movements laterally.

Anatomy and physiology
The motor nuclei of the oculomotor nerve lie caudal to the parasympathetic nuclei of CN III, within the midbrain or mesencephalon, and innervate several specific eyeball muscles (Fig. 1.20).

The nuclei of the trochlear nerve are localised in the grey substance of the mesencephalon (Fig. 1.21).

The nuclei of the abducens nerve originate on the ventral floor of the fourth ventricle in the medulla and project their axons ventrolaterally to the pyramids (Fig. 1.22).

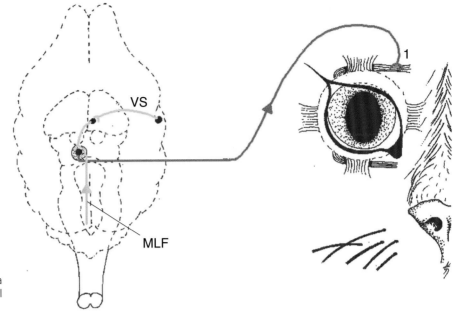

Fig. 1.21
Innervation of the dorsal oblique muscle (1) via
the trochlear nerve (red), the medial longitudinal
fasciculus (MLF) and vestibular system (VS).

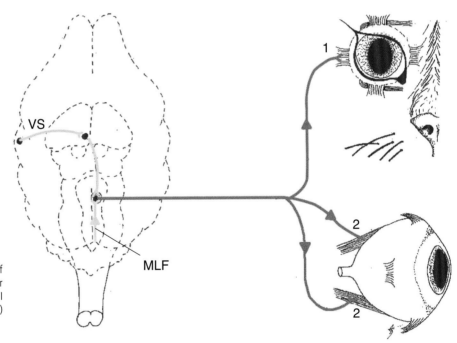

Fig. 1.22
Abducens nerve (red). Common innervation of
the lateral rectus muscle (1) and the retractor
bulbi muscle (2) via the abducens nerve and CN III
and IV, the medial longitudinal fasciculus (MLF)
and vestibular system (VS).

Examination and assessment

The eye movements are examined with the patient's head
initially at rest and then during movement. The position of
the eyes is observed and their ability to correct their position
in a particular axis is tested. The passive movement of the
head to the side, upwards or downwards simulates the active
tracking of an object and so leads to a **physiological nystagmus**. This is composed of two components, a slow and a
fast phase. The latter occurs in the direction of the head
movement.

Strabismus is the name given to abnormal eye position.
Knowledge of the anatomy and the innervation makes it possible to interpret the causative abnormalities (Fig. 1.23). As
the three above-mentioned nerves are responsible for the innervation of the seven main muscles which dictate the position of the eye, lesions of one or more of these CN leads to a
paralysis of one or more muscles resulting in an ipsilateral
strabismus. A lesion of CN III causes a ventrolateral strabismus +/− ptosis (paralysis of the levator palpebrae muscle) and
mydriasis (paralysis of the parasympathetic nerve).

1

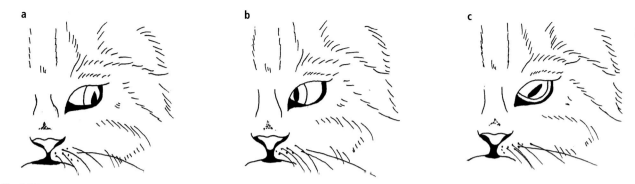

Fig. 1.23a–c
Abnormal positioning of the eyeball can occur due to lesions of the oculomotor nerve (ventrolateral, (a), the abducens nerve (medial, (b) or the trochlear nerve (rotation, c).

A rotational strabismus occurs with a lesion of CN IV. In this case, the dorsal part of the eyeball is pushed laterally. As cats have a slit-like pupil, this phenomenon is easier to detect than in the dog, where this condition can usually only be definitely diagnosed by using an ophthalmoscope and inspecting the retinal vascualture. The superior retinal vein is also shifted towards the temple. A lesion of CN VI leads to a medial strabismus with a loss in the animal's ability to retract the eyeball. Siamese cats can be affected by a congenital medial strabismus, which is not due to a paralysis of CN VI, but is related to an abnormal decussation of the optic tracts.

Incoordination of the eye movements, or more commonly a reduced to absent normal nystagmus, occur with a lesion in the vestibular system, cervical cord priorioception tracts or the medial longitudinal fasiculus in the brain stem,

V.   Trigeminal nerve

Anatomy and physiology
The trigeminal is a mixed cranial nerve, composed of three branches (ophthalmic, mandibular, maxillary). It contains both sensory and motor fibres (Fig. 1.24). The sensory fibres are important as the afferent portion of the corneal and palpebral reflexes.

Examination and assessment
All three sensory branches should be examined.
1. The ophthalmic branch is stimulated by tapping on the medial canthus of the eye. The normal reaction is closure of the eyelids. It also innervates the nasal mucosa.
2. The maxillary branch innervates the lateral canthal area, the muzzle and the nasal mucosa. The animal should show a behavioural defence reaction such as pulling its head away or trying to bite in response to a pinching of the lips, tapping the lateral canthus of the eye or stimulating the nasal mucosa. Tapping the lateral canthus of the eye also results in a reflex closure of the palpebral fissure.

3. The mandibular branch innervates the skin of the lower jaw. Pinching this area induces a behavioural defence reaction. Obtunded animals may demonstrate reduced reactions when they are stimulated over the head region.

In addition to the examination of the **sensory innervation of the head region,** an examination of the motor part of the trigeminal nerve should be performed. Passive opening of the mouth assesses jaw tone and palpation of the masseter and temporalis muscles assesses their degree of tone or atrophy. Testing the sensitivity to pain by palpating the skull in the region between the orbit and the zygomatic arch may cause a behavioural response in some patients with "headache" due to elevated intracranial pressure.

A lesion of the motor nucleus of CN V causes only masticatory muscle paresis or paralysis without any loss in sensation. In a one-sided lesion, muscle atrophy can be seen after 7 to 10 days. Asymmetry of the palpable masticatory muscles and possible dysphagia can be observed.

A lesion of the sensory nuclei results in a decrease or loss of pain perception with normal motor functions. With a focal lesion affecting a unilateral sensory cerebral cortex, the contralateral facial skin may have reduced pain perception. The animal can still feel stimulation of the nasal mucosa, but has a reduced reaction to facial skin stimulation.

VII.   Facial nerve (facial expression)

Anatomy and physiology
The reflex arc of the **palpebral reflex** is made up of an afferent part, (trigeminal nerve to brain stem), and an efferent part, the facial nerve (Fig. 1.25).

The neuroanatomical pathway of the **menace response** is made up of receptors in the retina, the optic nerve, optic chiasm, optic tract, lateral geniculate body, optic radiation,

Muscles of mastication

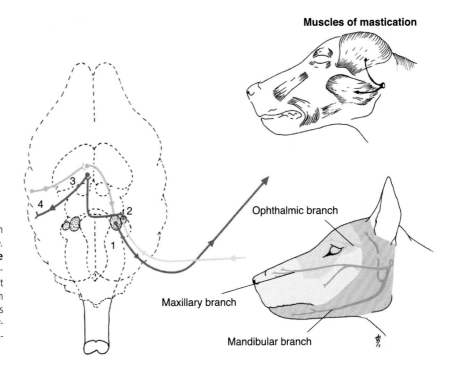

Fig. 1.24
Trigeminal nerve. The motor nucleus (1) lies within the pons at the level of the rostral cerebellar peduncle. The sensory part of CN V consists of the **pontine nuclei** (2), which receive information from mechanoreceptors and the **spinal nuclei**. The latter transmit information mainly from nociceptors. Projections from these nuclei run rostrally with the contralateral fibres of the **lemniscus** via the thalamus (3) to the cerebrum (4). Axons from both the pontine and spinal nuclei project to the facial nuclei.

Ophthalmic branch

Maxillary branch

Mandibular branch

Muscles of facial expression

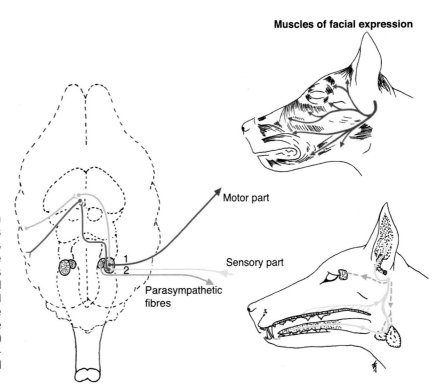

Fig. 1.25
Facial nerve. The nucleus (1) of the facial nerve lies in the rostral part of the medulla. The facial nerve enters the internal acoustic meatus with CN VIII and crosses over the facial canal. Its motor branches innervate the facial muscles and the caudal part of the diagastricus muscle. The cell bodies of its sensory neurons are found in the geniculate ganglion (2) in the petrous temporal bone. These innervate the caudal two-thirds of the tongue and the palate with the trigeminal nerve. The facial nerve innervates the stapedius muscle (inner ear) as the stapedius nerve. Its parasympathetic part innervates the nasal, mandibular, sublingual and lacrimal glands.

Motor part

Sensory part

Parasympathetic fibres

1

the visual cortex, descending crossing tracts to the brain stem, the cerebellum and the facial nerve.

Taste is conveyed via special taste receptors in the rostral two thirds of the tongue through the facial nerve. The receptors in the caudal third of the tongue are innervated by the glosso-pharyngeal nerve. The parasympathetic portion of the facial nerve is responsible for lacrimal gland stimulation.

Examination and assessment

A complete lesion of the facial nerve manifests itself clinically in many ways. Facial paralysis is characterised by a drooping of the ear and lip, a widening of the palpebral fissure, asymmetry of the nostrils and a loss in the sense of taste. As a secondary consequence, there can be damage to the cornea due to desiccation from a lack of tear production and the loss of the protective blink reflex. Inadequate closing of the lips can cause salivation or drooling on the affected side. A partial lesion of the facial nerve can be associated with one or more clinical signs.

The palpebral reflex is stimulated by touching the skin around the eyes and results in a closure of the eyelids. The corneal reflex is instigated by a gentle touching of the cornea. A closing of the eyes is again to be interpreted as a normal reaction to both of these tests, whereas lesions of the facial nerve result in the eyes not being closed in either test.

Additionally, the tear production test (Schirmer tear test) can help with the localisation of a lesion in this reflex arc. Intracranial-extramedullary lesions usually disturb all of the nerve's functions. A lesion in the petrous portion of the temporal bone, depending on its degree, affects one or more functions of the facial nerve. Additionally with such a lesion localisation, vestibular symptoms can be seen such as head tilt, nystagmus and positional strabismus.

The sense of taste can be tested with atropine. Healthy animals react quickly to atropine's bitter taste with immediate licking movements and salivation.

VIII. Vestibulocochlear nerve (balance and hearing)

Vestibular Nerve

Anatomy and physiology

The vestibular system is responsible for the static and dynamic position of the head. The CNS is informed about a change in the head's position by both labyrinths. The labyrinth of the inner ear contains the ampulla with its three semi-circular canals lying at right angles to each other, and the macula, another receptor system, that is found in the utricule and saccule. The organs of balance are stimulated by changes in position, acceleration or gravity. The resulting depolarisation is transferred via the vestibular neurons within CN VIII.

Examination and assessment

An examination of a patient in the acute phase of a vestibular syndrome is often difficult as the patient exhibits disorientation and is sometimes, obtunded. Head tilt, ataxia and nystagmus are the important cardinal signs of vestibular disease. It is important both for the therapy and the prognosis to determine between a central or peripheral cause of the vestibular dysfunction.

The postural and placement reactions and the direction of the nystagmus can help to localise the disease.

There are different types of nystagmus. Spontaneous nystagmus occurs without any movement of the head and is always pathological, comprised of rapid and slow phases, and defined according to the direction of its rapid phase. The three directions of nystagmus are vertical, rotary and horizontal, with the slow phase towards the diseased side. Pendular nystagmus does not have alternating rapid and slow phases, and can be elicited by a lesion in the cerebellum. Lesions of the peripheral vestibular apparatus mainly cause a horizontal or rotary nystagmus, where the direction of the nystagmus remains constant.

Normal nystagmus can be induced temporarily when the position of the animal's head is suddenly passively changed. Pathological nystagmus does not require head movement but may be elicited by certain head positions. In healthy animals the eye remains in the middle of the palpebral fissure when the head moves dorsally. In comparison, a vestibular (positional) strabismus occurs with vestibular lesions, whereby the eye becomes positioned downwards towards the damaged side when the head is moved dorsally.

As infections of the inner ear are frequently associated with a middle ear lesion, an otoscopic examination should always be undertaken in cases with vestibular symptoms.

Cochlear Nerve

Anatomy and physiology

Hearing is a complex process (Fig. 1.26).

Examination and assessment

A sudden acoustic stimulus (e.g. whistling, clapping) outside of its visual field causes a reaction in the healthy animal, whereby it turns its head in the direction of the sound. The localisation of a lesion within the auditory pathway is not possible with simple tests; only special and painstaking electrodiagnostic methods (auditory evoked potentials) are capable of achieving this.

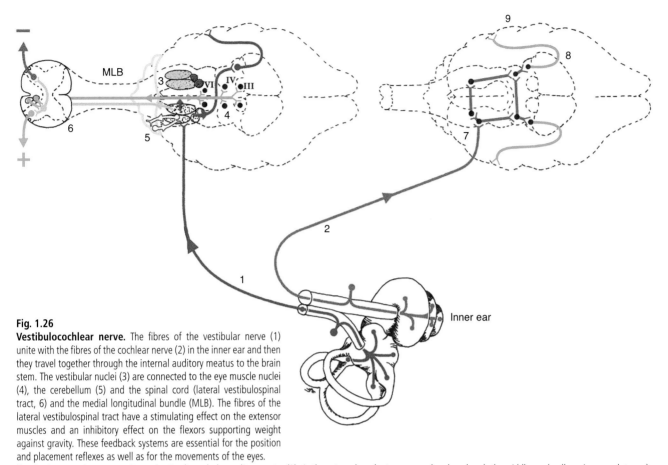

Fig. 1.26
Vestibulocochlear nerve. The fibres of the vestibular nerve (1) unite with the fibres of the cochlear nerve (2) in the inner ear and then they travel together through the internal auditory meatus to the brain stem. The vestibular nuclei (3) are connected to the eye muscle nuclei (4), the cerebellum (5) and the spinal cord (lateral vestibulospinal tract, 6) and the medial longitudinal bundle (MLB). The fibres of the lateral vestibulospinal tract have a stimulating effect on the extensor muscles and an inhibitory effect on the flexors supporting weight against gravity. These feedback systems are essential for the position and placement reflexes as well as for the movements of the eyes.

Hearing is a complex process. Acoustic stimuli reach the auditory cortex (9) via the external ear (outer ear canal and eardrum), the middle ear (malleus, incus and stapes), inner ear with its specialised receptor organs in the petrous temporal bone, the acoustic part of CN VIII (2), the cochlear nuclei (7), the superior olive, the midbrain and the thalamus (8).

IX.   Glossopharyngeal nerve } **(swallowing)**
X.   Vagus nerve

Anatomy and physiology

The glossopharyngeal nerve is responsible for the sensory innervation of the caudal tongue, pharynx and larynx, and also for the motor innervation of the pharynx, the soft palate and the oesophagus. It conveys parasympathetic fibres to the parotid and zygomatic salivary glands (Fig. 1.27).

The vagus nerve innervates the pharynx, larynx and palate with motor and sensory fibres; additionally, it supplies parasympathetic fibres to all of the thoracic and abdominal viscera except for the urinary bladder and the pelvic canal, which are innervated by the sacral parasympathetic nerves. The recurrent laryngeal nerve leaves the vagus and goes to the upper third of the oesophageal musculature and the larynx.

Examination and assessment

The swallowing reflex helps in the examination of both nerves. It can be elicited internally (by touching the mucosa of the pharynx with the finger; wear gloves!) or externally (by a light stimulation of the pharyngeo-laryngeal area. A swallowing motion is the normal reaction.

The clinical signs of a lesion in CN IX and/or X are dysphagia, including problems with swallowing, asymmetry of the pharynx or larynx, as well as regurgitation.

Whilst a complete paralysis causes an inability to swallow, a one-sided lesion leads to one-sided problems in swallowing and regurgitation of food; with the latter even occurring through the nose.

Bradycardia, an increase in bronchial secretion, a reduction in peristalsis and the production of gastrointestinal juices all occur with vagotonia (hyperexcitability of the vagus nerve).

Always consider rabies in any patient presenting with swallowing problems.

1

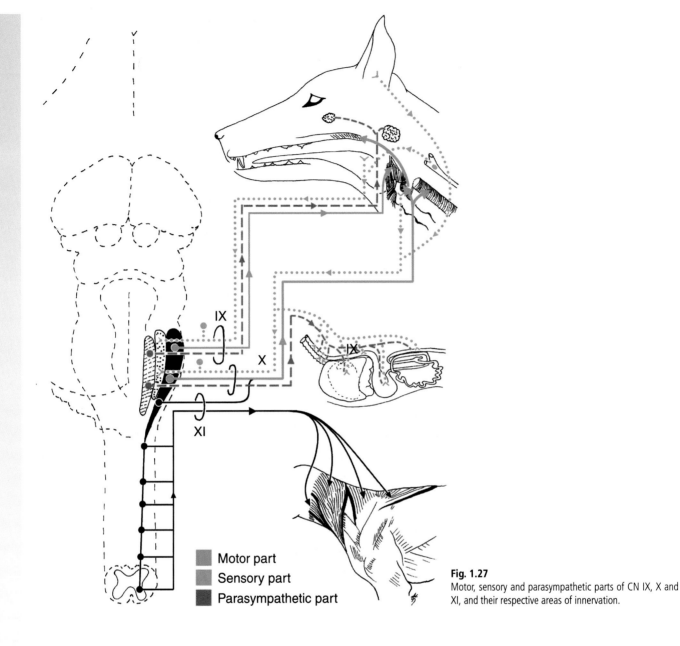

Motor part
Sensory part
Parasympathetic part

Fig. 1.27
Motor, sensory and parasympathetic parts of CN IX, X and XI, and their respective areas of innervation.

XI. Accessory nerve (neck muscles) ⎯⎯⎯⎯

Anatomy and physiology
The motor nucleus of CN XI is found between the spinal segments C1 and C6. The nerve fibres run cranially to the trapezius muscle, parts of the brachiocephalicus muscle and the sternocephalicus muscle (Fig. 1.27).

Examination and assessment
Disturbances of the motor innervations of these muscles are difficult to diagnose. Neurogenic muscle atrophy can be ascertained by a careful palpation of the neck musculature. The function of CN XI can be ascertained from the posture of the head and neck, which may be deviated toward the affected side in chronic cases.

XII. Hypoglossal nerve (tongue movements) ⎯⎯

Anatomy and physiology
The hypoglossal nerve is responsible for tongue function (Fig. 1.28).

Examination and assessment
Inspection of the symmetry of the tongue and its movements, observing intake of water and food as well as passive manipu-

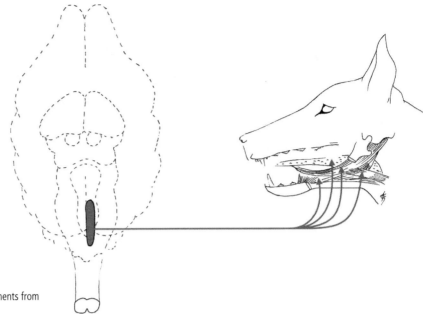

Fig. 1.28
Hypoglossal nerve. The innervation of tongue movements from
the nucleus of CN XII in the caudal medulla.

lation of the tongue should be included in the examination.
Difficulties in the intake of water and food as well as in chewing and swallowing are signs of a lesion of CN XII. If the
tongue hangs out of the mouth, then it is usually drawn to the
side of the lesion in chronic cases and away from the side of
the lesion in acute cases.

> **Disturbances in the last four cranial nerves may be
> difficult to differentiate from one another.**

1.4.6   Spinal reflexes

The spinal reflexes depend on intact motor and sensory nerve
function, the effector muscles and the grey substance of the
respective spinal segments. By testing the reflexes, it is possible to directly and simply examine the function of a specific
segment of the grey substance in the spinal cord, and its associated nerve roots and nerves. There are two types of reflexes to be differentiated in the practical neurological examination: the **tendon reflexes** and the **withdrawal reflexes**.

In the tendon reflexes, the muscles, and so their neuromuscular spindles, are passively stretched by hitting them with a reflex hammer, whereby a signal is elicited that is transferred
over the sensory nerves to the grey substance of the respective
spinal segment (reflex centre) and then on via the motor
nerves to instigate a reflex contraction of the muscle. More

precisely, the dorsal horns of the spinal cord receive the sensory stimuli via the sensory nerve fibres, dorsal roots, and spinal ganglia. The stimuli are then transferred to the target
muscle via the ventral horn cells, motor root and ventrally the
spinal nerves. This reflex arc can be modulated by afferent and
efferent pathways coming from the brain (UMN).

In the withdrawal reflex, stimulation of the skin leads to a
contraction of the muscle. This flexor reflex is elicited by, for
example, pressure on the foot pads or the skin between the
toes.

The possible results of such reflex investigations are (i) normal
reflex activity, (ii) areflexia (loss of reflex), (iii) hyporeflexia
(reduction), or (iv) hyperreflexia (increase) and clonus (repetitive flexion and extension of the distal limb after a single
stimulation). The spinal reflexes should be investigated with
the animal in lateral recumbency. The animal is tested first on
the uppermost side and then turned over and evaluated on the
other side. It is important that the animal is **relaxed** during
the reflex examination and its limbs are as loose as possible. A
lesion in the LMN leads to a reduction or loss of a reflex. In
contrast, a lesion in the UMN is associated with either a normal or increased reflex activity.

1.4.6.1   Pelvic limb reflexes

The reflexes of the pelvic limbs can be tested before those of
the thoracic limbs and then the two sets of limbs are compared

1

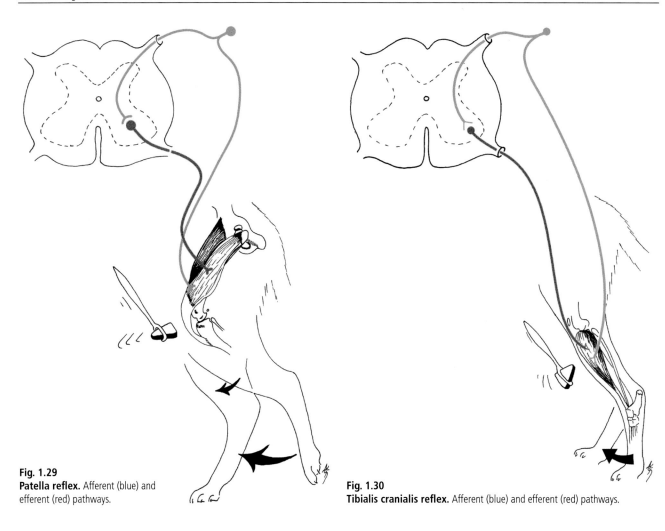

Fig. 1.29
Patella reflex. Afferent (blue) and efferent (red) pathways.

Fig. 1.30
Tibialis cranialis reflex. Afferent (blue) and efferent (red) pathways.

Patellar reflex (femoral nerve)

The reflex centre lies between L4–L6. The middle patella tendon is tapped whilst the animal is in lateral recumbency and the leg loosely supported. A reflex contraction of the quadriceps muscle and a forwards movement of the lower limb is to be expected (Fig. 1.29).

Cranial tibial reflex (peroneal nerve)

The reflex centre lies between L6–S1. Hitting the cranial tibial muscle (dorsolateral in the upper third of the lower leg) causes flexion of the tarsus (Fig. 1.30).

Flexor reflex (sciatic nerve)

The reflex centre lies between L4–S3. Pinching the toes, pads of the feet or the skin between the toes causes a sudden flexion of the whole limb; all joints must be seen to flex (Fig. 1.31).

1.4.6.2 Thoracic limb reflexes

Extensor carpi radialis reflex (radial nerve)

The reflex centre lies between C7–T1. The limb is supported under the elbow. A light tapping of the extensor carpi radialis muscle below the elbow causes a slight extension of the carpus (Fig. 1.32).

Triceps reflex (radial nerve)

The reflex centre lies between C6–T1. The thoracic limb is drawn slightly forwards and the shoulder is gently pushed outwards with the elbow flexed. A tap on the triceps tendon just above the olecranon causes an extension of the elbow and of the carpus (Fig. 1.33).

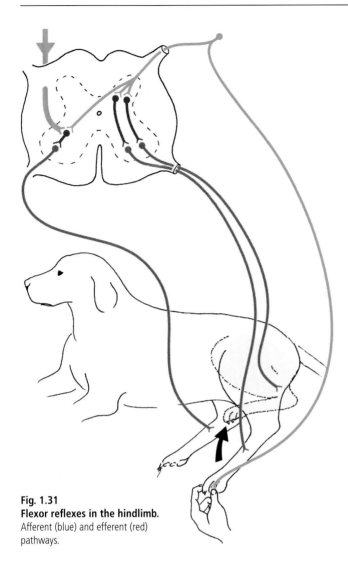

Fig. 1.31
Flexor reflexes in the hindlimb.
Afferent (blue) and efferent (red)
pathways.

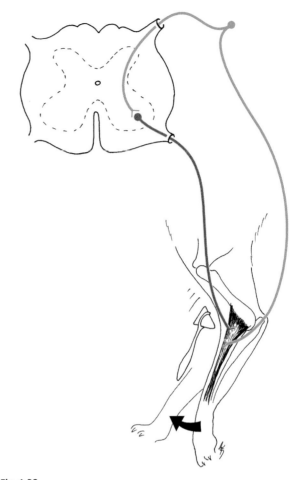

Fig. 1.32
Extensor carpi radialis reflex. Afferent (blue) and efferent (red) pathways.

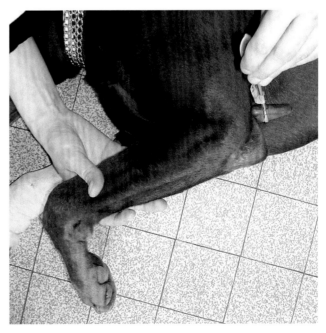

Fig. 1.33
Triceps reflex.

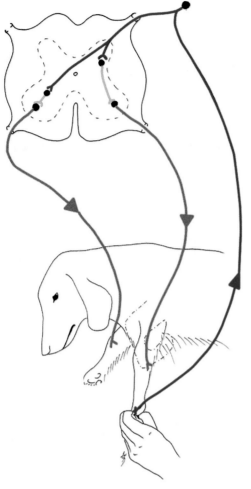

Fig. 1.34
Flexor reflexes in the forelimb. Afferent (dark blue), interneuron (light blue) and efferent (red) pathways.

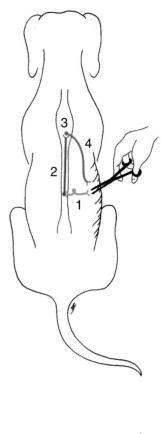

Fig. 1.35
Panniculus reflex. The stimuli are transmitted via afferent sensory fibres (1) to the spinal cord and along ascending pathways (2) to the motor reflex centre C8–T2 (3). The motor nerves (thoracic nerves, 4) arise from this centre and innervate the skin muscles.

Flexor reflex (musculocutaneous nerve, axillary nerve, median nerve, ulnar nerve and radial nerve)

The reflex centre lies between C6–T1. Pinching of the toes, pads or the skin between the toes causes a sudden flexion of the whole limb (Fig. 1.34).

1.4.6.3 Other reflexes

Cutaneous trunci (Panniculus) reflex

Pinching or touching the skin with a pointed object over the dorsal spinous processes from the caudal lumbar region to just below the shoulder blades causes a bilateral contraction of the skin muscles. The skin's nociceptors in specific dermatomes are stimulated. The function of this reflex not only depends on intact afferent and efferent nerves, but also on the ascending tracts between L4 and C8. These ascending tracts are situated on the grey and white matter border. As with all other reflexes, the left and right sides of the animal should be com-pared. The cutaneous trunci reflex may be absent caudal to a thoraco-lumbar spinal lesion (Fig. 1.35).

Perineal reflex

This reflex depends on the sensory and motor innervation occurring through the pudendal nerves and spinal cord segments S1–S3. Touching the anal or perineal area causes a contraction of the anal sphincter and flexion of the tail, with the latter mediated by the caudal nerves (Fig. 1.36).

Vulvourethral reflex

The neuroanatomy responsible for this reflex is as for the perineal reflex. Touching the vulva causes it to be slightly contracted and displaced dorsally (Fig. 1.37).

Bulbocavernosus reflex

The reflex centre lies between S1–S3. A slight pressure above the bulbocavernosus causes a contraction of the anus.

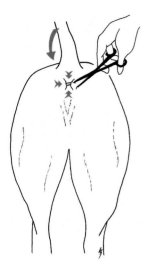

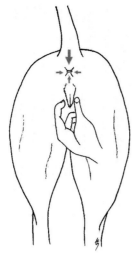

Fig. 1.36
Perineal reflex.

Fig. 1.37
Vulvourethral reflex.

1.4.6.4 Abnormal reflexes

Crossed extensor reflex
This reflex is part of the normal supportive mechanism of the animal; when one limb is flexed, the contralateral limb must extend to bear the weight. This should not occur when the animal is recumbent. The flexor reflex sensory fibres of L4–S3 (pelvic limbs) or C6–T1 (thoracic limbs), send collaterals to interneurons on the opposite side of the spinal cord, which excite extensor motor neurons. When the patient is in lateral recumbency, pinching the toes, footpads or between the toes stimulates a sudden flexion of the stimulated limb and an extension of the contralateral limb. This reflex occurs when there is a lesion of the spinal cord cranial to the reflex centre.

Mass reflex
Occasionally, severe spinal cord damage leads to a generalised dysinhibition of the reflex activity. The stimulation of a single reflex causes a struggling of all the limbs, a wagging of the tail and uncontrolled defensive movements.

1.4.7 Sensory system

Two types of sensory system are differentiated based on the location of the receptors: the superficial receptors (touch, temperature, pain, pressure) and the deep receptors (proprioception). The latter receptors inform the higher centres about the position of the different parts of the body with respect to each other and within space. The sensory system also forms the afferent component of the reflex arc (Fig. 1.38).

As sensitivity to pressure and temperature are difficult to test and/or determine in small animals, pain sensitivity is the only practically useable component of the superficial sensory receptor system. Proprioception is examined using postural and placement reactions. Deep pain receptors are evaluated by noxious stimulation of deep digital structures such as periosteum.

Anatomy and physiology
The sensory fibres of the internal organs, joints, muscles and skin run via the dorsal nerves into the spinal cord. The fibres that are responsible for superficial pain sensation continue in the dorsal cord cranially and the majority are to be found on the contralateral side. The fibres responsible for deep pain sensation run somewhat differently. They have many intersegmental and suprasegmental connections, which is the reason why they are arranged in a bilateral and diffuse manner in the ascending pathways. Pain transmission ends either in the **thalamus** or some of the pain impulses are projected on to the **cortex**. From here, the respective behavioural reactions such as defence, avoidance and biting are initiated.

A dermatome is a piece of skin which is innervated by one or more nerves. Each dermatome is made up of large differently sized areas of skin (Figs. 1.39, 1.40).

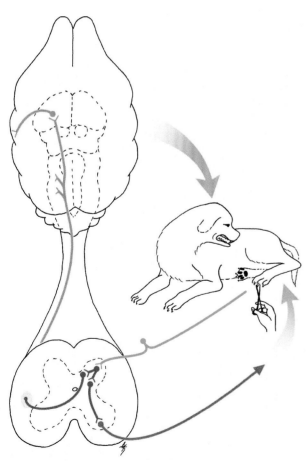

Fig. 1.38
Nociception.

1

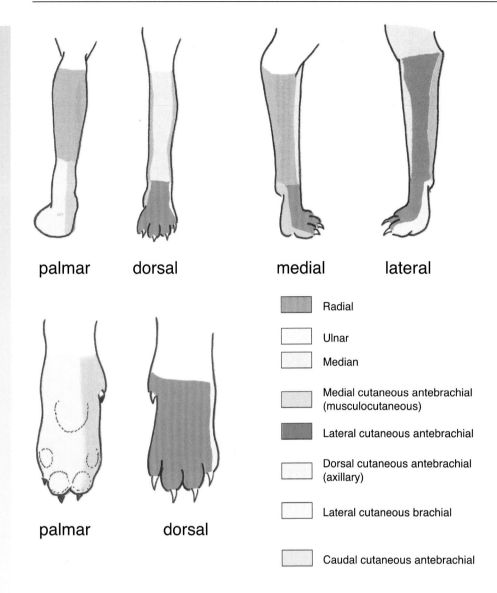

palmar   dorsal   medial   lateral

palmar   dorsal

Radial

Ulnar

Median

Medial cutaneous antebrachial (musculocutaneous)

Lateral cutaneous antebrachial

Dorsal cutaneous antebrachial (axillary)

Lateral cutaneous brachial

Caudal cutaneous antebrachial

Fig. 1.39
Forelimb dermatomes.

Examination and assessment

In the assessment of sensation, the presence and localisation of pain, the presence of superficial pain sensitivity and the presence of deep pain sensitivity are all examined. By careful palpation of the area to be investigated and by targeted, careful pressure from dorsal and lateral areas with increased pain appreciation (hyperaesthesia) and areas with reduced pain sensation (hypalgesia) can be determined. As a lesion in the CNS results in hypalgesia caudal to the lesion, the limbs should be examined in a distal to proximal direction. The pelvic region and the rump are palpated in a caudiocranial direction.

The haemostat test gives the examiner a general impression of the pain appreciation on the rump and limbs. Stimulation of the skin with a haemostat at different places causes different reactions, either a change in behaviour in the form of defence reactions such as vocalizing, and biting (only reactions that show that the stimulus has been consciously appreciated

should be considered as true pain) or a reflex reaction made up of a local skin or muscle contraction, which is not appreciated consciously. A systematic examination of the pain response is especially important when absolute motor dysfunction is present. When superficial pain appreciation is present then deep pain will be present. If the superficial pain reaction is missing, then the skin should be tested with a hemostat to stimulate the deep pain response. Breed specific and individual differences in temperament can make the interpretation of these tests difficult. Many animals overreact to the slightest touch while in others stimuli of a similar intensity are barely noticed.

It should be noted that the flexion of a limb away from a pain stimulus is a reflex reaction and not the expression of a conscious pain response. The deep pain response is the last one to disappear with spinal lesions and is therefore important for the animal's prognosis.

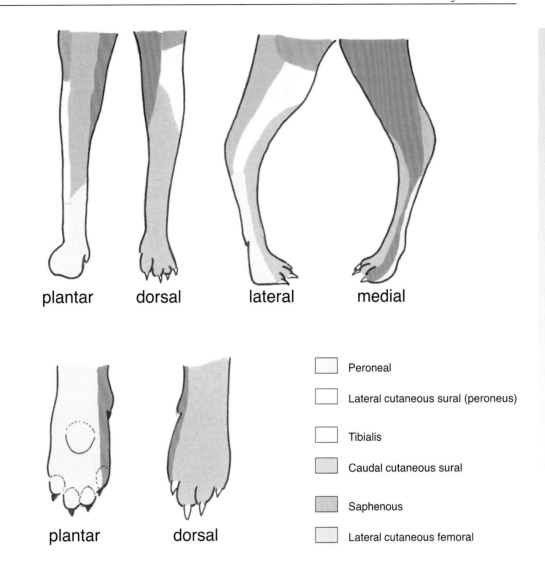

plantar   dorsal   lateral   medial

**Fig. 1.40
Hindlimb dermatomes.**

plantar   dorsal

☐ Peroneal

☐ Lateral cutaneous sural (peroneus)

☐ Tibialis

▨ Caudal cutaneous sural

▨ Saphenous

☐ Lateral cutaneous femoral

1.4.8　Localisation

To ensure a definite or suspected diagnosis, the examiner must delineate the pathological process using the neurological examination and its subsequent interpretation. Localisation is based on a neurophysiological interpretation of the clinical signs and the results of the neurological examination. Clinical neurological abnormalities may result from dysfunction of a specific anatomical area; i.e., facial paresis is seen with lesions of the facial nerve (CN VII). However, some clinical signs may result from dysfunction of more complex neuroanatomy or neuroanatomical interactions; i.e., ataxia may result from lesions of cerebellum, spinocerebellar tracts or the vestibular system. Clinical signs with a simple or complex physiology must be differentiated. The former are easy to localise and are the consequence of a lesion of the afferent or efferent nerves or their reflex centres (flaccid paralysis, loss of spinal reflexes and cranial nerve function, etc.). The picture found with clinical signs associated with complex physiological processes are indeed very characteristic of particular anatomical regions; for example, generalised ataxia and hypermetria with lesions in the cerebellum.

The nervous system is divided into seven regions for practical and clinical purposes. Lesions can be localised to one of these following regions:
- Peripheral nerves and nerve roots
- Muscles / neuromuscular junctions
- Spinal cord
- Brain stem
- Vestibular system
- Cerebellum
- Cerebral cortex (including thalamus, hypothalamus and the basal ganglia)

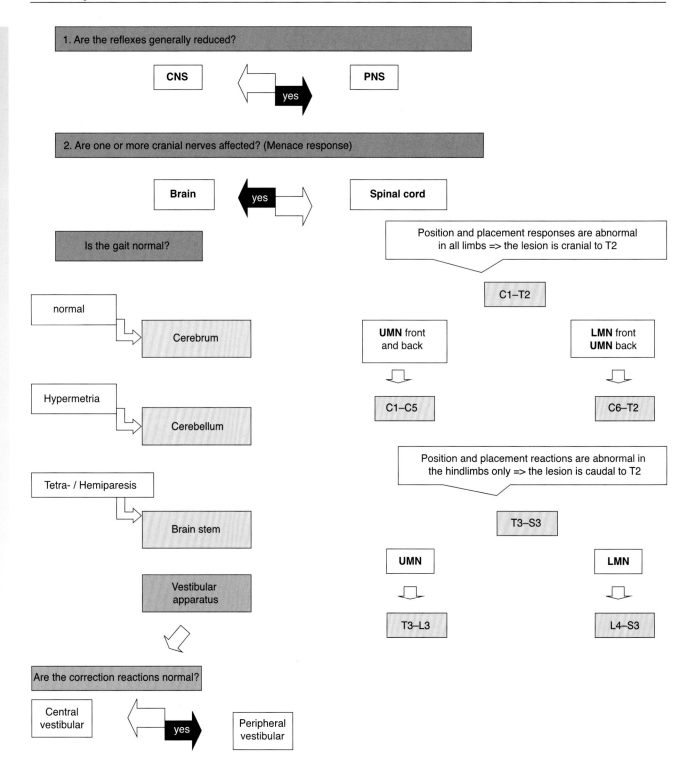

Fig. 1.41
Algorithm for the localisation of neurological disturbances.

The peripheral nerves can be subdivided into thoracic limbs, pelvic limbs, cranial nerves and the sacral nerves. The spinal cord can also be subdivided into the C1–C5 cervical cord, the cervical enlargement (C6–T2), the thoracolumbar cord (T3–L3), the lumbar enlargement (L4–S2) and the sacral cord (S1–S3). Within each region, the right or left side can be affected.

The first step in establishing localisation is the classification of the clinical signs based on whether they originate from a dysfunction of the peripheral nervous system (PNS), the central nervous system (CNS) or extraneural systems. The anamnesis and the results of the neurological examination can help with this classification (Fig. 1.41).

1.4.8.1 Peripheral nervous system

When spinal reflexes, i.e. flexors and extensors, in one or all four limbs are reduced, then the lesion affects the PNS. The majority of the diseases of the PNS affect the limbs. If all limbs are involved, this clinically represents a generalised lower motor neuron (LMN) disease. The LMNS consists of the α-motor neurons, the nerve roots, the peripheral nerves, the neuromuscular endplate and the muscles. The clinical signs depend on the extent of the lesion as well as its chronicity. Paresis, loss of proprioception, reduced muscle tone and muscle atrophy can all be observed. Disease of the LMN of a single limb or cranial nerve is relatively easy to localise.

1.4.8.2 Central nervous system

If the spinal reflexes are not reduced, then the lesion must be in the CNS. To further refine the CNS localisation, it can be divided into an intra- or extracranial lesion. **If one or more cranial nerve functions are affected and/or the menace response is abnormal, then the lesion is localised intracranially (brain).** In addition, the postural and placement responses in all four limbs may be abnormal. These tend to be more one-sided with focal processes. **Abnormalities of the gait** can help to classify intracranial lesion(s) as affecting the cerebrum, cerebellum, brain stem or vestibular apparatus. Lesions of the cerebrum can induce a wandering, aimless gait, or compulsive pacing. Additionally, obtundation and/or changes in behaviour or seizures can be observed. Hypermetria and intention tremors usually indicate a lesion in the cerebellum. Other abnormalities are also to be expected with a localisation in this region.

A multifocal, disseminated or diffuse disturbance should be considered when numerous regions of the nervous system are affected at the same time.

In addition to observing the gait and testing of the spinal reflexes, postural and placement reflexes, palpitation of the limbs and the dorsum are very helpful in localising hyperaesthesic regions. During the manipulation, the examiner should observe whether signs of pain, e.g. resistance to movement or increased tension in the musculature occur. When the examiner places one hand on the abdomen of the animal while pressing each vertebral segment with the other, an increase in tension in the abdominal muscles is an indicator of a pain response. Pain in the cervical region can also be determined by palpation or manipulation of the neck, followed by lateral and dorsoventral flexion.

Cerebrum

Clinical signs of a lesion in the cerebral cortex include abnormal behaviour and levels of consciousness, seizure activity, head turn, circling and a wandering gait, abnormal postural and placement responses, loss of vision, with an intact pupillary light reflex and reduced nasal sensation. The abnormalities are mainly apparent on the **contralateral** side.

Brain stem

Impairments in consciousness such as obtundation, stupor or coma, disturbances in gait from hemi- to tetraparesis, ipsilateral abnormal postural and placement responses, and dysfunction of cranial nerves are all typical clinical signs of a lesion in the brain stem.

Cerebellum

The cerebellum is a regulatory organ and is involved in the modulation of movement, muscle tone and balance. This organ facilitates well-rounded and fluid movements.

The majority of diseases affecting the cerebellum are diffuse lesions which result in a characteristic collection of clinical signs, most notable of which is **cerebellar ataxia**. The other clinical signs include normal behaviour; a wide-legged stance; standing with the tendency to fall forwards, to the side or backwards; abnormal head movements (intention tremor), manifested as a nodding of the head and dysmetria (hypermetria).

A **delay in initiation** is obvious in postural reactions which are then exaggerated. The cranial nerve examination is normal apart from the menace response which may be absent on the ipsilateral side or there may rarely be nystagmus. The fact that the head is also affected by ataxia helps in the differentation between a cerebellar and a spinal lesion. Focal lesions are rarer and also more difficult to recognise. Abnormal movements with hypermetria on the side of the lesion can be seen. In the acute case of cerebellar disease, another clinical syndrome can be seen: there is increased extensor tone in the

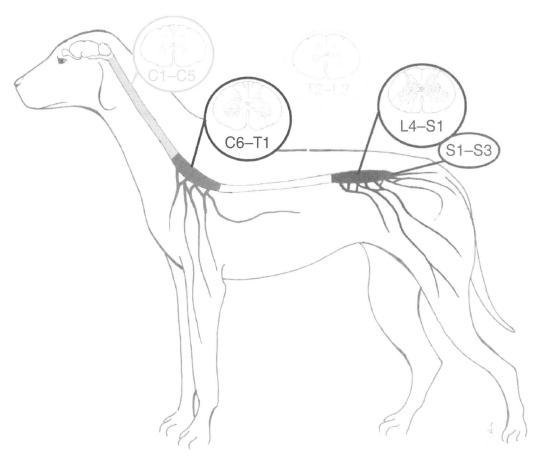

Fig. 1.42
Division of the spinal segments C1–S3 according to abnormalities in the positioning and placement reactions or the spinal reflexes.

thoracic limbs, flexion of the pelvic limbs, and opisthotonus (dorsal extension of the head and neck). Lesions in the flocculonodular lobes of the cerebellum and cerebellar peduncles cause similar clinical signs to those found in vestibular disease, but usually cause a contralateral head tilt (paradoxical vestibular disease)

1.4.8.3 Spinal cord
The spinal cord can be split into four sections: cranial cervical (C1–C5), caudal cervical (C6–T2), thoracolumbar (T3–L3) and the lumbosacral (L4–S3). In the lumbar region, the spinal cord is markedly displaced cranially with respect to the vertebral column (ascensus medullae). As a consequence, the lumbar enlargement lies over the L3–L4 vertebrae and the sacral grey matter over L5. Abnormalities in gait are noticeable with diseases of the spinal cord. Damage to the descending motor pathways (UMN) or of the α-motor neurons (LMN) leads to a paresis or a plegia depending on the severity of the lesion.

With damage to the afferent pathways, an incoordination of the limbs occurs (proprioceptive ataxia).

The localisation of a lesion in one of the above sections of the spinal cord can be determined by an assessment of the **spinal reflexes** as well as the **postural and placement reactions**. Lesions that occur cranial to T3 change the postural and placement reactions in all four limbs. Lesions caudal to T2 cause abnormal postural and placement reactions only in the pelvic limbs. In order to allocate a lesion to one of the four spinal cord segments, one must differentiate between the UMN and LMN by assessing the **reflex activity** of all limbs. UMN lesions cause increased spinal reflex activity, while lesions in the LMNs result in reduced spinal reflexes.

If the postural and placement reactions are abnormal in all four limbs, then the lesion is cranial to T3 (Fig. 1.42). Whether or not it lies in the cranial or caudal cervical spinal cord is determined by the assessment of the spinal reflexes.

Normal to increased reflexes in the thoracic or pelvic limbs (UMN) when all four limbs are affected by a gait abnormality mean that the lesion is in the cranial cervical region (C1–C5). Reduced reflexes in the thoracic limbs (LMN) and normal to increased reflexes in the pelvic limbs (UMN) implies a lesion in the caudal cervical region (C6–T2).

If the postural and placement reactions are abnormal only in the pelvic limbs, then the lesion is caudal to T2. Normal to increased reflexes in the pelvic limbs implies a lesion in the thoracolumbar area (T3–L3) and reduced reflexes implies a lesion in the lumbosacral region (L4–S3).

The presence of Horner's syndrome, and an assessment of the panniculus reflex or the perineal reflex can further help in the localisation of a spinal lesion.

Localisation T3–L3
Typical examination results:

Pelvic limb signs: paraparesis, paraplegia, increased or normal reflexes, abnormalities in the postural and placement reactions, possible urinary incontinence, the cutaneous trunci reflex may be absent caudal to the lesion, and there is a loss of deep pain response in the most severe cases.

Localisation L4–L7
Typical examination results:

Pelvic limb signs: flaccid paraparesis to paraplegia, hyporeflexia, areflexia, abnormalities in the postural and placement reflexes, reduced muscle tone, and possible urinary incontinence.

Localisation S1–S3
Typical examination results:

Paresis or paralysis of the urinary bladder and urethral spincters, colon, anal sphincter and tail; analgesia of the perineal and tail regions is present; no disturbances in gait with focal processes.

1.4.8.4 Vestibular system
A differentiation must be made between the peripheral and the central vestibular system for localisation purposes. The peripheral vestibular system consists of inner ear receptors and the vestibulocochlear nerve. The receptor organ is made up of three semi-circular canals lying at right angles to each other. The receptors within these canals measure changes in acceleration and deceleration. The **classical clinical signs** of a lesion in the vestibular system are a head tilt to one side, an ataxia to one side with a tendency to fall, circle, drift, roll over, a pathological nystagmus, **positional strabismus** and abnormal righting reactions.

Table 1.2: Localisation of a vestibular lesion

	Peripheral	Paradoxical	Central
Consciousness	Normal-depression	Normal-depression	Depression-stupor
Behaviour	Normal	Normal	Abnormal
Posture			
Head tilt	Ipsilateral	Contralateral	Ipsilateral
Muscle tone	Abnormal	Abnormal	Abnormal
Gait			
Falling down	Possibly	Possibly	Possibly
Drifting	Possibly	Possibly	Possibly
Ataxia	Usually	Yes	Yes
Cranial nerves	VII (V) (ipsilateral)	Multiple (ipsilateral)	Multiple (ipsilateral)
Horner's syndrome	Yes	No	Very rare; possibly
Nystagmus	Yes	Yes	Yes
■ Horizontal	Yes	Yes	Yes
■ Rotary	Yes	Yes	Yes
■ Vertical	Very rare / no	Yes	Yes
■ Positional	Possible / rare	Yes	Yes
■ Pendulous (tremor)	No	Yes	No
Strabismus	Ventral (ipsilateral)	Ventral (contralateral)	Ventral (ipsilateral)
Postural and placement reactions			
Hopping	Abnormal	Abnormal	Abnormal
Righting	Abnormal	Abnormal	Abnormal
Wheelbarrow	Abnormal	Abnormal	Abnormal
Correction of hindlimbs	Normal to slightly delayed	Abnormal	Abnormal
Reflexes			
Normal to increased	Yes	Yes	Yes
Pain appreciation	Normal	Normal	Normal to reduced

1

The central vestibular system contains the vestibular nuclei in the brainstem (medulla oblongata), the caudal cerebellar peduncle, and the descending vestibulospinal tracts. The vestibulospinal tract modulates the muscle tone of the trunk and the limbs. This is important for balance, posture, tone and movement. The medial longitudinal fasciculus is responsible for the connection between the vestibular nuclei and the motor nuclei of the extrinsic eye muscles, (III, IV and VI). These tracts are integral for normal nystagmus. A lesion in the central vestibular system causes signs similar to those of a lesion in the peripheral vestibular system: however, differences include possible dysfunction of a number of cranial nerves, an absence of Horner's syndrome and deficits in ipsilateral proprioception. The most reliable point for differentiation between the two systems, is that a normal postural reaction is most indicative of a peripheral lesion and an abnormal one indicative of a central lesion. It is **essential** to differentiate a peripheral lesion from a central one for the purposes of the differential diagnosis and prognosis (Table. 1.2).

Lesions in the caudal cerebellar peduncle can lead to a paradoxical vestibular syndrome, in which the head tilt is to the contralateral side of the lesion (see Fig. 15.1)

Further reading

JAGGY, A., TIPOLD, A. (1999): Die neurologische Untersuchung beim Kleintier und beim Pferd. Opuscula Veterinaria.

JAGGY, A. (1997): Neurologische Notfälle beim Tier, Enke Verlag, Stuttgart.

VANDEVELDE, M., JAGGY, A., LANG, J. (2001): Veterinärmedizinische Neurologie, 2. Aufl., Parey Verlag, Berlin.

OLIVER, J., LORENZ, K., KORNEGAY, J. (1997): Handbook of Veterinary Neurology, 3rd ed., Saunders, Philadelphia, pp.3–73.

1.5 Ophthalmological examination

Bernhard Spiess

The experienced examiner can assess all twelve cranial nerves during an eye examination. The pupillary light reflex, in addition to the testing of vision, is important as a part of a general patient examination. In comparison to human beings, the examination of the visual field is not as important. The assessment of the position, mobility and movements of both eyes as well as the tear production are of neuro-opthalmic importance.

1.5.1 Examination of vision

The assessment of vision requires the patient's cooperation and is not always easy in companion animals.

1.5.1.1 Menace response test

The simplest and most commonly used test of vision is the menace response test or menace response. A "menacing" movement with the hand is made a short distance away from the eye to be tested. The other eye is covered so that each eye can be tested individually. It is essential that no draught is caused by the hand movement otherwise this could cause the patient to blink. Touching of the long vibrissae in the cat should also be avoided for the same reason.

The menacing movement is recognised in the healthy animal and it responds by blinking. Sometimes a moderate defence reaction can be expected (1).

The afferent arm of this response is the optic nerve (CN II), while the closing of the eyelids occurs due to the orbicularis oculi muscles, which are innervated by the facial nerve (CN III). Integration of the afferent and efferent impulses takes place in the contralateral cerebral cortex.

It should be remembered that the menace response is not a reflex as it is a learned response to a menacing action. Puppies up to the age of 12 weeks do not show a reaction to the menace test (2). Sight should be tested in another manner in such young animals.

1.5.1.2 Dazzle reflex

The dazzle reflex is a subcortical reflex elicited by a strong light. When strong light is shone into an eye, then a slight blinking will occur in both eyes, with the reaction on the contralateral side tending to be weaker (3). The afferent arm is the optic nerve, while the efferent arm of this reflex must have an intact facial nerve. This reflex can be used to determine whether the animal has an intact retina and optic nerve when there are opacities in the eye (cataract, etc.) or when there is no menace response. Although investigations in the decerebrate cat have shown that this reflex remains intact, the dazzle reflex can still be used to provide valuable information about a patient's potential ability to see.

1.5.1.3 Cotton ball test

A useful test for judging vision is the so-called "cotton ball" test. In this test, how the patient's eyes follow a moving object is observed. In young and playful dogs and cats, a small beam of light can be moved backwards and forwards on the floor in the animal's field of vision.

Also, small rolling balls quickly catch the attention of such animals. As a rule, one usually only uses the cotton ball test, whereby a small ball of cotton wool is thrown from behind the animal into its field of vision. A cotton ball is especially suitable for this test as it does not make a sound when falling. A patient with normal eyesight will follow the cotton ball with its eyes and possibly make a corresponding movement of its head. In placid animals, just a slight twitching of the ears is the only indication that the cotton ball has been seen. As with the other tests, the cotton ball test should be repeated a number of times to exclude the possibility of a chance reaction. Each eye should be tested separately using this test (2).

This test is positive in puppies before the menace response is functional.

1.5.1.4 Obstacle course

Under certain circumstances, the previous ophthalmological tests are not adequate for testing any slight impairment in sight. To test a dog's ability to see under different lighting conditions, the animal can be made to go around an obstacle course (3). In this test, a number of different obstacles (e.g. chairs, wastepaper baskets, plastic bags, etc.) are placed in a room unknown to the animal. The dog is held on one side of the room and then is called over to the other side by its owner. It is easy to observe whether the dog can move confidently around the obstacles or if it hesitatingly feels around the objects with its head bent to the floor. This test can be done first of all in strong light and then repeated with the light turned down. Dogs with retinal degeneration are affected, in the initial stages, by a night blindness. In the obstacle course test, such dogs have no difficulty when the room is well lit, but they are obviously slow and uncertain in their movements in semi-darkness, and may even bump into the obstacles. It is often desirable to do this test for each eye separately, but to do this the other eye must be well covered. Not every animal will allow this and they often refuse to move at all or will only move when the "irritating" eye cover is removed. The obstacle course test usually cannot be effectively carried out in the cat.

1.5.2 Examination of the pupillary light reflex and the size of the pupils

The pupillary light reflex (PLR) is a most important neuro-ophthalmological test.

First of all, the symmetry of both pupils is assessed. It is best to judge the dog from a distance of about 1 m through a direct ophthalmoscope. The light reflected from the tapetum luci-

dum makes the pupils shine brightly, enabling the size of each pupil to be compared exactly. This should be done at first in a bright room and then when the room is darkened. Certain anisocorias are better seen in a bright light and disappear in the dark, and vice versa.

The PLR is always determined in a darkened room. The direct PLR is tested in the eye into which the light is shone and the consensual, indirect PLR is evident in the opposite eye (1). A strong, focal light source is necessary for this test. The anatomy of the PLR is shown in Fig. 1.43.

The quickest and most reliable way of testing the PLR is the so-called pendulum or swinging light test. A focal light is shone in one eye for a few seconds, whereby the direct PLR can be judged. Then the light source is quickly changed over to the other eye. In the healthy animal, this pupil is already narrowed (positive indirect PLR) and remains so (direct PLR). Now when the light source is shone back into the first eye, the pupil in that eye is still narrowed (indirect PLR) and remains so (direct PLR) (2). The PLR allows a localisation of the lesion in unilateral visual deficits. In this (normal) case one talks of a **negative** pendulum light test. With a **positive** pendulum light test, the direct PLR on the unaffected side is physiological, meaning that the pupil narrows on direct illumination. When the light is then shone in the affected eye, its pupil is initially narrowed (positive indirect PLR), but it then dilates under the direct illumination (negative direct PLR). If the light is then changed back to the unaffected side, its pupil is initially dilated (negative indirect PLR) and then narrows when the light hits the eye. The positive pendulum test is pathognomonic for one-sided changes in the retina or unilateral prechiasmatic lesions of the optic nerve (4).

The lateral and medial sections of the retina can be illuminated separately with a good focal light source, and so their respective PLRs can be assessed. In this manner, the visual field can be approximately tested.

1.5.3 Palpebral reflex

The palpebral reflex tests the sensory innervation of the palpebrae by the trigeminal nerve and the motor innervation of the orbicularis oculi muscle via the facial nerve. This reflex is elicited by a light tapping of the medial and lateral canthi, testing the ophthalmic and maxillary branches of CN V respectively.

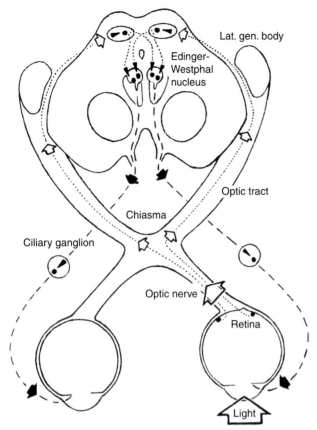

Fig. 1.43
The afferent arm of the PLR runs from the retina via the optic nerve, the optic chiasm and the optic tract to the pretectal nucleus. From there, it travels to the Edinger-Westphal nucleus of CN III. Then some of the axons cross over either in the area of the chiasm or the caudal commissure. The efferent parasympathetic fibres run to the ciliary ganglia together with the motor fibres of the oculomotor nerve. They then travel from there as short, caudal ciliary nerves to the pupillary sphincter muscle.

1.5.4　Corneal reflex

The innervation of the cornea (ophthalmic branch CN V) is tested by touching the surface of the cornea. The cornea should be gently touched by a sterile cotton bud on the side in such a manner that it cannot be seen by the patient, just felt. The innervation of the cornea can be determined in a semi-quantitative manner using an aethesiometer (5).

All the reflexes which result in a closing of the eyelids (i.e. menace response, dazzle reflex, palpebral and corneal reflexes) require an intact facial nerve.

1.5.5　Tear production

The basal and reflexive tear production is controlled afferently by the trigeminal nerve and efferently via fibres that originate in the parasympathetic nucleus of the facial nerve. Lesions of the afferent or efferent pathways lead to a neurogenic keratoconjunctivitis sicca (KCS) (3). Tear secretion is measured using the Schirmer tear test (6). Tear secretion must be tested in dogs with paresis or paralysis of the facial nerve (7).

1.5.6　Eyeball position

The normal and symmetrical position of both eyeballs should be assessed. Strabismus is relatively rare in small animals. A congenital esotropia has been described in the Siamese cat (8) and an acquired fibrosing esotropia occurs in the Shar Pei (1).

1.5.7　Normal vestibular nystagmus

Horizontal and vertical head movements induce impulses in the vestibular portion of the vestibulocochlear nerve (CN VIII). The resulting nystagmus has its rapid phase in the direction of the head movement. This type of nystagmus stops immediately when the head movement ceases. The recti muscles are innervated by three cranial nerves (CN III, IV and VI) and can be examined by eliciting vestibular nystagmus (1).

1.5.8　Electrophysiological examinations

Valuable additional information about blindness or disturbances in vision can be acquired by using the electrophysiological tests which belong in routine ophthalmological examinations.

1.5.8.1　Electroretinography (ERG)

The function of the retina can be tested using ERG. In this test, the retina is stimulated by a single flash of light and the mass response of the outer retinal layers are collected by two electrodes, enhanced and recorded. All the retinal cells with the exception of those in the ganglia are involved in the biogenesis of the ERG. As such the ERG is not a sight test per se; it is just a test of the retinal function. Despite this, the ERG allows the diagnosis of various forms of retinal degeneration and can help in the differentiation between ocular and retrobulbar forms of blindness (Fig. 1.44) (9). The rods and cones can be examined separately using suitable stimuli, which is important in the early diagnosis of retinopathies.

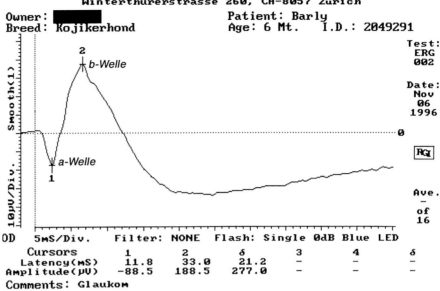

Fig. 1.44
Physiological ERG in a dog. An a-wave (generated by the photoreceptors) and a b-wave (which originates in the inner granular layer, mainly in the bipolar cells) are differentiated from each other.

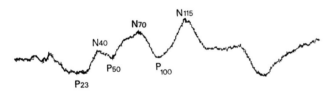

Fig. 1.45
Physiological VEP in a dog. The individual components are named according to their polarity and their peak time. While the amplitudes are subjected to relatively large fluctuations, the peak times are reproducible.

1.5.8.2 Visual evoked potentials (VEP)

VEP are the stimulus-correlated potentials which can be filtered out of the stochastic background "noise" of an EEG by the production of an electronic mean. The potentials are generated in areas 17 to 19 of the cerebral cortex, the so-called visual cortex. The retina is stimulated by flashes of light or patterned stimuli and the biosignals are recorded from the respective areas of the cerebral cortex.

Changes in the transmission of the stimuli, the so-called latency period, and in the amplitudes of the different signals can indicate lesions in the optic nerve, optic radiations and the visual cortex (Fig. 1.45) (9). The amplitude of these signals tends to be very small and variable, whereas in comparison, the latency period remains constant.

Literature

1 SCAGLIOTTI, R. (1999): Comparative Neuro-ophthalmology. In: Gelatt, K. (ed.): Veterinary Ophthalmology, 3rd ed., Lippincott Williams & Wilkins, Philadelphia.

2 SLATTER, D. (1990): Fundamentals of Veterinary Ophthalmology. 2nd ed. Vol. 1., W.B. Saunders, Philadelphia.

3 GELATT, K. (2000): Essentials of Veterinary Ophthalmology, Lippincott Williams & Wilkins, Philadelphia.

4 ENYEDI, L.B., DEV, S., COX, T.A. (1998): A comparison of the Marcus Gunn and alternating light tests for afferent pupillary defects. Ophthalmol. **105** (5): 871–873.

5 BARRETT, P., SCAGLIOTTI, R.H, MERIDETH, R.E, JACKSON, P.M, LAZANO ALACRON, F., (1991): Absolute corneal sensitivity and corneal trigeminal nerve anatomy in normal dogs. Vet Comp Ophthalmol. **1** (4): 245–254.

6 SPIESS, B. (1998): Der Schirmer Tränen Test (STT). Kleintierkonkret, **3**: 14–18.

7 KERN, T.J. ERB, H.N. (1987): Facial neuropathy in dogs and cats: 95 cases (1975–1985). J Am Vet Med Assoc. **191** (12): 1604–1609.

8 BLAKE, R., COOL, S.F., CRAWFORD, M.L., (1974): Visual resolution in the cat. Vision Res., **14**: 1211–1271.

9 SPIESS, B. (1994): Elektrophysiologische Untersuchungen des Auges bei Hund und Katze. Enke Copythek, Stuttgart.

2 Principles of Neuropathology

Thomas Bilzer
Marc Vandevelde
André Jaggy

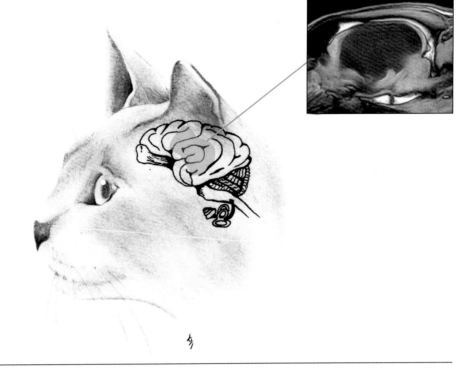

2.1 General neuropathology

2.1.1 Histopathology

2.1.1.1 Neuron

Neurons develop from the neuroectoderm and are highly differentiated somatic cells with unique characteristics. Despite having different sizes and forms (motor neurons, autonomic ganglion cells, Purkinje cells, interneurons, etc.), their metabolic, cytoarchitectural and functional characteristics are more or less the same. They are asymmetric and polarised. They all have a slightly peripheral nucleus that contains little chromatin and one or two nucleoli. Their mitochondria, lysosomes, Golgi apparatus and rough endoplasmic reticulum are collected together in the Nissl bodies in the perikaryon (1). Most of a neuron's mass consists of cytoplasmic processes: the dendrites and axons (Fig. 2.1). To overcome the enormous transport functions undertaken by these structures, neurons have a special cytoskeleton made up of microtubules, intermediary filaments and microfilaments. Neurons are in contact with each other and their peripheral target organs via synapses. Very many different types of molecules are necessary for transportation, supply and the processing of information, so that over 50% of all the body's genes are expressed only in the neurons.

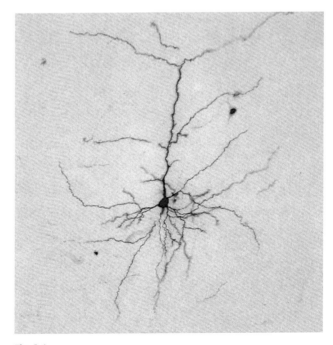

Fig. 2.1
Neurons. Pyramidal cell in the neocortex showing a long axonal section and many dendrites. Immunohistochemical staining with tyrosine hydroxylase (5-year-old dog).

2

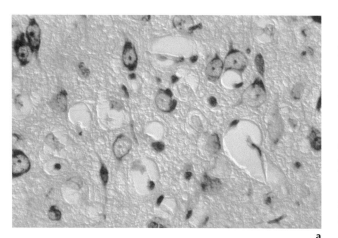

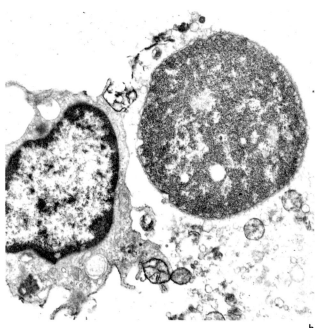

Fig. 2.2a, b
Neuronal death. (a) Spongiform encephalopathy with many nerve cells beginning to undergo necrosis due to a persistent virus infection (cerebral cortex, rat; cresyl violet stain). (b) Apoptosis of a neuron (condensation of the nucleus, dissolution of the cell membrane and cytoplasm; right) in contact with a microglial cell (cerebral cortex, 5-year-old dog; electron microscopy).

Neuronal cell death

After the end of proliferation and migration during brain development, surplus neurons are eliminated by programmed cell death (apoptosis; see below). Afterwards, two types of cells remain: fully differentiated post-mitotic neurons and adult stem cells arranged in nests. As neurons – with exception of the olfactory cells – can not proliferate, the possibility of CNS regeneration subsequent to a lesion is limited. However, recently there have been more and more indications that adult stem cells can play a part in the renewal of neurons.

Neuronal cell death can – depending on the noxious agent – occur in a number of different forms such as apoptosis, apoklesis (withering of the nerve cells, e.g., after axotomy), dark degeneration or ischemic cell necrosis. The different forms of cell degeneration as well as the artificial and transient intravital changes that occur in neurons are often difficult to differentiate from each other (2).

Apoptosis

Apoptosis or programmed cell death is described as the simultaneous a) decay of the cell membrane with b) condensation of the plasma and c) karyorrhexis. It is the classical form of normal cell degeneration in growing tissues elicited by internal gene activation. The different gene cascades that cause apoptosis in neurons and glial cells are also observed during neurodegenerative processes (3) (Fig. 2.2a).

Nerve cell necrosis

Nerve cell necrosis is a form of cell death that occurs in response to a number of exogenous noxious stimuli (heat, toxins, ischemia / hypoxia) and in which various indications of cell degeneration can be seen (4). Frequently, shrinkage of the nucleus is the most obvious sign, accompanied by dissolution of the Nissl bodies and an intensive eosinophilia of the cytoplasm. Such cells are dyed a dark blue-violet with cresyl violet (Fig. 2.2b). Often changes in the mitochondria are also apparent. Due to membrane damage, there is an influx of calcium leading to cell death. In contrast to apoptosis, cell clusters are affected rather than individual cells. Subsequently, microglial cells / macrophages group around the dying neurons and phagocytose them (neuronophagy).

Neuronal inclusion bodies, vacuoles, storage products

Characteristic and sometimes pathognomonic intra-cytoplasmic and/or intranuclear inclusion bodies can be seen with viral diseases (2, 5). In comparison, neuronal vacuolation is non-specific and occurs in response to different noxious stimuli, such as cytotoxic oedema or following axotomy. A special form of neuronal vacuolation seen in connection with nerve cell loss and astrocyte gliosis occurs in infectious spongiform encephalopathies such as Scrapie, Bovine Spongiform Encephalopathy and Creutzfeld-Jakob disease (6). A deposition of pigment (e.g. lipofuscin, neuro-melanin), glycogen or fat occurs in nerve cells either normally due to age or in storage diseases (see below).

2.1.1.2 Astroglia, ependymal cells, plexus epithelium

Astrocytes are the most important cells involved in metabolism within the nervous system. They also provide the structure to the system in conjunction with the neurons. As with the neurons, astrocytes originate from the neuroectoderm. They are connected by their processes on the one side to capillaries and on the other, to neurons. Astrocytes produce proteins of the extracellular matrix, adhesion molecules, neurotropic factors, growth factors and cytokines (2). It is possible that astrocytes, like the microglial cells, act as antigen-presenting cells (7).

The astroglia comprise a heterogenic group of cells that differ both functionally and morphologically, and which consists of cells with many specialised subtypes and complex interactions. Classically, they are differentiated morphologically into protoplasmic and fibrous astrocytes, with the protoplasmic types occurring more often in the grey matter and the fibrous in the white.

Reactive glial cells
One of the earliest and most frequent phenomena after a CNS lesion is astrocytic oedema. It can occur after ischemia / hypoxia, hypoglycaemia, neurotoxicosis, inflammation, epilepsy or trauma. The swelling of the astrocytes is the main parameter of so-called cytotoxic brain oedema. The formation of reactive astrocytes occurs regularly in pathological changes in the CNS (8). They are mainly distinguished by an increase in glial fibrillary acidic protein (GFAP) (Fig. 2.3a). Such hypertrophic astrocytes can be observed in subacute or chronic processes (i.e. close to tumours, abscesses or other focal processes). They may also be seen in diffuse changes such as oedema of the medullary layer, leukodystrophies and encephalitis. A "carpet" of astrocytes is formed after larger lesions, the so-called glial scar.

Ependymal cells and plexus epithelial cells
The ependymal cells cover the surface of the brain's ventricles and the central canal of the spinal cord. The plexus epithelial cells surround the blood vessel plexi in the ventricles and are involved in the production of the cerebrospinal fluid (CSF). Little is known about the reaction of the ependymal and plexus epithelial cells to pathological occurrences apart from that they can atrophy and degenerate or become neoplastic – just like other neuroectodermal cells. As a rule, defects in these cell layers are repaired by astroglia.

2.1.1.3 Oligodendroglia / Schwann cells

Myelin pathology
Similar to the astroglia, the oligodendrocytes and Schwann cells (which also originate from the neuroectoderm) are metabolically very active and, in particular, nourish the myelin sheath. They often lie close to the perikaryon of the nerve cells as satellite cells, or as cells of the myelin sheath they lie close to the axon in the neuropil. In damaged areas, these cells undergo cell hypertrophy and possibly cell division. Injury to the oligodendroglia results in vacuolisation, inclusion bodies, increased production of microtubules and changes in myelinogenesis (2).

Demyelination of varying degrees is a consequence of numerous noxious stimuli such as trauma, tumour, viral infection (9), immunopathological reactions against myelin protein or intoxication. This leads to the formation of vesicles (honey-

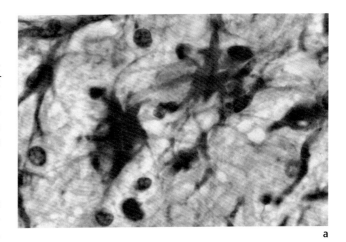

a

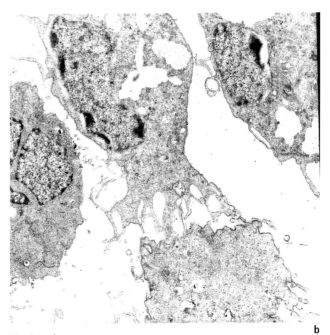

b

Fig. 2.3a, b
Glial cells. (a) Reactive astrocyte in the periphery of a tumour. Immunohistochemical staining of glial fibrillary acidic protein (GFAP; cerebral cortex, 8-year-old dog). Microglial cell (middle) in contact with virus-infected astrocytes (rat cell structure; electron microscopy).

combing), fragmentation and finally dissolution (Fig. 2.4). Even with a severe loss of myelin, axons can remain intact over prolonged periods of time. Remyelination starts quickly afterwards, especially when the endemic astrocytes and neighbouring oligodendroglia have not been injured. After myelin damage, immature oligodendrocytes are recruited and wander into the destroyed region.

The most common form of central myelin damage is vacuolisation, the so-called spongiform degeneration, which occurs as a consequence of intoxication, viral infection (e.g. distemper) and autoimmune disease.

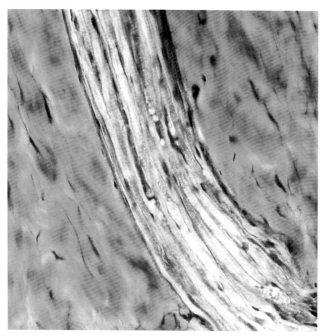

Fig. 2.4
Demyelination. Peripheral nerve fibre in a polyneuropathy (4-month-old Dogo Argentino; Gomori trichrome stain according to Engel).

2.1.1.4 Microglia

Microglial cells are nowadays unanimously considered as being the CNS's resident macrophages (2). Their behaviour is comparable to that of the macrophages, with whom they are classified in the so-called monocytic phagocyte system. They originate from the mesenchyme and form approx. 20% of all glial cells. They are distinguished by their typically differentiated morphology (rod glia). In the healthy adult brain, the microglia are mainly found disseminated evenly as so-called resting microglia. They form a network of immune accessory cells that react even to the subtlest changes in the microenvironment of the brain and spinal cord. With larger lesions, a wide-spread stimulation of the microglia occurs. The activated microglia proliferate, express / present antigens on their cell surface (e.g. MHC antigen) and synthesise numerous cytokines (10). They can differentiate further towards macrophages and are the main players in the mobile resorption of dead neural tissue (Fig. 2.3b).

2.1.1.5 Neuropil, blood-brain barrier

The collection of neurons and glial cells which is permeated by blood vessels is called the neuropil. The neuropil contains only very narrow extracellular spaces. It has no interstitial connective tissue lymphatics, though it communicates with the cervical and abdominothoracic lymphatic system via the CSF. This fact is very important for understanding the development of inflammatory reactions in the CNS, which is otherwise protected by the blood-brain barrier.

Brain capillaries are different to other blood vessels due to the existence of the blood-brain barrier, which can be better understood as a functional cooperation of the blood vessel endothelium, pericytes and astrocytes (11). This barrier protects the neural tissues from penetration by many different types of macromolecular substances and infectious agents.

2.1.1.6 Envelope cells

The meninges, comprised of the pia mater, arachnoidea and dura mater, are formed by mesenchymal cells. The dura is tightly bound to the periosteum of the skull in the head, though it runs as a loose tube through the spinal canal The subarachnoid space lying between the pia mater and the arachnoidea contains the CSF. Funnel-shaped layers of meningeal cells fuse with the perineural nerve sheaths at the roots of the spinal nerves, while at the roots of the cranial nerves these meningeal cell layers fuse with the dura. The enveloping tissue is rich in blood vessels and reacts earlier than the neural tissues to inflammation (2).

2.1.1.7 Neuronal degeneration / regeneration

Neuronal degeneration and regeneration affects both neurons and glial cells. Every nerve fibre (nerve cell process) in the CNS is enclosed by oligodendrocytes, while in the PNS, the fibre is covered by Schwann cells in a myelin sheath or it is enclosed within myelin-poor or myelinless Remak cells.

Axotomy, pro- and retrograde degeneration, axonal dystrophy

Damage to the axon caused by trauma, crushing, inflammation or tumour growth leading to a break in its continuity results in characteristic reactions (12). The proximal stump of the axon remains intact, while in the peripheral segment there is a swelling of the perikaryon, peripheral displacement of the cell nucleus and dissolution of the Nissl substance. In addition, the surrounding glial satellite cells are activated. Synonyms such as primary stimulation, axonal reaction and retrograde reaction or degeneration are used in connection with these changes (2).

The part of the axon lying distal to the lesion degenerates (prograde or Wallerian degeneration): dissolution of the axon and myelin sheath, phagocytosis and Schwann cell proliferation are seen. The Schwann cells form Büngner's bands (an alignment of the Schwann cells along the long axis of the nerve), which act as guide rails for the regenerating axon.

The complex and multi-functional axonal transport system is very sensitive to numerous noxious stimuli, especially mechanical lesions and oxygen deficiency. Such disturbances affect the neurofilament and microtubular systems resulting in problems in transportation, the building up of organelles, axonal swelling and tearing, which all result in axonal degeneration (12).

Neuroaxonal dystrophy is a condition in which there is enormous swelling of the axons (up to a diameter of $120\,\mu$) with the production of so-called axonal spheroids. This occurs primarily as an inherited disease, for example, in neuroaxonal dystrophy of the Rottweiler or secondarily in various degenerative diseases and toxicoses.

Neuronal regeneration

Neuronal regeneration occurs only to a limited extent in the CNS; most lesions are replaced by a gliosis. How far adult stem cells are capable of replacing defects still remains largely unclarified (2). Axonal growth can be induced in the area of lesions by blocking inhibitory molecules produced by the oligodendroglia and by applying neurotrophins at the same time. Doing this, for example, enables motor neurons of the spinal cord and the medulla oblongata as well as ganglion cells in the PNS to produce new axons. Basically, the PNS can regenerate well as long as there is the possibility of a structural and anatomical connection between the budding axon and its peripheral target.

2.1.2 Disturbances in development / malformations

2.1.2.1 Brain development – Pathogenesis of malformation

Malformations are an expression of disturbed morphogenesis, whereby the main points of resulting concern are cell form, migration, proliferation, differentiation and apoptosis (13). The pathogenesis of malformations is understood as a sequence of molecular, cellular and tissue changes, which lead to the development of a pathological phenotype. The interaction of primary gene defects or those caused by viruses, toxins or radiation induce a disturbance in cell differentiation and play an important role as aetiological factors. The understanding of the aetiology and pathogenesis of disturbances in brain development has been greatly transformed by the identification of a number of genes and cellular and molecular mechanisms that steer embryonic and foetal development,

The embryonal development of the CNS is very complex and there are numerous disorders which can affect each phase. Severe chromosome defects lead to conspicuously complex malformations (e.g. Turner's syndrome), whereas individual genetic mistakes cause smaller structural and functional disturbances. The latter remain undiscovered unless they are associated with behavioural disturbances, difficulties in learning, etc. Only a few of the real brain malformations are compatible with life. These are confined to two groups: disturbances in the closure of the neural tube (dysraphias) and disturbances in the development of the cortex.

2.1.2.2 Defects of the neural tube: dysraphias

In addition to genetic defects, virus infections play the greatest role in neural tube abnormalities (e.g. Parvoviruses: panleucopaenia in the cat; Togaviruses: Swine fever, Bovine viral diarrhoea). Depending on the stage of development, defects of differing dimensions occur (13):

- **Anencephaly** (brain congenitally absent) and **amyelia** (spinal cord is congenitally absent). Both of these can occur independently of each other and are usually concurrent and always associated with defects of the skull or spine (craniorachischisis).
- **Porencephaly** – defect in the brain substance which provides a connection between the ventricular system and the surface of the brain. This sometimes occurs in association with cavitation of the brain.
- **Hydranencephaly** is an extreme form of porencephaly (14), which occurs together with arthrogryposis (abnormal positioning of the limbs) in the calf.

Different forms of "herniation" of the brain or spinal cord tissue through bony defects can be seen to accompany some of these defects. These are leptomeningeal (covered in epidermis and fluid-filled) sacs that project out of an incompletely closed skull or spinal canal. If neural elements are contained in the sac then it is called an **encephalo-** or **myelomeningocele,** if not then it is a **meningocele**.

Syringomylia (syrinx: Greek for flute) represents the development of an extensive fluid-filled cavity in the spinal cord. It is frequently noticed first in adulthood (14). This condition should be separated from **hydromyelia**, the presence of a widened central canal, although even with advanced imaging, this distinction can be difficult and so the disorder is sometimes named syringohydromyelia

2.1.2.3 Constitutional hydrocephalus
(See Chap. 18.4.4.1)

2.1.2.4 Anomalies of the cortex: microgyria, macrogyria, lissencephaly

During the development of the brain from the neural tube, the neuroblasts lying close to the tube's lumen have to wander out to the periphery. If disturbances in this migration take place, then anomalies will occur in the cortex (13). Often changes in the cerebellar cortex and medulla oblongata occur in association with such disturbances in the cerebral cortex. In the most common developmental disturbance, **microgyria** (micro-polygyria), there is, in addition to an abnormal layering of the cortex, a fine folding of its surface that is reminiscent of street paving. An abnormal cortical structure is also found in **macrogyria** (pachygyria), though here the layers penetrate deep into the medulla and the sulci are so flattened in places that the gyri seem to fuse with each other.

Lissencephaly (agyria) is an extreme form of macrogyria in which the gyri seem to be completely missing. In contrast, the brain in **micro-encephaly** is often well proportioned as there is an associated microcephaly.

2.1.2.5 Malformations of the cerebellum

Both inherited diseases (e.g. in the Gordon Setter or St. Bernard) and viral diseases (e.g. panleucopaenia in the cat) play an important role in these malformations. They lead to **cerebellar aplasia** or **hypoplasia** (14), in which the cortex is thinner than normal or even missing (see Chap. 16.4.1). The development of the medulla can also be disturbed (**hypomyelinogenesis**).

2.1.2.6 Hypo- and dysmyelinogenesis

Disturbances in the development of the white matter in the spinal cord, brain and peripheral nerves occurs to different extents and have been described for a number of dog breeds (14). This type of disturbance is more likely to be due to an abnormality in the formation of myelin – possibly due to inadequate maturation of the oligodendrocytes rather than a degenerative disturbance. Both genetic defects and exogenous causes (viral infections, nutritional deficiencies) have been considered. The main breeds which are affected are the Chow Chow, Springer Spaniel, Samoyed, Weimaraner, Berner Sennenhund and Dalmatian (see Chap. 14.1.7).

2.1.3 Mechanical and physical disturbances

2.1.3.1 Increased brain pressure

The brain is a relatively flexible structure, which can adapt to moderate changes in pressure. Trauma, intracranial bleeding, inflammation, tumours, increased CSF or blood pressure and brain oedema can lead to a life-threatening increase in intracranial pressure (16).

2.1.3.2 Space-occupying processes/acquired hydrocephalus

Each space-occupying process within the inflexible skull causes an increase of intracranial pressure. The effect of such a process depends on its location and pathology: A rapidly growing invasive malignant glioma, a florid encephalitis or an expanding haemorrhage are all more difficult to control than, for example, a slow-growing meningioma. The quicker and more progressive the course, the lesser the chance the nerve tissue has for compensation (e.g. reduction of CSF production) and the more severe the consequences. Tumours, inflammatory processes and parasites can cause disturbances in CSF drainage leading to the development of an acquired internal hydrocephalus.

2.1.3.3 Swelling of the brain and brain oedema

A significant additional complication of trauma or space-occupying processes is the swelling/oedema of the brain. As the skull cavity is not expandable, it is possible that areas at a distance from the lesion are affected; for example, a shifting of the cerebellum into the foramen magnum (cerebellar hernia). Brain oedema is divided into **vasogenic** (disturbances in the blood-brain barrier; e.g. by focal processes such as trauma, abscess, tumour), **cytotoxic** (disturbances in the Na/K pump, e.g. in hypoxia/ischemia), **hydrostatic** (caused by blood pressure), **hypoosmolar** (e.g. in hyponatraemia) and **interstitial** (increase CSF pressure; e.g. in hydrocephalus) (16).

2.1.3.4 Infarct/cartilaginous emboli

Infarcts of the brain and the associated "stroke" play a subordinate role in animals unlike in people. Different to the primary thrombotic infarcts due to arthrosclerosis found in human beings, infarcts in animals are usually due to emboli from diseases such as endocarditis. Ischemia and the subsequent infarction and necrosis of the spinal cord occur in connection with vascular abscessation, atherosclerosis, arteriosclerosis, thrombosis, parasitic emboli, foreign bodies, severe intervertebral disc prolapse and cartilaginous emboli (17). The latter occur in all dog breeds and cats of every age, and may or may not be associated with with a disc herniation (see Chap. 14.1.1); as a consequence, the pathogenesis has not been fully elucidated. Infarcts and necrotic regions form resulting in a reactive inflammation with the immigration of microglia/macrophages. The clinical signs are peracute with the cervical and lumbar intumescences most commonly affected. In these cases, the reflexes and muscle tone are reduced; paralysis, hyperaesthesia or anaesthesia occurs and pain is rarely seen.

2.1.3.5 Haemorrhage

Massive haemorrhage in domestic animals is usually the result of trauma (Fig. 2.5). Bleeding from aneurysms, telangiectasis or angiomas is just as rare as are the consequences of diseases associated with hypertension. **Petechial bleeding** due to damaged capillary walls is caused by septic, allergic, chemotoxic, traumatic, physical and thermal stimuli.

2.1.3.6 Trauma

The process of craniocerebral trauma can be divided as follows: (1) primary injury; (2) aftereffects; (3) secondary lesions; and (4) recovery and restoration of function (18, 19).

The primary lesion is determined by the type, localisation and extent of injury and is also affected by the patient's age, nutritional status, constitution, condition and genetic predisposition. Skull fractures resulting from head trauma can cause primary injury to the brain; however, whether the fractures are **open or closed** does not seem to relate to the severity of the inciting lesion. When the skull or vertebral canal is opened by trauma, tearing, deformation and infection of the tissues are more likely to occur. Also independent of the severity of the trauma, (1) **concussion**; (2) **contusion or compression**; and (3) **laceration** of the nervous tissue can occur. Mild damage to the tissues occurs with concussion, which is usually only local and occurs in association with oedema. A temporary loss of consciousness and a loss or reduction of cranial nerve reflexes can also occur. Normally, there is no long-term damage incurred. With contusion / compression of the brain, severe tissue damage takes place, often in association with haemorrhage and oedema. Laceration is a coarse disturbance in the brain's structure, which leads to severe clinical symptoms and is often not compatible with life (see Chaps. 5.1.1 and 10.2.2).

The secondary injury processes of craniocerebral trauma have been extensively investigated in recent years and are known to include the formation of free radicals, accumulation of intracellular calcium and inflammation. These secondary injury processes result in cerebral lesions due to the resultant local ischemia, increased intracranial pressure, or brain oedema,

2.1.4 Metabolic disturbances

Disturbances in electrolyte balance, endocrinopathies and organ failure can lead to disturbances in energy metabolism, destabilisation of cell membranes, hypoxia or endotoxicosis within the CNS. These are also called metabolic encephalopathies (20).

2.1.4.1 Ischemia / hypoxia / hypoglycaemia

The lack of oxygen and hypoglycaemia caused by ischemia rapidly lead to disturbances in brain function due to the brain's limited endogenous reserves. If this situation is not rapidly treated or compensated for, then there will be nerve cell necrosis and spongiform encephalomalacia in the neocortex and allocortex (hippocampus). Early warning signs include adrenergic symptoms such as muscle shaking, weakness and restlessness. Later, ataxia, collapse and seizures may occur (21). Quite commonly, the cause is a tumour (insulinoma as well as non-endocrine tumours such as hepatic tumours, haemangiosarcomas, lymphosarcomas and adenosarcomas of the lungs or mammary glands). Another cause can be insulin over-dosage. Transient hypoglycaemia in puppies can occur in association with gastrointestinal diseases such as parasite burdens (see Chap. 18.4.5.2).

2.1.4.2 Hepatic encephalopathy

Severe liver dysfunction in either acute or chronic liver failure or a portocaval shunt can lead to the release of toxic metabolites (ammonia, phenylalanine, tryptophan, tyrosine, short-chain fatty acids, biogenic amines) in the circulation and the development of hepatic encephalopathy (22). Glutamine is formed from ammonia and accumulates intracellularly in the brain cells, which may induce brain oedema affecting large parts of not only the cerebral cortex, but also the cerebellum and brain stem. Changes in behaviour, staring, peculiar vocalisation, hyperactivity and aggression are obvious symptoms of this condition (see Chap. 18.4.5.3).

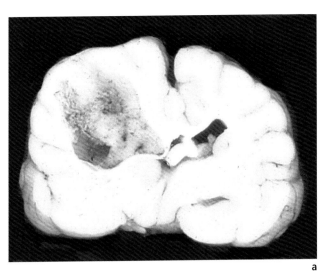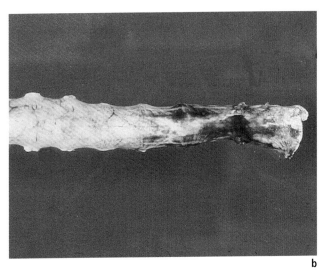

a · b

Fig. 2.5a, b
Haemorrhage / trauma. (a) Intracerebral haemorrhage in a 3-year-old Boxer with a glioma (tumour haemorrhage). (b) Subdural haemorrhage after spinal trauma at the level of the caudal thoracic vertebrae (12-year-old cat).

2.1.4.3   Uraemic encephalopathy

Acute or chronic renal insufficiency can lead to an impairment of the CNS. In the acute condition, seizures and myoclonus occur, while in the chronic form dementia develops (23). The pathogenesis of this encephalopathy is unclear though intracerebral hypoxia / reduced oxygen turnover and increased calcium values appear to play a part. The changes in the brain tissue are non-specific (see Chap. 18.4.5.4).

2.1.4.4   Hypernatraemia (salt poisoning)

Changes in the sodium balance of the cells can lead to brain oedema followed by intracranial haemorrhage, which in turn results in severe disturbances in brain function. The causes are excessive loss of water / inadequate water uptake and/or increased salt uptake (20).

2.1.4.5   Hyponatraemia

Hyponatraemia with hyposmolarity (true hyponatraemia) is usually a consequence of renal failure (20). Hyponatraemia with normal to hyperosmolarity of the serum (isomolar pseudohyponatraemia) occurs in connection with parenteral hyperglycaemia (or mannitol administration), urea nitrogen and toxins. It is often found in association with hyperlipidaemia and hyperproteinaemia.

True hyponatraemia can be divided into:
- Hypervolaemic hyponatraemia (in congestive cardiomyopathy, liver failure, nephrosis and hypoalbuminaemia),
- Normovolaemic hyponatraemia (renal failure, hypo-thyroidism, adrenocortical insufficiency and polydipsia) and
- Hypovolaemic hyponatraemia (renal or extrarenal syndromes, e.g. gastrointestinal disease).

Acute hyponatraemia leads to brain oedema and increased intracranial pressure.

2.1.4.6   Hypocalcaemia

Ionised calcium plays an important role in synaptic transmission. Hypocalcaemia leads to hyperreactivity, seizures, fever, ataxia, spasms and even tetany or epilepsy due to the loss of its stabilising effects. The main causes are hypoparathyroidism, hypovitaminosis D, renal failure, acute pancreatitis or intestinal malabsorption (20).

2.1.4.7   Acidosis and alkalosis

Severe acidosis and alkalosis can result in disorientation, changes in personality or even coma due to their association with an increase in intracranial pressure or brain oedema leading to a disturbance in CNS function (20).

2.1.4.8   Malnutrition

A general protein deficiency has an effect on the developing brain, but virtually none on the adult one. In comparison, hypo- and hypervitaminoses can lead to severe neurological disease. The majority of malnutrition diseases are rare nowadays due to modern feeding practices.

Cobalamin (Vitamin B12) deficiency

A deficiency of this essential enzyme co-factor occurs in Giant Schnauzers, Border Collies and Beagles as the result of an autosomal recessive or congenital malabsorption affecting the enterocytes of the ileum. Acquired cobalamin deficiency can occur in older animals due to malnutrition, malabsorption, exocrine pancreas insufficiency or bacterial overgrowth. The type and pathogenesis of the lesions in the neurological tissue have not been totally explained. In human beings, a spongiform degeneration of the dorsal horns in the spinal cord, the corticospinal tracts and the cerebral albi occurs in association with a peripheral neuropathy (24).

Hypervitaminosis A

An excessive intake of vitamin A over months or even years – mostly through the feeding of raw liver – causes a deformative cervical spondylosis in cats, which leads to a bony ankylosis that compresses and destroys the nerve roots. The mechanisms of this pathological change are not fully understood (24).

Thiamine (Vitamin B1) deficiency

A deficiency of thermolabile thiamine occurs sporadically and only when dogs and cats are fed solely on cooked (high temperatures) or thiaminase-rich (e.g., fish) food (see Chap. 15.5.1). Thiamine plays an important role in the oxidation of glucose in the Krebs cycle, which is why glucose-dependent organs such as the brain are particularly sensitive to a deficiency of this vitamin. Vitamin B1 deficiency leads to the development of a bilateral polioencephalomalacia (24).

2.1.4.9   Diabetes mellitus

Chronic hyperglycaemia can lead to ketoacidosis, hyperosmolarity, dehydration and electrolyte imbalance via an increased mobilisation and oxidation of fatty acids. Hyperosmolarity causes cerebral dehydration as with hypernatraemia, resulting in similar clinical signs (25). An acute onset can lead to seizures and coma. Late sequelae involve microangiopathies and neuropathies.

2.1.4.10   Hypothyroidism / hyperthyroidism

Many metabolic functions are hampered by a reduced production of thyroxin (T4) and triiodothyronine (T3). In the brain, the most important pathological effect is a myxoedema which can lead to coma. In addition, a peripheral neuropathy / myopathy can be produced (26). Hypothyroidism related nerve and muscle disease can occur in the dog (see Chap. 15.4.3).

Hyperthyroidism occurs almost exclusively in the cat. It can cause hyperkinesis / restlessness, changes in personality, seizures and in particular, neuromuscular disturbances associated with hypokalaemia.

2.1.4.11 Storage diseases
(See Chap. 18.8.)

2.1.4.12 Neurotoxicology
Many metals, pesticides, solvents, and medications as well as bacterial, animal, insect and plant poisons can be neurotoxic. The changes in the nervous system are not usually very specific. An extensive description of their effects is not possible within the framework of this chapter (see Chap. 18.4.5). A few examples are discussed in the following:

Lead is still contained in objects used in daily life (e.g. paint) and relatively often causes poisoning in dogs and cats (28). Lead inhibits a number of enzymes and prevents erythrocyte maturation. It causes nerve cell necrosis / spongiform changes with vascular and glial reactions especially in the frontal and parietal cortex as well as in the brain stem. In addition, the Purkinje cells of the cerebellum are affected. The PNS is less influenced than in human beings. Affected animals are usually conspicuous due to their extreme gastrointestinal and neurological symptoms.

Thallium is a commonly used rat poison that induces vomiting, bloody diarrhoea, salivation, anorexia, paralysis and dyspnoea. Death occurs within a few days. Thallium causes degenerative changes in the brain and the peripheral nerves (29).

Anticoagulants. Vitamin K antagonists are used in many rodenticides. Cumarin, a derivative of a plant glycoside, is a frequently used substance. It causes parenchymal bleeding, which can lead to ataxia, paresis and seizures.

Organophosphates are widely used as antiparasitic medications in veterinary medicine. Cats are especially sensitive to chlorpyriphos (30). Organophosphates are acetylcholine esterase inhibitors and due to the subsequent cholinergic and parasympathetic hyperstimulation cause salivation, urination, defaecation, bradycardia, narrowing of the pupils, muscle twitching / spasms, fear, restlessness, hyperactivity and seizures. The basis of an associated polyneuropathy is an axonal degeneration in the PNS.

Literature

1 SOTELO, C., TRILLER, A. (2002): The central neuron. In: Greenfield's Neuropathology, 7th ed., Graham D.I., Lantos P.L. (ed.) Arnold, London, pp. 1–74.

2 GÄBER, M.B., BLAKEMORE, W.F., KREUTZBERG, G.W. (2002): Cellular pathology of the central nervous system. In: Greenfield's Neuropathology, 7th ed., Graham D.I., Lantos P.L. (ed.) Arnold, London, pp. 123–191.

3 BECKER, E.B., BONNI, A. (2004): Cell cycle regulation of neuronal apoptosis in development and disease. Prog Neurobiol. **72**: 1–25.

4 YUAN, J., LIPINSKI, M., DEGTEREV, A. (2003): Diversity in the mechanisms of neuronal cell death. Neuron **40**: 401–413.

5 BRAUND, K.G. (2003): Inflammatory diseases of the central nervous system. In: Clinical Neurology in Small Animals – Localization, Diagnosis and Treatment. K.G. Braund (ed.) International Veterinary Information Service, Ithaca, New York.

6 MASTERS, C.L., RICHARDSON, E.P. Jr. (1978): Subacute spongiform encephalopathy (Creutzfeldt-Jakob disease). The nature and progression of spongiform change. Brain **101**: 333–344.

7 BECHER, B., PRAT, A., ANTEL, J.P. (2000): Brain-immune connection: immuno-regulatory properties of CNS-resident cells. Glia **29**: 293–304.

8 CHEN, Y., SWANSON, R.A. (2003): Astrocytes and brain injury. J Cereb Blood Flow Metab. **23**: 137–149.

9 GRIOT, C., VANDEVELDE, M., SCHOBESBERGER, M., ZURBRIGGEN, A. (2003): Canine distemper, a re-emerging morbillivirus with complex neuropathogenic mechanisms. Anim Health Res Rev. **4**: 1–10.

10 NELSON, P.T., SOMA, L.A., LAVI, E. (2002): Microglia in diseases of the central nervous system. Ann Med. **34**: 491–500.

11 VORBRODT, A.W., DOBROGOWSKA, D.H. (2003): Molecular anatomy of intercellular junctions in brain endothelial and epithelial barriers: electron microscopist's view. Brain Res Rev. **42**: 221–242.

12 BJARTMAR, C., WUJEK, J.R., TRAPP, B.D. (2003): Axonal loss in the pathology of MS: consequences for understanding the progressive phase of the disease. J Neurol Sci. **206**: 165–171.

13 HARDING, B.N., COPP, A.J. (2002): Malformations. In: Greenfield's Neuropathology, 7th ed., Graham D.I., Lantos P.L. (ed.) Arnold, London, pp. 357–384.

14 BRAUND, K.G. (2003): Developmental disorders. In: Clinical Neurology in Small Animals – Localization, Diagnosis and Treatment. K.G. Braund (ed.) International Veterinary Information Service, Ithaca, New York.

15 SARTIN, E.A., DORAN, S.E., RIDDELL, M.G., HERRERA, G.A., TENNYSON, G.S., D'ANDREA, G., WHITLEY, R.D., COLLINS, F.S. (1994): Characterization of naturally occurring cutaneous neurofibromatosis in Holstein cattle. A disorder resembling neurofibromatosis type 1 in humans. Am J Pathol. **145**: 1168–1174.

16 IRONSIDE, J.W., PICKARD, J.D. (2002): Raised intracranial pressure, oedema and hydrocephalus. In: Greenfield's Neuropathology, 7th ed., Graham D.I., Lantos P.L. (ed.) Arnold, London, pp. 193–231.

17 BRAUND, K.G. (2003): Degenerative and compressive structural disorders. In: Clinical Neurology in Small Animals – Localization, Diagnosis and Treatment. K.G. Braund (ed.) International Veterinary Information Service, Ithaca, New York.

18 GRAHAM, D.I., GENARELLI, T.A., MCINTOSH, T.K. (2002): Trauma. In: Greenfield's Neuropathology, 7th ed., Graham D.I., Lantos P.L. (ed.) Arnold, London, pp. 823–898.

19 BRAUND, K.G. (2003): Traumatic disorders. In: Clinical Neurology in Small Animals – Localization, Diagnosis and Treatment. K.G. Braund (ed.) International Veterinary Information Service, Ithaca, New York.

20 BRAUND, K.G. (2003): Endogeneous metabolic disorders. In: Clinical Neurology in Small Animals – Localization, Diagnosis and Treatment. K.G. Braund (ed.) International Veterinary Information Service, Ithaca, New York.

21 BAGLEY, R.S. (1996): Pathophysiologic sequelae of intracranial disease. Vet Clin North Am. (Small Anim Pract.) **26**: 711–733.

22 WOLSCHRIJN, C.F., MAHAPOKAI, W., ROTHUIZEN, J., MEYER, H.P., VAN SLUIJS, F.J. (2000): Gauged attenuation of congenital portosystemic shunts: results in 160 dogs and 15 cats. Vet Q. **22**: 94–8.

23 JACOB, F., POLZIN, D.J., OSBORNE, C.A., NEATON, J.D., LEKCHAROENSUK, C., ALLEN, T.A., KIRK, C.A., SWANSON, L.L. (2003): Association between initial systolic blood pressure and risk of developing a uremic crisis or of dying in dogs with chronic renal failure. J Am Vet Med Assoc. **222**: 322–329.

24 BRAUND, K.G. (2003): Nutritional disorders. In: Clinical Neurology in Small Animals – Localization, Diagnosis and Treatment. K.G. Braund (ed.) International Veterinary Information Service, Ithaca, New York.

25 SIEBER, F.E., MARTIN, L.J., BROWN, P.R., PALMON, S.C., TRAYSTMAN, R.J. (1996): Diabetic chronic hyperglycemia and neurologic outcome following global ischemia in dogs. J Cereb Blood Flow Metab. **16**: 1230–1235.

26 CIZINAUSKAS, S., BILZER, T., SRENK, P., PILLOUD, C., BLEY, T., JAGGY, A. (2000): Hypothyroid-associated gait abnormalities in the dog. Schweiz Arch Tierheilkd. **142**: 251–256.

27 BRAUND, K.G. (2003): Storage disorders. In: Clinical Neurology in Small Animals – Localization, Diagnosis and Treatment. K.G. Braund (ed.) International Veterinary Information Service, Ithaca, New York.

28 MORGAN, R.V., MOORE, F.M., PEARCE, L.K., ROSSI, T. (1991): Clinical and laboratory findings in small companion animals with lead poisoning: 347 cases (1977–1986). J Am Vet Med Assoc. **199**: 93–97.

29 KENNEDY, P., CAVANAGH, J.B. (1977): Sensory neuropathy produced in the cat with thallous acetate. Acta Neuropathol. (Berl) **39**: 81–88.

30 HOOSER, S.B., BEASLEY, V.R., SUNDBERG, J.P., HARLIN, K. (1988): Toxicologic evaluation of chlorpyrifos in cats. Am J Vet Res. **49**: 1371–1375.

31 BRAUND, K.G. (2003): Neurovascular disorders. In: Clinical Neurology in Small Animals – Localization, Diagnosis and Treatment. K.G. Braund (ed.) International Veterinary Information Service, Ithaca, New York.

32 KOESTNER, A., BILZER, T., FATZER, R., SCHULMAN, F.Y., SUMMERS, B.A., VAN WINKLE, T.J. (1999): Histological Classification of the Tumors of the Nervous System of Domestic Animals. WHO, Armed Forces Institute of Pathology, Washington.

2.2 Classification of neurological diseases: VITAMIN D

Marc Vandevelde

After an attempt at localising the problem, further elucidation of a disease is based on additional information from the signalment, anamnesis, disease progression, general examination and diagnostic tests. The clinician must have a wide knowledge of the most common diseases or lesions, so that a systematic strategy of determining which disease is responsible can be constructed.

Neurological diseases can be divided into groups according to their pathoanatomical aspects; they are characterised according to their specific tissue changes and pathological processes. These common pathologies are reflected to some extent in their clinical picture which encompasses signalment (age group, species, breed), the rate of onset and course of the clinical symptoms, disease symmetry and the results of the general examination and specific neurodiagnostic tests.

In order for a comprehensive list of differential diagnoses to be developed, we use the acronym "VITAMIN D" classification system: **v**ascular disease, **i**nflammation, **t**rauma / **t**oxicity, **a**nomalies, **m**etabolic diseases, **i**diopathic diseases, **n**eoplasia / **n**utritional and **d**egenerative diseases.

2.2.1 V = Vascular disease

Malformation of the blood vessels, embolization of blood vessels, coagulopathies, blood vessel tumours or inflammatory-necrotic changes in blood vessel walls can all lead to damage of the endothelial walls and subsequent bleeding. A spontaneous massive haemorrhage has a space-occupying effect and can lead to an increase in intracranial pressure (ICP).

The obstruction of large arteries can cause local ischemia and the production of infarcts in the affected area. Such infarcts are impressive as they are well demarcated regions with softening and cyst formation. Damage also quickly occurs in end-artery regions, such as around the internal capsule, with general hypoxic conditions or global perfusion disturbances (e.g. cardiac failure).

Cerebrovascular diseases are quite rare in animals. A special case is that of spinal cord infarction caused by fibro-cartilaginous emboli. Infarcts and bleeding can occur at every age and usually provoke peracute clinical signs that develop abruptly within minutes. The clinical signs remain stable for some time and can regress to a certain extent during the next days or weeks.

Extraneural symptoms can occur when vascular lesions in the CNS are due to a cardiovascular disease.

As spontaneous haemorrhaging and infarcts are well demarcated processes, the associated neurological symptoms are usually extremely focal. Often a marked lateralisation is seen with lesions in the brain and spinal cord.

The CSF is usually severely affected with an increase in protein and sometimes an increase in cell content if haemorrhage occurs in the subarachnoid space; otherwise, ischaemic lesions are accompanied by normal to mild inflammatory CSF. If there is suspicion of acute haemorrhage in the brain, an atlanto-occipital tap should not be performed until a coagulopathy has been investigated.

2.2.2 I = Inflammatory and infectious diseases

Viruses, bacteria, protozoa, rickettsia, fungi, and parasites can penetrate the nervous system via the blood, nerves or by direct expansion from the surrounding tissues. They destroy CNS tissue by their direct effects and instigate an immune response which is recognisable by the invasion of inflammatory cells around the blood vessels and in the subarachnoid space (encephalitis – myelitis – neuritis – meningitis – ependymitis). This inflammatory reaction is primarily aimed at the infectious agent, but it may lead to additional damage to the neural parenchyma (immunopathological complications). Some infections cause the formation of granulomas or abscesses.

Viruses have a predilection for specific types of cells, e.g. nerve cells in the grey matter of the spinal cord (poliomyelitis), glial cells in the white matter, endothelial cells (vasculitis) and generally provoke a mononuclear (lympho-plasmocytic) inflammatory reaction.

Bacteria cause purulent inflammatory reactions in the subarachnoid space: purulent meningitis – ependymitis – choroiditis or in the epidural space (empyema). Other bacteria

can penetrate the brain parenchyma via the blood system as septic thromboemboli. Certain bacteria cause abscessation. Mycotic and parasitic agents often induce focal changes with the production of granulomas, but they can also cause an acute necrotising encephalitis.

Rickettsial infections may cause meningitis and encephalitis in addition to vasculitis and haematological disorders. Protozoal infections can be responsible for uveitis, retinitis, myositis, and encephalitis; the muscles and CNS are the most common sites of infection. Animals affected with *Neospora* typically develop non-suppurative encephalomyelitis, polyradiculoneuritis, and myositis.

Inflammatory changes in the PNS are often related to immune dysfunction. Sterile inflammatory lesions in the CNS arising from "immunological derailment" are even more common and often present a diagnostic conundrum

The epidemiology of cases of encephalomyelitis must also be considered. Certain diseases occur in particular geographical areas or in a particular seasons. Clinicians should keep themselves informed about the current animal epidemic disease situation in their region.

Infectious inflammatory diseases occur in every age group, though young animals tend to be more susceptible to infection. Inflammation is often an acute process, which develops within a few days and progresses quickly. Subacute diseases that develop over the course of weeks can also occur. A chronic course over several months can be seen with a few inflammatory diseases. Diseases with an intermittent course are very rare in the CNS, though they are more often "the rule" in inflammatory, autoimmune processes in the PNS.

Many infectious organisms affect only the nervous system, while others also affect other organ systems, which can be recognised during the general examination. Fever frequently accompanies bacterial disease, though it is not always seen in viral conditions. Changes in the CBC are not frequent with isolated inflammatory processes in the CNS.

Disseminated or multifocal lesions occur in many inflammatory diseases. Although only roughly half of such cases show evidence of clinical signs arising from more than one localisation, region-specific symptomology is possible. Clinical signs such as pain, opisthotonus, hyperalgesia and myoclonus are not uncommon with inflammatory disease.

An increase in cells and protein within the CSF is observed in the majority of infectious diseases affecting the CNS. A cytological analysis of the CSF may enable conclusions about the aetiology to be reached (e.g. mononuclear pleocytosis in viral disease or polymorphonuclocytes in bacterial disease). The direct demonstration of the causal agent is sometimes possible using specific reagents.

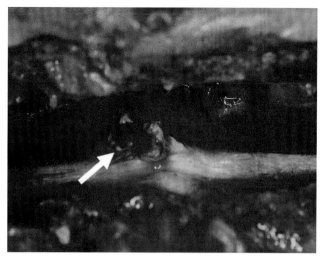

Fig. 2.6
Dorsal view of the spinal cord in a Dachshund after laminectomy (T12–T13). The neurological symptoms occurred acutely: paraplegia without pain sensation. The spinal cord was totally perforated at the site of the disc herniation and parenchyma can be seen protruding through the surface at this position (arrow).

2.2.3   T = Toxic diseases

A common facet of this group of diseases is a disturbance in neurological function, without any observable morphological changes in the CNS tissues. Functional disturbances can be caused by a multitude of exogenous poisons (e.g. tetanus toxin [Fig. 2.8], botulinum toxin, metaldehyde).

Exogenous intoxications predominantly have a peracute onset of clinical signs, which may then slowly regress.

With many different types of intoxication extraneural symptoms can also be seen.

As there are no morphological changes present in this group of functional disturbances, the CSF remains unchanged.

2.2.3.1 T = Trauma

As a consequence of external force, the brain can be injured at the place of impact by the displacement of the surrounding tissues, especially the bones of the skull (*coup*). The brain can also be injured indirectly (*contrecoup*) in a number of different places by being rapidly moved about within the skull due to a sudden acceleration or braking because it is suspended in the CSF and is only attached to the skull in a few places. In addition to direct mechanical injury to the parenchyma, there can be damage to the blood vessels causing bleeding. Large haemorrhages or haematomas, either in the parenchyma or on the surface of the brain act as space-occupying processes and cause compression and other perfusion disturbances, leading to oedema and an increase in ICP. Additionally, a series of biochemical processes are activated that are responsible for the actual tissue damage (excitotoxicity, reactive oxygen radicals). Similar mechanisms can occur in the spinal cord as it is suspended in the vertebral column – a rigid bony tube. Finally, damage can be delayed, whereby nerve cells and fibres progressively degenerate months after the trauma.

A special form of trauma is endogenous compression of the spinal cord associated with an absolute or relative stenosis of the spinal canal, e.g. disc herniation and vertebral instability.

Trauma is associated with peracute neurological symptoms, which can slowly regress over days to months. When active and massive haemorrhage occurs, the clinical signs quickly progress. Progressive, intermittent clinical signs can be observed with chronic, endogenous trauma to the spinal cord due to unstable vertebrae or disc compression.

Trauma can produce a focal lesion with localised clinical signs. Severe cranial trauma results in extensive or multifocal lesions and symptoms. With massive CNS trauma, there is frequently damage to other body systems and related symptoms are apparent.

Collection of CSF is contraindicated in head trauma. Trauma to the spinal cord rarely significantly affects the CSF. A significant increase in protein, and possibly in cell count, in CSF occurs in severe, extensive myelomalacia (Fig. 2.6).

2.2.4   A = Anomalies

Many different types of brain and spinal cord malformations are known. They can be divided according to their embryological-anatomical or genetic aspects. Clinically significant are partial malformations which affect only a section of the nervous system with the animal still being capable of life; for example, porencephaly (Fig. 2.7), hydrancephaly, cerebellar hypoplasia, spina bifida and syringomyelia.

Some malformations are inheritable and so occur more commonly in certain breeds. On the other hand, malformations can be caused by intrauterine infections or intoxications during certain phases of pregnancy (e.g. cerebellar hypoplasia in the cat caused by the panleucopaenia virus). Malformations usually manifest themselves shortly after birth and are static processes. The clinical signs are apparent at birth and remain stable. Depending on the degree and the localisation of the malformation, the animal can partially compensate so that the neurological symptoms slowly regress. As anomalies usually affect specific parts of the CNS, they mainly induce focal symptoms. One example of this is cerebellar ataxia associated with cerebellar defects.

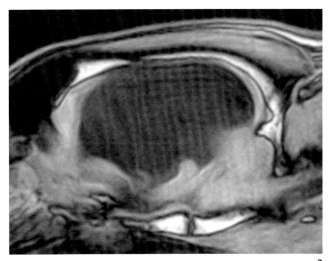

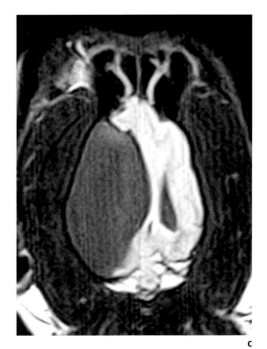

Fig. 2.7a–c
Eight-month-old Airedale Terrier with porencephaly. Sagittal T1w (a), transverse T2w (b) and dorsal FLAIR (suppression of CSF; c). Cystic malformation in the region of the right cerebrum and lateral ventricles corresponding to the vascular system of the medial cerebral artery. The cyst is space-occupying: the midline is displaced towards the left and there is an enlarged calvarium on the right (b). The cyst contents have the same characteristics as CSF as shown in the fluid-suppressed sequence (c) and as seen in the contents of the left lateral ventricle (Figure courtesy of.: Johann Lang, Bern)

As malformations are not usually accompanied by active destruction of tissue or reactive processes, there are no changes in the CSF, unless there is neural compression which may cause increased protein levels

2.2.5   M = Metabolic diseases

Metabolic diseases of the nervous system can be subsequent to systemic health issues or even crises such as hepatic disease, hypoglycaemia or hypoxia, They can also be related to specific inborn errors of cerebral metabolism with no systemic abnormalities notable. Both types of metabolic disease can lead to substrate deficiencies, and / or as endogenous toxin accumulations, leading to acute dysfunction of specific regions of the nervous system, which is usually distributed bilaterally and symmetrically. Metabolic diseases can have a very acute progression, developing within hours and reaching their maximum intensity very quickly. The clinical signs can slowly regress over the next few days and a partial recovery takes place. In several metabolic diseases, extraneural symptoms are also present. Diseases of extraneural organs often produce fluctuating, intermittent symptoms so that periods of neurological signs are interspersed with periods of normality.

Specific and mild neuropathological changes can be seen in relation to the substrate deficiencies or endogenous toxin accumulations, which are often degenerative in nature. More severe neuropathological changes such as malacia or visible "softening", whereby large parts of the tissue are replaced by cavitation and cyst production, can infrequently occur with inborn errors of metabolism. In some of these diseases, the grey matter is primarily affected (polioencephalomalcia); others affect the white matter (leucoencephalomalacia), and some attack both types of tissue. In some processes, the

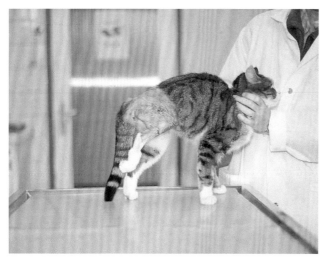

Fig. 2.8
Four-year-old female cat with a focal tetanus of the right hindleg after surgical stabilisation of the femur. The neurological abnormalities occurred three days after the operation. The cat was given physiotherapy under deep sedation and recovered after 2 months.

walls of the blood vessels are obviously damaged resulting in disturbances in their permeability and blood constituents extravasate into the brain parenchyma. There are vague similarities between this disease group and specific types of neurodegeneration.

The minor destructive changes associated with these diseases, which are also associated with disturbances in permeability, can cause mild changes in the CSF (mild to moderately increased protein content but rarely pleocytosis).

2.2.6   N = Neoplasia

Primary tumours in the CNS are either gliomas (neuronal cell tumours) developing from neuroectodermal elements or are of mesenchymal origin developing from the meninges (meningiomas) or blood vessels. Hypophyseal tumours often cause endocrine symptoms but can also be responsible for neurological dysfunction because they grow via the rudimentary diaphragma sellae, usually in a dorsal direction, up into the hypothalamus. Finally, metastases from tumours in other organs and local extension of tumours originating in surrounding tissues such as bone, can also affect the nervous system.

Neoplasia damages the CNS by invasive destructive growth and / or by displacement and compression. Their space-occupying effect leads to a destruction of the perfusion of the brain parenchyma resulting in vascular stasis, disturbances in blood vessel permeability, oedema and an increase in ICP.

The obstruction of CSF drainage channels can result in hydrocephalus.

Neoplasia is a sporadic disease. In the dog particular types of tumours are more common in specific breeds; for example, gliomas are more common in Boxers, Boston Terriers and English Bulldogs. Gliomas also occur less frequently in the cat than the dog, while meningiomas are more common in the former. The majority of tumours affect older animals, though some tumours are seen in very young ones (medulloblastoma). The disease course is usually subacute to chronic-progressive over a period of weeks or months. An acute deterioration can result when circulatory disturbances and oedema occur. After the compensatory ability of the intracranial tissues has been exhausted, the severity of the clinical signs rapidly increases.

With metastatic tumours, clinical signs resulting from the primary tumour may or may not be apparent. Tumours usually cause focal, often lateralised clinical signs determined by their localisation.

In many cases, a slight to obvious increase in protein within the CSF can be seen, indicating the presence of a disturbance in permeability. More rarely pleocytosis occurs. Cytological methods can sometimes be used to show the presence of tumour cells, although they are infrequently identified

2.2.7   D = Degenerative diseases

These diseases are characterised by a progressive destruction of neuronal tissue. They can be age related or be induced by congenital gene defects that as yet in many cases have not been elucidated. In the **storage diseases**, the defect lies in the catabolic enzyme systems, whereby the enzyme substrate is not degraded and collects in the cells, leading to the ultimate degeneration of the cell (e.g. accumulation of GM1 ganglioside with a deficiency of the enzyme β-galactosidase).

Storage diseases affect the brain usually in a diffuse manner, whereby all its regions are more or less involved. In other diseases, specific nerve cell populations degenerate; e.g. the motor neurons in the spinal cord or the purkinje cells of the cerebellum. With certain defects, the axons of specific nerve cell populations die back (neuroaxonal dystrophies). Demyelination and leucodystrophies are characterised by a destruction of the white matter. In many cases, this destruction affects only certain parts of the CNS or PNS (e.g. spinal cord in Afghan myelopathy). Demyelinating diseases can actually cause a destruction of the myelin sheath whilst the axon remains intact.

In addition to the sporadic occurrence of degenerative disease in all breeds, neurodegeneration is often inheritable and is known to occur in a whole series of specific breeds. Many of these diseases manifest themselves during the first months of life, some later on. Therefore, apart from a few exceptions, degenerative diseases usually affect predominantly the very young or young adult animals. The disease usually slowly progresses over a course of weeks or months.

In general, these diseases are specific to the CNS. Some storage diseases can, in comparison, affect more than one organ system (most common symptom: hepatomegaly), although as a rule the CNS disturbances are the most evident clinical abnormalities.

As certain regions of the nervous system are specifically affected, regional symptoms occur. Degenerative changes are often bilateral when due to enzymatic and/or biochemical defects, and often symmetrical. However, other examples of degenerative disease, for instance degenerative myelopathy, may be asymmetrical.

As the degeneration of the nervous tissue tends to be slow, i.e. takes places in tune with the "clearing up" processes, little change in the CSF is to be expected, besides an elevation of the protein levels.

Further reading

SUMMERS B.A, CUMMINGS J.F, de LAHUNTA A. (1995): Veterinary Neuropathology. Mosby, St. Louis.

2.3 Investigation of the cerebrospinal fluid (CSF)

André Jaggy

Most of the CSF is produced by ultrafiltration from the blood by the choroid plexi into the ventricles. The CSF flows out of the ventricles to the central canal caudally. It leaves the ventricular system and passes into the leptomeningeal space at the level of the fourth ventricle. CSF is resorbed into the blood partially via the arachnoid villi and partially via the subarachnoid veins, though most of it leaves the leptomeningeal space along the sheaths of the spinal nerves though the local lymphatic system.

Pathological changes can affect the composition of the CSF to a greater or lesser degree. This is why examination of the CSF plays an integral part in neurological investigations. The atlanto-occipital (AO) cisternal tap (Fig. 2.9) is more important than the lumbar tap when evaluating brain disease (Fig. 2.10). Both techniques require practise, otherwise serious compli-

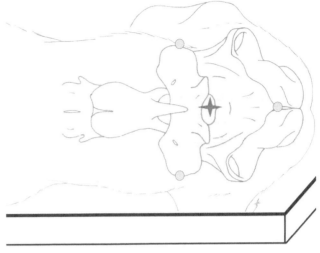

Fig. 2.9
Cisternal tap. The sedated animal is placed in lateral recumbency. The skin in the occipital area is shaved and disinfected. The head is bent ventrally to give an angle of 60° to the vertebral column. The site for needle insertion lies in the middle of the triangle formed by the occipital crest and the wings of the atlas.

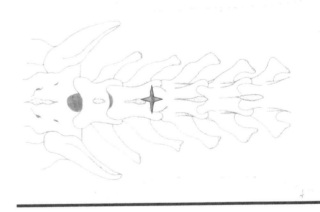

Fig. 2.10
Lumbar tap. The sedated animal is placed in lateral recumbency. The skin over the lumbar spine is shaved and disinfected. The point of the needle is moved forwards along the roof of the sixth lumbar vertebra until the intervertebral space between L5/L6 is reached. The needle is pushed in to just above the floor of the vertebral canal; in favourable circumstances, CSF flows out of the needle.

cations may arise which can include paraplegia or complete paralysis, and respiratory arrest. The risk of the CSF sample being contaminated with blood, thereby making it useless, is more of a problem with the lumbar tap than with the AO one.

The CSF sample should be taken to the cytology laboratory immediately after collection. The division of the CSF sample for the different investigations must occur within the first half hour before the cellular components begin to degenerate. If the amount of CSF is very small, the cell count takes priority over the cytological analysis. Cell count and protein level evaluations are undertaken on the supernatant, while cytology is done on the sediment.

Firstly, the macroscopic appearance of the CSF is assessed. Normal CSF is a clear water-like fluid. Yellowish discoloration of the CSF usually indicates the presence of a chronic haemorrhage or it could be secondary to icterus. If there is a high fibrin content, then the CSF may clot rapidly after collection.

Secondly, the protein and cell contents are determined. The normal protein content in the dog varies between 11–25 mg/dl and that in the cat between 8–20 mg/dl with the lumbar sample having a slightly higher protein level than the AO sample. A simple semi-quantitative method of measuring protein is the Pandy reaction. An increase in protein content causes cloudiness in the CSF: the more protein present, the more the cloudiness (+ to ++++). As the amount of protein in the CSF is about 200 times lower than in the serum, a refractometer used for serum protein cannot be used for its analysis. Urine test strips maybe used if there is more than 30 mg/dl of protein.

The number of cells in normal CSF is very low. The cells are normally counted using a standard blood cell counting chamber (haemocytometer) or a Fuchs-Rosenthal counting chamber. The normal cell count in the dog is 0 to 5 mononuclear cells/mm³ and 0 to 3 in the cat. Usually, all the cells in the counting chamber are counted. An increase in cell number (pleocytosis) of more than 5 cells per mm³ is pathological. Increased cell counts are most commonly encountered with inflammatory disease but can also occur in association with neoplasia, vascular disease and trauma (Table 2.1). It is important to pay attention to the cell morphology in such cases. This is possible to a certain extent in the counting chamber, but it is usually necessary to use special methods to concentrate the cells. For this, a sedimentation chamber can be used or a cytocentrifuge in which the cells are placed directly on a microscope slide (e.g. membrane filtration). The morphology of at least 250 cells should be determined where possible, when judging cytological preparations. The cells are classified into lymphocytes, monocytes, neutrophilic granulocytes, eosinophilic granulocytes, (rarely tumour cells), and other elements such as myelin. The CSF cell picture correlates to some extent with the type of disease process; e.g. mononuclear cells are predominantly found in viral infections.

Of all the enzymes that can be analysed in the CSF, CK is most probably the only useful one. An increased CK can indicate that organic damage to the CNS has taken place. The glucose content of CSF is reduced in bacterial infection. The latter type of disease can also be proven by isolation of the causal agent with culture. Immunoflorescence or PCR can be used to detect small amounts of foreign nucleic acids (e.g. neosporosis, distemper). The measurement of particular metabolites, for example γ-aminobutyric acid (GABA), is useful in certain situations (e.g. to confirm a diagnosis of idiopathic epilepsy). The albumin content of the CSF is an indicator of the permeability of the blood-brain barrier. The detection of intrathecal Ig synthesis is suggestive of an inflammatory infectious disease within the nervous system and this is especially useful in chronic cases when an obvious pleocytosis is present.

Table 2.1: VITAMIN D

	Age	Course	Extraneural symptoms	Localisation	CSF
V	All	Peracute, possible improvement	May be present	Focal	Protein + to +++, possibly blood
I	All	Acute to subacute, rarely chronic progressive	May be present	Focal-multifocal	Cells + to ++++, protein + to ++++
T	All	Peracute, possibly progressive, possible improvement	May be present	Focal-multifocal	CSF tap contraindicated
A	Neonates, young animals	Stationary, possible improvement	None	Focal	None
M	All	Acute, quickly progressive	Usually none	Focal-diffuse	Protein + to +++, cells − to ++
I	All	Acute, fluctuating, paroxysmal	None	Focal-diffuse	None
N	Old, rarely young	Subacute to chronic progressive	Usually none	Focal	Protein + to ++, tumour cells
D	Mainly young or young adults	Chronic progressive	None	Focal-diffuse	Protein − to +

Further reading

SCHATZBERG, S.J., HALEY, N.J., BARR, S.C., deLAHUNTA, A., OLBY, N., MUNANA, K., SHARP, N. (2003): Use of a multiplex polymerase chain reaction assay in the antemortem diagnosis of toxoplasmosis and neosporosis in the central nervous system of cats and dogs. Am J Vet Res. **64**: 1507–13.

BIENZLE, D., MCDONNELL, J.J., STANTON, J.B. (2000): Analysis of cerebrospinal fluid from dogs and cats after 24 and 48 hours of storage. J Am Vet Med Assoc. **216**: 1761–1764.

CHRISMAN, C.L. (1992): Cerebrospinal fluid analysis. Vet Clin North Am Small Anim Pract. **22**: 781–810.

HURTT, A.E., SMITH, M.O. (1997): Effects of iatrogenic blood contamination on results of cerebrospinal fluid analysis in clinically normal dogs and dogs with neurologic disease. J Am Vet Med Assoc. **211**: 866–867.

ABATE, O., BOLLO, E., LOTTI, D., BO, S. (1978): Cytological, immunocytochemical and biochemical cerebrospinal fluid investigations in selected central nervous system disorders of dogs. Zentralbl Veterinärmed B. **45**: 73–85.

WRIGHT, J.A. (1978): Evaluation of cerebrospinal fluid in the dog. Vet Rec. **103**: 48–51.

KOUTINAS, A.F., POLIZOPOULOU, Z.S., BAUMGAERTNER, W., LEKKAS, S., KONTOS, V. (2002): Relation of clinical signs to pathological changes in 19 cases of canine distemper encephalomyelitis. J Comp Pathol. **126**: 47–56.

DI TERLIZZI, R., PLATT, S.R. (2006): The function, composition and analysis of cerebrospinal fluid in companion animals: Part I – function and composition. Vet J. **172** (3): 422–431.

DI TERLIZZI, R., PLATT, S.R. (2008): The function, composition and analysis of cerebrospinal fluid in companion animals: Part II – Analysis. Vet J. [Epub ahead of print].

2

3 Genetic Neurological Diseases and Breed Predisposition

Claude Gaillard

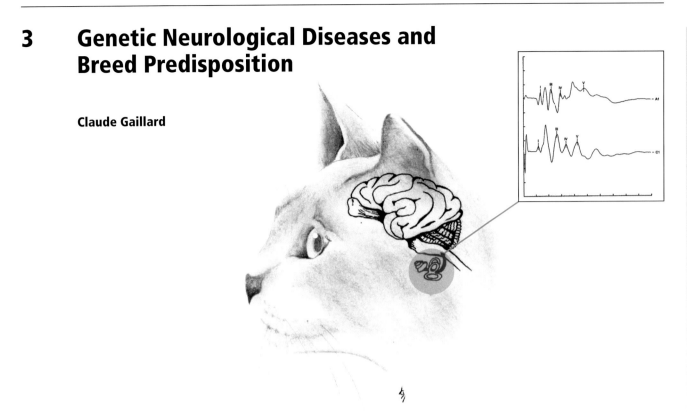

With a few exceptions, the development of pathological conditions is very complicated as they involve interactions between genetic and non-genetic factors. The non-genetic factors, also called environmental factors, can be as different as the influence of sex, nutrition and husbandry, climate or stress factors, etc. Part of the pathological conditions can be strongly or sometimes completely attributed to such environmental factors. If in a family the same malformation and/or disease occurs repeatedly, a genetic background could be involved. But one has to be aware of the fact that a common environment shared by members of a family may fake a genetic origin. This means that the aetiology now and then can be very confusing.

In the following, pathological conditions have been divided into two groups. There are pathological conditions:
- which are not or only minimally affected by environmental factors and inherited in a rather simple manner (e.g. genetic defects) and those
- which are affected by both genetic and environmental factors to a greater or lesser degree (e.g. genetic diseases).

3.1 Genetic defects

Genetic defects are formal defects that lie outside of the normal biological variation found within a species. Besides macroscopically visible defects, they include abnormalities which can only be detected histologically, immunologically or biochemically. Genetic defects can also be grouped according to the time of their manifestation in embryonic, post-embryonic or postnatal genetic defects. The genetic defects which are present in the embryonic stage lead, as a rule, to early embryonic death, which leads in multiparous animals, to smaller litter sizes. Postembryonal genetic defects often cause abortion or premature birth. Some genetic defects manifest themselves either at or just after birth, e.g. spina bifida. Other genetic disorders appear only during the development of the young animal or at a later stage of life, i.e. neuroaxonal dystrophy in cats (starts at approx. 6 months of age).

In the context of a genetic defect the concepts of incomplete penetrance and of expressivity have to be considered. Penetrance is the proportion of individuals of a particular genotype which show the expected pathological condition (manifestation frequency). If the penetrance is less than 100% some individuals remain unaffected although they carry the disease genotype (false negative diagnosis from a genetical point of view). The cause of incomplete penetrance may be a modification of the responsible gene by other genes (epistatic effects)

3

or environmental factors. An incomplete penetrance restricts the power of a pedigree analysis.

Expressivity describes the extent to which a defined genotype is expressed. The cause of a varying degree of expression can be genetic or nongenetic. For example, the abnormal gait in the Labrador Retriever myopathy can range from a slight ataxia to an inability to walk (1).

The phenotype is an observable trait of an organism that results from its genotype which may interact to a certain extent with the environment. A phenocopy is an environmentally induced phenotype that mimics the phenotype of a particular genotype. A false positive diagnosis can be considered as phenocopy too. If a dog suffers from epileptic seizures caused by organic causes, but still is diagnosed as having idiopathic or genetic epilepsy, this can be considered as a phenocopy. Obviously, such cases are undesirable in a pedigree analysis.

3.2   Inheritance

Dominant lethal genetic defects cannot be inherited as natural selection prevents their propagation. In a genetic defect with an incomplete dominant mode of inheritance, such as the Merle syndrome, the homozygous dominant genotype (M^MM^M; Fig. 3.1a) is characterised by an extensive lack of pigment in the hair coat and skin, in association with abnormalities of the eye and inner ear; the heterozygotes (M^MM^+) exhibit another phenotype, namely brindling. Most of the described genetic defects follow an autosomal recessive inheritance (see Appendices 2 and 3). Some genetic defects, such as X-linked recessive muscular dystrophy, have their gene on the X chromosome, which means that almost only males are affected (Fig. 3.1b). Only very rarely do genetic defects occur that are not anchored in the DNA of the cell nucleus but in the DNA of the mitochondria, for example mitochondrial myopathy in the dog. This kind of genetic defect can only be inherited from the mother.

Only a few defects are caused by a single gene. In most cases, probably a small number of loci (oligogenes) together with environmental factors are involved in the manifestation of their pathological conditions as pedigree analyses have often shown deviations from the expected Mendelian segregation.

There are a number of explanations, why genetic defects are propagated in a population and remain there. Sporadic de novo mutations obviously do not contribute, as the mutation rate is too small (10^{-5} to 10^{-6}). The founder effect could provide an explanation in many instances. Founder effect can be shown in populations where only very few individuals constituted the founders. For example, founder effects are present in a situation where a considerable part of the breeders mate their breeding females to the same champion male, whenever possible, over several years. Especially in small popu-

lations this mating policy can cause a dramatic increase in the frequency of unfavourable alleles. Another explanation is that in certain populations genetic defects are maintained because in the heterozygous form they give desired phenotypes, e.g. the Merle factor in the dog. In comparison to humans, only a small proportion of malformations found in companion animals have been investigated genetically. The neurological genetic defects listed in Appendices 2–4 originate from the following two sources: RUVINSKY and SAMPSON (2001), and Online Mendelian Inheritance in Animals (OMIA) (http://omia.angis.org.au/). These references often report a mode of inheritance that has to be considered tentative.

3.3   Demonstrating the mode of inheritance

To fight genetic defects and deficiencies using breeding measures, the mode of inheritance of the pathological conditions must be elucidated. Efficient selection strategies cannot be designed without having any knowledge about the mode of inheritance.

A genetic contribution to the aetiology of a pathological condition can at least be assumed when the incidence in certain families (breeds) is higher than in others. This empirical evidence cannot be accepted as proof as various interference factors can lead to a misinterpretation; e.g. common environmental factors, false diagnoses, unreported cases or false parentage. Intrauterine virus infections can mimic Mendelian inheritance; for example, the panleucopaenia virus in the cat can cause cerebellar hypoplasia (2). Another valuable indication that a genetic defect is indeed present is that the same disorder occurs both in domestic animals and humans. For example, the genetic defect α-fucosidosis occurs both in humans and the dog. In such situations, comparative medicine and comparative genetics play an important role in the elucidation of the genetic background.

If after the consideration of all possible alternatives, the suspicion of a genetic background still remains; an examination of the mode of inheritance is indicated. Ideally, a genealogical tree is drawn based on the family data (Fig. 3.1) and investigated with a segregation analysis to see if the trait belongs to one of the three following Mendelian models: autosomal recessive, autosomal dominant or sex-linked recessive. Such segregation analyses are based on genetic statistical models (3, 4).

In order to get reliable results, particular attention must be paid to the collection of the data. The information must be free of the above-mentioned interference factors. The way the data of families are collected also plays a role in the evaluation of the data. For example, if a genetic defect is inherited in an autosomal recessive way, often only families with one or more affected offspring are considered. This will lead to a dis-

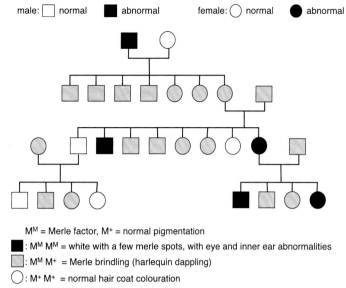

male: □ normal ■ abnormal   female: ○ normal ● abnormal

M^M = Merle factor, M^+ = normal pigmentation

■ : $M^M M^M$ = white with a few merle spots, with eye and inner ear abnormalities

▨ : $M^M M^+$ = Merle brindling (harlequin dappling)

○ : $M^+ M^+$ = normal hair coat colouration

Family tree 1: autosomal, incomplete dominant inheritance, e.g. Merle Syndrome in the Collie.

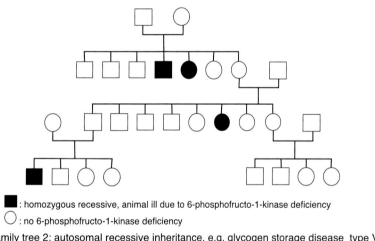

■ : homozygous recessive, animal ill due to 6-phosphofructo-1-kinase deficiency

○ : no 6-phosphofructo-1-kinase deficiency

Fig. 3.1a
Family trees with different forms of inheritance.

Family tree 2: autosomal recessive inheritance, e.g. glycogen storage disease type VII in the American Cocker Spaniel.

tortion of the results because heterozygous parents (genetic carriers) having only unaffected progeny will not be considered in the analysis. These families will therefore be missing in the calculation and the expected 3:1 ratio will not been reached. NICHOLAS (3) and WIENER and WILLER (4) have shown how to correct for this bias.

Often such simple segregation analyses are not feasible because of incomplete penetrance, age dependence of the phenotype or a non-monogenic inheritance which can be rather complex. In such cases, it is best to use a so-called complex segregation analysis (e.g. SAGE: http://darwin.cwru.edu/sage/; PAP: http://hasstedt.genetics.utah.edu//). It should be noted that these program packages require high-powered computers. In a complex segregation analysis on 357 clinically diagnosed Dalmatians, deafness was partially due to a recessive allele of a major gene (5). Two other independent studies of this type of deafness have obtained similar results (6, 7).

3

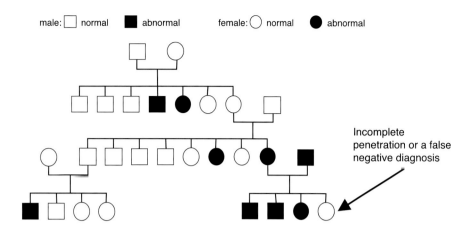

Family tree 3: autosomal, recessive inheritance with incomplete penetration.

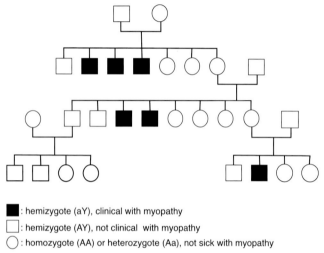

■ : hemizygote (aY), clinical with myopathy

□ : hemizygote (AY), not clinical with myopathy

○ : homozygote (AA) or heterozygote (Aa), not sick with myopathy

Family tree 4: sex-linked (X-chromosome) recessive inheritance,
e.g. X-linked myopathy in the Golden Retriever.

Fig. 3.1b
Family trees with different forms of inheritance (continued).

3.4   Testing for potential genetic carriers

The diagnosis of carriers of unfavourable alleles is a problem in case of a recessive inheritance. With dominant inheritance, the alleles are obvious as in the Merle syndrome in dogs or dominant white colouration in cats. Carriers are individuals having only one copy of the unfavourable allele and therefore are unaffected.

Whether or not an individual has an unfavourable allele can be investigated in a number of ways:
- Direct determination (gene test).
- Indirectly, using a marker (marker test).
- Using information on ancestors, siblings, and offspring.
- Specific test mating.

In a few instances, the causative mutation leading to a defect can be detected at the DNA level using molecular methods (8). For example, the following two tests for genetic defects are available: α-fucosidosis in the dog, which is caused by a deletion of 14 bp at the end of exon 1 (9); or glycogen storage disease type VII (phosphofructokinase deficiency), which is caused by a point mutation (10). The development of a gene test is very expensive. Most of the tests available in veterinary medicine have been developed based on knowledge from human medicine. Gene tests allow for a very efficient eradication of genetic disorders.

In certain enzymopathies, genetic carriers can be detected based on the gene dose phenomenon, which means that in heterozygotes about half the dose of the normal amount of enzyme can be measured. An example of this is the anaemia found in Basenji dogs due to a pyruvate kinase deficiency in the erythrocytes of affected animals (11).

Many polymorphic markers closely linked to specific genetic defects are known in humans and the mouse. The closer a marker is linked with the causative mutation, the more reliable is the diagnosis of the genetic defect (8). For example, carriers of the recessive copper storage disease in the Bedlington Terrier can be identified with a high degree of probability as the causing mutation is very closely linked to a microsatellite marker (marker test; 12).

If there is information available on the occurrence of a genetic defect in the ancestors, siblings and/or progeny of a proband, this information can be used to estimate the risk of the proband being a carrier (4). The reliability of such an estimation depends mainly on the completeness of the data, i.e. how far and exhaustive the cases of genetic defects have been registered.

For economic reasons, the identification of genetic carriers through test matings is only attempted for very valuable breeding animals that will have a large impact on their breed. This method is rarely used in companion animals. The test is done by mating the proband with suitable partners such as:
■ Affected animals (= recessive homozygotes who express the defect).
■ Known carriers (= individuals that have already produced at least one affected offspring).
■ Progeny of known genetic carriers or with the proband's own progeny (inbreeding test).
■ A representative sample of the population.

If the genetic defect occurs in one offspring of the test matings then the proband is recognised as being a carrier. If the proband goes through the test without producing an affected offspring, it can be attributed with a certain probability of not being a carrier of the unfavourable allele. The numbers of litters required for a certain probability listed in Table 3.1 only hold true if the genetic defect is monogenic, autosomal recessive and has complete penetrance – the ideal case. There-

fore, the number of litters indicated is to be taken as the minimum number needed. From Table 3.1 it can be seen that the mating of the proband to a randomly chosen group of individuals from the population is not suitable if the genetic defect is rare. Test matings with recessive homozygotes or known heterozygotes are much more efficient, provided that the necessary mating partners are available. The inbreeding test (e.g. father-daughter matings) is the only possible way of increasing test reliability in cases where the allele frequency is low. This method also allows the testing of more than one unfavourable allele in the proband at the same time, though it takes a long time before the results are available as one has to wait until puberty of the proband's progeny before starting.

3.5 Breeding methods to eradicate genetic defects

The control of genetic defects in a breeding population requires that those responsible for the breed must decide about the weight to be given to the genetic defect in the selection procedure and evaluate the effectiveness of the applied breeding methods. It is certainly not realistic to try and eliminate all genetic defects simultaneously, especially since there are other (important) traits forming part of the breeding goals for a given breed. The weight for selection depends, on the one hand, on the frequency and the degree of damage the genetic defect causes and on the other hand, on the possible alternative solutions that are available to alleviate or to correct the disorder (e.g. curative methods, simple surgery, the choice of breeding animals). Using model calculations, VAN VLECK (13) and HANSET (14) could show that breeding success can be achieved through consequent selection.

Success depends not only on the genetic parameters but especially on the chosen selection strategy. Breeding methods

Table 3.1: The required number of litters with normal progeny to show that a proband is not a genetic carrier with a given probability

The proband is mated with:	Number of progeny/litter	Required number of litters with a probability of		
		90%	95%	99%
Recessive homozygote	n = 3	2	2	3
	n = 6	1	1	2
Known heterozygote	n = 3	2	4	6
	n = 6	2	2	3
Descendents of known carriers or the proband's own descendents	n = 3	7	9	14
	n = 6	5	6	9
Sample from the population*	n = 3	41	53	82
	n = 6	26	34	52

* Frequency of the recessive allele in the population is 1%.

can only be effective if the breeders and the responsible breeding organisation are motivated to consequently implement the eradication programme.

3.6 Diseases due to multifactorial causes

In contrast to genetic defects, the genetic predisposition to disease is influenced by a large number of genes (polygenes), but also by environmental factors such as malnutrition, inbreeding or stress. The formation of these pathological conditions is therefore multifactorial and follows the same genetic model used in quantitative genetics. The difference to quantative traits, which are normally distributed, is that the phenotype is a so-called threshold trait. These are traits that can be divided into two or a few categories for the phenotype but their genotype is treated as normally distributed (Fig. 3.2). The X-axis shows the entirety of disease-causing aetiological factors; with the X value increasing from the left to the right the aetiological stress also increases, which means that the susceptibility (liability) increases. The factors can be genes, toxins, sex, age, stress and other environmental factors. Disease susceptibility is an example for a case where an invisible threshold has been overstepped; the phenotype changes from unaffected to affected, which means that the "resistance" is broken by the accumulation of unfavourable genetic and nongenetic factors. In this model, individuals with a higher genetic predisposition can, under favourable environmental conditions (lack of exposure), remain inconspicuous or unaffected; a lack of clinical signs is not to be equated with being free of the genetic predisposition for the disorder. FALCONER (15, 16) developed the population genetic approach for this type of assessment. The importance of the polygenes on the disease predisposition can be measured by the heritability (8). This value can range from 0 and 1. The greater the heritability, the more important are the genes in the development of the disease. For example, in an American investigation on Belgian Tervueren dogs, a very high heritability of 0.77 was calculated as their predisposition for epilepsy (17).

To reduce the disease susceptibility in a population, it is not possible to use the same methods applied for genetic defects. Breeding values are estimated for threshold traits instead of identifying carrier animals by threshold traits (8). The breeding value indicates how strongly an animal can pass on its "predisposition" to its progeny. This is why the breeding value is suitable as a basis for the selection against increased disease susceptibility. The requirements for the data for the estimation of breeding values are similar to those needed in the evaluation of carriers of genetic defects: a reliable diagnosis, correct pedigree information, a complete recording of the possible environmental factors as well as a large number of animals.

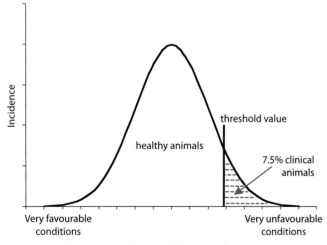

Fig. 3.2
Representation of threshold characteristics. In this population, the disease incidence is 7.5%. If the conditions in the population degenerate (e. g. through inbreeding), then the curve will be pushed towards the unfavourable side. As the position of the threshold value does not change, the curve to the right of the threshold increases meaning that the incidence of diseased animals increases.

Literature

1 BLEY, T., GAILLARD, C., BILZER, T.H., BRAUND, K.G., FAISSLER, D., STEFFEN, F., CIZINAUSKAS, S., NEUMANN, J., EQUEY, R., JAGGY, A. (2002): Genetic aspects of Labrador retriever myopathy. Res Vet Sci. **73**: 231–236.

2 KILHAM, L., MARGOLIS, G., COLBY, E.D. (1971): Cerebellar ataxia and its congenital transmission in cats by Feline Panleukopenia virus. J Am Vet Med Assoc. **158**: 888–901.

3 NICHOLAS, F.W. (1987): Veterinary genetics. Clarendon Press, Oxford, UK.

4 WIESNER, E., WILLER, S. (1993): Genetische Beratung in der tierärztlichen Praxis. Gustav Fischer Verlag, Jena.

5 MUHLE, A.C., JAGGY, A., STRICKER, C., STEFFEN, F., DOLF, G., BUSATO, A., KRONBERG, M., MARISCOLI, M., SRENK, P., GAILLARD, C. (2001): Further contributions to the genetic aspect of congenital sensorineural deafness in dalmatians. Vet J. **163**: 311–318.

6 FAMULA, T.R., OBERBAUER, A.M., SOUSA, C.A. (2000): Complex segregation analysis of deafness in Dalmatians. Am J Vet Res. **61**: 550–553.

7 JURASCHKO, K. (2000): Populationsgenetische Untersuchung der kongenitalen Taubheit beim Dalmatiner. Diss. vet. med., Hannover, Germany.

8 RUVINSKY, A., SAMPSON, J. (eds.) (2001): The genetics of the dog. CABI Publishing, Oxon, UK.

9 HOLMES, N.G., ACHESON, T., RYDER, E.J., BINNS, M.M. (1998): A PCR-based diagnostic test for fucosidosis in English Springer Spaniels. Vet J. **155**: 113–114.

10 SMITH, B.F., STEDMAN, H., RAJPUROHIT, Y., HENTHORN, P.S., WOLFE, J.H., PATTERSON, D.F., GIGER, U. (1996): Molecular basis of canine muscle type phosphofructokinase deficiency. J Biol Chem. **271**: 20070–20074.

11 ANDRESEN, E. (1977): Haemolytic anaemia in Basenji dogs. 2. Partial deficiency of erythrocyte pyruvate kinase (PK; EC 2.7.1.40) in heterozygous carriers. Anim Blood Gr Biochem Gen. **8**: 149–156.

12 YUZBASIYAN-GURKAN, V., BLANTON, S.H., CAO, Y., FERGUSON, P., LI, J., VENTA, P.J., BREWER, G.J., (1997): Linkage of a microsatellite marker to the canine copper toxicosis locus in Bedlington terriers. Am J Vet Res. **58**: 23–27.

13 VAN VLECK, L.D. (1967): Effect of artificial insemination on frequency of undesirable recessive genes. J Dairy Sci. **50**: 201–204.

14 HANSET, R. (1988): Gènes récessifs indésirables et insémination artificielle. Annales Méd. Vét. **132**: 677–686.

15 FALCONER, D.S. (1965): The inheritance of liability to certain diseases, estimated from the incidence among relatives. Ann Hum Gen. **29**: 51–76.

16 FALCONER, D.S. (1984): Einführung in die quantitative Genetik. Verlag Eugen Ulmer, Stuttgart.

17 FAMULA, T.R., OBERBAUER, A.M., BROWN, K.N. (1997): Heritability of epileptic seizures in Belgian Trevueren. J Small Anim Pract. **38**: 349–352.

3

4 Basic Laboratory Investigations

Frédéric Gaschen

4.1 Indications

The indications for investigating the blood and urine of neurological patients are multiple. Laboratory parameters are often of central importance in the exclusion method of determining the diagnosis of neurological disease in the dog and cat. After the signalment and anamnesis have been carefully noted, the general clinical examination, and especially the neurological examination, allows a localisation of the disease process. Subsequently, the possible causes are considered using the VITAMIN D principle (see Chap. 2.2.) and a list of differential diagnoses is made. At this point, laboratory investigations such as haematology with a complete differential blood count (CBC), blood chemistry and urine examination are indispensable, especially in diseases in which the nervous system is affected secondarily. Based upon these laboratory parameters, in addition to the signalment and anamnesis, the list of possible differential diagnoses can be reduced and ranked in probability on the way to achieving the final diagnosis.

Specific investigations for determining liver function (bile acids and/or ammonia concentration in the serum or plasma)

are very useful when there is suspicion of hepatic encephalopathy. A number of lysosomal storage diseases can be confirmed by determining the presence of abnormal metabolites in the urine (e.g. toluidine blue test in mucopolysaccharidosis; see Chap. 18.8). In addition to the purely diagnostic purposes, laboratory investigations are also indispensable in patients with neurological trauma or in the pre-anaesthetic assessment of elderly dogs and cats. This is useful to determine the extent of the trauma and any concurrent system damage in the former, and to identify subclinical problems before anesthesia in the latter (see Chap. 5.1).

Last, but not least, laboratory investigations are important in assessing the pharmacokinetics of therapeutic substances. The most common example of this, would be the determination of serum phenobarbital concentration in epilepsy patients. For further consideration of this theme, the reader is referred to the relevant chapters (see also Chap. 18.5).

In the following, only those laboratory parameters which are used in the explanation of neurological problems in the dog and cat are considered.

4

4.2 Haematology

Nowadays, a number of different mechanical analysers are available on the market that can be used for dog and cat haematology. They are affordable and provide good services for the engaged small animal practitioner. However, one should not forget that their results are not always reliable. The microscopic investigation of a blood smear still provides important information that cannot be expected from even the most expensive and high-performance machine. This is the reason why samples that have abnormal results with an automatic cell counter should be controlled using this simple method.

4.2.1 Anaemia

Anaemia can accompany certain diseases with neurological clinical signs. In some situations, anaemia can result in a noticeable physical weakness and must be differentiated from the general weakness caused by neurological disease.

Anaemia is defined as being a reduction in the number of erythrocytes in the circulation. In the haematological investigation, the haematocrit, erythrocyte count and haemoglobin content all fall below the reference values.

The clinical symptoms of anaemia are caused by the blood's reduced ability to transport oxygen and is characterised in the patient by pale mucous membranes, weakness, lethargy, tachypnoea and tachycardia. These clinical signs are normally more apparent in acute anaemia as a number of compensatory mechanisms come into effect in chronic cases. It can be difficult to recognise lethargy or weakness in the cat at an early stage, because a reduced ability to transport oxygen leads to a less active behaviour pattern and many cats normally sleep a lot during the day anyway. This means that the tachypnoea and/or dyspnoea are usually first recognised when the cat is forced to move itself. Surprisingly, again and again, it can be seen that chronically anaemic cats can survive with a haematocrit of 0.10 or less.

If anaemia is discovered in a dog or cat, then a systematic investigation should be undertaken to diagnose the primary cause of the problem. A complete haematological investigation allows a quantitative evaluation to be made (haematocrit, erythrocyte count and/or haemoglobin concentration). The erythrocyte indices MCV (mean corpuscular volume) and MCHC (mean corpuscular haemoglobin concentration) help to characterise the anaemia as microcytic, macrocytic, normochromic or hypochromic. These definitions can provide valuable information in the search for the cause of the anaemia.

The reaction of the bone marrow to the anaemia must be evaluated by doing a reticulocyte count. Reticulocytes are erythrocyte precursors. They do not have nuclei but have active mRNA in their cytoplasm. The RNA material precipitates forming a network with stains such as methylene blue, for example. A delay of at least three days must be taken into account between the onset of anaemia and an increase in reticulocytes in the peripheral blood. Reticulocyte counts are normally given in percentages, though one should always take the absolute or corrected reticulocyte count into consideration in order to make a correlation between the severity of the anaemia and the regeneration of the bone marrow (Table 4.1).

Cats cannot regenerate their erythrocytes as efficiently as dogs and so in this species an absolute reticulocyte count $> 40 \times 10^9/l$ already indicates that regeneration is taking place. Cats have two types of reticulocytes in their blood, which differ in the amount of granules they contain: (1) **punctate** reticulo-

Table 4.1: Reticulocyte counts and indices

Absolute reticulocyte count ($10^9/l$)	$10 \times$ reticulocytes (%) $\times$ erythrocytes ($10^{12}/l$)		
		Dog	Cat
	Non-regenerative	< 60[1]	< 15[1]
	Slightly regenerative	150[1]	50[1]
	Moderateley regenerative	300[1]	100[1]
	Very regenerative	> 500[1]	200[1]
Relative reticulocyte counts		Dog	Cat
	Non-regenerative	$< 1\%$	$< 0.4\%$
	Slightly regenerative	1–5%	0.4–2%
	Regenerative	5–20%	2–4%
Corrected reticulocyte count (CRC)	Reticulocytes (%) $\times \dfrac{\text{patient Hct}}{\text{normal Hct}}$[2]		
Reticulocyte production index (RPI)	$\dfrac{\text{CRC}}{\text{RMI}}$[3]		
	RPI	Dog and cat	
	Non-regenerative	< 1	
	Regenerative	> 2.2	
	Very regenerative (indicative of haemolytic anaemia)	> 3	

[1] According to WEISS, D., TVEDTEN, H. (2004): Erythrocyte disorders. In: WILLARD, M., TVEDTEN, H.: Small animal clinical diagnosis by laboratory methods. 4th ed. W.B. Saunders, St. Louis.

[2] Normal Hct: dog 0.45; cat 0.37.

[3] RMI = reticulocyte maturation index. The RMI takes into consideration the increased half-life of the reticulocytes in the circulation of anaemic patients. In the dog (in the cat): RMI = 1 when Hct is 0.45 (0.37); RMI = 1.5 when Hct = $\geq$ 0.35 (0.29); RMI = 2 when Hct = $\geq$ 0.25 (0.21); RMI = 2.5 when Hct = $\geq$ 0.15 (0.11).

cytes – these are older reticulocytes that have been in the circulation approx 3 weeks; and (2) **aggregate** reticulocytes that have just been released from the bone marrow and are less than one day old; they contain at least ten cytoplasmic granules. Aggregate reticulocytes are the best indicators of a regenerative anaemia in cats.

In emergency situations, the haematocrit and a microscopic examination of the blood smear provide important and quick information. If *Babesia* (dog) is prevalent in the area, it is essential that the blood smear is checked for this parasite. The cytological identification of *Haemobartonella* in cats is a much less sensitive method than determining the presence of the DNA of this organism using PCR. Other signs of a regenerative anaemia are anisocytosis and polychromasia. In addition, the presence of poikilocytes (erythrocytes with bizarre or abnormal shapes) can provide indications of the cause of the anaemia (e.g. spherocytes in autoimmune haemolytic anaemia, Heinz bodies in oxidative stress).

The anaemia found in chronic diseases is mild to moderate, nonregenerative, normocytic and normochromic. This form of anaemia can be caused by a number of different chronic inflammatory or infectious diseases as well as by trauma or neoplasia. Its pathogenesis is multifactoral and is induced by cytokines released during the inflammatory process. Some of the mechanisms involved are an increased storage of iron in the macrophage-monocyte system with reduced iron availability, a reduced life expectancy of the erythrocytes and insufficient erythrocyte production in the bone marrow. The treatment of this type of anaemia should always be aimed at the primary cause.

4.2.2 Polycythaemia

In comparison to anaemia, polycythaemia or erythrocytosis is a relatively rare abnormality. It can be primary or secondary. Primary polycythaemia occurs with an abnormal proliferation of the stem cells in the bone marrow (polycythaemia vera). Secondary forms are caused by an abnormal production of erythropoietin, which occurs mainly in tumours such as the renal carcinoma. Erythropoietin is a hormone that is normally produced in the kidney. It promotes the growth and differentiation of the bone marrow's stem cells, leading to an increase in the number of erythrocytes.

In affected dogs and cats, the increased number of erythrocytes (i.e. increased blood viscosity) causes the clinical signs of the disease. The mucous membranes are hyperaemic and there is a tendency for the animal to bleed. Polydipsia, polyuria and respiratory difficulties have been described. In addition, neurological symptoms, such as seizures, blindness, changes in behaviour and ataxia, can occur.

Diagnosis of a primary polycythaemia is based on the exclusion of secondary polycythaemia as well as the diagnosis of a low erythropoietin concentration in the blood in connection with an increased erythrocyte count. Therapy consists of removing the primary disease such as the tumour (secondary polycythaemia) or cytostatic chemotherapy (polycythaemia vera). Repeated bloodletting can help to lessen the clinical signs.

4.2.3 Leukocytosis

Leukocytosis is the most common change found in the leukocyte count. In the majority of cases, it involves a **neutrophilia** which arises either due to the release of neutrophils from the marginal pool (peripheral capillaries) in stress situations or as the result of an inflammatory process.

The so-called **stress leukogram** consists of a light to moderate neutrophilia (up to roughly twice the normal level) without a left shift, and a lymphopaenia (though lymphocytosis can occur in cats). These changes occur in stress situations due to different aetiologies (visit to vet, trauma, pain, etc.). Animals undergoing glucocorticoid therapy have a neutrophilia accompanied by a lymphopaenia, eosinopaenia and monocytosis.

With mild inflammatory reactions, a neutrophilia without a left shift can also be present. If, in comparison, there is a profound inflammatory reaction, then the neutrophils will be used up leading to an exhaustion of the neutrophil reservoir in the bone marrow and to the release of immature unsegmented neutrophils (**left shift**). In severe inflammatory reactions, even earlier stages are released (metamyelocytes, myelocytes). Sometimes the immature cells are more numerous than the segmented neutrophils, a condition known as a **degenerative left shift**. The causes of a neutrophilia with a left shift in patients with neurological symptoms are numerous. Local or systemic bacterial or parasitic infections as well as non-infectious inflammatory reactions or even autoimmune disease should be taken into consideration. In addition, haemolysis, massive tissue damage and tumour necrosis can lead to neutrophilia.

Leukocytosis can also occur due to neoplastic changes in certain leukocyte cell lines. Leukaemic forms of malignant lymphoma, acute or chronic lymphatic leukaemia and other types of leukaemia can all cause a profound increase in the leukocyte count.

4

4.2.4 Leukopaenia

Leukopaenia usually develops as a consequence of **neutropaenia**. Severe inflammatory processes (when the utilisation of neutrophils is higher than the rate of release from the bone marrow; often there is an obvious left shift, too) are some of the most frequent causes of neutropaenia; others include those which have a negative effect on the leukocyte production in the bone marrow. Bacterial sepsis and endotoxaemia are frequent inflammatory causes of neutropaenia. Both must be recognised as early as possible and treated as aggressively as possible. Hypoglycaemia is frequently involved in these conditions.

Diseases of the bone marrow can, in addition, lead to a reduced production of neutrophils with or without affecting other types of cells. In the dog, the average survival time for a neutrophil in the circulation is approx. 10 hours, that of thrombocytes approx. 10 days, and for erythrocytes it is roughly 120 days. This is why neutropaenia is often an early sign of bone marrow damage, followed by thrombocytopaenia. Known causes of bone marrow hypoplasia are medications such as cytostatics, oestrogen and chloramphenicol (in the cat); viral infections (FeLV, FIV in the cat) or Rickettsia (*Ehrlichia canis*, *Anaplasma phagocytophila*); or autoimmune diseases affecting the precursors of the different blood cells.

4.2.5 Thrombocytopaenia / thrombocytosis

The thrombocyte or blood platelet count can be determined exactly in the dog using an automatic counter. In contrast in the cat, as there is an overlapping between the diameter of the erythrocytes and the thrombocytes, mechanical counting is rather difficult. The thombocyte count can be done quickly and easily using a blood smear: when no aggregates of thrombocytes are visible in the periphery, then $10–15 \times 10^9/l$ thrombocytes can be expected for every platelet found in an oil immersion field.

Thrombocytopaenia can occur due to sequestration of the platelets in the spleen or consumption of the thrombocytes, for example with acute severe haemorrhage, disseminated intravascular coagulation, destruction by infectious agents (*Ehrlichia canis*, *Anaplasma phagocytophila*), or autoimmune reactions (autoimmune thrombocytopaenia). As long as the individual thrombocytes remain functional, clinical symptoms, such as mucosal haemorrhages (including epistaxis, haematuria, petechiae, etc.), are first seen with a massive reduction in platelet count ($< 40 \times 10^9/l$). Neurological abnormalities can arise due to CNS haemorrhage.

Thrombocytosis is a rare finding in the dog and cat. The most common causes are neoplasia, gastrointestinal disease and endocrinopathies, as well as treatment with glucocorticoids or antineoplastic drugs.

4.3 Biochemical blood parameters

Routinely, approx. 20 parameters are determined in serum **biochemical profiles**. These include electrolytes (Na, K, Cl, Ca, P), protein (total protein, albumin, globulins), lipid metabolism products (cholesterol, triglycerides) or carbohydrate metabolism products (glucose). In addition, parameters of renal function (urea, creatinine) or haemoglobin degradation (bilirubin) are also measured. Serum enzyme activity is additionally included in the chemical profile, whereby enzymes indicating liver activity (alanine aminotransferase [ALT], aspartate aminotransferase [AST], alkaline phosphate [AP], γ-glutamyl transferase [γ-GT] and glutamate dehydrogenase [GLDH]) and muscle breakdown (creatine kinase [CK]) are determined.

From the above list, it can be seen that the chemical profile provides information about different organ systems so that it can be used to determine many of the "metabolic" diseases which can be accompanied by neurological symptoms. The different blood parameters required for a clarification of the metabolic causes of epileptic seizures or lower motor neuron disease are listed in Tables 4.2 and 4.3, respectively. In the following, the different liver function tests needed to diagnose hepatic encephalopathy and the laboratory tests required to diagnose hypothyroidism will be discussed in more detail.

The **liver enzymes** (see above) provide information about the integrity of the liver cells and are known to be increased when the permeability of the hepatocyte cell membrane is increased or when hepatocytes die. Some other parameters of the biochemical profile are also suitable for determining liver function, i.e. albumin, urea and glucose; three substances which are synthesised in the liver and may be reduced in the serum in liver failure. Blood glucose is the least sensitive indicator of liver function. The determination of blood bilirubin is also useful in assessing the excretory ability of the liver; although prehepatic (massive haemolysis) and post-hepatic (disturbances in bile flow) reasons for hyper-bilirubinaemia should not be forgotten.

As most of the coagulation factors are synthesised in the liver, investigating them in a coagulation "screen" which includes the activated partial thromboplastin time (aPPT), D-dimers, anti-thrombin III and fibrinogen concentration should be done to test the patient's liver function, especially before an ultrasound and liver aspiration or biopsy is undertaken.

Table 4.2: Selected blood parameters that are important in the investigation of epileptic fits in small animals

Parameter	Change	Possible explanation (differential diagnosis as example)
Leukocyte count	Neutrophilia Neutropaenia Lymphopaenia Eosinophilia	Inflammatory / infectious diseases (aseptic meningitis, which responds to steroids) Viral diseases (distemper), bacterial diseases (sepsis) Viral diseases Protozoal diseases
Erythrocyte count	Anaemia (severe) Polycythaemia	Reduced oxygen flow to brain (parasites, blood loss due to immunological causes) Increased blood viscosity (erythropoietin-producing tumour, polycythaemia vera)
Thrombocyte count	Thrombocytopaenia	Intracranial bleeding due to failure of haemostasis (immunological, disseminated intravascular coagulation)
Sodium	Hypernatraemia	Hyperosmolar syndrome (adipsia)
Calcium	Hypercalcaemia (severe) Hypocalcaemia	Changes in the excitability of neuronal membranes (paraneoplastic as in malignant lymphoma, anal sac carcinoma, multiple myeloma) Changes in the excitability of neuronal membranes (puerperal eclampsia in small dog breeds)
Glucose	Hypoglycaemia Hyperglycaemia (severe)	Inadequate energy supply to the brain cells (insulinoma) Hyperosmolar syndrome possible (see hypernatraemia) (Diabetes mellitus)
Albumin	Hypoalbuminaemia	Suspicion of liver dysfunction (when renal or intestinal loss, or transfer into third space fluid have been excluded). Severe liver dysfunction can lead to a hepatic encephalopathy
Globulin	Hyperglobulinaemia (severe, monoclonal)	Hyperviscosity syndrome (paraneoplastic disturbances in connection with multiple myeloma in the dog)
Urea, creatinine	Azotaemia (severe)	Uraemic encephalopathy (chronic renal failure)
AP, ALT (AST)	Increased liver enzymes	Possible liver disease, use bile acids or ammonia as liver function test
Bile acids	Increased bile acids in serum	Indicates reduced liver function or the presence of a congenital or more than one acquired portosystemic shunt(s) with associated hepatic encephalopathy
Ammonia	Hyperammoniaemia	Indicates the presence of a congenital or more than one acquired portosystemic shunt(s) with associated hepatic encephalopathy
Cholinesterase	Reduced cholinesterase activity	Organophosphate poisoning
Specific antibody titres (IgG or IgM)	Increased (if necessary, two blood samples taken 2 to 4 weeks apart to show that the IgG titre has risen)	Toxoplasmosis

4

The investigation of plasma ammonia and serum bile acids are suggested in the diagnosis of hepatic blood vessel abnormalities (portosystemic shunts – congenital: single; acquired: multiple) or other severe liver diseases. The **plasma ammonia concentration** is very good for the diagnosis of such liver abnormalities in the dog and cat. Ammonia is produced in the colon due to bacterial degradation of poorly absorbed dietary protein, sloughed intestinal epithelium and digested bacteria. The ammonia travels via the portal vein system to the liver, where each ammonia molecule is degraded into two uric acid molecules. If there is a shunt between the portal vein and the vena cava, the ammonia goes straight into the circulation. The determination of plasma ammonia is less sensitive when there is just parenchymal liver damage.

The technical undertaking of this test can be problematic. Firstly, not all analysers are capable of providing useful results and secondly, the blood sample must be centrifuged within 30 minutes in a completely filled test tube. The plasma must be tested within an hour of the sample being taken or frozen. If questionable results have been achieved in an animal that has been starved overnight, then a "challenge" test can be undertaken. In this test, 100 mg/kg ammonium chloride (NH_4Cl) is given orally or per rectum as a 5% solution in water, or it is given in gelatine capsules (easiest method per os). Blood is taken 30 to 45 minutes before and after the ammonium chloride administration. In normal cases, the ammonia concentration may be no more than double the original value.

Table 4.3: Selected blood parameters for the clarification of lower motor neuron dysfunction in small animals

Parameter	Change	Possible differential diagnosis as examples
Glucose	Hyperglycaemia	Possibly diabetes mellitus; differential diagnosis: stress hyperglycaemia in the cat (diabetic polyneuropathy in cats)
Cholesterol	Hypercholesterolaemia	Possible hypothyroidism, hyperadrenocorticism
AP	Increased	Possible hyperadrenocorticism
Thyroxin	Reduced	Possible hypothyroidism
TSH	Increased	Primary hypothyroidism
Cortisol after ACTH stimulation	2nd value: > 550 nmol/l or > 20 µg/dl	Hyperadrenocorticism with possible myopathy
Cortisol after inhibition with low a dose of dexamethasone (0.01 mg/kg i.v.)	2nd value: > 40 nmol/l or > 1.5 µg/dl	Hyperadrenocorticism with possible myopathy
Cortisol after ACTH stimulation	No stimulation with respect to base value	Hypoadrenocorticism
Antinuclear autoantibodies (ANA)	Increased	Possibly systemic lupus erythematosus
CK, ALT (AST)	Increased	Possibly myopathy, myositis, muscle trauma
Anti-acetyl-cholinesterase antibody	Measurable	Myasthenia gravis
Antibodies against *Toxoplasma gondii*	Preferably two blood samples are taken 2–5 weeks apart to show a rise in titre	Toxoplasmosis
Antibodies against *Neospora caninum*	Abnormal titre	Neosporosis
Cholinesterase	Reduced	Organophosphate poisoning

The **serum bile acid concentration** also provides important information about liver function. All the bile acids are measured together. The bile acids are synthesised in the liver from haemoglobin and after conjugation, they are stored in the gall bladder. After eating, contraction of the gall bladder is instigated by cytokines, leading to a release of the bile acids into the duodenum, where they help in the absorption of fats. They are mainly resorbed in the ileum and return via the portal vein to the liver where they are removed from the blood (enterohepatic circulation). In the presence of a shunt or in many other diseases of the liver and bile ducts, increased amounts of bile acids bypass the liver and go directly into the vena cava.

Usually, this test is done on dogs and cats that have been fasted overnight (12 hours). The stimulation test enables the enterohepatic circulation to be checked more thoroughly: the bile acid concentration is measured before a meal and 2 hours after. According to various studies in the dog and cat with different types of liver disease, the specificity of the fasting value is 89% in the dog and 96% in the cat if a concentration of 15 µmol/l is chosen as the upper reference value or cut-off point. The sensitivity of the test under these conditions is roughly 70% and 54% in the dog and cat, respectively. If the bile acids are determined 2 hours after a meal, then setting the cut-off point at 15 µmol/l makes the test have a sensitivity of 82% and specificity of 89% in the dog. If the upper reference value is set higher at 25 µmol/l, then the specificity climbs to 100% but the sensitivity is slightly reduced to 74%. The postprandial determination in the cat has a sensitivity of 100% and a specificity of 80% when 20 µmol/l is used as the upper value. The differences between the pre- and postprandial serum bile acid concentrations do not provide any differentiation between the different liver diseases in the dog and cat. The test is therefore just an excellent screening method for investigating liver function.

Amongst the neurologically relevant endocrine diseases, hypothyroidism is the most common diagnostic challenge in the dog. The **serum thyroxine** (T_4) can be used to roughly evaluate thyroid function. Only very rarely are the T_4 values within the normal range in hypothyroid dogs. Accordingly, hypothyroidism is unlikely if there is a normal T_4 concentration. The main problem is that not all dogs with a subnormal T_4 value are hypothyroid. This is due to the influence of numerous diseases on the thyroxin level and the **hypophyseal-thyroid axis** (so-called euthyroid sick syndrome). The determination of the **free biologically active thyroxine fraction** (free T_4 or fT_4) in the serum can be of use. Equilibrium dialysis is the preferred method for this determination.

The differentiation between dogs with normal and reduced thyroid function is somewhat better with fT_4 than T_4. The determination of the **serum thyroid stimulating hormone** (TSH) level is also recommended. As false positives and false negatives are fairly common with this parameter, it should be interpreted in connection with the other two thyroid hormones (T_4, fT_4). A high TSH level with a reduced concentration of T_4 or fT_4 is a significant indication of primary hypothyroidism. As bovine TSH is no longer available for medical use, the only dynamic function test for stimulating the thyroid left available is TRH (thyrotropin releasing hormone). An increase in the level of T_4 of 6.4 nmol/l (0.5 µg/dl) above the basal value is expected when the animal is stimulated with 0.2 mg TRH. The basal value must lie within the laboratory's lower reference range. Sadly, the results of this test are difficult to interpret and rarely aid in giving a clear indication of thyroid function. Serological investigation of autoantibodies against either of the thyroid hormones can make it easy in certain cases to reach a diagnosis of hypothyroidism due to lymphocytic thryroiditis.

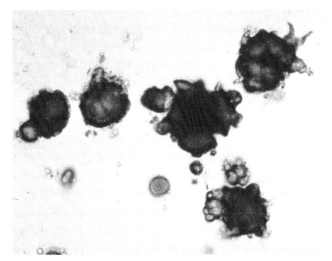

Fig. 4.1
Urinary sediment (magnification 100x). Ammonium biurate crystals as seen in animals with portosystemic blood vessel anomalies (with the kind permission of Hill's Pet Nutrition).

4.4 Urine investigations

An investigation of the urine is indispensable if there is suspicion of renal insufficiency or problems affecting the lower urinary tract (e.g. urinary incontinence). Collection of urine by bladder puncture or even catheterisation to collect spontaneously produced urine is preferable for certain investigations. Testing the **specific gravity of the urine** with a refractometer is used to assess the function of the renal tubules. This test is indicated if the serum concentration of urea and creatinine is increased (azotaemia) to differentiate between prerenal, renal and postrenal disease. First of all, a number of urinary parameters are investigated semiquantatively using **test strips**, which allow a diagnosis of bilirubinuria, glucosuria, ketonurea and haematuria to be made. Detailed qualitative information about the kidneys' ability to excrete certain substances (e.g. protein/creatinine ratio) can be acquired by determining specific indicators.

The investigation of the urinary sediment provides valuable information if there is suspicion of urinary tract infection or urolithiasis. Animals with a portosystemic shunt may have ammonium biurate crystals in their urine (Fig. 4.1) and the finding of such crystals is compatible with a shunt. A bacteriological investigation on the urine enables the causative agent to be isolated as well as a determination of which antibiotics it is sensitive to. For further details about urinary investigation, the reader is referred to textbooks of veterinary laboratory diagnosis.

Further reading

CENTER, S.A (1992): Serum bile acids in companion animal medicine. Vet Clin North Am. (Small Anim Pract.) **23**: 625–657.

DUNCAN, J.R., PRASSE, K.W., MAHAFFEY, E.A. (1994): Veterinary Laboratory Medicine, Clinical Pathology, 3rd ed., Iowa State University Press, Ames.

FAISSLER, D., GRIOT-WENK, M., FATZER, R., VON TSCHARNER, C., ABERLE THIERMANN, B., JAGGY, A. (1998): Krampfanfälle im Zusammenhang mit Polyzythämie, Literaturübersicht und Fallbeschreibung. Schweiz. Arch Tierheilk. **140**: 101–109.

GASCHEN, F. (1999): Paraneoplastische Syndrome. In KESSLER, M.: Kleintieronkologie, Diagnose und Therapie von Tumorerkrankungen bei Hunden und Katzen. Parey Buchverlag, Berlin, S. 29–47.

HAMMER, A.S. (1991): Thrombocytosis in dogs and cats: a retrospective study. Comp Haematol Int. **1**: 181–186.

KRAFT, W., DÜRR, U.M. (1999): Klinische Labordiagnostik in der Tiermedizin, 5. Aufl. Schattauer, Stuttgart.

KEMPPAINEN, R.J., BEHREND, E.N. (2001): Diagnosis of canine hypothyroidism. Perspectives from a testing laboratory. Vet Clin North Am Small Anim Pract. **31**: 951–962.

LEVEILLE-WEBSTER, C.R. (2000): Laboratory diagnosis of hepato-biliary disease. In ETTINGER S.J. und FELDMAN E.C: (ed.): Textbook of veterinary internal medicine. 5th ed. W.B. Saunders, Philadelphia, pp. 1277–1293.

MEYER, D.J., HARVEY, J.W. (1998): Veterinary Laboratory Medicine, Interpretation and Diagnosis, 2nd ed., W.B. Saunders, Philadelphia.

TESKE, E. (1999): Hämatopoietische Tumore. In KESSLER, M.: Kleintieronkologie, Diagnose und Therapie von Tumorerkrankungen bei Hunden und Katzen. Parey Buchverlag, Berlin, pp. 523–557.

WILLARD, M., TVEDTEN, H. (2004): Small Animal Clinical Diagnosis by Laboratory Methods, 4. ed. W.B. Saunders, St. Louis.

4

5 Anaesthesia

Gina Aeschbacher

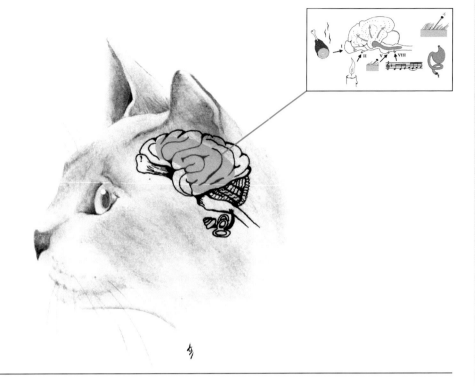

This chapter deals with the basics of sedation and general anaesthesia for diagnostic examination and surgery in the neurological patient. Complications that may occur during these procedures but are not directly associated with the anaesthesia are discussed. The necessity of pain control is mentioned, too (see also Chap. 9.3).

5.1 Basics of neuroanaesthesia

The different aspects of neuroanaesthetic care should be discussed before surgery by the neurologist, surgeon and anaesthetist. Such care varies according to the health status of the patient and the surgery planned. The discussion should encompass a number of aspects, for example, how the patient should be positioned; pre-, intra- and postoperative administration of medication (e.g. steroids, diuretics); increased intracranial pressure treatment; guidelines for the regulation of blood pressure, end-expiratory carbon dioxide, and body temperature. The anamnesis and the clinical examination play an important role in the anaesthetic protocol; the personal preferences of the veterinarian responsible for anaesthesia play a secondary role.

Prior to undertaking the anaesthesia, the risks associated with the anaesthesia and the examination or operation should be discussed with the patient's owner. Written permission for the procedures should be given and signed by the owner, citing where necessary the use of medication that is not licensed for use in the cat or dog. Independent of the health status of the animal and the invasiveness of the procedure, it is important at this stage to clarify what may be done with respect to resuscitation or euthanasia while the animal is still under general anaesthesia, should a crisis situation arise.

Preanaesthetic determination of the CBC, the biochemical parameters and the urine are only necessary in certain patients. In general, they help to ascertain the degree of anaesthetic risk and help in the intra- and postoperative nursing of the patient. In a young, healthy patient, electrolyte, glucose, blood urea and creatinine concentrations will usually suffice. When the anaesthesia has started and the additional results are available, the anaesthetic protocol (including, for example, the choice of anaesthetic, fluid therapy, postoperative monitoring) is adapted to the results.

The main aspects of anaesthesia in the neurological patient and the considerations leading to setting up the anaesthetic protocol are now discussed.

5.1.1 Control of intracranial pressure

The normal blood supply to the brain and spinal cord, i.e. the CNS, is subjected to autoregulation in the conscious healthy animal. Autoregulation is understood as being the ability of the CNS to maintain a relatively constant blood supply during moderate changes in perfusion pressure. The cerebral blood flow (CBF) is controlled by the arterial oxygen partial pressure (PaO_2), the arterial carbon dioxide partial pressure ($PaCO_2$), the mean arterial blood pressure (MAP) and the venous outflow from the brain. A rise in CBF can cause an increase in intracranial volume and consequently, an increase in intracranial pressure (ICP). In the case of a space-occupying lesion, an initial compensation is achieved by the displacement of CSF and venous blood from the intracranial to the extracranial space. As soon as this is no longer possible, even small changes in volume cause a great increase in ICP as the brain's volume is limited by the lack of elasticity of the surrounding bony cranium. The effect is either a reduction in the cerebral perfusion pressure (CPP) with resulting ischaemia or herniation of the brain. The probability of a significant rise in ICP increases with the presence of pathological processes (e.g. trauma, intracranial masses).

An important aspect of neuroanaesthesia is the need to influence the ICP. With a closed skull, it is necessary to ensure adequate brain perfusion (CPP = MAP – ICP) and/or prevent brain herniation. With an open skull, it may be important to achieve "relaxation" of the skull contents to provide better surgical access. The principles applied are similar to those used in the closed skull.

Independent of the cause of raised ICP, it is essential to focus on its reduction. The intracranial space is composed of cells (glia, neurons) and fluid (intracellular, extracellular, CSF, blood). The individual volumes of these compartments together form a dynamic system, whereby according to the Monroe-Kellie hypothesis an increase in one compartment leads to a reciprocal reduction in the others (1, 2, 3). A reduction in each of the different compartment volumes is possible in the following ways: the tissue mass by surgical means, intra- and extracellular fluid by pharmacological means using steroids and diuretics, and the CSF by drainage. The blood compartment is the easiest to manipulate. Accordingly, from the point of view of the anaesthetist, this is very important in the rapid treatment of raised ICP. The venous part forms 75% of this compartment and tends to be passive (4). A blockage, i.e. blocked venous drainage, is the most frequent cause of increased ICP, as is poor operative conditions. During anaesthesia and during periods of intensive nursing, the neck should routinely be placed in a neutral position and the head slightly raised – to prevent venous air emboli (5, 6). Cerebrovenous drainage problems due to extreme positioning of the head and/or compression of the jugular veins (e.g. surgical positioning, blood collection, placement of a jugular catheter, tight neck collars, etc.) should be completely avoided. It should not be forgotten that increased intrathoracic pressure

(e.g. kinked or blocked endotracheal tube, tension pneumothorax, coughing or inadequate depth of anaesthesia during intubation) can lead to disturbances in the venous drainage from the head/neck region. The arterial part of the blood compartment is just as important to ICP regulation. The effect of anaesthesia or the anaesthetic technique on cerebral perfusion is a vital aspect as any rise in CBF is associated with an increase in intracranial blood volume. The factors which affect the CBF are summarised in Table 5.1.

With increased ICP, the choice of anaesthetic becomes imperative. It would go beyond the aims and extent of this chapter to go into detail about every anaesthetic agent, but the most important aspects are discussed below.

Subsequent to CNS depression during general anaesthesia, there is a reduction in the metabolic rate of the nervous tissue and therefore, a reduction in the cerebral oxygen consumption (CMO_2). This is considered to be protective against the possibility of ischaemia developing during anaesthesia and neurosurgery. The autoregulation and reaction to carbon dioxide generally remains intact after injectable anaesthetics or inhalation anaesthesia (7).

Normally, intravenous anaesthetics induce a parallel reduction in CBF and cerebral metabolism and the intracranial compliance is not negatively influenced. Barbiturates are often used in neurosurgery due to their ability to reduce the CMO_2. The mechanisms responsible for this effect are, for example, a reduction in the calcium flux, blockade of the sodium channels, inhibition of the production of free radicals, increased activity of GABA, and inhibition of glucose transfer through the blood-brain barrier (8).

GOODMAN et al. (9) showed that there was less lactate, aspartate and glutamate in the extracellular space during barbiturate coma after head trauma with severely increased ICP.

Table 5.1: Factors that affect the cerebral blood flow

- Arterial oxygen tension
- Arterial carbon dioxide tension
- Cerebral metabolic rate
  - pain
  - epileptic seizures
  - body temperature
  - anaesthetics
- Blood pressure/condition of autoregulation
- Vasoactive substances
  - anaesthetics
  - medications that increase blood pressure
  - inotropic substances
  - vasodilators
- Blood viscosity

The excitatory effects of glutamate have been connected with ischaemic, anoxic, epileptic and traumatic damage to the neurons (10). Glutamate receptor antagonists have been shown to reduce anoxic, ischemic, and epileptic damage: thiopental has been shown to attenuate NMDA- and AMPA-mediated excitotoxicity whereas propofol has been shown to enhance NMDA-induced neuronal damage (10). However, it cannot be assumed that all barbiturates will behave in the same manner as thiopental (11).

In patients without any impairment in consciousness, high doses of the dissociative anaesthetics ketamine and tiletamine can lead to an increase in CBF (6, 12, 13). This has been shown to be caused by their sympathomimetic effect on the blood pressure (4).

Etomidate in its standard formula (dissolved in propylene glycol) should perhaps not be used in cats and dogs with intracranial pathology. In comparison to desflurane, the newest commercially available inhalation anaesthetic, an equivalent dose of etomidate induced a higher degree of hypoxia and acidosis of the brain tissue in human beings as well as obvious neurological symptoms (14).

All inhalation anaesthetics cause a degree of cerebral vasodilation depending on the dose, but its extent is also dependent on the active agent: halothane $\gg$ enflurane $>$ isoflurane $\sim$ sevoflurane $\sim$ desflurane (2, 15, 16, 17). Depending on the anaesthetic used, the net effect on the CBF is influenced by various factors such as concentration of the anaesthetic, combination with injectable anaesthetics (barbiturates, opioid antagonists), cerebral metabolic rate, changes in blood pressure and the carbon dioxide tension (7). Hyperventilation in cats or dogs anaesthetised with halothane, isoflurane, sevoflurane or desflurane causes a reduction in CBF (7).

Nitrous oxide (N_2O, nitrogen dioxide, laughing gas) induces an increase in cerebral metabolic rate, CBF and ICP (6, 8). These effects are strongest if N_2O is used alone, but are variable when it is used as a secondary anaesthetic with or without hyperventilation. Its effects in combination with narcotics, propofol or benzodiazepines are smaller than when combined with inhalation anaesthetics (6). However, N_2O also has a direct neurotoxic effect (8), but DRUMMOND and PATEL (6) have suggested that N_2O may be used in the majority of elective or emergency cerebral operations at a low concentration (inspiratory concentration lower than the minimal alveolar concentration [MAC]) in combination with inhalation anaesthetics. It appears that another method should be used in veterinary neuroanaesthesia. N_2O has a much smaller effect in animals than in human beings: MAC (= ED_{50}) in cats and dogs $>$ 200% and in human beings approx. 100% (18). This MAC value indicates that N_2O should not be used alone with oxygen for the anaesthesia of dogs and cats. As such, it appears to be appropriate to either completely desist from using N_2O in veterinary anaesthesia or at least to wait until the skull has been opened when the direct effect of

the anaesthesia on the brain can be judged. Inhaled anaesthetics are eminently suitable for anaesthesia in the majority of neurosurgical operations, although the potential effects of N_2O and potent inhaled anaesthetics should be taken into consideration when there is increased ICP and a restricted surgical field. In such situations, injectable anaesthetics are most advantageous.

Some muscle relaxants (e.g. atracurium) can induce the release of histamine. If needed, such relaxants should be given divided up into small doses. Suxamethonium chloride, a depolarising muscle relaxant, is used very rarely in the cat to aid intubation in laryngeal spasm as a slight and short-lived increase in ICP has been attributed to it (6).

5.1.2 Control of the carbon dioxide partial pressure

The $PaCO_2$ can be reduced (hypocapnia) by artificial respiration and hyperventilation. Due to the associated vasoconstriction, the cerebral blood volume, but not the CBF *per se*, is reduced (7). Accordingly, the ICP is reduced, resulting in a net effect of decreased brain volume and swelling which in turn makes surgical procedures easier.

In healthy brain tissue, the induced acute hypocapnia should not go below a $PaCO_2$ of 25–30 mmHg. It has been observed that a $PaCO_2$ of between 20–25 mmHg does not improve the effect on the brain's compliance. In contrast, hyperventilation can lead to brain ischaemia in the damaged brain as the CBF may already be reduced during the first 24 hours after the trauma; especially, for example, after head injuries (1, 6). Using artificial respiration, a moderate reduction in $PaCO_2$ down to 30–35 mmHg is aimed at in such patients (1). As with all therapeutic methods, the pros and cons of hyperventilation must be individually assessed for each patient. The indications for hyperventilation / hypocapnia are to reduce an increased or unknown ICP and / or the necessity of improving the operating conditions. Hyperventilation should be stopped once these indications no longer need to be fulfilled.

The influence of hypocapnia on the CBF is not continuous. At the start of hyperventilation, the pH of the CSF and the extracellular fluid increases and the CBF significantly drops. Due to a change in the function of carbonic anhydrase, the cerebral alkalinity is not maintained and the bicarbonate concentration in the CSF and the extracellular fluid is reduced. The pH of these compartments subsequently normalises over a period of 6 to 18 hours as does the CBF. At the end of a long period of hypocapnia, the artificial ventilation should be altered to ensure that the $PaCO_2$ slowly returns to its normal range. Although prolonged artificial respiration is very rarely implemented in veterinary medicine, hyperventilation should be principally maintained only as long as a reduced intracranial volume is necessary. In addition, the suggestion prevalent in human neuroanaesthesia that hyperventilation ought to be only used for the treatment of increased ICP which cannot be controlled by other methods should also be implemented (1, 7).

5.1.3 Control of blood pressure

It is important to maintain the cerebral perfusion pressure (CPP) in the upper (normal) range after acute brain damage and especially after head injury, as well as during most intracranial operations. CBF is often inadequate in damaged areas of the brain and the autoregulation response to this reduced blood pressure is not homogeneously intact. The maintenance of arterial blood pressure in areas of the brain compressed by surgical instruments is also of importance. Due to the pressure of the local tissues, the true perfusion pressure in such areas is reduced. Although only a little data is available, it appears sensible to maintain the blood pressure to the same degree in patients who have recently experienced a compression of the spinal cord as in those who are undergoing spinal surgery (6).

5.1.4 Pharmaceuticals

5.1.4.1 Steroids

The use of steroids serves to reduce oedema associated with tumours. The effect starts quite quickly but not rapidly enough to achieve an immediate improvement in an emergency during an operation. Intracranial operations should be undertaken at least 24 hours after steroids are given. An improvement in the clinical symptoms can be seen about 24 hours after the start of therapy, though it takes a further 1 to 2 days before the ICP falls (6). Steroids should be given both during and after the operation to maintain the preoperative effects (see Chap. 9.2.4).

At the moment, steroids are not used in human medicine in patients with head injuries as either there has been no success or adverse reactions and increased morbidity and mortality have been caused by using them (6, 19). This practise may be changed in the future with the use of fluoronated steroids (e.g. triamcinolone) (6).

5.1.4.2 Diuretics

Diuretics are often used to reduce the intracellular and, above all, the extracellular compartments of the brain. Loop diuretics (e.g. furosemide) are generally less effective (6). Due to this and due to the rapid onset and extent of effects (i.e. a reduction in ICP), mannitol is more commonly used. Mannitol is an osmotically active compound that reduces blood viscosity and so causes a narrowing of the cerebral blood vessels that in turn leads to a reduction in ICP (20). Mannitol's effects are dependant on an intact blood-brain barrier. Urea (an osmotic diuretic) is not used in veterinary medicine even though as a small molecule it has improved brain tissue penetration. Mannitol can also penetrate the brain tissue and has been found in the CSF. The use of mannitol in human medicine is considered to be ambivalent: oedema can be increased when mannitol is used in some cases (6). As suggested by DRUMMOND and PATEL (6) for human beings, empirical utilisation of mannitol appears to be most sensible, meaning that if mannitol leads to a reduction of the ICP or to improved surgical access then it should be used (possibly repeatedly) (see Appendix 5). Mannitol should be stopped if no effect is seen or if the serum osmolarity reaches approx. 320 mOsm/l (6).

Due to their synergism, it has been suggested that a loop diuretic should be combined with an osmotic diuretic. An osmotic gradient will be built up using mannitol to remove fluid from the brain tissue and furosemide will maintain this gradient as it accelerates the excretion of intravascular water. In addition, loop diuretics inhibit the homeostatic mechanisms for controlling cell volume in the neurons and glial cells (6). This mechanism can be of importance in so-called rebound brain swelling; this can occur when mannitol is used due to its concentration or because of general hyperosmolarity. The latter fact also suggests that hypertonic saline should not be used as an alternative therapy to diuretics (6).

5.1.4.3 Anticonvulsants

In general, any irritation of the cerebral cortical surface such as head injury or surgical incision in the cortex can lead to potential epileptic seizures (6). Postoperative epilepsy occurs in human medicine due to inadequate anticonvulsant prophylaxis (21). Electrolyte imbalance (e.g. hyper- / hyponatraemia), hypoxia and hypoglycaemia can also cause epileptic fits. Seizures must be halted as quickly as possible otherwise the ICP will increase, leading to a possible derailment of cerebral metabolism and blood flow as well as increased oedema (21). As long as there are no contraindications, anticonvulsants can be prophylactically used in animals as part of the premedication (see Chaps. 10.2.1.2 and 18.5). Surprisingly, ketamine has been shown to be successful in the suppression of self-sustaining status epilepticus in the rat and the dog (22).

5.1.4.4 Other pharmaceuticals

In addition to other methods used in human neuroanaesthesia, the prophylactic application of magnesium (which affects calcium influx), and the intra- and postoperative infusion of lidocaine (sodium channel blockade) have been suggested (8). Clinical investigations in the dog and cat are limited at present.

5.1.5 Positioning

Often neurosurgical operations involve prolonged periods of anaesthesia. Planning an operation and anaesthesia also involves discussion of the positioning of the patient. A vacuum mattress can be very useful. Not only must pressure points be recognised and well padded, but also pressure or pulling on limbs / nerves must be avoided. Optimal venous drainage is important: putting the head in a raised position by placing pads under the neck or extensive turning of the neck must be avoided. During operations on the spine (especially in the lumbar area), the caudal vena cava should not be compressed when the patient is in sternal recumbency. If the blood flow via the caudal vena cava is blocked, then the blood is diverted to the epidural plexus, thereby increasing the risk of bleeding during laminectomy (6, 23). Intraoperative blood loss is particularly common during operations involving time consuming work on more than one vertebra. Blood loss during operations in the thoracic or lumbar spine is greater than in the neck (24). Blood transfusions may even be necessary and should be considered prior to the type of surgery being performed.

Intraoperative swelling of the tongue or structures in the pharynx can lead to unexpected obstruction of the airway and respiratory distress once the endotracheal tube has been removed. The tongue should be maintained in a neutral position within the mouth by using, for example, tape on the upper and lower jaws to stabilise the patient's head. Unnecessary instrumentation should also not be used in the pharynx / larynx as the tubes and probes (oesophageal stethoscope, temperature probe, stomach tube, probes for transoesophageal echocardiography, etc.) placed in addition to the endotracheal tube could cause damage to these structures.

After placement of a CSF shunt, the patient should be positioned with the head only slightly elevated during the recovery phase and for the first 2 to 3 days after surgery so that the ventricles do not leak around the shunt or collapse too quickly (6).

5.1.6 Supervision of anaesthesia and hypothermia

Invasive methods of surveillance during anaesthesia and the recovery phase are often required in the neurological patient. This is particularly important during craniotomies, as the anaesthesia is usually maintained at a superficial level. Sudden changes in consciousness (waking up) are reflected in changes in arterial blood pressure.

Indications for intra-arterial pressure measurements are unstable circulation (e.g. after trauma), anticipated or potential blood loss (e.g. during tumour resection), light anaesthesia without muscle relaxants, etc. Additionally, intra-arterial pressure measurement is beneficial during the postoperative nursing phase.

Anticipated blood loss and fluid transfer (e.g. due to repeated administration of mannitol) and the assessment of the patient's normal capacity determine whether or not central venous blood pressure (CVP) should be measured during the anaesthesia and in the recovery phase.

Venous air emboli rarely occur in veterinary neuroanaesthesia, although the head in craniotomies often lays a number of centimetres above the level of the heart. Possibly this is because mass spectrometry used for measuring exhaled gases (25) and other such techniques are not commonly used in clinical veterinary anaesthesia due to financial reasons.

Body temperature should be measured continuously. At present, intraoperative hypothermia is not suggested for use in patients with head injuries. A prophylactic mild hypothermia of 1–3 °C under normal body temperature (26) has a neuroprotective effect (8).

Intraoperative (and also postoperative!) hyperthermia must be recognised immediately and treated, as in conjunction with brain ischaemia this can lead to the release of damaging excitatory amino acids (19).

5.1.7 Fluid therapy

Two principles dictate the type of fluid therapy to be used in neurosurgical patients: maintenance of circulating blood volume (normovolaemia) and the prevention of changes in serum osmolarity.

The maintenance of normal blood volume is a process in which the blood pressure is supported. Intravenous fluid therapy should not be restricted as this can lead to hypovolaemia, systemic hypotension, inadequate cerebral perfusion and brain damage. Intravenous fluid therapy serves to support an adequate MAP thereby ensuring optimal brain perfusion.

5

The second principle results from the consideration that reduced serum osmolarity leads to oedema in healthy and normal brain tissue. Fluids which provide free water cause a reduction in serum osmolarity when the infused amount is more than the body's requirement. These types of fluids include those which do not contain adequate amounts of glucose-free compounds and are not isoosmolar to blood. Fluids used for blood replacement should be, as far as possible, isotonic; for example, physiological saline (308 mOsm/l). Lactated Ringer's solution (272 mOsm/l) or similar is often used as a compromise. Generally, the difference between physiological saline and lactated Ringer's solution is minimal, but if it is necessary to infuse a large amount of fluid in a traumatised patient, then physiological saline is the better option. Infusion of large amounts of lactated Ringer's solution caused a drop in serum osmolarity leading to brain oedema in healthy experimental rabbits (27). The infusion of crystalloid solutions is adequate for the majority of elective craniotomies. The use of colloids in veterinary neurosurgery has been repeatedly suggested, but only very rarely do the relevant indications for their use arise (patient with multiple trauma including head injury). The use of hypertonic saline has also recently been suggested with its support of the whole circulation during resuscitation improving brain perfusion (6). The infusion of hypertonic saline increases serum osmolarity, which if not corrected will lead to the phenomenon of so-called rebound swelling of the brain (see Chap. 5.1.4.2).

Solutions containing glucose should be avoided if there is a possibility of underlying brain ischaemia. The massive availability of substrate during ischaemia promotes anaerobic metabolism leading to the production of lactate and pyruvate. This in turn causes acidosis, blood vessel paralysis and increased brain damage (4). Hyperglycaemia associated with head trauma seen in human beings has also been observed in the dog and cat (28). Insulin infusion may be necessary to regulate the blood glucose values but this has not been evaluated in dogs and cats (1).

5.1.8 Recovery period

A quiet recovery period without coughing, delirium-like behaviour and arterial hypertension is desirable in both patients with head injuries or after craniotomy; otherwise, haemorrhage, oedema and increased ICP can develop as complications. To overcome this risk, the use of opioids (for analgesia, sedation and cough reflex suppression), small doses of propofol (for maintenance of anaesthesia, once the inhalational anaesthesia has been stopped) and vasoactive substances (e.g. esmolol for the treatment of systemic hypertension) are indicated (Table 5.2). Hypoxia and hypercapnia lead to an increase in the catecholamine levels and must be excluded as being the cause of hypertension (21). Routine control of electrolytes, acid-base balance, glucose concentration and possibly the haematocrit and total protein is important.

The significance of controlling body temperature has already been mentioned in Chap. 5.1.6.

Adequate pain therapy is extremely important for the welfare of the cat and dog, and is instrumental in a complication-free recovery from anaesthesia and surgery (see Chap. 9.3 and Table 5.2).

5.2 Specific procedural techniques

5.2.1 CSF collection

Basics: short-term, relatively deep anaesthesia is necessary; no spontaneous movements; normally short length of anaesthesia; due to the extreme position of the head ensure patency of airways (Figs. 5.1 and 5.2) and consider possible hyperventilation; choice of anaesthetic generally depends on health status (see Chap. 2.3).

Suggested anaesthesia: controllable, short-acting or antagonisable substances; inhalational anaesthesia may be more suitable than injectable (29).
- Premedication: benzodiazepine; short-acting opioid possibly in combination with a small dose of acepromazine; medetomidine.
- Induction of anaesthesia: thiopental, propofol; cat: alphaxalone / alphadolone, possibly with ketamine; inhalational anaesthesia in oxygen by mask.
- Maintenance of anaesthesia: propofol, isoflurane, sevoflurane, O_2 (possibly with N_2O).
- Surveillance: oesophageal stethoscope; when available: capnography, pulse oximetry.

Recovery phase: intravenous catheter is left until complete recovery; surveillance dependent on health status.

Comments: endotracheal intubation is recommended; spontaneous respiration is advantageous; antagonising medetomidine with atipamezol is possible.

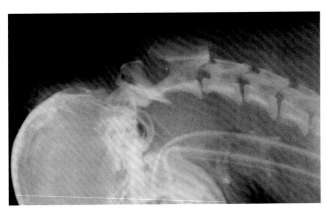

Fig. 5.1
Radiograph showing a kinked endotracheal tube caused by arching the neck into the correct position for the collection of cerebrospinal fluid.

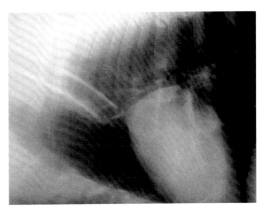

Fig. 5.2
Radiograph showing that the endotracheal tube has been pushed too far down the trachea after hyperextension of the head and neck.

5.2.2 Myelography

Basics: complications arising from the injection of contrast are rare nowadays, though they are more frequent following AO cisternal puncture; cardiovascular depression, cardiac arrhythmias (mainly bradycardia), hypotension, rarely cardiac arrest, initial increase in respiratory rate followed by respiratory depression, respiratory arrest lasting a few seconds to 15 minutes; an intravenous dose of emergency medication (e.g. atropine) should be given beforehand and possibly drawn up ready in a syringe; manual respiration (without stopping anaesthesia) may be necessary; spasms during anaesthesia and in the recovery phase are possible and are dependent on injection site (AO > lumbar) and contrast medium (old medium: metrizamide > new medium: iopamidol, iohexol); prevent epileptic seizures through choice of anaesthetic; prevent contrast agent flowing towards head; promote excretion of contrast agent; securing the airways using intubation is indispensable; adequate ventilation important; adequate depth of anaesthesia without spontaneous movement at the time of dural puncture; intravenous catheter for fluid infusion (10 ml/kg/h) and emergency therapy if necessary.

Trauma patients: transport and position very carefully. Avoid muscle relaxants and hyperextension during intubation; timely application of potent analgesic in painful situations and/or before operation; hypothermia is often a complication of prolonged operations; prevent loss of body temperature at the appropriate time (see Chap. 6.3.2).

Suggested anaesthesia: choice of anaesthetic depends on the health status of the patient but the possible aforementioned complications are more important considerations. The main consideration is to prevent seizure activity; this can be done by avoiding the concurrent use of certain medications (phenothiazines and butyrophenone, ketamine, tiletamine, etomidate and enflurane), using anaesthetics with anticonvulsant effects, and enhancing the excretion of the contrast agent.

- ■ Premedication: benzodiazepine, barbiturates, opioids, medetomidine.
- ■ Induction of anaesthesia: thiobarbiturate, propofol; cat: alphaxolone / alphadolone; inhalational anaesthetic with oxygen using a mask.
- ■ Maintenance of anaesthesia: isoflurane; O_2 (possibly with N_2O); dog: propofol as continuous infusion, possibly with fentanyl.
- ■ Surveillance: continual surveillance of respiratory function, cardiovascular system and body temperature.

Recovery phase: continuous surveillance because of possible seizures (±muscle spasms), generally more frequent in the dog than the cat; have anticonvulsant and spasmolytic preparations (e.g. diazepam) at the ready and give in individual doses; position head high; regularly control body temperature (hypothermia and hyperthermia are possible); leave intravenous catheter in place until complete recovery; evaluate pain status in trauma patients and those with disc disease, and treat accordingly.

Comments: if removal of the endotracheal tube is required by the radiologist for the purposes of radiographic investigation, then the materials for re-intubation including medication for increasing the depth of the anaesthesia should be at hand. The length of anaesthesia should be prolonged if the time between the injection of contrast medium and extubation is less than 20 minutes.

Table 5.2: Sedatives, anaesthetics and analgesics (see also Chap. 9.3)

Medication	Classification	Indication	Dosage (mg/kg) route, interval	Comments
Acepromazine	Phenothiazine	■ Sedation ■ Premedication	0.0005–0.03 IM, IV, SC	■ Other phenothiazines: propiopromazine, chlorpromazine ■ Controversial: as premedication for myelography (especially of neck vertebrae or cisternal contrast injection) and in patients affected by epileptic fits
Alphaxolone/ Alphadolone	Steroid anaesthetic	■ Induction/maintenance of anaesthesia	3–9 IV 12 IM	■ Only for cats
Atracurium	Curare-type muscle relaxant	■ Anaesthesia adjuvant: muscle relaxation	0.2–0.5 IV q 20–40 min	■ Metabolism via Hofmann degradation ■ Artificial respiration necessary
Atropine	Anticholinergic	■ Bradycardia	(0.01–) 0.02 IV 0.04 IM	
Buprenorphine	Partial opioid antagonist	■ Analgesia ■ Premedication ■ Sedation	0.005–0.02 IM, IV, SC q 6–10 h	■ Slight respiratory depression ■ With ↑ ICP: dose analgesic to effect
Butorphanol	Opioid agonist/ antagonist	■ Analgesia ■ Premedication ■ Sedation	0.2–0.6 IM, IV, SC q 1–3 h	■ Slight respiratory depression ■ With ↑ ICP: dose analgesic to effect
Carprofen	NSAID	■ Inflammation ■ Analgesia	2 SC, IV q 12 h	■ Contraindication: shock, ↓ renal function, bleeding, combination with other steroidal or non-steroidal anti-inflammatory drugs
Diazepam	Benzodiazepine	■ Sedation ■ Epileptic seizures	0.2–0.5 IV	
Esmolol	Beta-1-adrenergic inhibitor	■ Tachycardia (supraventricular, ventricular)	0.25–0.5 IV 0.02–0.05 IV/min	■ Bolus, then continuous infusion ■ Side-effects: bradycardia, hypertension
Etomidate	Imidazole	■ Induction of anaesthesia	1–3 IV	■ Avoid in epileptic seizures
Fentanyl	True opioid antagonist	■ Analgesia ■ Premedication	0.001–0.01 IV 0.001–0.005 IV/h	■ Respiratory depression ■ With ↑ ICP: dose analgesic to effect
Glycopyrrolate	Anticholinergic	■ Bradycardia	(0.005–)0.01 IV	
Ketamine	Cyclohexanone (disassociative anaesthetic)	■ Induction of anaesthesia ■ Analgesia (multimodal, chronic)	3–10 IV	■ Stimulates CNS ■ Contraindication: head trauma, epileptic fits, intracranial space-occupying processes, before myelography ■ Tiletamine is more potent than ketamine

5.2.3 Hemilaminectomy, dorsal laminectomy, ventral slot, subluxation and fracture stabilisation

Basics: see comments for myelography; endotracheal intubation and intravenous catheter for fluid therapy (10 ml/kg/h) and intraoperative medication (e.g. analgesics) are imperative; control respiration during cervical vertebral surgery (positioning and physical restraint of the patient may reduce the respiratory volume); vagal stimulation and cardiac rhythm disturbances may occur during a ventral approach to the cervical vertebrae; in trauma, instability and disc disease of the cervical spine: avoid hyperextension of the neck during intubation; depending on cause (disc, tumour, etc.), pain therapy should be initiated pre- and postoperatively (see Chap. 9.3); prevent temperature loss at the appropriate time; correct positioning of the body is very important: prevent tension on the limbs or nerves, prevent pressure on abdominal organs (to avoid heavy bleeding).

Table 5.2: Sedatives, anaesthetics and analgesics (continued) (see also Chap. 9.3)

Medication	Classification	Indication	Dosage (mg/kg) route, interval	Comments
Medetomidine	Alpha-2-adrenergic agonist	■ Sedation ■ Premedication ■ Analgesia	0.002–0.010 IM, IV	■ Dosage of all subsequent anaesthetics reduced by 30–80%. Muscle relaxation ■ Antagonistic reaction with Atipamezol
Meloxicam	NSAID	■ Inflammation ■ Analgesia	0.2 PO, IV q 24 h	■ Contraindication: shock, ↓ renal function, haemorrhage, corticosteroids and the combination with other NSAIDs
Methadone	True opioid agonist	■ Analgesia ■ Premedication	0.2–0.6 IM, IV, SC q 2–4 h	■ Respiratory depression ■ With ↑ ICP: dose analgesic to effect
Methohexital	Methylated barbiturate	■ Induction of anaesthesia	6–10 IV	■ Avoid in epileptic seizures
Midazolam	Benzodiazepine	■ Sedation ■ Epileptic seizures	0.2–0.5 IM, IV	
Morphine	True opioid agonist	■ Analgesia	0.2–0.6 IM, IV, SC q 2–4 h	■ Respiratory depression ■ With ↑ ICP: dose analgesic to effect
Neostigmine	Cholinesterase inhibitor	■ Antagonisation of muscle relaxation	0.05 IV	■ Give IV atropine or glycopyrrolate shortly before
Pentobarbital	Barbiturate	■ Sedation ■ Premedication ■ Coma induction	2–4 IM 2–16 slowly IV 0.2–1/h	■ Premedication: patient with epileptic fits or before myelography ■ Titrate according to effect (over ~20 min); barbiturate coma: intensive surveillance
Pethidine	True opioid agonist	■ Analgesia ■ Premedication	Dog: 3–8 IM Cat: 3–10 IM	■ Slight respiratory depression ■ With ↑ ICP: dose analgesic to effect
Phenobarbital	Oxybarbiturate	■ Premedication	2 IM	■ Premedication: patient with epileptic fits or before myelography
Propofol	Propylphenol	■ Induction of anaesthesia ■ Sedation	Dog: 4–6 slow IV TIVA: 0.1–0.5/h Cat: 6–8 slow IV	■ Not analgesic ■ Dog: total intravenous anaesthesia (TIVA)
Thiopental	Sulphur-containing barbiturate	■ Induction of anaesthesia	10–25 IV	

Suggested anaesthesia: choice of anaesthesia protocol depends on patient's health status.
■ Premedication: opioid; possibly acepromazine, medetomidine, or benzodiazepine.
■ Induction of anaesthesia: thiopental, propofol, etomidate; cat: ketamine, alphaxolone / alphadolone; possibly inhalation anaesthesia with oxygen per mask.
■ Maintenance of anaesthesia: isoflurane, O_2 (possibly with N_2O); dog: propofol as continuous infusion in combination with potent opioid (e.g. fentanyl).
■ Surveillance: continual surveillance of respiration, cardiovascular system and body temperature; check haematocrit and total proteins every 30 to 60 minutes if there is blood loss and compare with preanaesthetic values.

Recovery phase: regularly evaluate pain status; postoperative pain therapy over a number of days (3 to 7) is indicated; intravenous catheter should be left in place until complete recovery; with hypothermia, warm patient up slowly and check body temperature every 30 minutes until normal; after massive bleeding, check haematocrit and total proteins every 4 to 6 hours.

Comments: ensure that pain is controlled before physiotherapy.

5

5.2.4 Intracranial disease

- Inflammatory and vascular diseases of the brain
- Anomalous diseases of the brain
- Intracranial space-occupying processes, e.g., tumours
- Head injury
- Increased ICP

Basics: the critical patient should be examined and stabilised before anaesthesia as reduced consciousness, cardiopulmonary depression and increased ICP can be present; resuscitation (according to "A-B-C" of emergency treatment) is imperative, especially with head injuries; ICP should be reduced (mannitol, furosemide, possibly corticosteroids) before anaesthesia is started (see Chap. 5.1.1); premedication with a sedative is often not necessary or should only be given to effect as there may be CNS depression or a possible hypersensitivity to the sedative, and additional CO_2 retention is problematic; the use of anaesthetics for intubation may not be necessary in the semi-comatose or comatose patient as long as methods to reduce laryngeal sensitivity are employed; prepare drugs for cardiopulmonary and cerebral resuscitation in advance.

Suggested anaesthesia: principally attention must be paid to optimisation of the cerebral perfusion, prevention of cerebral ischaemia and avoidance of medications / techniques which will increase the ICP; all anaesthetics should be given to effect; avoid the use of N_2O, ketamine and tiletamine or induction of anaesthesia with inhalation anaesthetics by mask; keep anticholinergics such as glycopyrrolate and atropine (for the treatment of bradycardia) at hand; fluid therapy to stabilise the circulation; avoid respiratory depression, disturbances in venous drainage, coughing and defence reactions (e.g. when using a mask).

- Premedication: possibly not necessary; benzodiazepines on their own or in combination with a low dose of opioid.
- Induction of anaesthesia: thiopental, propofol; cat: alphaxolone / alphadolone.
- Maintenance of anaesthesia: continuous infusion of propofol (Total Intra-Venous Anaesthesia) combined with a potent short-term opioid and possibly a muscle relaxant; inhalation anaesthetic at a low dose combined with an opioid and possibly a muscle relaxant; as required, assisted or artificial respiration (hyperventilation with 100% O_2; end-expiratory CO_2 value 25–30 mmHg) to reduce the ICP and improvement of the ventilation; local anaesthesia for surgical field (e.g. lidocaine).
- Surveillance: intensity depends on potential blood loss; direct measurement of arterial blood pressure is advantageous; measurement of ICP for intraoperative management is not necessary (knowledge of the anaesthetics and their effects on ICP; direct intraoperative observation of the brain is possible); continual surveillance of the cardiovascular and respiratory parameters as well as body temperature; check haematocrit and total proteins every 30 to 60 minutes when there is blood loss and compare with preanaesthetic values; minimal haematocrit for optimal O_2 supply lies between 30 and 35%.

Recovery phase: intensive surveillance and nursing in padded cage in a room set especially aside for such patients; head placed slightly higher than body; continual surveillance of cardiovascular parameters (especially MAP; hypo- or hypertension), respiratory parameters (exclude hypoxia and hypercapnia) and body temperature (try to attain below normal range; above normal range should be avoided at all costs); seizure activity possible; have emergency medications at hand and calculate dosages beforehand; make arrangements for emergency intubation and / or artificial respiration; regular control of electrolytes, blood gases, glucose concentration, acid-base balance; regular evaluation of pain status; possibly supply oxygen.

Comments: due to possible disturbances in consciousness, the pain status after craniotomy is difficult to evaluate. Surgery that affects the hypothalamus may lead to hypertension, impaired consciousness and disturbances in water balance that start 12 to 24 hours after the operation. Avoid causing disturbances in consciousness and slow awakening (careful when using substances that bind to receptors such as opioids and benzodiazepines which may be responsible for these issues).

5.2.5 Electrodiagnostic investigations

Generally, dogs and cats lack cooperation and tolerance for electrodiagnostic investigations and so these need to be done under sedation or general anaesthesia. Although they cannot be avoided, these medications influence the nervous tissues throughout the body to a varying degree. The effects of anaesthetics on electrodiagnostic recording evaluations are variable dependent on the area of the nervous system under investigation (see Chap. 7).

5.2.5.1 Electroencephalography (EEG)

Basics: Recording of the EEG in the awake patient is the most ideal situation; anaesthetic substances affect the EEG in many different ways; experience with a single anaesthetic protocol is important for consistent and correct interpretation; short-acting and antagonisable substances are advantageous; aim for light sedation; use infiltration of the temporal muscles with a local anaesthetic (e.g. lidocaine) as alternative to general anesthesia or as additional medication; prevent hypothermia (see Chap. 7.2)

Artifacts caused by movements of the patient and by muscles in the region of the recording electrodes are a serious problem in awake patients and can limit the value of the EEG. Also, many dogs may remain fully aroused thus preventing recording during the various stages of sleep, which are important indicators of the health of the brain. Some EEG abnormalities, e.g. focal spikes, can be recorded from patients during general anaesthesia; however, some general anaesthetics induce spikes and thus can confuse interpretation. Importantly, general anaesthesia also prevents recording during physiological sleep. Sedative drugs, in doses just sufficient to render the animal drowsy when undisturbed, minimize or eliminate difficulties with movement and muscle artifacts. Sedation is used when necessary in restless patients or to induce sleep in human EEG patients and is not considered to detract from the value of the recordings obtained.

Light sedation can be used as follows: 15 minutes prior to placing the recording electrodes, dogs are given 5 mg/kg meperidine (IM or SC); 5 minutes prior to placing electrodes, 0.1 mg/kg acepromazine is administered IV (in a few instances only meperidine is given and in a few others, no sedation is administered). No physical restraint is used.

Further suggested anaesthesia:
- Premedication: none, possible medetomidine, possibly short-acting opioid.
- Induction of anaesthesia: propofol, thiopental; cat: alphaxolone / alphadolone; inhalation anaesthesia (isoflurane) by mask.
- Maintenance of anaesthesia: inhalation anaesthesia (isoflurane), O_2; dog: propofol (in small doses or continuous intravenous infusion).
- Surveillance: continual surveillance of the cardiovascular and respiratory parameters as well as body temperature.

Recovery phase: depending on the patient's health status (e.g. continual surveillance because of epileptic fits).

Comments: other electrical machines (e.g. pulse oximeter, ECG) and manual surveillance of the patient (e.g. stimulation of the palpebral reflex) can disturb the EEG recording; continue recording the EEG while the animal regains consciousness after the anaesthetic is finished or after the medetomidine or opioids have been antagonised.

5.2.5.2 Electromyography (EMG)
Basics: the choice of anaesthetic depends on the patient's health status; the use of peripherally active muscle relaxants (e.g. for making intubation in cats easier) is contraindicated. General anaesthesia is required to reduce spontaneous muscle contraction associated with movement and needle insertion as well as to reduce pain (see. Chap. 7.1.1).

Suggested anaesthesia:
- Premedication: alone or in combination: phenothiazines, opioids, medetomidine, benzodiazepines.
- Induction of anaesthesia: barbiturate, propofol, etomidate; cat: ketamine, alphaxolone / alphadolone; inhalation anaesthetic by mask or in chamber.

- Maintenance of anaesthesia: inhalation anaesthesia, O_2 (possibly with N_2O); dog: propofol; cat: ketamine, alphaxolone / alphadolone.
- Surveillance: continual surveillance of cardiovascular and respiratory parameters as well as body temperature.

Recovery phase: surveillance depends on patient's health status.

Comments: other electronic devices (e.g. pulse oximeter, ECG) can disturb the EMG recording. Sometimes muscle spasms occur after induction with propofol, which can last for several minutes and so disturb the recording. Increasing the depth of anaesthesia using inhalational anaesthetics or intravenous injection of diazepam does not alter this situation as a rule but will just increase the side effects such as hypotension or respiratory depression. Ketamine (1 mg/kg IV) helps in this situation.

5.2.5.3 Nerve conduction velocity studies
Basics: painful investigation which has to be done under general anaesthesia; choice of anaesthetic depends solely on patient's health status (see Chap. 7.1.2).

Suggested anaesthesia:
- Premedication: as single substance or in combination: phenothiazines, opioids, medetomidine, benzodiazepines.
- Induction of anaesthesia: barbiturate, propofol, etomidate; cat: ketamine, alphaxolone / alphadolone; inhalation anaesthetic by mask or in chamber.
- Maintenance of anaesthesia: inhalation anaesthesia, O_2 (possibly with N_2O); dog: propofol; cat: ketamine, alphaxolone / alphadolone.
- Surveillance: continual surveillance of cardiovascular and respiratory parameters as well as body temperature.

Recovery phase: surveillance depends on patient's health status.

Comments: other electronic devices (e.g. pulse oximeter, ECG) can disturb the recording.

5.2.5.4 Recording auditory and visual evoked potentials
Basics: anaesthetics can affect the recording of evoked potentials, with cortical potentials more affected than brain stem potentials. The techniques used in clinical anaesthesia have negligible or no effects on the auditory or visual evoked potentials (see Chaps. 1.5.8.2 and 7.1.3).

5

Suggested anaesthesia:
- Premedication: as single substance or in combination: phenothiazine, opioids, medetomidine, benzodiazepine.
- Induction of anaesthesia: barbiturate, propofol, etomidate; cat: ketamine, alphaxolone/alphadolone; inhalation anaesthetic by mask or in chamber.
- Maintenance of anaesthesia: inhalation anaesthesia, O_2 (possibly with N_2O); dog: propofol; cat: ketamine, alphaxolone/alphadolone.
- Surveillance: continual surveillance of the cardiovascular and respiratory parameters as well as body temperature.

Recovery phase: surveillance depends on the patient's health status.

Comments: The head, including the osseous bullae, may be radiographed before recording auditory evoked potentials if otitis media is suspected, and this will add to the length of the anaesthesia necessary. No special restrictions are placed on the anaesthetic protocol except to ensure that there are no spontaneous movements and there is adequate muscle relaxation. The positioning of the patient for lateral or dorsoventral views, or with open mouth can lead to a bending or movement of the endotracheal tube in any direction (intubation of a main bronchus, unintended extubation). An endotracheal tube that is strengthened by a metal spiral can be of assistance in maintaining ventilation. If removal of the endotracheal tube is required by the radiologist and/or is needed to ensure that the radiographic interpretation is unequivocal, then the equipment for re-intubation including medication for increasing the depth of the anaesthesia should be at hand.

5.2.5.5 Electroretinography, somatosensory and motor evoked potentials

The effects of clinical anaesthesia on these recordings in the dog and cat are not clear. Somatosensory evoked potentials are influenced by anaesthetics to different degrees.

5.2.6 Imaging using computed tomography (CT) and magnetic resonance imaging (MRI)

CT and MRI are becoming more important as imaging procedures in veterinary medicine. Both techniques are impressive due to their excellent resolution and clarity, but require patient immobility. As a consequence, general but light anaesthetia is required to prevent spontaneous movements. The choice of anaesthetic is dependent on the health status of the cat or dog. (Chaps. 1.5.8.1 and 7.1.2).

The ionising radiation in CT means that personnel may not be present during the examination. The surveillance of the anaesthetised patient is done at a distance using auditory signals (e.g. Doppler probe) or visual signals on a monitor (e.g. pulse oximetry, capnography, blood pressure).

The intense magnetic field associated with MRI causes special problems as it makes routine surveillance machines unusable. Ferromagnetic objects are drawn towards the magnet and become dangerous projectiles. Standard anaesthetic machines, machines for surveillance of normal parameters and those used for artificial respiration cannot be placed anywhere close to the magnet. MRI safe and compatible equipment is available. The anaesthetic protocol depends, therefore, on the monitoring machines available. Additionally, the patient is difficult to access throughout the procedures, MRI data collection takes a long time, and the anaesthetised patient can quickly become hypothermic.

Contrast agents are used both in CT and MRI to increase the resolution between tissues and identify vascularised abnormalities. The frequency of side-effects (in particular, changes in blood pressure, anaphylaxis) has not been documented in veterinary medicine. Despite this, necessary precautions should be taken. Therapy is restricted to supportive treatment.

The transport distances between practice/clinic and the CT/MRI unit may present a logistical problem (e.g. admission to a human hospital on an out of hours basis). All equipment, including an emergency kit, in case of the need for resuscitation, have to be taken with the patient to the unit. It is a prerequisite of inhalational anaesthesia that the gases expired by the patient are correctly scavenged. These can be discharged into a container in which the vaporised anaesthetics – but not N_2O – are absorbed onto granulate similar to soda lime. It is better not to use N_2O and to use isoflurane rather than halothane when an active exhaust system with disposal of the exhaled gases is not available outside of the clinic.

Literature

1 PROULX, J., DHUPA, N. (1998): Severe brain injury – Part II: Therapy. Comp Cont Educ. **20**: 993–1005.

2 HOWARD, R.A., MATJASKO, M.J. (1990): Management of intracranial hypertension in severe head injury. Problems in Anesthesia **4**: 477–491.

3 MOKRI, B. (2001): The Monro-Kellie hypothesis: applications in CSF volume depletion. Neurol. **56**: 1746–1748.

4 LAM, A.M., MAYBERG, T.S. (1995): Anesthetic management of patients with traumatic head injury. In: Anesthetic management of acute head injury. In: A.M. Lam (ed.), McGraw-Hill, Inc., New York, pp. 181–221.

5 DAYRELL-HART, B., KLIDE, A.M. (1989): Intracranial dysfunctions: stupor and coma. Vet Clin North Am. (Small Anim. Pract.) **19**: 1209–1222.

6 DRUMMOND, J.C., PATEL, P.M. (2000): Neurosurgical Anesthesia. In: Anesthesia. R.D. Miller (ed.), Churchill Livingstone, Philadelphia, pp. 1895–2240.

7 BRIAN, J.E. (1998): Carbon dioxide and the cerebral circulation. Anesthesiology **88**: 1365–1386.

8 COTRELL, J.E. (2001): Brain protection in neurosurgery – dos and don'ts. American Society of Anesthesiologists' Annual Meeting Refresher Course Lectures pp. 142./1–7.

9 GOODMAN, J.C., VALADKA, A.B., GOPINATH, S.P., CORMIO, M., ROBERTSON, C.S. (1996): Lactate and excitatory amino acids measured by microdialysis are decreased by pentobarbital coma in head-injured patients. J Neurotrauma **13**: 549–556.

10 ZHU, H., COTRELL, J.E., KASS, I.S. (1997): The effect of thiopental and propofol on NMDA- and AMPA-mediated glutamate excitotoxicity. Anesthesiology **87**: 944–951.

11 DRUMMOND, J.C., PATEL, P.M., COLE, D.J. (1996): Cerebral protection: are all barbiturates created equal? Anesthesiology **85**: 1504–1505.

12 DAWSON, D., MICHENFELDER, J.D., THEYE, R.A. (1971): Effects of ketamine on canine cerebral blood flow and metabolism: modification by prior administration of thiopental. Anesth Analg. **50**: 443–447.

13 PABLO, L.S., BAILEY, J.E. (1999): Etomidate and Telazol. Vet Clin North Am. (Small Anim Pract.) **29**: 779–792.

14 HOFFMAN, W.E., CHARBEL, F.T., EDELMAN, G., MISRA, M., AUSMAN, J.I. (1998): Comparison of the effect of etomidate and desflurane on brain tissue gases and pH during prolonged middle cerebral artery occlusion. Anesthesiology **88**: 1188–1194.

15 MCPHERSON, R.W., TRAYSTMAN, R.J. (1988): Effects of isoflurane on cerebral autoregulation in the dog. Anesthesiology **69**: 493–499.

16 TODD, M.M., DRUMMOND, J.C. (1984): A comparison of the cerebrovascular and metabolic effects of halothane and isoflurane in the cat. Anesthesiology **60**: 276–282.

17 MILETICH, D.J., IVANCOVICH, A.D., ALBRECHT, R.F., REIMANN, C.R., ROSENBERG, R., MCKISSIC, E.D. (1976): Absence of autoregulation of cerebral blood flow during halothane and enflurane anesthesia. Anesth Analg. **55**: 100–109.

18 HORNBEIN, T.F., EGER, E.I. II, WINTER, P.M., SMITH, G., WETSTONE, D., SMITH, K.H. (1982): The minimum alveolar concentration of nitrous oxide in man. Anesth Analg. **61**: 553–556.

19 PROUGH, D.S. (2001): Perioperative management of traumatic brain injury. American Society of Anesthesiologists' Annual Meeting Refresher Course Lectures, pp. 144./1–7.

20 SMITH, T.S. (1991): Care of the patient with brain injury. Anesth Clin North Am. **9**: 347–358.

21 OSBORN, I. (1994): The neurosurgical patient. Baillière's Clinical Anaesthesiology **8**: 855–871.

22 BORRIS, D.J., BERTRAM, E.H., KAPUR, J. (2000): Ketamine controls prolonged status epilepticus. Epilepsy Res. **42**: 117–22.

22a SERRANO, S., HUGHES, D., CHANDLER, K. (2006): Use of ketamine for the management of refractory status epilepticus in a dog. J Vet Intern Med. **20** (1): 194–197.

23 HARVEY, R.C., SIMS, M.H., GREENE, S.A. (1996): Neurologic disease. In: Lumb and Jones' Veterinary Anaesthesia. J.C. Thurmon, W.J. Tranquilli, G.J. Benson (eds.), William and Wilkins, Baltimore, pp. 775–785.

24 BLACK, S. (2001): Anesthesia for spine surgery. American Society of Anesthesiologists' Annual Meeting Refresher Course Lectures, pp. 236./1–7.

25 MATJASKO, J., PETROZZA, P., MACKENZIE, C.F. (1985): Sensitivity of end-tidal nitrogen in venous air embolism detection in dogs. Anesthesiology **63**: 418–23.

26 MOSS, E. (2001): The cerebral circulation. Br J Anaesthesia CEPD Review **1**: 67–71.

27 TOMMASINO, C., MOORE, S., TODD, M.M. (1988): Cerebral effects of isovolemic hemodilution with crystalloid or colloid solutions. Crit Care Med. **16**: 862–868.

28 SYRING, R.S., OTTO, C.M., DROBATZ, K.J. (2001): Hyperglycemia in dogs and cats with head trauma: 122 cases (1997–1999). J Am Vet Med Assoc. **218**: 1124–1129.

29 CELLIO, B.C. (2001): Collecting, processing, and preparing cerebrospinal fluid in dogs and cats. Comp Cont Educ. **23**: 786–792.

Further reading

PADDLEFORD, R.R. (1999): Anesthetic considerations in patients with preexisting problems or conditions. In: Manual of small animal anesthesia. R.R. Paddleford (ed.), Saunders, Philadelphia, pp. 267–317.

TRANQUILLI, W.J., GRIMM, K.A., LAMONT, L.A. (2000): Pain management for specific conditions and procedures. In: Pain Management. W.J. Tranquilli (ed.), Teton NewMedia, Jackson WY, pp. 73–104.

5

6   Neuroradiology

Johann Lang
Gabriela Seiler

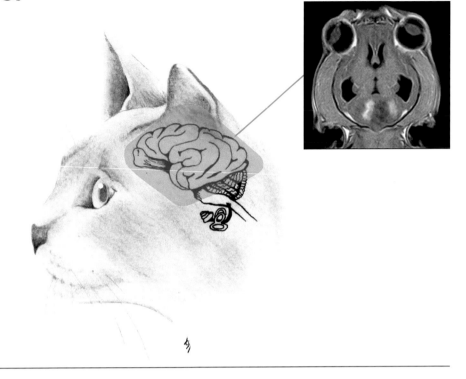

6

The upsurge of neurology and especially neurosurgery in the past few decades is closely related to the development of modern imaging techniques. The introduction of computed tomography (CT) in 1972 by GOTTFRIED NEWBOLD HOUNSFIELD (1) provided new possibilities for diagnosis and therapy, which have led to a virtual revolution in neurosurgery. Previously, all the radiography methods at the centre of diagnostic examinations had been invasive, such as many of the contrast investigations (myelography, discography, epidurography, ventriculography, thecography) and the angiographic techniques. All these methods have the same weaknesses: they are based on conventional radiography and are therefore summation pictures, meaning that a superimposition-free imaging of neural structures is not possible with any of them. In contrast, CT and to an even greater degree magnetic resonance imaging (MRI), provide a good degree of multiplanar localisation and tissue contrast resolution (Fig. 6.1). Additionally, the use of contrast in either of these methods, can greatly increase their diagnostic capabilities. CT and MRI can provide information about the blood supply to the nervous system which can be used to differentially visualise specific tissues. One example is the pituitary, which with its complex blood supply of arteries and its portal system can be differentiated using a dynamic contrast enhanced CT (2). As the availability of CT and MRI in veterinary medicine increases, especially for small animals, these techniques will become increasingly important. Conventional radiology and myelography still play an important role in imaging of the vertebral column and therefore they will be discussed in detail below. Other examination methods are only considered briefly within the framework of their respective indications.

6.1   Indications

Only rarely, for instance, with large peripheral nerve sheath tumours, can peripheral neuropathies be visualised using conventional radiography. Since the advent of CT, and to an even greater extent MRI, the imaging of diseases effecting the cauda equina, the brachial plexus, lumbosacral plexus and peripheral nerves has become possible (Fig. 6.2). The neural structures, many of their pathologies and the muscle, can be imaged using suitable MRI sequences. CT can provide information about neural compression in the vertebral canal at the level of the foraminae. Traumatic neuropathies are often associated with fractures in the pelvis or long bones. CT methods can also provide reliable information about the nature of such fractures. Larger nerves in certain locations can be directly visualised using MRI and so this may be a useful investigative technique for traumatized patients with peripheral nerve dysfunction.

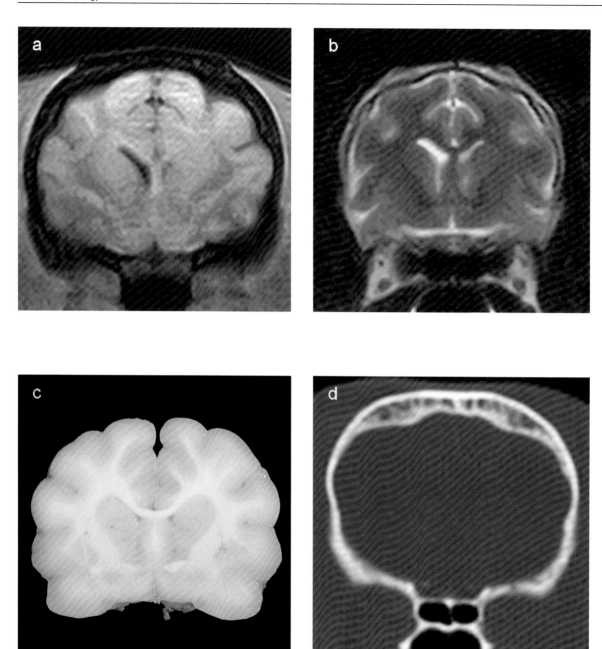

Figure 6.1a–d
MRI, macroscopic and CT sections of a normal cat brain. This is an example taken from the comparative atlas of the cross-sectional anatomy of the dog and cat brains in Appendix I.
The T1w MRI sequence (a) depicts the morphology of the brain, while the T2w sequence (b) preferentially portrays the CSF spaces. The information from the MR images can be easily compared with the macroscopic section (c). The CT image (d) depicts the osseous boundaries of the brain.

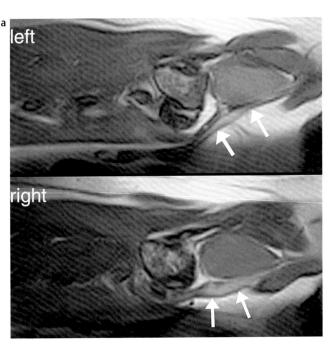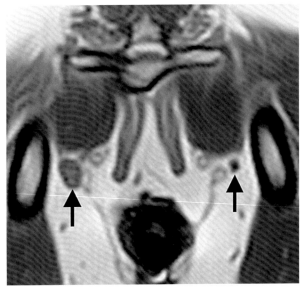

Fig. 6.2a, b
Tumour of the sciatic nerve: (a) sagittal and (b) transverse T1w sequences. Right and left sagittal T1w sequence at the level of the sacral wings with the sciatic nerve running along the ventral surface of the sacrum (arrows). On the right, the nerve has an obvious spindle-shaped thickening. This thickening and the increased signal intensity is especially obvious in the transverse image (arrows). The signal from the normal nerve is hypointense.

Diseases of the spinal cord and vertebral column are the most common indications for a neuroradiological examination. Malformations (congenital and acquired), metabolic disturbances, traumatic, inflammatory (infectious), degenerative and neoplastic diseases often lead to changes in the vertebral column, which can be depicted to a certain extent using conventional radiography. The visualisation of diseases of or affecting the spinal cord and the meninges require the more advanced imaging techniques of myelography, CT or MRI.

Disturbances of the cerebrum can not usually be visualised radiologically. Exceptions are infections and tumours of the middle ear, fractures with misalignment of the fragments, tumours of the calvarium and congenital malformations. Nevertheless, the sensitivity of a radiographic investigation is relatively low in these diseases. Visualisation of organic diseases of the brain and meninges requires the use of CT or MRI, which are becoming increasingly available in veterinary practise. Nuclear medical imaging techniques, such as PET and SPECT, have little current significance in veterinary practice, but they are being increasingly used in tumour research and investigations on regional brain function and perfusion.

6.2 Examination methods

6.2.1 Radiology

The specific requirements of the x-ray equipment necessary to produce high quality images of the head and vertebral column are described in detail elsewhere. The most important and standard aspects of the radiographic technique are: (i) generators with a power of 100 kV/300 mA; (ii) an examination table with a tiltable surface and a Potter-Bucky grid. A stationary linear parallel grid with a ratio of at least 10:1 and 40 lines/cm can be used as a substitute for the latter. The x-ray head should be freely movable to allow oblique and horizontal beam images to be taken.

The radiological examination of the head and vertebral column should take place under adequate **sedation or anesthesia**. Complete muscle relaxation may be necessary for the precise positioning required for investigations of the head and cervical vertebrae, as well as for the many different specific projections that may be required. Animals with a history of trauma are usually exceptions to this rule. These animals are normally examined without sedation or anesthesia to prevent unwanted cardiovascular effects – hypotension with resultant CNS ischemia – or muscle relaxation with resultant destabilisation of the vertebral column. Examinations under anaes-

6

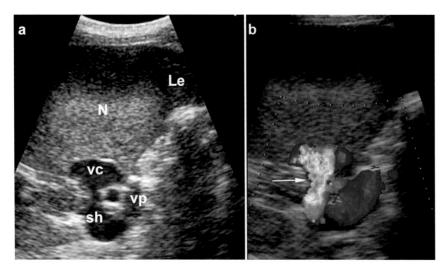

Fig. 6.3
B-mode (a) and Doppler (b) images of a portoventricular shunt. Dorsal plane with the transducer coupled ventrally directly below the lumbar muscles (Le). The curved course of the shunt vessel (sh) can be seen running from the portal vein (vp) to the caudal vena cava (vc). The highly turbulent blood flow (arrow) in the shunt's outlet at the level of the cranial pole of the right kidney (N) is depicted in the Doppler image.

thesia are only indicated in such traumatised patients if the clinical signs and / or the radiographic evidence make a subsequent surgical operation likely or necessary.

Definitive changes in osseous structures that help diagnosis and prognosis are often very subtle; therefore, **fine film-screen combinations** must be used. Exceptions to this are for large dogs, in which at times a quicker system has to be used. The screens available nowadays have an emulsion made of rare earth or a UV system and have a higher resolution than that available with calcium wolframate screens. Systems with a flat gradation are preferred. A **grid** is used to improve the contrast in images of objects with a diameter of 12 cm or more.

6.2.2 Radiological tomography (linear tomography)

Linear tomography is a very old method and is based on the principle of blurring the images outside a focal plane. The x-ray head is moved in an arc over the object during exposure and the x-ray cassette is moved in the opposite direction. The position of the beam (slice selection) can be freely chosen. It is the only section that is in focus; all the other structures of the object are blurred. This method requires the necessary technical equipment and still can provide a good alternative in the examination of complex structures such as the vertebral column and skull, even though it cannot compete with the modern tomographic techniques.

6.2.3 Ultrasonography

As ultrasonography allows a non-invasive examination of the brain, neurosonography is used in human medicine to investigate the CNS in foetuses, neonates and children. It also plays a role in human beings in determining brain death. This technique is only effective in the dog and cat when open or persistent fontanelles are present, or when it is used as an intraoperative technique after an acoustic window has been opened up by surgery. Intracranial structures such as the falx cerebri, lateral and third ventricles, mesencephalon, brain stem and cerebellum can be identified and visualised. The size of the lateral ventricles can be measured in congenital internal hydrocephalus as this can be associated with persistent fontanelles (3). Brain tumours can be localised intraoperatively and biopsied under ultrasonography. Ultrasonography can also be used to examine the spinal cord, but only intraoperatively or after a laminectomy: haemorrhage, other space-occupying processes and remnants of disc material can be localised. Doppler examination of intracranial and spinal vessels can provide information about their morphology and the vitality of the tissues, e.g. after trauma, suspicion of infarct or thrombus and the determination of high ICP (4, 5, 6).

Ultrasonography also plays an important role in the clarification of neurological disturbances due to systemic disease; for example, screening of the abdomen if there is suspicion of neoplasia or the investigation of the liver and the portal vein system when there is suspicion of a portosystemic shunt (PSS) (Fig. 6.3). Dependent on the experience of the investigator, the sensitivity of ultrasonographic determination of PSS is 90% (7).

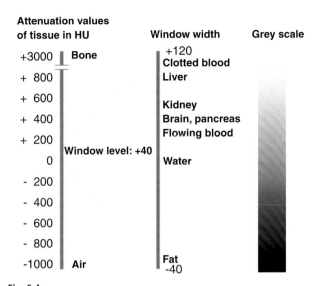

Fig. 6.4
Window technique. In CT, the attenuation values of the tissue are given in HOUNSFIELD UNITS (HU) on a scale from −1000 (air; black) to +3000 (cortical bones; white) and are classed according to their different shades of grey. The contrast can be improved when only a particular section of the grey scale (window width) is depicted with a suitable window level. In this example, all tissues with an absorption value lower than fat are shown as black, while all tissues with an absorption greater than clotted blood are white.

6.2.4 Computed tomography and magnetic resonance imaging

6.2.4.1 Computed tomography (CT)

CT works like radiography with ionising radiation (8). The x-ray beam weakened by its passage through the "object" is registered by a detector system that is either static or rotates in unison with the x-ray head. After the subsequent digitalisation of the data and picture reconstruction, a grey matrix is formed in the computer. In the CT machines used in clinics nowadays, the data for the determination of the attenuation values are logarithmised before reconstruction and ultimately put together as a two-dimensional image. For a better comparison, the reconstructed attenuation values are referenced with those of water. The relative attenuation values of the tissues are given in Hounsfield units (HU); water has the value 0, bone 400–3000 (white), air −1000 (black) (Fig. 6.4). The grey contrast can be improved by choosing a window width set to a suitable HU range depending on the tissues being studied (e.g. soft tissues or bone) (Figs. 6.4 and 6.5). CT is distinguished by its high contrast resolution of bone and soft tissues.

Certain disadvantages such as relatively long investigation times are no longer a problem with modern spiral or multislice CT machines. In the spiral CT, in comparison to standard CT, the x-ray head turns continually with the detector around the patient, while the patient is continuously pushed through the machine. The advantages are obvious: multiple slices per tube rotation are imaged, so that a greater volume can be investigated in a given time (9).

The combination of direct cross-sectional pictures, 2-D reformation in other levels and 3-D reconstructions provides precise information about the localisation and size of specific structures and their relationship to neighbouring anatomical features. With spiral CT machines, these reconstructions show a quality that is barely inferior to the original acquired tomography images. This information is a prerequisite for targeted and successful operations such as biopsy, excision or even radiation therapy of a tumour (Fig. 6.6). In the latter, the exposure plan is frequently developed from CT-based calculations. Even surgical operations can be exactly undertaken based on CT images and can even be done under computed tomographic guidance.

CT can be used to measure the volume of normal soft tissue structures (e.g. ventricle), in the diagnosis of intracranial masses, infarcts, haemorrhage and acquired hydrocephalus. In comparison to other methods, CT has the greatest utility and sensitivity in imaging the skull and vertebral skeleton. These anatomically complex structures can be depicted without any superimposition. CT's high contrast resolution allows the differentiation of fat from neural and other soft tissues. Vertebral, foraminal and lumbosacral stenosis due to disc material, fibrosis, bony exostoses or tumours can also be visualised. In the diagnosis of compressive spinal cord disease, the significance of CT can be improved by combining it with myelography, although this may not always be necessary (see Fig. 14.5).

CT investigations are undertaken with or without the administration of intravenous contrast media (10). Areas with increased or reduced perfusion as well as processes which lead to a pathological change in the blood-brain barrier can be determined and differentiated. Neoplasms, granulomas, abscesses and haematomas are often different in their depiction and can frequently be differentiated, although definitive diagnosis is not possible without pathology. As intra-axial processes can be differentiated from extra-axial processes, it is not uncommon that the type of tumour can at least be suggested.

The weakness of CT lies in its inadequate depiction of diffuse processes that cause neither a mass effect, a change in tissue density, or a change in the blood-brain barrier. In addition, the visualisation of soft tissues in approximation to very dense bone is difficult due to the physical qualities of x-rays. Due to the absorption of x-rays in the area of the caudal cranial fossa and the base of the skull, artefacts associated with cerebellar and brain stem imaging are to be expected. The high radiation dose in CT in comparison to radiology plays only a small role in veterinary medicine, and this is more than compensated for by the diagnostic information achieved using this method.

6

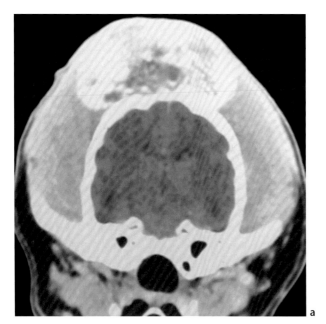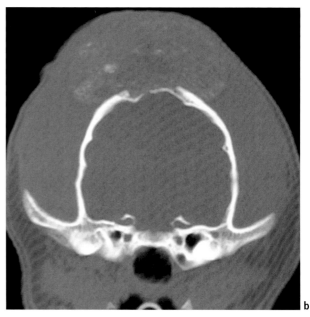

Fig. 6.5a, b
CT images of a skull with a multilobular osteochondrosarcoma. (a) The brain and ventricles are shown in the soft tissue window. The bones of the skull and the tumour appear mainly white. The bone structure is not shown. Fat and air are black on the chosen grey scale. (b) The destruction of the skull bones is recognisable on the bone window. The sarcoma exhibits the ice-flow-like mineralisation typical of this type of tumour. The brain tissue and the fluid space cannot be differentiated. Fat, in comparison, appears dark grey, air black. See also Fig. 6.6.

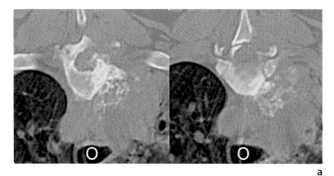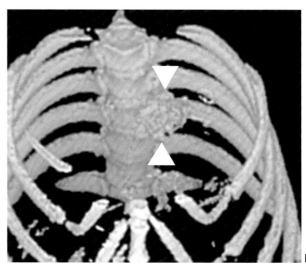

Fig. 6.6a, b
Transverse section through (a) T12 and (b) a three-dimensional reconstruction of the caudal chest cavity in a dog with a chondrosarcoma. The transverse sections (bone window) show an aggressive lesion of the bone with osteolysis and bone proliferation, including considerable intrathoracic soft tissue components ventrally. The oesophagus (O) depicted just below the aorta contains air. The three-dimensional picture shows the spatial relationships between the tumour (arrowheads), T12 and the ribs from a cranioventral direction. The last vertebra which is shown is L1, recognisable due to its lateral processes. (Pictures: Barbara Kaser-Holz, Zurich).

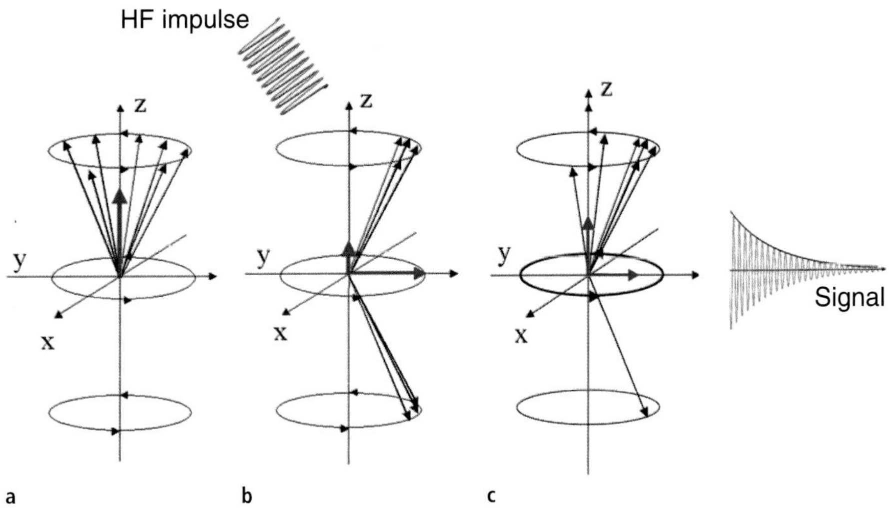

HF impulse

Signal

Fig. 6.7a, b
Basics of MRI. Signal production. (a) Free protons organise themselves parallel and anti-parallel in a strong magnetic field and spin (precision) with a particular frequency (Larmor frequency) around their pole. (b) Energy is transferred to the nuclei (resonance) by the application of a pulse of high frequency (HF) energy that has the same frequency as they do. As a result, their nuclear spin is transferred to a higher energy level and at the same time brought into phase. (c) Once the HF pulse has ceased, the nuclei return to their original situation in the magnetic field (longitudinal relaxation, T1 effect) and are dephased (transverse relaxation, T2 effect). A signal is released during both of these processes, which can be used to produce an image. The blue arrows represent the direction and relative strength of the magnetisation.

a   b   c

6

6.2.4.2 Magnetic resonance imaging (MRI)

Both PURCELL and BLOCH described nuclear magnetic resonance (NMR) independently of each other in 1946. In 1973, LAUTERBUR (11) made the first pictures based on this technique. As NMR does not use ionising radiation, it is an ideal non-invasive imaging method that provides much global and regional information about the morphology and pathology of organs. In this method, certain physical characteristics (nuclear magnetism) of electrically charged nuclear particles are used to form images. As the magnetic dipole moment of a nuclear particle can only work externally and be registered when an odd number of nuclear particles are present in the nucleus, only nuclei with an uneven number of nuclear particles can be used to form the image. The most common atom, and the one most commonly used in MRI, is hydrogen. According to quantum theory, hydrogen nuclei act like rotating gyroscopes which have a dipole moment about their rotational axis, the so-called nuclear spin. This causes the generation of a magnetic field. The rotational axis of the nuclear spin has a random and disorganised orientation at rest. When the nuclear spin is placed in a strong magnetic field (up to 30 000 times the earth's magnetic field), then the rotational axes of the nuclear spin are polarised – they align themselves parallel or anti-parallel along the field lines of the static magnetic field (Fig. 6.7). In magnetic resonance, the polarised nuclear spin is given a short high frequency pulse of energy. The previously polarised nuclear spin is excited by this pulse of energy and is knocked out of its original position and precesses with a frequency proportional to the static magnetic field. The nuclear magnetism of the rotating nuclei causes a magnetisation perpendicular to the direction of the main polarisation. This perpendicular magnetisation can induce a voltage in a receiver antenna, which can then be amplified, measured and analysed according to its frequencies. One talks about magnetic resonance because the energy transmission to the nuclear spin can only take place when the high frequency pulse has the same frequency as the nucleus. This resonance frequency is called the Larmor frequency. Different atoms have different Larmor frequencies, which are influenced by the field strength of the static magnetic field.

At the end of the high frequency pulse, the protons try to attain their original situation. One talks of relaxation, whereby basically two phenomena are differentiated: the T1 and the T2 relaxations. In the T1 relaxation, the protons straighten themselves out of their oblique position and line themselves up along the magnetic lines of the static magnetic field. T1 is therefore also called longitudinal relaxation. The length of T1 relaxation is called the T1 relaxation time. The length of time depends on the magnetic flux, the temperature and the quality of the relaxing substance: for fluids it lies in the range of seconds, and for soft tissues it is in tenths of seconds.

The nuclear spin is not only knocked over by the high frequency pulse but it is also brought into phase. A rapid dephasation takes place afterwards, the T2 relaxation. As the dephasing of the nuclear spin occurs transverse to the magnetic field, this process is called transverse relaxation. It is finished when the spins of the individual nuclei completely neutralise each other. The T2 relaxation time, like the T1 relaxation time, has a great influence on the signal intensity and image contrast. In T2-weighted (T2w) images, tissues with short T2 relaxation times such as brain tissue have comparatively low signal intensity. CSF, in comparison, has a long T2 relaxation time and so in T2w images, it has a high signal intensity (12, 13, 14).

6

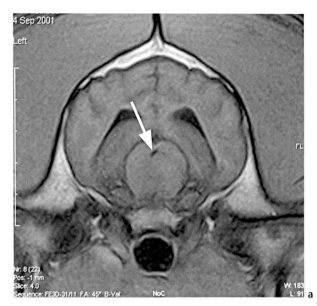 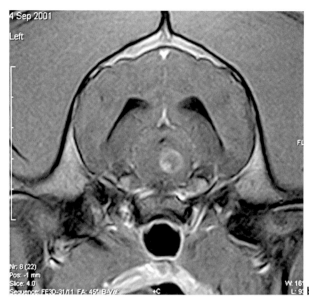

Fig. 6.8a, b
MRI investigation of a skull before and after contrast agent. (a) In the T1w pre-contrast study, only a discrete dorsal and right displacement of the fourth ventricle can be seen (white arrow). The actual lesion is isointense with the surrounding tissue. (b) After the administration of a contrast agent, the tumour (in this case a glioma) exhibits a strong ring-shaped area of contrast enhancement.

As described above, MRI provides excellent soft tissue contrast due to the different numbers of free protons and their diverse chemical interactions present in the various tissues. Direct sagittal, transverse (axial) or dorsal sequences make image reconstruction, as is necessary in CT, usually superfluous. In the nervous system, this method allows the direct and anatomically exact reproduction of grey and white matter, the ventricular system with its CSF, the spinal cord, the spinal nerves, the vertebral discs and the surrounding fat. Only the resolution of bony structures is poor with MRI (14).

Similar to CT, the significance of a MRI investigation can be improved with the injection of a contrast agent. Paramagnetic substances are used, such as intravenously applicable gadolinium diethylenetriaminepenta-acetic acid (gd-DTPA), which was first used clinically in 1984. Paramagnetic means that the hydrogen protons close to the gadolinium have been exposed to a strong magnetic field so that the energy exchange during magnetic resonance is speeded up and the T1 relaxation time of the hydrogen protons is shortened. This leads to an increase in signal intensity and increased contrast in comparison to tissues without contrast medium enhancement. Using contrast during the MRI examination of cranial lesions, it is possible to show the lack of a blood-brain barrier or the presence of blood-brain barrier disturbance due to a shortening of the T1 relaxation time. A normal blood-brain barrier prevents the loss of contrast into the extracellular space and contrast enhancement in healthy brain tissue does not occur, apart from certain areas without a barrier such as the pituitary and the choroid plexus. The contrast between diseased and healthy tissue is increased due to the uptake of contrast agent in diseased tissues (Fig. 6.8). In other tissues there is nothing comparable to the blood brain barrier, so contrast administration can lead to an increased signal intensity in many different areas of the body as well as in pathological changes (e.g. inflammation). Additional information about blood perfusion, vascularisation and vessel permeability can be acquired using modern measurement methods after the injection of a bolus of contrast agent (MR angiography) (15, 16).

6.2.4.3　Comparison of the examination methods
The physical differences between CT and MRI are shown in Table 6.1. Both methods must be undertaken with the patient under general anaestheisa. The animals can be positioned stably in either sternal or dorsal recumbency with their heads in the horizontal plane; whereby sternal recumbency is obviously preferred. During CT of the head, the forelegs should not be placed beside the head. If metal implants are present, then it must be ensured before doing MRI that these implants are not magnetic. Nevertheless, all implants (including transponders for identification and instruments such as the pulse oximeter) lying within the examination field will cause artefacts. Very radiopaque implants or foreign bodies will also lead to artefacts on CT images.

Table 6.1: Physical differences between computed tomography and magnetic resonance imaging

CT	MRI
■ Scanning imaging modality using ionising radiation.	■ Scanning imaging modality without ionising radiation.
■ Based on attenuation of x-rays, dependent on the number of protons and physical thickness of the tissue.	■ Signal depends on the proton concentration and chemical composition of the tissue.
■ Normally scanning is only possible from one angle.	■ Direct imaging from every angle is possible.
■ High contrast, method of choice for the imaging of bones. Very sensitive in detecting haemorrhages.	■ Excellent contrast. Method of choice for imaging neural structures such as brain, spinal cord and nerve roots. In addition, provides information about CSF and blood flow, tissue perfusion, tissue diffusion and chemical composition. Little information provided about compact bones.
■ Artefacts due to concentration of the x-ray beam close to very compact bones (e. g. caudal cranial fossa in the dog).	■ Artefacts due to pulsation in brain, fluid spaces and large blood vessels.

6

Transverse slices have proven to be most useful as the primary CT or MRI slice selection for the skull. Repositioning the animal or changing its head position enables other planes to be investigated with CT (e.g. dorsal slices). Only transverse slices can be made of the vertebral column with CT; the sagittal view is the primary projection with MRI, followed by transverse, dorsal or any other necessary views. The recordable parameters for CT are restricted to the choice of region to be investigated, the thickness of the slice, the movement of the table and to a small degree, the slope of the gantry. MRI protocols are much more complex; the basic examination consists of the T1w (read as T1-weighted) and T2w sequences. In addition, the Pw (proton-density-weighted) or FLAIR (Fluid Attenuated Inversion Recovery) sequences are used for the suppression of the signal from free fluid.

As mentioned above, contrast examinations are an important part of both techniques. Iodised contrast agents are used in CT (see Chap. 6.3.2) at a dosage of 600 mg iodine/kg bwt intravenously. In MRI, paramagnetic substances such as gd-DPTA are used at a dosage of 0.1 mmol/kg bwt (15). Dynamic investigations can be used in the examination of the pituitary for example, but they are also useful in the differentiation of pathological processes if there is a suspicion of neoplasia (2, 17). The significance of CT investigations on the spinal cord can be improved using myelography (for technique see Chap. 6.3.2). A myelographic effect can be achieved in MRI by using very strong T2w sequences instead of a contrast medium.

6.2.4.4 Principles of interpretation

The high spatial resolution and good contrast present with tomographic techniques has allowed the direct visualisation of the brain and of the spinal cord, both enclosed within an osseous casing. Over and above the imaging of normal macroscopic anatomy and pathology, blood and CSF flow in addition to tissue perfusion studies can also be undertaken, especially with MRI. Normal and pathological tissue diffusion and chemistry can be depicted by using suitable equipment and appropriate sequences.

These imaging potentials, whose development has far from been concluded, present new demands on radiologists. Their anatomical, pathophysiological and neuropathological knowledge must be sufficient to classify the morphological structures as being either normal or pathological, and to understand their significance in a clinical setting. In particular, slice-based anatomy must be relearned. Text-books such as the MRI and CT atlas from ASHEUER and SAGER (18) are helpful. The difficulty lies in the fact that anatomical structures in all of the three standard slice directions (sagittal, transverse and dorsal) are only depicted two-dimensionally and in different forms and sizes; the investigator must be able to reconstruct these three-dimensionally in his or her head. The dimensions of a structure play an important role in the choice of projection utilised: it is usual that the projection in which the structure has its greatest dimension is most helpful.

In MRI, signal intensity interpretation is also a challenge for the radiologist; e.g., the signal intensity of nervous tissue changes postnatally due to myelination and so an in-depth understanding of "normal" is essential. In T1w images, tissues with short T1 relaxation times such as fat (also structures which concentrate contrast agents) have a high signal intensity. Substances with a long T1 such as CSF have by comparison a low signal intensity. As the medullary (white matter) layer in the brain has a shorter T1 than the cortex, the medullary layer is depicted more intensely in T1w images. This effect is dependent on the sequence evaluated: inversion recovery (IR) sequences increase this effect, so that the contrast between the grey matter and the CSF is reduced. Pathological changes in tissues usually cause a prolongation of the T1 relaxation time and so are more hypointense than normal tissues on T1w sequences.

6

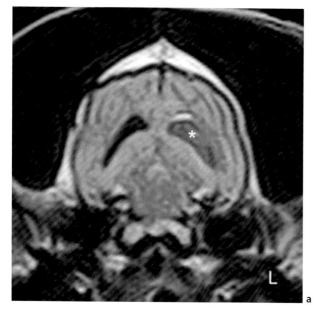 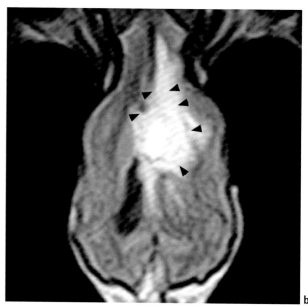

Fig. 6.9a, b
FLAIR sequence to suppress normal CSF. This is a transverse (a) and dorsal (b) T2w sequence in which the normal CSF signal is suppressed by an inversion impulse (time dependent on the strength of the magnetic field). The constituents of the CSF in the left ventricle are changed (especially the protein content) in this dog affected by abscessation and pyocephalus (*). The signal of the changed CSF is therefore not suppressed (signal intensification) and can so be differentiated from the normal contents of the right lateral ventricle. The dorsal image (b) demonstrates perilesional oedema (arrowheads). (Figure from Seiler et al. 2001 [201] with kind permission of Blackwell Publishing).

As mentioned above, brain tissue has a comparatively lower signal intensity than CSF on T2w images due to the longer T2 relaxation time of CSF. The contrast of the white to grey matter is the reverse of that in T1w sequences: the grey matter is more hyperintense than the white on T2w images. In addition on T2w sequences, the basal cranial arteries can be visualised owing to the high degree of contrast between the hyperintense fluid spaces and the reduction to absence of signal associated with blood flow in the vessels. Pathological changes in tissues, as a rule, lead to a prolongation of the T2 relaxation times and are therefore more hyperintense on T2w images than normal tissues.

In summary, T1w sequences are excellent for depicting the anatomy of brain tissues due to the good contrast between white and grey matter, whereas T2w sequences are good at depicting iron-containing structures such as the basal ganglia and nuclei in the brain stem and cerebellum, as well as fluid containing structures, such as the ventricles. Special sequences and images using contrast agents can selectively increase the contrast between different tissues (Fig. 6.9). Details of the interpretation of these images are described under the respective diseases discussed below.

Due to their different characteristics, described previously in the sections on CT and MRI, MRI is superior to CT in the diagnosis of many diseases of the brain (e.g. tumours, in-farcts). MRI also has advantages in the imaging of the spinal cord, nerve roots, cauda equina and the spinal nerves as the contrast between the CSF, spinal cord, nerves and fat can be selectively increased. Due to the sensitivity of MRI in the diagnosis of spinal cord lesions, it has largely superseded the use of myelography in human medicine.

6.2.5 Methods used in nuclear medicine

The examination methods used in nuclear medicine in human beings, such as scintigraphy; ECT (emission computed tomography), in which the gamma camera is replaced by a rotating detector system; SPECT (single photon emission computed tomography) which demonstrates CNS perfusion; or PET (positron emission computed tomography) which aids in the visualisation and quantification of CNS metabolic processes and microcirculation, have only a very limited current significance in small animal neurology. In the context of this book, only bone scintigraphy for the detection of bone metastases or the causes of spinal pain or lameness (Fig. 6.10) and scintigraphy of the thyroid have specific importance. PET is used in veterinary medicine, primarily as a research tool, for investigations of clinical tumours (10, 19).

6.3 Spine

6.3.1 Radiography

The region of spine with the supposed lesion must always be visualised using (at least) two views: lateral and ventrodorsal (VD). A lateral view alone can just be used for a rough initial overview. To prevent geometric artefacts and overlapping, especially at the intervertebral spaces, it must be ensured that the cassette or the field covered by the x-ray beam is no larger than 30 cm, even in large dogs. The different sections of the spine are then radiographed separately. This means that in large dogs, a separate radiograph is taken for the upper and lower neck, the chest and the lumbar region as well as the transitional regions between the thoracic and lumbar vertebrae, and the lumbar vertebrae and the sacrum.

The two standard views are often not enough for a detailed depiction of the vertebral column. The intervertebral foraminae are radiographed using additional VD views with the x-ray head rotated 30° to the animal's longitudinal axis. The exact degree of rotation depends on the species, breed and the section of spine. The odontoid process (dens) of the axis is best shown by a lateral view with the head slightly rotated around its longitudinal axis (Fig. 6.11). Frontal views through an open mouth (dog, cat) should be done extremely carefully due to the over-flexion of the neck. Stress views of the neck with flexion to prove the existence of instability is an infrequent method due to the danger of damaging the cervical spinal cord. In comparison, caudal cervical and lumbosacral spondylopathies with suspicion of concurrent instability often require radiographs taken in ventral or dorsal flexion (extension), which in combination with myelography provide important diagnostic and prognostic information (Fig. 6.27). Views obtained under traction help to differentiate disc protrusion from disc extrusion in the neck, which has therapeutic consequences. Caution is necessary when using "stress" radiographs: in the presence of instability of the cervical vertebrae, the use of force can increase compression on the underlying spinal cord, thereby exacerbating the neurological clinical signs even to the extent of causing tetraplegia.

A precise positioning of the spine to prevent projection and overlapping artefacts is necessary for radiography of the vertebral column. Due to the large differences in diameter between the individual regions of the body, the head, neck and lumbar regions must be supported with cushions, as should the limbs be, to prevent rotation artefacts.

The positioning of animals on their back is easiest with foam rubber cushions in various sizes. The nasal bone is supported in dorsal recumbency to prevent overlapping of the occipital bone with the atlas and axis. For an artefact-free image of the intervertebral spaces of the caudal spine, the x-ray head must be tilted 10° cranially. A lordosis of the thoracic and lumbar spine due to positioning is prevented by not extending the hindlimbs backwards. The intervertebral space at the transi-

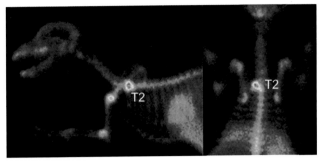

Fig. 6.10
Bone scintigraphy of head, neck, thorax and forelimbs in a five-year-old West Highland White Terrier with a slight monoparesis in the right forelimb and a severe pain syndrome. Radiography and myelography of the vertebral column were negative. Bone scintigraphy with Tc99m-HDP showed a highly active zone on the right in the second thoracic vertebra (T2) compatible with a primary bone tumour or a bone metastasis. The histopathology showed an osteosarcoma.

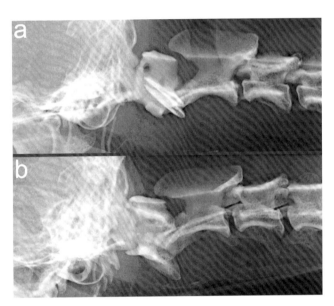

Fig. 6.11a, b
Projection of the dens axis. (a) On the lateral view, the wings of the atlas and the dens axis overlap. (b) By rotating the head, the dens can be imaged without any overlapping.

tion between the thoracic and lumbar spine can be radiographed in an orthograde manner by slightly turning the x-ray head cranially.

A detailed view of the spine and its structures without any overlapping requires the use of CT or MRI. It is possible to visualise the spinal skeleton in transverse slices on a CT. The contrast of the skeletal structures (bone window) or the soft

6

tissues (soft tissue window) can be optimised by using the correct window width and level. A longitudinal depiction requires computer-generated reconstruction in the sagittal or dorsal plane. The new generation of CT machines (spiral or multislice) enable a reconstruction to be made with the same quality as the original slices. Other reconstruction projections and three-dimensional reconstruction are important aids in the understanding of normal and pathological anatomy in CT. While CT is the most important instrument for depicting the spine and its pathology, MRI is the method of choice for depicting neural structures, especially the nerve roots and cauda equina (20, 21).

6.3.1.1   Principles of interpreting spinal images
An important prerequisite for the interpretation of spinal images is knowledge of the anatomy and anatomical variation, as well as of the peculiarities of particular regions or projections. In addition, a systematic assessment of the image is necessary (20, 22).

The following anatomical features in the dog and cat should be taken into consideration:
- The transverse processes of the vertebrae are very large.
- There are lucencies in the area of the vertebral body and vertebral canal due to overlapping of the base of each of the transverse processes. These are most obvious at C5 and C6, and when associated with a number of blood vessel foraminae (transverse foramina).
- In the region of the mid-thoracic vertebrae and about L6, there is a reasonably obvious overlapping of the intervertebral foraminae with the accessory processes (dependent on image and projection).
- T11 is classed as the anticlinal vertebra as the direction of its spinous process changes from caudal to cranial.
- The intervertebral space between T10–T11 is normally narrower than the neighbouring ones.
- Due to the overlapping of the ilium between L7 and S1, the intervertebral space appears to be overshadowed; it is wide and usually slightly wedge-shaped.
- The lumbosacral angle is very variable, dependent on flexion or extension.
- The ventral contours of L3 and L4 are vague due to the insertion of the lateral crura of the diaphragm.
- In VD views, without correction of the projection angle, the vertebral spaces of the caudal cervical spine, the cranial thoracic spine and the transitional area between the thoracic and lumbar spine are all depicted more narrowly than they really are.

A systematic examination is essential if important changes are not to be overlooked. The individual elements are judged, for example, from cranial to caudal, from ventral to dorsal (lateral view) and with respect to symmetry (VD view). The examination protocol should contain an assessment of the soft tissues; number of vertebrae; form and contours of the spine; form, size and contours of the individual vertebrae; bone density; width and form of the intervertebral spaces and foramina; the vertebral canal; and the articular and other vertebral processes.

6.3.1.2   Soft tissues
The soft tissues can provide important indications about disease processes affecting the spine. In addition, changes outside of the axial skeleton are often concomitant to spinal disease, especially in traumatic injuries or even neoplastic or infectious processes. Between 40% and 60% of dogs and cats with spinal injury show changes in their soft tissues and as such, attention should be paid to structures within the thorax and abdomen. Soft tissue tumours such as **malignant lymphoma** or **tumours of the nerve roots** may be associated with extraskeletal metastases (23).

Tumours can communicate with the vertebral canal via the intervertebral foramina or infiltrate the bone (Figs. 6.6. and 6.30). In the former, expansion of individual foramina may be seen, while in the latter osteolysis may be present. Lymphadenomegaly of the iliohypogastric nodes can be an indicator of metastatic disease in association with prostatic, urinary bladder or other tumours, or even infections of the hypogastric and perineal regions. Tumours are often associated with irregular vertebral contours that are indicative of infiltrative processes. Other concomitant clinical signs are dystrophic mineralisation or osteoneogenesis with tumours, or gas inclusions (emphysema) with injury or abscessation. Calcinosis circumscripta is a tumour-like process in the soft tissues with amorphous mineralisation that occurs over bony processes, especially in the neck. Similar radiological and histological changes have been described rarely as occurring between the vertebral arches of the atlas and axis. They can cause extradural compression of the cervical spinal cord (24, 25).

6.3.1.3   Shape and course of the vertebral column
The normal spine has a curved form. The gentle dorsal curvature of the cranial cervical spine is replaced by a marked but physiological lordosis in the area between the cervical and thoracic vertebrae. The thoracic and lumbar segments of the spine are more or less straight, or slightly curved. The lumbosacral area again exhibits a normal mild lordosis. There is usually no step down or up between one vertebra to the next. Abnormal curvature (Table 6.2) such as **kyphosis** (dorsal), **lordosis** (ventral) or **scoliosis** (lateral) can be seen for example in congenital abnormalities and are often associated with **wedge-shaped or fused vertebrae** (Fig. 6.12). Depending on the type of wedge-shaped vertebra, either a marked kyphosis or scoliosis occurs.

Fractures, luxations and subluxations can affect every part of the spine. Predelicted sites in small animals are the transitions between head / neck, neck / chest, and in the thoracolumbar and lumbosacral spine. The body and the lateral and spinous processes of the vertebrae, are affected most commonly (26). Marked deviations from the spinal axis are found particularly with fractures of the lumbar spine and less so with fractures of the thoracic vertebrae (see Figs. 10.25–10.28). The exact imaging of fractures with conventional methods is often difficult and requires views from different angles. If there is suspicion of a fracture, the radiographs should be taken without anaesthesia or sedation to prevent further destabilisation or the occurrence of unwanted vascular (local hypotensive) effects. Examination under anaesthesia is indicated when the neurological condition of the patient or the radiological results suggest that a surgical operation is subsequently necessary. Deviation of the fracture from the vertebral axis at the time of examination is often slight and does not necessarily reflect what happened during the application of force at the time of injury (27). As a consequence, a radiograph which looks relatively normal on first impression cannot be used to assume that the spine is stable. Fractures and luxations are often accompanied by traumatic disc herniations and hemorrhage. Narrow vertebral spaces should be looked at closely. Muscle contraction and paresis (nerve root syndrome) as well as pain around the spine or abdominal pain are other causes of abnormal posture and shape of the spine.

Atlantoaxial subluxation can be induced by **agenesis** and **hypoplasia**, lack of fusion or fracture of the odontoid process (dens) of the axis, or rupture of the ligaments between the occiput, C1 and C2 (28). In the healthy animal, the large spinous process of C2 towers above the dorsal arch of C1 or lies immediately caudodorsal to it. The straight odontoid process lies ventrally in the midline and can be depicted by slightly rotating it around its longitudinal axis. For further information see the chapters on specific spinal lesions. **Occipito-atlantoaxial malformations** are very rare in small animals (cat). CT and especially MRI are sensitive methods of examining the ligamentous structures associated with the osseous anatomy (29, 30).

Cervical spondylomyelopathy (malformation malarticulation or Wobbler syndrome) leads to deviation from the longitudinal axis and subluxations of individual vertebrae causing a disturbance in the continuity and contours of the vertebral canal (see. 13.4). In its most renowned form (Great Dane, Doberman), usually more than one of the caudal cervical vertebrae between C4 and C7 are almost always affected (31). There is also an inheritable form of cervical instability between C3 and C4 to be found in Bassets and Bulldogs. The following changes can be found either individually or in combination in cervical spondylomyelopathy: malformed vertebrae with rhomboid or triangular shapes, dorsal subluxation of the often slanted endplates of the vertebrae, mineralised intervertebral discs and narrowed intervertebral spaces due to disc prolapse. In the lateral view, the vertebral canal above the

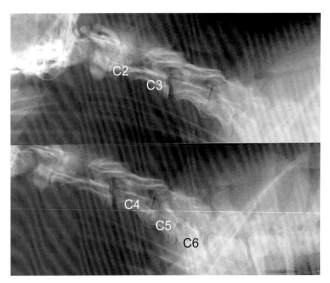

Fig. 6.12
Multiple malformations of the cervical spine in a five-month-old Flat-coated Retriever. The atlas is shortened and deformed. C2 and C3 have formed a fused vertebra. C4–C6 are partially fused and asymmetric forming wedge-shaped vertebrae, leading to a scoliosis of the neck.

Table 6.2: Causes of abnormal forms of the spine: kyphosis, lordosis, scoliosis, vertebral displacement

■ Anomalies such as hemivertebra, lumbosacral transitional vertebra
■ Atlantoaxial subluxation: congenital or acquired
■ Cervical and lumbosacral malarticulation / malformation
■ Luxation / subluxation
■ Fractures and abnormal fracture healing
■ Postural
■ Syringohydromyelia

affected vertebrae is narrowed in a caudiocranial direction. This is caused by the malformed pedicle of the vertebral arch which leads to a flattening and narrowing of the cranial part of the vertebral canal. Often the facet joints are malformed too, or they may be deformed due to osteoarthritic changes. Degenerative spondylitic exostoses are frequent accompaniments. The dorsal luxation can be static or dynamic (32). Dynamic changes are accentuated by flexion of the affected part of the neck. The dynamically increased compression of the spinal cord can be visually appreciated using myelography with a respective dynamic examination (flexion, extension, traction) of the affected part of the neck.

Compression of the cauda equina in the dog can be due to a number of causes: congenital, developmental, inflammatory, traumatic, neoplastic or degenerative.

6

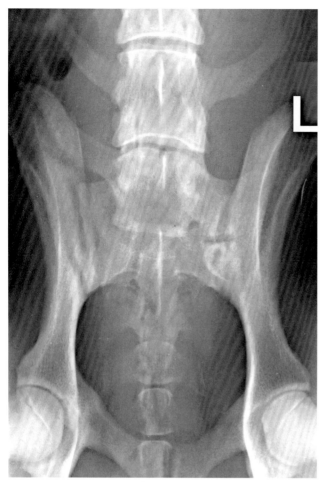

Fig. 6.13
Lumbosacral transitional vertebra. The left transverse process of L7 is articulated with the ilium (sacralisation). The right transverse process has developed as a normal lateral process. Lop-sided and asymmetrical intervertebral spaces lie between L6–L7 and L7–sacrum.

The most common and clinically most important disease of the lumbosacral area is degenerative lumbosacral stenosis (DLSS), often seen in large breeds of dogs (33, 34, 35, 36, 37, 38, 39). In the literature, lumbosacral instability is a purported cause, similar to the aforementioned cervical spondylomyelopathy. This is characterised by a dynamic ventral subluxation with the formation of a "step" between L7 and the sacrum. The ventral displacement induces a translational movement, which is largest during severe extension and flexion. It is unclear whether this is the cause or the effect of an earlier herniated disc as is seen most commonly in German Shepherds. In contrast, **spondylolisthesis** is the most frequent form of instability in human beings. Here L5 slides forwards slowly over the sacrum (or L4 over L5). This is mainly caused by a defect in the region of the articular processes (isthmus effect). Due to their posture, such a ventral displacement of L7 can only occur in the dog after facetectomy or trauma with fracture of the lumbosacral articular processes.

A lumbosacral transitional vertebra is considered as being a predisposing factor for DLSS (40). Spondylosis, a narrowed or collapsed intervertebral space (with obvious vacuum phenomenon under extension; Fig. 6.19), dynamically increased ventral subluxation of the sacrum, deformation and/or sclerosis of the sacral endplate or a free fragment in osteochondrosis are all considered to be pathologies associated with lumbosacral spondylopathy. For further information, see the chapter on degenerative lumbosacral stenosis.

6.3.1.4 Number of vertebrae

Variations in the number of vertebrae (C7, T13, L7, S3, Cd20) are frequent, especially in the number of tail vertebrae. Variations can occur due to additional vertebrae (e.g. 8 lumbar vertebrae) or a reduced number. Such variation is usually of no clinical importance in either the dog or cat, and it is known to occur in a number of other species, too. A false impression is given when there is agenesis or hypoplasia of the ribs of T13, or when there are additional ribs attached to L1. **Transitional vertebrae** in the lumbosacral region are very common in the dog (Fig. 6.13). There can either be a symmetrical or asymmetrical (one-sided) fusion of L7 with the sacrum (sacralisation) or a freeing of S1 from the sacrum (lumbarisation). Asymmetrical transitional vertebrae can cause a deviation from the longitudinal axis or a rotational displacement of the pelvis. In addition, lumbosacral transitional vertebrae appear to be a risk factor in the development of DLSS (40, 41, 42). Lumbosacral transitional vertebrae are most commonly found in the German Shepherd, Rhodesian Ridgeback, Doberman, Labrador Retriever and St. Bernard. Belgian Sheepdogs appear also to be frequently affected. Deviation from the normal number of vertebrae should, therefore, be taken note of when a surgical operation is being planned.

Agenesis and dysgenesis of the tail vertebrae and the sacrum is found in dogs and cats (Manx cat, English Bulldog, Brittany Spaniel, Bobtail, Entlebuch Cattle Dog). **Sacrococcygeal dysgenesis** can be associated with other malformations such as spina bifida, meningocele, meningomyelocele or syringomyelia (43). The lack of tail vertebrae can also be an indication of trauma, amputation for medical reasons, or cosmetic tail amputation (forbidden in some countries).

6.3.1.5 Size, shape and contours of individual vertebrae

Congenital abnormalities

Changes in the shape and size as well as abnormal contours can be found in congenital malformations such as **wedge-shaped, butterfly** or **fused vertebrae** (Fig. 6.12). Fused vertebrae occur when there is an incomplete or lack of segmentation of the vertebrae with loss of discovertebral contact, or even as a consequence of discospondylitis.

Depending on the cause, wedge-shaped vertebrae may be missing either their dorsal or ventral part. If the malformation is not compensated for by a neighbouring vertebrae, a kyphosis or lordosis may develop; or if the defect is asymmetrical to the right or left, it can lead to a scoliosis. A one-sided development in the form of a triangular vertebra occurs with a metameric segment displacement, which is pushed between two vertebrae as a **transitional vertebra** (44). With a butterfly vertebra, there is a sagittal split due to a lack of fusion of the two halves of the vertebra. A complete cleavage of the spine and the spinal cord (rhachischisis and myeloschisis, respectively) is not compatible with life. Milder forms of spina bifida in which only the vertebral arches and spinous processes are not fused (seen as double spinous processes on a radiograph) can occur either isolated and clinically insignificant, or in combination with a meningocele or meningomyelocele (see Fig. 14.9). These are more commonly found in brachycephalic breeds, the Entlebuch Cattle Dog and Manx cats.

Fusion of the spinous processes, lateral processes or of the ribs with the transverse processes can also induce obvious changes in shape like those seen with transitional vertebrae.

Primordial dwarfism, for example, due to somatotropin deficiency leads as a rule to proportionate dwarfism. Chondrodystrophies, such as hypochondrodystrophy, lead to disproportionate dwarfism with foreshortened limbs (micromelia, rhizomelia) and, depending on the type, to deformation of the skull and shortened vertebrae. Congenital metabolic disturbances such as the different kinds of mucopolysaccharidosis or congenital hypothyroidism often lead to severe changes in the shape and contour of the vertebrae. Congenital **hypothyroidism** is associated with dwarfism, and delayed or lack of skeletal maturation with irregularly wide epiphyses and bone endplates, asymmetrical intervertebral spaces, exostoses on the vertebral bodies and delayed fusion of the epiphyses to the vertebral column and the limbs. The deformations found on the limb bones are overlaid by later degenerative changes (45). Compression of the spinal cord is rare.

Different types of **mucopolysaccharidosis** (lysosomal storage disease) are known to occur in the dog and cat. The degree of skeletal changes depends on the type and can be very variable. The typical characteristics are short, pressed in nose and a domed, prominent skull cap; on the VD view, a markedly widened cervical spine with vertebrae of different sizes and shapes can be seen; the vertebrae may also be partly fused. There is often stenosis of the vertebral canal. In the region of the chest and abdominal spine, irregularly sized vertebrae, exostoses, intervertebral spaces with irregular widths and forms are conspicuous. Dysplasia of the hip joints and often severe deformation of the limb joints complete the picture (46).

In cervical spondylopathies in large breeds of dogs, rhomboid or even triangular vertebrae have been often observed. Compression fractures, spontaneous fractures due to disturbances in metabolism or tumours can lead to a shortening of a vertebral body. Changes in shape are regularly found with spondylosis, bone tumours, callus formation and discospondylitis.

Acquired abnormalities

Fractures, tumours, infections, hypervitaminosis A, degenerative changes and previous surgical operations can all lead to reasonably obvious changes in the shape and contours of the vertebrae.

Radiologically obvious changes, such as displaced fracture fragments and wide fracture lines, are often present with **fractures**, though discrete radiographic signs like changes in the shape or form of a vertebra and breaks in the contour of a vertebra, the vertebral canal or of vertebral processes may also be present. The formation of dorsal or ventral "steps" and narrow wedging or collapse of intervertebral spaces can also be indicative of trauma, as are some soft tissues changes (e.g. pneumothorax). CT is the method of choice to correctly visualise complex fractures.

The most common spinal **vertebral tumour**, by far, is the **osteosarcoma**, although metastases to the vertebrae are mainly carcinomas. Rhabdomyosarcoma can directly infiltrate the vertebral skeleton. Primary bone tumours of the spine are mostly monostotic – in contrast to metastatic ones that can occur as monostotic or polystotic. **Multiple myeloma** and **malignant lymphoma** (particularly in young animals; Fig. 6.14) show special behaviour patterns and can build disseminated polystotic foci in the limb bones (47, 48) (see below). As with the limb skeleton, large breeds of dogs are more commonly affected by spinal tumours than small breeds or cats. The majority of primary and secondary metastatic spinal tumours can, by their expansive growth, cause a massive distension of the affected vertebra and usually present themselves as predominantly radiolucent destructive osteolytic lesions. Primarily proliferative or mixed forms can also occur. Periosteal reactions in the surrounding soft tissues (rarely with osteoneogenesis) lead to abnormalities in the shape and contours of the vertebrae. Sclerotic boundaries, often present with osteomyelitis, are lacking due to the tumour's invasive and usually rapid rate of growth.

The joints of the vertebrae are never or only rarely affected by osteosarcoma and the joint spaces are not crossed by the tumours. Primary neoplasms can be differentiated from most other aggressive diseases, such as osteomyelitis or discospondylitis, due to their radiographic appearance. Spontaneous fractures (pathological fractures) are usually compression fractures and lead to a shortening of the vertebra with a break or bend in its contour. This can be seen particularly with destructive tumours. Severe neurological disturbances in association with metastatic vertebral tumours (which often appear

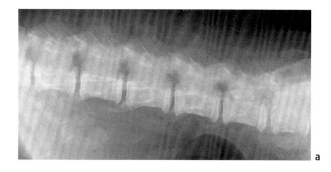

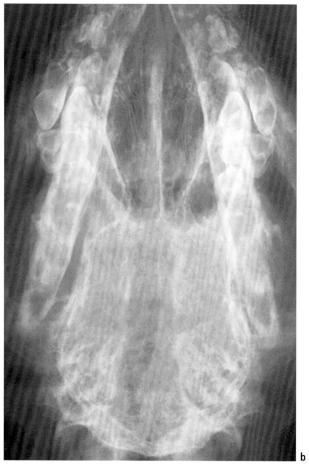

Fig. 6.14a, b
Views of the spine (a) and skull (b) of a six-month-old dog with juvenile lymphoma. Patchy bone structure of all parts of the spinal skeleton, ribs (a) and the bones of the head (b) due to a generalised aggressive bone lesion. Mainly osteolytic, confluent foci with only very few proliferative changes.

as poorly demarcated lytic foci) are an indication of extension into the vertebral canal. Confirmation is achieved using CT or MRI. Local metastases of neoplastic retroperitoneal lymph nodes (prostate carcinoma, urinary bladder and vaginal tumours, etc.) exhibit a different behaviour pattern. The ventral boundary of the spine is roughened by the invasive growth and later proliferative processes may ensue. The sublumbar lymph nodes are almost always enlarged; NB: the ventral contour of L3 / L4 is often blurred due to the insertion of the diaphragmatic crura. In **malignant lymphoma** and **multiple myeloma**, the neoplastic foci are often disseminated, well demarcated and have a small diameter ("moth-eaten"). Compression of the spinal cord with malignant lymphoma is mainly caused by epidural growth (myelography, CT, MRI). Cats and more rarely (young) dogs can be affected. As with tumours of the nerve roots, malignant lymphomas can grow through the vertebral foramen and into the paravertebral soft tissues.

Multiple cartilaginous exostoses occur in most species. A hereditary basis has been proven in human beings and a family predisposition is known to occur in dogs. Multiple cartilaginous exostoses appear as well-demarcated exostoses, particularly on the limbs, ribs and spine. The expansive growth can take on amazing proportions. They develop during the growth period in the dog, whereby the metaphyses form the starting point. In the cat, in comparison, they occur at every age, and there is a correlation with FeLV infection. Cartilaginous exostoses appear to have a preference for the cervical and thoracic spine. Later malignant transformation is known to occur, especially in human beings (49, 50). Whether or not a tumour causes compression of the spine depends less on the type of tumour than on its location, size and rate of growth. All neoplasms in the area of the spine can lead to an extradural compression of the spinal cord: malignant primary or metastatic tumours due to expansive and invasive growth; benign and malformation tumours (cartilaginous exostosis, osteochondroma or calcinosis circumscripta) by expansion (Fig. 6.15).

Osteomyelitis (spondylitis) and discospondylitis are other causes of changes in the shape and contour of the spine. An alteration in its radiopacity is also typical for these processes. In comparison to primary bone tumours, these are not usually monostotic foci. The cause can be either bacterial or fungal infections. Migrating grass awns can play a major role but are geographically restricted. Additionally, haematogenous dissemination of infection from the urogenital tract, teeth or other organs is an important mechanism for the development of vertebral infection. Acute osteomyelitis presents radiologically as a poorly demarcated, often extremely discrete area of osteolysis. Any associated soft tissue swelling can possibly be seen with ultrasonography, but it is rarely visible on a radiograph. At a later stage, these lytic foci are replaced or bordered by reasonably well-defined broad bands of sclerosis; the transition to normal bone is blurred. Irregular periosteal osteogenesis progressing to massive proliferation may affect the contours of the affected skeletal structure. A specific infection of the epiphyses has also been described. In this infection, the endplates and vertebral discs are not affected. It can cause a collapse of the affected region and apparently has a predilection for the caudoventral part of the vertebral body.

Discospondylitis also causes a massive change in the shape and contours of the vertebrae. In the initial stages, it can be seen as a narrowed and irregular intervertebral space because of the osteolysis of the neighbouring endplates. The osteolysis of the endplates can then expand and finally effect the vertebral body. In chronic cases, an increasing sclerosis of the vertebral body that circumscribes the osteolysis can be seen and is an indication of "healing" or disease resolution. Irregular and initially fine periosteal reaction and osteophyte production can lead to a bridging of the affected intervertebral space. The changes are often most profound on the ventral surface, but they can also be seen dorsally within the vertebral canal (51).

Spondylosis or spondylosis deformans often regularly leads to changes in the shape of a vertebra and is the most common degenerative change in the spine. Only rarely is it responsible for neurological clinical signs and, as such is a coincidental finding, apart from exceptional cases. In its hypertrophic form, where there is a band-like ankylosis of whole sections of the spine ("bamboo spine"), movement abnormalities and clinically often poorly localised pain have been described. However, when the spondylotic exostoses reach the intervertebral foraminae, they can cause compression or irritation of the nerve roots. Spondylosis is often described as an idiopathic disturbance, but it can be the expression of a ventral disc herniation, trauma or inflammation. Hereditary forms have been shown to occur in human beings and it is assumed that hereditary forms also occur in animals due to an increased incidence in certain breeds (Boxer) or families. In the young Boxer, an extensive ossification of the ventral longitudinal ligament is defined as syndesmitis ossificans. In a number of countries, a breeding programme designed to reduce the prevalence of this is being undertaken on the basis of radiographic evidence and mass selection. In addition to dogs, other domestic animals such as horses, cats and cattle, can show spondylotic changes. In the dog, such changes have been associated with instability of the lumbosacral joint.

Radiologically, spondylosis is seen as an osteophytic reaction on the ventral, lateral and sometimes dorsolateral edges of the vertebral body. Only in exceptional cases is it associated with stenosis of the foramenae. MORGAN (52) has divided spondylosis into five grades in the dog. Grade I is of a purely ligamentous nature and is not recognisable on a radiograph. Grades II–V present different degrees of osteoneogenesis from beak-like osteophytes along the edge of the vertebrae to stable bony bridges. Osteophyte formation, at least in the Boxer, occurs intermittently and can start very early in life. It can be seen in all ages from one year upwards. The caudal thoracic and cranial lumbar vertebrae are most commonly af-

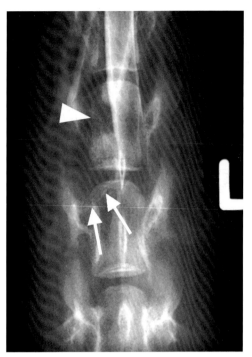

Fig. 6.15
Myelography of the neck in a young Siberian Husky with cartilaginous exostoses. The medial contour of the caudal part of the right pedicle of the vertebral arch is missing in C4 (arrowhead); the pedicle appears to be widened. A shell-like mineralised proliferation extends over C5 (arrows) with extradural compression and displacement of the spinal cord to the left.

fected, in addition to L7–S1. In predisposed breeds, spondylosis occurs in combination with cervical spondylomyopathies of the caudal cervical vertebrae. **Spondyloarthrosis** of the facet joints with superimposing hypertrophic changes occur, not uncommonly, with spondylosis deformans in the dog.

Extensive osteoneogenesis along a number of vertebrae with osteophyte production on the vertebral joints and pseudoarthrosis of the spinous processes is also known as disseminated idiopathic skeletal hyperostosis or DISH (53). The intervertebral spaces are not narrowed and the intervertebral discs show no obvious signs of degeneration, such as mineralisation or vacuum phenomena. These changes occur early in life, especially in large dog breeds (Fig. 6.16).

Spondylosis should not be confused with the radiologically similar changes that can occur in conjunction with *Spirocera lupi* or *Hepatozoon canis* infections, which are rarely seen in Europe. In the former infection, signs of spondylitis of the middle thoracic vertebrae can be seen in addition to space-occupying lesions in the caudal mediastinum (54). In *H. canis*

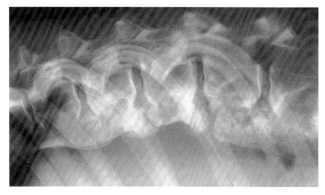

Fig. 6.16
Spondylosis in a four-year-old male Boxer. Grade IV spondylosis of T10–L3, with bridging in some places. The osteophytes lie mainly ventral, though on T13–L1 they lie along the endplate and extend into the neural foraminae. No neurological deficits were noted.

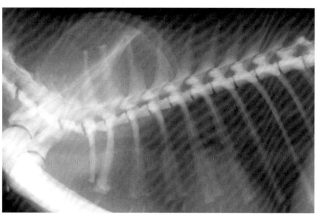

Fig. 6.17
Osteoporosis in a cat. Extremely radiopaque skeleton that is reminiscent of frosted glass. The bone structure is blurred, the trabeculae are not recognisable and the medullary cavities are filled in. Osteoporosis, associated with FeLV infection.

infections, periosteal osteophyte production on the vertebral bodies, ribs, pelvis and long bones can be found. Metabolic disturbances such as mucopolysaccharidosis (see above) and **hypervitaminosis A** in the cat often lead to a band-like ossification of the paravertebral soft tissues and to ankylosis of the spine. A resulting near complete stenosis of intervertebral foraminae can lead to neurological clinical signs. Mineralisation and ossification of the cervical, thoracic and lumbar spine can be seen, and sometimes affects the long bones and joints of the limbs (55).

6.3.1.6 Radiopacity

If there is a generalised change in the radiopacity of the whole spine, one must first ensure that the exposure (kV and mAs) was correct. Over- or underexposure and too low or too high kV inevitably cause changes in radiopacity, which can be misinterpreted as pathological. The contrast and radiopacity can also be influenced by the proximity of the animal to the x-ray head.

A generally **increased radiopacity** is rare and can be found with osteosclerosis or osteopetrosis in connection with diseases such as hypercalcitonism, myelofibrosis, viral infections (FeLV), congenital (very rare) or can be idiopathic (cat) (56, 57). Its characteristics are an increase in the density of the vertebral body cancellous bone with reduced contrast when compared to the endplates (Fig. 6.17). The trabecular structure is blurred with increasing density and in extreme cases appears porcelain-like and lacking in structure. A focal sclerosis can be seen in fractures due to superimposition or in callus production with osteomyelitis or discospondylitis; it can also be an indication of a bone infarct or tumour. An expansion and thickening of the vertebral endplates can be an indication of chronic disc disease or discospondylitis. The over-

lapping of spondylotic spikes and bridges with vertebral bodies leads to "shadows" on the radiograph.

The most common group of causes for **reduced radiopacity** are metabolic diseases such as hyperparathyroidism, hypothyroidism, Cushing's disease and diabetes mellitus, as well as age-related and inactivity-related osteoporosis. All these diseases appear the same on a radiograph: osteomalacia, osteoporosis and osteopaenia cannot be differentiated radiologically. The trabecular structure is "loosened", the often thin endplates contrast highly with the vertebral body. Focal osteolysis can be seen with infections as well as primary and secondary tumours (58). Osteosarcomas are usually monostotic. Multiple lymphoreticular tumours such as myeloma and malignant lymphoma can be both monostotic and metastatic. Soft tissue tumours can be polystotic or generalised and form disseminated foci.

6.3.1.7 Intervertebral spaces and intervertebral foraminae

This normally clearly defined space between two vertebrae requires its own chapter because it has a prominent position in the diagnosis of different diseases, in particular degeneration, protrusion and extrusion of the intervertebral disc. Each intervertebral space must be assessed in comparison with its neighbouring spaces.

In general, the space reflects the thickness of the intervertebral disc, though strictly speaking only if the radiographs are not taken under anaesthesia. Lack of muscle tone can make an intervertebral space appear to be wider than it really is, even after extrusion of its disc. The width of the intervertebral spaces slightly increases from C2 to C7 in the normal animal. The intervertebral space between T10 and T11 is always narrower than the neighbouring spaces (Fig. 6.18). The spaces between C7–T1 and L4–L6 also often appear to be slightly narrowed. The lumbosacral intervertebral space appears to be widened due to its thick disc, though at the same time, the width of this intervertebral space is difficult to assess due to an overlapping of the pelvis and the sacro-iliac joint. The situation is similar in the thoracic spine due to overlapping of the ribs. The intervertebral foraminae in the neck open ventrolaterally and can only be assessed on suitably angled views. The assessment of the intervertebral spaces in the VD view is difficult due to the physiological curvature of the spine.

NB: Only those intervertebral spaces that lie close to the centre of the beam will be depicted orthogonally

Narrowed intervertebral spaces. Narrowed intervertebral spaces and foraminae are an important radiographic sign of disc disease, whether it is due to degeneration with loss of water (osteochondrosis intervertebralis) (59), protrusion or extrusion. For more information concerning this topic see chapter 14.1.7. Malformations due to different causes, discospondylitis and trauma should also be considered. An intervertebral space which is narrowed due to a disc extrusion can appear normal under anaesthesia due to a relaxation of the musculature.

Widened intervertebral spaces are mainly caused by trauma. After traumatic "tearing" of the nerve roots, especially in the region of the cervical enlargement, the intervertebral space can be widened in a wedge-shaped manner on the VD view due to a one-sided (ipsilateral) loss of muscle tone. In acute discospondylitis, the intervertebral space appears widened due to osteolysis of the endplates. A one-sided widening of an intervertebral foramen is almost always caused by tumours such as those of the nerve roots or malignant lymphoma which communicate with the paravertebral soft tissues through the foraminae. Bilateral widening is sometimes seen with luxations.

Degeneration of the disc with mineralisation leads to an overshadowing of the intervertebral space. This mineralisation is used as a marker for disc degeneration in the Dachshund and similar chondrodystrophic breeds. Mineralised discs have a greater risk of extruding. They can also disappear without extruding, which is thought to occur because of an inflammatory reaction. Foraminae that are overshadowed by mineralised disc material are an important pathognomic sign for a disc extrusion. Bony stenosis of a foramen is the consequence of degenerative conditions, in particular those of the articular processes. They are rarely due to malformations and are most commonly seen in the neck and lumbosacral region. Osteophytes and fracture fragments can overlap the foraminae and so cause overshadowing.

Small, demarcated radiolucencies (same lucency as gas) indicate the presence of degeneration, necrosis or extrusion of the disc. This phenomenon is known as the "vacuum sign" and in

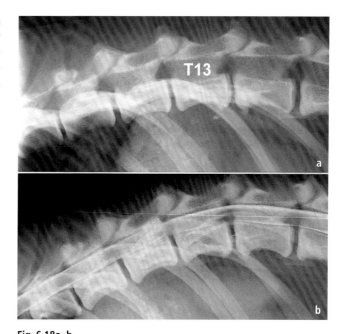

Fig. 6.18a, b
(a) Plain radiograph and (b) myelogram of a dog with a disc herniation at T12–T13. There are narrowed intervertebral spaces between T10–T11 and T12–T13. The intervertebral space at the level of the anticlinal vertebra is physiologically narrow. Between T12–T13, there is an extrusion of the disc with compression of the spinal cord. The spondylotic exostoses on T13 and L1, ventrally sclerosed endplates, narrowed intervertebral space and neural foramina are all indicative of a chronic discopathy without any demonstrable compression of the spinal cord.

reality shows the extrusion of nitrogen from the surrounding tissues (Fig. 6.19). Extension of the spine can instigate this phenomenon or enhance it (60).

6.3.1.8 Vertebral canal

The vertebral canal is formed by the upper dorsal laminae, the lateral pedicles and the ventral body of the vertebrae. Its diameter varies greatly. It is very wide at the level of C1 and C2, in the caudal cervical region and the region of the lumbosacral swelling. In comparison, it is narrower in the thorax and cranial lumbar region with, therefore, less spatial reserve for space-occupying processes. The ratio of the diameter of the vertebral canal to the spinal cord is also variable and depends on the species. In the dog, it also depends on the size and so on the breed. In breeds such as the Dachshund and the Cavalier King Charles Spaniel, the vertebral canal is narrowed due to in-breeding (40, 61). For details of the vertebral canal, see Chap. 6.3.2.4.

Congenital stenosis of the vertebral canal can sometimes be found in connection with wedge-shaped and transitional vertebrae. A congenital lumbosacral stenosis with corresponding

6

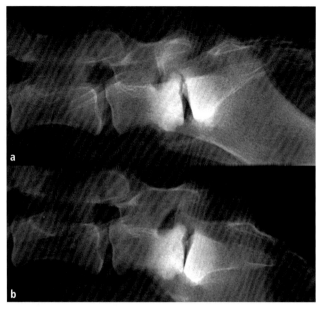

Fig. 6.19a, b
(a) Flexion and (b) extension views of a ten-year-old Dalmatian with chronic discopathy and vacuum phenomenon. Picture of a chronic discopathy (intervertebral osteochondrosis) with loss of the intervertebral disc: collapsed lumbosacral intervertebral space with smooth sclerotic endplates and vertebral bodies, and ventral spondylosis. The radiodensity of the intervertebral space is reduced especially in the extension view (b) due to the extrusion of nitrogen from the surrounding tissues (vacuum phenomenon). The mobility of the joint is obviously reduced.

clinical symptoms has been described in small dog breeds. Cervical spondylomyelopathy has already been discussed. It leads to a reduction in the VD diameter of the affected vertebral canal segment as does degenerative lumbosacral stenosis. Stenosis of the vertebral canal has also been described in the thoracic and thoracolumbar spine. It can be due to chronic disc disease, scarring or osteoneogenesis after trauma. Plain radiographs do not allow a precise assessment of the spatial relationships; this is only possible using contrast radiographic examination or to a greater extent, with CT or MRI.

A widened vertebral canal can be the consequence of a space-occupying lesion expanding at a slow growth rate in the vertebral canal; for example, intramedullary tumours such as astrocytoma or ependyoma. Luxation can lead to vertebral displacement, fractures and interruption of the contours, while tumours can cause a loss of normal vertebral canal contours by destroying bone (vertebral body and arch) (23).

Ossification of the dura (known previously as pachymeningitis ossificans) causes a linear shadowing of the vertebral canal known as an "auto-myelogram". Bone fragments (fractures) and prolapsed discs can also be the cause of such mineral-dense shadows (62).

6.3.1.9 Facet joints and other vertebral processes

Changes in the small vertebral joints are to be expected with malformations, disc prolapses (increased overlapping) and especially in degenerative processes such as spondyloarthrosis. Arthritis of these joints is rare. Spinous, lateral and accessory processes can be fractured (often the only sign of trauma) (see Fig. 10.24). Their contours, structure and density can be disturbed by tumours. The transverse processes may be missing from transitional vertebrae either uni- or bilaterally. Spina bifida can lead to a sagittal splitting of the spinous process.

6.3.2 Myelography

Myelography is still the most commonly used method of depicting spinal cord compression. Nevertheless, with the increasing availability of CT and MRI in small animal medicine, it is likely to lose significance in the future.

The principles of myelography are simple: the subarachnoid (leptomeningeal) space can be made visible on radiographs by using suitable contrast agents. Space-occupying processes lead to changes in the length, width and shape of this space. The image is dependent on whether the process is intramedullary, intradural-extramedullary or extradural.

Myelography is an invasive method with a small but definite risk of complications. It requires a clear indication for its use and the correct technique employed. The examination is indicated when the results on plain radiographs are not conclusive, when the radiological and clinical-neurological examination results are not compatible, or to confirm or exclude compression of the spinal cord. The necessity of surgery for a spinal patient's treatment is in part determined by the results of myelography. The affected segment of the spinal cord, the position of the pathological process with respect to the spinal cord and its extent should be investigated with this imaging technique, with the aim to provide further information about the nature of the problem. Diseases which have no influence on the shape, position and width of the subarachnoid space and/or the spinal cord cannot be visualised using myelography.

6.3.2.1 Contrast agents
A good myelographic contrast agent must be water soluble and mix with the CSF to achieve an even distribution throughout the subarachnoid space. It should also provide a high degree of contrast. It should not be neurotoxic and be absolutely inert chemically. It must remain long enough in the subarachnoid space to enable the undertaking of a prolonged (i.e. 30 to 60 minutes) investigation, but it should ultimately be completely resorbed and excreted. The second-generation monomer non-ionic contrast agents come close to these prerequisites; e.g. iopamidol (Niopam®, Merck, Iso-

vue®, Bracco; Solutrast®, Byk Gulden) and iohexol (Omni-paque®, Nycomed), both of which exhibit a low neurotoxicity ($<$ 5%) when they are used at a concentration of 180–300 mg iodine/ml and are injected slowly at body temperature. The water solubility, fluidity and contrast of these agents are good. Non-ionic contrast agents of the third generation such as iotrolan (Isovist®, Schering) and iodixanol (Visipaque®, Nycomed) are dimer non-ionic contrast agents. They are isotonic in the applied formulations and are therefore safe myelographic contrast agents. The molecule-to-iodine ratio of 1:6 (monomers 1:3) is very good. As they have a relatively high viscosity in comparison to monomer contrast agents, it is imperative that they are injected at body temperature.

Due to the high degree of contrast achieved with CT myelography, the contrast agent is diluted to give a solution of 1:10 to 1:20 to prevent artefacts.

6.3.2.2 Techniques

The technique of myelography has already been described elsewhere in detail. In this chapter, the most important basic principles will be summarised.

Myelography is always undertaken after plain radiographic views have been performed. The contrast agent is administered under aseptic conditions whilst the patient is under general anaesthesia (see Chap. 5.2.2). The contrast agent is warmed to body temperature and injected using a spinal needle (22 gauge) in the subarachnoid space either via the cisterna magna or the caudal lumbar region (L5–L6 in dogs and L6–L7 in cats and small dogs). Performance of the technique cranial to L5 in the lumbar region is problematic as there is an increased risk of filling the central canal with contrast agent. Reports in the literature have documented a greater risk of neurological damage when doing this (63), which is consistent with our own observations.

The basic principle is that contrast administration should be done as close as possible to the lesion but not in the region of the lesion itself. Lumbar injection should be preferentially used with a high cervical lesion, and cisterna magna injection may be considered when a caudal lumbar or lumbosacral lesion is present. The best results with thoracic or thoracolumbar lesions are produced by lumbar administration of contrast (61, 64). As the dural sac is a "cul-de-sac" and the injection of a contrast agent requires gentle pressure, the contrast can be forced to pass an obstructive lesion and so outline it. With a cervical injection, the contrast agent flows craniocaudally due to the tilted positioning of the animal.

Neither cisterna magna nor lumbar contrast administration provide any great technical problems, though collection of CSF is easier following a cistern magna (AO) tap. Although infrequent, injury to the spinal cord and brainstem is possible during a cistern magna injection and so great care should be taken with this procedure. Technical problems are to be mostly expected with obese animals. Two techniques have been described for lumbar contrast administration. The paramedial approach is technically easier than the medial one and the risk of an epidural injection of contrast is lower due to the flatter positioning of the needle's bevel in the subarachnoid space. Contrast can be injected in the subarachnoid space dorsal or ventral to the spinal cord in the lumbar site. The ventral positioning of the needle is easier. Even though in this technique the spinal cord is perforated, the risk of contrast being injected into the spinal cord in the area of the conus medullaris is less than with a dorsal injection. Also the clinical signs following such perforation are far less problematic than those arising from an injection of contrast within the spinal cord. The risk of contrast agent flowing into the epidural space is, at least in theory, reduced with a dorsal injection, as the subarachnoid space is only penetrated once. Multiple attempts at puncture of the subarachnoid space also increase the risk of extravasation of contrast. Epidural contrast agent makes interpretation of a radiograph difficult or sometimes impossible (Fig. 6.20).

After the required amount of CSF has been removed for examination, the warmed contrast agent is given slowly (1–3 ml/10–15 seconds in small animals) at a dosage of 0.2 (lesion close to injection site) to 0.3 ml/kg bwt. A higher dosage is rarely necessary, but can sometimes be required in animals which have a very "thin" spinal cord with respect to their subarachnoid space. A flexible adaptor attached to the needle hub prevents unwanted movement of the needle during the injection of contrast and reduces the risk of damaging the spinal cord (22). In cervical myelography, the needle is immediately removed after injection and the animal is positioned in a tilted craniocaudal position. Lateral radiographs are taken immediately and depending on the speed of flow, repeated after intervals of 5 to 10 minutes. Suspicious sections of the spine require both a lateral and a VD view. Insufficient contrast agent and also a high flow speed can lead to incomplete filling and an unsatisfactory contrast study of the spinal cord, especially in the cervical region. For imaging of the region between C5 and T2, it is suggested to initially raise the head and cranial cervical spine.

Rotating the animal around its longitudinal axis and redistributing the contrast agent by raising the head, the neck or the pelvic region can be used to "pool" the contrast agent in the region of the caudal cervical spine. If the animal is positioned on its stomach, then the caudal cervical spine is the lowest point and so, the dorsoventral (DV) view will lead to better results than the VD view, especially in large dogs.

In lumbar myelography, control and direction of the needle's position with either radiography or fluoroscopy using an image intensifier is suggested. This is done by injecting a small test amount of contrast agent through the needle. Further injection of contrast agent should only then take place if no contrast agent can be seen within the spinal cord nor is there

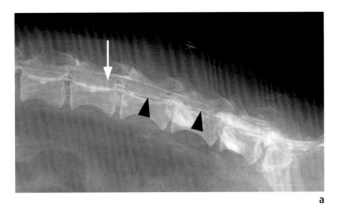

a

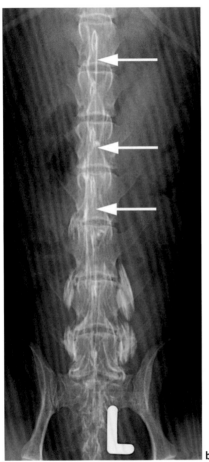

b

Fig. 6.20a, b
Canalo- and epidurogram after lumbar myelography. Epidural contrast agent lies close to the floor of the vertebral canal and so appears wavy. The dorsal displacement of the contrast agent column over the intervertebral space reflects the normal anatomy of the discs and dorsal longitudinal ligament, and cannot be confused with a disc herniation (a). The subarachnoid space is also filled with contrast (arrowheads). The drainage of epidural contrast along the nerve roots appears as stripes of contrast outside the intervertebral foraminae. In addition, a very straight line of contrast running centrally through the vertebral canal is present on both views; this is due to filling of the central canal (white arrows [b]).

any evidence of extravasation. To prevent pressure-induced drainage, the radiographs should be taken either during the injection of contrast or immediately afterwards especially in cases of acute processes (trauma, disc extrusion), oedema or haemorrhage (65).

Additional oblique views with the animal rotated around its longitudinal axis can demonstrate dorso- or ventrolateral disease which cannot be seen with the two standard views. Flexed and extended or traction views assist in cervical spondylomyelopathy and DLSS, and sometimes in other compressive lesions, to differentiate between a static or dynamic compression (66).

6.3.2.3 Restrictions, technical problems, artefacts and complications

Myelography can only depict space-occupying lesions which lead to changes in the length and width of the subarachnoid space. Accordingly, diseases that cause neither a widening nor a compression of the spinal cord and/or the subarachnoid space cannot be recognised (Table 6.3). Diseases in the region of the intervertebral foraminae can only be depicted in exceptional cases, and compression of the cauda equina is usually either not or unsatisfactorily visualised.

Artefacts can have many causes. In addition to overlapping and filling defects due to asymmetrical fat deposits in the spinal canal, dural adhesions can lead to blockage of the contrast agent flow and subsequent misinterpretations. If the contrast agent is injected by mistake in the virtual space between the dura mater and the arachnoid (subdural filling) (Fig. 6.21), this can lead to a very irregular and delayed contrast flow with many filling defects. It seems that this artefact tends to become less frequent with increasing experience of the examiner (67, 68). Extravasation of contrast agent following lumbar injection also causes an uninterpretable or misinterpreted myelogram. Extradural lesions, for example, can erroneously be interpreted as intradural-extramedullary. Air bubbles can get into the subarachnoid space forming round to oval filling defects if the injection needle is not completely filled with CSF or the syringe and its connector/adaptor piece are not totally filled with contrast agent. Air bubbles, in contrast to tumours or thickened nerve roots are mobile, which can be shown by an additional injection of contrast or oblique positioning of the animal.

One must pay attention to performing a perfect technique to minimalise complications. This also includes surgical preparation of the injection site. Injection injuries of the first segments of the cervical spinal cord or intramedullary injection of contrast lead to severe neurological signs and must be avoided. Subarachnoid haemorrhage due to injection is, by comparison, virtually impossible to avoid, but has no clinical significance. A rapid suboccipital injection can lead to apnoea, which can be overcome in the intubated animal by manual or mechanical artificial respiration. Complications

Table 6.3: Diseases associated with a normal myelogram

- Congenital and metabolic myelopathies
- Degenerative myelopathies
- Ischaemic myelopathies
- Myelomalacia, haematomyelia
- Myelitis, meningomyelitis

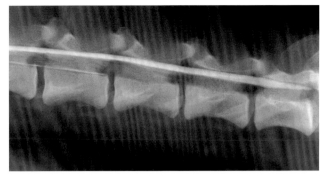

Fig. 6.21
Subdural contrast agent after cisternal myelography. Wide dorsal and very fine, broken ventral columns of contrast. This abnormal distribution is to be taken as an artefact and is due to a subdural injection of contrast agent. With the introduction of a needle, the dura can be separated from the arachnoidea and the normally virtual space between them is opened up. This leads to a sequestration of the contrast agent in this space with often wavy and irregular lines of contrast.

arising from the contrast itself have become rare since the introduction of disassociative agents (1–5%) and are usually easy to control. Such complications include seizures during the recovery period which can be controlled by intravenous injection of diazepam at a dosage of 0.2–0.5 mg/kg bwt or in severe cases with phenobarbital. Severe complications such as malignant hyperthermia or death are extremely rare. Following cisterna magna injection, contrast agent frequently flows into the skull (within the basal cisterns and sometimes the ventricles), and following lumbar injection it is not rare for contrast to be seen within the central canal (Fig. 6.20); neither of which has been connected with a higher rate of complications. Injection of contrast within the central canal can occur more frequently with injections cranial to L5. When the central canal communicates with the subarachnoid space in the region of the conus medullaris, contrast agent may flow into it, too. A fine line of contrast agent in the centre of the spinal cord is usually clinically insignificant. A dilatation of the central canal can be found with hydromyelia, sometimes following trauma and other destructive processes, and also after a forceful injection of contrast agent (63).

6.3.2.4 Principles of interpretation

A good knowledge of the normal anatomical relationships of the spinal cord, the meninges and the central canal are the most important prerequisites for a correct interpretation of the results of myelography. With cisterna magna administration, the speed with which the contrast agent flows depends on the body size and spatial relationships. On average it takes approximately 10 minutes until the contrast has reached the dural sac. In large dogs, contrast flow is rapid as a rule as the vertebral canal is wide in comparison to the spinal cord and so the subarachnoid space is wide, too. The contrast agent flows slower in small dogs and cats as the spinal cord is relatively wide and the subarachnoid space narrow (69). The ventral column of contrast appears slightly wavy in such animals as it takes on the contours of the vertebrae and the discovertebral junctions. The subarachnoid space is widest between C1 and C2, and so the contrast column is wide here as well. At the level of C2–C3, the cross-section of the spinal cord is round, its diameter is narrower and the contrast-filled subarachnoid space appears as two parallel radiopaque lines (contrast columns) extending caudally down the canal. The spindle-like swellings of the cervical (C5–C7) and lumbar (L4–L5) enlargements cause the contrast columns to transiently alter their shape. These swellings are most prominent

in the cat where the contrast columns are displaced to the periphery of the vertebral canal.

The position of the spinal cord within the vertebral canal depends on the shape of the respective spinal vertebrae. It lies ventrally within the canal of a kyphotic area and dorsally within the canal of a lordotic area. This is the reason why the ventral subarachnoid column over C2–C3 is relatively thin and is compensated for by a broader dorsal subarachnoid column. The situation is reversed in the caudal cervical spine. The conus medullaris narrows from spinal segments L5–L6 onwards (with breed and species differences), which is seen as a convergence of the two columns of contrast. The dural sac ends in the cat and in approximately 80% of dogs in the sacrum. In large breeds, however, it can end between L6–L7, with considerable variation in its size and shape. (40, 66, 70). Normal anatomical filling defects frequently occur in the area of the ventral subarachnoid column at the level of C1–C2 and in the lumbar region, too (due to blood vessels). The spinal nerves can also be seen as linear filling defects between their exit from the spinal cord to where they leave the dural tube (22, 71).

Lesions visualised by myelography can be classified according to their position in the vertebral canal: **extradural, intradural-extramedullary** and **intramedullary** (Table 6.4). The criteria for the assessment of such lesions are their location, the associated width of the contrast column, associated filling defects, the rate of flow of the contrast agent around the lesion, and the diffusion of contrast into the spinal cord and central canal.

The column of contrast in **extradural compression of the spinal cord** is displaced and compressed towards the centre of the vertebral canal. The opposite column is pushed to the

Table 6.4: Differential diagnosis of spinal cord lesions that can be seen on myelography

Extradural compression of the spinal cord	Intradural-extramedullary compression of the spinal cord	Intramedullary lesions of the spinal cord	Contrast agent in the medulla or central canal
■ Normal variations (e. g. ventral over C2–C3), artefacts (excessive fat deposits in epidural space) ■ Hansen type I disc herniation ■ Hansen type II disc herniation, Protrusion / hypertrophy of the fibrous ring or the ligaments (yellow ligament – dorsal compression) ■ Extradural neoplasia – primary or metastatic bone tumours – neurofibroma – meningioma – lymphoma – other soft tissue tumours, possibly paraspinal ■ Bony lesions ■ Malformations ■ Trauma: fracture / luxation ■ Hypervitaminosis A ■ Mucopolysaccharidosis ■ Haematoma, haemorrhage – trauma – coagulopathy ■ Infection – abscess, discospondylitis ■ Post-operative scarring ■ Changes in the small vertebral joints – spondyloarthrosis – synovial or ganglial cysts ■ Aneurysm of the venous sinus ■ Calcinosis circumscripta ■ Extradural foreign bodies	■ Neoplasia – neurofibroma, schwannoma – meningioma – neurofibrosarcoma – lymphoma – nephroblastoma – myxoma / myxosarcoma ■ Disc prolapse with rupture of the dura ■ Subdural haemorrhage ■ Intra-arachnoid cyst, meningocele ■ Artefact (air)	■ Normal at the level of the cervical and lumbar enlargements of the cat ■ Neoplasia – ependymoma – glioma – astrocytoma – neurofibroma – lymphoma – metastases ■ Granuloma (FIP) ■ Haemorrhage (oedema) ■ Acute infarct, myelomalacia ■ Granulomatous meningoencephalitis (rare) ■ Hydromyelia / syringomyelia	■ Iatrogenic ■ Perforation of the spinal cord, e.g. due to explosive disc prolapse ■ Myelomalacia

edge of the vertebral canal and can also be compressed (Figs. 6.22 and 6.23). The diameter of the spinal cord lying between the contrast columns narrows in the area of the compression. On the orthogonal views, the lines of contrast are compressed and pushed to the periphery of the vertebral canal by the "flattened" spinal cord. A complete obstruction of flow of contrast can occur due to the compression.

An **intradural-extramedullary compression** is characterised by a gradual broadening of the subarachnoid space and therefore of the contrast column, which is abruptly obstructed by the lesion. The lesion itself can be seen as a filling defect (so-called "golf tee"). On the orthogonal view, an intradural lesion is seen as a filling defect and depending on the size of the lesion, the spinal cord may be wider than normal (Figs. 6.22 and 6.31). The flow of contrast may even be completely blocked. Differentials for this pattern include tumours of the nerve roots which frequently also have an extradural component and may communicate with the extraspinal area via a widened intervertebral foramen. Additionally, arachnoid "cysts" can be considered intradural-extramedullary lesions, in which the contrast-filled subarachnoid space gradually widens from cranial to caudal. The edge of the cyst is rounded and the spinal cord is compressed from more than one side (see Fig. 14.8).

The myelographic pattern for all **intramedullary lesions** is similar. Typical for these lesions is a spindle-shaped widening of the spinal cord, which as a consequence leads to a displacement of the contrast columns to the periphery of the vertebral canal, seen on all views. Depending on the size of the swelling, there is either reduced contrast flow or a complete obstruction (Figs. 6.22 and 17.5).

As the spinal cord has an exceptional ability for compensation, intra-medullary tumours may have already achieved an amazing size when they are first diagnosed. Infrequently, an inappropriately small spinal cord, characterised by a widening of the contrast columns on all sides can be documented with myelography (see Fig. 14.11). In addition to congenital causes, loss of spinal cord substance can be due to vascular insult and chronic compression.

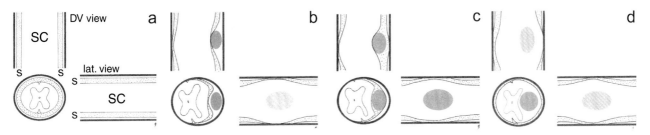

Fig. 6.22a–d
Schematic representation of a normal myelogram (a) compared to myelograms showing (b) extradural, (c) intradural-extramedullary and (d) intramedullary space-occupying lesions. (a) Normally the contrast agent is shown in the subarachnoid space (s) as parallel radiopaque lines apart from around the cervical and lumbar enlargements, and the conus medullaris. SC = spinal cord. (b) With extramedullary space-occupying lesions, the column of contrast is displaced toward the middle of the vertebral canal over the lesion and at the same time it is compressed. The column on the opposite side is pushed to the edge of the vertebral canal and is also compressed. In the perpendicular (here lateral) view, the columns of contrast are displaced to the edges of the vertebral canal due to the flattened spinal cord.
(c) The tangential view of an intradural-extramedullary lesion shows a gradual widening of the columns of contrast both cranial and caudal to the lesion. The columns are interrupted by the lesion which is shown as a filling defect (golf tee). Typically, intradural lesions are seen as filling defects, which compress the spinal cord to a varying degree depending on their size. This causes the columns of contrast to be pushed to the periphery and compressed.
(d) A spindle-shaped widening of the spinal cord is typical of focal intramedullary space-occupying lesions. As a result there is displacement of the columns of contrast to the periphery of the vertebral canal that can be seen on all views.

As mentioned above, penetration of contrast into the spinal cord or central canal may be iatrogenic. Explosive disc extrusion can tear through the meninges thereby allowing the contrast agent to get inside the cord. A discolouring or blanching of the spinal cord with contrast may occur after traumatic transection and with diffuse myelomalacia (Table 6.4). The prognosis of such spinal injuries is unfavourable.

6.3.3 Discography

Discography has acquired practical importance in the diagnosis of DLSS in the dog. In combination with epidurography, it is considered to be a very precise method of depicting lumbosacral discs and lumbosacral stenosis. In the discography of lumbosacral discs, a needle (24 gauge) is introduced dorsally through the lumbosacral foramen, the vertebral canal and the annulus fibrosus (resistance can be appreciated at this point) into the nucleus pulposus of the disc.

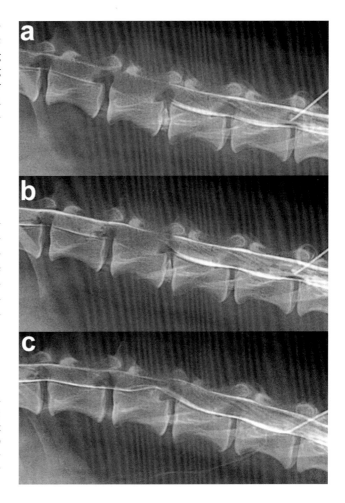

Fig. 6.23a–c
Disc extrusion at L3–L4 with severe compression of the spinal cord in a four-year-old Dachshund cross. View (a) was taken after the first injection of contrast agent; views (b) and (c) were taken during the injection of contrast. (a) Mineralised disc and divergence of the caudoventral contrast column. Only during the injection (b and c) could the severe degree of extradural compression be visualised. Divergence of the contrast column can occur with small central or dorsolateral disc extrusions.

The position of the needle is controlled using either radiography or a fluoroscopic image intensifier. Then a dissociative contrast agent (see Chap. 6.3.2.1) is injected through the needle. Little or no contrast can be injected into a normal disc and a high resistance can be felt with as little as 0.1 ml contrast agent. A multiple of this amount can be injected when degenerative disc changes are present. If the anulus fibrosus is ruptured, then the contrast agent will flow into the surroundings and in some cases back into the vertebral canal. In the method combining discography and epidurography, the needle is withdrawn into the vertebral canal when once the injection into the disc is complete and contrast agent is then injected into the epidural space (72).

6.3.4 Epidurography

In this technique, the same dosage of contrast agent used for myelography is injected dorsally through the lumbosacral foramen or an interarcuate space of the proximal tail vertebrae into the epidural space (73). Lateral views are taken immediately after the injection, both in flexion and extension. Due to the inhomogeneous distribution of the contrast agent which usually quickly disperses, little information is provided by VD views. This method is almost only utilised for depicting compression of the cauda equina, either on its own or in combination with discography. It is considered by some authors as a precise conventional method for imaging lumbosacral compression, while others prefer to use myelography as the primary conventional method, followed by epidurography if an obvious lesion is not identified. However, none of these conventional methods achieve the sensitivity or specificity of CT or MRI (74, 75). Since the availability of CT and MRI in small animal practise has recently increased, conventional methods of imaging lumbosacral disease will soon belong to the past.

Angiographic techniques such as sinus venography have been described as methods for depicting space-occupying lesions in the area of the cauda equina and sacral nerves, but they have not been able to establish themselves in veterinary medicine (76, 77).

6.4 Specific diseases

6.4.1 Degenerative diseases

6.4.1.1 Disc degeneration and herniation

Disc degeneration is common in the dog and is clinically the most important degenerative disease of the spine in this species. In comparison, the clinical manifestation of disc disease in the cat is rare (78). In diagnostic imaging, it is important to be able to differentiate between disc degeneration with the disc *in situ* and disc protrusion or extrusion. A **miner-**alised nucleus pulposus is a sign of advanced disc degeneration and a reduction of its function as a shock absorber (Fig. 14.12). Calcification usually starts in the centre of the nucleus pulposus and extends from there to the periphery. The annulus fibrosus can be independently calcified. The most important significance of a mineralised disc is that there is a distinctly higher risk of extrusion than with an unmineralised one. However, it should not be forgotten that an unmineralised disc as seen on a radiograph can still be degenerate. Radiography relies on mineralisation as the sign for degeneration and so is less sensitive than MRI. Degenerate and mineralised discs can occur throughout the spine. In a number of large dog breeds and the Dachshund, it has been seen that degenerate discs tend to occur more in the middle of the thoracic spine (T4–T9), in addition to other locations. Despite this, disc herniation is rarely observed between T2 and T10. This phenomenon may be explained by the thick dorsal intercapital ligament in this region, strengthened by the transverse conjugal ligaments coupled with the low degree of mechanical stress applied to this region. A good summary of this issue can be found in COATES (79).

Disc protrusion or extrusion is a disease that particularly affects those segments of the spine that are very mobile and are exposed to high mechanical stress. The intervertebral spaces in the neck are frequently affected (between 13.9% and 25.4% of all herniations) with the C2–C3 disc having the highest risk, though the thoracolumbar region is affected most frequently (between 66% and 80%). It seems that the disc between T12–T13 has the highest risk, though in large, non-chondrodystrophic breeds L1–L2 is especially at risk (80, 81, 82, 83).

With respect to disc herniation, a distinction is made between protrusion and extrusion. Chondrodystrophic breeds are subjected to **disc extrusion** with chondroid metaplasia and subsequent necrosis, with dystrophic calcification of the disc. An extrusion is the release of material from the nucleus pulposus through a ruptured annulus fibrosus into the vertebral canal. With an explosive extrusion, the dura can be damaged and disc material can be found within the dural tube. The degree of mechanical damage and compression of the spinal cord – and so the clinical signs – depends mainly on the dynamics of the rupture, the size of the herniation and the spatial relationships within the vertebral canal. Disc extrusion predominantly leads to a significant extradural compression of the spinal cord that can be seen with myelography (Figs. 6.23 and 14.12).

Disc protrusion is a "swelling" of the dorsal aspect of the disc caused by an overexpansion of the annulus fibrosus with dorsal "bulging" of the nucleus pulposus. This type of disc herniation is often associated with cervical spondylomyelopathy and degenerative lumbosacral stenosis. It is mainly a disease of non-chondrodystrophoid animals with fibroid metaplasia of the discs. In this form, compression is generally mild and exists directly over the affected intervertebral spaces.

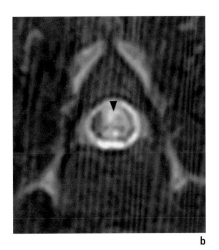

a

b

Fig. 6.24a, b
Perforation of the spinal cord in a Flat-coated Retriever after a car accident. (a) Lumbar myelography L6–L7 after a non-diagnostic suboccipital injection. The spinous processes of L5 and L6 are split. The dorsal line of contrast over L4 and L5 is thin and irregular (subarachnoid haemorrhage) (arrow). The focal collection of contrast in the vertebral canal at the level of L4–L5 is a consequence of the perforation of the dura and the spinal cord due to explosive expulsion of disc material. (b) The transverse T2w sequence demonstrates focal myelomalacia as a focal homogeneous increase in signal intensity (arrowhead).

The differentiation and ascertainment of the diagnosis is done using myelography, CT or MRI. At the moment, myelography is the most common method used in the dog and cat with a suspicion of spinal cord compression.

■ Extradural spinal cord compression can be revealed on a myelogram. The contrast columns and the spinal cord over the herniation are pushed towards the middle of the vertebral canal. Determining the exact position of the herniation often requires multiple views taken with the animal rotated around its longitudinal axis (see Fig. 14.12).

■ The contrast columns are compressed both on the side of the lesion and on the opposite side. With a high degree of compression, the flow of contrast agent can be obstructed. Due to this reason, the lumbar technique is preferred for cases of thoracolumbar extrusion, whereby the contrast agent can be forced past a large compression with the application of light pressure. Under certain conditions, the compression can only be clearly seen when radiographs are taken during the injection of contrast (Fig. 6.23). The type and dynamics of the herniation determine how the image appears: extruded pieces of disc can lie compactly looking like a "pillow" over the intervertebral space or they can be disseminated over a large area. A ventrolateral and a slight midline compression leading to a "forking" or divergence of the contrast columns can be also seen.

■ Extensive extradural haemorrhaging, oedema and swelling of the spinal cord can extend over three or more vertebrae and totally obliterate the subarachnoid space over a long distance. As a consequence, the exact localisation of the cause of compression can be made difficult or totally impossible.

■ Direct injury of the cord due to disc material, intraparenchymal haemorrhage or oedema can cause a widening of the spinal cord, which can be seen on a myelogram. The extravasation of spinal cord into the extradural space and penetration of the spinal cord are compatible with a direct laceration of the cord and indicate a grave prognosis (Fig. 6.24). These are considered to be signs of an explosive incident with subsequent perforation and damage to the spinal cord. In myelomalacia, the spinal cord may be diffusely "blanched" by contrast agent (84).

The sensitivity of a myelographic investigation varies widely. The correct localisation of the affected intervertebral space has a sensitivity of between 90% and 100%. In comparison, the determination of the side of herniation can be difficult; the documented sensitivity ranges from very low (40–60%) up to 100% (34, 64, 85, 86, 87). Technical reasons such as site of injection or rate of injection have been given as being the cause of such variation. The position of the affected disc material in the vertebral canal is another limiting factor.

A disc extrusion can only be depicted on a myelogram if it compresses the subarachnoid space and spinal cord. A dorsolateral extrusion with sequestration of disc material into a foramen often cannot be appreciated using myelography. The same difficulties arise in the region of the dural sac, especially between L7 and the sacrum.

Both CT and, to an even greater degree, MRI are superior to myelography in the diagnosis of diseases of the discs and

6

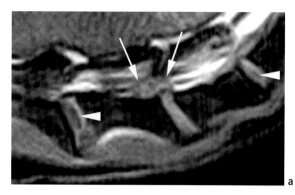 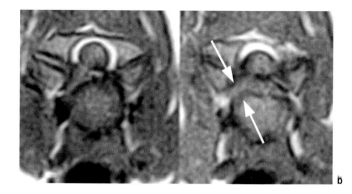

Fig. 6.25a, b
Extrusion and migration of the C5–C6 disc with stenosis of the right foramen. (a) T2w sagittal sequence, paramedian. Slightly narrowed intervertebral disc spaces at C5–C6 and C6–C7. Mushroom-shaped material lies over the intervertebral space and the body of C5, which has an identical signal intensity as the nucleus pulposus (arrows). Note the loss of signal intensity in the centre of the neighbouring disc (arrowheads). (b) The transverse T1w sequence at the level of the neural foramina (left) and the disc (right) shows a broad-based dorsolateral extrusion with stenosis of the right neural foramen (arrows).

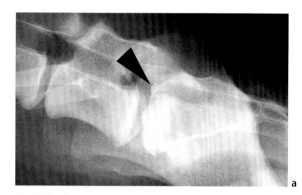 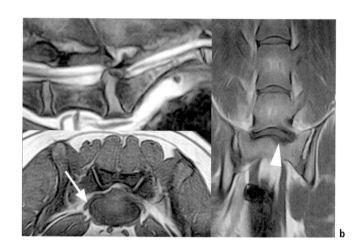

Fig. 6.26a, b
(a) Lateral radiograph and (b) MRI demonstrating osteochondrosis of the sacrum. (a) The dorsally slanted sacral endplate and fragment (arrowhead) lying apparently free in the vertebral canal are typical signs of OCD. The intervertebral space is too narrow and appears butterfly-shaped. Massive sclerosis and apparent broadening of the sacral endplate. (b) Sagittal CBASS, transverse T1w and dorsal T2w sequences of the lumbosacral disc. Defect in the sacral endplate (arrowhead), reduced signal intensity in the dorsal area, disc extrusion with hypointense bone fragment lying in the extruded material, high-grade stenosis of the right vertebral canal and neural foramen. The left nerve root lies free within the foramen (arrow).

spinal cord. As a consequence, these methods will supersede myelography in veterinary medicine in the not so distant future.

The prerequisite for a successful CT investigation is a very exact clinical examination and localisation. Compared with myelography or MRI, this method can be more time-consuming in an extensive investigation of the spinal cord for compression. The combination of CT with myelography can increase the sensitivity of the investigation but may not be necessary. Transverse slices can be supplemented with a sagittal reconstruction.

MRI is the most sensitive method for the diagnosis of degenerative discs and disc herniation (Figs. 6.25 and 6.26). Disc degeneration is a very complex process which leads to changes in the nuclear matrix (proteoglycans and glycosaminoglycans) with a reduction in its water-binding capacity (88, 89). The loss of water can be seen on T2w sequences as a loss of signal in the normally hyperintense nucleus pulposus. The degenerate nucleus pulposus finally takes on the same signal intensity as the normally hypointense annulus fibrosus (90, 91). At least two different planes of imaging are used in MRI: a sagittal T2w sequence can be combined with a T1w sequence in the sagittal and transverse planes with the slices parallel to the intervertebral spaces. It is recommended to utilise

3-D volume techniques with high local resolution and a narrow slice thickness in small animals due to their small volumes and structures.

Bulging of the disc into the spinal canal, an increase in soft tissue density associated with a loss of epidural fat, displacement and compression of the dural tube and spinal cord are all signs of a disc herniation (75, 92).

The disc material can be displaced proximally or distally under the dorsal longitudinal ligament. If the disc material is fragmented, it is known as sequestration, if not then migration (59).

A great advantage of MRI when compared to myelography is in the depiction of foraminal stenosis on transverse or cross-sectional images caused by osseous "lipping", synovial and ganglion cysts or sequestered disc material (Fig. 6.25). If atrophy of the spinal cord is observed in spondylomyelopathy, it may be a prognostically poor sign (93).

6.4.1.2 Degenerative lumbosacral stenosis

The most common and clinically most important disease of the lumbosacral region is degenerative lumbosacral stenosis (DLSS) in large dog breeds (33, 34, 35, 36, 37, 38, 39). Until the introduction of CT and MRI in veterinary medicine, diseases of this area presented a great diagnostic challenge due to the spatial anatomical relationships of the lumbosacral vertebrae, ileosacral joints and the pelvis. In large breeds of dog in particular, the dural sac can be very thin in this area or end just cranial to it; this has been shown in a comparison between Dachshunds and German Shepherds (40). Due to this inconsistency, epidurography, discography and sinus venography have been used in conjunction with myelography for the diagnosis of the cauda equina syndrome (35, 66, 94, 95). Discography and epidurography are methods that can be easily undertaken and have a low morbidity. They have a sensitivity of between 75% and 90% (34, 37, 72, 94, 96, 97). However, since CT and MRI have been introduced, they have set new standards for the diagnosis of cauda equina compression negating the need for these more antiquated imaging techniques.

Plain radiographs rarely provide significant results when investigating this disease. The presence of a lumbosacral transitional vertebra or osteochondrosis of the sacral endplate are considered as being predisposing factors (38, 41, 98). Osteochondrosis of the sacrum can be seen as a defect on a plain radiograph with bevelling and sclerosis of the dorsal part of the cranial sacral endplate (Fig. 6.26). Whether an ossified fragment is demonstrable in the vertebral canal depends on the size of the fragment and the radiographic technique used (slice CT images are useful).

Degenerative osseous changes may be present in the young animal and can lead to a degeneration of the lumbosacral disc with compression of the cauda equina due to extensive tissue proliferation (98). Spondylosis, narrowed or collapsed intervertebral disc spaces, vacuum phenomenon, ventral subluxation of the sacrum, deformation and/or sclerosis of the endplate of the sacrum and osteoarthritis of the facet joints are all signs of a chronic degenerative process of the vertebral junctions. These results, however, are not sufficient for the diagnosis of a compressive disease (38, 97, 99, 100, 101). The presence of a stenosis of the vertebral canal or a foramen must be proven using special methods. Stress views in flexion and extension are undertaken to measure the degree of movement and to see whether there is instability of the lumbosacral joint with respect to a translational movement (Fig. 6.27). The significance of this investigation without the use of contrast is, however, limited. It has been found that the degree of movement is highest in female animals and that lumbosacral instability has been found in clinically normal animals (100). For these reasons, it is best to do a dynamic study in combination with the application of a contrast agent (myelography or epidurography). Myelography is done via a cisterna magna injection as the assessment of a lumbar myelogram can be made difficult if there is any extradural contrast agent. The examination is dynamic, with the views in flexion being done first. Typically there is a ventral, lateral and sometimes dorsal compression with displacement and compression of the dural sac. The compression of the dural sac is often accentuated during extension.

In large dog breeds, the dural sac may often be too short or too thin (in approx. 20%) to allow for myelographic diagnosis, even when there is a complete stenosis of the vertebral canal. In addition, the stenosis may lie in the area of the nerve root as it exits the canal and so cannot be depicted by myelography at all. Other methods of using contrast, such as epidurography or combined discography-epidurography, show a high sensitivity with respect to DLSS, but they cannot depict changes cranial to L7–S1 or foraminal stenosis. The method of choice for diagnosis of foraminal stenosis is CT or MRI. Both of these imaging techniques have a greater sensitivity and specificity than conventional methods. Mass effect within the vertebral canal is visualised as a displacement of the epidural fat on CT and MR images. MRI also allows direct imaging of the cauda equina and the nerve roots. The position and condition (signal intensity) of the discs can also be analysed at the same time (see Chap. 6.4.1.1).

6.4.1.3 Other degenerative diseases

Cervical spondylomyelopathy (cervical malformation-malarticulation or Wobbler syndrome) is most common in the Doberman and Great Dane. The caudal cervical spine (C5–C7) is classically affected. In the Doberman, the changes are seen in middle-aged dogs and comprise abnormal rhomboid or triangular vertebral bodies which may be subluxated dorsally (tipping). Hansen type II disc protrusion, hyper-

6

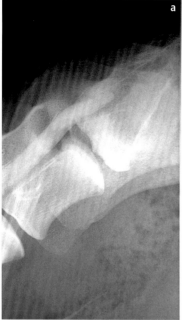

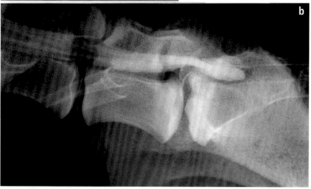

Fig. 6.27a, b
Dynamic investigation in flexion (a) and extension (b) of degenerative lumbosacral stenosis caused by OCD of the sacrum in a two-year-old German Shepherd. A broadened dural sac that reaches far into the sacrum can be seen. In flexion, the dural sac is displaced dorsally but is normal in width. In extension, the sac is compressed by more than 50%. In addition, characteristic changes of the sacral endplate typical of OCD can be seen.

ligament is enhanced by dorsal flexion of the neck and is lessened by a ventroflexion (see Fig. 14.6). A slight traction on the neck can also reduce the degree of compression and may help determine if a distraction-type of surgery is necessary. Additional information about the exact location, degree of spinal cord compression and atrophy can be acquired by a myelo-CT scan or MRI. A relative broadening of the subarachnoid space at the site of a disc protrusion is a sign of spinal cord atrophy and is a prognostically poor sign (93).

MRI also enables excellent visualisation of the soft tissues, which is especially important in the region of the small vertebral joints in this disease. Dorsolateral compression of the spinal cord often develops as a consequence of an increase in soft tissue, facet hypertrophy or the presence of synovial or ganglion cysts (102). These cysts can be seen as hyperintense round structures associated with the joint on T2w sequences. In addition, intramedullary lesions such as gliosis or oedema can also be detected (103).

The significance of radiological and myelographical investigations in dogs with **degenerative myelopathy** lies with the exclusion of other diseases, especially those causing compression. The MRI appearance of degenerative myelopathies in human beings similar to canine degenerative myelopathy has been described as hyperintense in T2w sequences and iso- or hypointense in T1w sequences (104).

Ossification of the dura mater is occasionally seen in older large breed dogs. It has no clinical significance, but it can take on the function of a myelogram (auto-myelogram) as it naturally follows the course of the spinal cord.

6.4.2 Tumours

Tumours of the spine can be divided into primary tumours and metastases. Primary tumours include all those tumours which develop from normal bone, namely osteosarcomas, chondrosarcomas, fibrosarcomas, haemangiosarcomas, undifferentiated sarcomas and solitary plasma cell tumours. The tumours which metastasise to the spine include different types of carcinoma, multicentric lymphoma, multiple myeloma, osteosarcoma of the appendages and other sarcomas (23).

Primary bone tumours of the spine can demonstrate bone destruction, partial cyst-like appearance and, less frequently, osteogenesis. The most common tumour of the spine is osteosarcoma. These are usually monostotic, but they can also affect neighbouring vertebrae (105). The small vertebral joints are practically never affected and are not traversed. On a plain radiograph, osteosarcomas can be detected as very discrete osteolytic lesions, but they can also produce markedly "distended" vertebral bodies. Periosteal reactions are often present, as is, although more infrequently, osteogenesis of the soft tissues.

trophy of the yellow ligament, osteophytes and malformed pedicles of the vertebral arch all lead to a narrowing of the vertebral canal and the cranial vertebral foramen in particular. The disease starts earlier in the Great Dane and is characterised by stenosis of the vertebral canal with degenerative changes in the small vertebral joints and hypertrophy of the ligaments (31, 32). A diagnosis can be achieved using myelography. Radiographs in flexion and extension are used for the differentiation between static and dynamic compression of the spinal cord (Fig. 6.27). Compression due to hypertrophy of either the dorsal longitudinal ligament or the yellow

The poorly defined lesions on a plain radiograph can be more clearly shown using linear tomography. Neurological clinical signs occur when the tumour expands within the vertebral canal. Myelography can demonstrate an extradural (Fig. 6.28) or intradural-extramedullary compression. Although they are rare, benign aneurismal bone cysts must be included in the differential diagnosis of lytic changes in the vertebrae (106).

Metastases of urogenital tract carcinomas can occur in the spine or in the proximal long bones. Typically, more than one vertebra is affected in contrast to primary neoplasms (107). Bone scintigraphy is an excellent method of screening for metastases (Fig. 6.10). The radiological image is very similar to that of a primary tumour (23). Infiltration of the bone by neoplasms of the surrounding soft tissues is possible, too. Damage to the blood supply of the vertebrae can lead to bone necrosis, visible as sclerosis (108).

Plasma cell carcinomas occur primarily in bones with active haemopoesis; in approx. 25% of cases the vertebrae are affected. Two types of plasma cell carcinoma are known to occur in the spine: the disseminated form or multiple myeloma and the rare solitary plasma cell tumour. The typical changes on a radiograph are discrete well-defined lytic lesions without sclerosis of the surrounding bone. A larger percentage of patients demonstrate a generalised osteopaenia at the time of diagnosis. If there is suspicion of multiple myeloma, radiographic overviews of the predilection sites should be made (spine, pelvis, skull, ribs). Scintigraphy is not suitable in this case for screening as purely lytic lesions will not be visible (109). Solitary plasma cell tumours appear as lytic lesions within the vertebrae, but can progress to a disseminated form later (48). Atypical forms with lytic and proliferative lesions, and spinous process involvement have also been described (110). Infiltration of bone by a multicentric lymphoma is seen as a disseminated osteolysis, with proliferations on the ribs and spine, and sometimes with pathological fractures (47) (Fig. 6.14).

A **vertebral angiomatosis** has been described in the thoracic spine in young cats, but it may also affect the cervical spine. This disease is a benign proliferation of blood vessels which leads to lytic and proliferative changes in the vertebrae (especially of the pedicle) and compression of the spinal cord (Fig. 6.29). The prognosis appears to be very good after surgical removal, though relapses are possible (111).

Primary soft tissue tumours of neural origin such as astrocytoma, ependymoma, oligodendroglioma, medulloepithelioma and sarcoma are mainly intramedullary. On a plain radiograph, they can rarely be seen as a focal widening of the vertebral canal and lysis of the pedicle of the vertebral arch due to pressure atrophy of the bone. Usually tumours of the spinal cord can initially be visualised with myelography as focal intramedullary lesions. CT due to its better osseous resolution is more sensitive at showing regional osteolysis or osteogenesis (58), but it is limited in its visualisation of the spinal cord.

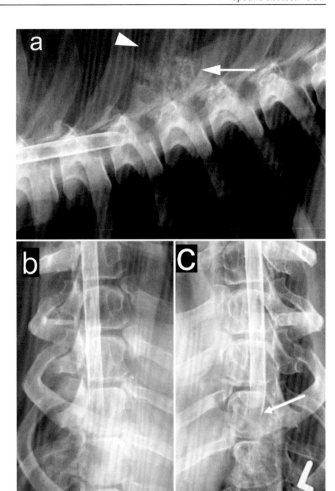

Fig. 6.28a–c
Osteosarcoma of the spine (T6): myelography. (a) Massive lytic and proliferative changes on the spinous process of T6 causing pressure atrophy of the spinous process of T7 (arrow). There are amorphous areas of osteoneogenesis (arrowhead) in the surrounding tissues. (b, c) The roof of the vertebra is broken and a soft tissue component of the tumour has presumably penetrated through this into the vertebral canal. It can be seen on the myelograms as an extradural compression coming from the left (arrow) and dorsally.

The method of choice for visualising tumours of the spinal cord is MRI. T1w and T2w sequences as well as T1w sequences after contrast agent administration should be routinely undertaken. At least two projections are needed to differentiate intramedullary from extramedullary lesions. The structures involved and the degree of spinal cord compression as well as the relationship of the spinal cord to the tumour can all be precisely visualised by MRI. At the moment, minimal

6

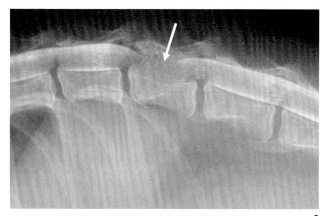

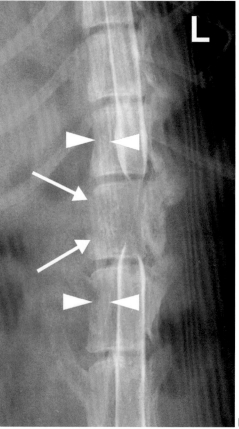

a

b

Fig. 6.29a, b
Myelography of vertebral angiomatosis of L1 in a cat. (a) Dorsal extradural compression is shown in the lateral view (arrow). The bone structure of the widened vertebral roof appears to be broken up. (b) In the slightly oblique VD view, both pedicles of the vertebral arch are widened in comparison to the normal ones (arrowheads). They are also poorly demarcated and appear as a dispersed, sponge-like bone structure (arrows). A severe hour-glass-shaped compression is present.

information has been published in veterinary literature about the appearance of the different tumours with MRI. Different signal intensities and contrast enhancement can narrow down the list of differential diagnoses but they do not allow a definitive diagnosis. Also the extent of the lesion is difficult to judge as the MRI images and surgical findings do not always agree (112). Changes in the surrounding tissues are difficult to differentiate from the tumour tissue itself; for example, the signal intensity of bone varies greatly depending on its fat content. Fat-suppressed STIR sequences are used to differentiate between bone marrow containing fat and tumour infiltration. In comparison, there is more information available about the MRI appearance and behaviour of spinal cord tumours in human medicine. The most common primary cord tumours are ependymomas which are typically located in the neck (within the centre of the spinal cord). They are often intimately associated with large cysts. Neighbouring regions with reduced signal intensity can represent haemosiderin deposits due to chronic haemorrhaging (113). Astrocytomas are usually eccentric in position, poorly demarcated and show an inhomogeneous enhancement with contrast. They also sometimes contain cystic components (112). The injection of contrast allows the differentiation between a reactive lesion and oedema in nervous tissues (114).

Tumours of the nerve roots (schwannoma, neurofibroma / neurofibrosarcoma) and **meningiomas** are the most common intradural-extramedullary tumours (Figs. 6.30 and 6.31). They can cause changes such as widening of the intervertebral foraminae, which can be seen on plain radiographs. Intradural, intramedullary or extradural lesions can be visualised on myelography, though the depiction of such lesions is difficult in the cervical spine due to the overlapping of the osseous structures. As the tumours, or a large part of them, often lie outside the vertebral canal, MRI and CT are examination methods of choice. Space-occupying lesions in the region of the brachial plexus can be visualised using ultrasonography (115). With MRI, tumours of the nerve roots typically appear as hyperintense structures on T2w sequences and isointense structures on T1w sequences. Such tumours can be extradural, intradural-extramedullary or even partially intramedullary; a clear anatomic delineation is not always possible. Transverse sequences and sequences demonstrating the high signal intensity typical of CSF (MR-myclogram) are the most useful in this respect. The majority of tumours developing from nerve roots have a distinct contrast enhancement (114).

Meningiomas are usually well demarcated from the spinal cord and have variable signal intensity on T1w sequences and a slightly increased signal intensity on T2w sequences, with obvious contrast enhancement (116).

Nephroblastoma (neuroectodermal tumour of young dogs) should be considered if an intradural-extramedullary compression at the level of T10–L2 is found in young large breed dogs (117).

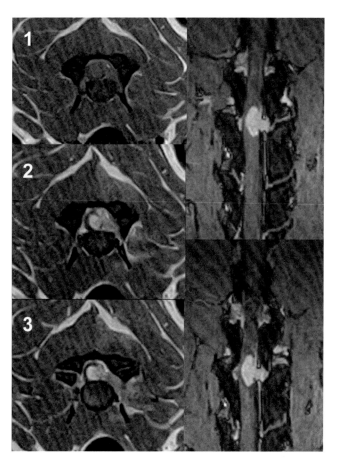

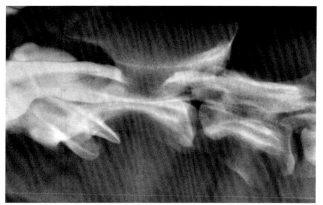

a

6

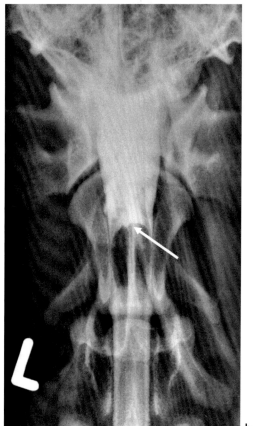

b

Fig. 6.30
MRI images of a nerve root tumour. Left: transverse images both before (1) and after (2, 3) the injection of contrast. Right: dorsal images. Muscle atrophy of the left neck muscles, whose increased signal intensity in comparison to normal muscle indicate the presence of fatty deposits. The left neural foramen is enlarged. On the plain image, the tumour is isointense to the normal spinal cord. The tumour shows a very intense and homogenous contrast enhancement. Contrast enhancement can also be seen outside of the neural foramen. The spinal cord is slightly broader than normal, although it has mostly been replaced by tumour tissue – a sign of infiltrative growth.

Fig. 6.31a, b
Meningioma in an eight-year-old Newfoundland with tetraparesis. (a) Dorsal broad-based, intradural-extramedullary lesion developing from the dura with 50% compression of the cervical spinal cord at the level of C2. (b) On the VD view, there is a large filling deficit (arrow) with laterally displaced and compressed contrast columns.

6

Metastatic soft tissue tumours can either infiltrate the spinal cord or compress it. Tumour metastases with purely soft tissue components, such as malignant lymphoma (more frequent in cats) or malignant histiocytosis (in the dog), are often localised to the epidural space. Intramedullary metastases of lymphomas or lipomas have been described. Lipomas can be identified with MRI due to the high signal intensities typical of fat which can be measured on both T1w and T2w sequences.

6.4.3 Anomalies

Congenital atlantoaxial instability is a developmental disturbance found in diverse miniature dog breeds. It can also occasionally occur in larger dog breeds and cats. The possible causes include agenesis (in cats with mucopolysaccharidosis), hypoplasia or lack of fusion of the odontoid process (dens) with the body of C2, or a lack of ligamentous support between the occiput, atlas and axis.

Hereditary factors have been purported with respect to the different miniature breeds, e.g. Yorkshire Terrier, Toy Poodle and Pekingese. Acquired atlantoaxial instability can be induced by fracture of the dens or rupture of its apical ligament, the lateral alar ligaments or the transverse ligament of the atlas.

Atlantoaxial instability is seen on radiographs as a greater distance than normal between the roof of the atlas and the spinous process of C2; this should not be more than 2–3 mm in small breeds. Other characteristics are a disrupted longitudinal axis between C1–C2 with dorsal displacement of the dens (see Fig. 14.4). A stump-like, shortened or fragmented dens is also characteristic. In some cases, there can be a bone fragment lying between the shortened dens and the occiput. Quite often there is a hypoplastic C1 associated with a very thin atlas arch, which makes dorsal surgical stabilisation a logistical problem (28). Stress radiographs (mild flexion) may only be done with great care. Rostrocaudal views with an open mouth for visualising the dens are dangerous and rarely indicated. It is better to use a lateral view with the head slightly rotated around its longitudinal axis so that the dens is not covered by the wings of the atlas. Both CT and MRI are sensitive methods for investigating this condition, particularly with respect to abnormalities of the ligaments, cord compression and associated parenchymal damage such as haemorrhage.

Occipitoatlantoaxial malformations are rare in small animals (cats). They are characterised by a fusion of the atlas with the occiput, hypoplasia of the atlas with rudimentary transverse processes, and hypoplasia of the spinous process and dens (29, 30).

Cartilaginous exostoses are cartilage-covered bony proliferations. They form on the metaphyses of bones that develop from endochondral ossification. The vertebrae, ribs and limbs are mainly affected.

Solitary exostoses are called osteochondromas, while multiple lesions are known as osteochondromatosis or multiple cartilaginous exostoses (MCE). Their appearance in the dog and cat are completely different. Exostoses in the dog occur during endochondral ossification and once this is finished, they do not increase in size; although malignant transformation to osteosarcoma or chondrosarcoma is possible (118). Malignant transformation to chondrosarcoma is shown on a radiograph or CT as a 2- to 3-cm thick, irregular layer of cartilage on the surface of the lesion (119). Another form of this disease involving symmetrical ring-shaped osteo chondromas in association with shortened and deformed limbs has been described in a litter of mixed-breed dogs (120). In the cat, MCE develop in young adults after the maturation of the skeleton and grow continuously. They occur mainly on flat bones such as the scapula, skull, ribs and vertebrae. An association with the FeLV virus has been purported.

Exostoses appear on a radiograph as well-demarcated bony proliferations with a smooth attachment to the original bone, but without any periosteal reactions or signs of osteolysis (121). Neighbouring vertebrae may show changes in shape and sclerosis. Cartilaginous inclusion bodies give the lesion an inhomogeneous appearance. Neurological clinical signs occur when the exostoses cause a narrowing of the vertebral canal (Fig. 6.15). Myelography, CT or MRI examinations are necessary to reveal compression of the spinal cord (49, 50).

Calcinosis circumscripta can lead to extradural spinal cord compression if it is localised, for instance, between C1 and the spinous process of C2. On a radiograph, this disease appears as a space-occupying lesion with ice-flow-like mineralisation and without any attachment to a bone (24, 25, 50).

Anomalies of the vertebrae result from a lack of development in a part of the vertebra (mainly the body) during embryogenesis. Different forms are possible and depending on their shape are known as wedge-shaped vertebrae or hemivertebrae, butterfly vertebrae or – in the case of incomplete or lack of segmentation of two vertebrae with a loss of the intervertebral junction – as fused vertebrae. They cause abnormal angulation of the spine, which depending on the form and number of vertebrae involved leads to kyphosis, lordosis or scoliosis. Hemivertebrae have a normal bone structure, smooth cortices and endplates. The neighbouring vertebrae can develop compensatory changes and there may be a widening or narrowing of the intervertebral spaces. However, osteophytes can be formed on the vertebral bodies due to the mechanical stresses within the spine.

Anomalies of the spine are usually without any clinical significance though compression is possible. The presence and extent of compression cannot be adequately judged on a plain radiograph and a myelographic or CT / MRI examination is necessary. All of the spine should be examined in each case as vertebral malformations can occur in conjunction with other problems such as dysraphia or arachnoid cysts. Fused vertebrae can lead to disc degeneration or even herniation in neighbouring segments as it causes a relative rigidity of a longer segment of spine (44).

Transitional vertebrae are easy to recognise and usually have no clinical significance. One exception is a lumbosacral transitional vertebra (lumbarisation of S1 or sacralisation of L7), which predisposes the animal to developing degeneration of the lumbosacral disc and compression of the cauda equina (41).

Spinal column defects, such as **spina bifida,** are the result of a lack of fusion of the vertebral laminae and sometimes of the nervous tissue, too (see Fig. 14.9). A breed-specific predisposition to this disease has been shown to occur in the English Bulldog, Entlebuch Cattle Dog and the Manx cat (43). On a radiograph, the spinous process is doubled, has an abnormal shape or is missing; this is most common in the lumbar or sacral vertebrae. Cystic meninges or nervous tissue can protrude through the dorsal deficit as meiningoceles or meningomyeloceles, respectively. In order to visualise these changes, contrast examinations such as myelography, CT-myelography or MRI are indicated. A contrast-filled protrusion of the subarachnoid space can be seen in cases of meningocele, while in meningomyeloceles the spinal cord also protrudes into the defect. MRI examinations have the advantage that not only is the lesion itself well visualised (signal intensity is that of normal CSF), but that associated diseases such as arachnoid cysts or syringohydromyelia can also be recognised (49).

Hydromyelia is defined as a dilatation of the central canal, which is lined with ependyma. **Syringomyelia**, in comparison, develops outside of the central canal and does not have an ependymal lining. A differentiation between hydromyelia and syringomyelia is not possible with imaging methods and the term **syringohydromyelia** is, therefore, often used. However, if the fluid-filled cavity lies eccentrically in the spinal cord, then it tends to indicate that it is a syringomyelia (122). MRI is the method of choice when there is suspicion of syringohydromyelia (see Figs. 14.8, 14.9, and 17.5). The fluid in the cavities of a syringohydromyelia has the same signal intensity as CSF, if not slightly increased on T2w images. Hypo-intense cavities (black) are seen instead of the central canal on T1w sequences, which are hyperintense (white) on T2w sequences. Connections to the ventricular system can be demonstrated using MRI. Congenital malformations affecting the cerebellum such as Chiari-like malformation with displacement of the cerebellum through the foramen magnum or Dandy-Walker syndrome with cerebellar hypoplasia, cysts in the fourth ventricle and hydrocephalus, often occur in combination with syringohydromyelia. The cause is thought to be related to obstruction of the CSF pathways. Cystic tumours can be definitively differentiated from syringohydromyelia due to their different signal intensities and contrast enhancement of their more solid or tissue components.

Larger cavities within the spinal cord can also be demonstrated using CT. Small lesions, however, are only detectable when they are joined to the subarachnoid space and can then be filled with contrast agent.

A non-specific indicator of syringohydromyelia on a plain radiograph is a widening of the vertebral canal. On myelography, a broadening of the spinal cord with a narrowed subarachnoid space is visible. The dorsal subarachnoid space can be so narrow that CSF only flows following a spinal tap when the central canal has been punctured. In such cases, contrast agent can be unintentionally injected into the central canal (canalogram) (122, 123, 124).

Meningeal or arachnoid cysts (subarachnoid cysts) are more frequent in young large dog breeds (e.g., Rhodesian Ridgeback and Rottweiler) and in older smaller dog breeds (such as the Schipperkee and Pug) as well as in cats. The predilection sites are the highly mobile spinal segments such as the upper neck (C1–C4) in the large breed dogs and the thoracolumbar junction in the small breeds; though the middle thoracic spine and the caudal neck are frequently affected. Plain radiography is usually unhelpful, but in some cases a widening of the vertebral canal may be visible. Arachnoidal cysts are seen on myelography as club-shaped cul-de-sacs of the dorsal subarachnoid space with a virtually complete obstruction of the contrast agent; a tendency for the cyst to be lateralised is not common. The spinal cord lying under the "sac" or diverticulum is narrowed. The majority of these cysts fill with contrast after cisterna magna contrast administration, but some can only be filled retrogradely after lumbar puncture. CT can provide additional information about the caudal borders of the cyst as well as to which side it lies (see Fig. 14.8). An increased density of the spinal cord at the level of the compression has been described as an indication of parenchymal pathology possibly related to associated compression (125). As meningeal cysts can occur in combination with syringohydromyelia, MRI examination before operating is sensible. Connections to the central canal can be visualised, which is, above all, important for the prognosis and surgical therapy (126). Arachnoid cysts are hypointense on T1w sequences and hyperintense on T2w sequences (as with CSF) and contrast distinctly with the spinal cord. Arachnoid cysts have been described in cats, but they are rare in this species (127).

The **dermoid sinus** is a defect of the neural tube and develops due to an incomplete separation of the skin and neural tube during embryonal development (see Fig. 14.9). Single or multiple lesions occur in the cervical, cranial thoracic and more rarely the sacrococcygeal regions. The neurological symptoms depend on the depth of the sinus and the involvement or infection of nerve tissue. The most commonly affected breed is the Rhodesian Ridgeback (128, 129).

6

6.4.4 Trauma

Fractures, luxations and subluxations occur most commonly at the junctions between the mobile and immobile segments of the spine: e.g., atlantoaxial, atlantooccipital, cervicothoracic, thoracolumbar and lumbosacral junctions. The forces that can affect the spine are bending, torsion and compression; the lesions resultant depend on the predominant type of force applied.

The first radiographs taken in a traumatised patient should be lateral views with the patient lying on its side without sedation or anaesthesia, as muscle relaxation can decidedly increase any instability of the spinal column and manipulation can lead to further damage to the spinal cord. In addition, the drop in blood pressure and reduced perfusion experienced during anaesthesia can lead to even more damage to the spinal cord. For oblique and VD views, the animal must be very carefully repositioned with the help of stabilising supports; to avoid this manipulation, a horizontal beam radiograph is frequently advised.

The radiographic signs of trauma to the spine are changes in the shape and size of a vertebra; its density can be increased (compression fracture) or reduced (fracture of a bone fragment). In addition, fracture lines, fragments, dorsal or ventral step formation, and rotations may be found. A narrow or collapsed, wedge-shaped intervertebral space can be an indicator of a herniated disc.

Hyperflexion of the spine usually leads to a dorsal displacement of the vertebrae and extrusion of the nucleus pulposus through a tear in the annulus fibrosus. Compression fractures of the vertebrae can occur with hyperflexion in combination with compression. Hyperextension is less common and leads to fractures of the small vertebral processes and possible ventral extrusion of the nucleus pulposus. Combinations of bending and rotation are common and may lead to subluxation or luxation, which can occur in combination with fractures. It should be taken into consideration that during trauma, the movement of the individual vertebral bodies and so the resultant spinal cord damage is far greater than can be seen from the results on the radiograph (26).

To assess its instability, the spine is divided into two compartments (or three depending on the operator). The vertebral bodies and discs with the dorsal and ventral longitudinal ligaments belong to the ventral compartment. The dorsal compartment is composed of the vertebral arches including the pedicles, small vertebral processes and the spinous processes with their associated ligaments (see Fig. 10.24). The spine is considered to be unstable if there is any injury to either of the compartments, and it must be stabilised surgically or conservatively.

Appraisal of the prognosis for recovery based on the structural lesions present in the spinal cord after trauma can best be done using MRI (130). In human medicine, it has been shown that patients with oedema of the spinal cord have a better prognosis than those with haemorrhage or spinal cord necrosis. Oedema is seen as a diffuse, poorly defined region with increased signal intensity on T2w sequences, but normal signal intensity on T1w sequences. There is also a slight swelling of the spinal cord. Reduced signal intensity in the grey matter on T1w sequences and increased signal intensity on T2w sequences is associated with severe damage to the spinal cord. This may indicate myelomalacia and at a later date, "cyst" development (104, 131) (Fig. 6.24).

6.4.5 Metabolic diseases

Metabolic diseases such as hyperparathyroidism or Cushing"s disease often lead to changes in the radiopacity of the skeleton, but they are rarely associated with neurological clinical signs.

Hypervitaminosis A is characterised by bony proliferation and ossification of the soft tissues along the spine. It is also sometimes seen affecting the limbs, whereby ligamentous insertions are often involved. Massive osseous "bridge" formation occurs especially in the cervical spine, leading to ankylosis in the final stages. The proliferations can cause a narrowing of the intervertebral foraminae and compression of the nerve roots (55).

Different forms of **mucopolysaccharidosis** (a **lysosomal storage disease)** can affect dogs and cats. Type VI is most common in cats. The radiopacity of the complete skeleton is reduced and it has a coarse trabecular structure with thin cortices. The vertebrae have different sizes, are shortened or partially fused, and show widened metaphyses. Degenerative changes in the joints of the spine, shoulder and hip typically occur. The dens is mostly hypo- or aplastic, though it may be fragmented or even have inadequate ossification. Stenosis of the vertebral canal with compression of the spinal cord or nerve roots due to proliferative spondylosis frequently occurs in this disease (46).

Dwarfism, delayed formation and closure of the epiphyses throughout the skeleton and shortened vertebrae are the most important radiographic signs of **congenital hypothyroidism.** Irregularly widened epiphyses and endplates of the vertebrae have been described, but compression of the spinal cord rarely occurs. The cranial sutures remain open longer than normal and the affected animals have a short, wide skull (45).

6.4.6 Vascular diseases

The predilection sites for **infarction** of a segment of the spinal cord following the blockage of a blood vessel by nucleus pulposus material are the cervical and lumbar enlargements. Young dogs from large non-chondrodystrophic breeds are mostly commonly affected. Radiography and myelography serve to exclude acute compressive spinal cord lesions such as disc extrusion or haemorrhage. Usually no changes can be found on a plain radiograph or with myelography, though sometimes disc degeneration and narrowed intervertebral spaces can be observed within the area of the lesion; however, these are non-specific (132). Swellings in the region of the infarct are rarely visible. Diagnosis with MRI is possible: changes in the intramedullary signal intensity are to be expected (133).

Haemorrhage within the spinal cord or epidural space is usually secondary. Coagulation disturbances, trauma (explosive disc extrusion, vascular malformations [arteriovenous fistula, aneurysm]) or neoplasia such as haemangiosarcoma or lymphoma can play a part in the cause (134). Haemorrhage in the epidural space can be seen on a myelogram as an extradural spinal cord compression extending over a number of spinal segments. In comparison, intramedullary haemorrhage is seen as a very discrete swelling of the spinal cord on myelography and the true degree of change can only be assessed with MRI (Fig. 6.32). Explosive extruded discs can concuss or perforate the spinal cord and lead to a haemorrhagic myelomalacia. Extravasation of contrast agent in the extradural space and possible entry of the contrast into the spinal cord or the central canal are important and grave prognostic indices (135).

Extradural haemorrhage usually occurs in conjunction with disc herniation and leads to irregular contrast column contours or their complete disappearance over long stretches of the spine.

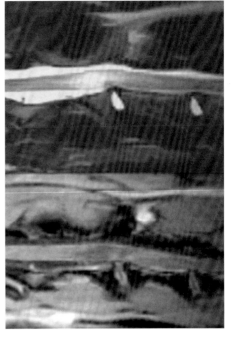

Fig. 6.32
Acute, severe spinal cord oedema of unknown origin – MRI. On the T2w sequence (top) there is focal spinal cord swelling with poorly demarcated areas of increased signal intensity. These have reduced signal intensity in the T1w sequence (bottom). Acute infarction with oedema formation frequently has space-occupying characteristics and is hypointense on T1w sequences and hyperintense on T2w ones.

6.4.7 Inflammatory diseases

Plain radiographs are usually diagnostic in **discospondylitis, physitis** and **osteomyelitis**. The earliest changes to be seen with discospondylitis are discrete radiolucencies in the endplates of two neighbouring vertebrae and possibly swelling of the soft tissues. With progression of the disease, the lysis of the endplates and vertebral bodies increases and band-like sclerosis of the vertebral bodies either surrounds or replaces the lytic zones. A sequestration of the endplate is also possible. The intervertebral space can be irregularly wide or collapsed. In the chronic stage, the intervertebral space is usually collapsed and bridged ventrally by spondylosis. Fusion of the vertebrae means healing has taken place. More than one intervertebral space can be affected (Fig. 6.33). It should be realised that the radiological changes lag behind the clinical signs. In early or uncertain cases, CT or MRI can be used for diagnosis. The CT changes reflect the radiographic picture, with irregular osteolysis of the endplates, sclerosis and bony proliferations on the vertebrae (136). MRI is considered to be

the most sensitive method (Fig. 6.34). In comparison to the other modalities, soft tissue changes and extension of the infection to other structures (myelitis, arthritis of the small vertebral joints) as well as possible spinal cord compression, can be assessed. On T2w sequences, a strong increase in the signal intensity of the nucleus pulposus, endplates and neighbouring vertebral bodies can be seen. The signal intensity on T1w sequences is reduced and the affected tissues show an irregular enhancement with contrast (136, 137).

Lysis and reaction of the bone centred on the growth plates of the vertebral body without any changes in the intervertebral space or erosion of the neighbouring endplates is called **physitis**. It has mainly been described in young dogs, whereby a haematogenous infection is presumed to be the cause (138). The lysis can lead to a collapse of the vertebrae and kyphosis of the spine. Sequestration of a bone fragment after physitis is another possible complication (139).

Osteomyelitis of the vertebrae can be caused by the migration of a grass awn (predilection site: L1–L4). Periosteal

6

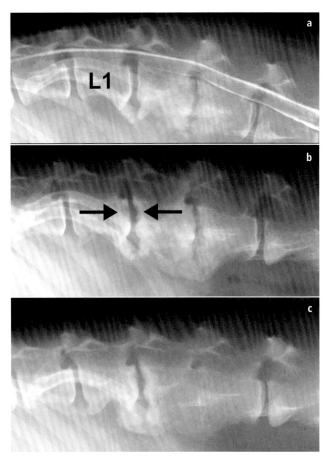

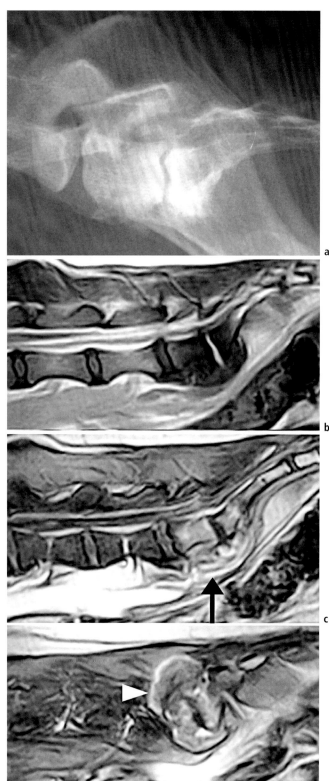

Fig. 6.33a–c
Radiographic monitoring of discospondylitis. Figure (a) shows a narrow and irregular intervertebral space between L2–L3, with osteolysis of the neighbouring endplates and sclerosis of the vertebral bodies; there is also ventral osteophyte formation and spondylosis of L1–L2. The myelograms demonstrate only mild displacement and narrowing of the ventral column of contrast. (b) Three weeks later: the sclerotic changes are predominant, with ventral consolidation of the osteophytes associated with a very small neural foramen. New foci have developed between L1–L2 with osteolysis of the endplates that is demarcated from the normal bone by a sclerotic edge (arrows). (c) Again one month later: the focus at the level of L2–L3 has healed, and the vertebrae are fused. The proliferative changes are now predominant at L1–L2 (Fig.: Tuez, Tenniken).

Fig. 6.34a–d (right)
Radiograph (a) and MRI images (b–d) of chronic discospondylitis. (a) The radiograph demonstrates a narrowed, irregular intervertebral disc space, massive sclerosis of the neighbouring vertebral bodies and a periosteal reaction on the ventral vertebral contours. (b) The sagittal CBASS MRI sequence prior to contrast administration reveals the collapsed lumbosacral intervertebral disc space. Both vertebrae show a loss in signal and extensive bridging on their ventral surfaces. The massively increased signal intensity of the disc is typical of inflammatory reactions. (c, d) The T1w sequences after contrast show extensive distinct contrast enhancement in both vertebrae, and in the reactive proliferation ventral to L7 (arrow) and the sacrum, as well as in the ileosacral joint (arrowhead).

reaction ventral to the vertebrae has been described on MRI in association with increased signal intensity and contrast enhancement in the sublumbar musculature (140). *Nocardia* infections (141) and infections with *Spirocerca lupi* (predeliction site: T8) can lead to similar lesions of the vertebrae.

Other inflammatory diseases. Inflammatory diseases of the spinal cord and the meninges rarely require radiological investigation as the diagnosis usually relies on the clinical and CSF results. **Feline infectious peritonitis** (FIP) can lead to meningitis or the formation of granulomas and ependymitis in the central canal (142). These lesions appear as intramedullary space-occupying structures on myelography (Fig. 6.35). MRI reveals increased signal intensity on T2w sequences and reduced signal intensity on T1w sequences with contrast enhancement. If a lesion is located within the central canal, it can lead to a blockage of the canal and the ventricular system.

Abscesses in the epaxial muscles can, in rare cases, expand into the epidural space and lead to spinal empyema with a rapidly progressive myelopathy (143).

6.5   Skull

Radiography of the skull and contrast examinations such as theco- or cisternography, ventriculography or cerebral angiography all currently play a very limited role in the investigation of neurological disease in small animals. Radiography is used for the initial examination predominantly in patients with an anamnesis of trauma, tumours of the face and skull, certain congenital malformations or suspicion of a peripheral vestibular disturbance. In order to gain the best results and as changes can only be recognised by comparing both sides of the skull, it is important to pay attention to using optimal radiographic techniques, especially with respect to positioning the animal. The animal should be examined under anaesthesia to ensure symmetrical positioning – except for animals with acute craniocerebral trauma. Cushions, bandages and other aids should be used to fix the animal in position; holding the animal by hand should not be done due to the health and safety implications of dealing with radiation.

The standard views used include lateral, VD and DV. Due to the complex anatomy of the skull, specialized views are needed to visualise individual regions of the head (Table 6.5). Imaging of other structures belonging to the viscerocranium such as lower jaw, teeth or nasal cavities requires other projections which are described in the literature.

In the past, the main indication for cerebral angiography was for the depiction of blood vessel architecture when a space-occupying lesion (i.e., tumour) was suspected. For a number of reasons, this method never acquired any great significance in veterinary medicine. In contrast, CT and MRI imaging of

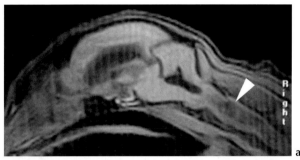

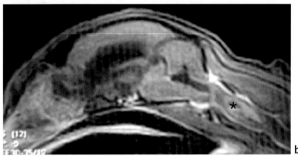

Fig. 6.35a, b
FIP granulomas in the cervical spinal cord with secondary hydrocephalus in a cat. Sagittal T1w sequence (a) plain and (b) after gadolinium IV. In the plain image, the spinal cord in the region of C2 is thickened with a large hypointense intramedullary focus (arrowhead). Cranial to this, there is dilatation of the central canal and the ventricles. The granulomas show a distinct contrast enhancement with a central hypointense focus (necrosis *).

Table 6.5: The most important views / projections for the radiographic examination of the skull

	Position	Projection
Nasal passages, nasal cavities including frontal sinus	Dorsal recumbency	VD: mouth open
Frontal projection for depicting the frontal sinus, only sometimes possible in cats and brachycephalic breeds
	Sternal recumbency	DV: imaging device placed intraorally
Middle ear, tympanic bulla	Lateral recumbency	Lateromedial projection: head rotated by 15–20°
	Dorsal recumbency	Frontal projection with open mouth. Angle of beam centre – hard palate:
■ dolichocephalic dogs: 0–5°
■ mesaticephalic dogs: 10–15°
■ brachycephalic dogs: 25°
Foramen magnum	Dorsal recumbency	Frontal projection with head bent forwards and the x-ray head aimed 25–40° caudally

6

blood vessels have gained increasing significance in veterinary diagnosis and therapeutic planning.

The anatomical details of the brain surface can be visualised using cisternography; e.g., the sulci and gyri of the cerebrum and cerebellum, the basilar blood vessels (basal artery, arterial circle of the brain), pituitary and optic nerves. The contrast agent can be injected into the cisterna magna. Both negative and positive contrast agents can be used (see Chap. 6.3.2.1). Ventriculography, performed by injecting contrast into a lateral ventricle has been used to visualise the size and position of the ventricles. Both of these methods have been largely replaced by CT and MRI.

6.5.1 Principles of interpreting imaging examinations

A precise knowledge of the complex anatomical structures of the skull and brain is the basis for radiological investigation. A range of anatomy books and radiography atlases are available. Assessment of the structures of the skull is based on very precise positioning of the animal for the various views (lateral, symmetrical positioning for VD, DV and frontal views) and the comparison of every structure with its counterpart on the opposite side of the skull. The criteria for examination include bone density, contrast in relation to surrounding tissues, and the architecture. This is especially important in the examination of the nasal passages, sinuses, the ethmoid turbinates and the conchae, as well as the middle and inner ear. Neurological diseases with radiographic abnormalities of the skull are rare (Table 6.6). Brain tumours, infarcts, inflammation, etc. require CT or MRI. These methods are the mainstay of cerebral imaging diagnostics and provide the basics for targeted therapy. The criteria for the systematic assessment of intracranial lesions are summarised in Table 6.7.

6.5.2 Viscerocranium

6.5.2.1 Nasal passages and sinuses

Diseases of the nasal passages and sinuses only lead to neurological symptoms when destructive processes, such as tumours, penetrate the frontal and sphenoidal sinuses or the ethmoids, and enter the rostral cranial fossa.

The potential consequences include compression of the rhinencephalon and frontal lobes by tumours, or infection causing meningitis / meningoencephalitis. The majority of nasal cavity tumours are malignant in the dog (80%) and cat (> 90%). In the dog squamous cell carcinomas, adenocarcinomas, and undifferentiated carcinoma are common (60–75% of all nasal tumours combined) (144). Other tumours include fibrosarcomas, chondrosarcomas and lymphoma, which is the

Table 6.6: Diseases of the skull that can be seen on a radiograph

Congenital and inherited diseases	■ Malformation of the skull ■ Internal hydrocephalus ■ Occipital dysplasia (Arnold Chiari Malformation, dog) ■ Occipitoatlantoaxial malformation ■ Craniomandibular osteopathy (dog)
Metabolic disease (congenital or acquired)	■ Leukocyte adhesion protein deficiency (LAD; dog) ■ Mucopolysaccharidosis ■ Hyperparathyroidism
Tumours	■ Primary and metastatic tumours of the cranial skeleton ■ Tumours of the nasal passages and sinuses ■ Sometimes tumours of the middle ear ■ Sometimes meningioma (cat) based on overlying hyperostosis
Trauma	■ Fractures ■ Gun shot wounds ■ Luxation of the temporomandibular joint
Infections	■ Osteomyelitis ■ Otitis media: empyema and osteitis of the bulla ■ Nasal passages, sinuses

Table 6.7: Intracranial lesions – assessment criteria CT / MRI

a) Origin and anatomical location
■ Cranial fossa
■ Intra-axial:
  – tumours of neuroepithelial origin: astrocytoma, oligodendroglioma
  – metastases
■ Extra-axial:
  – Tumours of intra- or extracranial origin: meninges, pituitary, nerve roots, bone

b) Form
■ Ovoid, broad-based, plaque-like

c) Contours
■ Smooth to irregular
■ Well to poorly demarcated

d) Mass effect
■ Displacement of ventricles and midline, compression

e) CT number / Signal intensity (MRI)
The majority of tumours are:
■ On CT: isodense to slightly hyperdense
■ On MRI:
  – iso- to hypointense in T1w sequences
  – iso- to hyperintense in T2w sequences

f) Contrast enhancement: intensity and pattern
■ –/+/++/+++
■ Uniform
■ Nonuniform
■ Ring-like

g) Other findings
■ Oedema, hydrocephalus
■ Necrosis
■ Mineralisation
■ Osteolysis
■ Bone sclerosis
■ Bone proliferation

most common nasal tumour in the cat. Adenocarcinomas of the nasal cavities often develop in the ethmoid region (145). Nasal tumours can be very destructive, breaking through the nasal septum and penetrating the internal surface of the frontal bone via the cribriform plate, or the rostral cranial fossa via the sphenoidal sinus. Penetration of the orbit is also not uncommon.

Radiographic investigation or CT can differentiate a destructive rhinitis from a neoplastic process extremely well; although a diagnosis acquired by either method must be confirmed using biopsy or other tests (146, 147). Focal and multifocal abnormalities with increased soft tissue density, or variably sized lytic foci that are often well demarcated in the region of the nasal cavity tend to indicate an infectious cause. Typical features of a tumour are homogeneous unilateral soft tissue shadowing of the nasal cavity with extensions in the frontal sinus, and an overshadowing or destruction of the turbinates, conchae or ethmoids (148, 149). The most important single sign which speaks for a rhinitis is a lack of change in the frontal sinus, whereas an encroachment on the bony borders of the nasal cavities indicates a neoplastic process. The position of the lesion in the nasal cavity, uni- vs. bilateral changes, or mineralisation have no significance in forming a differential diagnosis (147).

Radiography can visualise nasal tumours with a high degree of sensitivity, but the extension of the tumour in the surrounding skeletal structures is inexactly depicted, even with multiple views. In contrast to radiography, CT (Fig. 6.36) and MRI can accurately visualise the exact location and extension of pathological changes, two factors which are fundamental principles for targeted therapy. As radiotherapy of tumours in the nose and within the cranium has become more relevant in recent times, CT and MRI investigations are being done with increasing regularity (146, 150, 151, 152, 153, 154).

Aspergillosis, as shown by CT, is seen as a destruction of the turbinates with variable degrees of soft tissue reaction, thickening of the frontal sinus mucosa, maxillary recess and nasal cavities as well as surrounding osseous reactions. The changes can be uni- or bilateral (155).

The destruction of bony structures, such as the cribriform plate, by tumour infiltration, is shown with a high degree of sensitivity using MRI. MRI allows precise representation of the expansion of a tumour in the surrounding soft tissues and cranial cavity due to the different signal intensities of tumour tissues, necrosis, haemorrhage and perilesional oedema. Typically, a tumour is shown as a hyperintense object on T2w sequences. Mass effect with displacement and compression of normal structures such as the lateral ventricles, and perilesional oedema – also hyperintense on T2w sequences – are typical findings. Adenocarcinomas cause an increase in signal intensity on T1w sequences following contrast enhancement (150, 156).

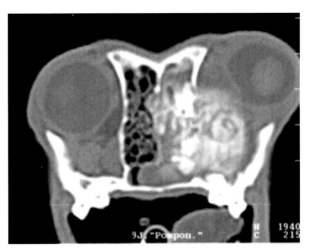

Fig. 6.36
Transverse CT at the level of the ethmoturbinates. Squamous cell carcinoma in a nine-year-old Berger des Pyrenees with exophthalmus. The tumour has arisen from the left nasal cavity causing destruction of the endoturbinates of the ethmoid, the septum and the ventral part of the basal ethmoid plate and the vomer. Tumour tissue lies in the meatus and the nasopharynx. The medial wall of the orbit has been penetrated and a large amount of mineralised tumour tissue is lying within the orbit.

6.5.2.2 Eye

Pathology of the orbit such as soft tissue tumours (including meningiomas of the optic nerve), abscesses and granulomas, are rarely identified by radiography. Sometimes lytic or proliferative changes in the bones in the region of the orbit can occur with infections and tumours (e.g. tumours of the nasal cavities). More sensitive methods of orbital imaging include ultrasonography, CT (Fig. 6.36), and especially MRI. The sensitivity of ultrasonography in retrobulbar disease associated with exophthalmus is quite high, although false negative and false positive results have been described. Deformation of the eyeball, disturbances of the normal architecture of the retrobulbar tissues with changes in the echogenity and definable space-occupying lesions are indicators of inflammatory or neoplastic processes (157). Ultrasonography rarely provides specific results (e.g. foreign body), though it enables ultrasonography-guided tissue biopsies to be undertaken. An assessment of the bony borders of the orbit is, however, difficult.

The CT and MRI anatomy of the orbit is well described (158, 159). Both methods can reveal the anatomy of the orbit and its surrounding structures. CT and, to an even greater extent, MRI are able to precisely image and differentiate pathological processes in this region with a very high degree of resolution. CT allows the scanning of transverse slices with subsequent reconstruction of sagittal and dorsal images, while MRI enables transverse, sagittal and dorsal sequences to be imaged directly. In MRI, T2w and T1w sequences both before and after injection of a paramagnetic contrast agent are evaluated (Fig. 6.37). In a series of 25 dogs and cats with signs

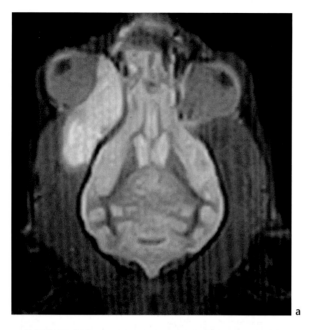

a

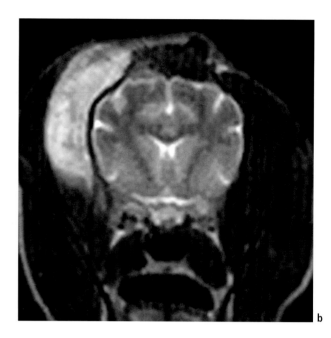

b

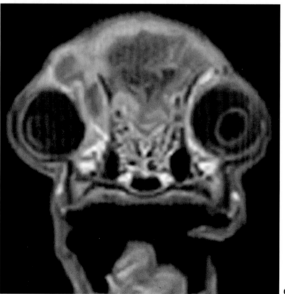

c

Fig. 6.37a–c
MRI of an adenocarcinoma in a dog with exophthalamus. (a) The fat-suppressed sequence in the dorsal projection (STIR) reveals a strongly hyperintense tumour, which extends from the orbit into the temporal musculature. (b) The T2w transverse sequence reveals extension of a patchy hyperintense tumour into the temporal musculature. (c) The cranial bones are intact.

of orbital disease, a correct diagnosis was possible in 22 cases based on the MRI results alone. Solid space-occupying processes with mass effect, with or with- out osteolysis of the surrounding bones, including the sinuses, maxillary recess, cribriform plate, presphenoid, palatine bones, and cranial fossa have all been described with tumours. This study and a series using 26 dogs and cats (159b), which had been examined using CT, demonstrated that involvement of orbital bone in the pathology is characteristic of a tumour. Contrast enhancement after intravenous gadolinium (MRI) administration or an iodine-containing contrast agent (CT) is not specific for

neoplasia and has been described as also occurring with inflammatory processes. The latter reveal themselves as diffuse, often very inhomogeneous areas in the region of the retrobulbar fat, eye musculature, adnexal structures and sometimes the mastication muscles. Fluid-filled pockets with ring-shaped contrast enhancement are indications of an abscess; usually the bony borders of the orbit remain intact. Visualisation of foreign bodies may be as easily achieved with ultrasonography as with MRI, but the extent of soft tissue reaction will be seen more accurately with MRI (160, 161).

6.5.3 Cranial cavity

The radiologically depictable processes in this region are confined to infections and tumours of the cranium, congenital malformations, disturbances in development, and fractures.

6.5.3.1 Middle and inner ear

Both species and breed specific differences must be taken into consideration in the assessment of the ear. In the cat, the osseous bulla has two compartments, whereas in brachycephalic dogs, it often appears small and deformed. The most common indication for an imaging investigation of the middle and inner ear is otitis media or otitis media / interna. Tumours of the middle and inner ear are very rare and these mainly involve invasion of tumours from the external auditory canal. Calcification and dystrophic ossification in the wall of the outer auditory canal are the sequelae to a chronic otitis externa. A narrow and irregularly demarcated auditory canal can be an indication of otitis or a tumour. Acute **otitis media / interna** is usually not depictable with conventional methods. With optimal radiographic techniques and by the comparison of both sides, a unilateral process can, in exceptional cases, be identified as a discrete diffuse increase in radiodensity (Fig. 6.38). Reduced contrast in comparison to the soft tissues, of the normally air-filled osseous bullae, can be seen in empyema, granulomatous processes, otopharyngeal polyps or tumours. Chronic inflammatory processes (see Fig. 15.2a) lead to sclerosis and roughened contours due to periosteal proliferation, occasionally with very extensive osteoneogenesis in the surrounding soft tissues. In destructive forms, osteolysis can predominate and destroy the wall of the bulla. Very extensive osteolysis, not only of the osseous bulla, but also of the base of the cranium and the zygomatic process, is more indicative of a tumour than an inflammatory process.

CT and MRI are the imaging modalities of choice for investigating the middle and inner ear; both are reasonably sensitive and specific for infections and tumours (see Figs. 6.39 and 15.2b). The bony structures of the middle and inner ear can be visualised in detail with CT (162). MRI signs indicative of otitis media / interna include: bulla filled with material that is isointense with its surroundings on T1w sequences but hyperintense on T2w sequences; the lining of the bulla may show a ring of contrast enrichment on the T1w sequence after contrast administration (163, 164) (Fig. 6.39). This is less obvious on CT due to the neighbouring radiopaque bone, although a fluid-filled bulla or one filled with soft tissue can be visualised with great certainty. NB: the thickness of the bone can be overestimated on CT when imaging a fluid-filled bulla; this phenomenon is especially obvious with large slice thicknesses and in the soft tissue window (165). Destruction of the bulla or hyperostosis can be seen in advanced cases (see Fig. 15.2). The membranous part of the labyrinth is normally seen as a Z-shaped hyperintense structure on transverse T2w sequences. In the dorsal sequence, the labyrinth can be seen as circular hyperintense structures (Fig. 6.39b). The lack of this

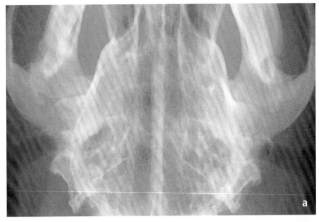
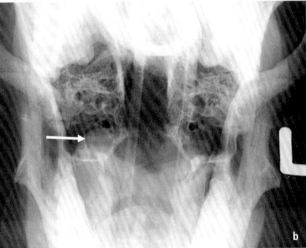

Fig. 6.38a, b
Acute otitis media (right) in a young crossbreed. (a) Dorsoventral and (b) frontal views. Apart from a discrete increase in density in the area of the right bulla (arrow), there are no other changes visible.

characteristic structure and contrast enhancement of the petrosal bone in T1w sequences are indications of otitis interna (Figs. 6.39b, c). Otitis media / interna can lead to destruction of the petrosal bone or it can penetrate the caudal cranial fossa via the internal auditory meatus. In such cases, imaging signs of meningitis or focal intracranial hyperintense lesions can be seen in the area of the brain stem or cerebellopontine angle on the T2w sequence (163).

6.5.3.2 Craniomandibular osteoarthropathy

Craniomandibular osteoarthropathy (CMO) is found more frequently in dog breeds such as the West Highland White, Scottish and Cairn Terriers, though it has also been described in other breeds such as the Boston Terrier, Bull Terrier, Doberman, Labrador Retriever and Great Dane. It is equivalent to human infantile hyperostosis. It rarely causes neurological symptoms but it can cause pain and osteoneogenesis in the

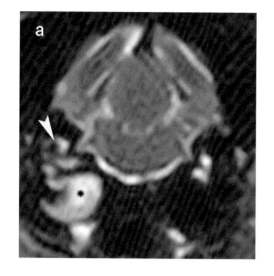

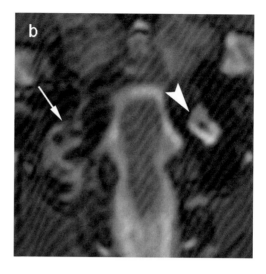

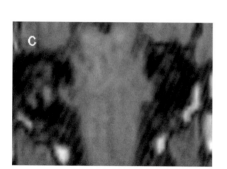

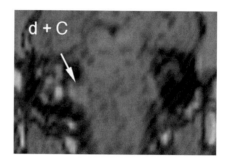

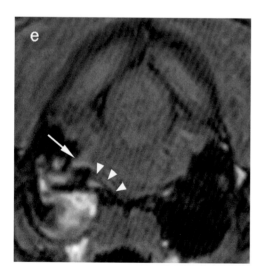

Figure 6.39a–e

Otis media and interna depicted by MRI. (a) In the T2w sequence, the right inner ear has a reduced signal intensity (white arrowhead). The ventral and caudal parts of the right bulla are filled with a hyperintense substrate (black star). (b) In the BASG – a fluid-sensitive sequence – the normal left bulla appears to have no signal, while the semicircular canals of the inner ear are signal rich (white arrowhead). The fluid-filled right bulla evinces a high signal intensity, while the semicircular canals appear to be signal poor (white arrow). (c, d) In the dorsal FE3DT1 MPR both the inner ear and the vestibulocochlear nerve have taken up an increased amount of contrast. A slight increased contrast uptake is also present focally in the meninges (only around the origin of the nerve; white arrow). (e) Transverse T1w sequence after the administration of contrast. The white arrow indicates the uptake of contrast by the inner ear, vestibulocochlear nerve, and the neighboring meninges (white arrowheads). The right bulla shows a high signal intensity.

area of the tympanic bulla and the lower jaw leading to a life-threatening "lock-jaw". The main imaging changes described include palisade-like osteoneogenesis in the region of the osseous bulla and the cranial calotte, which then regresses once growth has been completed. The long bones can also show periosteal deposits, which due to their position on the diaphysis must be differentiated from hypertrophic osteodystrophy (166, 167, 168).

A similar disease has been described in five- to ten-month-old Bull Mastiffs and has been designated as idiopathic hyperostosis of the cranial cavity. Irregular (sub)periosteal thickening of the frontal, temporal and occipital bones, including the bullae are seen on radiography. This disease is similar to CMO in that it is self-limiting (169). It should be differentiated from leukocyte adhesion protein deficiency (LAD), a deficiency in the immune system that leads to a similar radiological picture in the Irish setter.

6.5.3.3 Tumours of the calvarium

Tumours of the calvarium are not common. Osteosarcoma of the roof of the skull (10–15% of all osteosarcomas found on the skull) generally have osteoblastic characteristics. They are well demarcated and lead to proliferations that have a bony consistency. In comparison, in the region of the base of the skull, they are typically associated with more osteolytic changes; as a consequence of this and due to the complex anatomical relationships present in this area, they are difficult to depict using radiography. In other areas of the skull they behave as they do in the limbs.

Other primary tumours of the skull are rare and have only a minor significance. Osteomas are very radiopaque. Osteochondromas are the same as those found on the rest of the skeleton. Fibrosarcomas, chondrosarcomas and soft tissue tumours lead to focal lucency, although osteoneogenesis has also been observed with these types of tumour.

The multilobular osteochondrosarcoma is a tumour that more commonly affects larger dog breeds; it is rare in cats. This is known under a number of different names: multilobular osteoma, calcifying or juvenile aponeurotic fibroma or chondroma rodens. The tumour prefers the temporooccipital region, although other regions of the skull can be affected. It has a low metastasis rate. The animals affected are on average 7 years old (15 months to 12 years). Multilobular osteochondrosarcoma often appears on a radiograph as a large lobulated structure with a frost-like pattern of soft tissue mineralisation. The cranial bones lying under the tumour can demonstrate signs of osteolysis. CT and MRI (103) are the methods of choice for depicting the characteristic structure of this tumour, the extent of the osteolysis and the portion of the tumour that lies intracranially and which can lead to significant compression of the brain. The tumour strongly contrast enhances in its unmineralised areas (Figs. 6.5 and 6.40).

6.5.3.4 Metabolic disturbances

Metabolic diseases can lead to changes in the radiopacity and conformation of the skull. Different forms of **mucopolysaccharidosis** have been described in both species (cat and dog) and in different breeds (e.g. Type IV in the Siamese cat, Type I in the domestic cat). Independent of the type, these diseases cause neurological symptoms and varying degrees of deformation of the skull. The typical changes are short, wide maxillae with aplastic or hypoplastic frontal sinuses, sphenoidal sinuses and conchae (46).

A generalised reduced radiopacity is mainly due to a metabolic disturbance of the bones such as **osteofibrosis** as a consequence of hyperparathyroidism. Typical for this disease is a loss in trabecular structure, a broadening of the cortical bone, and an increase in fibrous tissue. The porosity of the bone leads to a so-called "salt and pepper" image.

6.5.3.5 Trauma

The radiographic diagnosis of **skull fractures** can be difficult. The extent and severity of the lesion are usually underestimated. Although fractures of the base of the skull are rarer than those of the dorsal skull bones, they have a greater clinical significance and are more difficult to depict radiologically. The exceptions to this are depressed fractures and comminuted fractures, e.g. due to bites. Fractures form straight, jagged or curved lines of radiolucency, which may be confused in the adult animal with open fontanelles and sutures. Skull fractures are often associated with damage to the soft tissues, intracranial haemorrhage and brain trauma, which can only be visualised using CT or MRI (Fig. 6.41). CT is a very sensitive method for imaging craniocerebral trauma. In most hospitals, CT is the imaging method of choice for the acute stage of head trauma due to its high sensitivity for fractures and the short acquisition times On the other hand, MRI has the same sensitivity for haemorrhage as CT, but it is much better than the latter in depicting diffuse axonal injuries. Axonal rupture occurs in human beings after trauma at the boundary of grey and white matter in the region of the corpus callosum, cerebrum, basal ganglia and the rostral brain stem (170).

Extradural haematomas form between the skull bones and the dura. With arterial bleeding, the dura separates from the underlying bone and leads to a concurrent compression of the brain. In CT, extradural haemorrhage can be seen as a biconvex lesion between the bones of the skull and the dura or brain. They are initially hyperdense a few hours after their start. Within 1 to 2 weeks, haemorrhage becomes iso- to hypodense and begins to shrink. The signal characteristics of haemorrhage on MRI depends on the concentration of haemoglobin and methaemoglobin, which alters with time.

Subdural haemorrhages behave similarly on CT and MRI. As they form in the virtual space between the dura and pia / arachnoidea, they are flatter than extradural haemorrhages. A

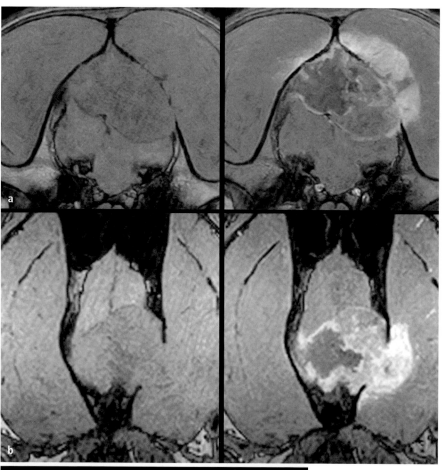

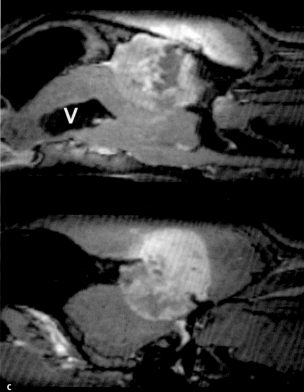

Fig. 6.40a–c
(a) Transverse and (b) dorsal MPI sequences before (left) and after gadolinium (right). (c) Reconstruction in the sagittal projection, paramedian. Giant lobulated temporal tumour with destruction of the cranial bones compatible with a multi-lobular osteochondroma; both extra- and intracranial tumour components are demonstrable. The tumour has a well-demarcated surface with irregular but strong contrast enhancement. Massive compression of the brain and dilatation of the left ventricle (V) due to obstruction of the ventricular system is also apparent.

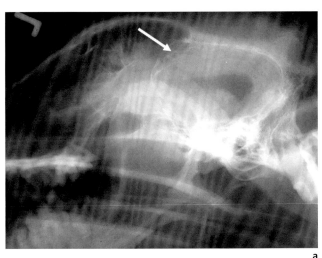
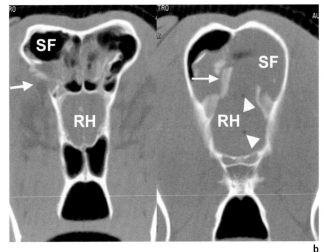

Fig. 6.41a, b
Cranial fracture and encephalitis: lateral radiography and CT of a Bernese Cattle Dog one month after trauma. (a) The radiograph shows an overshadowing of the frontal sinus which has the density of soft tissue and osteolysis of the inner surface of the frontal bone (arrow). The lateral ventricle is filled with gas. (b) The CT shows multiple fractures (arrows) in the region of the frontal sinus (SF) with a connection of the sinus to the rhinencephalon (RH). Soft tissue overshadowing of the frontal sinus with gas inclusions (arrowheads) in the region of the rhinencephalon. The pathological investigation revealed purulent-necrotising sinusitis and encephalitis.

6

recent sub-arachnoidal haemorrhage looks like hyperdense sulci and cisterns on CT. MRI is more sensitive for subacute and chronic haemorrhage (171). Further details on the imaging of haemorrhage with CT and MRI can be found in Chap. 6.5.5.2 and Table 6.8.

It is always advisable to examine the cervical vertebrae especially in an animal with severe neurological symptoms after head trauma, as concurrent fractures and luxations of the spine can substantially influence the prognosis.

6.5.3.6 Congenital malformations

Malformations of the skull can lead to changes in its shape and/or size. Hydrocephalus and malformations of the occipital region are the most common congenital malformations in the dog, but are both rare in cats. Some radiographic char-

acteristics are typical of **congenital hydrocephalus**: an enlarged intracranial volume; an obviously domed cranium; pronounced "flattening" of the back of the head; "compressed" frontal sinuses; the base of the skull is flattened and elongated; and the roof of the skull is thin. Additionally, the rugae that normally give the cranial cavity its characteristic shape are flattened, which gives it a uniform, frosted-glass-like appearance (Fig. 6.42). The fontanelles and sutures may still be open. On the VD view, the temporomandibular joints appear to be displaced medially. These changes are most obvious in congenital hydrocephalus; in acquired hydrocephalus these signs may not be present if the disease started after skeletal growth has stopped. The diagnosis and characterisation of the different types of hydrocephalus is possible with CT or MRI. If the fontanelles are open, then ultrasonography can be used and the size of the ventricles can be measured.

Table 6.8: MRI imaging of intracranial haemorrhage on spin echo sequences using 0.5T magnets

	Time post-haemorrhage	Iron localisation	T1w sequence	T2w sequence
Oxyhaemoglobin	A few hours	Intracellular	Slightly hypointense	Hyperintense
Deoxyhaemoglobin	Hours to day	Intracellular	Slightly hypointense	Very hypointense
Methaemoglobin	A few days	Intracellular	Very hyperintense	Very hypointense
Haemolysis	Days to months	Extracellular	Very hyperintense	Very hyperintense
Ferritin and haemosiderin	a few days to open-ended			
– centre		None	Hypointense	Hyperintense
– edge		Extracellular	Hypointense	Very hypointense

6

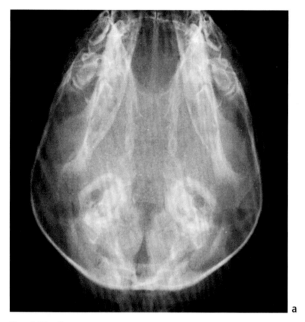

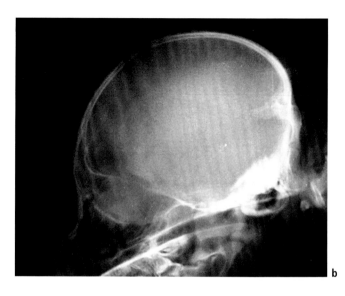

Fig. 6.42a, b

(a) Ventrodorsal and (b) lateral radiographs of severe congenital hydrocephalus. The cranium has a huge volume with compression of the frontal sinuses, straight base of the skull and frosted-glass-like bone structure (b). On the VD view, the middle ear region and the temporomandibular joints have been pushed medially. Open fontanelles and sutures can be seen.

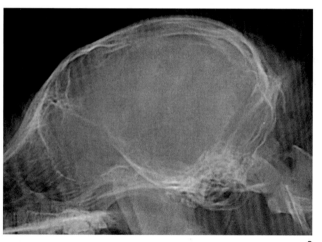

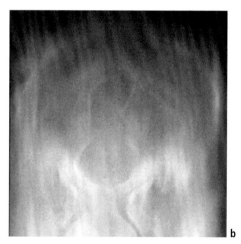

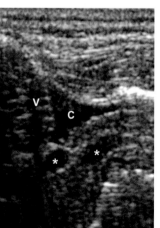

Fig. 6.43a–c

Occipital dysplasia in a Yorkshire Terrier. (a) Short caudal cranial fossa. (b) The foramen magnum is elongated and keyhole-shaped; it has been depicted using a modified frontal projection. (c) The ultrasonography scan in the sagittal section shows the cisterna magna (C), the vermis cerebelli (V) and syringohydromyelia (*).

Occipital dysplasia is malformation of the foramen magnum which occurs in various toy breeds such as the Yorkshire Terrier, Chihuahua and Toy Poodle. It is characterised by an elongated, key-hole-shaped foramen magnum, which can be visualised using a modified frontal radiographic projection. Disturbances in CSF flow may occur in association with this condition due to cerebellar herniation leading to a secondary obstructive hydrocephalus and syringohydromyelia (Fig. 6.43). However, although occipital dysplasia appears to be widely disseminated in small dog breeds, it is usually clinically silent (29).

Chiari malformation in human beings, describes caudal displacement of the cerebellum and syringohydromyelia, which may be accompanied by hydrocephalus. There is a comparable disease described in several small breeds of dog, most commonly the Cavalier King Charles Spaniel (see Fig. 17.5). A malformation of the occiput (occipital hypoplasia) results in an inappropriately small cranial fossa with caudal displacement of the cerebellum and medulla oblongata through the foramen magnum (herniation). This leads to obstruction of the cisterna magna, causing hydrocephalus and syringohydromyelia, most obviously in the cranial and caudal cervical and cranial thoracic regions. Dorsal angulation of the odontoid process has also been described in one Cavalier King Charles Spaniel. It remains unclear whether this was a part of the Chiari-like malformation or if it was an independent malformation of the dens or its ligaments (172, 173, 174). Malformation of the skull and cervical skeleton can be identified with CT, as can the dilated CSF spaces. Enlarged CSF spaces can be best seen on T2w sagittal MRI sequences, while the cerebellar herniation is better visualised on T1w sequences.

6.5.4 Intracranial tumours

6.5.4.1 General considerations
Intracranial tumours are rarely visible using conventional imaging methods. In cats, meningiomas occasionally cause thickening and sclerosis of the cranium overlying a superficial tumour. Enlarged and increased blood vessel outlines representing dilated meningeal arteries have been described. Rarely, osteolysis occurs with invasive forms of neoplasia. Mineralised opacities in the cranial cavity may indicate the presence of these tumours on radiographs. The information provided by a radiograph is, however, inadequate for precise diagnosis, prognosis and therapeutic planning.

CT and MRI are, at present, the most sensitive methods for the depiction of anatomical changes in the meninges, brain, ventricles, cranial nerves or blood vessels (see Chap. 6.2.4). CT and MRI can identify intracranial tumours based on their specific imaging characteristics (Table 6.7). Such characteristics include displacement and compression of normal structures due to mass effect, changes in the physical tissue density,

Table 6.9: The different types of intracranial space-occupying processes

Neoplastic	Non-neoplastic
■ Neuroepithelial tumours	■ Granuloma (GME)
■ Tumours of the nerve roots	■ Cyst
■ Pituitary tumours	■ Abscess
■ Meningioma	■ Infarct
■ Teratoma	■ Haematoma
■ Metastases	
■ Lymphoma	
■ Others	

oedema, damage to the local blood-brain barrier and a tendency for haemorrhage. MRI is better than CT in the diagnosis of brain disease due to its high resolution, which can be increased by choosing the most suitable sequences. Pathological cellular infiltrates can influence the signal intensity in the different sequences, such that even the presence of minimal oedema can be identified. However, there are lesions which are isointense to the surrounding tissues on practically all sequences and they can only be visualised following contrast administration.

For a lesion to be visualised using CT, it must affect the absorption of the x-ray beam. Before the application of contrast, the majority of tumours are isodense to normal brain tissue. However, CT can fail to identify some slow-growing tumours, such as infiltrative gliomas, because the tumour remains isodense following contrast administration due to an intact blood-brain barrier. Very small tumours can also remain undiscovered. Concentration of the CT x-ray beam in areas of very dense bone makes assessment of the brain stem, cerebellum and medulla oblongata very difficult. The following summary of tumour characteristics on CT and MRI is based not only on the general literature, but also on the descriptions given by KRAFT and GAVIN (174), THOMAS et al. (175, 176) and MOORE et al. (177). It should be noted that not all space-occupying lesions are of neoplastic origin: malformations, inflammations or vascular diseases can also be associated with mass effects (Table 6.9).

The **assessment criteria** used to determine the presence of tumours include the number of lesions, their origin, anatomical position, shape, contours, density (CT number) or signal intensity, their effects on the surrounding tissues (mass effects, oedema) and their behaviour after the application of an intravenous contrast agent (Tables 6.7 and 6.10).

CT and MRI results
The majority of primary tumours arising in the brain are solitary; exceptions to this are the meningioma in the cat and lymphomas, which can be multiple. Brain metastases of other tumours can form individual foci or multiple lesions. Meningeal infiltrations (leptomeninges and dura) may be seen with intracranial metastases of lymphosarcomas.

Table 6.10: Differential diagnosis based on the signal intensity after administration of an intravenous contrast agent

Type of tumour	Contrast enhancement	
Meningioma	+++	Uniform or ring-shaped
Plexus papilloma	+++	Uniform
Astrocytoma, glioma	+ to +++	Uniform or ring-shaped
Nerve root tumours	++ to +++	Uniform
Pituitary adenoma	+ to +++	Uniform or ring-shaped
Pituitary carcinoma	+ to +++	Nonuniform
Tumour of the nasal cavities	+ to +++	Nonuniform
Granuloma	+ to +++	Variable

6

The classification of brain lesions based on their localisation is disputed in the veterinary medical literature. NYKAMP et al. (65) reject the frequently used classification of intra- and extra-axial lesions and use intra- and extramedullary instead. The latter terms are, however, of little use in intracranial disease. The authors of this book follow the classification of KRAFT and THOMAS (174, 175, 176), whereby intracranial tumours are differentiated according to their location as either intra- or extra-axial tumours. Intra-axial tumours are neuroepithelial tumours arising from the brain tissue, such as astrocytoma (see Fig. 18.25) oligodendroglioma (Figs. 6.8 and 6.44), and medulloblastoma. They all develop from a point within the brain and grow outwards. In comparison, extra-axial tumours such as meningioma, pituitary tumours, and nerve sheath tumours or choroid plexus tumours (see Fig. 18.27) either grow inwards from the outside of the brain or compress it from the outside. The exceptions to this generalisation are ependymomas and choroid plexus tumours, which are technically extra-axial tumours but which grow outward in most cases, especially when they have a lateral ventricle origin. Metastases are often intra-axial tumours.

The anatomical location of a tumour in the cranial cavity often provides important information about its origin. The most common tumours of the ventricular system are ependymomas or choroid plexus tumours; those in the hypophyseal fossa are pituitary tumours, meningiomas or nasal tumours that have penetrated the cribriform plate and which have components both inside and outside of the cranial cavity. Extra-axial, well-demarcated, space-occupying lesions in the cerebellopontine angle are commonly meningiomas, choroid plexus tumours or nerve sheath tumours of the trigeminal nerve (see Fig. 17.3). Widening of the canal of the trigeminal nerve and a unilateral atrophy of the temporalis and masseter muscles are important and usually obvious indicators of the latter tumours (178).

However, the anatomical location is obviously not 100% indicative of the type of tumour present; meningiomas can occur in virtually all regions of the cranium. They can often be difficult to differentiate from pituitary tumours (Fig. 6.45) and choroid plexus papillomas. In addition to the convexities,

frequent origins of meningiomas include the diaphragma sellae and the tentorial notch. Metastases and lymphoma are other types of tumour which may occupy any anatomical location (Table 6.11).

The **shape of a tumour** can be described as oval, broad-based or plaque-like, and this can also indicate a tumour's origin. A broad-based or plaque-like tumour sitting on the base of the skull is often a meningioma, especially when it has a contrast-enhanced extension into the surrounding meninges (so-called dural tail) (179) (Fig. 6.46). Pituitary tumours have a round or oval shape in a characteristic location. Ependymomas and choroid plexus tumours are well-demarcated, round to irregularly shaped tumours with connections to the ventricular system. Astrocytomas, oligodendrogliomas and lymphosarcomas have variable shapes – from well demarcated and round to totally amorphous and not demarcated.

The growth of a tumour depends on its type and dynamics. This can best be visualised using MRI. Tumours that grow slowly and expansively, such as meningiomas or plexus tumours, lead to a displacement and compression of the neighbouring structures, whereas aggressive grade IV astrocytomas or nasal adenocarcinomas infiltrate the brain tissue and replace it. Accordingly, a tumour can be identified as a structure that is well demarcated from normal brain tissue, as abnormal brain architecture, or only as an abnormal signal intensity on MRI.

CT number and MRI signal intensity. On CT, the majority of tumours are isodense to normal brain tissue prior to the administration of contrast. Due to their higher physical density, they can be differentiated from tissue necrosis or surrounding oedema, which appear hypodense. Other secondary signs of neoplasia include haemorrhage and mineralisation, which appear hyperdense on CT. On MRI, many tumours are hypointense in T1w sequences and hyperintense in T2w sequences. This is particularly true of aggressive tumours that originate in the brain and metastases as they are strongly hyperintense in T2w sequences. Exceptions to this rule are the more benign extra- and intra-axial tumours, which are isointense on T1w sequences without contrast and so are not as easily visualised.

Space-occupying lesions in the brain usually lead to changes in the surrounding parenchyma. **Mass effect** is characterised by oedema, displacement and compression or destruction of neighbouring anatomical structures. Oedema is hypodense on CT, hypointense on T1w MRI sequences and hyperintense on T2w sequences. It can be differentiated from CSF and other fluids (e.g. cyst fluid) by using specific inversion recovery sequences (e.g., FLAIR). The extent of the oedema can vary greatly with the type of space-occupying process, and less so with the size of the lesion.

Metastases often have significant peri-lesional oedema despite their modest size, just like some nonneoplastic processes such as brain abscesses (Figs. 6.9, 6.47 and 6.50). Cysts can be as-

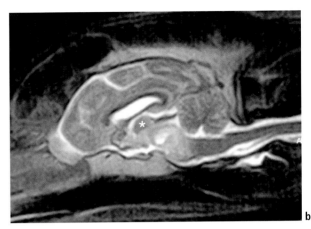

Fig. 6.44a, b
Brain stem glioma. (a) Sagittal T1w sequence after gadolinium and (b) T2w sequence (same case as in Fig. 6.8). On the T1w plain study (Fig. 6.8), the intra-axial lesion is isointense to the surrounding brain tissue. After contrast, the glioma shows a strong, ring-shaped area of contrast enhancement on the T1w sequence. On the T2w sequence, there is extensive perifocal oedema revealed as a diffuse hyperintensity of the hypothalamus going up and into the pons. Due to the lesion's mass effects the interthalamic adhesion (*) is deformed and the third ventricle is compressed.

sociated with many different types of tumours (most commonly with meningiomas) and can be well defined by CT or MRI. Tumours anywhere in the ventricular system can lead to hydrocephalus. Haemorrhage is hyperdense on CT, but on MRI their characteristics depend on the age of the haemorrhage (Table 6.8) and on the type of the magnet used. Mineralisation can be demonstrated well with both techniques, as can bony proliferation, sclerosis or osteolysis secondary to tumour growth.

Contrast investigations are an integral part of a CT examination as many pathological processes can only be seen with contrast enhancement. Contrast agents also play an important role in MRI as the grade and type of contrast enhancement give an indication about the nature of the tumour. The blood-brain barrier prevents the penetration of contrast agents into the brain tissue and so stops the increase in density or signal intensity on CT or MRI, respectively. In many tumours and some nonneoplastic processes, the blood-brain barrier is disturbed and allows the uptake of contrast. Tumours follow certain rules with respect to their contrast enhancement; however, there are many exceptions. As extra-axial tumours arise from tissues which do not have a blood-brain barrier, they usually show very strong contrast enhance-

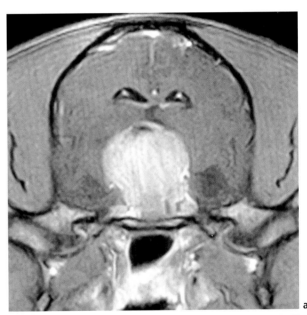

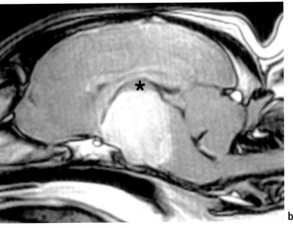

Fig. 6.45a, b
Pituitary adenocarcinoma in an eight-year-old male dog. (a) Transverse and (b) sagittal T1w sequences after gadolinium. The broad-based, semi-spherical extra-axial tumour lies over the bone above the central cranial fossa and extends laterally and caudally over the sella. On the plain sequence (not shown), the tumour is hypointense, but after contrast it demonstrates strong contrast enhancement and is sharply demarcated. There is no oedema around the tumour. Mass effect is present with displacement and compression of the hypothalamus, thalamus, third ventricle and the interthalmic adhesion (*).

Table 6.11: CT and MRI characteristics of common brain tumours

a) Meningiomas
- Solitary (multiple) extra-axial – intracranial
- Arise from dura including cerebral falx (hypophyseal fossa, ventricle)
- Smooth or irregular contours, demarcation good to poor
- Broad-based, plaque-like, rarely round
- Mass effect: oedema +/–
- CT: iso- to hyperdense
- MRI: T1w = isointense; T2w = iso- to hyperintense
- Signal increase after contrast: ++, uniform, sometimes ring-shaped

b) Pituitary tumours
- Solitary
- Arise from hypophyseal fossa
- Smooth or irregular, well demarcated
- Round (adenoma) or broad-based (adenocarcinoma)
- Mass effect: oedema +/–
- CT: iso- to hyperdense
- MRI: T1w or T2w = iso- to hyperintense
- Signal increase after contrast: +++, homogenous in adenoma, irregular in adenocarcinoma. Dynamic contrast examination: behaviour dependent on vascularisation (arterial or portal system)

c) Glioma, astrocytoma
- Intra-axial, diencephalon and cerebrum, often in the frontal lobes
- Well demarcated and round to very irregular and poorly demarcated
- Mass effect: oedema +/–
- CT: iso- to hyperdense
- MRI: T1w = hypointense, possibly inhomogeneous; T2w = hyperintense, inhomogeneous
- Extreme contrast enhancement may be an indicator of high degree of malignancy

d) Choroid plexus tumours, ependyoma
- Localised in ventricle system, most commonly in fourth ventricle. Can lie extra-axially in the lateral aperture of the fourth ventricle
- Demarcation good to poor
- MRI: T1w = hypointense; T2w = hyperintense
- Compression of fourth ventricle may lead to hydrocephalus

e) Medulloblastoma
- Cerebellum, cerebellopontine angle
- Young animals

f) Metastases
- Intra-axial
- Round, well demarcated
- Mass effect: often extreme oedema
- MRI: T1w = hypointense; T2w = hyperintense
- Multiple lesions possible

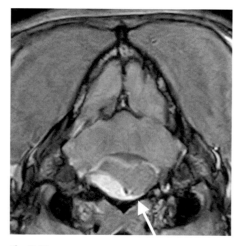

Fig. 6.46
Transverse T1w sequence after contrast (gadolinium): a dural tail (arrow) is present in this basally located meningioma.

Microadenomas of the pituitary also demonstrate a typical contrast enhancement pattern. Due to their unique blood supply, they have a slightly delayed uptake of contrast in comparison to normal pituitary tissue. This was seen in earlier imaging methods as a filling defect due to the dynamic imaging process.

The degree and pattern of contrast enhancement is very variable in intra-axial tumours. Benign variants can show every degree of enhancement from none to strong. The aggressive forms of such tumours usually demonstrate a very inhomogeneous uptake due to the presence of necrosis, haemorrhage or cysts, or they may have ring enhancement. Ring-shaped contrast enhancement is neither specific for a particular type of tumour nor is it indicative of a tumour. Table 6.12 lists the most important differential diagnoses for a ring-shaped pattern. Inflammatory or neoplastic infiltration of the meninges (e.g. by lymphosarcoma metastases) can also result in an increase in contrast enhancement, for which MRI is more sensitive than CT.

Unique imaging characteristics have been seen in association with meningio-angiomastosis, a disease that has only been described in four dogs. This is a benign, space-occupying process with expansile growth, located in the cerebrum or brain stem. It is not clear whether this is a dysontogenetic tumour such as a haemangioma, a leptomeningeal meningioma or a vascular malformation (180). In contrast to the infiltrative meningioma however, the brain is not infiltrated by this disease. These tumours can be clearly depicted both with CT and MRI (hyperintense on T2w sequences). They can be partially mineralised and have perifocal oedema. They also show contrast enhancement. Specific differentiation from meningiomas and other tumours based on the CT and MRI results is not possible.

ment; but this is not always uniform, and inhomogeneous, patchy patterns are quite common. Meningiomas can demonstrate a ring-shaped uptake of contrast even without the formation of cysts (Tables 6.10 and 6.12). A linear area of contrast in the dura adjacent to an extra-axial space-occupying lesion is known as a dural tail and occurs primarily with meningiomas, though it can occasionally be seen with inflammatory processes or other types of neoplasia (Fig. 6.46). The cause of this sign has been explained as being a migration of tumour cells into the dura or possibly an excessive vascular reaction (179).

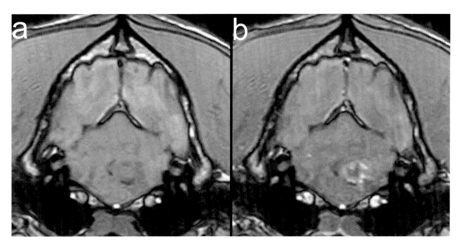

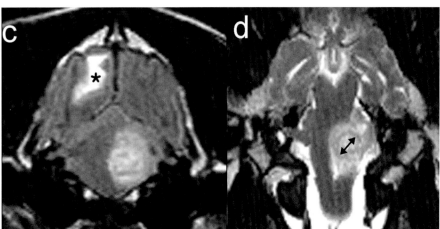

Fig. 6.47a–d
Metastases of a haemangiosarcoma with extensive perifocal oedema in a ten-year-old Setter. Transverse T1w sequence before (a) and after (b) gadolinium; transverse FLAIR (c) and dorsal T2w sequences (d). A hypointense focus in the brain stem can be seen on the plain T1w sequence (a), which takes on a ring of contrast appearance (b) after gadolinium. In the white matter of the right cerebrum there is a markedly hyperintense region that represents oedema (c, *). Extensive perifocal oedema is also present in the brain stem and the cerebellum, and can be seen as a hyperintense band (arrows) around the tumour on the dorsal T2w sequence (d).

Other sporadic malformation tumours include (*inter alia*) dermoid and epidermoid cysts as well as craniopharyngiomas. Dermoid and epidermoid cysts are iso- to hypodense on CT and cannot be differentiate from one other. They can be differentiated using MRI based on the difference in their contents. The contents of epidermoid cysts have a signal intensity similar to that of CSF, while dermoid cysts have fatty contents which are hyperintense on T1w sequences. In addition, the latter have a heterogenous structure and due to their lack of vasculature, they do not take up any contrast (181, 182).

Table 6.12: Differential diagnosis of ring-shaped increases in signal intensity after administration of a contrast agent

- Abscess
- Astrocytoma
- Cyst
- Granuloma
- Meningioma (rarely)
- Metastasis
- Oligodendroglioma

6.5.5   Non-neoplastic diseases of the brain

Acquired space-occupying lesions of non-neoplastic origin such as hydrocephalus, cysts, haemorrhage / haematomas, infarcts, granulomas (GME) and abscesses can be depicted with CT and MRI, but not with conventional radiography. Many of these conditions cause characteristic changes which enable a definitive diagnosis to be made.

6.5.5.1   Malformations
Congenital malformations of the brain, such as internal and external hydrocephalus, can be visualised with CT and MRI independent of the cause (obstructive / non-obstructive). However, there is great variation in the size of the lateral ventricles in the dog. The normal differences between the individual breeds and head shapes make differentiation between clinically and non-clinically significant enlargement of the ventricular system difficult. There are large differences between the absolute and relative sizes of the ventricles (as a percentage of the brain surface) between breeds; however, the

6

exact size at which a ventricle can be called abnormal in animals of the same breed is unknown (183).

Measurements of the lateral ventricles are usually undertaken in transverse CT or MRI slices at the level of the interthalamic adhesion. The ventricle size is most often given as the ratio between the ventricular diameter and the brain diameter. A relative ventricular diameter of 0–14% is considered normal; 15–25% as moderate and > 25% as severe hydrocephalus (184). Significant differences between the right and left lateral ventricles can occur in various breeds (e.g. Labrador Retriever) that are without any clinical consequence and are not associated with the inheritable epilepsy found in these breeds (185).

Hydrocephalus *ex vacuo* represents brain atrophy with dilated ventricles and a dilated subarachnoid space (external hydrocephalus). In obstructive hydrocephalus, the portion of the ventricular system rostral to the obstruction is dilated; however, obstructive hydrocephalus can only be confirmed when the obstruction itself is proven, e.g. in the form of an aqueductal stenosis due to a neoplastic or inflammatory process (ependymitis) (Fig. 6.35). Acute obstructive hydrocephalus with increased intra-ventricular pressure can lead to periventricular oedema, which can be seen on MRI as hypointense on T1w sequences and hyperintense in T2w and FLAIR sequences. In experimentally induced hydrocephalus, this oedema starts along the dorsolateral contours of the lateral ventricles (186, 187). The well-known complications of hydrocephalus in human beings of chronic haemorrhaging and subdural haematomas have recently been described in a two-month-old Newfoundland (65). The relative ventricular diameter was 80% in this dog; the septum pellucidum was missing and both lateral ventricles communicated with each other. The haematomas were seen as large, broad-based convex structures sitting on the cranium causing mass effect. These structures did not show any contrast enhancement and did not have any relationship to the skull sutures.

Dandy-Walker Malformations of different types occur in human beings, dogs and other animals. Typical for this condition in humans is an enlargement of the caudal cranial fossa, but this has not been described in the dog. In comparison, hypoplasia of the cerebellar vermis, cystic dilatation of the fourth ventricle and very small hypoplastic cerebellar hemispheres have also been described in the dog. CT and MRI can visualise these specific changes with great sensitivity. Other sporadically occurring malformations are of little clinical significance.

Intracranial intra-arachnoid cysts are known to occur in the dog and cat. They are dysontogenetic malformations. They frequently occur in the area of the tentorium cerebelli. An arachnoid cyst is a thin-walled, well-demarcated, fluid-filled cavity which often has a triangular cross-section. The fluid is isodense to CSF in CT and it has a very similar signal intensity to CSF in all sequences on MRI. The capsule does

not frequently take up contrast. The degree of compression of neighbouring structures depends on the size of the cyst and this may or may not be associated with clinical signs. If compression of the CSF channels accompanies the presence of a cyst then hydrocephalus may develop (188, 189).

Holoprosencephaly (lack of or inadequate lateral division of the proencephalon) can appear as a "mono"-ventricle if there is complete lack of the septum pellucidum. Hydranencephaly and porencephaly are other rarely seen malformations that lead to an abnormal collection of CSF. In contrast to hydrocephalus, there is destruction of the cerebral cortex in hydranencephaly. The cystic malformations seen in porencephaly are most probably due to intrauterine ischemic necroses.

Cerebellar hypoplasia in the cat caused by an intrauterine infection with the panleucopaenia virus is the best described but not only form of cerebellar hypoplasia. In the dog, it is presumed that in addition to intrauterine infections, inheritable factors are also involved. Cerebellar hypoplasia can lead to a "flattening" of the caudal cranium, which can be seen on a radiograph. CT and MRI can depict the abnormally small cerebellum or even its absence, as well as the CSF filling the residual cavity in the cranial fossa (see Fig. 16.7).

Malformations of cranial blood vessels have been described in both the dog and cat, whereby they are mostly arterial in nature. Clinical symptoms occur mainly when such malformations lead to haemorrhage. Such haemorrhages can be depicted using CT or MRI (see Chap. 6.5.5.2). Contrast investigations can help to directly visualise the malformation. Depending on the sequence, circumscribed foci may occur in MRI either without any signal (signal or flow void) or with massively increased signal intensity. Venous, capillary or cavernous malformations are rare. In the latter, focal hyperdense regions with variable mineralisation and only slight contrast enhancement can be seen on CT. In MRI, the focus presents with mixed signal intensity (methaemoglobin), surrounded by hypointense rings (due to ferritin and haemosiderin). Large and tortuous blood vessels are always an indicator of vessel malformation, though these signs may be missing due to thrombosis or compression of the vessels.

6.5.5.2 Haemorrhage and haematomas

Intracranial haemorrhage and haematomas can have various causes. CT and MRI are not only sensitive in proving the presence of a haemorrhage, but they can also classify it as extradural, subdural, subarachnoidal, intraventricular or intracerebral. The most sensitive method for an acute haemorrhage is CT. The attenuation of the x-ray beam increases linearly with the haematocrit. With a haematocrit of 46%, the attenuation is roughly 56 HU. The grey matter has, in comparison, an attenuation of 37–41 HU, and the white matter 20–34 HU. An acute haemorrhage in a patient with a normal haematocrit, therefore, is seen as hyperdense. During the next 72 hours, the density increases and then decreases from the periphery inwards due to lysis and resorption until after about 1 month, when it is isodense to the brain tissue. An acute haemorrhage is often surrounded by a hypodense region: an area of oedema. Mass effect can also be present. Contrast investigation of acute haemorrhage is not indicated, although it can help to identify the cause of the haemorrhage, e.g. tumour-associated bleeding. In the resorption phase, a ring of contrast enhancement can be observed between approx. weeks 2 and 6 (190, 191).

The signal in MRI images depends on various factors such as age of the hemorrhage, its origin (arterial or venous), its localization, and the cause of the hemorrhage. In addition, the signal is also affected by the strength of the magnetic field and the chosen sequence. Gradient echo sequences are now standardly performed in most MRI protocols as acute haemorrhage will result in a signal void which can help in its differentiation from other mass lesions. The chemical form and type of bonding of the iron in the erythrocytes that have left the blood vessels also determines the type of signal. Oxyhemoglobin is converted via deoxyhemoglobin and methemoglobin into ferritin and hemosiderin and this significantly influences the various effects responsible for the type of signal (e.g. paramagnetism). A detailed discussion of these effects and their consequences would be outside the bounds of this book; however, a good discussion can be found in THOMAS (175). Table 6.8 shows the results of these effects on the images in T1w and T2w sequences.

The differentiation of tumour-associated haemorrhage and other causes is often not easy. Contrast administration can reveal the presence of a tumour. A secondary effect which often accompanies a tumour is the presence of persistent oedema. However, oedema due to other causes is resorbed during the subacute to chronic phases. The hypointense edge, indicative of a subacute or chronic haematoma, is missing with tumour-induced haemorrhage due to the continual disturbance of the blood-brain barrier by the tumour. The images of such haemorrhages also tend to be more heterogeneous. Follow-up investigations can therefore provide important information about the cause of any haemorrhage.

6.5.5.3 Infarcts

Infarcts can be visualised by CT or MRI independent of their origin. Within hours of the insult, oedema develops in many cases which can be seen on CT as a hypodense region with a slight mass effect. This reaches a maximum after 3 to 5 days and is resorbed within 2 to 3 weeks. A peripheral, ring-shaped region of contrast enhancement that represents the ingrowth of capillaries without a blood-brain barrier can occur from 1 to 7 days after the infarct, and usually persists for weeks. It seems that haemorrhagic infarcts tend to show contrast enhancement more often than nonhaemorrahgic ones. In the chronic phase, after approx. 3 to 4 weeks, the infarct becomes more demarcated due to the resorption of necrotic tissue. The final stage of many infarcts is reduction in

volume with a widening of the neighbouring sulci or ventricle. Within an hour of a vessel being blocked by embolus or thrombus, an infarct can be seen due to the associated increased signal intensity in T2w, Proton-weighted or FLAIR sequences on MRI (see Fig. 18.6). Small infarcts and ones in the brain stem are better visualised with MRI compared to CT. Within 24 hours, the signal intensity on T2w and proton-weighted sequences will continue to increase, while it is slightly reduced on the T1w sequence. Oedema and mass effect increase during the first 3 to 7 days. Contrast enhancement appears after 3 to 4 days and may last up to approx. 3 to 4 weeks after the vascular obstruction. Infarcts are often wedge-shaped corresponding to the area supplied by the affected blood vessel(s).

Due to reperfusion of damaged blood vessels following an ischemic infarct, **haemorrhagic infarcts** can occur, which are hyperdense on CT. However, due to signal summation with associated hypodense oedema, neutralisation of the CT signal can result in a lesion which appears isodense to the surrounding brain tissue. The mass effect of the associated oedema, however, can reveal the presence of the lesion. A massive haemorrhage leads to a hyperdense centre with a hypodense "halo". On MRI, haemorrhagic infarcts are similar to intracerebral haemorrhage in that they have a mixed signal intensity. Infarcts are often restricted to the dependent territory of a blood vessel. Reduction in volume of the lesion during the chronic phase of recovery also helps to differentiate an infarct from tumour-associated bleeding (192, 193).

6.5.5.4 Polio- and leukoencephalomalacia

Ischemia due to an accumulation of cytotoxic substances, disturbed brain metabolism and/or perfusion during prolonged epileptic seizures can lead to foci of necrosis in various areas of the brain. The hippocampus, brain stem nuclei, piriform lobe and the frontal lobes appear to be most commonly affected. These lesions are apparently reversible (193).

Polioencephalomalacia can be a consequence of lead or cyanide intoxication, thiamine deficiency, hypoglycaemia, distemper, cardiac arrest or the ligation of portosystemic shunts. It often remains unclear whether polioencephalomalacic foci are the cause or consequence of epileptic seizures. The foci develop as described above for oedema formation on MRI, i.e. first of all they are iso- or slightly hypointense on the T1w sequence and hyperintense on the T2w sequences. After 11 to 19 days, the lesions become slightly hyperintense on T1w sequences, though they remain hyperintense in the T2w ones. The lesions also show contrast enhancement after the application of a paramagnetic contrast agent. Cortical lesions remain hyperintense on the T1w and T2w sequences, and show a variable degree of contrast enhancement.

These characteristics on the T1w sequence can persist for months before they "fade". Deep subcortical lesions of the white matter can be seen as hypointense foci on T1w se-

6

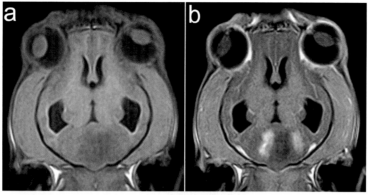

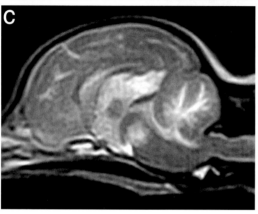

Fig. 6.48a–c
Necrotising encephalitis in a Yorkshire Terrier. Dorsal T1w sequence, before (a) and after (b) gadolinium as well as a sagittal T2w sequence (c). Poorly demarcated hypointense lesion in the mesencephalon on the T1w sequence (a), which shows peripheral foci of contrast enhancement after the intravenous administration of gadolinium, which also makes the hypointensity in the centre of the lesion more prominent (b). Markedly hyperintense foci without any recognisable mass effect are seen on the T2w sequence. The dilated lateral ventricle is most probably congenital and has no clinical significance. Note the very hyperintense cerebellar *arbor vitae*.

quences and hyperintense on T2w sequences after 3 to 4 weeks, which become even stronger with time. Proton-weighted sequences can strengthen the contrast of cortical lesions. The hyperintensity seen on the T1w sequence in the chronic stage may be due to so-called gitter cells (lipid-filled macrophages) or increased protein content.

6.5.5.5 Inflammation and infection

Changes in the brain and meninges due to infectious and other inflammatory diseases can be visualised using CT or MRI. The most important ones clinically are meningitis, encephalitis and granulomas due to different causes as well as bacterial encephalitis / brain abscess. Experimentally induced **meningitis** in the dog has a similar picture as bacterial meningitis in human beings. Both CT and MRI are usually normal prior to the application of contrast. A slight dilatation of the CSF-filled spaces and cerebral oedema have been described in association with severe meningitis, but they are non-specific findings that can also occur with other diseases of the brain. Contrast enhancement of the meninges can be seen with meningitis which is better visualised with MRI than CT (195). A differentiation of the dura and arachnoidea from the pia mater is possible as the pia lies close to the brain surface and within the sulci between the individual gyri. A re-

cent study in 15 dogs and 3 cats described contrast enhancement of the pia in five cases and of the dura in 13 cases. The causes included meningitis in 5 cases (bacterial, cryptococcal and plasmacytic), otitis which had broken through into the cranial cavity in 4 cases, GME in 2 cases, FIP in 1 case and 6 cases of tumour (5 with lymphosarcomas / leukaemia). Depending on the cause and severity, the contrast enhancement varied from a fine line to a very strong, almost patchy increase (196).

Chronic **distemper encephalitis** can be seen on CT as hypodense foci, especially in the white matter; however, the lesions are not specific for this disease. In MRI, the foci are hypointense on T1w sequences and hyperintense on T2w sequences. The lesions take up contrast either homogenously or in a ring. There may be oedema at the edge of the lesions and mass effect can be seen.

The central form of **FIP** leads to pyogranulomatous lesions in the ependyma, choroid and meninges.

Ependymitis can lead to a disturbance in the CSF drainage in the area of the aqueduct and fourth ventricle, with the development of an internal hydrocephalus, which can be depicted on both CT and MRI. The ependymitis, choroiditis and

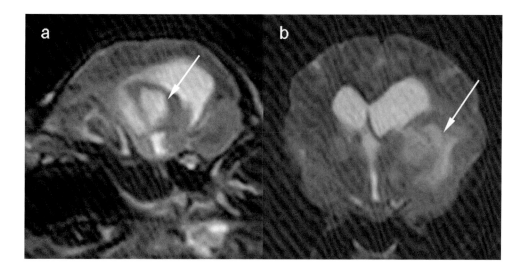

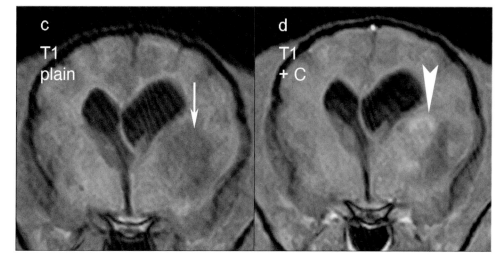

6

Figure 6.49a–d
Three-year-old Yorkshire Terrier with dilated lateral ventricles and granulomatous meningoencephalitis. (a, b) Multiple hyperintense foci are present in the cerebrum (mainly on the left), thalamus (bilateral), and in the left brain stem (white arrows) in these T2w sequences.
(c) In the native T1w sequence, the foci are hypointense to isointense (white arrow) with a slight mass effect. (d) After the administration of contrast, the foci appear as inhomogeneous, patchy areas of contrast (white arrowhead).

meningitis can be seen on the T2w sequence on MRI as a hyperintense border on the brain parenchyma that shows contrast enhancement after gadolinium administration

The acute stage of **necrotising encephalitis** found in the Pug, Maltese Terrier, Yorkshire Terrier and Chihuahua is seen as rather unspecific changes like acute infarcts or other forms of encephalitis. The foci are hypodense on CT and are mainly located in the cerebral hemispheres. A CT investigation of three Yorkshire Terriers revealed no mass effect or contrast enhancement associated with the lesions (197). On MRI, the acute stage appears hyperintense on T2w or inversion recovery sequences, and hypointense on the T1w sequence. The contrast enhancement seen is usually minimal. Initially, the mass effect can be significant due to peri-lesional oedema. In the chronic form, necrotising and cystic foci dominate. These are hypodense and similar to CSF on CT, whereas they are highly hyperintense in T2w and proton-weighted sequences, and just as obviously hypointense in the

T1w sequence. The lesions are usually found periventricular in the white matter – and additionally, often in the brain stem (in the Yorkshire Terrier, Fig. 6.48). Contrast enhancement is rare, though in positive cases it can be ring-shaped. Mass effect is no longer present and due to the loss in brain volume, the opposite effect may occur as shown by a widening of the CSF-filled spaces. Such lesions should be differentiated from chronic infarcts. In contrast to infarcts, these foci are not just associated with the territories supplied by blood vessels (198).

In the disseminated form of **GME**, multiple, poorly demarcated foci are formed in the parenchyma and meninges. They are associated with a poorly demarcated contrast enhancement. Some foci may be associated with mass effect and oedema (Fig. 6.49).

The focal form of GME leads to the formation of hyperdensities in the cerebrum and in the transitional area between the cerebellum and medulla. These can present as iso-

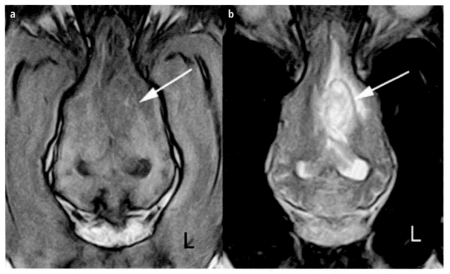

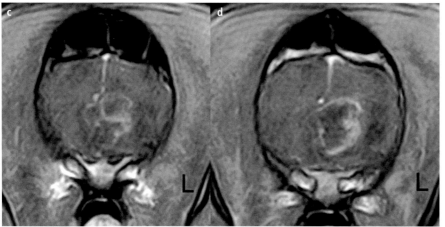

Fig. 6.50a–d
Brain abscess. Dorsal T1w (a) and T2w (b) sequences; transverse T1w sequences after contrast (c, d). (a) Extensive hypointense focus in the left forebrain in the T1w sequence with moderate mass effect. Weakly hyperintense capsule-like structure (arrow) is shown, which is hyperintense on the T2w sequence (b, arrow). The abscess shows a ring of contrast enhancement (c, d). In these sequences, the central necrosis and the extensive perifocal oedema is especially obvious. See also Fig. 6.9.
(Figures from SEILER et al. 2001 [201]; with kind permission from Blackwell Publ.)

or hyperdense on CT, whereas they are hypo- or isointense on T1w MRI sequences and hyperintense on T2w (see Fig. 17.2) and proton-weighted sequences. Contrast enhancement after the administration of a paramagnetic contrast agent is very variable: from no increase to homogeneous increase to a ring of contrast. Mass effect and oedema can occur as with other space-occupying processes (tumours and inflammation) (199).

The development stages of a bacterial encephalitis into an **abscess** can be followed using either CT or MRI (Figs. 6.9 and 6.50). Acute encephalitis appears on CT as an irregular, poorly demarcated and hypodense focus. The dynamic contrast enhancement after the administration of an intravenous contrast agent shows a characteristic behaviour pattern. In the early sequences, there is a ring-shaped area of contrast enhancement. With time, the contrast diffuses into the centre of the lesion until the lesion is completely filled. On MRI, the signal intensity on T2w sequences is hyperin-

tense and irregular with blurred and irregular contours. It can only be differentiated from the somewhat more homogeneous oedema with great difficulty. A space-occupying effect is usual. The contrast enhancement is diffuse and irregular. Later, central necrosis occurs and the formation of a capsule with an ingrowth of blood vessels takes place. An abscess is typically hypointense on T1w sequences, and isointense or slightly hyperintense on T2w sequences. The centre of the abscess can consist of a number of concentric rings, which may represent the different layers of cell populations and necrotic tissue. This layer phenomenon is typical of an abscess. The signal characteristics of the capsule (hypointense on T2w sequences and hyperintense in T1w sequences) is not normally found with tumours. An abscess is normally accompanied by a profound peri-lesional oedema, which is markedly hyperintense on the T2w sequence. A ring of contrast enhancement can be seen with abscesses but this can also be seen with other pathological processes. Rupture of the abscess with penetration of a ventricle is a complication that leads to pyocephalus. This can be recognised by an increase in signal intensity within the affected ventricle. In inversion recovery sequences, this effect can be particularly well visualised (200, 201).

Fungal and parasitic infections tend to be rare in Central Europe but are widespread throughout the rest of the World. Cryptococcal infections leading to meningitis and purulent / granulomatous encephalitis or encephalomyelitis can be visualised in the dog and cat using CT, or even better with MRI. Focal or multifocal contrast enhancement of the dura or nod-

ular areas of contrast enhancement in the brain can be depicted on T1w sequences. Without contrast, these lesions are hypointense on T1w sequences and hyperintense on T2w sequences. In one case, a nodule showing contrast enhancement in the cerebellum and a dilated fourth ventricle was found (197, 202). In individual cases, changes on CT or MRI in connection with larval migration (*Cuterebra*) and cysts due to *Coenurus* have been described (175, 203, 204). In contrast to arachnoid cysts, these types of cysts lie within the brain parenchyma.

Literature

6

1 HOUNSFIELD, G.N. (1973): Computerized transverse axial scanning (tomography). 1. Description of system. Br J Radiol. **46**: 1016–1022.

2 LOVE, N.E., FISHER, P., HUDSON, L. (2000): The computed tomographic enhancement pattern of the normal canine pituitary gland. Vet Radiol Ultrasound **41**: 507–510.

3 SPAULDING, K.A., SHARP, N.J.H. (1990): Ultrasonographic imaging of the lateral cerebral ventricles in the dog. Vet Radiol Ultrasound **31**: 59–64.

4 FUKUSHIMA, U., SASAKI, S., OKANO, S., OYAMADA, T., YOSHIKAWA, T., HAGIO, M., TAKASE, K. (2000): Non-invasive diagnosis of ischemic brain damage after cardiopulmonary resuscitation in dogs by using transcranial Doppler ultrasonography. Vet Radiol Ultrasound **41**: 172–177.

5 HUDSON, J.A., FINNBODNER, S.T., COATES, J.R., et al. (1995): Color Doppler imaging and Doppler spectral analysis in the spinal cord of normal dogs. Vet Radiol Ultrasound **36**: 542–547.

6 HUDSON, J.A., BUXTON, D.F., COX, N.R., FINNBODNER, S.T., SIMPSON, S.T., WRIGHT, J.C., WALLACE, S.S., MITRO, A. (1997): Color flow Doppler imaging and Doppler spectral analysis of the brain of neonatal dogs. Vet Radiol Ultrasound **38**: 313–322.

7 LAMB, C.R. (1998): Ultrasonography of portosystemic shunts in dogs and cats. Vet Clin North Am Small Anim Pract. **28**: 725–753.

8 CURRY, T.S., DOWDEY, J.E., MURRY, R.C. (1990): Computed Tomography. in Christensen's Physics of Diagnostic Radiology, Philadelphia, pp. 289–322.

9 DOEHRING (2001): Radiologische Bildgebende Verfahren. Uni Magdeburg, Germany.

10 TUCKER, R.L., GAVIN, P.R. (1996): Brain imaging. Vet Clin North Am Small Anim Pract. **26**: 735–758.

11 LAUTERBUR, P.C. (1973): Image formation by induced local interactions: examples employing nuclear magnetic resonance. Nature **242**: 190

12 SANDER, B. (2001): Informationen zur Magnetresonanz – Magnetresonanz-Grundlagen. http://www.mrx.de/mrpraxis/praxis.html

13 REISER, M., SEMMLER, W. (1997): Magnetresonanztomographie. Springer.

14 THOMSON, C.E., KORNEGAY, J.N., BURN, R.A. (1993): Magnetic resonance imaging: a general overview of principles and examples in veterinary neurodiagnosis. Vet Radiol Ultrasound **34**: 2–17.

15 KURIASHKIN, I.V., LOSONSKY, J.M. (2000): Contrast enhancement in magnetic resonance imaging using intravenous paramagnetic contrast media: a review. Vet Radiol Ultrasound **41**: 4–7.

16 BONGARTZ, G. (1997): MR-Angiographie. in Magnetresonanztomographie **2**: 432–453.

17 GRAHAM, J.P., ROBERTS, G.D., NEWELL, S.M. (2000): Dynamic magnetic resonance imaging of the normal canine pituitary gland. Vet. Radiol Ultrasound **41**: 35–40.

18 ASSHEUER, J., SAGER, M. (1997): MRI and CT Atlas of the Dog. Blackwell Science Ltd.

19 PEREMANS, K., DE, W.F., JANSSENS, L., DUMONT, F., VAN, B.H., DIERCKX, R. (2002): An infected hip prosthesis in a dog diagnosed with a 99mTc-ciprofloxacin (infecton) scan. Vet Radiol Ultrasound **43**: 178–182.

20 LOVE, N.E., BERRY, C.R. (2002): Interpretation Paradigms for the Axial Skeleton – Small and Large Animal. In: Textbook of Veterinary Diagnostic Radiology, 4th ed., Philadelphia 57–71.

21 MIDDLETON, D.L. (1993): Radiographic positioning for the spine and skull. Vet Clin North Am Small Anim Pract. **23**: 253–268.

22 LANG, J. (2001): Neuroradiologie. In: Veterinärmedizinische Neurologie, 2. Auflage, Berlin 69–97.

23 MORGAN, J.P., ACKERMAN, N., BAILEY, C.S., POOL, R.R. (1980): Vertebral tumors in the dog: a clinical, radiologic, and pathologic study of 61 primary and secondary lesions. Vet Radiol Ultrasound **21**: 197–212.

24 BICHSEL, P., LANG, J., VANDEVELDE, M., HAENI, H.J., OETTLI, P. (1985): Solitary cartilaginous exostosis associated with spinal cord compression in three large-breed dogs. J Am Anim Hosp Assoc. **21**: 619–622.

25 LEWIS, D.G., KELLY, D.F. (1990): Calcinosis circumscripta in dogs as a cause of spinal ataxia. J Small Anim Pract. **31**: 36–38.

26 BAGLEY, R.S. (2000): Spinal fracture or luxation. Vet Clin North Am Small Anim Pract. **30**: 133–vii.

6

27 THACHER, C. (1993): Biomechanics of cranial fractures, spinal fractures, and luxations. in Disease Mechanisms in Small Animal Surgery **2**.: 999–1009.

28 DENNY, H.R., GIBBS, C., WATERMAN, A. (1988): Atlanto-axial subluxation in the dog: a review of thirty cases and an evaluation of treatment by lag screw fixation. J Small Anim Pract. **29**: 37–47.

29 WATSON, A.G., DE LAHUNTA, A., EVANS, H.E. (1988): Morphology and embryological interpretation of a congenital occipito-atlanto-axial malformation in a dog. Teratology **38**: 451–459.

30 WATSON, A.G., HALL, M.A., DE LAHUNTA, A. (1985): Congenital occipitoatlantoaxial malformation in a cat. Comp Cont Ed Pract Vet. **7**: 245–254.

31 TROTTER, E.J., DELAHUNTA, A., GEARY, J.C., BRASMER, T.H. (1976): Caudal cervical vertebral malformation-malarticulation in Great Danes and Doberman Pinschers. J Am Vet Med Assoc. **168**: 917–930.

32 LINCOLN, J.D. (1992): Cervical vertebral malformation./malarticulation syndrome in large dogs. Vet Clin. North Am Small Anim Pract. **22**: 923–935.

33 DENNY, H.R., GIBBS, C., HOLT, P.E. (1982): The diagnosis and treatment of cauda equina lesions in the dog. J Small Anim Pract. **23**: 425–443.

34 McKEE, W.M. (1993): Differential diagnosis of cauda equina syndrome. In Practice **15**: 243–250.

35 NESS, M.G. (1994): Degenerative lumbosacral stenosis in the dog: A review of 30 cases. J Small Anim Pract. **35**: 185–190.

36 PALMER, R.H., CHAMBERS, J.N. (1991): Canine Lumbosacral Diseases. Part I. Anatomy, Pathophysiology and Clinical Presentation. The Compendium 61–79.

37 SISSON, A., LECOUTEUR, R., INGRAM, J., PARK, R., CHILD, G. (1992): Diagnosis of cauda equina abnormalities by using electromyography, discography, and epidurography in dogs. J Vet Intern Med. **6**: 253–263.

38 JAGGY, A., LANG, J., SCHAWALDER, P. (1987): [Cauda equina syndrome in the dog]. Schweiz Arch Tierheilkd. **129**: 171–192.

39 SCHULMAN, A.J., LIPPINCOTT, C.L. (1988): Canine cauda equina syndrome. Compendium **10**: 835–844.

40 MORGAN, J.P., ATILOLA, M., BAILEY, C.S. (1987): Vertebral canal and spinal cord mensuration: a comparative study of its effect on lumbosacral myelography in the dachshund and German shepherd dog. J Am Vet Med Assoc. **191**: 951–957.

41 MORGAN, J.P., BAHR, A., FRANTI, C.E., BAILEY, C.S. (1993): Lumbosacral transitional vertebrae as a predisposing cause of cauda equina syndrome in German shepherd dogs: 161 cases (1987–1990). J Am Vet Med Assoc. **202**: 1877–1882.

42 MORGAN, J.P. (1999): Transitional lumbosacral vertebral anomaly in the dog: a radiographic study. J Small Anim Pract. **40**: 167–172.

43 LEIPOLD, H.W., HUSTON, K., BLAUCH, B., GUFFY, M.M. (1974): Congenital defects on the caudal vertebral column and spinal cord in Manx cats. J Am Vet Med Assoc. **164**: 520–523.

44 BAGLEY, R.S., FORREST, L.J., CAUZINILLE, L., HOPKINS, A.L., KORNEGAY, J.N. (1993): Cervical vertebral fusion and concurrent intervertebral disc extrusion in 4 dogs. Vet Radiol Ultrasound **34**: 336–339.

45 SAUNDERS, H.M., JEZYK, P.K. (1991): The radiographic appearance of canine congenital hypothyroidism: skeletal changes with delayed treatment. Vet Radiol Ultrasound **32**: 171–177.

46 KONDE, L.J., THRALL, M.A., GASPER, P., et al. (1987): Radiographically visualized skeletal changes associated with mucopolysaccharidosis IV in cats. Vet Radiol. Ultrasound **28**: 223–228.

47 DHALIWAL, R.S., REED, A.L., KITCHELL, B.E. (2001): Multicentric lymphosarcoma in a dog with multiple-site skeletal involvement. Vet Radiol Ultrasound **42**: 38–41.

48 RUSBRIDGE, C., WHEELER, S.J., LAMB, C.R., PAGE, R.L., CARMICHAEL, S., BREARLEY, M.J., BJORNSON, A.P. (1999): Vertebral plasma cell tumors in 8 dogs. J Vet Intern Med. **13**: 126–133.

49 BAILEY, C.S., MORGAN, J.P. (1992): Congenital spinal malformations. Vet Clin North Am Small Anim Pract. **22**: 985–1015.

50 VANHAM, L.M., VAN BREE, H.J., TSHAMALA, M., THOONEN, H. (1995): Use of computed tomography and computed tomographic myelography for assessment of spinal tumoral calcinosis in a dog. Vet Radiol Ultrasound **36**: 115–118.

50a WALKER, M.C., PLATT, S.R., GRAHAM, J.P., CLEMMONS, R.M. (1999): Vertebral physitis with epiphyseal sequestration and a portosystemic shunt in a Pekingese dog. J Small Anim Pract. **40** (11): 525–528.

51 SHAMIR, M.H., TAVOR, N., AIZENBERG, T. (2001): Radiographic findings during recovery from discospondylitis. Vet Radiol. Ultrasound **42**: 496–503.

52 MORGAN, J.P. (1967): Spondylosis Deformans in the Dog. Acta Ortopaedica Scandinavica Supplementum **96**: 6–88.

53 MORGAN, J.P., STAVENBORN, M. (1991): Disseminated idiopathic skeletal hyperostosis (DISH) in a dog. Vet Radiol. Ultrasound **32**: 65–70.

54 DVIR, E., KIRBERGER, R.M., MALLECZEK, D. (2001): Radiographic and computed tomographic changes and clinical presentation of spirocercosis in the dog. Vet Radiol. Ultrasound **42**: 119–129.

55 CHO, D.Y., FREY, R.A., GUFFY, M.M., LEIPOLD, H.W. (1975): Hypervitaminosis A in the dog. Am J Vet Res. **36**: 1597–1603.

56 JOHNSON, K.A., WATSON, A.D.J. (2000): Skeletal Diseases. in Textbook of Veterinary Internal Medicine **5**.: 1887–1918.

57 KRAMERS, P., FLÜCKIGER, M.A., RAHN, B.A., CORDEY, J. (1988): Osteopetrosis in cats. J Small Anim Pract. **29**: 153–164.

58 DROST, W.T., LOVE, N.E., BERRY, C.R. (1996): Comparison of radiography, myelography and computed tomography for the evaluation of canine vertebral and spinal cord tumors in sixteen dogs. Vet Radiol Ultrasound **37**: 28–33.

59 FARDON, D.F., MILETTE, P.C. (2001): Nomenclature and classification of lumbar disc pathology. Recommendations of the Combined task Forces of the North American Spine Society, American Society of Spine Radiology, and American Society of Neuroradiology. Spine **26**: E93–E113.

60 WEBER, W.J., BERRY, C.R., KRAMER, R.W. (1995): Vacuum phenomenon in twelve dogs. Vet Radiol Ultrasound **36**: 493–498.

61 LAMB, C.R. (1994): Common difficulties with myelographic diagnosis of acute intervertebral disc prolapse in the dog. J Small Anim Pract. **35**: 549–558.

62 LAMB, C.R., GUTHRIE, S. (1995): Radiology corner – a rare example of an automyelogram. Vet Radiol Ultrasound **36**: 383–383.

63 KIRBERGER, R.M., WRIGLEY, R.H. (1993): Myelography in the dog: review of patients with contrast medium in the central canal. Vet Radiol Ultrasound **34**: 253–258.

64 KIRBERGER, R.M., ROOS, C.J., LUBBE, A.M. (1992): The radiological diagnosis of thoracolumbar disc disease in the dachshund. Vet Radiol Ultrasound **33**: 255–261.

65 NYKAMP, S.G., SCRIVANI, P.V., KENNEDY, S., BLISS, S.P. (2001): What is your diagnosis? Attenuation of the dorsal and lateral columns of contrast material and slight ventral deviation of the dorsal column at T12–T13 and T13–L1. J Am Vet Med Assoc. **218**: 1417–1418.

66 LANG, J. (1988): Flexion-extension myelography of the canine cauda equina. Vet Radiol Ultrasound **29**: 242–257.

67 SCRIVANI, P.V., BARTHEZ, P.Y., LEVEILLE, R., SCHRADER, S.C., REED, S.M. (1997): Subdural injection of contrast medium during cervical myelography. Vet Radiol Ultrasound **38**: 267–271.

68 PENDERIS, J., SULLIVAN, M., SCHWARZ, T., GRIFFITHS, I.R. (1999): Subdural injection of contrast medium as a complication of myelography. J Small Anim Pract. **40**: 173–176.

69 FOURIE, S.L., KIRBERGER, R.M. (1999): Relationship of cervical spinal cord diameter to vertebral dimensions: a radiographic study of normal dogs. Vet Radiol Ultrasound **40**: 137–143.

70 PARDO, A.D., MORGAN, J.P. (1988): Myelography in the cat: a comparison of cisternal versus lumbar puncture, using metrizamide. Vet Radiol Ultrasound **29**: 89–95.

71 WIDMER, W.R., THRALL, D.E. (2002): Canine and Feline Intervertebral Disc Disease, Myelography, and Spinal Cord Disease. in Textbook of Veterinary Diagnostic Radiology 4th ed. Philadelphia, pp. 110–126.

72 BARTHEZ, P.Y., MORGAN, J.P., LIPSITZ, D. (1994): Discography and epidurography for evaluation of the lumbosacral junction in dogs with cauda equina syndrome. Vet Radiol Ultrasound **35**: 152–157.

73 FEENEY, D.A., WISE, M. (1981): Epidurography in the normal dog: technic and radiographic findings. Vet Radiol Ultrasound **22**: 35–39.

74 JONES, J.C., SORJONEN, D.C., SIMPSON, S.T., et al (1996): Comparison between computed tomographic and surgical findings in nine large-breed dogs with lumbosacral stenosis. Vet Radiol Ultrasound **37**: 247–256.

75 ADAMS, W.H., DANIEL, G.B., PARDO, A.D., SELCER, R.S. (1995): Magnetic resonance imaging of the caudal lumbar and lumbosacral spine in 13 dogs (1990–1993). Vet Radiol Ultrasound **36**: 3–13.

76 BLEVINS, W.E. (1980): Transosseous vertebral venography: a diagnostic aid in lumbosacral disease. Vet Radiol Ultrasound **21**: 50–54.

77 KOBLIK, P.D., SUTER, P.F. (1981): Lumbo-sacral vertebral sinus venography via transjugular catheterization in the dog. Vet Radiol Ultrasound **22**: 69–77.

78 BAGLEY, R.S., TUCKER, R.L., MOORE, M.P., HARRINGTON, M.L. (1995): Radiographic diagnosis – intervertebral disk extrusion in a cat. Vet Radiol Ultrasound **36**: 380–382.

79 COATES, J.R. (2000): Intervertebral disk disease. Vet Clin North Am Small Anim Pract. **30**: 77–110.

80 GOGGIN, J.E., LI, A.S., FRANTI, C.E. (1970): Canine intervertebral disk disease: characterization by age, sex, breed, and anatomic site of involvement. Am J Vet Res. **31**: 1687–1692.

81 CUDIA, S.P., DUVAL, J.M. (1997): Thoracolumbar intervertebral disk disease in large, nonchondrodystrophic dogs: a retrospective study. J Am Anim Hosp. Assoc. **33**: 456–460.

82 HOERLEIN, B.F. (1978): Intervertebral Disks. in Canine Neurology Diagnosis and Treatment 3rd ed. Philadelphia, pp. 470–560.

83 GAGE, E.D. (1975): Incidence of clinical disc disease in the dog. J Am Anim Hosp Assoc. **11**: 135–138.

84 LU, D., LAMB, C.R., TARGETT, M.P. (2002): Results of myelography in seven dogs with myelomalacia. Vet Radiol Ultrasound **43**: 326–330.

85 SCHULZ, K.S., WALKER, M., MOON, M., WALDRON, D., SLATER, M., MCDONALD, D.E. (1998): Correlation of clinical, radiographic, and surgical localization of intervertebral disc extrusion in small-breed dogs: a prospective study of 50 cases. Vet Surg. **27**: 105–111.

86 LUBBE, A.M., KIRBERGER, R.M., VERSTRAETE, F.J.M. (1994): Pediculectomy for thoracolumbar spine decompression in the dachshund. J Am Anim Hosp Assoc. **30**: 233–238.

87 OLBY, N.J., DYCE, J., HOULTON, J.E.F. (1994): Correlation of plain radiographic and lumbar myelographic findings with surgical findings in thoracolumbar disc disease. J Small Anim Pract. **35**: 345–350.

88 BRAY, J., BURBIDGE, H. (1998): The canine intervertebral disk. Part one: structure and function. J Am Anim Hosp Assoc. **34**: 55–63.

89 BRAY, J., BURBIDGE, H. (1998): The canine intervertebral disk. Part two: degenerative changes – nonchondrodystrophoid versus chondrodystrophoid disks. J Am Anim Hosp Assoc. **34**: 135–144.

90 TERTTI, M., PAAJANEN, H., LAATO, M., AHO, H., KOMU, M., KORMANO, M. (1991): Disc degeneration in magnetic resonance imaging. A comparative biochemical, histologic, and radiologic study in cadaver spines. Spine **16**: 629–634.

91 SCHIEBLER, M.L., GRENIER, N., FALLON, M., CAMERINO, V., ZLATKIN, M., KRESSEL, H.Y. (1991): Normal and degenerated intervertebral disk: in vivo and in vitro MR imaging with histopathologic correlation. Am J Roentgenol. **157**: 93–97.

6

6

92 DE HAAN, J.J., SHELTON, S.B., ACKERMAN, N. (1993): Magnetic resonance imaging in the diagnosis of degenerative lumbosacral stenosis in four dogs. Vet Surg. **22**: 1–4.

93 SHARP, N.J.H., COFONE, M., ROBERTSON, I.D., DECARLO, A., SMITH, G.K., THRALL, D.E. (1995): Computed tomography in the evaluation of caudal cervical spondylomyelopathy of the doberman pinscher. Vet Radiol Ultrasound **36**: 100–108.

94 DE RISIO, L., THOMAS, W.B., SHARP, N.J. (2000): Degenerative lumbosacral stenosis. Vet Clin North Am Small Anim Pract. **30**: 111–32.

95 WHEELER, S.J. (1992): Lumbosacral disease. Vet Clin North Am Small Anim Pract. **22**: 937–950.

96 SELCER, B.A., CHAMBERS, J.N., SCHWENSEN, K., MAHAFFEY, M.B. (1988): Epidurography as a diagnostic aid in canine lumbosacral compressive disease. V.C.O.T. **2**: 97–103.

97 MORGAN, J.P., BAILEY, C.S. (1990): Cauda equina syndrome in the dog: Radiographic evaluation. J Small Anim Pract. **31**: 69–77.

98 LANG, J., HÄNI, H., SCHAWALDER, P. (1992): A sacral lesion resembling osteochondrosis in the German Shepherd Dog. Vet Radiol Ultrasound **33**: 69–76.

99 LENEHAN, T.M. (1983): Canine cauda equina syndrome. Comp Cont Ed Pract Vet. **5**: 941–951.

100 SCHMID, V., LANG, J. (1993): Measurements on the lumbosacral junction in normal dogs and those with cauda equina compression. J Small Anim Pract. **34**: 437–442.

101 WATT, P.R. (1991): Degenerative lumbosacral stenosis in 18 dogs. J Small Anim Pract. **32**: 125–134.

102 DICKINSON, P.J., STURGES, B.K., BERRY, W.L., VERNAU, K.M., KOBLIK, P.D., LECOUTEUR, R.A. (2001): Extradural spinal synovial cysts in nine dogs. J Small Anim Pract. **42**: 502–509.

103 LIPSITZ, D., LEVITSKI, R.E., CHAUVET, A.E., BERRY, W.L. (2001): Magnetic resonance imaging features of cervical stenotic myelopathy in 21 dogs. Vet Radiol Ultrasound **42**: 20–27.

104 SILBERSTEIN, M., HENNESSY, O. (1993): Implications of focal spinal cord lesions following trauma: evaluation with magnetic resonance imaging. Paraplegia **31**: 160–167.

105 MOORE, G.E., MATHEY, W.S., EGGERS, J.S., ESTEP, J.S. (2000): Osteosarcoma in adjacent lumbar vertebrae in a dog. J Am Vet Med Assoc. **217**: 1038–40, 1008.

106 SHIROMA, J.T., WEISBRODE, S.E., BILLER, D.S., OLMSTEAD, M.L. (1993): Pathological fracture of an aneurismal bone cyst in a lumbar vertebra of a dog. J Am Anim Hosp Assoc. **29**: 434–437.

107 COOLEY, D.M., WATERS, D.J. (1998): Skeletal metastasis as the initial clinical manifestation of metastatic carcinoma in 19 dogs. J Vet Intern Med. **12**: 288–293.

108 MOON, M.L., SAUNDERS, G.K., MARTIN, R.A. (1990): Vertebral osteosclerosis in a cat secondary to rhabdomyosarcoma. Vet Radiol Ultrasound **31**: 39–41.

109 LAMB, C.R. (1987): Bone scintigraphy in small animals. J Am Vet Med Assoc. **191**: 1616–1622.

110 JERGENS, A.E., MILES, K.G., MOORE, F.M. (1990): Atypical lytic proliferative skeletal lesions associated with plasma cell myeloma in a dog. Vet Radiol Ultrasound **31**: 262–264.

111 KLOC, P.A., SCRIVANI, P.V., BARR, S.C., REESE, C.J., TROTTER, E.J., FOREST, T.W., POOL, R. (2001): Vertebral angiomatosis in a cat. Vet Radiol Ultrasound **42**: 42–45.

112 BALERIAUX, D.L. (1999): Spinal cord tumors. Eur Radiol. **9**: 1252–1258.

113 MIYAZAWA, N., HIDA, K., IWASAKI, Y., KOYANAGI, I., ABE, H. (2000): MRI at 1.5 T of intramedullary ependymoma and classification of pattern of contrast enhancement. Neuroradiology **42**: 828–832.

114 KIPPENES, H., GAVIN, P.R., BAGLEY, R.S., SILVER, G.M., TUCKER, R.L., SANDE, R.D. (1999): Magnetic resonance imaging features of tumors of the spine and spinal cord in dogs. Vet Radiol Ultrasound **40**: 627–633.

115 PLATT, S.R., GRAHAM, J., CHRISMAN, C.L., COLLINS, K., CHANDRA, S., SIRNINGER, J., NEWELL, S.M. (1999): Magnetic resonance imaging and ultrasonography in the diagnosis of a malignant peripheral nerve sheath tumor in a dog. Vet Radiol Ultrasound **40**: 367–371.

116 LEVITSKI, R.E., LIPSITZ, D., CHAUVET, A.E. (1999): Magnetic resonance imaging of the cervical spine in 27 dogs. Vet Radiol Ultrasound **40**: 332–341.

117 McCONNELL, J.F., GAROSI, L.S., DENNIS, R., SMITH, K.C. (2003): Imaging of a spinal neprhoblastoma in a dog. Vet Radiol Ultrasound **44**: 537–541.

118 GREEN, E.M., ADAMS, W.M., STEINBERG, H. (1999): Malignant transformation of solitary spinal osteochondroma in two mature dogs. Vet Radiol Ultrasound **40**: 634–637.

119 SILVER, G.M., BAGLEY, R.S., GAVIN, P.R., KIPPENES, H. (2001): Radiographic diagnosis: cartilaginous exostoses in a dog. Vet Radiol Ultrasound **42**: 231–234.

120 MOZOS, E., NOVALES, M., GINEL, P.J., PEREZ, J., POOL, R.R. (2002): A newly recognized pattern of canine osteochondromatosis. Vet Radiol Ultrasound **43**: 132–137.

121 CAPORN, T.M., READ, R.A. (1996): Osteochondromatosis of the cervical spine causing compressive myelopathy in a dog. J Small Anim Pract. **37**: 133–137.

122 KIRBERGER, R.M., JACOBSON, L.S., DAVIES, J.V., ENGELA, J. (1997): Hydromyelia in the dog. Vet Radiol Ultrasound **38**: 30–38.

123 TAGA, A., TAURA, Y., NAKAICHI, M., WADA, N., HASEGAWA, T. (2000): Magnetic resonance imaging of syringomyelia in five dogs. J Small Anim Pract. **41**: 362–365.

124 BAGLEY, R.S., GAVIN, P.R., SILVER, G.M., MOORE, M.P., KIPPENES, H., CONNORS, R. (2000): Syringomyelia and hydromyelia in dogs and cats. Comp Cont Ed Pract Vet. **22**: 471–479.

125 GALLOWAY, A.M., CURTIS, N.C., SOMMERLAD, S.F., WATT, P.R. (1999): Correlative imaging findings in seven dogs and one cat with spinal arachnoid cysts. Vet Radiol Ultrasound **40**: 445–452.

126 MILHORAT, T.H., JOHNSON, W.D., MILLER, J.I., BERG-LAND, R.M., HOLLENBERG-SHER, J. (1992): Surgical treatment of syringomyelia based on magnetic resonance imaging criteria. Neurosurgery **31**: 231–244.

127 VIGNOLI, M., ROSSI, F., SARLI, G. (1999): Spinal subarachnoid cyst in a cat. Vet Radiol Ultrasound **40**: 116–119.

128 CORNEGLIANI, L., JOMMI, E., VERCELLI, A. (2001): Dermoid sinus in a golden retriever. J Small Anim Pract. **42**: 514–516.

129 PRATT, J.N., KNOTTENBELT, C.M., WELSH, E.M. (2000): Dermoid sinus at the lumbosacral junction in an English springer spaniel. J Small Anim Pract. **41**: 24–26.

130 GOPAL, M.S., JEFFERY, N.D. (2001): Magnetic resonance imaging in the diagnosis and treatment of a canine spinal cord injury. J Small Anim Pract. **42**: 29–31.

131 OHSHIO, I., HATAYAMA, A., KANEDA, K., TAKAHARA, M., NAGASHIMA, K. (1993): Correlation between histopathologic features and magnetic resonance images of spinal cord lesions. Spine **18**: 1140–1149.

132 ABRAMSON, C.J., GAROSI, L., PLATT, S.R., DENNIS, R., McCONNELL, J.F. (2005): Magnetic resonance imaging appearance of suspected ischemic myelopathy in dogs. Vet Radiol Ultrasound **46**: 225–229.

133 GRUNENFELDER, F.I., WEISHAUPT, D., GREEN, R., STEFFEN, F. (2005): Magnetic resonance imaging findings in spinal cord infarction in three small breed dogs. Vet Radiol Ultrasound **46**: 91–96.

134 APPLEWHITE, A.A., WILKENS, B.E., MCDONALD, D.E., RADASCH, R.M., BARSTAD, R.D. (1999): Potential central nervous system complications of von Willebrand's disease. J Am Anim Hosp Assoc. **35**: 423–429.

135 ROUSH, J.K., DOUGLASS, J.P., HERTZKE, D., KENNEDY, G.A. (1992): Traumatic dural laceration in a racing greyhound. Vet Radiol Ultrasound **33**: 22–24.

136 KRAFT, S.L., MUSSMAN, J.M., SMITH, T., BILLER, D.S., HOSKINSON, J.J. (1998): Magnetic resonance imaging of presumptive lumbosacral discospondylitis in a dog. Vet Radiol Ultrasound **39**: 9–13.

137 GONZALO-ORDEN, J.M., ALTONAGA, J.R., ORDEN, M.A., GONZALO, J.M. (2000): Magnetic resonance, computed tomographic and radiologic findings in a dog with discospondylitis. Vet Radiol Ultrasound **41**: 142–144.

138 JIMENEZ, M.M., O'CALLAGHAN, M.W. (1995): Vertebral physitis: a radiographic diagnosis to be separated from discospondylitis. Vet Radiol Ultrasound **36**: 188–195.

139 WALKER, M.C., PLATT, S.R., GRAHAM, J.P., CLEMMONS, R.M. (1999): Vertebral physitis with epiphyseal sequestration and a portosystemic shunt in a Pekingese dog. J Small Anim Pract. **40**: 525–528.

140 FRENDIN, J., FUNKQUIST, B., HANSSON, K., LONNEM-ARK, M., CARLSTEN, J. (1999): Diagnostic imaging of foreign body reactions in dogs with diffuse back pain. J Small Anim Pract. **40**: 278–285.

141 MITTEN, R.W. (1974): Vertebral osteomyelitis in the dog due to Nocardia-like organisms. J Small Anim Pract. **15**: 563–570.

142 FOLEY, J.E., LEUTENEGGER, C. (2001): A review of coronavirus infection in the central nervous system of cats and mice. J Vet Intern Med. **15**: 438–444.

143 CHERRONE, K.L., EICH, C.S., BONZYNSKI, J.J. (2002): Suspected paraspinal abscess and spinal epidural empyema in a dog. J Am Anim Hosp Assoc. **38**: 149–151.

144 BRODEY, R.S. (1970): Canine and feline neoplasia. Adv Vet Sci Comp Med. **14**: 309–354.

145 BRIGHT R.M., BOJRAB M.J. (1976): Intranasal neoplasia in the dog and cat. J Am Anim Hosp Assoc. **12**: 806–812.

146 BURK R.L. (1992): Computed tomographic imaging of nasal disease in 100 dogs. Vet Radiol Ultrasound **33**: 177–180.

147 RUSSO, M., LAMB, C.R., JAKOVLJEVIC, S. (2000): Distinguishing rhinitis and nasal neoplasia by radiography. Vet Radiol Ultrasound **41**: 118–124.

148 SULLIVAN, M., LEE, R., JAKOVLJEVIC, S., SHARP, N.J.H. (1986): The radiological features of aspergillosis of the nasal cavity and frontal sinuses in the dog. J Small Anim Pract. **27**: 167–180.

149 SULLIVAN, M., LEE, R., SKAE, L.A. (1987): The radiological features of sixty cases of intra-nasal neoplasia in the dog. J Small Anim Pract. **28**: 575–586.

150 VOGES, A.K., ACKERMAN N. (1995): MR evaluation of intra and extracranial extension of nasal adenocarcinoma in a dog and cat. Vet Radiol Ultrasound **36**: 196–200.

151 TASKER, S., KNOTTENBELT, C.M., MUNRO, E.A., STONEHEWER, J., SIMPSON, J.W., MACKIN, A.J. (1999): Aetiology and diagnosis of persistent nasal disease in the dog: a retrospective study of 42 cases. J Small Anim Pract. **40**: 473–478.

152 CODNER, E.C., LURUS, A.G., MILLER, J.B., GAVIN, P.R., GALLINA, A., BARBEE, D.D. (1993): Comparison of computed tomography with radiography as a noninvasive diagnostic technique for chronic nasal disease in dogs. J Am Vet Med Assoc. **202**: 1106–1110.

153 THRALL, D.E., ROBERTSON, I.D., MCLEOD, D.A., HEIDNER, G.L., HOOPES, J., PAGE, R.L. (1989): A comparison of radiographic and computed tomographic findings in 31 dogs with malignant nasal cavity tumors. Vet Radiol Ultrasound **30**: 59–66.

154 PARK, R.D., BECK, E.R., LECOUTEUR, R.A. (1992): Comparison of computed tomography and radiography for detecting changes induced by malignant nasal neoplasia in dogs. J Am Vet Med Assoc. **201**: 1720–1724.

155 SAUNDERS, J.H., ZONDERLAND, J.L., CLERCX, C., GIELEN, I., SNAPS, F.R., SULLIVAN, M., VANBREE, H., DONDELINGER, R.F. (2002): Computed tomographic findings in 35 dogs with nasal aspergillosis. Vet Radiol Ultrasound **43**: 5–9.

6

156 MOORE, M.P., GAVIN, P.R., KRAFT, S.L., DE HAAN, C.E., LEATHERS, C.W., DORN, R.V. (1991): MR, CT and clinical features from 4 dogs with nasal tumors involving the rostral cerebrum. Vet Radiol Ultrasound **32**: 19–25.

157 MORGAN, R.V., ZANOTTI, S.W. (1989): Horner's Syndrome in dogs and cats: 49 cases (1980–1986). J Am Vet Med Assoc. **194**: 1096–1099.

158 FIKE, J.R., LECOUTEUR, R.A., CANN, C.E. (1984): Anatomy of the canine orbital region: multiplanar imaging by CT. Vet Radiol Ultrasound **25**: 32–36.

159 MORGAN, R.V., DANIEL, G.B., DONNELL, R.L. (1994): Magnetic resonance imaging of the normal eye and orbit of the dog and cat. Vet Radiol Ultrasound **35**: 102–108.

159a DENNIS, R. (2000): Use of magnetic resonance imaging for the investigation of orbital disease in small animals. J Small Anim Pract. **41** (4): 145–155.

159b CALIA, C.M., KIRSCHNER, S.E., BAER, K.E. et al. (1994): The use of computed tomography scans for the evaluation of orbital disease m cats and dogs. Vet Comp Ophthal. **4**: 24–30.

160 DENNIS, R. (2000): Use of magnetic resonance imaging for the investigation of orbital disease in small animals. J Small Anim Pract. **41**: 145–155.

161 MATTOON, J.S., NYLAND, T.G. (2002): Eye. In Small Animal Diagnostic Ultrasound 2nd ed. Philadelphia, pp. 305–324.

161a HARTLEY, C., MCCONNELL, J.F., DOUST, R. (2007): Wooden orbital foreign body in a Weimaraner. Vet Ophthalmol. **10**(6): 390–393.

162 RUSSO, M., COVELLI, E. M., MEOMARTINO, L., LAMB, C.R., BRUNETTI, A. (2002): Computed tomographic anatomy of the canine inner and middle ear. Vet Radiol Ultrasound **43**: 22–26.

163 GAROSI, L.S., DENNIS, R., PENDERIS, J., LAMB, C.R., TARGETT, M.P., CAPPELLO, R., DELAUCHE, A.J. (2001): Results of magnetic resonance imaging in dogs with vestibular disorders: 85 cases (1996–1999). J Am Vet Med Assoc. **218**: 385–391.

164 DVIR, E., KIRBERGER, R.M., TERBLANCHE, A.G. (2000): Magnetic resonance imaging of otitis media in a dog. Vet Radiol Ultrasound **41**: 46–49.

165 BARTHEZ, P.Y., KOBLIK, P.D., HORNOF, W.J., WISNER, E.R., SEIBERT, J.A. (1996): Apparent wall thickening in fluid-filled versus air-filled tympanic bulla in computed tomography. Vet Radiol Ultrasound **37**: 95–98.

166 RISER, W.H., PARKES, L.J., SHIRER, J.F. (1967): Canine craniomandibular osteopathy. Vet Radiol Ultrasound **8**: 23–31.

167 WATSON, A.D.J., ADAMS, W.M., THOMAS, C.B. (1995): Craniomandibular osteopathy in dogs. Comp Cont Educ Pract Vet. **17**: 911–922.

168 MUIR, P., DUBIELZIG, R.R., JOHNSON, K.A., SHELTON, G.D. (1996): Hypertrophic osteodystrophy and calvarial hyperostsis. Comp Cont Educ Pract Vet. **18**: 143–151.

169 PASTOR, K.F., BOULAY, J.P., SCHELLING, S.H., CARPENTER, J.L. (2000): Idiopathic hyperostosis of the calvaria in five young bullmastiffs. J Am Anim Hosp Assoc. **36**: 439–445.

170 PARIZEL, P.M., OZSARLAK, VAN GOETHEM, J.W., VAN DEN, H.L., DILLEN, C., VERLOOY, J., COSYNS, P., DE SCHEPPER, A.M. (1998): Imaging findings in diffuse axonal injury after closed head trauma. Eur Radiol. **8**: 960–965.

171 PARIZEL, PM., MAKKAT, S., VAN MIERT, E., VAN GOETHEM, J.W., VAN DEN, H.L., DE SCHEPPER, A.M. (2001): Intracranial hemorrhage: principles of CT and MRI interpretation. Eur Radiol. **11**: 1770–1783.

172 KIRBERGER, R.M., JACOBSON, L.S., DAVIES, J.V., ENGELA, J. (1997): Hydromyelia in the dog. Vet Radiol Ultrasound **38**: 30–38.

173 BYNEVELT, M., RUSBRIDGE, C., BRITTON, J. (2000): Dorsal dens angulation and a Chiari-type malformation in a Cavalier King Charles Spaniel. Vet Radiol Ultrasound **41**: 521–524.

174 KRAFT, S.L., GAVIN, P.R. (1999): Intracranial neoplasia. Clin Tech Small Anim Pract. **14**: 112–123.

175 THOMAS, W.B. (1999): Nonneoplastic disorders of the brain. Clin Tech Small Anim Pract. **14**: 125–147.

176 THOMAS, W.B., WHEELER, S.J., KRAMER, R., KORNEGAY, J.N. (1996): Magnetic resonance imaging features of primary brain tumors in dogs. Vet Radiol Ultrasound **37**: 20–27.

177 MOORE, M.P., BAGLEY, R.S., HARRINGTON, M.L., GAVIN, P.R. (1996): Intracranial tumors. Vet Clin North Am Small Anim Pract. **26**: 759–777.

178 CIZINAUSKAS, S., LANG, J., MAIER, R., FATZER, R., JAGGY, A. (2001): Paradoxical vestibular disease with trigeminal nervesheath tumor in a dog. Schweiz Arch Tierheilkd. **143**: 419–425.

179 GRAHAM, J.P., NEWELL, S.M., VOGES, A.K., ROBERTS, G.D., HARRISON, J.M. (1998): The dural tail sign in the diagnosis of meningiomas. Vet Radiol Ultrasound **39**: 297–302.

180 LORENZO, V., PUMAROLA, M., MUNOZ, A. (1998): Meningioangiomatosis in a dog: magnetic resonance imaging and neuropathological studies. J Small Anim Pract. **39**: 486–489.

181 TARGETT, M.P., MCINNES, E., DENNIS, R. (1999): Magnetic resonance imaging of a medullary dermoid cyst with secondary hydrocephalus in a dog. Vet Radiol Ultrasound **40**: 23–26.

182 PLATT, S.R., GRAHAM, J., CHRISMAN, C.L., ADJIRI-AWERE, A., CLEMMONS, R.M. (1999): Canine intracranial epidermoid cyst. Vet Radiol Ultrasound **40**: 454–458.

183 ESTEVE-RATSCH, B., KNEISSL, S., GABLER, C. (2001): Comparative evaluation of the ventricles in the Yorkshire Terrier and the German Shepherd dog using low-field MRI. Vet Radiol Ultrasound **42**: 410–413.

184 VULLO, T., KORENMAN, E., MANZO, R.P., GOMEZ, D.G., DECK, M.D., CAHILL, P.T. (1997): Diagnosis of cerebral ventriculomegaly in normal adult beagles using quantitative MRI. Vet Radiol Ultrasound **38**: 277–281.

6

185 DE HAAN, C.E., KRAFT, S.L., GAVIN, P.R., WENDLING, L.R., GRIEBENOW, M.L. (1994): Normal variation in size of the lateral ventricles of the Labrador Retriever dog as assessed by magnetic resonance imaging. Vet Radiol Ultrasound **35**: 83–86.

186 NAIDICH, T.P., SCHOTT, L.H., BARON, R.L. (1982): Computed tomography in evaluation of hydrocephalus. Radiol Clin North Am **20**: 143–167.

187 DRAKE, J.M., POTTS, D.G., LEMAIRE, C. (1989): Magnetic resonance imaging of silastic-induced canine hydrocephalus. Surg Neurol. **31**: 28–40.

187a MATIASEK, L.A., PLATT, S.R., SHAW, S., DENNIS, R. (2007): Clinical and magnetic resonance imaging characteristics of quadrigeminal cysts in dogs. J Vet Intern Med. **21** (5): 1021–1026.

188 VERNAU, K.M., KORTZ, G.D., KOBLIK, P.D., LECOUTEUR, R.A., BAILEY, C.S., PEDROIA, V. (1997): Magnetic resonance imaging and computed tomography characteristics of intracranial intra-arachnoid cysts in 6 dogs. Vet Radiol Ultrasound **38**: 171–176.

189 MILNER, R.L., ENGELA, J., KIRBERGER, R.M. (1996): Arachnoid cyst in cerebellar pontine area of a cat – diagnosis by magnetic resonance imaging. Vet Radiol Ultrasound **37**: 34–36.

190 ENZMAN, D.R., BRITT, R.H., LYONS, B.E. (1981): Natural history of experimental intracerebral hemorrhage: sonography, computed tomography and neuropathology. Am J Neuroradiol. **2**: 517–526.

191 WOLF, M., PEDROIA, V., HIGGINS, R.J., KOBLIK, P.D., TURREL, J.M., OWENS, J.M. (1995): Intracranial ring enhancing lesions in dogs: a correlative CT scanning and neuropathologic study. Vet Radiol Ultrasound **36**: 16–20.

192 THOMAS, W.B., SORJONEN, D.C., SCHEULER, R.O., KORNEGAY, J.N. (1996): Magnetic resonance imaging of brain infarction in seven dogs. Vet Radiol Ultrasound **37**: 345–350.

193 GAROSI, L., McCONNELL, J.F., PLATT, S.R., BARONE, G., BARON, J.C., DE LAHUNTA, A., SCHATZBERG, S.J. (2206): Clinical and topographic magnetic resonance characteristics of suspected brain infarction in 40 dogs. J Vet Intern Med. **20**: 311–321.

194 MELLEMA, L.M., KOBLIK, P.D., KORTZ, G.D., LECOUTEUR, R.A., CHECHOWITZ, M.A., DICKINSON, P.J. (1999): Reversible magnetic resonance imaging abnormalities in dogs following seizures. Vet Radiol Ultrasound **40**: 588–595.

195 MATHEWS, V.P., KUHARIK, M.A., EDWARDS, M.K., D'AMOUR, P.G., AZZARELLI, B., DREESEN, R.G. (1989): Dyke award. Gd-DTPA-enhanced MR imaging of experimental bacterial meningitis: evaluation and comparison with CT. Am J Roentgenol. **152**: 131–136.

196 MELLEMA, L.M., SAMII, V.F., VERNAU, K.M., LECOUTEUR, R.A. (2002): Meningeal enhancement on magnetic resonance imaging in 15 dogs and 3 cats. Vet Radiol Ultrasound **43**: 10–15.

197 DUCOTE, J.M., JOHNSON, K.E., DEWEY, C.W., WALKER, M.A., COATES, J.R., BERRIDGE, B.R. (1999): Computed tomography of necrotizing meningoencephalitis in 3 Yorkshire Terriers. Vet Radiol Ultrasound **40**: 617–621.

198 VON PRAUN, F., MATIASEK, K., GREVEL, V., ALEF, M., FLEGEL, T. (2006): Magnetic resonance imaging and pathologic findings associated with necrotizing encephalitis in two Yorkshire terriers. Vet Radiol Ultrasound **47**: 260–264.

198a CHERUBINI, G.B., PLATT, S.R., ANDERSON, T.J., RUSBRIDGE, C., LORENZO, V., MANTIS, P., CAPPELLO, R. (2006): Characteristics of magnetic resonance images of granulomatous meningoencephalomyelitis in 11 dogs. Vet Rec. **159** (4): 110–115.

199 LOBETTI, R.G., PEARSON, J. (1996): Magnetic resonance imaging in the diagnosis of focal granulomatous meningoencephalitis in two dogs. Vet Radiol Ultrasound **37**: 424–426.

200 SEILER, G., CIZINAUSKAS, S., SCHEIDEGGER, J., LANG, J. (2001): Low-field magnetic resonance imaging of a pyocephalus and a suspected brain abscess in a German Shepherd dog. Vet Radiol Ultrasound **42**: 417–422.

201 KLOPP, L.S., HATHCOCK, J.T., SORJONEN, D.C. (2000): Magnetic resonance imaging features of brain stem abscessation in two cats. Vet Radiol Ultrasound **41**: 300–307.

202 TICHES, D., VITE, C.H., DAYRELL-HART, B., STEINBERG, S.A., GROSS, S., LEXA, F. (1998): A case of canine central nervous system cryptococcosis: management with fluconazole. J Am Anim Hosp Assoc. **34**: 145–151.

203 GLASS, E.N., CORNETTA, A.M., DELAHUNTA, A., CENTER, S.A., KENT, M. (1998): Clinical and clinicopathologic features in 11 cats with Cuterebra larvae myiasis of the central nervous system. J Vet Intern Med. **12**: 365–368.

204 SMITH, M.C., BAILEY, C.S., BAKER, N., KOCK, N. (1988): Cerebral coenurosis in a cat. J Am Vet Med Assoc. **192**: 82–84.

7 Electrodiagnostics

Petr Srenk
Gaby Flühmann
Anne Muhle
Luciana Bergamasco
André Jaggy

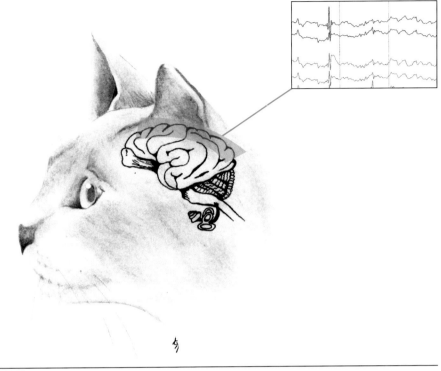

The nervous system is specialised for conducting changes in the membrane potentials of its cells. The recording of these changes in potential utilizing specialized equipment is the physiological basis of electrodiagnosis. At present, measurements of electrical processes in both the CNS and PNS are used diagnostically in veterinary neurology. The indications, measurement methods and evaluation of the most commonly used methods are discussed in this chapter.

The indications for an electrodiagnostic investigation can be divided into two groups: firstly, lesions of the lower motor neuron system (LMNS), which may be generalised or focal; secondly, lesions in the CNS, particularly cerebrocortical or brain stem lesions.

The results of the electrodiagnostic measurements for the purposes of anatomical localisation are often definitive when investigating the LMNS; specifically when it comes to the differentiation of focal and generalised LMN diseases. Polyneuropathies can manifest clinically as mono neuropathies and their exact localisation can only be ascertained using an electrodiagnostic investigation. Focal changes can be found with focal lesions of the nerve roots (tumour, trauma, haemorrhage, discospondylitis, disc herniation) or in focal lesions of the peripheral nerves (trauma, neoplasia). A diffuse distribution of abnormalities indicates, in comparison, the presence of a polyneuropathy or a poly myopathy. The exact ana-

tomic classification and distribution of the lesion between the musculature (myopathies, myositis, myotonia), neuromuscular endplates (myasthenia gravis, botulism, organophosphate and carbamate poisoning), myelin and axon (metabolic neuropathies, neuritis) is also possible thanks to these types of investigations. The indications for a targeted nerve/muscle biopsy are made more precise with electrodiagnosis (see Chap. 7.3). Abnormalities revealed during spontaneous and evoked electromyographical investigations indicate a myopathy or a neuropathy with axonopathy and or demyelination. The size of the compound muscle action potential (CMAP) is important in patients with normal electomyographic findings, but with reduced motor nerve conduction velocity. A normal CMAP coupled with a reduced conduction velocity is an indication of demyelination; similarly, when the CMAP and conduction velocity are reduced, one must consider axonopathy and demyelination. In diseases of the neuromuscular junctions, needle electromyography and motor nerve conduction velocity are normal, but repetitive nerve stimulation may reveal abnormalities. The methods used to determine the anatomical location of dysfunction and the interpretation of results are summarised in Fig. 7.1 for the LMNS.

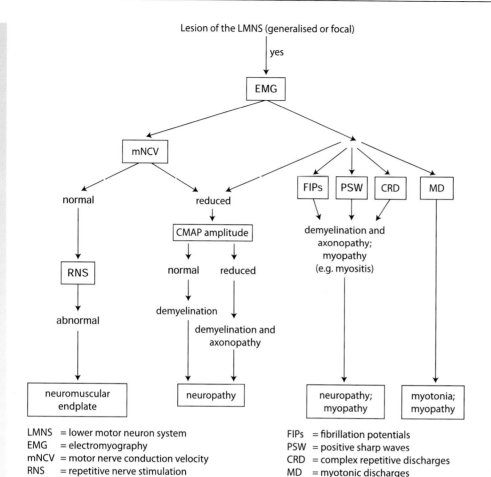

Lesion of the LMNS (generalised or focal)

LMNS = lower motor neuron system
EMG = electromyography
mNCV = motor nerve conduction velocity
RNS = repetitive nerve stimulation
CMAP = compound muscle action potential

FIPs = fibrillation potentials
PSW = positive sharp waves
CRD = complex repetitive discharges
MD = myotonic discharges

Fig. 7.1
Electrodiagnostic methods for investigating diseases of the peripheral nervous system (LMNS).

7

Animals are usually anaesthetised for electrodiagnostic investigations because voluntary and involuntary movement falsify the results. The advantages of anaesthesia include the fact that the procedures may be undertaken accurately, calmly and without causing pain (see Chap. 5.2.5). Due to this need for anaesthesia, the physiological stimulation of a nerve must be imitated by an electrode in electroneurography.

7.1 Electrodiagnosis of the peripheral nervous system (PNS)

The smallest functional motor unit of the PNS consists of an α-motor neuron cell body, a ventral nerve root, a nerve fibre, a synapse and a muscle fibre. The sum of all motor units in the body forms the LMNS, which is equivalent to the efferent part of the PNS.

The afferent system originates in the specialised receptors in the ligaments, muscles and skin. The dorsal ganglia of the spinal cord and the brain stem contain the nerve cells of the peripheral sensory nervous system. The sensory ganglia are bipolar. This term is based on the fact that the sensory nerve cells are connected to the receptors via one of their axons and they provide information to the CNS via their second axon.

The autonomic nervous system is made up of a parasympathetic and a sympathetic section. The parasympathetic innervation takes place within cranial nerves III, VII, IX and X, and the pelvic nerve. The sympathetic innervation runs via the cervical and the thoracolumbar sympathetic trunk.

At the cellular level, the most important structures are the neurons with their axons, the Schwann cells and the synapses. The peripheral nerves originate from the motor nerve cells in the spinal cord and the brain stem, in conjunction with the sensory nerve cells in the dorsal ganglia of the spine and head regions. They form and maintain the string-like processes known as axons. The neurons work as metabolic centres. Protein synthesis takes place here; due to a continuous but slow production of cytoskeleton parts (neurofilaments, microtubules, mitochondria, endoplasmic reticulum and vesicles), the ordered construction and regeneration of the axon is assured. The neurons are the starting point for the cell's rapid antegrade energy transport to the periphery of the nerve and they also process the waste products that are brought via the retrograde axoplasmic flow back to the neuron. The function and integrity of the sometimes very long axons can only be maintained by the normal activity of the neurons.

The Schwann cells play an important role in nerve conduction. They produce the myelin which is bound in spirals around the axon. The myelin sheath is divided into segments by Ranvier's nodes. Myelin is an important prerequisite for efficient and rapid nerve conduction. Electrical action potentials travel along the nerve. The electrical activity is generated mainly with help of an avalanche-like sodium influx through the axon's cell membrane into the cell. In nerves which do not have a myelin sheath, these action potentials travel slowly along the axon. If the nerve fibres have a myelin sheath, the action potential can jump from Ranvier's node to Ranvier's node, which massively increases the velocity of the signal conduction. This so-called saltatory nerve conduction is important for efficient signal transmission. The greater the diameter of the axon, the greater the distance between the Ranvier's nodes and the quicker the nerve conduction.

Another important station for signal transmission is the synapse. This is the contact point between the axon and the musculature, glands or other nerve cells. It consists of a presynaptic nerve ending, a synaptic space and a postsynaptic membrane with receptors. Simply said, in a synapse electrical nerve impulses are partially transformed into chemical energy. Electrical signals activate the release of neurotransmitters from vesicles which are attached to the presynaptic membrane. The released molecules diffuse to the postsynaptic membrane and bind to specific receptors, which in turn initiate electrical signals towards the effector organ. The most important neurotransmitter in the PNS is acetylcholine.

In muscle cells, the action potential spreads out over the whole of the muscle membrane. The so-called T-tubules allow the impulse to penetrate into the depths of the muscle fibre. The release of calcium from the sarcoplasmic reticulum into the muscle fibres enables the connection between actin and myosin. Muscle contraction and muscle relaxation are processes that are heavily dependent on an adequate supply of energy.

7.1.1 Electromyography (EMG)

Three different types of muscle activity can be measured using EMG: activity due to electrode insertion, the spontaneous activity of the relaxed muscle, and the activation due to volitional or reflex movements. In human medicine, EMG is normally undertaken on the conscious patient, whereby volitional muscle contractions induce a recruitment of additional motor units, and an interference pattern with increased muscle contraction can be seen. With the evaluation of our patients under anaesthesia, this method is not possible (see Chap. 5.2.5.2). The assessment of the insertion activity and spontaneous muscle activity, however, still provides adequate information (3).

7.1.1.1 Measurement methods

The basic EMG equipment consists of electrodes, an amplifier, oscilloscope and a loudspeaker. Abnormal spontaneous muscle activity is usually an irregularly occurring phenomenon with diffuse scattering of its localisation. Accordingly, the sensitivity of EMG increases with increasing number of evaluations in a particular muscle independent of which type of electrode is used. The potentials recorded via the electrodes are amplified up to a million-fold. The oscilloscope assists with the visualisation of the electromyographic signals, with the amplitude provided in volts and the time in milliseconds. The loudspeaker is important as the different EMG signals make typical noises.

Normal muscle activity

Completely relaxed normal musculature (i.e., under general anaesthesia) shows no spontaneous activity – it is electrically silent. Activity can only be seen in connection with (a) the insertion of the needle and (b) the positioning of the electrode close to a neuromuscular junction.

a) The insertion activity, also called **insertion potential**, is caused by mechanical damage of the muscle fibres resulting from the movement of the needle. Independent of the speed and length of time with which the needle is moved, a spontaneous outbreak of electrical activity is stimulated, which ceases when the needle is in its end-position. The insertion potentials last between 5 and 300 ms, and have an amplitude of $100\,\mu V$. The amplitudes have a monophasic or biphasic form. With diseases of the muscle membrane, e.g. denervation or myositis, the insertion activity can be prolonged. Muscle denervation increases the insertion potentials within 4 to 10 days to an amplitude of $100–650\,\mu V$ with a time of 2 to 4 seconds and a frequency of 50–200 Hz. In severe muscle atrophy or fibrosis, the potentials can also be reduced due to a lower number of contributing muscle fibres. A lack of insertion potentials is one of the typical electomyographic signs in ischemic muscle lesions.

7

7

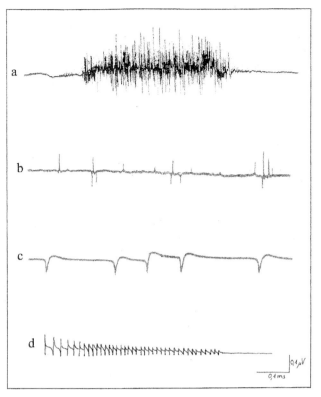

Fig. 7.2
Electrophysiological abnormalities. (a) Prolonged insertion potentials; (b) fibrillation potentials (Fibs); (c) positive sharp waves (PSW); (d) myotonic potentials (MP).

b) An arbitrary but continual release of acetylcholine leads to a depolarisation of the postsynaptic membrane. If the electrode is placed close to a neuromuscular junction, **endplate potentials** can be registered. Diseases such as myasthenia gravis which involve reduced binding of acetylcholine to the postsynaptic membrane, demonstrate a reduced amplitude but a normal frequency of the endplate potentials (see Chap. 7.1.2.3). The summation of these potentials results in endplate noise. They appear as rapid, irregular mono- or biphasic fluctuations of the basal line and start with a negative value. Their amplitude is from 3–60 μV, their frequency is 600–1000 Hz and they last for 1–1.5 ms; their sound is a moderate hiss. It is very important that this recording is not confused with pathological fibrillation potentials (1, 2, 3).

Pathological spontaneous activity

Fibrillation potentials (Fibs) and **positive sharp waves (PSW)** arise from the same basic pathological changes (Fig. 7.1). They only differ in their morphological appearance with respect to their orientation to the recording electrode at the moment of electrical discharge. Both occur due to spontaneous firing of individual hypersensitive muscle

fibres as a result of a destabilisation of their sarcolemma. This can occur with denervation, polymyositis, muscular dystrophy or other myopathies. Fibs are considered to be pathological if they occur at more than two insertion sites outside of the endplate region (Fig. 7.2). Fibs can be found regularly in the interosseus muscle in healthy animals. They consist of bi- or triphasic waves with an initial positive (downwards) deviation from the basal line or a negative deviation when they are recorded in an endplate region. Their amplitude lies on average between 100–300 μV, though in exceptional cases they can be in the range of 20–500 μV. Fibs last for 1–5 ms and appear as collections of amplitudes with a regular rhythm of approximately 13 Hz. They sound like frying eggs or raindrops falling on a tin roof. A significant reduction in the Fibs is an indication of the start of successful motor nerve reinnervation, although this phenomenon can also occur with fibrosis (1, 2).

Positive sharp waves (PSW) are spontaneous potentials with a typical triangular shape, which means that they have an initial steep positive deviation from the basal line and a subsequent slow negative fluctuation (Fig. 7.2). They show different amplitudes ranging from 50–4 μV and have a deeper sound than Fibs. PSW can be recorded in places where excitation transmission is blocked and therefore count as denervation potentials. In animals, they may not be seen until 10 to 20 days after a lesion, but this is variable and they are not a sign of poor prognosis. In the reinnervation phase, spontaneous activity is reduced a few weeks before volitional activity can be recorded (2, 3).

Pseudomyotonic potentials, formerly known as bizarre high frequency discharges, are now termed complex repetitive discharges (CRD). These discharges occur with muscular dystrophy, myositis, metabolic myopathies (e.g. Cushing's syndrome in the dog) and, more rarely, in neurogenic damage. It should be noted that they have nothing to do with true myotonia. The discharges are polyphasic, repetitive waves with a uniform frequency of 5–100 Hz and amplitudes in the range of 50–1 μV. CRD represent spontaneous discharges of roughly synchronised discharging muscle fibres. Typically they show a sudden appearance, with a constant discharge rate over a short time and then abruptly stop. The rat-tat-tat of a machine gun can be heard over the loudspeaker (1).

Myotonic potentials (MP) are independent, repetitive discharges from individual injured muscle fibres (Fig. 7.2). The characteristic "dive bomber" noise created is due to the typical increase and decrease in the amplitude of the potential, and the discharge frequency. The frequency lies between 20 and 80 Hz. MP are characteristic for myotonia (e.g. congenital myotonia of the dog or cat). A blockage of the neuromuscular endplate with curare or the motor axon with a local anaesthetic cannot stop these discharges. Reduced chloride permeability of the muscle membrane is currently being discussed as a possible cause for this type of potential (2).

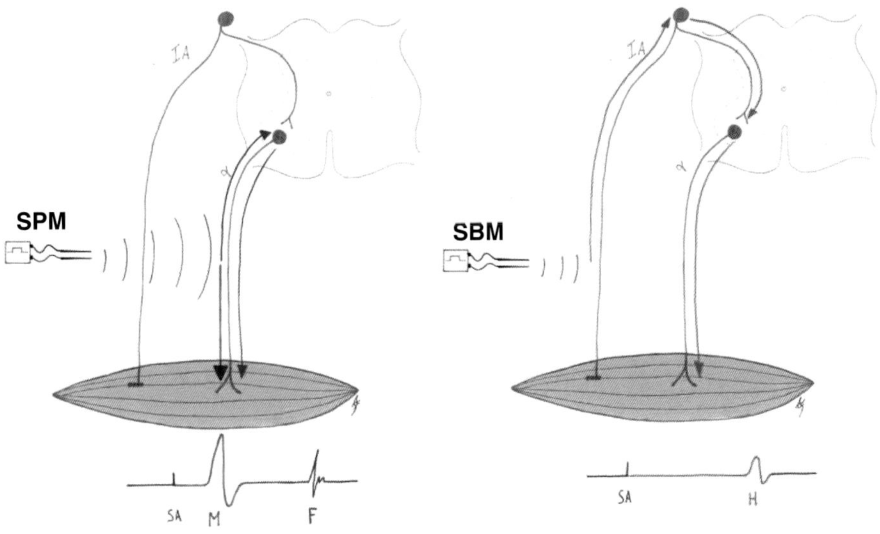

Fig. 7.3
Evoked muscle action potentials. SA = stimulation artefacts (M, F and H waves); SPM = supramaximal stimulation; SBM = submaximal stimulation.

7

Fasciculations occur with mechanical or inflammatory damage of the ventral nerve root and in peripheral nerve lesions. Where they come from has not been totally elucidated. Superficial fasciculations can be seen by the naked eye in contrast to fibrillations. Deep fasciculations are far more common, but they can only be recorded using EMG. Their transmission is caused by a spontaneous contraction of the muscle fibres within a motor unit. They can differ greatly in both their type and shape. They make a sharp crackling sound that bears no relationship to exertion (1, 2, 3).

7.1.2   Electroneurography

The principles of signal amplification and the visualisation of the recording in EMG are also used in electroneurography (see Chap. 5.2.5.3). The electrodiagnostic evaluation of peripheral nerve conduction velocity (PNCV) contains a motor and a sensory component. In individual cases, the cranial nerves can also be assessed. All wave forms are induced with supramaximal stimuli so that the complete pool of axons in a particular nerve can be assessed independent of its diameter and spatial relationship to the electrode. The information about the functionality of the peripheral nerve is invaluable in the clarification of traumatic nerve lesions and in polyneuropathies with different aetiologies. PNCV is normal in myopathies, greatly reduced in demyelination, while in axonal degeneration it is either normal or slightly reduced.

7.1.2.1   Motor nerve conduction velocity (mNCV).

Motor nerve conduction is the most common evaluation of the peripheral nerves performed in small animals. The test allows assessment of the measurement of the mNCV, as well as the amplitude, duration and area of the provoked MAPs. The provoked MAPs are made up of the individual potentials from many motor units that lie within the range of the electrode. They can be divided into the so-called M and F waves. The **M wave** (Fig. 7.3) is the summation of those potentials which are formed from motor units when they are orthdromically stimulated (in the physiological direction). The **F wave** is the response to antidromic activation of the motor neuron, resulting in the motor units stimulated a second time and a potential being registered with a 10–30 ms greater latency than the M wave. In the dog, the maximal amplitude of the F wave is 3% of the amplitude of the M wave (200–300 µV). No F waves can be recorded when there is a lesion of the ventral root, in contrast to those seen with a severing of the dorsal root. Changes in the F waves as found with proximal neuropathies (e.g. polyradiculoneuritis) often occur long before any other EMG or NCV abnormalities. **H waves** represent the passage of conduction through the dorsal nerve root, into the spinal cord and out through the ventral nerve root. The nerves which are most commonly tested on the forelimbs are the radial and ulnar nerves; less often the median nerve.

The sciatic-tibial and the peroneal nerves are the most frequently tested on the hindlimb. The cranial nerves can only be subjected to a limited evaluation due to their inaccessibility, e.g. recurrent laryngeal nerve and facial nerve.

7

Insertion of the stimulating needle electrodes close to the nerve under scrutiny causes a local depolarisation due to a flow of electricity between the cathode and the anode. The evoked potentials are recorded from the muscle by EMG. To calculate the **mNCV**, the nerve is stimulated at two different sites so that two different latencies can be measured in the same muscle. The latency is the time between the onset of stimulation and the beginnings of the M wave response. The mNCV is the distance between the two stimulation points divided by the latency difference. It is not possible to measure a single latency as it consists of three components: (1) generation time of the nerve action potential, (2) the nerve conduction time from the site of the stimulus to the end of the nerve and (3) the neuromuscular transmission time including the time necessary for the generation of a cMAP. The measurement of the latency difference excludes (1) and (3), so that the actual conduction velocity can be determined. In normal nerves, the NCV should **not be below 50 m/s**. It should be noted that excessive stimulation intensities can lead to the production of erroneously short latencies and so falsify the calculations.

The age of an animal has a significant influence on the mNCV. Dogs attain their adult values between the ages of 6 and 12 months. There is a tenfold increase in velocity during the maturation of myelin, with the largest increase occurring between birth and the fifth week of life. There is stability in the value between 1 and 7 years of age, followed by a gradual slowing. At 10 years old, the mNCV appears to be reduced by 10–15%. Cats attain their normal values at approx. 3 months old. An age-associated reduction has not been found with any certainty in this species. Every reduction in limb temperature by 1°C leads to a reduction in the mNCV by 1.7–1.8 m/s. It is, therefore, important to maintain the body and limb temperatures above 36°C during anaesthesia. The mNCV is also affected by the length of the limb; the longer the limb, the slower the velocity, while the amplitude of the MAP is smaller and it has a greater duration.

Neuropathy of the distal nerves and the intramuscular nerve branches is best calculated using the **residual latency**. The residual latency is a measurement of the collective delay of the fine intramuscular, motor branches and the neuromuscular endplate. The amplitude of the evoked MAPs is a measurement of the number of activated nerve fibres. **Area calculations** are theoretically a better index for the number of available functional axons because this takes into account the average cMAPs and so includes the slow motor part (1, 2, 3, 4).

Abnormal motor nerve conduction velocity
In general, an axonal lesion leads to a loss in the cMAP amplitude, whilst demyelination increases the conduction time. The most important abnormalities associated with motor nerve conduction studies are discussed in the following.

(1) A **reduction in the amplitude** of the cMAPs without any scatter indicates a generalised axonopathy (e.g. Coonhound paralysis), a severe myopathy (e.g. polymyositis) or reduced neuromuscular transmission (e.g. botulism).

(2) A **slow mNCV** without any significant reduction in the M wave amplitude indicates demyelination (e.g. diabetes mellitus in cats). Severe demyelination can result in a time-associated scatter and polyphasic M waves (desynchronisation) due to the different diameters of the myelinated fibres. An axonopathy with complete loss of the fast-conducting fibres can also cause a slow conduction velocity. In this case, there is a recordable concomitant reduction in amplitude of the cMAPs of about 50%.

(3) A reduction in the proximal M wave amplitudes in comparison to the distal ones without any time-associated scatter and polyphasic waves are characteristic of a **conduction block**. Conduction blocks occur when segmental demyelination along a nerve is larger than two internodes in length. This can be seen, for example, in cats with diabetic neuropathy. Independent of the amplitude, a conduction velocity of less than 60% of the normal value is indicative of a peripheral nerve disease. Serial electrophysiological investigations can indicate the possible course of a particular disease; they are very valuable for prognosis (3, 4).

7.1.2.2 Sensory nerve conduction velocity

Sensory fibres only degenerate when the lesion lies distal to the sensory ganglia (dorsal root). The presence of the distal sensory potentials serves, therefore, as a diagnostic criterion; for example, for the differentiation between a root lesion and a plexopathy. The amplitude, form and duration of the evoked nerve potentials are determined in addition to the NCV. In contrast to the motor latency, the sensory latency consists of only the nerve activation and conduction velocity from the stimulation site to the recording electrode. It is recommended despite this to calculate the NCV from a number of different sites. Two methods are used, the orthodrome and the antidrome assessment of the NCV. The orthodrome measurement stimulates the sensory nerve endings distally and transmits it proximally, i.e. in the physiological direction. The action potentials of the sensory nerves have smaller amplitudes than the muscle potentials and, therefore, it is more difficult to differentiate them from background noise than the latter.

Sensory fibres with large diameters have a lower threshold and conduct faster (up to 10%) than the antidromic motor conduction within a mixed nerve. As a consequence, these are recorded using a stimulus which is submaximal for the motor fibres. This means, therefore, that the recorded potentials from mixed nerves (e.g. tibial and ulnar nerves) have a quicker NCV than the antidromic motor fibres. The NCV of sensory fibres is calculated from the latency divided by the distance between the stimulating cathode and the recording electrode.

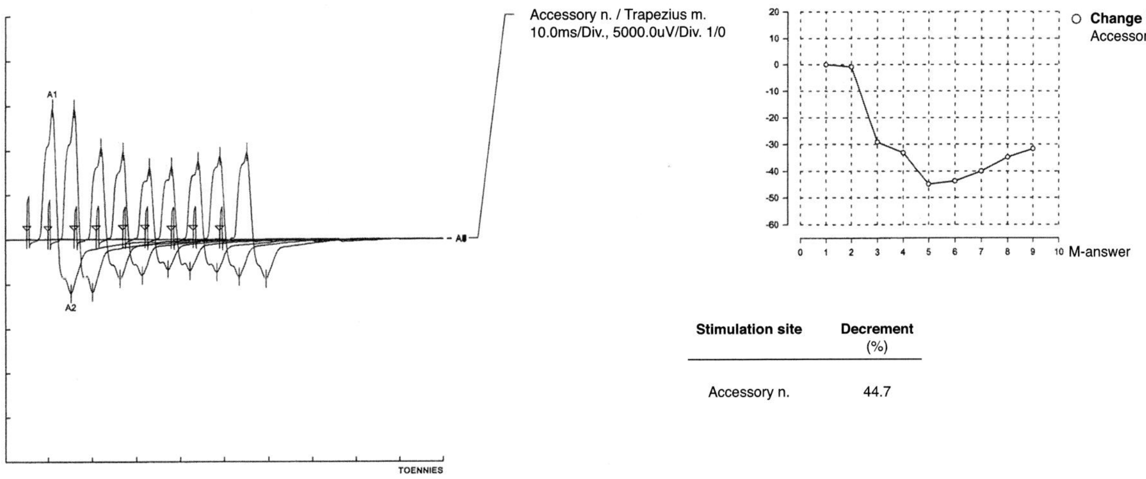

Accessory n. / Trapezius m.
10.0ms/Div., 5000.0uV/Div. 1/0

○ **Change in amplitude -> M1**
Accessory n.

M-answer

Stimulation site	Decrement (%)
Accessory n.	44.7

Fig. 7.4
Repetitive supramaximal nerve stimulation at a frequency of 5 HZ in a young Doberman with suspicion of myasthenia gravis. There is an obvious decrement of 44.7%. The patient additionally had a significantly high antibody titre against ACh receptors and was tensilon positive.

The latency is normally measured from the start of the stimulus artefacts to the initial positive displacement (displacement downwards). In dogs older than 9 years, there is usually a reduction in the sensory conduction velocity of approximately 10 m/s. HECKMANN could never elicit an antidromal nerve summation potential in the dog by using a submaximal stimulation. He is of the opinion that only the orthodrome method is of any significance in this species.

The abnormalities described under motor nerve conduction can be principally used for the sensory conduction, too. A severe reduction in the sensory nerve conduction indicates the presence of demyelination, while axonotmesis leads to a reduction of the amplitude of the nerve action potentials (1, 2, 3, 4, 7).

7.1.2.3 The electrophysiological assessment of the neuromuscular endplate

Many relaxed muscle fibres exhibit a spontaneous subliminal activity: the miniature endplate potentials (MEPP). They represent depolarisations of the postsynaptic membrane caused by the continual but random presynaptic release of individual acetylcholine quanta or packages. If a needle is placed close to an endplate, then such MEPP can be registered. A small dose of curare reduces their amplitude, whilst equivalent doses of neostigmine (prostigmine) increase it. MEPP cannot be recorded after either denervation or local anaesthesia of the nerve. An action potential arriving at the pre-synaptic membrane causes a synchronised release of acetylcholine, which results in a summation of many MEPP and the induction of an endplate potential. The size of the endplate potential de-

pends on the acetylcholine quanta that are immediately available and the potential-dependent calcium concentration within the end of the axon. A neuromuscular block takes place when the endplate potential is not able to overcome its threshold value. A subthreshold endplate potential can be due either to an insufficient release of acetylcholine from the end of the axon or due to a reduced sensitivity of the neuromuscular endplate.

Repetitive supramaximal nerve stimulation is the most commonly used method of evaluating diseases of the neuromuscular junction, such as botulism or congenital and acquired forms of myasthenia gravis. The method consists of the stimulation of a peripheral nerve with a series of impulses and the concomitant recording of the evoked cMAPs. The most obvious amplitudes or changes in area (under the curve) of these muscle potentials can be found if the first potential is compared with the subsequent ones (e.g. waves 3 to 5 and 10). The amplitudes and areas of these later potentials are measured and formulated as a percentage reduction of the first potential. A reduced response using a high stimulation frequency (e.g. 30 Hz) is characteristic for every normal endplate, therefore stimulation rates greater than 5 Hz should not be used in diagnostic evaluations. A stimulation of 2–3 Hz is enough to immediately empty the acetylcholine store, while it is slow enough to prevent the neurosecretory mechanisms that can strengthen the neuromuscular transmission.

In patients with myasthenia gravis, there is a reduction of the amplitudes by more than 10% in comparison to the first potential (usually to the first five potentials; Fig. 7.4). With a series of stimuli, the threshold potential is reached in fewer

7

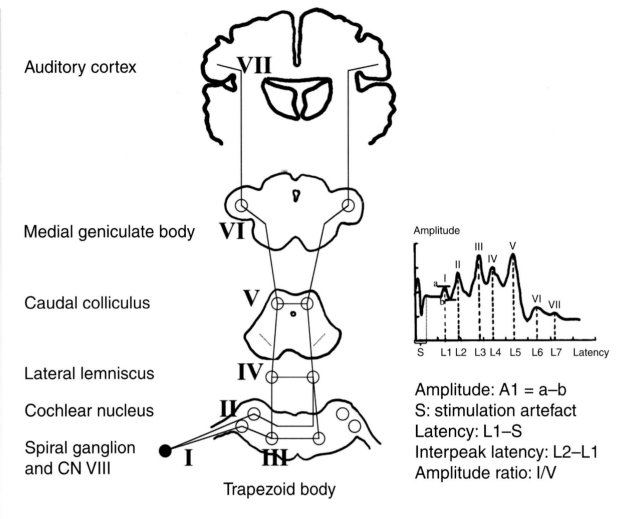

Auditory cortex

Medial geniculate body

Caudal colliculus

Lateral lemniscus

Cochlear nucleus

Spiral ganglion
and CN VIII

Trapezoid body

Amplitude

S   L1 L2 L3 L4 L5 L6 L7   Latency

Amplitude: A1 = a–b
S: stimulation artefact
Latency: L1–S
Interpeak latency: L2–L1
Amplitude ratio: I/V

Fig. 7.5
Anatomical structure of the brain stem as pertaining to auditory function.

and fewer fibres leading to a reduction in the compound muscle action potential. A reduced MEPP amplitude suggests a reduced number of acetylcholine molecules per quantum, a loss in diffusion through the synaptic space or a reduced sensitivity of the acetylcholine receptors. The function of the neuromuscular junction is age-dependent. Its maturation seems to occur in dogs at an age of 2 months. The same criteria as in the adult dog are, therefore, used in young dogs and puppies older than 8 weeks with a suspicion of congenital myasthenia gravis.

In comparison to myasthenia gravis, which typically demonstrates a reduced response to repetitive stimuli, botulism can induce an increased or a decreased response. An increased response is seen because the repetitive nerve stimulation counteracts the complete block caused by the botulinum toxin causing excessive release of acetylcholine. The destruction of areas of the postsynaptic membrane, seen as a side-effect of some myopathies (e.g. myositis), can induce a reduced potential response. The differentiation between polymyositis and myasthenia gravis can be made by observing the initial amplitudes of the cMAPs. Animals with myasthenia gravis initially produce a normal cMAP amplitude, whereby animals with polymyositis have initial cMAPs with low amplitudes. Medications such as aminoglycosides (neomycin, kanamycin) not only induce the release of acetylcholine but also directly interfere with postsynaptic transmission and subsequently affect the EMG evaluation (1, 2, 3).

7.1.3 Auditory evoked potentials (AEP)

AEP represent the brain activities induced by an auditory stimulus and reflect the electrophysiological processes in the sensory cells of the entire auditory tract. AEP consist of positive and negative potential differences with a very low amplitude (μV). They are, therefore, often hidden by other factors such as muscle twitching. Due to repetitive time-locked acoustic stimulation, the stimulus-correlated potentials are added together, averaged and shown as summated action potentials. The early potentials, recorded within 10 ms after stimulation, are generated in the auditory nerve and brain stem (see Chap. 5.2.5.4). They are therefore called **b**rain stem **a**uditory **e**voked **p**otentials (BAEP) (11, 32, 36, 37).

7.1.3.1 Indications

The recording of AEP is mainly done for an objective diagnosis of deafness. Other indications include the recognition of diseases of the brain stem (e.g. space-occupying lesions). A disturbance in auditory function is caused by disturbances in sound conduction (conductive deafness) or sound sensation (sensorineural deafness). Abnormal sound conduction occurs when the transmission of sound is disturbed, e.g. obstruction of the auditory canal (exudative otitis externa, foreign body), ear drum rupture or middle ear pathology. Cochlear defects (cochlear/sensorineural deafness) lead to a disturbance in sound sensation. The causes of cochlear defects include congenital disease, infections, tumours, ototoxic medications or senile degenerative changes (15, 17, 22, 26, 37, 40, 41, 42, 43, 45).

Animals can be tested once their hearing has completely developed (Fig. 7.5). Hearing begins to function in kittens at the age of five days, in puppies from day 10 to 11 post partum and is mature by approx. 5 weeks of age (16, 20, 24, 35, 43). Animals with bilateral deafness can be tested for their hearing by making a loud noise whilst they are sleeping, although this is quite subjective. In central deafness, the cerebral hemispheres and/or auditory tracts are damaged by disease. These animals often therefore have other neurological deficits, which can be severe, especially in brain stem lesions. With unilateral deafness, it is not possible to decide whether the animal is deaf or is just not listening. AEP is a widely used and established objective method of recognising such animals. The advantage of this method is that cooperation from the patient is not necessary; it can also be undertaken on the sedated animal (14, 25, 31, 39, 48).

7.1.3.2 Measurement methods

The equipment setup is shown in Fig. 7.6. The stimulation unit generates an acoustic signal of a defined frequency and strength, which is transferred to the ear being tested by an earplug or headphones. The other ear is provided with white-noise which keeps background noises at bay. The acoustic stimulus is an electrical rectangular signal with a wide frequency spectrum and short duration; it is called a "click". The evoked potentials arise due to the electrical potentials in the nerve fibres, which are induced by the transmission of the sensory stimulus. The change in potential is measured via an electrode placed at the bottom of each ear. A third electrode situated on the vertex is used as the reference. Other electrode set-ups or "montages" are also described. An electrical waveform is recorded after each click and is checked for artefacts by the computer. The individual sequences following each click are added together and averaged. The summation potentials are depicted on an output machine (oscilloscope) (11, 32, 37).

7

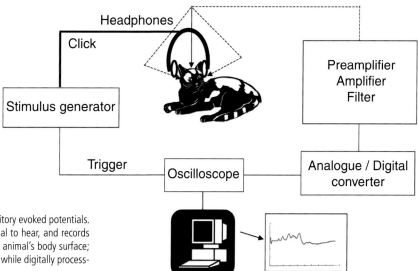

Fig. 7.6
Schematic diagram of the instruments used to record auditory evoked potentials. The equipment generates an acoustic signal for the animal to hear, and records these which are represented as induced potentials on the animal's body surface; the equipment also filters and reinforces these potentials, while digitally processing the potentials' signals.

7

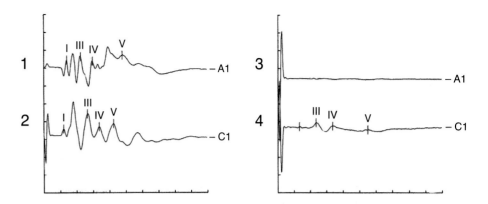

No.	Stimulus site / Recording site	ms/Div	uV/Div	Cycles	Stimulus (dB)
1/A1	right / right ipsi	1.0	2.0	2000	75.0
2/C1	left / left ipsi	1.0	2.0	2000	75.0
3/A1	right / right ipsi	1.0	2.0	2000	100.0
4/C1	left / left ipsi	1.0	2.0	2000	100.0

Fig. 7.7
Examples of a normal bilateral hearing function test (1 and 2), congenital sensorineural deafness on the right (3) and conductive deafness (4) (ipsi = ipsilateral).

7.1.3.3 Description and anatomical classification of the AEP

The summation potentials consist of up to seven waves, which are designated from I to VII according to when they appear on the time scale, and are described due to their polarity as being either positive (P) or negative (N). A series of experimental studies have been done to designate each AEP wave to a specific anatomical structure (Fig. 7.5). The generators of the first two AEP waves have been identified. Due to the anatomical and functional complexity of the auditory brain stem structures, it has not been possible to accurately associate the later AEP waves (III–VII) with any particular structure. Many auditory brain stem structures are activated simultaneously by an auditory stimulus and the AEP wave form depends on the summation of all of the positive and negative activities.

The response threshold to a stimulus is described as being the lowest stimulation intensity at which recordable AEP are induced. The hearing threshold lies in general under the potential threshold, though it can hardly be differentiated from the EEG background. The individual waves are characterised according to their amplitude, latency or interpeak latency, and amplitude ratios (Fig. 7.7).

Wave I appears after a latency of approx. 1 ms and has the greatest amplitude in the dog (Fig. 7.7: 1 and 2). In the cat, wave II is larger than wave I. Wave I and V are easy to identify, but waves III and IV in the dog are very variable and can "merge" together to form one wave; in the cat, these are usually separate from each other. Wave VII is not always present. The latency and amplitude are dependent on the intensity and rate of acoustic stimulation: the higher the stimulation intensity, the shorter the latency and the higher the

amplitude (12, 18, 22, 28, 29, 30, 38, 44). The average values for a six-week-old, healthy, anaesthetised (medetomidine; Domitor®) Dalmatian puppy are shown below. The measurements were undertaken with a Multilinear Neuroscreen Plus (Jaeger / Toennies) with ear plugs (EARTONE, Aero Company) using a stimulus intensity of 90 db, 14 Hz frequency and every 2000 cycles. The average body temperature during the measurements was 37.5°C.

Wave I	Wave II	Wave III	Wave V	Wave VI
A (µV)	A (µV)	A (µV)	A (µV)	A (µV)
L (ms)	L (ms)	L (ms)	L (ms)	L (ms)
3.7	1.6	3.1	2.5	0.9
1.1	1.3	1.9	3.2	4.3

A = amplitude
L = latency

The morphology of the AEP waves are influenced by various factors (21, 36, 37, 46, 47), which include the following:
- Species and breed of patient (27, 34)
- Age and postnatal maturation (16, 23, 35, 44)
- Position or montage of the electrodes (19)
- Stimulus: intensity, rate, type and polarity (33)
- Body temperature of the patient (13)
- Anaesthetic used (14, 25, 31, 39, 48)

The aim of the AEP investigation is to determine the presence and severity of deafness (uni- or bilateral) and the localisation of the lesion (central / peripheral auditory tracts) (Fig. 7.7: 3 and 4).

7.2 Electrodiagnostic examinations of the CNS

7.2.1 Electroencephalography

Luciana Bergamasco
André Jaggy

Electroencephalography (EEG) measures the spontaneous electrical activity of the brain (49). This non-invasive investigation can be used to investigate neurological diseases such as malformation (hydrocephalus), inflammatory disease (encephalitis), brain tumours, vascular disease, craniocerebral injuries, and especially epilepsy. Localised changes in the electrical activity recorded from the brain can be used to locate cerebral diseases. The quantification of the brain's electrical activity using spectral analysis of the frequency patterns, so-called q-EEG or brain mapping, enables a better clinical understanding of most of the different types of cerebral disease (50).

7.2.1.1 Physiological principles

With the aid of the EEG, spontaneous changes in the electrical activity of the cerebral cortex can be recorded using superficial electrodes. These are usually placed over the frontal, parietal, temporal and occipital lobes (49). Recording with superficial electrodes can be understood on the basis of the volume conductor theory. According to this theory, the changes in neuronal membrane potential are transferred to the extracellular fluid. For this to happen, the cerebral surface must be at least 6 cm^2 and have a depth of approx. 5 mm. The measured differences in potential are produced by the postsynaptic potentials of thousands of neurons lying under the electrodes. The pyramidal cells, lying perpendicular to the surface and parallel to each other, appear to produce more of the EEG activity than the glial cells. In comparison to the postsynaptic potentials, action potentials play only a negligible part in the total electrical activity due to their short duration and small summation.

7.2.1.2 Method

The EEG has been standardised so that positive differences in potentials are shown by a displacement of the basal line downwards; the displacement is upwards with negative differences in potential. The polarity depends electrophysiologically on whether it is an excitatory (EPSP) or an inhibitory (IPSP) postsynaptic potential, and in which layer of the cerebral cortex it occurs. If EPSPs occur in the deeper layers of the brain then a positive or downward displacement of the EEG is seen; IPSP cause the opposite effect. The response is vice versa with superficial EPSP and IPSP.

Each amplitude is caused by a number of simultaneously active neurons. A high amplitude with a low frequency is known as a synchronised EEG, i.e. all the neurons are acting together. A low amplitude with a high frequency is known as a desynchronised EEG.

The frequency of potential changes in EEG depends on the activity of both the medial nuclear area in the thalamus and the reticular formation, both of which are connected to the cortex. The measured values lie between 0.5 and 50 Hz, whereby normal values are between 0.5 and 30 Hz. The normal amplitude is from 20–200 µV. Some predominant rhythmic frequencies can be observed: δ (0.5–4.0 Hz), θ (4.0–8.0 Hz), α (8.0–12.0 Hz) and β (12.0–30.0 Hz).

The optimal measuring conditions can be achieved in a quiet, darkened and electrically screened room. The measurements can be undertaken on an animal while it is unsedated (51), sedated (52) or anaesthetised (53). The main advantage of the latter method is the possibility of preventing movement and muscle artefacts (54). In addition, pathological activity such as focal spikes often cannot be recorded in animals when they are awake (54). Independent of the mode of sedation, there is a dose-dependent slowing of the main EEG frequency. With different medications, however, various dominant EEG frequencies and special EEG patterns can be elicited (55). Some anaesthetics induce spikes and/or burst suppression patterns; others suppress the spike activity and therefore make diagnosis difficult (56, 57). An obvious reduction in the general and artificial paroxysmal brain activity can be achieved by sedating with medetomidine/propofol (see Chap. 5.2.5.1) (58).

7.2.1.3 Equipment

A classical EEG machine allows the bioelectrical signal to be collected, amplified and printed (e.g. with a needle printer). Digital saving of the data is not possible. With the use of a digital recording system, the data can be saved for further processing, especially for spectral analysis (q-EEG), which provides information about the harmonic content of the signals. Short recording periods using digital equipment (60 phases with 2 seconds) provide the same information as a prolonged recording with standard polygraphic EEG (59).

7.2.1.4 Electrodes and their placement

Small needle electrodes are placed subcutaneously under the skin of the head. These are simple and quick to use in comparison to other electrodes, but they usually have a high impedance, which may lead to an unwanted distortion of the basal line. Alternatively, small silver chloride electrodes are glued to the skin or miniature alligator clips are clipped to the skin. In bipolar recording, the electrodes are placed in a longitudinal (rostrocaudal) and/or transverse arrangement. Each "channel" records the difference in potential between the two active electrodes. Unipolar recording occurs between an electrode in the skin of the head and an electrically inac-

7

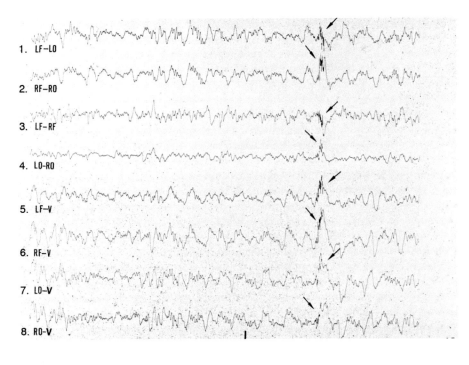

Fig. 7.8
EEG recordings from a five-year-old male Golden Retriever with idiopathic epilepsy. Bipolar (recordings # 1–4) and monopolar (recordings # 5–8) with prominent spike activity (arrows). Basal frequency: 15 Hz with 75 µV; paroxysmal activity 5–6 Hz with 70–150 µV.

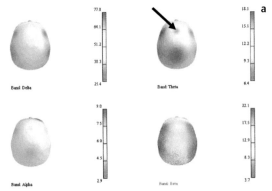

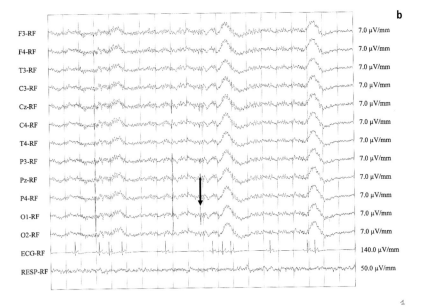

Fig. 7.9
Giant Schnauzer, three years old, with idiopathic epilepsy under medetomidine sedation. Paroxysmal activity is obvious in all the recordings in both the q-EEG (a = colour intensity based on EEG activity) and the routine EEG (b = spike activity).

tive, so-called reference electrode on the bridge of the nose, ear lobe or neck. These reflect the actual electrical activity of the neurons under the electrode.

In veterinary medicine, a number of different electrode sites or montages (set up of two or more electrodes) are used enabling different standard recording deviations to be undertaken. The most commonly used montage consists of five electrodes (60) and eight recording deviations. Other montages are based on the international 10 to 20 system used in human beings (61), with up to 21 electrodes being placed in a standardised manner. The recording time takes between 10 and 20 minutes.

7.2.1.5 Interpretation

In the visual inspection of an EEG, the frequency, amplitude and the pattern of the amplitude, topography, symmetry and synchronisation of the potential differences are assessed

(Fig. 7.8). Frequency is understood to be the frequency of the change in potential from negative to positive; the units are Hertz (Hz). The amplitude is the total displacement from wave to wave, i.e. negative-positive; the units are microvolts (μV). The morphology describes the course of the curve, e.g. sharp, rounded, etc. The topography is the spatial classification of an EEG recording, i.e. frontal, parietal, etc. One talks of a symmetrical EEG when the signals have the same wave length, amplitude and duration in both hemispheres.

Furthermore, transient electrical occurrences can be differentiated from the so-called background rhythms. The latter has a frequency which ranges between 10–30 Hz (α and β) and an amplitude of 10–30 μV (62). During sleep, the frequency falls to 1–3 Hz (d) and the amplitude increases to 150–300 μV. Young animals have a lower frequency and a higher amplitude than older animals, though the amplitude also decreases with age. Brachycephalic breeds have a lower amplitude than other breeds. The electrical background ac-

7

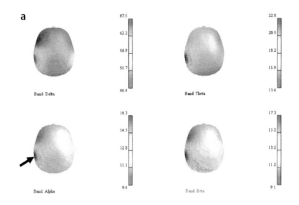

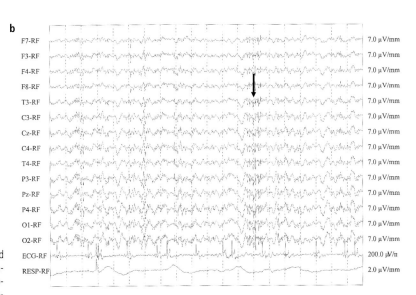

Fig. 7.10
Finnish Spitz, one year old, under medetomidine sedation and phenobarbital therapy. The q-EEG recordings (a = colour intensity based on EEG activity) and the routine EEG (b = repetition of polyspikes and wave complexes as well as synchronised sharp waves) show different paroxysmal activities.

tivity in sedated patients is a synchronous slow frequency and an increased amplitude. The previously mentioned anaesthesia protocol with medetomidine / propofol results in an EEG with a frequency of 1.8 Hz and an amplitude of 28 μV (63). Additionally, a so-called low voltage pattern of 14 μV can also be recorded.

Transient occurrences are changes in EEG which last for only a few seconds. They can be transposed on the background activity or they can completely replace it. They can be normal or pathological. Many artefacts also appear as transient occurrences and must be differentiated from real ones. In the sedated animal, spindle activity, K complexes and sharp vertex and occipital signals can often be observed. These resemble the results of non-REM sleep in human beings (49). Spindles are repetitive sinus waves of 8–12 Hz, which are most prominent in the fronto-central channel and can be recorded from the median sagittal electrodes. K complexes appear spontaneously and are often provoked by acoustic stimulation. They are characterised by their large amplitude (on average 50 μV) and their biphasic pattern, on which spindles may also arise. The sharp vertex waves consist of one or repeated waves with an average frequency of 9.6 Hz. They can be best recorded over the vertex. Their amplitude is less than 100 μV. The positive sharp waves in the area of the occiput are individual waves with a much higher amplitude and a lower frequency; these waves are preferentially found in the vertex and the caudal cranial areas.

Generalised abnormal EEG activity is usually due to a diffuse disease of the cerebrum. Changes that are confined to one channel usually have a focal or multifocal cause. As a rule, a change in both frequency and amplitude are seen with pathological processes (64). The combination of low amplitude and high frequency (low voltage, fast activity; LVFA) is characteristic of inflammatory processes. So-called spikes can be found in connection with LVFA; these are pointed waves with a duration of less than 80 ms. So-called sharp waves with a duration of 80–200 ms can also be present. High amplitudes in combination with a low frequency (high voltage, slow frequency; HVSF) are a sign of chronic cerebral disease and neuronal degeneration.

In patients with **hydrocephalus**, the EEG results are substantially dependent on the ICP. HVLF (1–5 Hz and 100–300 μV) with superimposed waves of 10–20 Hz are typical of this disease. In addition, LVFA waves with a combination of high frequencies and high amplitudes may be recorded (65).

Short sections of electrical inactivity are characteristic for **inflammatory processes,** the so-called "burst suppression" in conjunction with slow waves (5–10 Hz and 20–50 μV), complexes with spikes and slow waves such as sharp waves, and HVSF (1–4 Hz and 100–200 μV) (66, 67). KLEMM found pathological spindle activity with bacterial or viral encephalitis (53). Dogs experimentally infected with distemper showed HVSF waves with superimposed LVFA of 8–12 Hz, whereby the latter activity was associated with lesions in the affected animals which lead to clinical signs of epilepsy (Fig. 7.8) (68). Independent of the type of causative encephalitis, a characteristic paroxysmal EEG activity with a high amplitude (average 106.3 μV) and fast frequency (8.5 Hz) is seen in patients with relapsing epilepsy (69).

Other suddenly occurring depolarisations such as spikes, polyspikes, complexes with sharp waves, and complexes with sharp waves and spikes can be recorded in **epilepsy** patients either during a seizure or as interictal events in the conscious or sedated dog (Figs. 7.9 and 7.10) (54, 70). This epileptiform activity can be generalised or focal. In a retrospective study on idiopathic epilepsy in the dog, two typical interictal EEG patterns could be found (71). They consisted of a pattern with a low frequency (1–2.5 HZ) and a high amplitude (10–90 μV), superimposed by a second pattern with a higher frequency of 7–18 Hz and a low amplitude (4–20 μV). In addition, a widely disseminated spindle activity of 12 Hz and differing amplitudes has been described in dogs with an inheritable form of epilepsy (63).

Brain tumours can also cause changes in the EEG. Continuous or intermittent HVSA, spikes and sharp waves can be recorded (72, 73). These results are not specific for a brain tumour, and are only to be considered as indications of a destructive brain lesion. **Vascular diseases** can also have the same EEG patterns. The presence of a q-rhythm is a frequent but not typically pathognomonic sign for patients with **hepatoencephalopathy** (74).

Literature

1 KIMURA, J. (2001): Electrodiagnosis in Diseases of Nerve and Muscle, 3rd ed., Oxford University Press.

2 LUDIN, H.-P. (1981): Praktische Elektromyographie, 2. Auflage, Enke, Stuttgart.

3 CUDDON, P.A. (2002): Electrophysiology in Neuromuscular Disease, Vet Clin North Am Small Anim Pract. **32**: 31–61.

4 HECKMANN, R. (1989): Grundlagen und Methodik zu klinisch-neurophysiologischen Untersuchungen beim Hund, Enke, Stuttgart.

5 ALEXANDER, C.-S. (2001): Physikalische Therapie für Kleintiere, Parey, Berlin.

6 LUDIN, H.-P. (1977): Pathophysiologische Grundlagen elektromyographischer Befunde bei Neuropathien und Myopathien, 2. Auflage, Thieme, Stuttgart.

7 LUDIN, H.-P. (1979): Sensible Neurographie, Thieme, Stuttgart.

8 LENMAN, J.A.R., RITCHIE, A.E. (1977): Clinical Electromyography, 2nd ed., Pitman medical.

9 OLIVER, J.E., LORENZ, M.D., KORNEGAY, J.N. (1997): Handbook of Veterinary Neurology, 3rd ed., Saunders, Philadelphia.

10 VANDEVELDE, M., JAGGY, A., LANG, J. (2001): Veterinärmedizinische Neurologie, 2. Auflage, Parey, Berlin.

11 AMINOFF, J. M. (1999): Electrodiagnosis in Clinical Neurology. 4th ed., Churchill Livingstone, Philadelphia.

12 BIACABE, B., CHEVALLIER, J.M., AVAN, P., BONFILS, P. (2001): Functional anatomy of auditory brainstem nuclei: application to the anatomical basis of brainstem auditory evoked potentials. Auris Nasus Larynx **28**: 85–94.

13 BODENHAMER, R.D., HUNTER, J.F., LUTTGEN, P.J.(1985): Brainstem auditory-evoked responses in the dog. Am J Vet Res. **46**: 1787–1792.

14 COHN, M.S., BRITT, R.H. (1982): Effects of sodium pentobarbital and halothane, and chloralose on brainstem auditory evoked responses. Anesth Analg. **61**: 338.

15 EGER, C.E., LINDSAY P. (1997): Effects of otitis an hearing in dogs characterised by brainstem auditory evoked response testing. J Small Anim Pract. **38**: 380–386.

16 EGGERMONT, J.J. (1985): Evoked potentials as indicator of auditory maturation. Acta Otolaryngol. **421**: 41–47.

17 FISCHER, A., OBERMAIER, G. (1994): Brainstem auditory-evoked potentials and neuropathologic correlates in 26 dogs with brain tumors. J Vet Int Med. **8**: 363–369.

18 HOLLIDAY, T.A., NELSON, H.J., WILLIAMS, D.C. (1992): Unilateral and bilateral brainstem auditory-evoked response abnormalities in 900 Dalmatian dogs. J Vet Int Med. **6**: 166–174.

19 HOLLIDAY, T.A. and TESALLE, M.E. (1985): Brain stem auditory-evoked potentials of dogs: Wave forms and effects of recording electrode positioning. Am J Vet Res. **46**: 845–851.

20 HOSKINS, J. D. (2001): Veterinary Paediatrics, 3rd ed., W. B. Saunders, Philadelphia.

21 HUANG, C. M. and BUCHWALD, J. S. (1978): Factors that affect the amplitudes and latencies of the vertex short latency acoustic responses in the cat. Electroencephalograph Clin Neurophysiol. **44**: 179–186.

22 JAGGY, A., OLIVER, J.E., FERGUSON, E.A. (1994): Neurological manifestations of hypothyroidism: A retrospective study of 29 dogs. J Vet Int Med. **8**: 328–336.

23 JEWETT, D. L., ROMANO, N. (1972): Neonatal development of auditory system potentials averaged from the scalp of rat and cat. Brain Res. **36**: 101–115.

24 KAWASAKI, Y., INADA, S. (1992): Effects of analog filtering on brain stem auditory-evoked potentials in dogs. Am J Vet Res. **53**: 1096–1100.

25 MARSHALL, A.E. (1985): Brainstem auditory-evoked response of nonanesthetized dog. Am J Vet Res. **46**: 966–973.

26 MARSHALL, A.E. (1986): Use of brainstem auditory-evoked response to evaluate deafness in a group of Dalmatian dogs. J Am Vet Med Assoc. **188**: 218–222.

27 MEJI, B.P., VENKER-VAN HAAGEN, A.J., VAN DEN BROM, W.E. (1992): Relationship between latency of brainstem auditory-evoked potentials and head size in dogs. Vet Quart. **14**: 121–126.

28 MELCHER, J.R., KNUDSON, I.M., FULLERTON, B.C. (1996): Generators of the brainstem auditory evoked potential in cat. I. An experimental approach to their identification. Hearing Res. **93**: 1–27.

29 MELCHER, J.R., GUINAN, J.J., KNUDSON, I.M., KIANG, N.Y.S. (1996): Generators of the brainstem auditory evoked potential in cat. II. Correlating lesion sites with waveform changes. Hearing Res. **93**: 28–51.

30 MELCHER, J.R., KIANG, N.Y.S. (1996): Generators of the brainstem auditory evoked potential in cat. III. Identified cell populations. Hearing Res. **93**: 52–71.

31 MEYERS, L.J., REDDING, R.W., WILSON, S. (1985): Reference values of the brainstem auditory evoked response of methyoxyflurane anesthetized and unanesthetized dogs. Vet Res Communic. **9**: 289–294.

32 MÜHLAU, G. (1990): Neuroelektrodiagnostik. 1. Aufl. VEB Gustav Fischer Verlag, Jena.

33 PONCELET, L., COPPENS, A., DELTENRE, P. (2000): Brainstem auditory evoked potential wave V latency-intensity function in normal dalmatian and beagle puppies. J Vet Intern Med. **14**: 424–428.

34 POOK, H. A., STEISS, J. E. (1990): Correlation of brain stem auditory-evoked responses with cranium size and body weight of dogs. Am J Vet Res. **51**: 1779–1783.

35 PUJOL, R., HILDING, D. (1973): Anatomy and physiology of the onset of auditory function. Acta Otolaryng. **76**: 1–10.

7

7

36 SHIU, J.N., MUNRO, K.J., COX, C.L. (1997): Normative auditory brainstem response data for hearing threshold and neuro-otological diagnosis in the dog. J Small Anim Pract. **38**: 103–107.

37 SIMS, M.H. (1988): Electrodiagnostic evaluation of auditory function. Vet Clin North Am Small Anim Pract. **18**: 913–944.

38 SIMS, M.H. (1990): Evoked response audiometry in dogs. PVN **1**: 275–283.

39 SIMS, M.H., HOROHOV, J.E. (1986): Effects of xylazine and ketamine on the acoustic reflex and brain stem auditory-evoked response in the cat. Am J Vet Res. **1**: 102–109.

40 STEFFEN, F., JAGGY, A. (1998): Taubheit und ihre Diagnose bei Hund und Katze. Schweiz Arch Tierheilk. **140**: 397–404.

41 STEISS, J. E., COX, N. C., HATHCOCK, J. T. (1994): Brain stem auditory-evoked response abnormalities in 14 dogs with confirmed central nervous system lesions. J Vet Int Med. **8**: 293–298.

42 STEISS, J.E., WRIGHT, J.C., STORRS, D.P. (1990): Alterations in the brain stem auditory evoked response threshold and latency-intensity curve associated with conductive hearing loss in dogs. PVN **1**: 205–211.

43 STRAIN, G.M. (1991): Congenital deafness in dogs and cats. The Compendium **13**: 245–251.

44 STRAIN, G.M., TEDFORD, B.L., JACKSON R.M. (1991): Postnatal development of the brain stem auditory-evoked potentials in dogs. Am J Vet Res. **52**: 410–415.

45 STRAIN, G. M. (1996): Aetiology, prevalence and diagnosis of deafness in dogs and cats. Br Vet J. **152**: 17–36.

46 STOCKARD, J.J., STOCKARD, J.E., SHARBROUGH, F.W. (1978). Nonpathologic factors influencing brainstem auditory evoked potentials. Am J Electroencephalograph Technol. **18**: 177–209.

47 STOCKARD, J.E., STOCKARD, J.J., WESTMORELAND, B.F. (1997): Brainstem auditory-evoked responses. Normal variations as a function of stimulus and subject characteristics. Arch Neurol. **36**: 823.

48 TOKURIK, M., MATSUNAMI, K., UZUKA, Y. (1990): Relative effects of xylazine-atropine, xylazine-atropine-ketamine, and xylazine-atropine-pentobarbital combinations and time-course effects of the latter two combinations on brain-stem auditory-evoked potentials in dogs. Am J Vet Res. **51**: 97–102.

49 NIEDERMEYER, E., LPES DA SILVA, F. (1987): Electroencephalography: basic principles, clinical applications and related fields. Urban and Schwarzenbeck, Baltimore-Munich.

50 DUFFY, F.H. (1986): Topographic mapping of brain electrical activity. Butterworths, Boston.

51 CROFT, P.G. (1962): The EEG as an aid to diagnosis of nervous diseases in the dog and cat. J Small Anim Pract. **3**: 205–213.

52 REDMAN, H.C., WILSON, G.L., HOGAN, J.E. (1973): Effect of chlorpromazine combined with intermittent light stimulation on the electroencephalogram and clinical response of the Beagle dog. Am J Vet Res. **34**: 929–936.

53 KLEMM, W.R. (1968): Electroencephalograms of anaesthetized dogs and cats with neurological diseases. Am J Vet Res. **29**: 337–340.

54 KLEMM, W.R. (1989): Electroencephalography in the diagnosis of epilepsy. Problems in Vet Med. **1**: 535–557.

55 PRYNN, R.B., REDDING, R.W. (1968): Electroencephalographic continuum in dogs anaesthetized with methoxyflurane and halothane. Am J Vet Res. **29**: 1913–1928.

56 JOAS, T.A., STEVENS, W.C., EGER, E. (1971): Electroencephalographic seizure activity in dogs during anaesthesia. Br J Anaesth. **43**: 739–745.

57 TOMODA, K., SHINGU, K., OSAWA, M. (1993): Comparison of CNS effects of propofol and thiopentone in cats. Br J Anaesth. **71**: 383–387.

58 JAGGY, A., HEYNOLD, Y. (1998): Idiopathic epilepsy in the dog. Europ J Comp Anim Pract. *VIII*: 51–57.

59 BERGAMASCO, L., ACCATINO, A., PRIANO, L. NEIGER-AESCHENBACHER, G., JAGGY, A. (2003): Quantitative electroencephalographic findings in beagles anaesthestized with propofol. Vet. J. **166**: 58–66.

60 REDDING, R.W. (1987): Electrophysiologic diagnosis. In: OLIVER, J.E., HOERLEIN, B.F., MAYHEW, I.G. (eds) Veterinary Neurology. W.B. Saunders, Philadelphia, p. 111.

61 BERGAMASCO, L., ACCATINO, A., JAGGY, A. (1999): Methodical approach to digital electroencephalography and its use in veterinary medicine. Veterinaria **13**: 7–22.

62 PAMPIGLIONE, G. (1963): Development of cerebral function in the dog. Butterworths, Washington.

63 SRENK, P., JAGGY, A. (1996): Interictal electroencephalographic findings in a family of golden retrievers with idiopathic epilepsy. J Small Anim Pract. **37**: 317–321.

64 KLEMM, W.R., HALL, C.L. (1974): Current status and trends in veterinary electroencephalography. J Am Vet Med Assoc. **164**: 529–532.

65 KLEMM, W.R., HALL, C.L. (1971): Electroencephalogram of anaesthetized dogs with hydrocephalus. Am J Vet Res. **32**: 1859–1863.

66 REDDING, R.W., PRYNN, R.B., WAGNER, J.L. (1966): Clinical use of electroencephalogram in canine encephalitis. J Am Vet Med Assoc. **148**: 141–149.

67 CROFT, P.G. (1970): Electroencephalography in canine encephalitis. J Small Anim Pract. **11**: 241–244.

68 ACCATINO, A., JAGGY, A., GAILLARD, C., AESCHBACHER, G. (1997): Electroencephalographic findings in beagle dogs experimentally infected with canine distemper virus. J Vet Med. **44**: 39–48.

69 MARISCOLI, M., JAGGY, A. (1997): Clinical and electroencephalographic findings of inflammatory and infectious diseases of the central nervous system in dogs: a retrospective study. J Vet Med. **44**: 1–18.

70 WIEDERHOLT, W.C. (1974): Electrophysiologic analysis of epileptic beagles. Neurology **24**:149–155.

71 JAGGY, A., BERNARDINI, M. (1998): Idiopathic epilepsy in 125 dogs: a long-term study. Clinical and electroencephalographic findings. J Small Anim Pract. **39**: 23–29.

72 CROFT, P.G. (1972): Electroencephalographic and space-occupying lesions in small animals. J Small Anim Pract. **13**: 175–179.

73 STEISS, J.E., COX, N.R., KNECHT, C.D. (1990): Electroencephalographic and histopathologic correlation in eight dogs with intracranial mass lesion. Am J. Vet Res. **51**: 1286–1290.

74 BUNCH, S.E. (1991): Hepatic encephalopathy. PVN **2**: 287–296.

7.3   Biopsy

Tim Bley

As in the other organ systems, biopsy techniques are used for definitive diagnosis of nervous system diseases. Brain biopsies have been described in the dog, but without image-guided technology, they are infrequently performed. However, nerve and muscle biopsy investigations are a very useful aid in neuromuscular disease. Muscle and nerve biopsies require, in most cases, an initial electrodiagnostic investigation to localise the pathologically affected muscle or nerve (see Fig. 7.1).

7.3.1   Muscle biopsy

These are best coordinated with EMG investigation when the animal is already under anaesthesia and the affected muscles have been localised. The biopsies should be taken at standardised sites, whose normal anatomical consistencies are well known (NB: the site of biopsy should not be at a site where EMG was performed). In chronic diseases with extreme muscle wasting and fibrosis, samples should be taken from the less severely affected muscles. Different methods for muscle biopsy have been described, which will be discussed in the following section.

The most commonly chosen invasive surgical method is the open biopsy (1, 2). A basic set of surgical instruments is required. The procedure can be described as follows: a 4-cm incision is made with a scalpel in the skin at the surgically prepared operation site. The dermis and subcutis are incised and the muscle fascia is revealed by blunt dissection of the subcutaneous fat. The muscle tissue is revealed by a 3-cm incision through the fascia. Retention sutures are placed in the muscle at a distance of 1–2 cm from each other. These serve to carefully manipulate the biopsy, which is excised as a 1-cm diameter cylinder in the direction of the muscle's longitudinal axis. After the biopsy has been removed, a subcutaneous-fascia suture should be used to close the defect. The skin should be closed using a number of individual sutures.

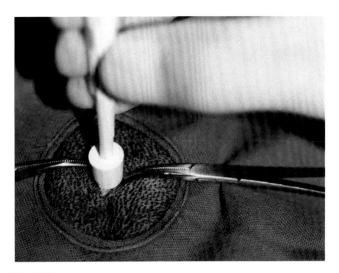

Fig. 7.11
The biopsy punch is pushed down into the tissue with a smooth turning motion to collect the muscle sample.

Another, less commonly practised method is the percutaneous needle biopsy in which a modified 11- or 14-gauge needle (3, 4) is used. The method of taking a muscle sample under local anaesthesia with subcutaneous lidocaine 2% and epinephrine injection is well described (3). The outer skin and the muscle fascia are incised and the biopsy needle is pushed into the muscle until the lateral cutting "window" of the needle lies at a depth of 0.5–0.75 cm. By inducing a slight vacuum, muscle tissue is sucked laterally into the lumen and the aspirate is parted from the rest of the tissue by a stilette within the biopsy needle. This procedure is repeated after rotating the needle and a second sample is collected.

Some advantages are gained by using a biopsy punch consisting of a hollow metal cutting cylinder with a diameter of 0.8 cm. The operation is undertaken under short-term anaesthesia. The skin incision is 1.5 cm long and the muscle fascia is incised with a scalpel for a length of approx. 1 cm. The edges of the fascia are held to the side with artery forceps enabling a direct approach to the muscle. The biopsy punch is placed perpendicular to the muscle body and it is pushed with a fluent turning motion in one direction, into the muscle under light pressure until the white plastic collar is just about touching the muscle (Fig. 7.11). The sample must then be cut away close to the base of the rest of the muscle.

The biopsy is kept fresh in a fluid medium (e.g. on a piece of gauze soaked in physiological saline) and sent as quickly as possible to a specialised laboratory, where cryostat sections can be produced and investigated using a variety of special stains.

7

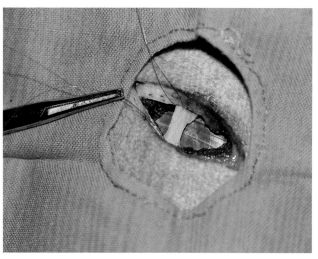

Fig. 7.12
After being dissected free and held using retention stitches, a 1-cm-long biopsy is taken from the peroneal nerve which is roughly a third of the nerve's diameter.

7.3.2 Nerve biopsy

Nerve biopsies are also undertaken at the end of an electro-diagnostic investigation in which a nerve with reduced conduction velocity has been localised. The technique of choice is the so-called fascicular biopsy (see Chap. 10.5.4.1). Roughly 30–50% of a branch of a nerve for a distance of approx. 2 cm is removed parallel to the nerve fibres with a scalpel from the surgically prepared nerve. This fascicle is then cut through at both ends with a scalpel and placed in 3% glutaraldehyde solution and sent immediately to the laboratory.

Literature

1 BOJRAB, M.J. (1998): Technique of skeletal muscle biopsy. In: Current Techniques in Small Animal Surgery. Williams & Wilkins, Baltimore, 4th ed., pp. 91–94.

2 WHEELER, S.J. (1995): Manual of Small Animal Neurology, 3rd ed., BSAVA, London.

3 REYNOLDS, A.J., FUHRER, L., VALENTIN, B.A. (1995): New approach to percutaneous muscle biopsy in dogs. Am J Vet Res. 56: 982–985.

4 MAGISTRIS, M.R., KOHLER, A., PIZZOLATO, G., MORRIS, M.A. (1998): Needle muscle biopsy in the investigation of neuromuscular diseases. Muscle Nerve. 2: 194–200.

5 BLEY, T., BILZER, T., NEUMANN, J., JAGGY, A. (2001): Muskelbiopsien mit der Biopsiestanze – Entnahmetechnik, Versand und Beurteilungsfähigkeit. Schweiz Arch Tierheilk. 143: 405–409.

8 Rehabilitation

Iris Challande-Kathmann
André Jaggy

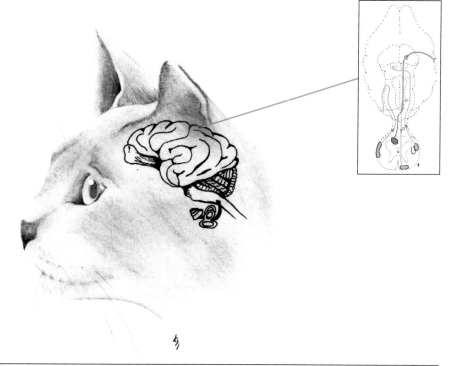

A well-designed physiotherapy programme is the prerequisite for successful rehabilitation. Rehabilitation is an important part of the treatment of neurological disease in small animal medicine. The aim of physiotherapeutic exercises is to maintain the functional muscle mass of the animal and to prevent / slow down disuse atrophy or neurogenic muscle atrophy. Different physiotherapeutic methods, each with their own indications, are used in rehabilitation: massage, hydrotherapy, thermotherapy and electrotherapy, all in combination with kinesiotherapy (2). Initiation and the choice of a suitable physiotherapy programme depends on the disease, the treatment (surgical or medical), the size and cooperation of the animal, and the stage of healing (1, 6).

At the same time as physiotherapy, secondary complication prevention plays an important part in rehabilitation; for example, decubitus prophylaxis, bladder management and the promotion of the patient's motivation through personal attention. It is also important to examine the patient at regular intervals to recognise any changes in their health status, to undertake necessary changes in the rehabilitation programme, or to start additional therapy. Pain must be adequately treated as it can severely negatively affect both the re-attainment of function and the animal's motivation (1, 6).

This chapter provides an overview of the different physiotherapeutic and adjunct methods employed in the treatment or rehabilitation of neurological disease in the dog and cat. In Fig. 8.1, the course of a rehabilitation programme is provided using the example of a tetraplegic dog (i.e. one that at the start of the programme had been surgically treated for disc prolapse at the level of C7–T1).

8.1 Physiotherapy

Physiotherapy consists of the application of physical stimuli to various tissues to effect recovery. In the following, hydrotherapy, massage, kinesiotherapy, electrotherapy, thermotherapy and magnetic field therapy are described more fully. The indications and contraindications of these therapies are summarised in Table 8.1.

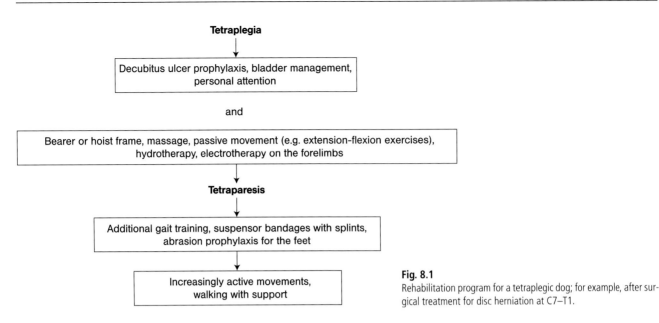

Fig. 8.1
Rehabilitation program for a tetraplegic dog; for example, after surgical treatment for disc herniation at C7–T1.

8

8.1.1 Hydrotherapy

Hydrotherapy provides the optimal conditions for the recovery of normal movement. Swimming in warm water (37–39°C) or in a whirlpool, or training on an underwater treadmill maintains joint movement, stimulates the blood circulation in atrophied muscles, relaxes the muscles, and keeps the patient clean. Good kinetics are achieved with relatively little expenditure of muscle strength due to the buoyancy of the body and the reduction of its effective weight on the joints, so that weakened patients are encouraged to undertake active movements. In addition, the animal's instincts cause it to move in water. This self-preservation behaviour can be implemented in unmotivated patients or in the assessment of the degree of motor deficits. Depending on the individual, water can also be frightening; this should be taken into consideration in the treatment plan to prevent negative effects such as stress or the loss of the patient's cooperation. Due to the animal's buoyancy in water, the tonic afferent impulses from the skin are inhibited, which leads to relaxation of the musculature. The water's viscosity causes a constant friction that allows isotonic muscle work under reduced gravity. The biochemical effect of hydrotherapy consists of a reduction in the blood concentrations of catecholamines, renin-angiotensin and vasopressin, leading to diuresis.

Indications for hydrotherapy are **plegia**, severe **paresis** or **degenerative joint disease**. Cardiac or respiratory insufficiency, infected skin lesions, seromas and hydrophobia are all contraindications for its use. Swimming training should be done for approx. 5 minutes at least two to three times a day. If there is no initiation of extremity movement during the pro-

cedure, then only a couple of minutes are necessary. Support of the animal is often required; for example in the tetraparetic or tetraplegic patient, this can consist of a sling wrapped around the thorax, or a flotation device (Fig. 8.2). In paraparesis or paraplegia, just holding up the animal by its tail may provide enough support (Fig. 8.3). The swimming training should be stopped with the first signs of tiring in the patient. New scars or sutured wounds should be covered with a water-repellent ointment (e.g. zinc ointment). The cardiovascular status should be checked before letting the patient swim in very warm water (> 38°C) (1, 3, 6).

8.1.2 Massage

Massage is defined as being a manual or mechanical application of pressure or traction to the skin, subcutis and musculature. The aims of a massage are to control the nutrient and oxygen transport to the tissues and the removal of metabolites. Due to the mechanical effects of massage, adhesions especially between muscle fibres and the connective tissues can be broken down. Pressure on the tissues causes fluid perfusion through the tissues and the lymph flow is accelerated. This leads to increased diuresis and oedema can be reduced. The blood circulation in the tissues is enhanced and a local hyperaemia occurs that also affects the muscles. Massage can increase the blood circulation in tissues by up to forty fold.

The analgesic effect of massage takes place at different levels. It is a very potent pain therapy due to a summation of the following effects:

Table 8.1: Indications and contraindications of different physiotherapeutic treatment methods

	Indications	Contraindications
■ **Hydrotherapy**	Especially in plegia and severe paresis. Patients with additional degenerative joint disease.	Cardiac or respiratory insufficiency, infected skin lesions, panic-reactions to water
■ **Massage**	Hypertonus or hypotonus of the muscles, muscle pain, scars and neoplasia (no massage in affected area).	Coagulopathies, acute thrombosis, dermatitis.
■ **Kinesiotherapy**	**Passive:** plegia or severe paresis (spastic or flaccid); shortening of tendons, muscle atrophy. **Active:** last phase of rehabilitation in every patient with neurological disease.	**Passive:** primary diseases of joints, ligaments or bones (no treatment in affected areas); acute disease; acute inflammation; instability of the spine **Active:** same as for passive.
■ **Electrotherapy**	**Selective stimulation:** flaccid paralysis in LMN lesions. Electrostimulation cannot replace the active exercising of the muscles! **TENS:** pain due to neuralgia, neuritis, peripheral nerve lesions, myopathies; degenerative diseases of the spine; postoperative pain.	Patients with pacemakers. pregnancy, paralysis due to inflammation (start once inflammation has disappeared).
■ **Thermotherapy**	**Warmth:** muscle tension or pain after other physical treatments (massage, kinesiotherapy). **Cold:** pain; flaccid paralysis.	**Warmth:** cardiovascular insufficiency, arthritis. **Cold:** none.
■ **Magnetic field therapy**	Pain reduction; fractures (effective through plaster cast); arthritis; contusions.	Sepsis, acute viral or other infections, pregnancy.

8

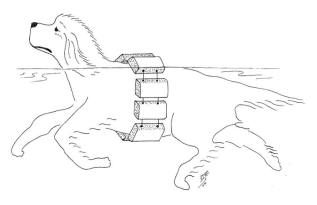

a

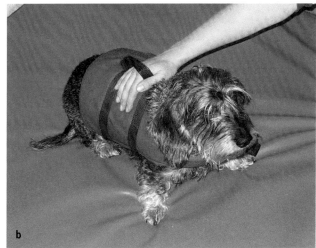

b

Fig. 8.2a, b
(a) Hydrotherapy of a tetraplegic patient using a Styrofoam® aid. (b) Dachshund with a life jacket.

■ Stimulation of the mechanoreceptors increases the activity of the afferent fibres, which causes a segmental pain inhibition at the level of the spinal cord (masking effect).

■ Due to the effect of massage on tissue perfusion, pain-stimulating substances such as histamine and prostaglandin are washed out of the tissues with the fluid.

■ Endorphins (endogenous opioid peptides) are released during massage; their half-lives are approx. 6 to 8 hours.

■ The psychological effects of massage should not be forgotten. It is not only the tissues which relax on being massaged but also the psyche, which leads to a further reduction in pain due to muscle tension.

Muscle tone can be altered reflexively by massage. It is increased due to massage's stretching stimulus, but if the muscle is affected by hypertonia, then the muscle tone is reduced. The stretching stimulus due to massage induces the intrinsic myotatic reflex of the muscle via the muscle spindles.

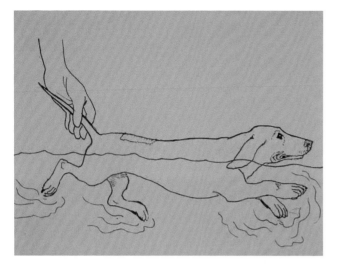

Fig. 8.3
Hydrotherapy of a paraparetic patient supported by holding up its tail.

8

Table 8.2: Different massage grip techniques

Effleurage (stroking) Used in taking up contact to the patient and to finish massage.	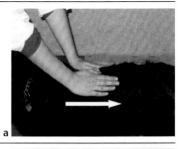 a
Petrissage (kneading) Used to lift up and dissolve adhesions. Stimulates the lymph flow	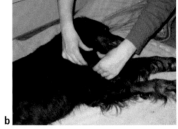 b
	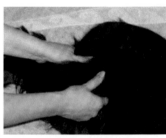 c
Friction (rubbing) Stimulates perfusion of the skin.	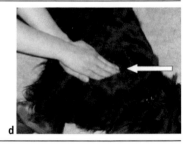 d
Vibration (shaking) Induces general and muscle relaxation.	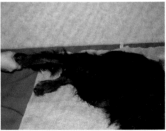 e
Tapotement (tapping) If done strongly this induces hyperaemia of the skin and stimulates muscle tone.	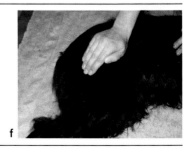 f

The indications for massage are **muscle hypertonia** and **hypotonia**, **muscle pain**, **paresis** and **plegia**. Contraindications are coagulopathies, recent thrombosis, dermatitis, scarring and neoplasia. A massage frequency of two to three times a day is ideal, with a duration of approx. 10 minutes. Five different massage techniques have been described: effleurage (stroking), petrissage (kneading), friction (rubbing), vibration (shaking) and tapotement (hitting) (Table 8.2). Massage machines are used mainly for vibration. All these techniques can be used to increase or decrease muscle tone. Due to the enormous increase in perfusion, massage is strenuous for the animal and no longer than 30 minutes should be used for massaging the whole body (1, 5, 6).

8.1.3 Kinesiotherapy

Depending on the degree of neurological symptoms, the patient is prescribed either passive and/or active kinesiotherapy. The encouragement of independent movement is most important.

In passive movement, the joints are moved without muscle contraction by the application of an external force. The active form is, by definition, a movement caused by active muscle contraction. Contraindications for kinesiotherapy are acute inflammation and other acute processes, as well as instability of the spine (1, 6).

8.1.3.1 Passive movement

Passive movement is mainly used for the **prophylactic treatment of atrophy and contraction**.

Joint mobility and mechanical elasticity of the musculature is maintained and the nutrition of the cartilage improved. In addition, the blood perfusion is stimulated, pain is partially reduced and most importantly, the sensation of movement is maintained. It has been shown that through continual passive movements post-traumatic muscle atrophy can be restricted due to joint proprioceptor stimulation (muscle spindles and the tendon receptors [Golgi organs]) leading to a stimulation of the α-motor neurons.

The patient should be treated in a normal body position. All the joints of paralysed limbs must be manipulated every day, otherwise tendon shortening will occur with time due to a lack of movement. Depending on the disease, slow and fluent passive movement of a joint should be done up to ten times in all directions in which it moves naturally. Depending on the joint, such movements are flexion/extension (Table 8.3.a), abduction/adduction, and supination/pronation. The muscles responsible for the movement of the carpus and tarsus are often the last ones to be reinnervated and so these joints often stiffen up. The affected joint should be held in extension 10 to 15 minutes a day as prophylaxis for maintaining the elasticity of the tendons. A support bandage with splints can be applied to allow the animal to walk without buckling (Table 8.3b). However, the splint may only be put on the animal for a few hours per day otherwise the blood supply of the muscle will be compromised. In any case, the splint must be removed for the night. Animals that cannot stand on their own should be stood up on their feet every day to elicit proprioceptive stimuli. Tetraplegic patients are put in a hoist frame for 2 to 4 hours a day (Table 8.3.c). In such a frame, the patient regains an awareness of its normal body stance and the normal positioning of its limbs with respect to its body. The limbs must be returned to their normal position or temporarily bound in the correct position.

The combined flexion-extension exercises performed with the animal in standing have proven to be very effective in the treatment of spastic paralysis. By bending and picking up a limb, the contralateral side is presented with more weight. In addition, pressure is placed on the sacrum using the palm of the hand forcing the limbs to flex against the resistance of the extensor muscles (Table 8.3d). When the pressure is removed, the patient can again actively flex its muscles (Table 8.3e). The other side is exercised after five to ten repetitions depending on the staying power of the patient (1, 3, 5, 6).

8.1.3.2 Active supported movement

So that the muscles are rebuilt and the patient's original strength is regained, a targeted daily workout is necessary. Active movements are also important for the training of coordination and facilitation through proprioceptive impulses. All forms of kinesiotherapy serve to improve the patient's balance reactions and voluntary movements, as well as give it a renewed sensory and motor appreciation of its body. Suitable movements in open spaces increase the patient's motivation. Cats, therefore, should be placed in a large box (Table 8.4a). The first step consists of gait training with supported movements. The paraparetic patient is supported by a sling (i.e., made of cloth [Table 8.4b]) that is placed under the abdomen; the tetraplegic patient is also supported under the thorax. To give the patient a feeling for the physiological processes involved in moving, it can be helped with every step by binding a gauze bandage to the neurologically affected leg (e.g. in a monoparetic animal), like a "pulley" system which aids the limb to move properly instead of it being dragged behind. The muscles of the affected limbs can be forced to do more work by applying exercise weights to the limb. At first an approx. 150-g weight is attached to the leg using tape or bandages (Table 8.4c). The weight is applied for approx. 30 minutes during each walk. Later, the weight can be increased depending on the size of the animal up to a maximum of 300 g. The advantage of this method is that the animal is forced to use those limbs which it would not otherwise use. With lesions in the neck area, a body harness must be used instead of a collar for walks on a leash. The muscle re-building exercises usually takes 4 to 6 weeks. Different technical appliances such as a treadmill can be used to progressively increase the animal's endurance (Table 8.4d). Active kinesiotherapy is the last phase of every patient's rehabilitation (1, 3, 5, 6).

8.1.4 Electrotherapy

In electrotherapy, electrical currents are used for medical purposes usually on a specific area of the body. Electrotherapy is generally indicated in **lesions of the LMNS** such as flaccid paralysis due to inflammation (e.g. polyradiculoneuritis) or trauma (e.g. damage to a peripheral nerve). Contraindications are cardiac pacemaker, pregnancy and paralysis due to inflammation (the electrotherapy should be started once the inflammation is under control) (1, 2, 6, 8).

8.1.4.1 Functional electrical therapy (FET)

During FET, paralysed muscles are selectively stimulated until there is an arbitrary contraction. The paralysed muscle is subjected to single impulses (Fig. 8.4).

The duration of the impulse and intervals between them depend on the degree of muscle involvement, which should be determined by EMG before starting the therapy. Healthy muscle can adapt better to an impulse than damaged ones, and it reacts with a contraction only when there is a significant increase in the threshold current strength. This adaptability is known as accommodation. The paretic muscle already reacts to impulses with a much lower current intensity than healthy

Table 8.3: Passive movement

Flexion / Extension

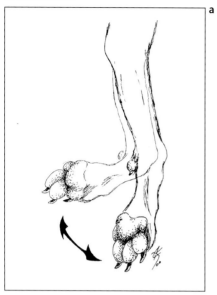

a

Splint support dressing

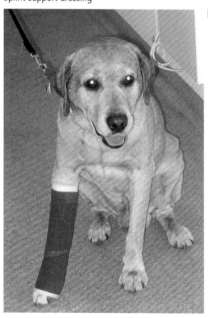

b

Wheeled frame

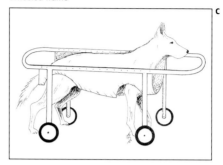

c

Flexion-extension exercise

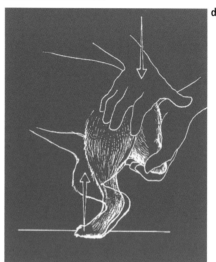

d

Extension-flexion exercise

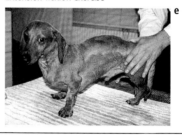

e

muscle. As a consequence, paralysed muscles can be selectively stimulated while the intact muscle remains relaxed. Due to the selective stimulation current, muscle atrophy can be prevented or at least delayed. In addition, muscle degeneration and fibrosis can be reduced and the muscle's ability to regenerate itself is maintained.

The exponential current can cause unpleasant sensations, therefore the applied impulse is biphasic and bipolar.

The indication for FET is **flaccid paralysis** associated with LMN lesions seen with complete or partially denervated muscles and peripheral nerve lesions (e.g. post-traumatic, operative). Contraindications include lack of regeneration prospects (root avulsion) or denervation that has lasted for longer than one year (1, 6, 8).

Table 8.4: Active movement

Cat in large box

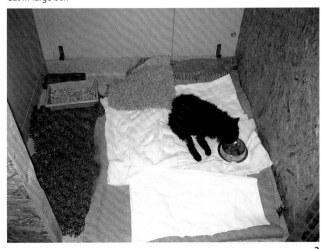

a

Bandage with lead strip

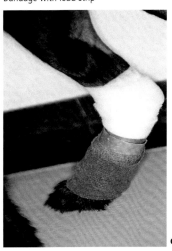

c

Walking aid using a sling

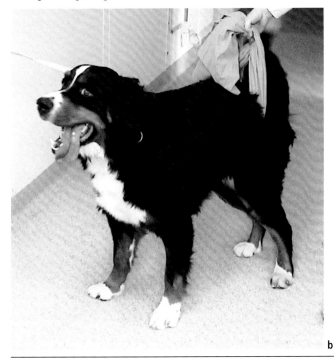

b

Treadmill

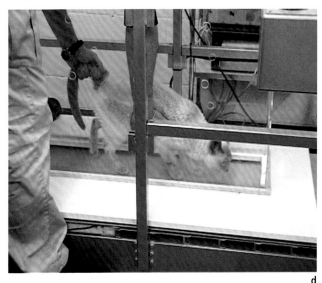

d

8.1.4.2 Transcutaneous electrical nerve stimulation (TENS)

TENS is a method of electroanalgesia. Mechanoreceptors in the skin are stimulated by specific stimuli.

These stimuli are transmitted to the spinal cord via the fast-conducting sensory fibres (A-β-nerve fibres); there then follows a blockage of the interneurons. Pain impulses that are transported by the slow-conducting nerve fibres cannot find a "doorway" and therefore cannot be transmitted to the sensory cortex. Indications for TENS are neuritis, peripheral traumatic nerve lesions, myopathy, degenerative diseases of the spine and postoperative pain.

Not all patients show a good reaction initially, though good results can mostly be attained with long-term therapy (1, 2, 6).

8

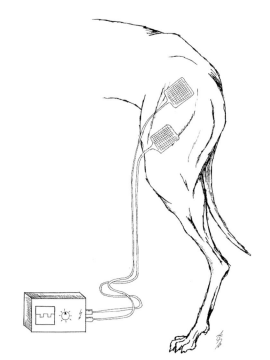

Fig. 8.4
Electrotherapy (Illustration: KATHMANN et al. 2001 [6])

8.1.5　Thermotherapy

Thermotherapy is the name for heat-related treatment. It is differentiated into therapies using an application of heat or ones involving the removal of heat. It should be ensured both in the application of warmth or cold, that there is no direct skin contact. Regular patient vital parameters should be taken and the temperature of the therapy should be adapted accordingly. Hot or cold packing should never be fixed to the patient (1, 6, 8).

8.1.5.1　Application of heat
The local application of heat (warm packs, electrical pads, water bottles and lamps) causes hyperaemia, which increases the supply of nutrients and oxygen in the heated area, leading to an increase in its metabolism. Prolonged application leads to pain reduction, the muscles are relaxed and the elasticity of the connective tissues is increased, improving the mobility of the joints. Unwanted side-effects can be an increase in oedema, inflammation, increased tendency for bleeding and / or disturbances in blood circulation. The beneficial effects of applying heat are pain reduction, anti-inflammatory in states of chronic inflammation, reduction in muscle tone, increase in elasticity of the collagen fibres, increased circulation, increased local defence and a decrease in the synovial viscosity (Fig. 8.5).

Increased muscle tone or pain are both indications for heat treatment. In the first 72 hours postoperatively, heat treatment is used to treat swelling, pain and muscle spasm in the area of the operation. This type of treatment also augments the effectiveness of other physical treatments such as massage, kinesiotherapy and electrotherapy. In contrast, heat is contraindicated with arthritis and cardiovascular insufficiency (1, 6, 8).

8.1.5.2　Removal of heat (Cryotherapy)
Cryopacking using ice bags can reduce inflammation by inhibiting the mediator activity and reduce pain by inhibiting the nocioceptors. A short application of cold can stimulate the muscle spindles leading to an increase in muscle tone. The cold packing should be applied for 5 to 10 minutes, two to three times a day. The treatment should not be longer than 30 minutes, otherwise vasodilation occurs leading to oedema. Cryotherapy is especially beneficial in the first 12 to 48 hours after an operation.

Indications for cryotherapy are **pain** and **muscle spasm** (1, 6, 8).

8.1.6　Magnetic field therapy

Electromagnetism is produced by conducting electricity through a coil, which is bound by a suitable conducting material. The number of impulses per second (= frequency) determines the biological effect. Magnetic field therapy has an effect on cells, improves vascularisation and reduces pain. The cells' superficial potentials appear to be more quickly regained, and therefore so is their function. The treated tissue exhibits an increase in perfusion and oxygen partial pressure, which also supports the healing process. With some frequencies, a definite reduction in the appreciation of pain can be attained.

8.2　Adjuvant therapeutic measures

8.2.1　Bladder management

Disturbances in the function of the urinary bladder such as incontinence, urine retention, cystitis and bladder atony occur with many neurological diseases (see Chap. 14.2). Lesions of the lumbar enlargement are associated with a flaccid bladder and reduced sphincter tone; the bladder can only be partially emptied. Due to continual dribbling of urine, there is a great danger of ascending urinary tract infection. Lesions in the thoracolumbar spine can also lead to disturbances in micturition. With these, an overfilled bladder occurs due to increased

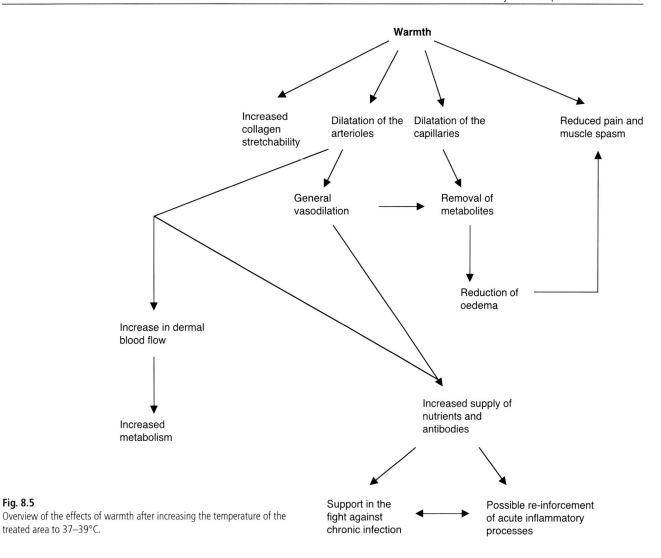

Fig. 8.5
Overview of the effects of warmth after increasing the temperature of the treated area to 37–39°C.

8

sphincter tone and reduced detrusor muscle contractility. The spastic bladder can barely be expressed manually. A method for treating this condition is described in Fig. 8.6.

The bladder should be emptied at least three times a day. This can be done manually by pressing on the bladder wall or by using a catheter (Fig. 8.7). In addition, different medications can be used. Urethral resistance is increased with phenylpropanolamine and reduced with phenoxybenzamine. Bethanechol increases and propantheline reduces detrusor contractility (Fig. 8.8). In patients that spontaneously urinate, the degree of bladder emptying should be evaluated and monitored by palpating it manually or using ultrasound, as the danger of bladder wall damage or cystitis increases with residual urine.

The risk for urinary tract infection is always high with disturbances of micturition; infections should be treated with a suitable antibiotic based on culture and sensitivity results (1, 4, 6, 7).

8.2.2 Decubitus prophylaxis

The best prophylaxis for decubitus is soft and dry bedding as well as regular turning of the patient (every 2 to 4 hours) (Fig. 8.9).

A water bed is a good method of providing an especially soft bed and it reduces pressure on those parts of the body that are

Spastic bladder

Dog moving freely outside on grass 10 min ⟶ Urination

↓

No urination

↓

Try to carefully empty bladder by squeezing ⟶ Urination

↓

No urination

↓

Buprenorphine 0.005 mg/ kg IV. Wait 20 min

↓

Dog again outside on grass ⟶ Urination

↓

No urination

↓

Try to carefully empty bladder by squeezing ⟶ Urination

↓

No urination

↓

Diazepam 0.2 mg/kg. Wait 5–10 min;
reduced tone of urethral muscle (striated muscle)

↓

Dog again outside ⟶ Urination

↓

No urination

↓

Try to carefully empty bladder by squeezing ⟶ Urination

↓

No urination

↓

Catheterise bladder, remove catheter once bladder is empty

Fig. 8.6
Treatment suggestions for a spastic/upper motor neuron bladder; repeat every 8 hours.

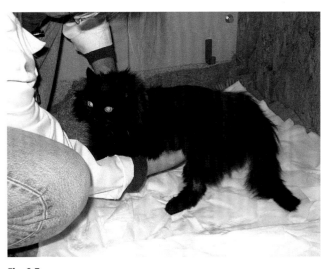

Fig. 8.7
Manual emptying of the bladder.

Disturbances in micturition with spinal problems

Bladder is difficult to squeeze; increased tone of the urethral sphincter muscle

↓

Phenoxybenzamine 5–15 mg, SID, PO

↓

α-adrenergic effect; reduced sphincter tone

Continuous dripping of urine; bladder easy to squeeze; reduced detrusor contractility

↓

Bethanechol 2.5–25 mg, TID, PO (additionally phenoxybenzamine 5–15 mg, SID, PO)

↓

Cholinergic effect; increased detrusor contractility

Improvement in urination
after 1 to 2 weeks at the latest

Yes: continue medication until normal urination occurs

No: medication not effective

Fig. 8.8
Medication used to treat urination disturbances.

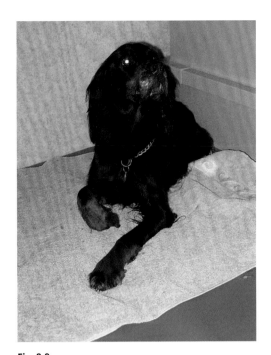

Fig. 8.9
Soft bedding is important in decubitus ulcer prophylaxis.

prone to decubitus. Skin areas which are often unavoidably damp such as the inner surface of the thighs, scrotum and perineal area should be protected with an ointment containing zinc oxide (Fig. 8.10). If the patient does develop decubitus, then the respective areas must be shaved and regularly cleansed and disinfected. The bedding must be kept clean and as aseptic as possible. Paralysed animals and especially large dog breeds are particularly at risk of wound infections, respiratory tract infections and urinary incontinence.

Spontaneous knuckling and dragging of the paws can lead to severe injuries to the digits (Fig. 8.11). Skin infection and osteomyelitis can be the consequences. The endangered areas of the limbs should be protected using a leather or plastic shoe, or bandaging to prevent abrasions (Fig. 8.12). During healing, itching or tingling / prickling can arise due to the regeneration of sensory nerves. The affected animals can self-mutilate and protection using bandages or an Elizabethan (cone) collar can be necessary. The patient's nails should be regularly cut to prevent injury and to enable the animal to place its foot down properly (1, 6).

8

8.2.3   Individual attention

In every patient, but especially in the very frightened or aggressive animal, it is important to gain its friendship and cooperation. The patient's motivation can be stimulated using

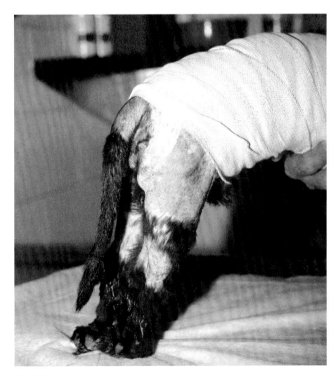

Fig. 8.10
Dermatitis due to continual urinary incontinence.

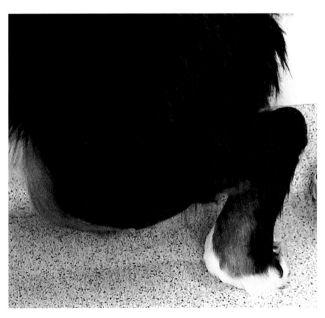

Fig. 8.11
Spontaneous knuckling.

8

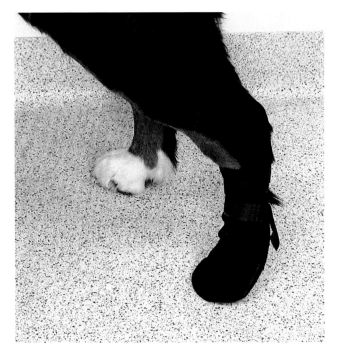

Fig. 8.12
Abrasion prophylaxis using a plastic shoe.

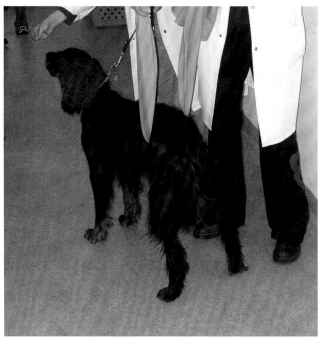

Fig. 8.13
Motivation using edible treat during gait training.

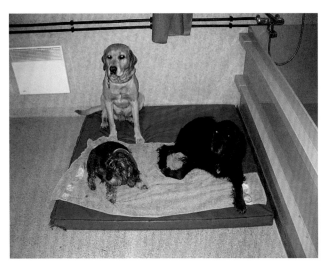

Fig. 8.14
Canine patients are more motivated in the company of other dogs.

aids such as toys and edible treats (Fig. 8.13). Social contact with other animals and the owner is indispensable for the well-being and motivation of the patient (Fig. 8.14). The recovery time in a cooperative and motivated patient is much reduced (1, 6).

Literature

1 ALEXANDER, C.-S. (2001): Physikalische Therapie für Kleintiere. Parey Buchverlag, Berlin.

2 BROMILEY, M.W. (1995): Physiotherapie in der Veterinärmedizin. Enke Verlag (Vetprax), Stuttgart.

3 GÖDDE, T., JAGGY, A. (1993): Thorakolumbaler Bandscheibenvorfall beim Dackel (Diagnose und Therapie). Prakt. Tierarzt **7**: 653–663.

4 JAGGY, A. (1997): Neurologische Notfälle beim Kleintier. Enke Verlag (VET special), Stuttgart.

5 JERRAM, R.M., HART, R.C., SCHULZ, K.S. (1997): Postoperative management of the canine spinal surgery patient – Part 1. The Compendium **19**: 147–160.

6 KATHMANN, I., DEMIERRE, S., JAGGY, A. (2001): Rehabilitationsmassnahmen in der Kleintierneurologie. Schweiz Arch Tierheilk. **10**: 495–502.

7 VANDEVELDE, M., JAGGY, A., LANG, J. (2000): Einführung in die veterinärmedizinische Neurologie. Parey Buchverlag, Berlin, 2000.

8 WERNER, G., KLIMCZYK, K., RUDE, J. (1997): Physikalische und Rehabilitative Medizin. Georg Thieme Verlag, Stuttgart, New York.

9 Neuropharmacology

Tony Glaus
Claudia Reusch
Gina Aeschbacher

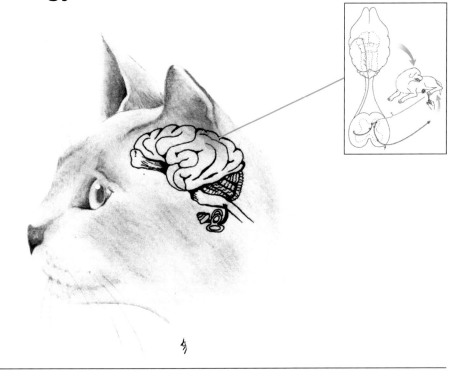

9.1 Antibiotic therapy in neurological disease

Tony Glaus

Antibiotics are used to treat neurological diseases with different localisations and infectious aetiologies (Tables 9.1 and 9.2). The indications for the use of antibiotics are not only the treatment of infectious neurological diseases, but also the treatment of extraneural complications (for example, aspiration pneumonia arising from megaoesophagus).

In order to achieve a successful result with antibiotic therapy, various aspects must be taken into consideration. It is, for example, ideal to know the causative agent and its antibiotic sensitivity. As it is not always possible to determine the causative agent (time) due to the localisation of the disease, the choice of antibiotic must be based on the knowledge of the range of potential causative agents. As many antibiotics do not (or only poorly) penetrate the CNS, this within sufficient quality must also be taken into consideration.

In this chapter, the rational use of antibiotics for infectious neurological diseases will be presented. In addition, the spectrum of activity of the standard antibiotics used in veterinary medicine and their penetration into the CNS will be explained; finally, the recommended choice of antibiotic based on the neuroanatomical localisation of the infection is discussed.

9.1.1 Classes of antibiotics and their antibiotic spectra

9.1.1.1 Penicillins

Representatives of this class are the β-lactam antibiotics. Penicillin G is very effective against many gram-positive and anaerobic bacteria. However, many *Staphylococci* and gram-negative bacteria are resistant as they produce β-lactamase. Penicillin G must be given parenterally. Semisynthetic antibiotics such as ampicillin and amoxicillin can be given orally or parenterally. They also have a wider spectrum against gram-negative bacteria (*E. coli*, *Proteus* spp.), although they are sensitive to β-lactamase.

Newer penicillins like ticarcillin or imipenem have a wider spectrum with respect to gram-negative (especially against *Pseudomonas* spp.) and anaerobic bacteria.

Table 9.1: Possible infectious aetiologies based on their neuroanatomical localisation

Peripheral nerves	■ Subsequent to sepsis: gram-positive / gram-negative bacteria; aerobic / anaerobic
Musculature	■ *Toxoplasma gondii*, *Neospora caninum*
Spine: ■ Discospondylitis ■ Myelitis ■ Abscess (cat)	■ *Staphylococcus intermedius*, *E. coli*, Streptococci, *Brucella*, others ■ *Toxoplasma gondii*, mixed flora from the oral cavity after bite wounds ■ Anaerobic bacteria, *Pasteurella* spp., different types of gram-positive bacteria, *Actinomyces* spp.
Middle and inner ear	■ *Staphylococcus intermedius*, *Pseudomonas* spp., *Proteus*, Streptococci.
Brain stem, cerebellum and cerebrum	■ Streptococci, *E. coli*, *Klebsiella* spp., *Staphylococcus* spp., *Pasteurella* spp., various anaerobic bacteria ■ *Toxoplasma gondii*, *Neospora canium*, *E. canis*, systemic aspergillosis ■ Penetrating otitis interna: see above ■ Septic thrombus: bacteria associated with the primary lesion ■ (Bite) wounds: mixed flora of the oral cavity
Hepatoencephalopathy	■ Intestinal flora: Enterobacteriaceae, anaerobic bacteria
Aspiration pneumonia	■ Flora of the oral cavity (aerobic and anaerobic)

9

Table 9.2: Recommended choice of antibiotic for specific indications

Otitis media / interna*	Amoxicillin-clavulanic acid 10–20 mg/kg BID First-generation cephalosporin 20–30 mg/kg TID Enrofloxacin**, *** 10 mg/kg SID–BID
Discospondylitis	First-generation cephalosporin 20–30 mg/kg TID Amoxicillin-clavulanic acid 10–20 mg/kg BID
CNS injury / abscess	Amoxicillin 20–30 mg/kg TID + enrofloxacin**, *** 10 mg/kg SID Amoxicillin 20–30 mg/kg TID + cefotaxime 20–30 mg/kg TID Clindamycin 10 mg/kg BID + enrofloxacin**, *** 10 mg/kg SID
Bacterial meningo- encephalitis	Cefotaxime 20–40 mg/kg TID Sulphonamide-trimethoprim 15 mg/kg BID Metronidazole 10–15 mg/kg TID
Toxoplasmosis / Neospora	Clindamycin 20 mg/kg BID Sulphonamide-trimethoprim 15 mg/kg BID
Aspiration pneumonia	Amoxicillin 20–30 mg/kg TID + enrofloxacin**, *** 10 mg/kg SID Clindamycin 10 mg/kg BID + enrofloxacin**, *** 10 mg/kg SID
Hepatoence- phalopathy	Amoxicillin 20 mg/kg BID Metronidazole 10–15 mg/kg TID

  * The choice of antibiotic should be based on a bacterial investigation with sensitivity testing.

  ** Cat < 2.5 mg/kg BID.

*** Enrofloxacin has been associated with acute retinal blindness in cats.

The sensitivity of these antibiotics to β-lactamase can be suppressed by combining them with clavulanic acid, so that their spectrum against *Staphylococci* and gram-negative bacteria can be expanded. Amoxicillin + clavulanic acid (PO, IV) and ticarcillin + clavulanic acid (IV) are both very effective against many gram-positive, gram-negative and aerobic bacteria. The penetration of the penicillins in the CNS is mediocre.

9.1.1.2 Cephalosporins
The cephalosporins are β-lactam antibiotics like the penicillins but they are more potent against gram-negative bacteria. The spectrum of activity depends on the generation of the cephalosporin.

First-generation cephalosporins are mainly active against gram-positive bacteria with the exception of a few resistant *Staphylococci*. These antibiotics have a very good activity against gram-negative bacteria, but only a small activity against anaerobes. Their penetration into the subarachnoid space is poor. Important representatives of this group of antibiotics are cephalexin (PO), cefadroxil (PO) and cefazolin (IV).

Second-generation cephalosporins are very effective against gram-negative and anaerobic bacteria, but they are less effective against gram-positive bacteria. With the exception of a few of the third-generation antibiotics, the cephalosporins have little effectivity against pseudomonads. An important exception is cefotaxime, which penetrates the subarachnoid space well. Cefotaxime must be given intravenously. Its spectrum of activity includes *Streptococci*, *Staphylococci* (with or without β-lactamase), most Enterobacteriaceae and, with different degrees of effectivity, anaerobes. Cefotaxime is well suited for treating bacterial meningitis.

9.1.1.3 Aminoglycosides

In veterinary medicine, streptomycin and gentamycin are predominantly used from this group of drugs; amikacin is less frequently used. These antibiotics must be given parenterally to achieve a systemic effect as they are not well absorbed by the intestines. Their spectrum of activity primarily includes gram-negative bacteria, especially *Pseudomonas* spp., and *Staphylococcus intermedius*. They do not have any effect against anaerobes. As streptomycin has been used to a great extent in veterinary medicine, many bacteria have developed resistance to it. A greater problem in the use of aminoglycosides is their possible side-effects, in particular nephrotoxicity and ototoxicity (auditory and vestibular systems).

The penetration of aminoglycosides into the CNS and CSF is poor.

Due to their high potential for side-effects, aminoglycosides should only be used in exceptional cases. The use of gentamycin remains unchanged in the treatment of septic animals when other antibiotics cannot be used due to bacterial resistance or because of cost. It should not be given for more than 5 days and at a dosage of < 6 mg/kg, SC. Another rational use for this antibiotic is in the treatment of bacterial pneumonia, where the inhalation of gentamycin results in high concentrations of the antibiotic in the respiratory tract with little systemic resorption.

Another often described indication for aminoglycosides is the oral application of neomycin to reduce the number of enteral bacteria in hepatic encephalopathy (HE). Nowadays, however, amoxicillin or metronidazole are mainly used instead.

9.1.1.4 Chloramphenicol

Chloramphenicol has a very wide spectrum against various gram-positive, gram-negative and anaerobic bacteria. It is also effective against mycoplasma and *Ehrlichia* spp. The brain tissue penetration of chloramphenicol is excellent.

Chloramphenicol inhibits hepatic microsomal enzymes and so delays the elimination of drugs that are metabolised in the liver. For example, the concomitant application of chloramphenicol and phenobarbital can lead to an increased serum level of phenobarbital.

The biggest danger with the use of chloramphenicol is bone marrow suppression, which is idiosyncratic in human beings and potentially irreversible. In the dog and cat, bone marrow suppression is dose-dependent and reversible; though the cat is more sensitive than the dog. Due to the potential intoxication of humans with this antibiotic, chloramphenicol is now only rarely used in veterinary medicine. Its main indi-

cations are pneumonia and otitis when other antibiotics are not effective or contraindicated.

9.1.1.5 Tetracyclines

Tetracyclines also have a broad spectrum against aerobic and anaerobic bacteria, spirochetes, mycoplasma and *Ehrlichia* spp. Doxycycline has a higher effectivity against anaerobes than tetracycline. Tetracyclines penetrate most tissues well, including the brain.

Doxycycline, in particular, can develop an immune-modulating and inflammation-inhibitory effect in addition to its antibiotic effect. A clinical improvement with the application of doxycycline, therefore, does not always mean that an infectious disease is present.

9.1.1.6 Macrolides

Some representatives of this chemical group are erythromycin, azithromycin, clarithromycin, tylosin and clindamycin. Clindamycin is most commonly used in veterinary medicine. Its spectrum mainly includes gram-positive aerobic and gram-positive and gram-negative anaerobic bacteria. In addition, clindamycin is very effective against *Toxoplasma gondii* and *Neospora caninum*. Clindamycin only weakly penetrates the brain or CSF.

9.1.1.7 Trimethoprim-Sulphonamides

This combination has a broad spectrum and is effective against gram-positive and gram-negative aerobes, but it has virtually no effect against anaerobes. *Toxoplasma gondii* is also sensitive to it. The combination has an excellent CNS penetration.

9.1.1.8 Quinolones

The two most important representatives of the second generation of quinolones often used in veterinary medicine are enrofloxacin and marbofloxacin. Their spectrum of activity covers gram-negative bacteria, including *Pseudomonas* spp., and gram-positive bacteria, including β-lactamase-producing *Staphylococci*. Anaerobes are mainly resistant. Quinolones can penetrate the CNS but only with high plasma concentrations. Other quinolones used include ciprofloxacin and orbifloxacin.

9.1.1.9 Metronidazole

This antibiotic mainly affects anaerobic bacteria, especially *Bacteriodes*. Metronidazole shows a good penetration of the CNS and CSF. Although metronidazole can be given intravenously, it is mainly given orally. Side-effects are extremely rare unless there is overdosage (as a rule only when > 60 mg/kg is given daily).

9

The most important side-effects are neurological, whereby central vestibular disturbances are predominant. Seizures have been infrequently reported in dogs but can occur in cats. The side-effects are usually reversible, but it may take weeks before they disappear.

The main indication for this antibiotic in neurology is in the supportive treatment of HE. As metronidazole is metabolised in the liver, no more than 30 mg/kg should be given in a day in HE patients due to the danger of neurological side-effects. This antibiotic is also a good choice in anaerobic CNS infections.

9.1.1.10 Four-quadrant antibiosis
This term implies a form of chemotherapy that is effective against all gram-positive and gram-negative, aerobic and anaerobic bacteria. Four-quadrant antibiosis is used when the animal is in a critical condition as a consequence of a supposed bacterial infection and the causative agent is (still) not known. Based on the above description, different combinations of antibiotics are possible.

Antibiotic combinations in the four-quadrant antibiosis:
- Amoxicillin + clavulanic acid
- Enrofloxacin + amoxicillin
- Enrofloxacin + clindamycin
- Trimethoprim-Sulphonamide-+ metronidazole
- First-generation + third-generation cephalosporin

In critical patients, the antibiotics should be given parenterally (intravenously).

9.1.2 Choice of antibiotic depending on neurological lesion localisation

Infectious disease of the nervous system can be located in the peripheral nerves, muscles, spinal cord, peripheral vestibular apparatus (inner ear), brain stem, cerebellum and cerebrum. The most important infectious causes of neurological disease are shown in Table 9.1 according to their neuroanatomical location. The logical selection of which antibiotic should be used is summarised in Table 9.2.

9.1.2.1 Peripheral nerves
Peripheral neuropathies are rarely due to bacterial infections. An extremely rare complication of sepsis is ischemic polyneuromyopathy, which may lead to tetraplegia. The therapy consists of general supportive treatment in conjunction with antibiotics. The choice of antibiotic is ideally based upon a bacterial culture and sensitivity test; the sample should be taken from the original focus of the sepsis. If the causal agent is not known, then four-quadrant antibiosis is indicated.

9.1.2.2 Polymyositis
The most important infectious causes of polymyositis are toxoplasmosis or neosporosis. The antibiotic of choice is clindamycin, 15–20 mg/kg, BID for at least 2 weeks.

9.1.2.3 Discospondylitis
The most important cause of this disease in the dog is *Staphylococcus* spp. Other important agents are *Streptococcus* spp. and *E. coli. Brucella canis* can be responsible but less frequently. Before antibiotic treatment is initiated, there should be an attempt to determine the causal agent, ideally from cultures of the urine, blood and in particular, from an aspirate of the affected disc taken under fluoroscopy (3). Until the results of such cultures are available, an empirical choice such as amoxicillin + clavulanic acid or a first-generation cephalosporin should be used. If there are signs of sepsis, the antibiotics should be given intravenously; otherwise they can be given orally. The duration of treatment is very long: as a rule 2 to 3 months is recommended. When there are no culture results available and if there is no improvement seen after a few days of treatment, then the antibiotic therapy should be changed.

Clindamycin is a good first choice in cats with compressive myelopathy due to a suspected abscess; alternatively, amoxicillin + clavulanic acid can be used.

9.1.2.4 Otitis media/interna
The bacteria most commonly found in this disease are *Staphylococcus intermedius, Pseudomonas* spp., *Proteus* spp. and *Streptococcus* spp. (4). If culture and sensitivity are not available, then clavulanated amoxicillin, first-generation cephalosporins or quinolones are sensible choices for treatment. If otitis externa is present, then concurrent topical treatment may be indicated.

9.1.2.5 Meningitis/encephalitis
Bacterial meningitis/encephalitis is rare in the dog and cat. In addition, when such an infection is present, frequently no bacteria can be cultured from the CSF. *Streptococci* have been most commonly isolated in dogs with meningitis or meningoencephalitis. Other possible bacteria include *Staphylococcus intermedius, Pasteurella multocida, Actinomyces* spp., *Nocardia* spp. and anaerobes (5, 6). Based on its spectrum of activity and its ability to penetrate into the CNS, cefotaxime is a good choice when there is suspicion of bacterial meningitis; alternatives are chloramphenicol or trimethoprim-sulphonamide and metronidazole. The antibiotics should be given intravenously if the patient is especially obtunded.

CNS toxoplasmosis or neosporosis can be treated with clindamycin. Penetration of clindamycin into the CNS is normally poor, but it has better penetration during meningitis due to the disturbed permeability of the blood-brain barrier found in this disease. Alternatively, trimethoprim-sulphonamide can be used.

Ehrlichia spp., *Rickettsia* spp., and *Anaplasma* spp., can all affect the nervous system causing meningitis, in addition to infecting other organ systems. Doxycycline or imidocarb are the treatments of choice for these infections. A recommended therapy scheme is the injection of imidocarb (5 mg/kg SC; repeat after 2 weeks) and the additional oral administration of doxycycline (10–20 mg/kg SID for 3 to 4 weeks). If the animals have not improved at the end of this treatment, other diseases have been excluded, or there is a persistently high serum *E. canis* titre, then treatment with doxycycline (5 mg/kg SID) may be necessary for several months. PCR has been suggested as another diagnostic method for the documentation of a persistent infection.

Itraconazole (5mg/kg SID to BID) can be used for the treatment of the rare CNS form of aspergillosis even though its penetration in the CNS is normally poor; the prognosis for the disease however is guarded to grave. Another anti-fungal with much better penetration into the CNS is fluconazole.

Although it is experimentally possible, the occurrence of naturally acquired CNS borreliosis in the dog has never been proven. Theoretically, ceftriaxone (a third-generation cephalosporin), amoxicillin, doxycycline, penicillin G and azithromycin should be effective.

Literature

1 GREENE, C.E. (2006): Infectious diseases of the dog and cat, 3rd ed. W.B. Saunders, Philadelphia.

2 PLUMB, D.C. (2005): Veterinary drug handbook, 5th ed. Iowa State University Press, Ames.

3 FISCHER, A., MAHAFFEY, M.B., OLIVER, J.E. (1997): Fluoroscopically guided percutaneous disk aspiration in 10 dogs with discospondylitis. J Vet Intern Med. **11**: 284–287.

4 COLE, L.K., KWOCHKA, K.W., KOWALSKI, J.J, HILLIER, A. (1998): Microbial flora and antimicrobial susceptibility patterns of isolated pathogens from the horizontal ear canal and middle ear in dogs with otitis media. J Am Vet Med Assoc. **212**: 534–538.

5 CIZINAUSKAS, S., TIPOLD, A., FATZER, R., BURNENS, A., JAGGY, A. (2001): Streptococcal meningoencephalomyelitis in 3 dogs. J Vet Intern Med. **15**: 157–161.

6 RADAELLI, S.T., PLATT, S.R. (2002): Bacterial meningoencephalomyelitis in dogs: a retrospective study of 23 cases (1990–1999). J Vet Intern Med. **16**: 159–163.

9.2 Steroid therapy

Claudia Reusch

The important basic aspects of steroid therapy will be discussed in the following sections. Information about the use of steroids in specific neurological diseases should be taken from the respective chapters in this book.

The adrenal hormones can be classified according to their biological effects: glucocorticoids, mineralocorticoids and androgens. Glucocorticoids comprise 95% of the activity.

Cortisol is the predominant natural glucocorticoid in the dog and cat. In comparison to the situation in human beings, its secretion is not circadian but rather episodic with a number of peaks spread throughout the day. The synthesis and secretion of glucocorticoids is stimulated by ACTH, whose own secretion is regulated by corticotrophin-releasing hormone (CRH) produced by the hypothalamus. There is a negative feedback system between the anterior lobe of the pituitary, hypothalamus and the higher centres, which influence the secretion of CRH via neurotransmitters, and the circulating glucocorticoids. Exogenous glucocorticoids also affect these regulatory mechanisms, whereby there are large individual differences with respect to the development of an iatrogenic adrenal insufficiency.

9.2.1 Chemistry, pharmacokinetics and clinical pharmacology

All substances with a mineralo- or glucocorticoid effect are derivatives of sterane and contain 21 carbon atoms. The synthetic derivates are all built on the basic model of the natural hormone. Due to a relatively slight change (e.g. introduction of another double bond, a methyl group or a fluorine atom), glucocorticoids have been developed with a much higher glucocorticoid effect and a reduced mineralocorticoid effect. Only cortisol, prednisone and prednisolone still have a mineralocorticoid effect; in the rest (e.g. methylprednisolone, triamcinolone, dexamethasone), this has been completely eliminated by chemical modification.

There is a great variation between the different glucocorticoids with respect to their strength. The reasons for this are, on the one hand, due to their differing affinities for the glucocorticoid receptor and on the other hand, due to their degree of binding to plasma proteins and how quickly they are metabolised. It should be noted that the differences in efficacy between these products are of a quantitative nature not a qualitative one. The glucocorticoid receptor reacts virtually identically once bound to by any of the different glucocorticoids. Accordingly, the spectrum of activity of the different

9

preparations is practically the same, and the same wanted and unwanted effects occur with all of them.

The potency of the different glucocorticoids is expressed as their anti-inflammatory activity and is related to that of cortisol, which has been given the arbitrary value of 1. For clinical use, these differences in potency mean that in order to obtain the same effect far less dexamethasone is needed than prednisolone. With respect to the duration of their effects, the synthetic glucocorticoids have been divided into three groups: cortisone and cortisol are short-acting; prednisone, prednisolone, methylprednisolone and triamcinolone are intermediate-acting; and flumethasone, betamethasone and dexamethasone are long-acting (Table 9.3).

There are three galenic forms available for parenteral application. The type of preparation affects when the product starts to work and how the preparation should be applied (IV versus IM or SC).

1. **Water-soluble esters** (liquid solutions). The most commonly used esters are succinate, hemisuccinate and phosphate. The most common formulations are prednisolone sodium succinate, prednisolone sodium phosphate, methylprednisolone sodium phosphate and dexamethasone sodium phosphate. As glucocorticoids are released from their binding to the ester within minutes of entering the body, they are immediately available for absorption and binding to the glucocorticoid receptor. They can be applied IV, IM or SC. Such preparations are used in acute disturbances such as spinal trauma, brain oedema or endotoxic shock.

2. **Free steroid-alcohol.** These preparations are only available for use in veterinary medicine, e.g. dexamethasone solution. The compound's solubility is made possible by the binding of polyethylene glycol. The glucocorticoid is available within minutes or hours. The administration can be done either IM or IV. However, as high intravenous doses of polyethylene glycol can cause CNS disturbances, preparations containing water-soluble esters should only be used when high doses of glucocorticoids are required in emergencies.

3. **Water-insoluble esters (suspensions).** These preparations are given intramuscularly or intralesionally. Acetate and diacetate esters are moderately insoluble; their efficacy lasts for days to weeks (e.g. methylprednisolone acetate). Acetenoid, pivalate and dipropionate esters are even more insoluble, and they remain effective for many weeks (e.g. triamcinolone acetenoid). The compounds in this group have the greatest potential of inducing unwanted side-effects. They should only be used when in all probability the inflammation is going to be persistent and the oral administration of glucocorticoids is not possible.

9.2.2 Physiological and pharmacological effects

Glucocorticoids stimulate gluconeogenesis, reduce the insulin sensitivity of peripheral tissues and have, therefore, a diabetogenic effect. They have proteolytic and lipolytic effects, which with high concentrations can be seen as muscle weakness, muscle atrophy, skin atrophy, delayed wound healing, osteoporosis, lipolysis and repositioning of fat deposits (android adiposity). Glucocorticoids increase the glomerular filtration rate and reduce the secretion and tubular effects of ADH. In higher concentrations, this leads to polyuria and polydipsia in the dog. Glucocorticoids have important functions in the cardiovascular system such as being involved in the maintenance of vessel tone and cardiac output. This effect is due to the permissive influence of glucocorticoids on different vasoactive substances and the sympathetic nervous system. Glucocorticoids are also of importance for normal brain function. How many of the observed changes in mood, behaviour and cognitive function seen in human beings in association with hypo- and hypercortisolism occur in dogs and cats is not well known. Glucocorticoids influence growth and cell division. In young individuals, pharmacological dosages of glucocorticoids can lead to a slowing or interruption of growth. Glucocorticoids inhibit intestinal resorption of calcium and increase its renal excretion. In healthy animals, this calcium-reducing effect is compensated for, though it can be used therapeutically to treat hypercalcaemia.

The therapeutic use of glucocorticoids exploits their anti-inflammatory and immunosuppressive effects. Independent of the underlying disease, glucocorticoids inhibit the early (oedema, fibrin deposition, capillary dilatation, leukocyte migration, phagocytic activity) and late (proliferation of capillaries and fibroblasts, collagen deposition, scarring) inflammatory reactions.

Their inflammatory and immunosuppressive effects are based on the following mechanisms:

- **Reduced migration of neutrophilic granulocytes into inflamed tissues**. In addition, glucocorticoids have an inhibitory effect on phagocytosis and the destruction of bacteria.
- **Reduction in the number of circulating lymphocytes**, whereby the T-lymphocytes are more affected than the B-lymphocytes. Glucocorticoids lead to a reduction in lymphocyte proliferation, lymphokine synthesis, transformation, antigen recognition and cytotoxic effects. B-lymphocytes are mainly influenced indirectly via the glucocorticoids' effects on the accessory cells (monocytes, macrophages). In therapeutic doses, the synthesis of specific antibodies is not inhibited; with increased doses, the IgG and IgA levels fall, and to a lesser extent, so do the IgM levels.
- **Reduced blood vessel permeability**. The stabilisation of microvascular integrity is therapeutically important, e.g. in brain oedema. Various factors induced by the glu-

cocorticoids are responsible for this effect: the suppressed neutrophil granulocytes, the reduced prostaglandin synthesis, the antagonistic effect against various vasoactive substances and the reduced synthesis of plasminogen activator by the macrophages.

■ **Reduced production of arachidonic acid metabolites**. Pharmacological doses of glucocorticoids lead to the synthesis of phospholipase-A inhibitory proteins (lipocortins), and subsequently to a reduction in the proinflammatory mediators (prostaglandins, prostacyclines, thromboxane, leukotrienes).

The anti-inflammatory effects of glucocorticoids are helpful in many situations and are often life-saving. However, the danger of a therapeutic disaster also lies in these effects. The use of glucocorticoids may suppress inflammation, which is a marker of an underlying disease process. A patient can therefore appear to be clinically better, but in reality the disease is progressing. Improper use of glucocorticoids can have catastrophic consequences for the patient.

9.2.3   Side-effects

No side-effects occur when glucocorticoids are administered at physiological doses. Unwanted effects are associated with the duration and dosage of glucocorticoids used. They can be divided into two groups:

Unwanted effects during glucocorticoid therapy. It should be noted that the frequency and severity of the side-effects differ between individuals. After 1 to 2 weeks of therapy, the majority of dogs develop polyuria, polydipsia and panting; in some cases, these clinical signs can start after only a few hours to days. Long-term therapy (weeks to months) can additionally result in alopecia, skin atrophy, poor wound healing, weakness and other clinical signs of Cushing's syndrome. It may not be possible to determine whether Cushing's syndrome is iatrogenic or endogenous based on the clinical signs alone. Cats are more resistant to these side-effects than dogs, as they only have approximately half as many glucocorticoid receptors.

Glucocorticoids can enhance the development of gastrointestinal ulcers. This usually occurs with the use of high doses or when NSAIDs are given at the same time. Patients that are especially at risk for severe gastrointestinal side-effects are those which have undergone spinal surgery. Numerous cases of ulcerative colonic perforation resulting mainly in death have been reported with the use of high doses of dexamethasone. The exact mechanism responsible is not known, although it is presumed that factors such as autonomic dysfunction, reduced intestinal motility and stress work together with a disturbed intestinal integrity due to the dexamethasone. The ulcers arising from the use of glucocorticoids may initially be subclinical, which makes it especially important to monitor

for this risk. Other potential side-effects are increased susceptibility to infection, sepsis and pancreatitis.

Unwanted effects during or after cessation of glucocorticoid therapy. After a rapid withdrawal of glucocorticoid therapy, acute adrenocortical insufficiency can occur due to the depression of the hypothalamus-pituitary-adrenal (HPA) axis. More often, there is a latent adrenocortical insufficiency which is first visible when stress situations such as trauma, severe infections or operations occur. Suppression of the HPA axis can occur both with the systemic or topical application of glucocorticoids. There are large individual variations of duration and degree of HPA axis suppression. In general, the higher the dosage and the longer its duration, the more likely it is for a suppression to occur. HPA axis suppression can last for months, especially when depot products have been be given repeatedly (e.g. methylprednisolone acetate). A single dose of 0.01 mg/kg dexamethasone can suppress the HPA axis for up to 16 hours; 0.1 mg/kg for up to 32 hours; 1–2 mg/kg prednisolone causes a suppression of 24 to 36 hours; 0.22 mg/kg IM triamcinolone acetonide causes suppression for up to 4 weeks; and 2.5 mg/kg IM methylprednisolone acetate causes suppression for up to 5 weeks.

In human beings, sudden cessation of glucocorticoids can lead to the so-called "glucocorticoid withdrawal syndrome" resulting in fever, muscle and joint pain, depression and a non-specific feeling of being unwell. Clinical experience has shown that this phenomenon also occurs in the dog.

9.2.4   Therapeutic uses

The glucocorticoid dosage used depends on the indication for its use. For the correct use of these substances, it is important be aware of the anti-inflammatory potency of the respective compounds and their equivalent dosages (Table 9.3).

9.2.4.1   Replacement therapy
Animals with chronic adrenocortical insufficiency require glucocorticoid replacement (0.1–0.2 mg/kg prednisolone SID). The equivalent dosage of cortisol is approx. 0.5–1.0 mg/kg; however, this must be given twice a day due to its shorter half-life. In times of great stress (trauma, operations), the patient's requirement increases greatly and the glucocorticoid dose should be increased by at least tenfold. For the dosage of mineralocorticoids and the treatment of acute adrenocortical insufficiency, the reader is referred to veterinary endocrinology and internal medicine textbooks.

9.2.4.2   Therapeutic use
Glucocorticoids are used therapeutically for their anti-inflammatory and immunosuppressive effects. Other indications for their use include neoplasia, and trauma. In addition, there are

9

Table 9.3: Relative potencies of glucocorticoids

Glucocorticoid	Anti-inflammatory potency	Mineralocorticoid potency	Equivalent dosage (mg)	Half-life in tissues (hours)
■ Short-acting				
Cortisone[1]	0.8		25	8–12
Cortisol (hydrocortisone)	1.0	2	20	8–12
■ Intermediate-acting				
Prednisone[1]	4.0	1	5	12–36
Prednisolone	4.0	1	5	12–36
Methylprednisolone	5.0	0	4	12–36
Triamcinolone[2]	40.0	0	1.3	12–36
■ Long-acting				
Flumethasone	15.0	0	0.5	35–54
Dexamethasone	40.0	0	0.5	35–54
Betamethasone	50.0	0	0.4	35–54

[1] Cortisone and prednisone have to be reduced in the liver to the active compounds cortisol and prednisolone.

[2] In some textbooks, triamcinolone is considered as being one of the long-acting glucocorticoids.

9

some endocrine and endocrine-related indications (insulinoma, hypercalcaemia) for glucocorticoid use.

Some important aspects of glucocorticoid anti-inflammatory and immunosuppressive therapy include:

■ Depot preparations (e.g. methylprednisolone acetate) should only be used in exceptional cases, namely when it is not possible to use compounds with a shorter half-life which can be better controlled (e.g. prednisolone). The main indications for methylprednisolone acetate are feline eosinophilic granuloma complex and idiopathic stomatitis-gingivitis.

■ Prednisolone (given PO) is the glucocorticoid of choice in most cases of long-term therapy.

■ Cats have approximately half as many glucocorticoid receptors as dogs and so need a higher dosage.

■ The recommended dosage is only a guideline as individual animals respond differently.

■ Anti-inflammatory dosages are approx. 10 times higher than physiological replacement dosages; immunosuppressive dosages are approx. twice as high as anti-inflammatory ones. Even higher dosages have been recommended in shock and spinal trauma; however, their duration must be limited to 1 to 2 days because of the associated risks.

■ If short- or intermediate-acting preparations are used for a period of 1 to 2 weeks, they can be stopped without a decremental reduction in dose. It is recommended that longer-lasting therapies should be tapered off.

The anti-inflammatory dosage of prednisolone in the dog is 1–2 mg/kg/day (0.15–0.3 mg/kg dexamethasone/day); in the cat it is approx. 2–4 mg/kg/day (0.3–0.5 mg dexamethasone/day). The immunosuppressive dosage of prednisolone in

the dog during the initial phase is 2–4 mg/kg/day; in the cat it is approx. 2–4 mg/kg/day. It does not appear to have any impact on the efficacy if the dose is given once a day or divided into two.

In immune diseases, it can take weeks before remission takes effect at which time, a dose reduction can be started. How this is done depends on personal preference. For example, the dosage can be reduced by 50% every 10 to 14 days. When the dosage has fallen to the normal level then the time between the doses can be increased to every two and then to every three days. Alternatively, after remission the same dosage of prednisolone can be given every second day instead of daily and if the patient's condition remains stable over the subsequent weeks, the dosage can be reduced slowly (approx. 50% every 10 to 14 days). In cases in which glucocorticoid therapy is necessary for more than 3 to 4 weeks, it should be attempted to maintain the therapy by giving the least effective dosage every second day instead of daily. In many cases, the pharmacological effect will last, whereas the extent of the side-effects and HPA axis suppression is reduced. It should be noted that due to its half-life, only prednisolone (or prednisone) is suitable for such alternate-day dosing.

9.2.4.3 Glucocorticoids in neurological diseases

Glucocorticoids are used in a number of neurological and neuromuscular diseases. A detailed description is given in the respective chapters. In many cases, the above-mentioned principles for the choice of preparation and the dosage have been used. One special situation is the therapy of brain and spinal cord trauma. Theoretically, glucocorticoids can achieve a favourable effect: they stabilise lysosomal membranes, inhibit lipid peroxidation and further expansion of the damage; they also reduce oedema formation and modulate the inflammatory reactions. However, their purported beneficial effects are controversial. The reason for this is that the favourable effects have mainly been shown in experimental studies, while in clinical studies, no significant differences have been seen.

The most commonly used preparation in recent times is methylprednisolone (as methylprednisolone sodium succinate), which at high doses is a better free radical scavenger than the other glucocorticoids. The time of administration of this preparation is the most decisive factor. A favourable effect is only potentially achieved if the patient is treated within the first 8 hours after trauma. Delayed administration can actually have negative effects. The recommended administration is as follows: initial IV bolus of 30 mg/kg methylprednisolone, followed by a second IV bolus 2 hours later of 15 mg/kg, which is repeated every 6 hours over 24 to 48 hours. This high dose schedule has not been proven to be effective as yet in dogs as currently a properly controlled clinical trial is lacking. With such a high dosage, the risk of side-effects, especially gastrointestinal ones, is relatively high. Until now it has not been proven that these gastrointestinal side-effects can be prevented by the application of H2-receptor blockers, proton pump blockers, sucralfate or misoprostol

Further reading

BEHREND, E.N., GRECO, D.S. (1995): Clinical applications of glucocorticoid therapy in nonendocrine disease. In: BONAGURA J.D: Kirk's Current Veterinary Therapy XII, Small Animal Practice. W.B. Saunders Company, Philadelphia, pp. 406–413.

CALVERT, C.A., CORNELIUS, L. M. (1990): The pharmacodynamic differences among glucocorticoid preparations. Symposium on the Use and Misuse of Steroids. Vet Med. 860–865.

CALVERT, C.A., CORNELIUS, L.M. (1990): Avoiding the undesirable effects of glucocorticoid hormone therapy. Symposium on the use and misuse of steroids. Vet Med. 846–856.

CALVERT, C.A., CORNELIUS, L.M. (1990): The most common indications for using corticosteroid hormones in veterinary practice. Symposium on the use and misuse of steroids. Vet Med. 826–845.

CALVERT, C.A., CORNELIUS, L.M. (1990): Corticosteroid hormones: Endogenous regulation and the effects of exogenous administration. Symposium on the use and misuse of steroids. Vet Med. 810–823.

CULBERT, L.A., MARINO, D.J., BAULE, R.M., KNOX, V.W. (1998): Complications associated with high-dose prednisolone sodium succinate therapy in dogs with neurological injury. J Am An Hosp Assoc. 34: 129–134.

HANSON, S.M., BOSTWICK, D.R., TWEDT, D.C., SMITH, M.O. (1997): Clinical evaluation of cimetidine, sucralfate, and misoprostol for prevention of gastrointestinal tract bleeding in dogs undergoing spinal surgery. Am J Vet Res. 58: 1320–1323.

JAGGY, A. (1997): Neurologische Notfälle beim Kleintier. Enke-Verlag, Stuttgart.

JOHNSON, J.A., MURTAUGH, R.J. (2000): Craniocerebral Trauma. In: BONAGURA J.D.: Kirk's Current Veterinary Therapy XIII, Small Animal Practice. W.B. Saunders Company, Philadelphia, pp. 178–185.

KEMPPAINEN, R.J., LORENZ, M.D., THOMPSON, F.N. (1981): Adrenocortical suppression in the dog after a single dose of methylprednisolone acetate. Am J Vet Res. 42: 822–824.

MACDONALD, J.M. (2000): Glucocorticoid therapy. In: ETTINGER, S.J., FELDMAN, E.C.: Textbook of Veterinary Internal Medicine, 5th ed., Vol. 1. W.B. Saunders Company, Philadelphia, pp. 307–317.

NEIGER, R., GASCHEN, F., JAGGY, A. (2000): Gastric mucosal lesions in dogs with acute intervertebral disc disease: characterization and effects of omeprazole or misoprostol. J Vet Intern Med. 14: 33–36.

OLBY, N. (1999): Current concepts in the management of acute spinal cord injury. J Vet Intern Med. 13: 399–407.

PAPICH, M.G., DAVIS, L.E. (1989): Glucocorticoid therapy. In: KIRK, R.W.: Current Veterinary Therapy X, Small Animal Practice. W.B. Saunders Company, Philadelphia, pp. 54–62.

ROMATOWSKI, J. (1990): Iatrogenic adrenocortical insufficiency in dogs. J Am Vet Med Assoc. 196: 1144–1146.

THOOMBS, J.P., GAYWOOD, D.D., LIPOWITZ, A.J., STEVENS, J.B. (1980): Colonic perforation following neurosurgical procedures and corticosteroid therapy in four dogs. J Am Vet Med Assoc. 177: 68–72.

9

9.3   Analgesics

Gina Aeschbacher

This section deals with the principles of analgesia in neurological patients: the knowledge of pain physiology is summarised, the significance of pain therapy is explained and possibilities for treating pain with medications are suggested (see also Chaps. 5 and 8). Many analgesics (e.g. certain opioids) are not licensed for use in the dog and cat. Their efficacy and tolerance have been proven by scientific publications and these have been substantiated by their clinical use. Despite this, it is recommended that before beginning treatment the owner of the animal should sign a consent form, which clearly states that compounds will possibly be used which are not licensed for use in dogs and cats. It is the job of the veterinarian to alleviate pain and so contribute to the patient's well-being.

9

9.3.1 Principles of pain physiology and therapy

The knowledge gained over the last 10 to 20 years in the area of pain physiology has greatly influenced the care of the veterinary patient. The reader is referred to the specialist literature on pain for an in-depth coverage of this subject. The processing of painful stimuli is simply summarised in the following text:

A noxious stimulus to the body surface is detected by so-called nocioceptors (free nerve endings) and changed into an electrical signal (**transduction**). The impulse is sent to the dorsal horn of the spinal cord (**transmission**) via afferent nerve fibres (A-d and C). The spinal cord has an important function as a relay centre: all information is collected, adapted and changed here (**modulation**), and then it is in part sent back to the initial entry point in the spinal cord via the descending nerve tracts. Additionally, the signal ascends centrally via the spinal tract up to the mesencephalon and finally up to the cortex (**perception**). Many different substances (e.g. substance P, arachidonic acid derivates, histamine, bradykinin, serotonin) play a role in the transfer of information and the production of the sense of pain.

Sensitization of the (peripheral and central) nervous tissues can occur when there is a continual transfer of peripheral and central impulses. This can cause a reduction in the pain threshold, extension of the perceived painful area and an interpretation of nonpainful stimuli as painful (wind-up). **Sensitization** remains for a significantly longer time than the causative pain stimulus: the nervous system therefore heals slower than the wound (1). Once sensitization has occurred (e.g. due to inadequate postoperative pain therapy or chronic pain), then successful pain therapy is difficult to achieve.

The **pathophysiological response** to acute pain is not just limited to the nervous system. It is accompanied by a "stress response" affecting the whole body: cardiovascular system (e.g. tachycardia, hypertension), respiration (e.g. hypercapnia, hypoxia, lung atelectasis), gastrointestinal tract (e.g. inappetence), urinary system (e.g. urinary retention), musculo-skeletal system (e.g. muscle pain, reduced movability), endocrine system (e.g. increased adrenergic activity, increased metabolism, increased oxygen requirements), CNS (fear, sedation, tiredness) and the immune system (reduced function) (1, 2). The extent and duration of this stress response depends on the degree of the tissue damage. It can last for many days and influence the morbidity of the patient. After a surgical operation, the stress response reaches a high postoperatively. Adequate analgesia is especially important during the recovery phase, as the increased well-being of the patient is involved in a quicker recovery and return of normal behaviour.

In the neurological patient, the treatment of acute (e.g. postoperative), chronic (e.g. tumour) and neuropathic (trauma to nervous tissue) discomfort is of importance, even when it is difficult to classify the mechanism of pain evolution in each patient. Due to this reason, it is improbable that a single analgesic given in a standard dosage will be successful in treating pain in all patients (2). For example, the pain associated with disc disease has both inflammatory and neuropathological components, and there may be both acute and chronic pain present at the same time. Accordingly, the following considerations and measures are of strategic importance in **pain relief**:

- **Individual therapy**. Differences with respect to pain threshold and pain intensity should be taken into consideration, and the analgesic treatment should be individually tailored to each patient. This involves regular monitoring of the patient including pain assessment or a determination of the success of the therapy (monitoring after treatment or pre-, intra- and postoperatively). Guidelines for pain therapy (e.g. analgesic dosage, interval between individual doses, duration of treatment, listing possible side-effects) should be present in every practise. The use of a scheme for the determination of pain can especially help the inexperienced observer.

- **Early initiation** of pain therapy. If analgesic substances are given before surgery (so-called pre-emptive analgesia) or as quickly as possible after a trauma, then the individually designed pain therapy will be easier to use (better pain reduction with the use of smaller dosages), the stress response of the body reduced and the possibility of nervous system sensitization is limited.

- **Multimodal pain therapy** (balanced analgesia). As many different substances and individual steps (transduction, transmission, modulation) play a role in the conduction of pain, it is possible to stop the transfer of pain and pain recognition at a number of places. The application of a high dose of a single analgesic for the treatment of acute pain is not recommended. It is better to concomitantly use a balanced mixture of various substances that cause pain suppression at different levels. With this multimodal form of pain therapy, a better reduction in pain is achieved despite the reduced dosage of each individual substance; the potential side-effects of the analgesics are also reduced (4). Multimodal pain therapy can also include non-pharmacological methods (e.g. acupuncture, physiotherapy).

- **Duration of pain therapy**. Pain treatment must be continued if inflammation affecting the tissue has not been significantly reduced, as this is responsible for the persistent repeated delivery of pain impulses (1). Even when the reasons for acute and chronic pain are no longer recognisable in the periphery, the nervous system may not have recovered from the damage (i.e. sensitization). Accordingly, treatment may be necessary for many days to weeks independent of the degree of pain. The adaptation of the therapy to the needs of the individual patient should be at the fore of all considerations. During tapering of pain therapy, the interval between treatments should not be changed prior to the dosage of each analgesic being reduced.

Different degrees of pain due to disease, injury or surgery are to be expected in the neurological patient (3, 5). For example:

- **Severe, agonising**: neuropathic pain (e.g. trapped nerve, cervical intervertebral disc herniation – additional chronic pain components are possible); after surgery with extensive tissue trauma and resulting inflammation; meningitis.
- **Moderate to severe**: intervertebral disc herniation in the thoracolumbar region; fractures; limb amputation; head injury; tumour; otitis; trauma and inflammation of soft tissues; post-radiation therapy; pain remission in previously mentioned conditions.
- **Mild to moderate**: mildly invasive surgery; pain remission in previously mentioned conditions.

Opioids and non-steroidal inflammatory substances (NSAIDs) are primarily used for pain relief in the neurological patient. Table 9.4 provides some suggestions for the dosages of the most commonly used analgesics in the cat and dog.

9.3.2 Opioids

Natural or synthetic opioids are used especially for acute pain and during the postoperative period. They are considered as being the best therapeutic options in the cat and dog (6), and are the first choice in the treatment of moderate and severe pain.

Opioids attach themselves to different receptors found peripherally, intraspinally and supraspinally in the body. The μ-receptor (OP3) is especially important for analgesia, as is the k-receptor (OP2). In general, activation of the opioid receptors inhibits impulse transmission in the synapses, whereby either the release of neurotransmitters is reduced or the production of action potentials in nerve cells is prevented.

Independent of their effects on the receptors, opioids are traditionally divided into agonists (e.g. morphine), partial agonists (e.g. buprenorphine), agonist-antagonists (e.g. butorphanol) or antagonists (e.g. naloxone). The analgesic effects of an opioid are influenced by different factors such as dosage and species, as well as the intensity, type and duration of the pain stimulus. Opioids dampen both peripheral and central transmission. They are mainly administered parenterally in the neurological patient (IM, IV administered as bolus or infusion, SC) or transdermally and rarely orally.

Some of the important unwanted side-effects of opioids include respiratory depression (which in contrast to human beings, is rarely a problem in dogs and cats), vomiting (especially with morphine), histamine release (especially after intravenous administration; pethidine > morphine), constipation (infrequent) and excitement (especially with overdosage; more often in cats than dogs). Respiratory depression leads to carbon dioxide accumulating in the blood, which induces an increase in cerebral blood flow and so an increase in intracranial pressure (see also Chap. 5.1.1).

As stated before, opioid-induced respiratory depression is not generally present as a clinical problem in the dog or cat (7, 8). However, even small doses of opioids can cause deterioration of a respiratory condition in dogs or cats with disturbances in consciousness (7, 9), and opioids in such cases should either be given to effect or not used at all. If consciousness is severely disturbed, if high doses are needed for pain relief, or if the treatment must be continued over a long period, then the use of NSAIDs should be considered (see Chap. 9.3.3). When severe respiratory depression does occur it can be treated with naloxone (0.01–0.04 mg/kg, IV, IM, SC) titrated according to effect. Analgesia and sedation are also reversed with this compound, which is why there may be a stimulation of the sympathetic system (release of catecholamines, dysrrhythmia, hypertension, death). Naloxone acts quickly and due to its short duration further injections may be necessary. Naltrexone and nalmefene are also true opioid antagonists.

Epidural administration of opioids (with or without local anaesthetic) is indicated when patients with head injuries need a greater degree of pain relief due to concomitant injury of the limbs. Although small doses of morphine injected epidurally rarely leads to respiratory depression, this can be relieved using naloxone without affecting the local analgesia (9).

The use (acquisition, storage, implementation, destruction) of opioids must be recorded and is controlled by regional dangerous drugs laws. As stated previously, opioids may not be licensed for use in the dog and cat. Table 9.4 gives guidelines for the use of opioids.

9.3.3 Non-steroidal anti-inflammatory drugs

Non-steroidal inhibitors of inflammation have been used for decades in the treatment of chronic pain. In comparison, their use for the relief of acute moderate to severe pain is new in veterinary medicine. Whether applied orally, intramuscularly, subcutaneously or intravenously, they all prevent the production of prostaglandins, particularly by inhibiting cyclo-oxygenases (COX-1, COX-2). Part of their analgesic effects can be explained by their influence on both inflammation in the periphery and the sensitisation effect of inflammation mediators on the peripheral nociceptors and nerves. In addition, nonsteroidal anti-inflammatory drugs (NSAIDs) possess a central effect, which reduces pain recognition and central hypersensitivity (10, 11). At present, an exact knowledge of the central mechanism of action is lacking. However, it appears that NSAIDs inhibit prostaglandin synthesis in the spinal cord (12), influencing transduction and modulation. Prostaglandins are to be found throughout the body and they play an important role in physiological processes in both health and sickness.

9

Table 9.4: Analgesics for the treatment of acute and chronic pain (see text and Chap. 5)
The dosages are always mg/kg unless otherwise specified (3, 6, 8).

Active agent	Classification	Indication	Dosage (mg/kg) Route, interval	Comments
Buprenorphine	Partial opioid antagonist	■ Light to moderate (postoperative) pain	0.005–0.02 IM, IV, SC q 4–8 h	■ Slow acting (30–60 min) ■ Slight respiratory depression ■ With ↑ ICP dose to effect
Butorphanol	Opioid agonist/antagonist	■ Light to moderate (postoperative) pain	dog: 0.2–0.5 cat: 0.2–0.8 IM, IV, SC q 1–3 h	■ Less analgesic potency than morphine ■ Slight respiratory depression, slight sedation, no histamine release ■ With ↑ ICP dose to effect
Carprofen	NSAID	■ Inflammation ■ Postoperative pain ■ Multimodal analgesia ■ Chronic pain	4.0 once then ≤ 2.0 SC, IV, PO BID	■ Effective after 30–60 min ■ Contraindication: shock, ↓ renal function, haemorrhage; concomitant use of corticosteroids or other NSAIDs
Etodolac	NSAID	■ Inflammation ■ Chronic pain	Dog: ≤ 10–15 PO SID	■ Effective after 30–60 min
Fentanyl	Opioid agonist	■ Severe postoperative pain	0.001–0.002 IV q 20–30 min IV infusion: 0.001–0.005/h 2–4 µg/kg/h transdermal	■ Quick acting (5 min) ■ Up to 100 times the analgesic effect of morphine ■ Respiratory depression, sedation, no release of histamine ■ With ↑ ICP dose to effect ■ Transdermal plaster (Duragesic®): dog: 3–10 kg: 25 µg/h; 10–20 kg: 50 µg/h; 20–30 kg: 75 µg/h: L 30 kg: 100 µg/h cat: 25–30 µg/h; effective after 8–24 h
Hydromorphone	Opioid agonist	■ Moderate to severe (postoperative) pain	0.1–0.4 IM, IV, SC q 2–4 h	■ Up to seven times analgesic effect of morphine ■ Respiratory depression, sedation, no release of histamine ■ With ↑ ICP dose to effect
Ketamine	Cyclohexanone (dissociative anaesthetic)	■ Multimodal analgesia ■ Chronic pain	1–4 IM, IV, SC 2–10 PO q 0.5 h	■ Stimulates CNS ■ Contraindications: cranial trauma, epileptic seizures but not status epilepticus, intracranial space-occupying lesions, before myelography
Ketoprofen	NSAID	■ Inflammation ■ Postoperative pain ■ Multimodal analgesia ■ Chronic pain	2.0 IM, IV, SC once, then for 5 days 1.0 IM, IV, SC, PO SID	■ Effective after 30–60 min ■ Contraindications: shock, ↓ renal function, haemorrhage, concomitant use of corticosteroids or NSAIDs
Keterolac	NSAID	■ Inflammation ■ Postoperative pain ■ Multimodal analgesia ■ Chronic pain	dog: 0.3–0.5 IM, IV cat: 0.25–0.3 SC q 12–24 h max. 1–2 doses	■ Effective after 30–60 min ■ Contraindications: shock, ↓ renal function, haemorrhage, concomitant use of corticosteroids or NSAIDs
Medetomidine	α2-adrenergic agonist	■ Multimodal analgesia ■ Chronic pain	0.001–0.010 IM, IV	■ Bradycardia, hypotension, muscle relaxation (careful with spinal fractures) ■ Antagonism with atipamezol
Meloxicam	NSAID	■ Inflammation ■ Postoperative pain ■ Multimodal analgesia ■ Chronic pain	≤ 0.2 once then ≤ 0.1 IV, SC, PO SID cat: only for 3 to 4 days	■ Effective after 30–60 min ■ Contraindications: shock, ↓ renal function, haemorrhage, concomitant use of corticosteroids or NSAIDs
Methadone	Opioid agonist	■ Moderate to severe (postoperative) pain	0.2–0.6 IM, IV, SC q 2–4 h	■ Up to 1.5 times the analgesic effect of morphine ■ Respiratory depression ■ No histamine release ■ With ↑ ICP dose to effect

9

Table 9.4: Analgesics for the treatment of acute and chronic pain (see text and Chap. 5) (continued)
The dosages are always mg/kg unless otherwise specified.

Active agent	Classification	Indication	Dosage (mg/kg) Route, interval	Comments
Morphine	Opioid agonist	■ Light to moderate (postoperative) pain	Dog: 0.2–1.0 Cat: 0.1–0.2 IM, SC, slow (!) IV q 2–4 h IV infusion 0.2/h	■ Effective after 20–30 min ■ Panting, respiratory depression, bradycardia (after high doses), vomiting, urinary retention, sedation ■ Histamine release with rapid IV injection ■ With ↑ ICP dose to effect
Nalbuphine	Opioid agonist/antagonist	■ Light to moderate (postoperative) pain	0.03–0.10 IM, IV, SC q 2–4 h	■ Less analgesic potency than morphine
Oxymorphone	Opioid agonist	■ Moderate to severe (postoperative) pain	0.03–0.10 IM, IV, SC q 3–4 h	■ Up to ten times analgesic effect of morphine ■ Same side-effects as for morphine but without histamine release ■ With ↑ ICP dose to effect
Pentazocine	Opioid agonist/antagonist	■ Light to moderate (postoperative) pain	1–3 IM, IV, SC q 2–4 h	■ Less analgesic potency than morphine
Pethidine	Opioid agonist	■ Moderate to severe (postoperative) pain	dog: 4–8 IM cat: 4–10 SC q 0.5–1.5 h	■ Effective after 5–10 min ■ Up to 10 times less analgesic effect than morphine ■ Less respiratory depression than with morphine ■ Release of histamine with IV injection ■ With ↑ ICP dose to effect

Key: ↑ increased; ↓ decreased; for others see Abbreviations.

9

NSAIDs have been attributed with a better effect in treating somatic rather than visceral pain (13). Their analgesic effect starts after 30 to 60 minutes. Depending on the substance, the maximum plasma concentrations are reached after 1 to 5 hours (14). As a consequence, opioids should be used initially to treat intra- and postoperative pain so that rapid pain relief is attained. NSAIDs work synergistically with other analgesics (e.g. opioids).

The general health status of a patient influences the decision of whether NSAIDs may be used or not (15). With today's knowledge, NSAIDs can only be recommended for cats and dogs under the following conditions: normal water balance, normal blood pressure, no disturbances in blood coagulation, no signs of or presence of stomach ulcers, no treatment with corticosteroids (15). According to MATHEWS (15), the use of NSAIDs before the induction of anaesthesia is only to be done with care as there is as yet insufficient data available about their use in this group of patients. Independent of how they are applied, NSAIDs can lead to generalised stomach ulcers. When given orally, they should always be taken with food to prevent the development of a local circumscribed ulcer (15). Meloxicam, carprofen and etodolac appear to hardly affect coagulation (15); however, in trauma patients, NSAIDs should not be used initially until haemorrhage and adequate blood perfusion of the organs has been achieved. Pain relief with opioids is better in such situations.

Absolute contraindications (14, 15) for the use of NSAIDs in the neurological patient include hypotension (e.g. shock and trauma patient), dehydration, actual or potential (e.g. acute disc herniation) haemorrhaging, coagulopathies, the concomitant use of more than one NSAID and/or corticosteroids, stomach ulcers or any other gastrointestinal disease, and renal or liver insufficiency. Stomach mucosa lesions occur frequently in dogs with acute disc herniations and corticosteroid treatment (16). Histamine-2-receptor antagonists (H2-antagonists, e.g. cimetidine) or proton pump inhibitors (antacids, e.g. omeprazole) have been suggested for the prophylaxis of stomach ulcers. In addition, sucralfate has been suggested for the treatment of an ulcer. H2-antagonists are not suitable for the prophylaxis of ulcers that have not been caused by NSAIDs (17). In an investigation by NEIGER (16), omeprazole (0.7 mg/kg, PO, SID) and misoprostol (0.002 mg/kg PO, TID) did not have a beneficial effect on anti-inflammatory associated stomach mucosal lesions. Sucralfate does not appear to be effective in the prophylaxis of ulcers in animals on corticosteroids or NSAIDs (17). Used in therapeutic doses, most NSAIDs do not influence either coagulation or bleeding time (7, 14). In patients with head injuries and possible haemorrhage or coagulation disturbances, PASCOE (9) advises not to use NSAIDs, but to treat the pain locally if possible. In dog breeds with a high probability of Von Willebrand disease (e.g. Doberman), NSAIDs should be used with care (14).

The concomitant administration of diuretics and NSAIDs should also be done with caution. SHARPE and THOMPSON (13) indicated that there is an increased risk of nephrotoxicity. The antihypertensive and diuretic effects of furosemide, a loop diuretic, are influenced to different degrees by the various NSAIDs. A reduction of furosemide's effects may occur and so they should be checked, and when necessary an increase in dosage should be given (18). The underlying mechanism for this is not known, but many complex processes appear to be involved (18).

9.3.4 Other medications and treatments used in pain relief

Local anaesthetics (e.g. lidocaine, bupivacaine, ropivacaine) block the reversible sodium channels. Local (e.g. infiltration) in the area of an incision or regional (e.g. epidural injection) administration methods may be used. Local anaesthetics inhibit the stimulation of nociceptors, the transmission of the stimulus and when used centrally, they also affect modulation. Local anaesthetics can also help in neurological pain situations (19). The intravenous infusion of small amounts of lidocaine can relieve pain and hyperalgesia (excessive sensitiveness to pain), while allodynia (pain evoked by non-painful stimuli) and dysaesthesia (spontaneous or evoked abnormal sensation) are reduced (19, 20, 21).

Alpha-2-adrenergic agonists (e.g. medetomidine, dexmedetomidine, xylazine) bind to the α2-receptors in the dorsal horn of the spinal cord and also supraspinally in different parts of the brain. Binding to the presynaptic α2-receptors leads to a reduction in the neurotransmitter norepinephrine and so a sympatholytic effect, while the activation of postsynaptic α2-receptors induces a more sympathomimetic result. Binding to central α2-receptors (reduction of norepinephrine release) results in an inhibition of impulse transmission causing sedation, analgesia and muscle relaxation. In addition, α2-agonists inhibit the cranial relaying (transmission, modulation) of the impulse or due to their sedative effects, the perception of pain.

For pain relief, these compounds are most commonly used in combination with local anaesthetics to prolong the blockade of sensory nerves (19). In cadiovascularly stable patients, small doses of medetomidine in combination with opioids can be used for the treatment of extreme or difficult to control pain.

The disassociative anaesthetic **ketamine** also inhibits the N-methyl-D-aspartate receptor and so is involved in the modulation of pain impulses in the spinal cord (22). Even in small doses, ketamine can improve pain relief as it prevents wind-up and sensitisation of the dorsal horn in the spinal cord. This is why ketamine is useful in chronic neurological pain conditions in which both opioids and NSAIDs are less successful. Ketamine can be given intramuscularly or intravenously (bolus, continual infusion). If a continual ketamine infusion is used, then it is recommended to give a sedative or an opioid at the same time (19). Amantadine is a similar drug and has recently been proven to be effective in dogs with refractory osteoarthritis pain.

General anaesthesia (e.g. halothane, isoflurane) lead to unconsciousness and therefore inhibit the processing (perception) of the impulses arriving in the brain. Transduction, transmission or modulation of the pain signals are not influenced; strictly speaking, therefore, general anaesthetics are not analgesics. As already discussed, it is particularly important to start analgesia before surgical operations (pre-emptive analgesia) and to undertake pain relief at different levels (multimodal analgesia).

Sedatives such as phenothiazines (e.g. ace[tyl]promazine) or benzodiazepines (e.g. diazepam) are often used with opioids for the relief of pain. Although, it does not have any analgesic effects of its own, acetylpromazine strengthens the effects of analgesics as it reduces the fear, stress and anxiety of the patient. In addition, diazepam reduces muscle tension (19).

Glucocorticosteroids (see Chap. 9.2) are not classed as analgesics. They have a local anti-inflammatory effect in damaged nerve tissue, though they can be used to relieve chronic and tumour-related pain (19).

Tricyclic antidepressants (e.g. amitriptyline) and **anticonvulsants** (e.g. gabapentin) appear to be very promising in the treatment of neuropathological pain (9, 19, 23), but at the moment they have not been evaluated in veterinary medicine.

As part of a multimodal therapy and so in addition to pharmacological pain relief, **non-medicinal methods** may be used. Until now, these alternatives have not been adequately clinically tested in cats and dogs. Even in human beings, further studies are necessary to definitely determine the efficacy of non-medicinal pain relief (24, 25). To improve the efficacy of non-medicinal methods, these forms of treatment should be started as early as possible (pre-emptive). Some of these alternative methods include acupuncture (see Chap. 11), transcutaneous or percutaneous electrical nerve stimulation (electroanalgesia; see Chap. 8.1.4.2) and magnetic field induction (see Chap. 8.1.6). Neurolytic techniques (laser, cold, radiation) are rarely used to reduce pain.

Attentive nursing of the patient is of particular importance. The individually tailored use of analgesics leads to a better tolerance and relaxation of the patient and facilitates the use of **physiotherapy**, **chiropractic methods** or **massage** (see Chap. 8) for further pain relief, and to support an early return of normal body functions.

Literature

1 ROWLINGSON, J.R. (2002): Acute pain management revisited. IARS Review Course Lectures, pp. 92–99.

2 LAMONT, L.A., TRANQUILLI, W.J., GRIMM, K.A. (2000): Physiology of pain. Vet Clin North Amer Small Anim Pract. **30**: 703–728.

3 MATHEWS, K.A. (2000): Pain assessment and general approach to management. Vet Clin North Amer Small Anim Pract. **30**: 729–755.

4 KEHLET, H., DAHL, J.B. (1993): The value of "multimodal" or "balanced analgesia" in postoperative pain treatment. Anesth Analg. **77**: 1048–1056.

5 TRANQUILLI, W.J., GRIMM, K.A., LAMONT, L.A. (2000): Pain management for specific conditions and procedures. In: TRANQUILLI, W.J., GRIMM, K.A., LAMONT, L.A. (eds.): Pain management for the small animal practitioner. Teton New Media, Jackson; pp. 73–103.

6 PASCOE, P.J. (2000): Opioid analgesics. Vet Clin North Amer Small Anim Pract. **30**: 757–772.

7 NOLAN, A.M. (2000): Pharmacology of analgesic drugs. In: FLECKNELL, P., WATERMAN-PEARSON, A. (eds.): Pain management in animals. W.B. Saunders, London; pp. 21–52.

8 NICHOLSON A., CHRISTIE, M. (2002): Opioid analgesics. In: MADDISON, J.E., PAGE, S.W., CHURCH, D. (eds.): Small animal clinical pharmacology. W.B. Saunders, London; pp. 271–292.

9 PASCOE, P.J. (2000): Problems of pain management. In: FLECKNELL, P., WATERMAN-PEARSON, A. (eds.): Pain management in animals. W.B. Saunders, London; pp. 161–177.

10 MALMBERG, A.B., YAKSH, T.L. (1992): Hyperalgesia mediated by spinal glutamate or substance P receptor blocked by spinal cyclo-oxygenase inhibition. Science **257**: 1276–1279.

11 LIVINGSTON, A. (2000): Mechanism of action of nonsteroidal anti-inflammatory drugs. Vet Clin North Amer Small Anim Pract. **30**: 773–781.

12 MØINICHE, S., KEHLET, H., DAHL, J.B. (2002): A qualitative and quantitative systemic review of preemptive analgesia for postoperative pain relief: the role of timing of analgesia. Anesthesiology **96**: 725–741.

13 SHARPE, P., THOMPSON, J. (2001): Non-steroidal anti-inflammatory drugs. The Royal College of Anaesthetists Bulletin **6**: 265–268.

14 MADDISON, J.E., JOHNSTON, K.A. (2002): Nonsteroidal anti-inflammatory drugs and chondroprotective agents. In: MADDISON, J.E., PAGE, S.W., CHURCH, D. (eds.): Small animal clinical pharmacology, W.B. Saunders, London; pp. 251–269.

15 MATHEWS, K.A. (2000): Nonsteroidal anti-inflammatory analgesics. Vet Clin North Amer Small Anim Pract. **30**: 783–804.

16 NEIGER, R., GASCHEN, F., JAGGY, A. (2002): Gastric mucosal lesions in dogs with acute intervertebral disc disease: characterization and effects of omeprazole or misoprostol. J Vet Intern Med. **14**: 33–36.

17 MADDISON, J.E., GUILFORD, G. (2002): Gastrointestinal drugs. In: MADDISON, J.E., PAGE, S.W., CHURCH, D. (eds.): Small animal clinical pharmacology, W.B. Saunders, London; pp. 429–448.

18 STOCKLEY, I.H. (1996): Drug interactions. The Pharmaceutical Press, London; pp. 385–387.

19 LAMONT, L.A., TRANQUILLI, W.J., MATHEWS, K.A. (2000): Adjunctive analgesic therapy. Vet Clin North Amer Small Anim Pract. **30**: 805–813.

20 TANELIAN, D.L., MACIVER, M.B. (1991): Analgesic concentrations of lidocaine suppress tonic A-delta and C fiber discharges produced by acute injury. Anesthesiology **74**: 934–936.

21 PANG, W.W., MOK, M.S., HUANG, S., HWANG, M.H. (1998): The analgesic effect of fentanyl, morphine, meperidine, and lidocaine in the peripheral veins: a comparative study. Anesth Analg. **86**: 382–386.

22 KOHRS, R., DURIEUX, M.E. (1998): Ketamine: Teaching an old drug new tricks. Anesth Analg. **87**: 1186–1193.

22a LASCELLES, B.D., GAYNOR, J.S., SMITH, E.S., ROE, S.C., MARCELLIN-LITTLE, D.J., DAVIDSON, G., BOLAND, E., CARR, J. (2008): Amantadine in a multimodal analgesic regime for alleviation of refractory osteoarthritis pain in dogs. J Vet Intern Med. **22** (1): 53–59.

23 ROSE, M.A., KAM, P.C.A. (2002): Gabapentin: pharmacology and its use in pain mangement. Anaesthesia **57**: 451–462.

24 WHITE, P.F. (2002): The role of non-opioid analgesic techniques in the management of pain after ambulatory surgery. Anesth Analg. **94**: 577–585.

25 LYNCH, L., SIMPSON, K.H. (2002): Transcutaneous electrical nerve stimulation and acute pain. BJA. CEPD Reviews **2**: 49–52.

9

Further reading

HANSEN, B. (1997): Pain: Semin Vet Med Surg (Small Anim) **12**(2).

MATHEWS, K.A. (2000): Management of Pain, Vet Clin North Amer Small Anim Pract. **30**(4), 2000.

FLECKNELL, P., WATERMAN-PEARSON, A. (2000): Pain management in animals, W.B. Saunders, London.

HELLEBREKERS, L. (2001): Schmerz und Schmerztherapie beim Tier, Schlütersche, Hannover.

ANIL, S.S., ANIL, L., DEEN, J. (2002): Challenges of pain assessment in domestic animals. J Am Vet Med Assoc. **220**: 313–319.

10 Neurosurgery

Ulrich Rytz
Franck Forterre
Hugo Schmökel
Cornelius v. Werthern

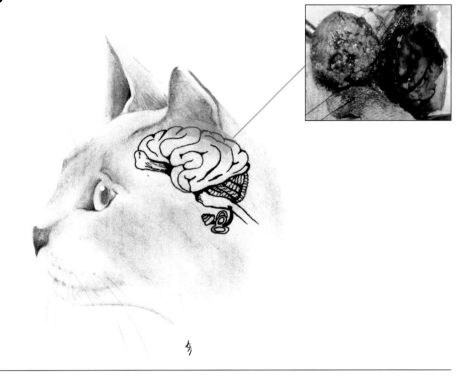

10.1 Instrumentation

Ulrich Rytz

The undertaking of neurosurgical techniques requires a precise knowledge of anatomy; an exact, atraumatic surgical technique; and a good surgical instrument set with some specialised neurosurgical instruments. Of course, each surgeon has his or her own preferences with respect to techniques and instrumentation. Suitable premises and good lighting conditions are essential for neurosurgery. An optical enlargement of the operating field with loupe eye-sets (2–3 × enlargement) or in special cases, with an operating microscope is very helpful.

Some specialised neurosurgical instruments are depicted in Figs. 10.1–10.10:
- Weitlaner retractors
- Gelpi retractors
- Periosteal elevators
- Electrocautery: monopolar, bipolar
- Small sharp osseous curettes
- Rongeurs and bone punches (Kerrison)
- Nerve root and dura hooks
- Pneumatic hand drill with ball-nosed and diamond bits
- Fine suction heads, blunt cannulas
- Bone wax, haemostatic cellulose (Lyostypt®), Gel foam®
- Polymethylmethacrylate (PMMA) cement

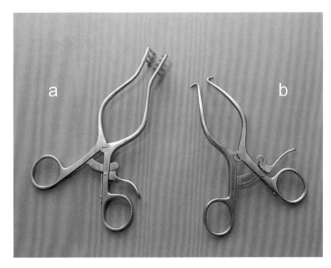

Fig. 10.1a, b
(a) Weitlaner and (b) Gelpi retractors are used as self-retaining wound retractors.

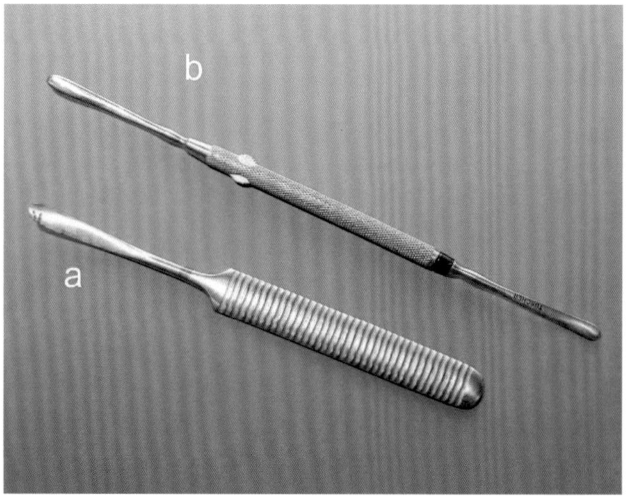

Fig. 10.2a, b
(a) Periosteal and (b) Freer elevators are used to detach the muscle from the vertebral bodies.

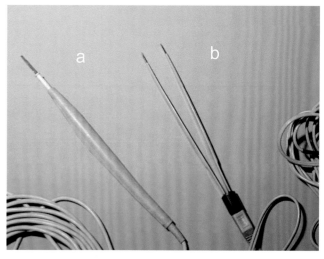

Fig. 10.3a, b
(a) Monopolar electrocoagulation is used to coagulate small blood vessels and to incise tissue at a distance away from nerve and muscle tissues. Only bipolar electrocoagulation (b) is used close to nerves or the spinal cord.

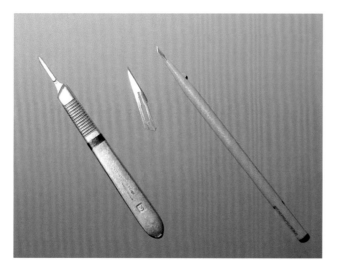

Fig. 10.4
A pointed scalpel blade (No. 11) or an eye / iris scalpel is used for the precise incision of the annulus fibrosus, ligaments or dura.

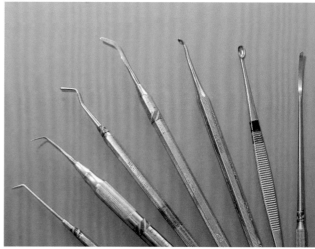

Fig. 10.5
Sharp spoons, small curettes and nerve root or dental hooks with different points are used for the removal of disc material from the vertebral canal.

10.2   Brain

Franck Forterre

The modern-day methods of imaging such as MRI and CT make it possible to accurately determine a diagnosis and treatment strategies. This was barely possible with standard radiography, angiography and ventriculography, as these techniques are less sensitive and specific. Previously, intracranial surgery in veterinary medicine was mainly done for experi-

mental reasons and rarely for therapeutic reasons. Accordingly, knowledge about intracranial surgery is based almost completely on experimental studies which were focussed on the principles of human neurosurgery. However, as CT and MRI has become more routinely used in veterinary medicine, more publications can be found in the literature about the surgical treatment of tumours, trauma and hydrocephalus in small animals.

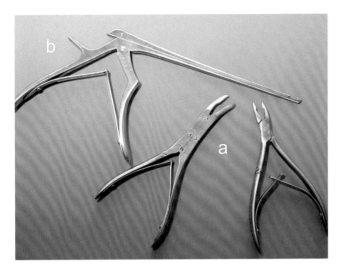

Fig. 10.6a, b
(a) Rongeurs and (b) Kerrison bone punches in different sizes are used to remove bone.

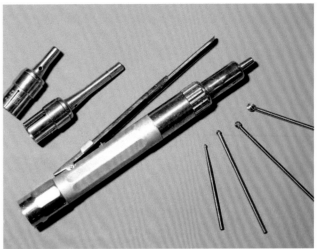

Fig. 10.7
A pneumatic hand drill with spherical drill bits of different diameters is used to remove bone.

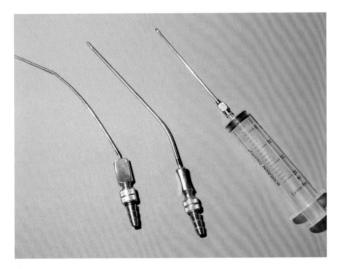

Fig. 10.8
Fine suction heads with overload protection to protect the tissues and a rinsing syringe with a blunt cannula are used to ensure a clear view of the operating field.

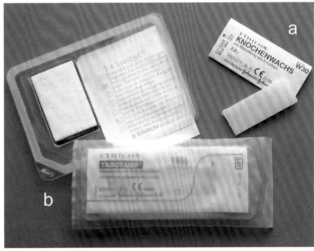

Fig. 10.9a, b
(a) Bone wax and (b) haemostatic cellulose are used for haemostasis in the operating field.

10

10.2.1 Brain tumours

10.2.1.1 General information

Brain tumours cause cerebral dysfunction due to primary effects such as infiltration or compression of their neighbouring anatomical structures, or due to their secondary effects such as the development of hydrocephalus. Other primary effects include disturbance of the cerebral circulation and local necrosis, which can lead to additional destruction of nervous tissue. The most important secondary effects of a brain tumour are an interruption in the CSF flow dynamics, an increase in ICP, cerebral oedema and herniation of the brain (5, 8).

The main aims of the treatment of intracranial neoplasia are the control of secondary effects such as increased ICP and brain oedema, and potentially, the complete removal of the tumour. The palliative treatment of brain tumours with glucocorticoids in the dog and cat is aimed at reducing brain oedema and in some cases, slowing down tumour growth. If anticonvulsive therapy is necessary, phenobarbital is the drug of choice for the control of generalised seizures.

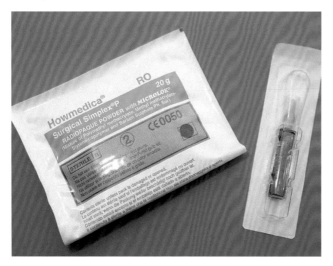

Fig. 10.10
Polymethylmethacrylate cement is used for the internal stabilisation of the spine with pins or screws.

10

The reduction of tumour size or its complete removal are the main factors which determine long-term survival. Four therapeutic methods are presently available for the treatment of brain tumours in the dog and cat: surgery, radiation therapy, chemotherapy and immunotherapy.

Surgery offers the chance for a rapid decompression of the intracranial cavity and the option of removing the tumour either completely or at least partially to improve the efficacy of adjunct therapies such as chemotherapy and / or radiation therapy. The surgical treatment of brain tumours in veterinary medicine has often been disappointing as the tumours could not be completely removed and severe damage to the brain tissues was caused by the operation itself and the effects of the anaesthesia. The reasons for this include inadequate experience in the choice of cases that were suitable for surgical intervention, and inadequate preoperative knowledge of the localisation, size and tissue type of the tumour.

CT, MRI and the further development of neurosurgical and anaesthetic techniques have allowed the number of successful intracranial operations done in the dog and cat to rise.

The localisation, size, type and invasiveness of the tumour all influence the resectability of an intracranial neoplasm. Meningiomas in the frontal and the caudodorsal regions of the cranial fossa are easy to reach and they can be surgically removed without any expectation of a functional disturbance of the brain. In comparison, the removal of a neoplasm from the ventral regions of the rostral and middle fossa is associated with a high morbidity and mortality. Resection of a neoplasm in the ventral regions of the caudal fossa cannot be done without the risk of severe damage to the medulla and the cranial nerves.

Partial resection of a brain tumour can enable not only its histology to be determined but can also reduce the secondary cerebral dysfunction caused by the tumour. In addition, better response with adjunctive therapies, such as radiation therapy, are attained as the tumour volume is reduced (8, 11, 12). Ideally, a biopsy should always be taken before chemotherapy or radiation therapy is commenced; however, due to the cost and morbidity of brain biopsy, there is a tendency not to always do this. Nowadays, CT-guided stereotactic biopsy is being used more frequently at several institutions in tumour diagnostics with minimal risk for the patient.

10.2.1.2 Premedication – Anaesthesia
If surgical removal of a brain tumour is planned then the peri- and intraoperative management of the patient determine the maintenance of brain function. Hyperosmolar solutions, diuretics and glucocorticoids are given to reduce the brain volume. The positioning of the patient and altering the carbon dioxide and oxygen partial pressures by artificial respiration can also influence the intracranial blood volume.

Preoperatively, 30 minutes before the induction of anaesthesia, mannitol (0.5–1.0 g/kg, IV over 15 minutes) and methylprednisolone succinate (30 mg/kg, IV) are given. The prophylactic application of a broad spectrum antibiotic (cephazolin 22 mg/kg, IV) is recommended, because of the risk of infection to the brain tissues, which is increased by long operating times. Anesthesia is induced with a benzodiazepine such as diazepam (0.1 mg/kg, IV) and a short-acting barbiturate or preferably, propofol. Anaesthesia is then continued with inhalational anaesthesia using isoflurane and oxygen or with constant rate infusions of propofol (see Chap. 5.2.4). After shaving the operation site, the patient is placed in sternal recumbency with its head raised at approximately 30° to the level of the table. Care should be taken that the jugular veins are not compressed so that venous drainage from the brain is maintained. The carbon dioxide partial pressure is kept low (approx. 30–35 mmHg) by intraoperative hyperventilation (4, 9).

10.2.1.3 Techniques
Craniotomy is performed using a pneumatic drill. During the drilling, the area should be continually flushed with isotonic saline. Excess saline and bone dust should be removed by aspiration. Bleeding from the cut edges of the bone and the diploid veins is arrested using bone wax. After removal of the bone (craniectomy), an attempt is made to reduce the ICP further via a durotomy and intraoperative loss of CSF. Further reduction in ICP can be achieved by puncture of the ventricle. Due to the loss of CSF, the brain starts to relax making its structures easier to assess and to dissect. After the dura has been opened, the brain can be manipulated with a tissue

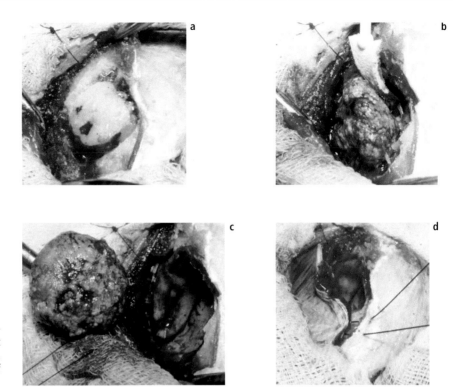

Fig. 10.11a–d
Meningioma resection. (a) Craniotomy after detachment of the temporalis muscle. (b) Blunt dissection of the meningioma after durectomy. (c) Situation after excision. (d) Re-apposition of the temporalis muscle.

10

spatula. During dissection of the tumour, bleeding from arterioles and venules should be immediately arrested using bipolar coagulation. The tumours found in the different topographical regions of the brain require an individual resection technique. The main principle is to make the tumour smaller which provides room for further manipulation and resection; at the same time, it causes decompression of the brain. During this procedure, the bulk of the tumour is enucleated in stages from the centre (inner tumour parenchyma). If bleeding arises during removal of the tumour then the blood is aspirated, the haemorrhage is carefully swabbed with neurosurgical swabs or gauze and the source repeatedly coagulated using bipolar coagulation (12). Additionally, it can be useful to use haemostatic substances such as oxidised cellulose or muscle tissue. After the excision of the tumour, the wound is closed in layers; the excised dura and cranial bone are usually discarded (Fig. 10.11) (1, 4, 8, 9) .

The patient is closely monitored during the first 48 hours postoperatively. The antibiosis (cephazolin 20mg/kg, BID IV or PO) is continued for a period of 5 to 7 days. It is also useful to give anti-inflammatory doses of glucocorticoids for 7 to 10 days. If seizures were noted prior to the operation, then they should be treated with phenobarbital (1–2 mg/kg, q 12 h PO or q 6 h IV).

The site of the craniectomy fills in with connective tissue within 6 to 8 weeks of the operation, and separates the brain tissue from the overlying muscle. This membrane is sufficiently strong enough to protect the brain after 2 to 3 months. The temporalis muscle sticks to the membrane but not to the brain (11).

10.2.1.4 Problems
Even when tumour resection in combination with chemotherapy and / or radiation therapy result in good long-term results, post-operative problems may remain. For a tumour to be completely removed, it must be easily imaged, visible to the naked eye or with magnification, and resectable. Ideally, the operation should be done under continual imaging but this is rarely possible in veterinary medicine. It should be noted that not all easily visualised tumours are easy to resect.

Last but not least, the successful resection of a tumour depends on its biological characteristics. These are manifested as the tumour's specific growth characteristics as well as its relationship to the surrounding tissues. A well-demarcated tumour seen with MRI can prove to be poorly demarcated during the operation.

10.2.2 **Cranial trauma** (Fig. 10.12)

10.2.2.1 **General information**

Road accidents and falling from a window / height are the most common causes of brain trauma in the dog and cat, respectively. Young animals are more commonly affected than older ones. The brain is so well protected by the relatively thick skull and the overlying muscle that only severe trauma can cause brain injury. Accompanying injuries occurring in the thorax (pneumothorax, lung contusion) and the jaw bones are frequent. Pathophysiologically, the external force causes a destruction of the blood-brain barrier and brain cells (vasogenic oedema). Extracellular hyperkalaemia occurs with the release of free radicals, which in turn leads to cytotoxic oedema. The swelling of the cells increases the ischemia and hypoxia. Oedema and the pooling of blood increases ICP, reduces the perfusion pressure and so extends the area of ischemia (2, 3).

The treatment of brain injury is focussed on the neurological symptoms, their time-related development, the neuro-anatomical localisation of the lesion, and the type of lesion (fracture, contusion, haematoma). If consciousness is disturbed, aggressive therapy should be started immediately. The aim of drug therapy is to prevent the development of oedema with any resulting increase in ICP, and as prophylaxis against infection. The drugs of choice are methylprednisolone (30 mg/kg, IV), mannitol (0.5–1 g/kg, IV over 15 minutes), furosemide (0.7 mg/kg, IV), cephalosporins (cephazolin, 22 mg/kg, IV) and oxygen. Diazepam (0.5–2 mg/kg, IV) and/or phenobarbital (5–10 mg/kg, initial slow IV to effect) are suitable for the treatment of spasms and/or seizures.

The aim of surgical treatment following head trauma is to remove compressive lesions (haematoma, fracture fragments) in order to reduce the ICP; this is, however, only performed when medical therapies have failed. Accordingly, the lesion must be precisely localised. Radiographs of the skull are sufficient in a few cases for the recognition of a fracture line and/or depressed bone fragment. CT and MRI are, however, much better imaging methods for diagnosing cranial trauma as both these methods allow the finest fracture lines to be seen (which usually remain hidden on a radiograph) and they are able to depict damage to the parenchyma and haematomas; therefore, following their use, the patient can be quickly given the most appropriate therapy. However, such imaging often requires anaesthesia which can destabilise a patient in the 72 hours following head injury.

10.2.2.2 **Techniques** (Fig. 10.13)

The procedures – premedication, anaesthesia and patient positioning – are the same as for brain tumour surgery. In a fracture with a depressed fragment or fragments, the fragment(s) should be carefully lifted up and/or removed taking care not to damage the underlying parenchyma. If a haematoma is present, any bleeding should be immediately arrested, and

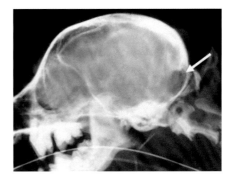

Fig. 10.12
Occiput fracture due to a bite wound in a Yorkshire Terrier (arrow).

then the lesion should be washed out well with isotonic saline. Stabilisation and reconstruction of the calvarium is rarely necessary.

A haematoma without a concurrent fracture is approached using a craniotomy or craniectomy in the area of the lesion. If the haematoma lies in the subarachnoid space, then the dura and the arachnoids are incised over the whole length of the lesion. The haematoma is carefully removed, any bleeding is arrested and the surgical site is flushed out well with isotonic saline. Epi- or subdural haematomas are dealt with in the same manner, though the dura remains closed with an epidural lesion, and the arachnoids remain closed with a subdural lesion. These are rare lesions in the dog and cat, unlike in humans. To close the wound, the muscles are reinserted, and the subcutis and skin are closed in the standard manner. If the dura has been incised, neither it nor the craniotomy wound are closed, so that there can be no build up of post-operative pressure (2, 3, 6, 11).

10.2.2.3 **Problems**

The prognosis depends on the severity of the neurological deficits, the extent of the lesion and the time of treatment. Patients with mild neurological disturbances and immediate therapy (i.e., within 8 hours after the trauma) have a good prognosis. With severe lesions, the assessment of consciousness, respiration, pupil size and response to light (modified Glasgow coma scale) can determine the prognosis. If the patient exhibits coma with mydriatic, non-responsive pupils then the prognosis is hopeless. However, the choice of adequate therapy for situations between the extremes of this situation and a more normal-appearing patient is difficult.

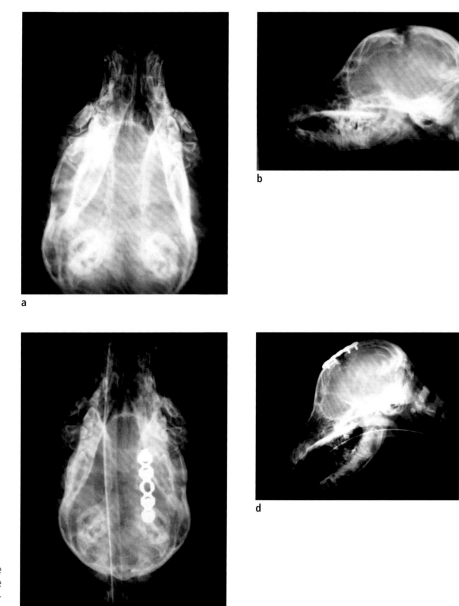

Fig. 10.13a–d
Unstable circular skull fracture in a young male mixed-breed dog. Stabilisation of the fracture with a face reconstruction plate. (a, b) Preoperative situation; (c, d) situation after stabilisation.

10

10.2.3 Hydrocephalus

10.2.3.1 General information

Hydrocephalus can be primarily congenital or secondary as a consequence of a disturbance in CSF flow. Where possible the causative disease is treated and the production of CSF is reduced by medication. Glucocorticoids and carbonic anhydrase inhibitors are usually not very effective treatments and they have side-effects when used for long-term therapy. Bearing this in mind, ventriculoperitoneal shunt surgery should be considered in many patients. This technique has become successful due to the development of a subcutaneously placed valve. In human medicine, there are a number of shunt systems available which mainly differ with respect to the pressure required to open the shunt valve. The shunt system is made up of an inlet tube with perforations, a valve unit and an outlet tube, which all have to be fitted together; although, recently so-called one piece uni-shunts are available for implantation. Until now, these shunt systems have only been sporadically used in veterinary medicine.

10.2.3.2 **Techniques**

Anaesthesia and premedication are similar to those used in brain tumour surgery. The operation is done in two phases. First of all, the valve unit and outlet tube are positioned subcutaneously. A number of skin incisions are normally required to enable the correct placement of the tunnel for the outlet tube, unless a large trochar can be used to guide the tube subcutaneously. The valve unit is usually placed between the shoulder blades and the head at the back of the neck. Afterwards, the valve unit and the outlet tube are joined together and filled with isotonic saline. In the second phase of the operation, a minimal opening to the enlarged lateral ventricle is made. This micro-craniotomy is done where the least amount of brain tissue covers the ventricle, which can be calculated from an MRI. The inlet tube is pushed into the ventricle through an incision in the meninges using a stylette; it is guided to a precise depth, again using the MRI and the appearance of fluid at the opening of the tube. It is then fixed on the cranium close to where it comes out of the skull, usually by use of a sterile anchoring device supplied with the shunt. The inlet tube is subsequently attached to the valve unit and secured with suture. Finally, the free end of the outlet tube (at least 25 cm) is inserted into the peritoneal cavity through a small incision in the lateral abdominal wall. The surgical wounds are closed routinely (7, 10).

10.2.3.3 **Problems**

Although this surgical operation is relatively simple, complications are not uncommon. Patency problems of the catheter due to blockage (blood clot, inflammatory cells, protein plugs), separation of the individual sections of the catheter, displacement of the tip of the catheter, and infection have been reported in human medical literature. The postoperative rate of infection can be as high as 38%. These complications can also negatively influence the long-term prognosis in veterinary medicine.

Literature

1 BAGLEY, R.S., HARRINGTON, M.L., PLUHAR, G.E., KEE-GAN, R.D., GREENE, S.A., MOORE, M.P., GAVIN, P.R. (1996): Effect of craniectomy/durotomy alone and in combination with hyperventilation, diuretics and corticosteroids on intracranial pressure in clinically normal dogs. Am J Vet Res. **57**: 116–125.

2 DEWEY, C.W., BUDSBERG, S.C., OLIVER, J.E. (1992): Principles of head trauma management in dogs and cats – Part I. Comp Cont Educ Pract Vet. **14**: 199–207.

3 DEWEY, C.W., BUDSBERG, S.C., OLIVER, J.E. (1993): Principles of head trauma management in dogs and cats – Part II. Comp Cont Educ Pract Vet. **15**: 177–184.

4 GORDON, L.E., THACHER, C., MATTHIESEN, D.T., JO-SEPH, R.J. (1994): Results of craniotomy for the treatment of cerebral meningioma in 42 cats. Vet Surg. **23**: 94–100.

5 GORDON, G.C. (1990): Genesis and pathology of tumors of the nervous system. Sem Vet Surg. **5**: 210–222.

6 HOPKINS, A.L., WHEELER, S.J. (1991): Subdural hematoma in a dog. Vet Surg. **20**: 413–418.

7 KESTLE, J., DRAKE, J., MILNER, R., SAINTE-CLOSE, C., CINALLI, G., BOOP, F., PIATT, J., HAINES, S., SCHIFF, S., COCHRANE, D., STEIBOK, P., MACNEIL, N. (2000): Long-term follow-up data from the shunt design trial. Pediatr Neurosurg. **33**: 230–236.

8 LECOUTEUR, R.A. (1993): Brain tumors in dogs and cats. Proceedings WSAVA, Berlin.

9 NIEBAUER, G. (1991): Evaluation of craniotomy in dogs and cats. J Am Vet Med Assoc. **198**: 89–95.

10 REKATE, H.L. (1994): Treatment of hydrocephalus. In: CHEEK, W., Pediatric neurosurgery. W.B. Saunders. Philadelphia.

11 SEIM, H.B. (2002): Surgery of the brain. In: FOSSUM, T.W. (ed.). Small Animal Surgery, 2nd ed. Mosby. St Louis.

12 YASARGIL, M.G. (1996): Microneurosurgery. Georg Thieme Verlag. New York.

10.3 **Spinal cord / Spine**

Ulrich Rytz

10.3.1 **Diseases of the intervertebral discs**

The spinal column and the spinal cord running protected through it, are both divided anatomically into the cervical spine (C1–C7), the thoracic spine (T1–T13), the lumbar spine (L1–L7) and the sacral spine (S1–S3). Accordingly, intervertebral disc diseases are subdivided into cervical, thoracolumbar and lumbosacral spinal cord compression. Spinal cord compression, as a consequence of intervertebral disc disease, is the most common neurological problem in the dog. Disc degeneration is due to senility of the disc material and leads either to extrusion (Hansen type I) or protrusion (Hansen type II). Chondroid degeneration of the nucleus pulposus occurs particularly in chondrodystrophic breeds (e.g. Dachshund, Pekingese, Poodle, Spaniel, etc.) in the first two years of life. Dehydration and mineralisation of the nucleus pulposus reduce the shock-absorber ability of the disc and weakens the fibres of the annulus fibrosus. Disc extrusion (Hansen type I) means that the anatomically thinner dorsal part of the fibrous ring ruptures and there is prolapse of degenerate disc material into the vertebral canal, usually between the third and sixth year of life in affected breeds. Fibrinoid degeneration occurs more often in non-chondrodystrophic dog breeds at a much older age, and leads to protrusion of the annulus fibrosus into the vertebral canal. This process is called disc protrusion (Hansen type II). The clinical symptoms associated with disc extrusion can be explained, on the one hand, by the mechanical compression of the spinal cord and nerve roots, and on the other hand, by the biochemical and inflammatory processes in the nervous tissues and or the disc. The clinical signs are determined not only by the extent of the compression (mass effect) but also the dynamic nature of the compression (slow protrusion or explosive disc prolapse).

The clinical symptoms therefore depend on the extent, dynamics and localisation of the compression. They can vary from just pain alone to pain in association with severe neurological dysfunction. The degree of neurological dysfunction ranges from ataxia to paraplegia with loss of nociception. The extent and the duration of these clinical symptoms are also important prognostic factors.

10.3.2 Diseases of the cervical intervertebral discs

Roughly 15% of all disc disease in the dog affects the neck (23). The most commonly affected intervertebral disc space is C2–C3. The clinical symptoms include pain in the neck region, stiff gait with an extended neck, head held low, avoidance of head movements, and depending on the degree of spinal cord compression, tetraparesis to tetraplegia. Localisation and type of disc protrusion / extrusion determine the clinical symptoms. Ventral midline disc protrusion, often accompanied by a reactive thickening of the dorsal longitudinal ligament, often results in isolated, acute or intermittent pain in the neck. Dorsolateral extrusion of disc material toward the nerve root causes compression and ischemia. The nerve roots C6–T2 supply the brachial plexus of the forelimbs and a compression of these roots can lead to marked neuropathic pain and monoparesis. A dorsal midline extrusion of disc material compresses the spinal cord and can lead to tetraparesis or rarely tetraplegia. The clinical tentative diagnosis of a cervical spinal cord compression must be confirmed and precisely localised using diagnostic imaging methods (radiography, contrast myelography +/− CT, MRI).

Therapy of cervical spinal cord compression depends on the severity of the clinical signs and can either be conservative or surgical. Conservative therapy consists of strict cage rest for 2 to 4 weeks followed by a gradual rehabilitation over the next 3 to 4 weeks (see also Chap. 8). The aim of surgical therapy of cervical spinal cord compression is both decompression of the cord by the removal of the prolapsed disc material, and where appropriate, stabilisation of an unstable cervical spine. The approach to the cervical spine can be ventral, dorsal or dorsolateral depending on the extent and localisation of the spinal cord compression. The techniques for decompression consist of **fenestration** of the intervertebral disc, followed by a partial removal of the neighbouring vertebral body in the form of a **ventral slot**. Fenestration alone is not generally considered adequate as a therapeutic measure for spinal cord compression. It is only indicated as a prophylactic measure for degenerate discs and those at risk of prolapsing so that a prolapse in the direction of the spinal canal can possibly be prevented. Dorsal or dorsolateral decompression is performed via **laminectomy** or **hemilaminectomy** of the spine. Various methods are available for stabilising an unstable cervical spine but this is usually only necessary following a trauma (see Chap. 10.4).

The positioning of the patient for the ventral approach to the cervical spine is dorsal recumbency with a small amount of extension of the cervical spine achieved by supporting it on vacuum cushions or towels. The forelimbs are tied pointing in a caudal position. The approach to the cervical spine is via a midline skin incision starting at the larynx and running caudal to the manubrium. The pairs of sternal muscles (sternohyoideus and sternocephalicus) are separated centrally. The oesophagus and the trachea are displaced towards the left, taking care not to damage the recurrent laryngeal nerve and the right trunks of the carotid artery and the vagal nerve. The structures are held in place with handheld retractors; Weitlaner or Gelpi retractors can be used, but only with extreme caution. The affected intervertebral space is identified using the prominent ventrally directed transverse processes of C6 and the intervertebral space between C1–C2 (atlas / axis). The fascia of the longus colli muscles is incised centrally when the appropriate intervertebral space has been identified, and the ligaments from the vertebral bodies forming the intervertebral space are cut or cauterized and held with Gelpi retractors. **Fenestration** of the intervertebral disc space is done by excising an oblong-shaped hole in the ventral annulus fibrosus with a No. 11 scalpel or an iris knife. Then the nucleus pulposus is removed using a small sharp osseous curette. A central, oblong window (**ventral slot**) is made in the neighbouring vertebral bodies using a pneumatic drill with a rose-headed burr of suitable size mounted on it (Fig. 10.14). The size of the slot should be no more than a third of the width of the vertebral body length to prevent instability or bleeding due to damage of the central venous plexus lying in the vertebral canal. The depth of the drilled slot can be judged according to the layers of the vertebral bone being drilled through (outer cortex, medullary bone, inner cortex), so that sudden penetration into the vertebral canal can be prevented. The last thin layer of the inner cortex before penetration of the vertebral canal is carefully removed with a fine rongeur or a bone punch (Kerrison). The dorsal longitudinal ligament is usually hypertrophic and is carefully picked up using fine ophthalmic forceps and cut with an iris knife.

The prolapsed disc material is carefully removed from the vertebral canal using nerve root hooks or fine curettes until the spinal cord can be seen ventrally and appears to be adequately decompressed (Fig. 10.15). In chronic disc prolapse with massive adhesions of the disc material to the dura, the ventral

10

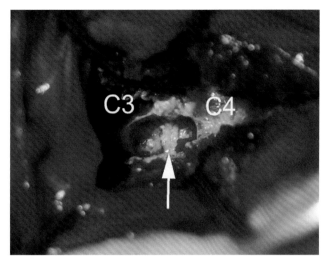

Fig. 10.14
Ventral slot: for the ventral decompression of the cervical spinal cord, a window-like partial removal of the neighbouring vertebrae next to the disc is undertaken (arrow). The size of the slot is $1/3$ of the length of the vertebral body and $1/3$ of its width.

10

venous plexus can be easily damaged leading to excessive bleeding, which can massively hinder the overview of the site and the operation. Such bleeding can be stopped by using ice-cold physiological saline, haemostatic cellulose or gauze. Bone wax can be used if bleeding appears to be originating from the medullary bone. In critical cases, with massive blood loss, a temporary ligature of the external carotid artery has been described; however, this is very rarely necessary. The operation site is closed by re-apposition of the ventral neck muscles, reposition of the trachea and the oesophagus in their normal positions, re-apposition of the sternal musculature and closure of the subcutis and skin. The application of a loose neck bandage with cotton wool padding for a few days prevents the formation of a ventral seroma and slightly immobilises the cervical spine.

The positioning of the patient for a dorsal or dorsolateral approach to the cervical spine is in ventral recumbency with a slight flexion of the cervical spine achieved by placing a vacuum cushion or towels beneath it. The approach to the cervical spine is via a midline skin incision from the occiput to the spinous process of the first thoracic vertebra. The neck muscles are separated through the central raphe down to the nuchal ligament, which starts at the caudal end of the spinous process of C2 (axis) and ends on the spinous process of T1. This band is held to one side and the dissection is continued past it down to the dorsal lamina of the vertebrae. The pairs of epaxial muscles are separated centrally down to the spinous process of the vertebrae. For a **dorsal laminectomy**, the muscles of the vertebrae supporting the affected intervertebral space are dissected free, down to the lateral joint processes on both sides, using a periosteal elevator. For a **dorsal hemi-**

laminectomy, one side of the vertebral body from the spinous process to the joint processes (and including these structures) is dissected free. A dorsal laminectomy involves the removal of the spinous process, the dorsal arch and the lamina of the vertebra down to the lateral joint processes using a pneumatic drill and rongeurs or bone punches. A dorsal laminectomy can be indicated when there are multiple ventral compressions of the spinal cord. Its advantage, when done over a number of vertebrae, is a generous decompression of the spinal cord; its disadvantage is that there is a very limited view of the ventral and lateral spinal cord. The dorsolateral hemilaminectomy involves the removal of the lamina on one side of the spinous process with the removal of the joint processes and a part of the lateral vertebral body wall, the pedicle. Indications for a hemilaminectomy include lateral, ventrolateral or ventral compression of the spinal cord and the nerve roots. After removal of the bony lamina, joint processes and the pedicle with a pneumatic drill and rongeurs or bone punches, the spinal cord and the nerve roots are carefully separated from the epidural fat using dental hooks or fine curettes. The intervertebral artery lying ventral to the foramen must be identified and protected to prevent massive arterial bleeding. The prolapsed disc material is removed carefully to decompress the spinal cord and nerve roots. The wound is closed in layers by re-apposing the separated neck musculature, and suturing the subcutis and the skin. The application of a loose neck bandage with cotton wool padding for a few days prevents the formation of a ventral seroma and slightly immobilises the cervical spine.

Post-operative treatment includes cage rest, and a daily evaluation of the neurological status and the bladder / bowel function. If spontaneous micturition does not occur, the bladder must be emptied manually 3 to 4 times daily until the patient has regained spontaneous emptying of the bladder or it must be catheterised (see Chap. 8.2.1). Physiotherapy and hydrotherapy should be started as soon as the status of the patient allows it. The prognosis is dependent on the preoperative neurological status. The prognosis for a re-attainment of full function is very good if proprioception is present, but with a loss of nociception of more than 24 hours, it is poor.

Spondylomyelopathy of the caudal cervical spine (**Wobbler syndrome**) is a multifactoral disease of the caudal cervical spine and discs, which causes a compression of the spinal cord. It is found in large breeds of dogs and occurs often in middle-aged to older Dobermans and in young Great Danes. The cause is unknown, though factors such as nutrition, trauma and inherited or acquired vertebral malformations can play a role. The pathophysiology is subdivided into five classes depending on the localisation of the compression within the vertebral canal (chronic degenerative disc disease, congenital bony malformation, dorsal displacement of the cranio-dorsal portion of the vertebra in the vertebral canal, hypertrophy of the yellow ligament and "hour-glass" compression of the spinal cord, which is due to dorsal and ventral cord compression by the other four processes).

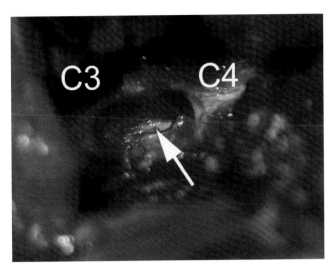

Fig. 10.15a
Ventral slot: after incision and removal of the dorsal longitudinal ligament, the compressive disc material (arrow) can be removed using a sharp curette.

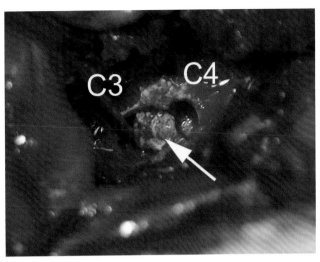

Fig. 10.15b
Ventral slot: the ventral side of the spinal cord (arrow) is visible after complete removal of the prolapsed disc material.

10

Chronic degenerative disc disease due to primary degeneration of the disc (disc protrusion, Hansen type II) or instability of the cervical spine result in ventral compression of the spinal cord as a consequence of hypertrophy of the dorsal longitudinal ligament, collapse of the intervertebral space and protrusion of the disc into the vertebral canal. This is a dynamic compression which is increased by extension (dorsi-flexion) of the neck, and is decreased by a ventral flexion and "stretching" of the dorsal longitudinal ligament. Congenital bony malformation of the vertebral bodies, facets, pedicle or vertebral arches can lead to a narrowing of the spinal canal and compression of the spinal cord. An association with calcium-rich diets and disturbances of endochondral growth (osteochondrosis) has been suggested in young Great Danes. Dorsal displacement of the craniodorsal part of the vertebral body in the vertebral canal (vertebral "tipping") compresses the spinal cord ventrally. Hypertrophy of the yellow ligament and malformation of the vertebral arches compress the spinal cord dorsally. The "hour-glass" compression occurs due to a dorsal, ventral and lateral compression of the spinal cord because of a combination of the aforementioned factors.

The clinical symptoms vary from isolated pain in the neck, to mild gait disturbances in the hindlimbs such as ataxia and paraparesis, to tetraparesis or rarely, tetraplegia. Compression of the nerve roots results in lameness of the forelimbs, muscle atrophy and pain. The diagnosis is confirmed and localised using diagnostic imaging techniques (radiography, contrast myelography, CT, MRI).

Spondylomyelopathy of the caudal cervical spine is a chronic, degenerative disease and conservative therapy with strict control of the patient's movements, the use of a chest harness instead of a collar, and the application of anti-inflammatory and analgesic drugs usually results in a temporary improvement of the clinical symptoms. The aim of surgical therapy is decompression of the spinal cord and stabilisation of the cervical spine. Different surgical techniques have been described. The choice of technique depends on the classification and localisation of the spinal cord compression, the extent of the clinical symptoms, the number of affected vertebrae and intervertebral discs, and the presence of a static or dynamic lesion. The most successful techniques are ventral decompression (ventral slot), ventral distraction-stabilisation, and dorsal decompression (dorsal laminectomy). The **ventral slot** is performed as described previously. The dorsal annulus fibrosus and the hypertrophic dorsal longitudinal ligament are generously resected to the sides, if possible without damaging the ventral venous plexus. Different successful techniques for **ventral distraction-stabilisation** have been described. Stabilisation with positive-threaded Steinmann pins and PMMA is favoured by a number of authors. A ventral slot, with or without penetration of the vertebral canal, is the first step in this technique. Due to the subsequent distraction of the affected intervertebral space, the hypertrophic dorsal longitudinal ligament is "stretched" and so loses its compressive effects on the spinal cord due to the stabilisation of the vertebral body. For the distraction, a Gelpi retractor is placed with a tip in each of the neighbouring vertebral bodies, via a pre-drilled hole and is spread as far as possible (without risk of subluxating the vertebrae).

The space created by the ventral slot is filled with autologous cancellous bone, collected from the proximal humerus, placed on top of a free fat graft. Two positively threaded Steinmann pins (e.g. IMEX, Longview, Texas, USA) with a suitable diameter are used for stabilisation. They are placed in the bodies of the neighbouring vertebrae, by screwing them into the middle of the ventral vertebral body surface at an angle of 30–35° towards the dorsolateral so that two cortical bone layers are potentially incorporated without damage to the spinal cord. The pins are cut approx. 2–3 cm above the bone surface and conjoined with a block of sterile PMMA cement. The heat released during the solidification of the cement block should be transferred away from the site by irrigating with cooled physiological Ringer's solution for 5–10 min. The Gelpi retractors are removed and the surgical site is closed routinely.

An alternative to ventral decompression and distraction stabilisation is a **dorsal laminectomy** performed over a number of vertebral bodies (i.e., C4–C7). The laminectomy is performed as described above, whereby its extent should be adapted to the scope of the decompression needed. If hypertrophic joint facets are present, then these should be removed on their inner side (including the joint capsule) with rongeurs or a bone punch. If stability is no longer ensured, the joint facets can be fixed on both sides using tension screws. The application of a loose neck bandage with cotton wool padding or a softcast bandage prevents the formation of a ventral seroma and slightly immobilises the cervical spine.

Post-operative treatment includes cage rest and a daily evaluation of the neurological status and the bladder / bowel function. If spontaneous micturition does not occur, the bladder must be emptied manually 3 to 4 times daily until the patient has regained spontaneous emptying of the bladder, or it must be catheterised (see Chap. 8.2.1). Physiotherapy and hydrotherapy should be started as soon as the status of the patient allows it. Patients that are unable to walk can be immobilised in ventral recumbency in a suspension rack.

The prognosis of Wobbler syndrome depends on its classification, the extent of the neurological damage, and on the number of affected vertebrae. Patients that are able to stand or walk with a single localisation can attain a success rate of 80%, while those that are not able to walk only have a success rate of 40%, when multiple sites are affected. The most common complications are a continual deterioration of the neurological status, implant failure, and the development of a compressive lesion at a neighbouring intervertebral space (domino effect).

10.3.3 Diseases of the thoracolumbar intervertebral discs

Roughly 66–83% of disc disease affects the thoracolumbar spine; over 50% are localised at T12–T13 or T13–L1, and approx. 75% between T11 and L2. The clinical symptoms can

Table 10.1: Classification of neurological deficits associated with thoracolumbar intervertebral disc disease

Grade	Symptoms, neurological deficits
1	Pain
2	Ataxia, proprioception disturbances, ambulatory paresis
3	Non-ambulatory paresis
4	Paraplegia
5	Paraplegia with urinary retention and overflow incontinence
6	Paraplegia with loss of nociception

be peracute, acute or chronic, and consist of spinal pain, neurological symptoms in the hindlimbs of differing severity and disturbances in micturition. The extent of the neurological disturbances dictates the therapy and the prognosis (Table 10.1).

The neuroanatomical localisation of the compression is done using the presence of intact (T3–L3) or reduced (L4–S3) spinal reflexes in the hindlegs and diagnostic imaging techniques (radiography, contrast myelography, MRI).

The therapy of thoracolumbar spinal cord compression can be conservative or surgical depending on the degree of neurological symptoms. An initial episode of Grade 1 (pain only) or 2 (ataxia, postural reaction deficits or ambulatory paraparesis) neurological dysfunction can be treated conservatively, whereby the success rate can be up to 82%. Animals that have more significant motor deficits (Grade 3 – non-ambulatory paraparesis) attain a success rate of up to 51% when treated surgically and success is considered as return to complete normality. The rate of relapse with conservative treatment can be as high as 50%. If conservative treatment does not help in Grades 1 and 2 or there is a progressive worsening of the symptoms through Grades 3–5 (paraplegia with intact nociception) or 6 (paraplegia with loss of nociception), then surgery is immediately indicated (as long as the loss of nociception has been for less than 24 to 48 hours). With a longer duration of nociception loss, the success rate is lower than 15%. The difficulty lies in being able to determine exactly when the loss in nociception has occurred.

The aim of surgical therapy is decompression of the spinal cord and the removal of the compressive disc material. The techniques for decompression of the thoracolumbar spinal cord include **laminectomy, dorsolateral hemilaminectomy** or lateral **pediculectomy** ("mini" hemilaminectomy). The thoracolumbar fenestration on its own does not have therapeutic effect. Fenestration of the most "at-risk" intervertebral spaces T11–L2 is recommended by some authors as a prophylactic measure for preventing further disc herniation subsequent to a laminectomy or hemilaminectomy; however, the beneficial effects remain controversial. Fenestration can be performed via a dorsolateral, lateral or ventral approach, based upon the amount of disc material that needs to be removed.

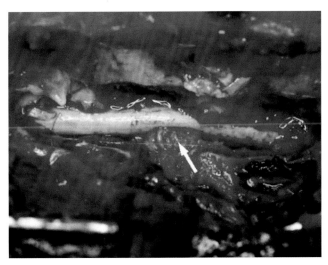

Fig. 10.16

Hemilaminectomy: compression of the spinal cord by prolapsed disc material (arrow) is visible after removal of the joint processes and the wall of the vertebral body.

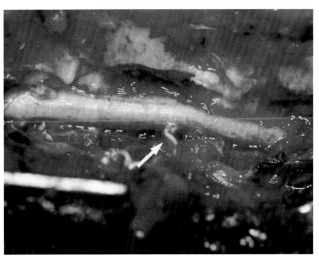

Fig. 10.17

Hemilaminectomy: after removal of the disc material with nerve hooks and curettes, the spinal cord appears to be decompressed and the nerve root is freed (arrow).

10

The positioning of the patient for a dorsal or dorsolateral approach to the thoracolumbar spine is in ventral recumbency with a slight flexion of the spine. For the dorsolateral approach, a slightly slanted positioning with a rotation of the body away from the side to be operated on has proven to be useful. A dorsal laminectomy includes the removal of the spinous process and the dorsal lamina of the affected vertebra down to the lateral joint processes. The incision is made on the midline over the affected vertebrae. The deep fascia around the spinous process is incised and the epaxial muscles are removed on both sides from the spinous processes and the lamina of the vertebral body down to the joint processes. The muscles are then retracted with Gelpis. The spinous processes of the affected vertebrae are removed using a rongeur. The lamina is removed with a pneumatic drill until the inner cortex is reached. The yellow ligament is cut using a No. 11 scalpel blade and the inner cortical layer and the periosteum is carefully removed with rongeurs or a bone punch. The epidural fat is removed with nerve hooks and careful suction until the dorsal surface of the spinal cord lies free. The degree of the dorsal laminectomy relies on the pathology. The standard laminectomy (Funkquist A), down to the joint processes, leaving the facets intact, can be done over a number of intervertebral spaces without causing instability of the vertebral column. The extension of the laminectomy to include the joint processes and part of the pedicle (Funkquist B) can destabilise the spine and should only be done over one intervertebral space. Even with a broad dorsal laminectomy, the approach to the ventral part of the spinal cord and the nerve roots is limited. As a consequence, it is recommended to do a dorsolateral hemilaminectomy when these areas need to be reached. **Dorsolateral hemilaminectomy** consists of the removal of the lamina on one side of the spinous process and the joint processes down to the accessory process. The skin incision is made slightly paramedian on the side of the spinal cord compression. The deep fascia is separated from the spinous process on this side and the epaxial muscles are separated from the lamina and the joint processes down to the accessory process and held with Gelpi retractors. The joint processes are removed with rongeurs. The lamina and the pedicle are removed down to the inner cortical layer with a pneumatic drill. The yellow ligament is cut and the inner cortical layer and periosteum are removed with rongeurs or a bone punch (Fig. 10.16). The compressive disc material is carefully removed from the spinal canal with nerve root hooks and fine curettes, leaving the spinal cord and the nerve roots free (Fig. 10.17). The ventral venous plexus should not be damaged. With chronic disc protrusion or extrusion, adhesions form between the disc material and the venous plexus and the dura, making the atraumatic removal of the material difficult. Bleeding from the venous plexus can be arrested by irrigating with cooled physiological solutions and haemostatic cellulose. The **lateral fenestration** of the intervertebral space via incision of the annulus fibrosus and removal of as much nucleus pulposus material as possible with fine curettes enables the decompression of chronically adhered disc protrusions and prevents a relapse due to further extrusion of disc material after an acute disc extrusion. For a **lateral pediculectomy** ("mini" hemilaminectomy), the joint processes are not removed.

The epaxial muscles are removed down to the transverse processes, and the intervertebral foramen is enlarged in a circular manner using a pneumatic drill and rongeurs whilst protecting the spinal nerves. The foramen is opened ventrally through to the bottom of the vertebral canal. This technique allows a minimally invasive removal of disc material that lies on the floor of the vertebral canal and around the nerve roots. Wound closure in all these techniques includes re-apposition of the epaxial musculature and closure of the deep fascia, subcutis and skin.

Post-operative treatment includes cage rest and a daily evaluation of the neurological status and the bladder / bowel function. If spontaneous micturition does not occur, the bladder must be emptied manually 3 to 4 times daily until the patient has regained spontaneous emptying of the bladder, or it must be catheterised (see Chap. 8.2.1). Physiotherapy and hydrotherapy should be started as soon as the status of the patient allows it.

10.3.4 Diseases of the lumbosacral intervertebral discs

Degenerative lumbosacral stenosis (Cauda equina syndrome) is the most common cause of lumbosacral disease, and it often requires surgical intervention. The cause is a compression of the lumbar, sacral and caudal nerves (cauda equina) and their ganglia by soft tissue and bony structures at L6–L7 and L7–S1, causing stenosis of the vertebral canal. The degenerative changes occur as a consequence of abnormal movement in this area, which include a ventrally displaced sacrum, sclerosis of the lumbosacral endplates, osteophyte formation on the joint facets, hypertrophy of the yellow ligament and protrusion of the dorsal annulus fibrosus. Large dog breeds, and especially the middle-aged males, are predisposed; the German Shepherd is the most commonly affected breed probably due to its anatomical conformation. The clinical symptoms include lumbosacral pain, paresthesia, and paresis of the tail with urinary and faecal incontinence. The diagnosis is confirmed with imaging techniques (radiography, contrast myelography, epidurography, discography, linear tomography, CT, MRI). Conservative therapy can be started in an early phase even when there are no neurological disturbances. Rest in the form of controlled walking on the lead, anti-inflammatory drugs (NSAIDs, steroids) and weight reduction can lead to an improvement in the clinical signs. Continual problems and neurological disturbances are an indication for surgical therapy.

The aim of surgical therapy is decompression of the cauda equina via **dorsal laminectomy**, unilateral or bilateral **facetectomy** or **foramenotomy**. Instability of the lumbosacral spine is treated using **distraction-stabilisation**, as for instability of the cervical spine, which is described above. However, in the lumbosacral spine, the fixation pins and cement are positioned dorsally, rather than ventrally, incorporating L7, S1 and the wings of the ilium.

The positioning of the patient is in sternal recumbency with the hindlimbs placed cranially to flex the intervertebral space L7–S1 and open it dorsally. The skin incision is performed on the midline over the spinous processes of L6–S3. The deep fascia is incised around the spinous processes. The epaxial musculature is removed from both sides of the spinous processes, the laminae and the joint processes of L7–S1 with a periosteal elevator; retraction is necessary with Gelpi retractors. The spinous processes from L7 and S1 are removed using rongeurs. The yellow ligament is excised with a # 11 scalpel. The lamina is removed from L7 and S1 down to the inner cortex using a pneumatic drill (Fig. 10.18). The length of the dorsal laminectomy should measure roughly half of the length of the vertebral body or S1. The width depends on the degree of compression. For a **dorsal laminectomy**, the lamina is removed to the joint processes. For a **foramenotomy**, the inner joint processes are also removed to decompress the nerve ganglia, while for a **facetectomy** all the joint processes are removed and the foramen is opened to completely decompress the nerve ganglia and the spinal nerves. A bilateral foramenotomy does not appear to influence lumbosacral stability, but a bilateral facetectomy requires stabilisation of the lumbosacral spine. With careful handheld retraction of the nerves of the cauda equina to one side, the dorsal annulus fibrosus ring is revealed. A window is cut in the annulus fibrosus with an iris scalpel and the disc material is removed with a fine curette (Fig. 10.19). If the lumbosacral spine is unstable then it should be stabilised (pin / PMMA, internal fixation, external fixation, transilial pins, etc.; see Chap. 10.4). Wound closure is performed by re-apposing the epaxial musculature and closure of the deep fascia, subcutis and skin.

Postoperative rest is necessary for 1 to 2 months after decompression and 2 to 3 months after stabilisation. A slow rebuilding of the musculature over a further 2 months is recommended via physiotherapy. Daily evaluation of the neurological status and bladder function is essential. The bladder must be manually emptied 3 to 4 times a day or it must be catheterised until the patient can urinate spontaneously (see Chap. 8.2.1). The prognosis for lumbosacral decompression alone or in combination with distraction fusion is good, and approx. 75% of the cases re-attain their full function again, unless urinary and or faecal incontinence has been present prior to surgery for over 6 weeks.

10.3.5 Tumours of the vertebral body, spinal cord and nerve roots

Tumours of the spine can arise from the spinal cord or the surrounding tissues. They are classified as primary tumours or metastatic tumours and can be located in the spinal cord, nerve roots, in the soft tissues or bone structures surrounding the spinal cord.

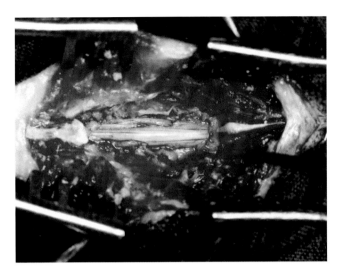

Fig. 10.18
Dorsal laminectomy: the vertebral arch is removed to the joint processes and the cauda equina is exposed.

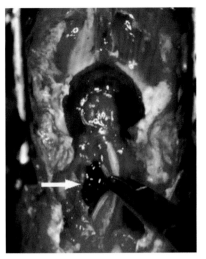

Fig. 10.19
Dorsal laminectomy: the prolapsed disc material with haemorrhage (arrow) can be seen after the cauda equina has been carefully displaced to one side.

Another classification refers to the location relative to the dura mater and is divided into extradural, intradural-extramedullary and intramedullary. About 40–50% of the spinal tumours are extradural and originate from the vertebral bones (e.g. osteosarcoma, chondrosarcoma, fibrosarcoma, multiple cartilaginous exostoses, multiple myeloma) or in the paraspinal soft tissues (e.g. lymphosarcomas, haemangiosarcomas, undifferentiated sarcoma). Roughly 35% of the tumours are found in an intradural-extramedullary location and arise from the meninges or the nerve roots (meningioma, schwannoma, neurofibroma, neurofibrosarcoma). Intramedullary tumours tend to be rather rare (15%) and they originate from glial cells (e.g. astrocytoma, ependymoma). The clinical symptoms are dependent on the localisation of the tumour, the degree of spinal cord compression, the tumour's growth rate and any secondary effects arising from the tumour. The localisation and the extent of the tumour are depicted using imaging techniques (radiography, contrast myelography, CT, MRI).

Drug therapy is aimed directly against the tumour's secondary effects rather than the tumour itself. At the fore of such therapies are corticosteroids (methylprednisolone sodium succinate) for the reduction of peritumoural oedema. The surgical visualisation of the tumour and, depending on its size and borders, the removal of an incisional or excisional biopsy is necessary for histological determination of tumour type and the planning of adjunct therapy.

The aims of surgery are to expose the tumour, resect as much as possible, decompress the spinal cord and nerve roots and if necessary, stabilise the spine. If complete resection of the tumour is not possible, the surgery is limited to biopsy and decompression. The surgical techniques used include **dorsal**

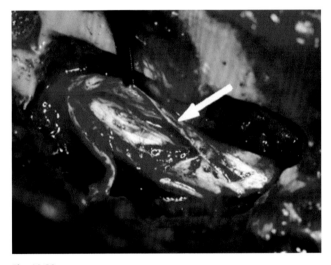

Fig. 10.20
Durotomy: the dura (arrow) is incised longitudinally enabling the assessment of the spinal cord with subdural discolouration and for the presentation and removal of intramedullary tumours.

laminectomy or **dorsolateral hemilaminectomy** with **facetectomy** or **foramenotomy**. The visualisation and excision of an intramedullary tumour requires a **durotomy** (Fig. 10.20). Stabilisation of the spine is necessary depending on the amount of vertebral tissue that has to be resected.

The stabilisation techniques are no different from the ones used for spinal fractures or luxations (K-wires +/− tension screws in the joint processes, Steinmann pins and PMMA, etc.).

The postoperative treatment is similar to that for other types of spinal surgery. Adjunct therapy is performed depending on the definitive diagnosis (radiotherapy, chemotherapy, immunotherapy). The prognosis depends on the localisation of the tumour, its extent and type, as well as the effects of the adjunct therapy. In general, malignant extradural tumours tend to have an unfavourable prognosis, while benign extradural tumours have a more favourable one. Malignant and benign intramedullary tumours have an unfavourable to poor prognosis, and intradural-extramedullary ones should be assessed with a guarded to unfavourable prognosis.

Literature

1 ANDERSON, S.M., LIPPINCOTT, C.L., GILL, P.J. (1991): Hemilaminectomy in Dogs without Deep Pain Perception. A Retrospective Study of 32 Cases. Calif Vet. **45**: 24–28.

2 BAGLEY, R.S., TUCKER, R., HARRINGTON, M.L. (1996): Lateral and foraminal disk extrusion in dogs. Comp Cont Educ Pract Vet. **18**:795–805.

3 BOJRAB, M.J. (1998): Current Techniques in Small Animal Surgery, 4th ed. Williams & Wilkins, Baltimore, pp. 793–864.

4 BRUECKER, K.A., SEIM, H.B., BLASS, C.E. (1989): Caudal cervical spondylomyelopathy: decompression by linear traction and stabilization with Steinmann pins and polymethylmetacrylate. J Am Anim Hosp Assoc. **25**: 677.

5 CHAMBERS, J.N., OLIVER, J.E., BJORLING, D.E. (1986): Update on ventral decompression for caudal cervical disk herniation in Dobermann Pinschers. J Am Anim Hosp Assoc. **22**: 775–778.

6 COATES, J.R. (2000): Intervertebral Disk Disease. Vet Clin North Am Small Anim Pract. **30**: 77–110.

7 DANIELSSON, F., SJOSTROM, L. (1999): Surgical treatment of degenerative lumbosacral stenosis in dogs. Vet Surg. **28**: 91.

8 DE RISIO, L., THOMAS, W.B., SHARP, N.J.H. (2000): Degenerative lumbosacral stenosis. Vet Clin North Am Small Anim Pract. **30**: 111–132.

9 DERNELL, W.S., VANVECHTEN, B.J., STRAW, R.C., LARUE, S.M., POWERS, B.E., WITHROW, S.J. (2000): Outcome following treatment of vertebral tumors in 20 dogs (1986–1995). J Am Anim Hosp Assoc. **36**: 245–253.

10 DHUPA, S., GLICKMAN, N., WATERS, D.J. (1999): Reoperative neurosurgery in dogs with thoracolumbar disk disease. Vet Surg. **28**: 421.

11 FOSSUM, T.W. (2002): Small Animal Surgery, 2nd ed. Mosby, St. Louis.

12 FITCH, R.B., KERWIN, S.C., HOSGOOD, G. (2000): Caudal cervical intervertebral disk disease in the small dog: Role of distraction and stabilisation in ventral slot decompression. J Am Anim Hosp Assoc. **36**: 68–74.

13 FRY, T.R., JOHNSON, A.L., HUNGERFORD, L. (1991): Surgical treatment of cervical disc herniations in ambulatory dogs. Ventral decompression vs. fenestration, 111 Cases (1980–1988). PVN **2**: 165–173.

14 GILL, P.J., LIPPINCOTT, C.L., ANDERSON, S.M. (1996): Dorsal laminectomy in the treatment of cervical intervertebral disc disease in small dogs: A retrospective study of 30 Cases. J Am Anim Hosp Assoc. **32**: 77–80.

15 JEFFERY, N.D. (1988): Treatment of acute and chronic thoracolumbar disc disease by mini-hemilaminectomy. J Small Anim Pract. **29**: 611–616.

16 LEVY, M.S., (1997): Spinal tumors in 37 Dogs: clinical outcome and longterm survival (1987–1994). J Am Anim Assoc. **33**: 307–314.

17 LIPSITZ, D., BAILEY, C.S. (1992): Lateral approach for cervical spinal cord decompression. Prog. Vet Neurol. **3**: 39–44.

18 LUBBE, A.M., KIRBERGER, R.M., VERSTRAETE, F.J.M. (1994): Pediculectomy for thoracolumbal spinal decompression in the Dachshund. J Am Anim Hosp Assoc. **30**: 233–238.

19 LYMAN, R. (1991): Wobbler Syndrome: Continuous dorsal laminectomy is the procedure of choice. Prog Vet Neurol. **2**: 143–151.

20 McKEE, W.M. (1992): A comparison of hemilaminectomy (with concomitant disc fenestration) and dorsal laminectomy for the treatment of thoracolumbar disc protrusion in dogs. Vet Rec. **130**: 296–300.

21 MUIR, P., JOHNSON, K.A., MANLEY, P.A. (1995): Comparison of hemilaminectomy and dorsal laminectomy for thoracolumbar intervertebral disc extrusion in Dachshunds. J Small Anim Pract. **36**: 360–367.

22 NESS, M.G. (1994): Degenerative lumbosacral stenosis in the dog: A review of 30 Cases: J Small Anim Pract **35**: 185–189.

23 TOOMBS, J.P. (1992): Cervical intervertebral disc disease in dogs. Comp Cont Educ Pract Vet. **14**: 1477–1402.

24 WHEELER, S.J., SHARP, N.J.H. (1994): Small animal spinal disorders. Mosby, St. Louis.

25 WILSON, E.R., ARON, D.N., ROBERTS, R.E. (1994): Observation of a secondary compressive lesion after treatment of caudal cervical spondylomyelopathy in a dog. J Am Vet Med Assoc. **205**: 1297–1299.

26 YOVICH, J.C., READ, R., EGER, C. (1994): Modified lateral spinal decompression in 61 dogs with thoracolumbar disc protrusion. J Small Anim Pract. **35**: 351–356.

10

10.4 Spinal fractures / luxations

Hugo Schmökel

Car accidents, falls and collisions between two animals during play or fights can lead to fractures or luxations of the spine (2, 4). A large majority of animals suffer a polytrauma with other fractures and injuries of the inner organs and the long bones and skull (4). A thorough initial examination and stabilisation of the respiration and circulation are, therefore, indispensable. If there is a suspicion of a lesion of the spine, the patient should be moved as little as possible (this is also important during transport; a flat board is advantageous). A neurological examination (see Chap. 1) should be done immediately in order to be able to assess the progression of disease. The mental state of the patient should be noted but it should be remembered that the presence of shock can severely influence the neurological results. A second examination after stabilisation of the respiration and circulation is necessary in such cases.

10.4.1 Emergency measures

Spinal luxations / fractures should always be considered as emergencies as time plays an important role in the prognosis (Figs. 10.21–10.23).

Imaging techniques are usually used after the initial examination and treatment of the patient to ascertain the definitive diagnosis. It should be noted that when the spinal column is unstable, the muscles will reflexively keep it "fixed". Therefore, with suspicion of a spinal injury, the patient should be sedated / anaesthetised in a place where any further treatment (i.e. surgery) is to be undertaken, to minimize vertebral movement when the muscles are relaxed. If this is not possible, then the patient must be transferred unsedated and secured to a flat carrying surface (with appropriate analgesia). In addition, sedation / anaesthesia leads to a drop in blood pressure which can exacerbate spinal cord ischaemia if this is present.

10.4.1.1 Primary and secondary damage to nervous tissue

Neuropathology classifies direct, primary damage of nerve tissue as being due to mechanical insult. Subsequently, there are changes at the cellular level which can then lead to further damage of the nervous tissues.

Primary trauma to nervous tissue causes changes in the local blood supply of the spinal cord, which leads to ischemia, oedema and the further destruction of nerve cells (3). As a consequence, the restoration and maintenance of normal peripheral blood pressure is extremely important (2).

Due to these local changes, chemicals are released (neurotransmitters, catecholamines and free radicals) which damage the nervous tissues even more (membranous lipid peroxidation). Changes in the ion concentrations within the nerve cells (especially calcium influx) can cause death of these cells (3, 5).

This chain reaction (secondary injury mechanisms) can damage the nervous tissue more than the original injury itself (2). An attempt should, therefore, be made to prevent any further mechanical injury to the spinal cord and lipid peroxidation should be inhibited by the restoration of adequate cord perfusion and possibly with the application of corticosteroids. Clinical data from human medicine and experimental studies have shown that only methylprednisolone sodium succinate (Solu-Medrol®, Upjohn) in high dosages has an inhibitory effect on the free radicals responsible for lipid peroxidation. However, the magnitude of its benefit when weighed against the risks have given rise to major controversy. In addition, the treatment should be started within the first eight hours after the trauma or else it may actually be detrimental. The recommended dosage is 30 mg/kg slowly over 5–10 mins IV, followed by 15 mg/kg slowly IV after 2 and 6 hours (2, 3).

The prognosis of the patient depends on the severity of both the polytrauma and the neurological deficits. As long as nociception is still present, a guarded to fair prognosis can be given if treatment is provided immediately; it should be noted that the further treatment of paretic / paralysed cats and small dogs is easier than in heavier animals. About 50% of dogs with a lack of nociception after disc herniation recover voluntary movement and urinary continence when they are surgically decompressed within 48 hours (1). This percentage is less after a trauma and when nociception has been absent for more than 48 hours, the prognosis for functional healing (i.e. ability to walk and voluntary micturition and defaecation) is very poor (2).

10.4.1.2 Diagnostic work-up

Fractures, luxations and subluxations occur mainly in the atlantoaxial, cervicothoracic, thoracolumbar and lumbosacral regions.

The forces which occur during trauma include bending, torsion and compression. Different lesion patterns occur depending on the main type of force applied to the vertebrae.

The first radiographs in a traumatised patient are performed in lateral recumbency without sedation / anaesthesia (including thorax and abdomen because of other possible injuries).

Depending on these images and the neurological status of the patient, it can often be decided whether or not the patient may be treated conservatively. It should be noted that an animal may suffer more than one spinal fracture (2, 4), and so, even when localisation of the trauma based on the neurologi-

10

10

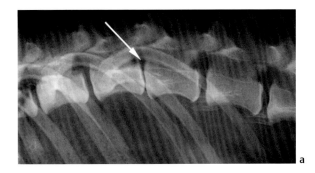

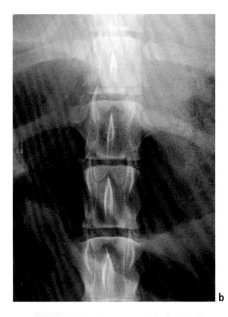

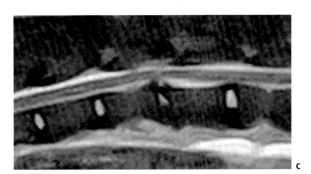

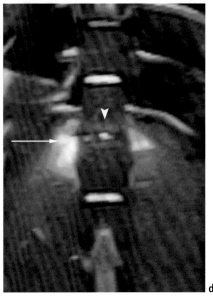

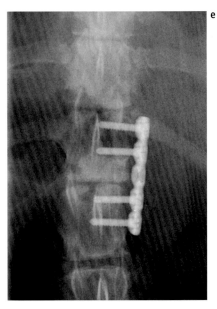

Fig. 10.21a–e
Five-year-old Border Collie with paraparesis after being kicked by a horse. (a) On the lateral radiograph, it can be seen that the intervertebral space T13–L1 is collapsed (white arrow) and L1 is subluxated ventrally.
(b) The intervertebral space between T13 and L1 is only slightly narrower than normal on the dorsoventral radiograph.
(c) In the sagittal T2w MRI sequence, the intervertebral space T13–L1 is narrowed and the intervertebral disc has an inhomogeneous signal intensity. L1 shows a slight displacement ventrally. The vertebral disc material has prolapsed dorsally and is touching the spinal cord, which has an increased signal intensity. There is an increased signal intensity in the areas dorsal and ventral to the spine.
(d) In the dorsal STIR MRI sequence extensive soft-tissue trauma can be seen surrounding the lesion (white arrow). The intervertebral disc and the neighboring endplates exhibit an inhomogeneously increased signal intensity (white arrowhead).
(e) On the postoperative radiograph, the internal fixation with a Unilock plate placed between T13–L1 can be seen with a minimal lateral subluxation. (Figure: Johann Lang, Bern, Switzerland)

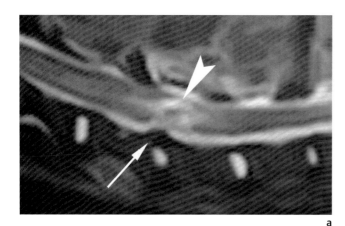

a

Fig. 10.22a–c
Tetraplegic four-year-old Yorkshire Terrier three weeks after a bite wound with a vertebral fracture at the level of C6 and an intramedullary lesion indicating a spinal cord injury with hemorrhage. (a) In the sagittal T2w MRI sequence, the nucleus pulposus of the intervertebral disc C6–C7 is reduced in size and it protrudes slightly dorsally, though apparently without causing any compression to the spinal cord (white arrow). However, the spinal cord appears to be swollen and has an inhomogeneously increased signal intensity (white arrowhead).
(b) In the transverse T1w sequence, the spinal cord lesion appears to be isointense to slightly hyperintense. It has not taken up any contrast (white arrow).
(c) The central area of the spinal cord has a severe increase in signal intensity in the T2* sequence (white arrowhead). The fracture of the right vertebral arch can be clearly seen (white arrow). (Figure: Johann Lang, Bern, Switzerland)

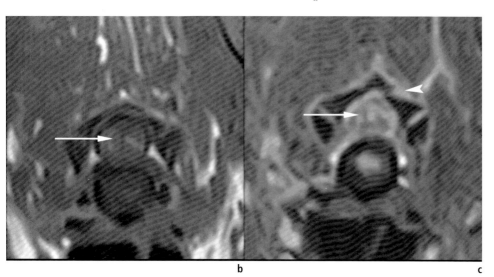

b   c

10

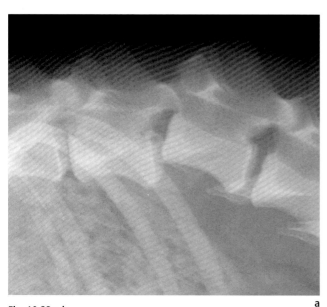

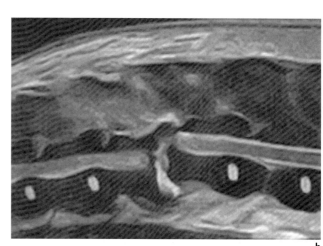

a   b

Fig. 10.23a, b
Four-year-old Bernese Mountain Dog with paraplegia after an accident. A lateral thoracolumbar spinal radiograph confirms dorsal luxation of the cranial aspect of the L2 vertebral body in relation to L1. In the sagittal T2w MRI sequence, the whole of L2 has been pushed dorsally so that the floor of the vertebral foramen of L2 is in contact with the roof of the vertebral foramen of L1. The spinal cord has been completely severed over the luxation. (Figure: Johann Lang, Bern, Switzerland)

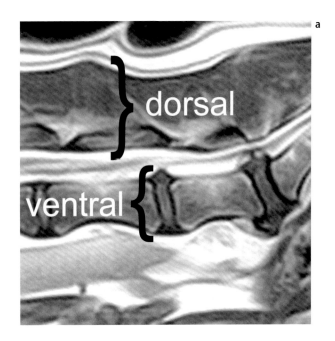

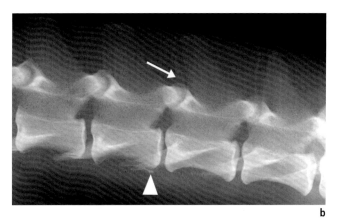

Fig. 10.24a, b
(a) The division of the spinal column into dorsal and ventral compartments. (b) Unstable spine: dog with an unusual longitudinal fracture of two spinous processes and an avulsion fracture ventral to the body of L4 (represents the insertion of the ventral longitudinal ligament); therefore, both the dorsal (spinous process; arrow) and ventral (vertebral body; arrowhead) compartments are involved.

10

cal examination fits with the localisation seen on the radiographs, a search should be made for other injuries.

The radiographic signs of a spinal injury include abnormal vertebral conformation and size, and an increased (compression fracture) or decreased (loss of a bone fragment) radiodensity. Furthermore, fracture lines, fragments, dorsal or ventral displacement or rotation may be seen. A narrowed or collapsed, wedge-shaped intervertebral space may be an indication of a traumatic disc prolapse.

Hyperflexion of the spine leads to vertebral displacement and the extrusion of the disc dorsally through a tear in the annulus fibrous. Hyperflexion in combination with compression leads to compression fractures of the vertebrae. Hyperextension is rare and leads to fractures of the vertebral joints and possibly to ventral disc extrusion.

A combination of bending and rotation is frequent and leads to luxation / subluxation (and fractures).

When assessing a radiograph, it should be taken into consideration that movement of the individual segments during the trauma may have been much greater than is appreciated on the image; therefore, spinal cord damage can be more severe than expected.

In order to assess its instability, the spinal column can be divided into two or three compartments: a ventral compartment which includes the vertebral body, discs and the ventral and dorsal longitudinal ligaments; and a dorsal compartment which includes the vertebral arch plus the pedicles, the small

vertebral joints and the spinous processes with their associated ligaments (Fig. 10.24). An injury to both compartments infers that the spinal column is unstable.

If conservative therapy is not indicated, then a preoperative myelogram is recommended as prolapsed disc material, haematomas or bone fragments may compress the spinal cord, even after correction of the fracture / luxation, making decompression of the spinal cord necessary. In addition, the presence of intramedullary swelling or extravasation of contrast provides an indication about the severity of the neurological trauma (see Chap. 6.3.2 and Fig. 6.22).

10.4.1.3 Conservative treatment

Not every vertebral fracture / luxation needs an operation for successful therapy. When the indications are correctly identified, the prognosis with conservative therapy may be equal to that of an operation (4, 7). Making a correct decision, however, is not always easy. In general, an ambulatory animal with no (or only slight) neurological deficits should be treated conservatively as an operation can lead to further trauma to the nervous tissues due to the anaesthesia and potential vertebral column manipulations; for example, cardiac arrest due to manipulation of the cervical spine is described as a possible complication during surgery (4). If the neurological status deteriorates during conservative therapy, then a myelogram and operation are indicated.

Radiologically visible displacement of the vertebrae or the presence of changes in the dorsal and ventral areas of the affected vertebrae (see Figs. 10.24b, 10.26a) all indicate the

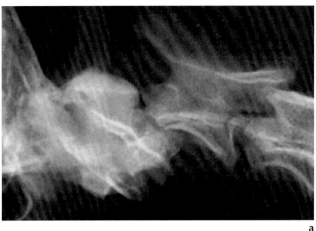
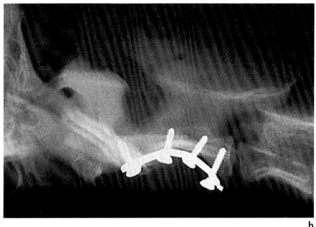

a

b

Fig. 10.25a, b
(a) Dog with a fracture of the vertebral body of C2 with avulsion of the dens. Dorsal dislocation of C2 with narrowing of the vertebral canal. (b) The fracture / luxation underwent open reduction and fixation with a ventral plate. Follow-up radiograph 6 weeks postoperatively: the fracture has been bridged by bone. (Fig. Johann Lang, Bern.)

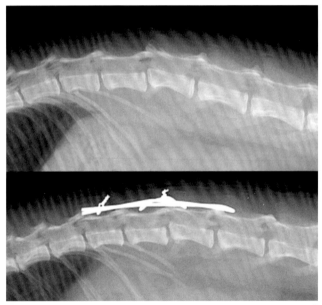
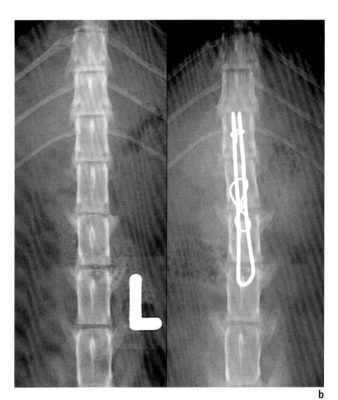

10

a

b

Fig. 10.26a, b
Thoracolumbar region in a cat with an unstable spine. (a,b) Lateral and ventrodorsal views, both pre- and postoperatively. L2 is subluxated dorsally to the right. Slight narrowing of the vertebral canal and intervertebral space L1–L2 is seen. Fixation by dorsal stapling has been undertaken.

presence of instability that is best treated surgically. If there is narrowing of the intervertebral space, compression of the spinal cord must be excluded by myelography before conservative therapy can be initiated.

Splinting of the spine can be a useful method of supporting the affected column especially in the neck region. Not every animal will tolerate such devices (especially cats) which may lead to the animal moving around more. Absolute cage rest for at least 3 weeks and the daily monitoring of micturition, defaecation and neurological status lead to good results in approx. 90% of the conservatively treated cases (4, 7).

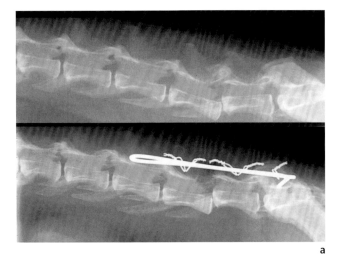

a

10.4.1.4 Surgical treatment

In the literature, there are many techniques for the stabilisation of a vertebral fracture / luxation. While the choice of operative techniques often reflects the education and the personal preferences of the surgeon, some general points can be adhered to. Fractures / luxations in the transitional areas of the cranio-cervical (approx. 70% of the cervical vertebral fractures affect C1 and C2), thoracolumbar and lumbosacral spine are particularly affected by large mechanical forces, so that an implant with high tensile strength is required. The thoracic vertebrae are, in comparison, stabilised by the rib musculature, which is lacking in the lumbar region.

Independent of the chosen technique, decompression must be performed if the myelogram indicates that the spinal cord is being compressed. Preferentially, a hemilaminectomy should be undertaken as it destabilises the spinal column less than the other methods.

To prevent further injury to the spinal cord, the damaged vertebrae should be manipulated as little as possible. Only **one** attempt at repositioning should be undertaken; the implant for the definitive or temporary fixation should then be put into position or prepared. Kirschner pins placed through the facet joints after repositioning are used in many cases as a temporary fixation.

A ventral approach is usually chosen when there is injury to the cervical spine (possibly combined with a dorsal approach for decompression). The vertebrae are stabilised with a ventral plate or pins and cement (Fig. 10.25) (9).

Dorsal stapling (tension band) has proven to be valuable in injuries of the thoracic vertebrae in the cats and small dogs (6, 8). This type of fixation is not completely rigid although the vertebrae are maintained in position (Fig. 10.26).

The lumbar spine can also be fixated with a dorsal tension band in the cat (Fig. 10.27). In addition, in cats it is difficult to place pins and plates due to their size.

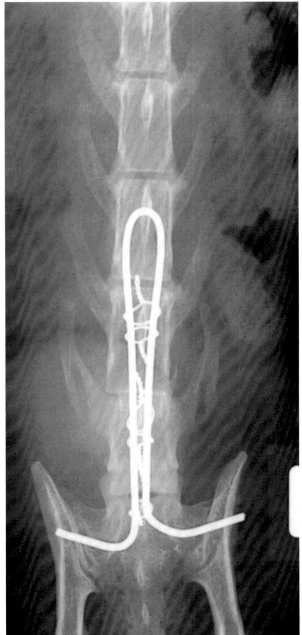

b

Fig. 10.27a, b
Lumbar spine in a cat with a luxation fracture L6–L7. (a) Lateral and (b) ventrodorsal views, both pre- and postoperatively. L7 is luxated dorsally and is rotated slightly around its longitudinal axis. The intervertebral space L6–L7 is collapsed. The caudal joint processes of L6 and its vertebral arch are fractured and displaced dorsally. Fixation and correction of the lordosis using a staple anchored into the wings of the ileum. The caudal joint processes of L6 were removed. (Fig. Johann Lang, Bern.)

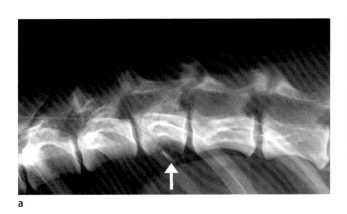

a

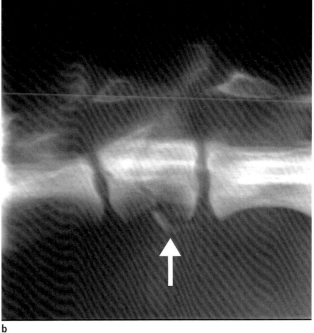

b

10

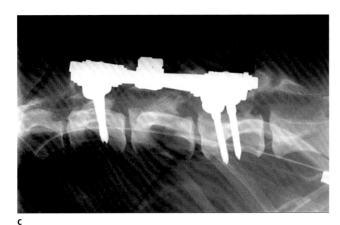

c

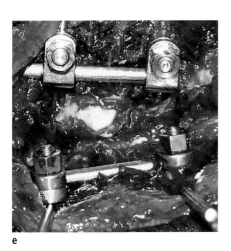

e

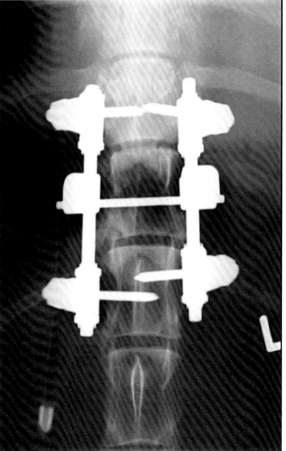

d

Fig. 10.28a–e
(a) Lateral view and (b) a thin slice image of a compression fracture of the body of T12 leading to kyphosis. The fragments (arrows) and fracture lines entering into the vertebral canal are especially obvious on the thin slice image. (c, d) After dorsal laminectomy, fixation was performed using two half pins in the body of T11 and T13. (e) Intraoperative view of the internal fixation device in the spine. (Fig. Johann Lang, Bern.)

The strain on the lumbar spine is so great in the dog that a semi-rigid tension band is often too weak, and so the techniques of choice are fixation with either an internal fixation device (pins with PMMA or metal clips) or an angled plate (Fig. 10.28). The advantages of internal fixation include a greater degree of stability. If metal clips are used to bind the bone pins, then there are no problems with heat production which occur with the use of PMMA (Fig. 10.28c). External fixation can also be used. The advantages of internal fixation include the possibility of postoperative modification and the easy removal of the implants. Its disadvantages lie in the necessary post operative nursing care and the risk that the patient will "tear" out the implant especially when it crawls under objects such as furniture.

Mechanical strain is also high in lumbosacral fractures / luxations in the dog, making internal fixation the method of choice here, too. In cats, such injuries leading to a ventral displacement of the sacrum can be fixed with a transilial pin; this method is not recommended in dogs, even in small ones.

10 Literature

1 ANDERSON, S.M., LIPPINCOTT, C.L., GILL, P.J. (1991): Hemilaminectomy in dogs without deep pain perception. Calif Vet. **45**: 24–32.

2 BAGLEY, R.S. (2001): Spinal fracture or luxation. Vet Clin North Am Small Anim Pract. **30**: 133–153.

3 COUGHLAN, A.R. (1993): Secondary injury mechanisms in acute spinal cord trauma. J Small Anim Pract. **34**: 117–122.

4 HAWTHORNE, J.C., BLEVINS, W.E., WALLACE, L.J., GLICKMAN, N., WATERS, D.J. (1999): Cervical vertebral fractures in 56 dogs: a retrospective study. J Am Anim Hosp Assoc. **35**: 135–145.

5 JEFFREY, N.D., BLAKEMORE, W.F. (1999): Spinal cord injury in small animals. 1. Mechanisms of spontaneous recovery. Vet Rec. **144**: 407–413.

6 KOCH, D.A., MONTAVON, P.M. (1998): Eine chirurgische Methode zur Stabilisation von traumatischen Subluxationen, Luxationen und Frakturen der Brust- und Lendenwirbelsäule bei Hunden und Katzen. Schweiz Arch Tierheilk. **140**: 413–418.

7 SELCER, R.R., BUBB, W.J., WALKER, T.L. (1991): Management of vertebral column fractures in dogs and cats: 211 cases (1977–1985). J Am Vet Med Assoc. **198**: 1965–1968.

8 VOSS, K.; MONTAVON, B.M. (2004): Tension band stabilization of fractures and luxations of the thoracolumbar vertebrae in dogs and cats: 38 cases (1993–2002). Am Vet Med Assoc. **225**: 78–83.

9 VOSS, K., STEFFEN, F., MONTAVON, B.M. (2006): Use of the Compal Unilock system for vetral stabilization produres of the cervical spine: a retrospective study. VLOT. **19**: 21–28.

10.5 Peripheral nerves

Franck Forterre

10.5.1 Principles of peripheral nerve surgery

The extent and localisation of the lesion should be as accurately defined as possible before an operation. After the clinical neurological examination, the diagnostic methods of choice include radiography and myelography (although nerve root / peripheral nerve lesions cannot be identified unless they compress the spinal cord), CT-myelography, MRI, and specifically, evoked EMG testing (electroneurography).

The patient should be in a stable condition for the operation. Nerve injuries which are not caused iatrogenically, due to accidental ligation (i.e., during perineal hernia repair) or "piercing" (following placement of intramedullary surgical wire), are not systemic emergencies and the vital functions of the patient are not usually an issue prior to the operation. The operation is performed under standard inhalation anaesthesia after intravenous induction. The patient is given a single dose of antibiotic (amoxicillin or cephazolin) as a prophylaxis 20 min. before the start of the operation. A good knowledge of the neuroanatomy and careful manipulation of the nerves are prerequisites for a successful operation (Fig. 10.29). Nerve suturing should be undertaken under a magnifying glass or, even better, under a microscope. The suture material should be 8–0 or 9–0 nonresorbable monofilament. Special instruments such as suture forceps, eye forceps and a pair of microscissors are required (4, 5, 6).

There should be no tension applied to a nerve suture. If this is not possible, then the limb must be immobilised in such a position for 2 to 3 weeks that the sutured nerve can be maintained in relaxation. However, a padded dressing for 5 to 7 days to protect the wound is usually adequate. Apart from surgical therapy, physiotherapy should be initiated after a few days as this is an important adjunct for the success of treatment.

10.5.2 Frequency

The indications for peripheral nerve surgery in veterinary medicine are limited. Diseases of the nerves occur in less than 0.5% of veterinary patients and only 50% of these are potential candidates for surgery. In order of frequency, the indications are transections (**neurotmesis**), followed by tumours and compressions. The radial and sciatic nerves are particularly affected by these pathologies, as is the brachial plexus. Another important indication in neurosurgery is biopsy for

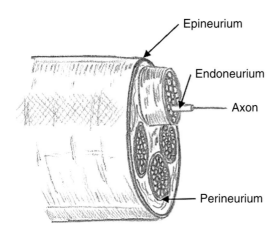

Fig. 10.29
Anatomy of a peripheral nerve.

the diagnosis of metabolic nerve disease (i.e. hypothyroidism). A biopsy is usually taken from the ulnar, median, tibial or fibular (most common site) nerves (7).

10.5.3 Problems

Problems associated with surgery are related to the physiology of nerve healing. Three different types of nerve lesion should be differentiated. In mild lesions (traumatic or iatrogenic), vascularisation disturbances can arise leading to temporary dysfunction of the nerve without anatomical disruption of the axon. This is called **neuropraxia**. Complete function recurs within 6 to 8 weeks. In the second form of nerve injury, **axonotmesis**, axons are structurally disrupted while the continuity of the nerve (myelin sheath) is retained. Functional improvement can be observed within 6 to 8 weeks in most patients. Whether or not complete function of the nerve returns often depends on the severity and localisation of the lesion. If axonotmesis is present, then the patient does not require surgery. If, however, the nerve is completely severed, the third form of nerve injury, **neurotmesis** is present and spontaneous healing is usually not possible as scar tissue can proliferate at the ends of the nerve, which may prohibit regeneration. The section of the nerve distal to the lesion degenerates completely within a week (Wallerian degeneration). The proximal part of the nerve demonstrates retrograde degeneration for an approx. length of three Ranvier's nodes. At this level, the nerve also starts to regenerate, which is due to a reorganisation of the synthesising capabilities of the nerve cells. If the lesion is very proximal (i.e., with nerve root avulsion), then it may lead to death of the nerve and regeneration will not be possible. Regeneration occurs at a speed of approx. 1 mm/day. However, the regeneration potential of the nerve cell is usually exhausted after 4 months. With respect to the prognosis, the distance between the lesion and the target

organ (i.e., muscle) must be considered, as the best chances for functional regeneration exist with distances under 15 cm (2, 3). As nerve injuries tend to lie very proximally (plexus avulsion, iatrogenic sciatic nerve injury, nerve tumours), the distance to the target organ is usually more than 20 cm in medium-to large-sized dogs. Further parameters which influence nerve healing are the mechanism of injury, the time between trauma and surgery, and the age and health status of the patient. Linear resection of nerves has a better prognosis for recovery than blunt injuries which cause a large amount of "crushing" nerve damage. Due to progressive atrophy and fibrosis of the target muscles, surgical treatment should be planned for between the sixth week and the eighth month after the trauma. After this time, neurotisation will be unsuccessful due to the poor state of the muscles. Young healthy patients have a quicker and more complete regeneration of an injured nerve than adult animals.

10.5.4 Techniques

10.5.4.1 Nerve biopsy

Indications
Typical indications for nerve biopsy include polyneuropathy, metabolic nerve disease and tumours without expansive growth (early stage or intraneural) which would be difficult to differentiate from fibrosis. A biopsy should always be taken from the neighbouring muscle at the same time.

With mononeuropathies, the biopsy site is determined by the localisation of the lesion. In polyneuropathies, the more anatomically accessible nerves are chosen (ulnar, median, fibular, tibial).

Method
A nerve can be easily identified due to its lipid sheath and its longitudinal blood vessels. Once the nerve is revealed, it is useful to place some easily visible support beneath it, such as a piece of Penrose drain or the packing from suture material. The epineurium should be incised for a length of approx. 1 cm so that the fascicles can be identified. Fine retention sutures (6–0) are helpful in isolating the nerve segment to be biopsied. The biopsy should be roughly 1 cm long and about a third of the width of the nerve. Resection and dissection are performed with a pair of microscissors. Manipulation of the nerve sample should only be performed by securing the epineurium with atraumatic microforceps. If there is suspicion of a tumour, the edges of the biopsy site should be marked with 8–0 nonresorbable suture material, so that the tumour may be more easily found for resection via a second operation. The sample can be placed in formalin and/or physiological saline and sent overnight to a specialised pathological institute. The surgery site is closed routinely.

10

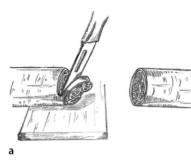
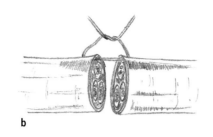
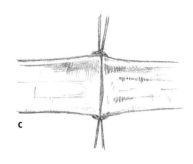
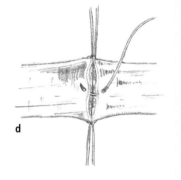
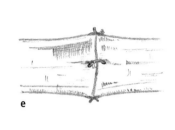

Fig. 10.30a–e
Neurorrhaphy. (a) The nerve end is cut back to healthy tissue using a new scalpel blade on a sterile wooden spatula. (b) The first suture is placed laterally; the ends of the suture are left long to move the nerve atraumatically. (c) A second suture is placed on the contralateral side. (d) Another epineural suture is placed between the first two sutures. Using traction on the long ends of the sutures, the back of the nerve can be brought forward and another suture can be placed here. (e) Four or five sutures are enough for a complete neurorrhaphy.

10

Comments

Nerve biopsies are infrequently performed. This is possibly due to the concern of inducing an iatrogenic loss of function. If the operation is performed correctly, and if the major nerves (radial and sciatic) are not biopsied, then an asymptomatic axonotmesis is all that is usually seen clinically.

10.5.4.2 Neurorrhaphy (Fig. 10.30)

Indications

Neurorrhaphy or nerve anastomosis is only indicated in traumatic or iatrogenic neurotmesis lesions. The most frequent indications are injuries of the radial nerve at the level of the distal third of the humerus or of the sciatic nerve, caudal to the femur.

Method

An extensive operating field should be shaved and sterilely prepared as the nerve ends can retract back for a great distance after a complete resection and subsequent isolation of the nerve "stumps" can be difficult. In the acute stage, haematomas and oedema make identification of the nerve endings difficult; later such difficulties are caused by scar tissue. The proximal and distal nerve segments are freed and mobilised so that a coaptation of the two ends can be performed without any tension. The nerve "stumps" are placed on a sterile wooden spatula and are scarified with a new scalpel until

healthy neural structures can be seen. The heavily oedematous nerve tissue should be excised if the trauma is recent; in the chronic stage, any scar tissue present should be removed. By mobilising the nerve ends, a defect of 2 cm can be bridged without any tension. The course of the vessels parallel to the longitudinal axis of the nerve is important to orientate the re-apposition of the nerve ends. A coloured background makes the job easier under a microscope. The epineurium of both nerve ends is freed of fat for a length of 1–2 mm. The sutures should only include the epineurium. The first two sutures are laid down diametrically opposite to each other and their ends are left long at first so that the nerve can be manipulated or rotated atraumatically. The anastomosis is finished with another two to three sutures. All the suture ends are shortened and the wound is closed routinely (3, 5).

Comments

A good result is not only dependent on the apposition of the nerve ends, but also on the localisation of the lesion. If the lesion is proximal, leaving more than 15 cm to the target muscle, it should be assumed that only a partial return of function is possible. Another limiting factor is that regenerating motor neurons can sometimes "bud" into sensory axons, and so the actual target organ (muscle) is never reached. Maximal potential regeneration of motor function is complete after one year and that of the sensory functions, after two years. The most important adjunctive measure to consider during the healing process is physiotherapy.

10.5.4.3 Neurolysis

Indications
External neurolysis is the first step in every nerve dissection. It consists of the freeing of the nerve from its surrounding fibrous and/or scar tissues. Even though nerve scarring is relatively rare in small animals, it can occur as a consequence of trauma or surgery. This form of nerve damage is, however, very rarely diagnosed.

Methods
Neurolysis can be done using a sharp scalpel (blade No. 15) or preferably bluntly with a small pair of Metzenbaum scissors. An important indication for clinically relevant perineural fibrosis is that the longitudinal nerve blood vessels cannot be clearly seen. After the nerve has been freed, the free segment is enclosed within a piece of narrow Penrose drain and the dissection is continued under slight tension. If there is fibrosis of the epineurium, it should be carefully resected to decompress the underlying nerve tissue. It is recommended that freely prepared nervous tissue should be embedded in a fat transplant to reduce the danger of a relapse. The wound is closed in the usual manner. Care should be taken that the sutures of the deeper layers do not compress the nerves (3).

Comments
Neurolysis is difficult and takes a lot of time. If it is undertaken successfully, improvement occurs within a few days, especially with respect to pain relief. Due to the typically small number of cases, it is difficult to discuss prognosis. Fibrosis secondary to a surgical implant tends to be more suitable for neurolysis than post-traumatic fibrosis, and relapse is more likely to recur with post-traumatic disease.

10.5.4.4 Neurectomy/rhizotomy

Indications
Nerve tumours are the main indication for neurectomy or rhizotomy (removal of a nerve root). If a major nerve is affected in the proximal area (radial, sciatic) or if more than one nerve (brachial plexus) is affected, then neurotisation (transfer of nerves for the restoration of function following injury) should be considered following neurectomy. A rather rare indication for this radical surgery is post-traumatic degeneration-induced fibrosis of a nerve below the elbow and/or knee joint. The resulting pain can lead to a treatment-resistant lameness. A sensory neurectomy can lead to abolition of the pain in these cases.

Methods
Nerve tumours can be palpable as a firm increase in the thickness of a nerve (neurofibroma, schwannoma) or visualized as a diffuse, "speckled" thickening of the nerve (lymphoma). If the tumour is diagnosed in its early stages, then it can often only be detected by careful palpation of the nerve due to its intraneural localisation. After exposure of the tumour, external neurolysis is recommended for a distance of approx. 3 cm proximal and distal, so that a surgically appropriate margin is ensured. The surgical wound is closed routinely. The proximal end of the resected nerve is marked with a suture, which enables the pathologist to determine in which direction the tumour is still present (proximal or distal), and so the rest of the tumour can be removed more easily during a second operation.

Comments
In many cases, the definitive diagnosis of a nerve tumour is only possible after surgical biopsy of the nerve, which is usually performed relatively late in the disease process. Accordingly, the diameter of the tumour may already be quite large. Peripheral nerve tumours are often very proximal and localised intradural-extramedullary, so that they can only be partially resected and relapse after a mean period of 2 to 9 months. Tumours which lie more distally are better to resect and so are prognostically more favourable. They are, however, very rare.

10.5.4.5 Neurotisation (Fig. 10.31)

Indications
Neurotisation consists of transposing a healthy nerve to the distal segment of a nerve that has been irreversibly damaged/transected proximally. The most frequent indications in veterinary medicine include injuries of the radial and sciatic nerves as well as plexus injuries.

Methods
The distal segment of the damaged nerve is exposed as close to the target organ (muscle) as possible and is dissected free from the surrounding tissues. The donor nerve is also exposed in the same manner and prepared so that a tension-free neurorrhaphy can be done. The donor nerves for brachial plexus reconstruction include the accessory nerve, phrenic nerve and intercostal nerves; those for radial nerve neurotisation include the median and ulnar nerves; the tibial nerve is used for fibular neurotisation and the sural and saphenous nerves can be used for sciatic neurotisation.

The donor nerve and the irreversibly damaged nerve are sectioned and the proximal portion of the donor nerve is anastomosed with the distal portion of the damaged nerve. The method is identical to that of neurorrhaphy. If the diameter of the donor nerve is too small (e.g., neurotisation of the radial nerve), then more than one nerve can be used as a donor (e.g., intercostal nerves). Surgical site closure is in the normal manner (1).

Comments
The principle of neurotisation is based on the plasticity of the nervous system. This means that the function of a nerve is determined by its target organ and is therefore adaptable. For example, after transposition to an extensor muscle, a nerve with flexion function takes on extensor functions. This

10

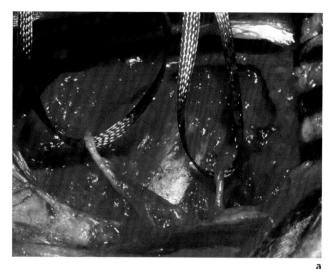
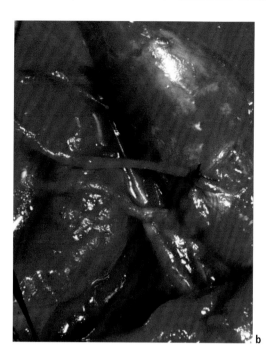

Fig. 10.31a,b
Neurotisation of the triceps muscle with intercostal nerves IC2 and IC3 after a plexus avulsion. (a) Freeing of IC2 and IC3 from the surrounding tissues. A loop of mersilene band is placed around each nerve. (b) Situation after neurotisation of the paralysed radial nerve with IC2 and IC3 at the level where it enters the muscle.

10

change is a process that is accompanied by a reorganisation in the brain, which takes 3 to 6 months. The choice of donor nerves must be well thought over. Donor nerves should be undamaged, lie anatomically in close proximity, have a high proportion of motor fibres and result in no relevant loss in function after transposition. The advantages of this technique include by-passing the physiological problems of nerve healing (especially regeneration distance) and restoration of important muscle function at the minimal cost of the function of the donor nerve. However, the donor nerves must be so chosen that any functional loss resulting from their use can be well compensated for clinically.

10.5.4.6 Nerve transplantation

Indications
The process of nerve healing means that nerve transplantation is rarely indicated. A nerve transplant serves to bridge a deficit of major nerve function (radial nerve, sciatic nerve), after tumour excision, for example, or after severe injury to a nerve. The saphenous and tibial nerves are the most common donor nerves.

Methods
The damaged nerve should firstly be exposed. The extent of the lesion and the length of the defect should be determined. A temporary skin suture is used to close this wound. If necessary the patient is repositioned so that the donor nerve can be exposed. Enough of the donor nerve should be prepared so that a segment 1 cm longer than the deficit can be excised. This wound is then closed surgically. The ends of the trans-

plant and the recipient nerves are "freshened up" and then the transplant is laid in the defect and anastomosed by neurorrhaphy, both proximally and distally. This wound is then also finally closed surgically (3).

Comments
Nerve transplantation is primarily indicated to treat pathologies of proximal nerves. The transplant serves as a biological mechanical splint for the regenerating axons from the proximal nerve segment. This splint has also trophic functions assisting regeneration, i.e. the provision of Schwann cells and the synthesis of nerve growth factors. However, the problem of regeneration distance remains unresolved, therefore the prognosis can only be poor to guarded.

Literature

1 FREY, M., GRUBER, H., HOLLE, J., FREILINGER, G. (1982): An experimental comparison of the different kinds of muscle reinnervation: nerve suture, nerve implantation and muscular neurotisation. Plast Reconstr Surg. 69: 656–667.

2 GORIO, A., MILLESI, H., MINGRINO, S. (1981): Posttraumatic peripheral nerve regeneration. Raven Press, New York.

3 KLINE, D.G., HUDSON, A.R., KIM, D.H. (2001): Atlas of peripheral nerve surgery. W.B. Saunders, Philadelphia.

4 RODKEY, W.G. (1993): Peripheral nerve surgery. In: BOJRAB, M.J. (ed.): Disease mechanisms in small animal surgery. Lea and Febiger, Philadelphia.

5 SEIM, H.B. (2002): Surgery of the peripheral nerves. In: FOSSUM, T.W. (ed.): Small Animal Surgery, 2nd ed. Mosby, St Louis.

6 SWAIM S.F. (1972): Peripheral nerve surgery in the dog. J Am Vet Med Assoc. 161: 904–911.

7 WELCH J.A. (1996): Peripheral nerve injury. Sem Vet Med Surg. 11: 273–284.

10.6 Surgery of the middle and inner ear

Cornelius v. Werthern

Opening the tympanic bulla as a surgical therapy of otitis media / interna is indicated when medical therapy has not resulted in long term success.

Otitis media / interna occurs secondary to extension of otitis externa via a compromised tympanum (which may still appear to be intact) (1). Micro-organisms may also ascend the eustachian tube into the bulla from the pharynx, or less frequently attain access to the bulla via haematogenous dissemination. Another indication for the surgical opening of the bulla is that of nasopharyngeal polyps, which can grow up through the eustachian tube, especially in young cats. An exploratory bulla osteotomy can be indicated as a diagnostic step for otitis media / interna, especially if it is refractory to medical therapy. Prior imaging evidence is usually necessary; ideally CT or MRI examination is advised as there are no radiological changes visible in 25% cases (2). An exploratory bulla osteotomy may also be necessary as a diagnostic step to confirm neoplasia of the middle / inner ear.

10.6.1 Anatomy of the middle and inner ear

Surgery of the tympanic bulla requires a precise knowledge of the regional anatomy in order to prevent complications. The ear consists of three parts: the outer ear (earlobe, vertical and horizontal auditory canals), the middle ear (tympanic cavity, ear drum, auditory ossicles), and the inner ear (cochlea, semi-circular canals and ducts); the latter two parts lie within the tympanic bulla.

The ear drum (tympanum) separates the outer ear from the middle ear. Medioventral to the horizontal auditory canal lies the tympanic bulla. In contrast to the dog, the cat's bulla is separated by the bulla septum into a dorsolateral and a some what larger ventromedial compartment (Fig. 10.32).

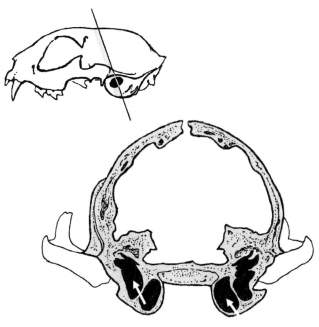

Fig. 10.32
Cross-section through the skull of a cat revealing the dorsolateral and ventromedial compartments of the bullae (arrows).

10

The facial nerve, responsible for facial movements (reflex closing of the eyelids, lip movements), runs ventrally from the area of transition between the external auditory meatus to the horizontal auditory canal. It exits caudally out of the stylomastoid foramen and runs rostroventrally. In chronic otitis, this nerve can frequently become involved in the calcified inflammatory tissue and be subsequently damaged. A preoperative neurological examination is necessary to determine the deficits already present (reduced blink reflex).

The auditory ossicles, the cochlea and the semi-circular canals are situated in the dorsal part of the tympanic bulla. This area must be avoided during an operation. If the infection has already extended to this area, then it may result in hearing loss. Preoperatively, the hearing of the patient should be tested in the presence of the owner. Sympathetic nerve fibres to the eye also run through the tympanic bullae, as does the tympanic chord and branches of the facial and minor petrosal nerves. These sympathetic fibres can be damaged during removal of the dorsal bulla in the cat as they cannot be seen intraoperatively. As a consequence, a post-operative Horner's syndrome (miosis, enophthalamus, ptosis, third eyelid protrusion) can occur, though it is usually transient. Damage to the tympanic chord can lead to keratoconjunctivitis sicca, which requires continual postoperative eye treatment. Excessive curettage over the promonotorium can lead to damage of the minor petrosal nerve and reduction of saliva flow.

10

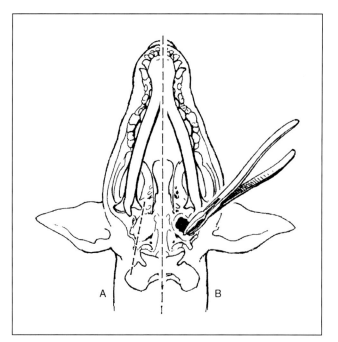

Fig. 10.33
Approach to a ventral bulla osteotomy (A). Ventral osteotomy of the tympanic bulla using a rongeur (B).

10.6.2 Techniques

10.6.2.1 Preoperative preparation and positioning

The surgical area is shaved from the level of mid-mandible along the ventral neck down to the sternum and prepared aseptically. If a complete ablation of the auditory canal has to be done, then the affected side of the face must also be prepared, as well as the inner and outer surfaces of the ear. The auditory canal is cleansed with warmed Ringer's solution and cotton buds. Antiseptic solutions should not be used if there is suspicion of ear drum rupture as they are often neurotoxic.

The patient is placed in dorsal recumbency with cushions placed under the neck. This makes the intraoperative palpation of the bulla easier. To keep the head in one position, the upper jaw is fixed to the operating table with a piece of tape. The forelimbs are extended caudally and tied down.

If a total ablation of the auditory canals is done to treat chronic otitis externa, then this must always be done in combination with a bulla osteomy, as the middle ear is almost always affected too. A bulla osteomy without ablation of the auditory canal is indicated when the disease is definitely restricted to the tympanic bulla (neoplasia, nasopharyngeal polyps). If both operations are done at the same time, the patient must be repositioned by 90 degrees during the operation. If the whole of the operating area is covered by sterile cloths at the beginning of the operation, then the patient can be repositioned sterilely.

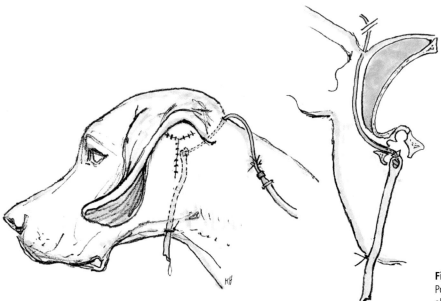

Fig. 10.34
Position of the drainage channels after auditory canal ablation and ventral bulla osteotomy.

10.6.2.2 Operation

A bulla osteotomy can be performed from a ventral or lateral approach. Patients treated with a lateral bulla osteotomy are often deaf postoperatively (3), while hearing ability after the ventral approach usually remains intact (4). The overview of the bulla is better intraoperatively following the ventral approach as is the location of the surgical site for postoperative drainage. The ventral bulla osteotomy is described below.

For the ventral approach, the skin is incised paramedian, from the angular process of the mandible caudally, to the wing of the atlas (Fig. 10.33A). After separation of the subcutaneous fascia, haemostasis is appropriately addressed. Blunt dissection is performed down between the lateral digastricus muscle and the stylohyoideus and hypoglossus muscles. Once the hypoglossal nerve lateral to the hypoglossal muscles has been found, a Gelpi retractor is placed to retract the muscles. The thin muscle lying ventrally over the bulla is incised with a scalpel blade (No. 15). The bulla is cleaned of periosteum ventrally with a elevator. A hole is bored in the bulla with a hand drill and a Steinmann pin (3.0 mm). The hole is then widened with rongeurs until approx. $2/3$ of the ventral bulla has been removed (Fig. 10.33B). A swab should be taken of the bulla contents for bacteriological and mycological culture. If there is suspicion of tumour or polyps, then a tissue sample should be examined histologically. The inner surface of the bulla is completely removed using a fine synovectomy rongeur, though the dorsomedial aspect (inner ear, auditory ossicles) should not be touched.

At the end of the operation, a drainage device is installed (Fig. 10.34). A small, approx. 30-cm-long feeding tube is placed under the skin caudal to the ear via a separate skin incision, with one end in the bulla. The outer end of the tube is knotted and two small holes proximal to the knot are cut into the tube. A Penrose drain is stuck over the end of the feeding tube and they are tied together with a suture so that both holes lie over the join. The distal end of the Penrose drain is removed ventrally out of the wound. Postoperatively, continual irrigation of the drainage system is performed via an infusion pump for at least 3 days. The wounds are covered with a loose neck bandage and an Elizabethan (cone) collar.

A ventral bulla osteotomy in the cat is performed as in the dog. The bulla is relatively large and is easy to palpate. After opening the bulla, the inner septum must be opened separately as nasopharyngeal polyps are mainly found in the dorso-lateral compartment. Care must especially be taken in the dorsal area of the septum as the sympathetic nerves cross the bulla in this region. Damage of these nerves can lead to Horner's syndrome. The dorsomedial part of the tympanic bulla (inner ear) should also be avoided. The wound can be passively drained by attaching a Penrose drain to the periosteum of the bulla with a resorbable suture.

10.6.2.3 Postoperative measures

Patients should remain hospitalised until the drainage has ceased. Animals which have been operated on because of otitis media / interna should be given appropriate antibiotics for 3 weeks. Neurological deficits such as facial nerve damage, Horner's syndrome and head tilt can partially resolve over the following weeks depending on the extent and duration of the damage.

If there is postoperative abscessation or fistula development, it is worth considering a renewed exploration of the bulla. However, a lateral bulla exploration is recommended in such cases for the removal of any remaining abnormal epithelium (5).

10

Literature

1 COLE, L.K., KWOCHKA, K.W., KOWALSKI, R.F. (1998): Microbial flora and antimicrobial susceptibility patterns of isolated pathogens from the horizontal ear canal and the middle ear in dogs with otitis media. J Am Vet Med Assoc. **212**: 534–542.

2 REMIDIOS, A.M., FOWLER, D.J., PHARR, J.W. (1991): A comparsion of radiographic versus surgical diagnosis of otitis media. J Am Anim Hosp Assoc. **27**: 183–192.

3 McANULTY, J.F., HATTEL, A., HARVEY, C.E. (1995): Wound healing and brain stem auditory evoked potentials after experimental total ear canal ablation with lateral tympanic bulla osteotomy in dogs. Vet Surg. **24**: 1–8.

4 McANULTY, J.F., HATTEL, A., HARVEY, C.E. (1995): Wound healing and brain stem auditory evoked potentials after experimental total ear canal ablation with ventral tympanic bulla osteotomy in dogs. Vet Surg. **24**: 9–14.

5 HOLT, D., BROCKMANN, D.J., SYLVESTRE, A.M., SADANAGA, K.K. (1996): Lateral exploration of fistulas developing after total ear canal ablations: 10 cases (1989–1993). J Am Anim Hosp Assoc. **32**: 527–530.

11 Acupuncture

Oliver Glardon

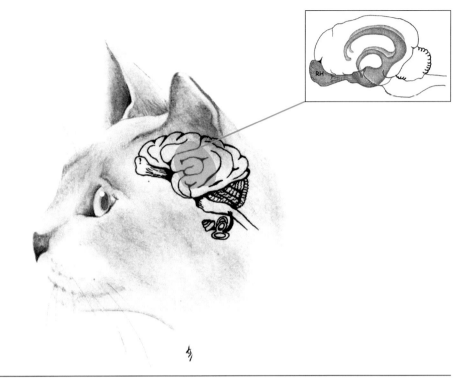

11.1 Introduction

To the outsider, acupuncture (ACP) as an empirical discipline has little to do with the highly technological field of neurology. Despite this, the interest of animal owners in this type of treatment has increased. Also veterinary surgeons feel the need to complement standard therapies in some neurological diseases (see Fig. 11.1). For these reasons, it seems appropriate to describe the **potential and limits** of ACP as a form of conservative therapy in neurological disease or painful processes, and to give some indications for its practical application.

11.1.1 Acupuncture in traditional Chinese medicine (TCM)

Basically, ACP is only a part of TCM. It is one possible method of treatment, which has been developed in this medical field over the ages. It can be defined as a **therapy of "functional" disturbances** by the stimulation of specific sites on the body (acupoints, which are classified into tracts or meridians).

According to Eastern practice, ACP has the following indications:
- Repair of "functional" disturbances
- Treatment of visceral pain
- Fever reduction
- Treatment of certain types of lameness
- Relief of neuromuscular pain.

11.1.2 The acupoints

In ancient Chinese documents, only the main points of stimulation (acupoints) are described in animals without any relationship to the meridians. For this reason, important additional acupoints were extrapolated from human anatomy for use in veterinary acupuncture; these were then either confirmed by clinical investigations or relocated.

No uniform definition of the histological structure of the acupoints or meridians has been achieved as yet. However, at all of these acupoints there are similar structures (neurovascular bundles, sensory receptors, afferent and efferent fibres of the autonomic nervous system, gland tissue, lymph vessels), which are sometimes found in greater numbers at such points relative to other sites within the skin.

In addition, many of the acupoints used in veterinary medicine have **characteristics in common with each other**; these not only allow a precise localisation on the sick animal but also a choice of stimulation type. Depending on the course of disease, signs of pain, swelling or even superficial inflammation are obvious at so-called "diagnostic points" (11). In some cases (but not in all species or points), changes in the skin resistance can be measured during the course of a disease (22).

These reactions are induced by **cutaneovisceral interactions**, which play an important role in the response of the body to the activation of acupoints (8). In part, these points are the same as those which have been known for a long time in Western medicine (Head's or Mackenzie zone, *clavier équin de Roger*), but which have not been used for therapy.

11.1.3 Choice of acupoints

Thanks to detailed investigations, a number of body and ear acupoints are available for both diagnostic and therapeutic purposes in veterinary ACP (4, 25).

In most cases, the body's reactions seem to be based on one or more of the following influences (11, 23, 27):
- Hormone production
- Local or central endorphin release
- Local hypalgesia (gate theory of pain)
- Skeletal muscle relaxation
- Smooth muscle relaxation
- Promotion of blood perfusion
- Local or general immunostimulation.

During the course of ACP therapy, different stimulation points are combined so that the whole spectrum of beneficial influences can be appreciated. The following possibilities or combinations are available:
- Local points
- Points on the meridian
- Points on a paired meridian
- Reactive points (so-called Ashi points)
- Master points (Mu in acute and Shu in chronic problems)
- Connection points between paired meridians
- Points with special effects
- Points along nerves which supply the affected area
- Auricular (ear) points

11.1.4 Activation of the acupoints

It is not only the correct choice of points which plays a major role in ACP treatment, but also the **type of stimulation**. TCM differentiates between different possibilities depending on the condition of the patient, the type of disease or even the weather conditions. Due to a lack of scientific investigation, it is difficult to set clear-cut guidelines for all indications. Despite this, the following types of activation (*inter alia*) are generally accepted for body ACP, which can be used depending on the disease, body region, age or condition of the patient (10, 18):

Simple needling. Bimetal (sterilisable) or disposable needles are inserted manually. The needles are left *in situ* or are continually manipulated with a turning motion.

Therapy: 10 to 20 minutes, three to five sittings at an interval of 3 to 7 days.

Massage or manual treatment of the points. This form replaces using needles at painful points in very young animals or when the treatment is going to be continued by the owner. This gives a weaker stimulation than a needle, but it has an additional effect on the surrounding muscles, which is useful in paresis or paralysis.

Therapy: a few minutes per point, use daily.

Injection of liquids (aquapuncture). Sometimes classical drugs, but mainly vitamin B12 or procaine, are used to cause stimulation of an acupoint. The solution is injected into the point or applied using a Dermojet (percutaneous high pressure injection). Aquapuncture causes a longer stimulation and is simple to use in uncooperative animals.

Therapy: three to five sittings at an interval of 3 to 7 days.

Heat (moxibustion). Lighted *moxa* (mugwort herb) rolls are either put on the needles or close to the skin at hairless sites. This causes a mild warming of the acupoint.

Therapy: as for needling.

Low frequency electrostimulation (electroacupuncture, EAP). In comparison to the transcutaneous electrostimulation (TENS) used in physiotherapy, EAP machines produce a biphasic oblong impulse. Frequencies between 8 and 50 Hz are mainly used, whereby a current of between 1 and 10 mA at 4–5 volts is set according to the reaction of the animal. EAP can be used not only for intra- or postoperative analgesia but also therapeutically in lameness.

Therapy: 10 to 20 minutes during three to five sittings at an interval of 2 to 3 days.

Laser (low level laser therapy). This consists of cold light in the infra red range (600–900 nm) from a gas (He-Ne) or a diode laser (GaAlAs). These types of light have photo-osmotic, photoionic and photoenzymatic effects. For body ACP, either a pulsating light emission (high intensity over a very short time) or a continual sinus radiation is applied. Empirically, a dosage of 4 J (Watt × second) per square centimetre is considered as being optimal for biostimulation.

Therapy: in most cases, dosages of 0.05–2.0 J per acupoint and 1.0–4.0 J per pain point are applied.

11.2 The use of acupuncture in neurological disease

11.2.1 Choice of therapy

As a medical treatment, ACP usage must follow similar rules and quality control as classical Western medical therapy (1). Accordingly, the acutherapist must have undergone a thorough education in this field. In addition, a general and a neurological examination of the patient according to Western principles are the prerequisites for an ACP therapy; only then can an indication for ACP be provided.

It is possible that an ACP treatment according to the principles of TCM can be undertaken without a prior diagnosis and "concrete" indication (a so-called cookery book approach to ACP). This manner of practising ACP limits, however, the efficacy of body ACP. Therefore before every ACP treatment, an examination and evaluation of the patient according to specific TCM criteria should be done (18).

The course of consultation and treatment can be summarised as in Fig. 11.1.

11.2.2 Possible indications for acupuncture

Problem-oriented medical case assessment is part of the standards of clinical work. For this reason, this system will be used here as the basis for determining indications for ACP (Table 11.1) (26). The information for the evaluation of ACP as a possible therapy is based primarily on data from specialist literature or papers, as well as personal experience. The following text should only be used as encouragement to look for further information about specific therapy in the literature (3, 6, 13, 16, 19, 21).

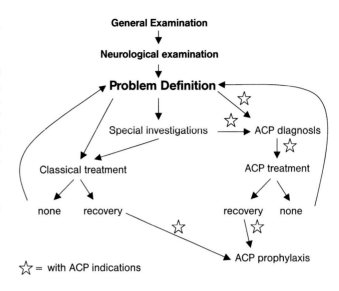

Fig. 11.1
Integration of acupuncture treatment.

11.2.3 Combined treatment

Acupuncture is rarely used as a monotherapy even in TCM. Plant medications are prescribed that complete the treatment in the spirit of TCM. In addition, a series of manual techniques are used which have been built into the Eastern medical system. In Western medicine, these methods include massage, physiotherapy, manual medicine or osteopathy. In this sense, the choice of treatment of neurological problems should not just be focussed on ACP; other therapeutic methods should be used which may then guarantee "healing" or at least an improvement in the status of the patient (14, 29). This is especially true in the postoperative rehabilitation of patients, where the highest aim is to attain a rapid improvement of the patient's condition and quality of life.

11.2.4 Acupuncture as a prophylactic measure

Tradition in China says that the doctor is paid for as long as the patient remains healthy. Without completely adopting this system, ACP provides a good potential for the prevention of relapses in patients with neurological problems. The regulatory influence on the neuromuscular structures and the pain-relieving effects of ACP promote optimal movement and help maintain a correct body or limb posture.

Its direct effects on the metabolism improve the patient's general condition and its quality of life. Acupuncture helps in the prevention of relapses, especially in neuromuscular problems.

11

Table 11.1: Acupuncture indications in common neurological problems

Problem	Possible localisation	ACP indication*	ACP treatment
■ **Gait disturbances**			
Lameness in an individual limb	Limb nerves	2–3	– Needling – EAP
Weakness and ataxia in the hindlimbs, lameness in both limbs	Spinal cord	2–3	– Needling – EAP
	Polyneuropathy	1	– Needling – EAP – Laser
■ **Seizures and convulsions**			
Convulsive partial or generalised seizures (epilepsy)	Cerebrum	1	– Needling – Laser – Ear acupuncture
Muscle twitching	Cerebrum	1–2	– Needling – Laser – Ear acupuncture
Tremors	Cerebrum	1–2	– Needling – Laser – Ear acupuncture
■ **Pain**			
Pain radiating down a limb with lameness / paralysis	Nerves of the affected limb (roots)	1–2	– Needling – Aquapuncture – Laser – Ear acupuncture
Pain in the cervical region, stiff neck	Cervical spinal cord	2–3	– Needling – Aquapuncture – Laser
Back pain, arching of the back, pain when the back is touched	Spinal cord (compressive lesion)	1–2	– Needling – Aquapuncture – Laser
Low back (sacroiliac) pain	Cauda equina	1–2	– Needling – Aquapuncture – Laser

EAP = electro-acupuncture
* 1: weak; 2: good; 3: very good

11.3 Acupunctural analgesia and postoperative pain relief

The use of ACP for surgical analgesia is a modern development in TCM. The discovery of the role of endorphins has promoted intensive research in this area, which has enabled the setting up of good acupoint combination and stimulation protocols (2). The most important aspect is the optimal combination of local acupoints, which can vary according to the operation, and acupoints that have a general or a long-distance effect.

Minor cutaneous operations and major abdominal surgeries have been undertaken in domestic animals using ACP to aid analgesia (7, 17). The animals could immediately eat after the operation, a factor which plays an important role in the recovery time. In small animals, the quality of ACP analgesia is not good enough for it to be used as a sole agent routinely for surgery (5, 15, 24).

The situation in the postoperative period appears to be different, as the effects of ACP do not stop with the removal of the needles but continue for some hours (analgesia) or days (immunosuppression). It is possible, thanks to pre- or intraoperative ACP analgesia, that the patient's well-being and recovery can be positively influenced after the period of intervention (12, 24). This is especially important in animals that are temporarily unable to walk properly or are more susceptible to infection due to abnormalities in their neurological function (bladder paralysis after disc herniation, faecal incontinence). The general immune-stimulating and anti-inflammatory effects of many ACP points play an important role in such situations (23).

Table 11.1: Acupuncture indications for common neurological problems (continued)

Problem	Possible localisation	ACP indication*	ACP treatment
■ **Head region**			
Cranial nerve dysfunction	Cranial nerves	1–2	– Needling – Laser
Head tilt (vestibular syndrome)	Inner / middle ear	1	– Needling – Aquapuncture – Moxibustion – Laser – Ear acupuncture
■ **Trauma**			
Tail paralysis	Sacral spinal cord, cauda equina	1–2	– Needling – EAP
Post-traumatic / postoperative pain	Mono- and polyneuropathies	2–3	– Needling – EAP – Laser
■ **Others**			
Behavioural abnormalities	Cerebrum	1–2	– Needling – Ear acupuncture
Micturition and defaecation abnormalities	Sacral spinal cord, cauda equina	1–2	– Needling – Aquapuncture – Moxibustion – EAP
Self-mutilation of the limbs	Polyneuropathy	1	– Needling – Aquapuncture – Laser
	Cerebrum (behavioural disturbances)	1	– Needling – Aquapuncture – Laser – Ear acupuncture

* 1: weak; 2: good; 3: very good

11

When there is an optimal choice of acupoints, it is possible to induce local pain relief (due to similar mechanisms as in TENS) as well as general analgesia (endorphin release) when the acupoints are stimulated by EAP or laser. Combined with physiotherapeutic manipulations, ACP represents a potent rehabilitation measure, especially when it is started at the beginning of the postoperative period (9).

Literature

1 ANON, P. (1996): Guidelines for alternative and complementary veterinary medicine. JAVMA **209**: 6–12.

2 ANON, P. (1979): AP anaesthesia of domestic animals. Research Group of AP Anaesthesia, Dept. of Animal Husbandry and Vet. Science, Huachung Agricultural College, Wuhan.

3 ALTMAN, S. (1995): Application of acupuncture to neurologic diseases. 20th Congress of the WSAVA, Yokohama.

4 AMBRONN, G. (1989): Die Ohrlokalisationen beim Hund. Der Akupunkturarzt./Aurikulotherapeut **7–8**: 168–172.

5 AUTEFAGE, A. (1975): Recherche de quelques points d'AP chez le chien, application à l'analgésie chirurgicale. Thèse doct. vét. Toulouse.

6 CHAN, W.W. (1996): A review of acupuncture therapy for canine paralysis and lameness. Vet Bulletin **66** (10): 999–1003.

7 CHO, S.W. (1998): Research on bovine electroacupuncture analgesia. 1: Investigation on the effect of dorsal acupoints. Proceedings of the World Buiatrics Congress, Sydney.

8 CRANENBURGH, B. (1987): Schema's Fysiologie. 2. druk. De Tijdstroom, Lochem. Cit in (1990): Segmental organisation of the nervous system and possible routes for cutaneo-visceral interactions, Proccedings of the 16th IVAS Congress, Noordwijk.

9 DEMONTOY, A. (1986): Effet antalgique de l'AP en clinique vétérinaire. Rec Méd Vét. **162**: 1371–1381.

10 FAO (1990): Methods of acupuncture and moxibustion. In: Handbook of Chinese Veterinary Acupuncture and Moxibustion. FAO Regional Office for Asia & the Pacific, Bangkok.

11 GLARDON, O.J. (1980): Effet de l'AP et de l'ACTH sur la sécrétion de cortisol chez le cheval, Diss. med. vet., Berne.

12 GLARDON, O. J. (1999): Etude expérimentale comparée des effets antalgiques de l'acupuncture en postopératoire. Proceedings of the 24th Congress of WSAVA, Lyon.

13 JANSSENS, L.A.A. (2001): Acupuncture for thoracolumbar and cervical disk disease. In: SCHOEN, A. M. (ed.): Veterinary acupuncture: Ancient art to modern medicine, 2nd ed. Mosby Inc., St Louis.

14 KATHMANN, I., DEMIERRE, S., JAGGY, A. (2001): Rehabilitationsmassnahmen in der Kleintierneurologie. Schweiz Arch Tierheilk. **10**: 495–502.

15 KLIDE, A.M., GAYNOR, J.S. (2001): Acupuncture for surgical anaesthesia and postoperative analgesia. In: SCHOEN A. M. (ed.): Veterinary acupuncture: Ancient art to modern medicine. 2nd ed. Mosby Inc., St Louis.

16 KLINE, K.L., CAPLAN, E. R., JOSEPH, R. J. (2001): Acupuncture for neurologic disorders. In: SCHOEN A. M. (ed.): Veterinary acupuncture: Ancient art to modern medicine, 2nd ed. Mosby Inc., St Louis.

17 KOTHBAUER, O. (1975): Kaiserschnitt bei einer Kuh unter AP-Analgesie. Wiener tierärztl Monatsschrift **82**: 10–11.

18 KROPEJ, H. (1977): Propädeutik der chinesischen Akupunktur. Haug Verlag, Heidelberg.

19 LOONEY, A.L (1998): Anaesthesia pain management: Use of acupuncture to treat psychodermatosis in the dog. Canine Pract. **23** (5): 18–20.

20 ROBINSON, N. G. (2001): Acupuncture and manipulative therapy: A perfect marriage. In: SCHOEN A. M. (ed.): Veterinary acupuncture: Ancient art to modern medicine, 2nd ed. Mosby Inc., St Louis.

21 SCHOEN, A. M. (1996): Acupuncture for canine musculoskeletal and neurologic conditions. Proceedings of the 10th North American Veterinary Conference, Orlando.

22 SCHUEPBACH, M. (1985): Thermographische Darstellung erwärmter Punkte und Zonen nach Reizung des Uterus beim Minipig, ihre Koinzidenz mit Orten erniedrigten Hautwiderstandes und der Nachweis ihrer Organbezogenheit durch hysterographische Untersuchungen nach AP. Diss. med. vet., Zürich.

23 STEISS, J. E. (2001): The neurophysiological basis of acupuncture In: SCHOEN, A. M. (ed.): Veterinary acupuncture: Ancient art to modern medicine, 2nd ed. Mosby Inc., St Louis.

24 STILL, J. (1994): Anaesthetic and post-anaesthetic effects of buprenorphine, auricular electroacupuncture and placebo in bitches ovariohysterectomised under halothane anaesthesia. Proccedings of the 19th Congress of WSAVA Durban.

25 STILL, J., KONRAD, J. (1988): Die Aurikulodiagnostik von Erkrankungen des Nerven- und Bewegungsapparates bei Hunden. Der Akupunkturarzt/Aurikulotherapeut **1**: 5–8.

26 VANDEVELDE, M., JAGGY, A., LANG, J. (2000): Einführung in die veterinärmedizinische Neurologie, 2. Auflage. Parey Buchverlag, Berlin.

27 ZOHMANN, A. (1990): Physiologische und pathophysiologische Grundlagen von Ohr-, Körperakupunktur und Neuraltherapie. Prakt Tierarzt **71**: 83–84.

11

12 Stabilization of the Neurological Emergency Patient

Nadja Sigrist
David Spreng

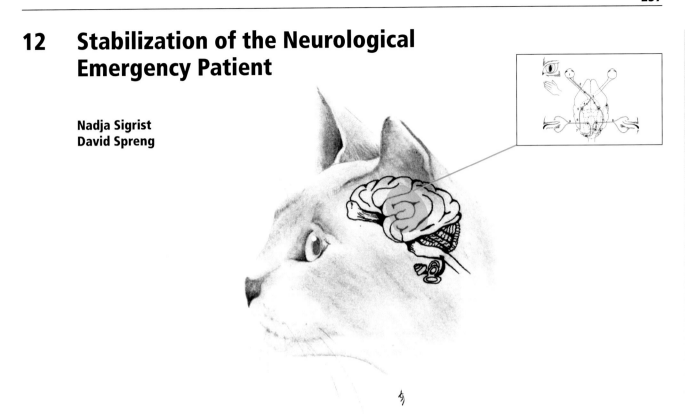

12.1 General aspects

12.1.1 Introduction

Stabilization of the neurological emergency patient follows the ABC principles: if the Airway is patent, Breathing must be ensured, and then the Circulation should be stabilized. This emergency treatment principle is followed by an assessment of the state of consciousness, interpretation and treatment of the level of pain, and the treatment of active hemorrhaging (Table 12.1).

These steps are all undertaken during the initial emergency examination. Only after stabilization is a complete clinical investigation performed, including orthopedic and neurological investigations.

12.1.2 The respiratory tract and artificial respiration

There are many causes of respiratory tract obstruction in the neurological patient: accumulation of vomitus in patients with a reduced level of consciousness or paralysis, traumatic hemorrhage, and laryngeal paralysis are the most common examples. Animals with respiratory tract stenosis exhibit inspiratory dyspnea and usually stridor or stertor. An obstructed respiratory tract is addressed using foreign-body removing forceps with / without swabs. If this is not possible, then a tracheotomy is necessary. Patients with respiratory arrest should be immediately intubated and ventilated after the upper respiratory tract has been cleared.

If the respiratory tract is patent (or has just been made patent), then the patient's respiration, i.e. the ventilation and the oxygenation, should be addressed. The assessment of the frequency and type of respiration as well as the results of auscultation make localization and treatment of respiratory problems possible in the majority of cases (Table 12.2).

Table 12.1: A(irway), **B**(reathing), **C**(irculation) **of the neurological emergency patient**

ABC	Assessment	Additional tests	Initial treatment
Airway	Oral cavity open? Inspiratory dyspnea?	Inspection of mouth	Intubation Tracheotomy
Breathing	Frequency Type Auscultation	SpO$_2$ Blood gas analysis	Oxygen supplementation
Circulation	Heart rate Pulse strength Colour of mucous membranes Capillary refill time	Measure blood pressure	Infusion therapy
Neurological status	Consciousness Pupils – size and reaction Menace reflex Muscle tone	Complete neurological investigation Ocular fundus	
Pain level	Heart rate Signs of pain		Analgesia (short-acting opioids)
Hemorrhage	Arterial vs. venous		Pressure bandage

SpO$_2$ = surface partial pressure of oxygen

12

Table 12.2: Localization; differential diagnosis and therapy of respiratory problems in the neurological emergency patient

Localization	Type of respiration	Auscultation	Differential diagnosis	Therapy
Extrathoracic upper respiratory tract	Inspiratory dyspnea	Stridor/stertor audible without stethoscope	Stenosis of the upper respiratory tract (foreign material, swelling, laryngeal paralysis, tracheal collapse)	O$_2$, intubation/tracheotomy
Intrathoracic upper respiratory tract (trachea, bronchus)	Inspiratory dyspnea	Possibly stridor is audible with stethoscope	Tracheal collapse, tracheal rupture with swelling	O$_2$, intubation
Lower respiratory tract (bronchi, bronchioles)	Expiratory dyspnea	Rhonchus	Lung oedema, asthma	O$_2$, bronchodilators
Lung parenchyma	Mixed dyspnea, superficial respiration	Intensified/moist lung sounds	Contusions, lung oedema (cardiogenic/noncardiogenic)	O$_2$, cardiogenic oedema: furosemide
Pleural space	Inverse respiration	Dampened dorsal/ventral intestinal sounds	Pneumothorax, pleural hemorrhage, diaphragmatic hernia	O$_2$, thoracocentesis
Chest wall	Superficial rapid respiration	Normal	Rib fractures, muscle tearing	O$_2$, analgesia
	Abnormal movements of the chest wall		Muscle paralysis	Artificial respiration

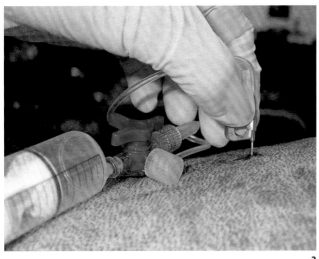 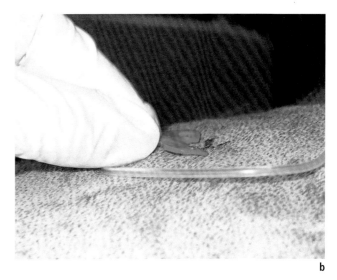

Fig. 12.1a, b
Thoracocentesis using a butterfly catheter. (a) The butterfly catheter is connected to a 20- to 60-ml syringe via a three-way tap. The sterile puncture is performed between the 7th–9th intercostal space vertically to the thoracic wall and under slight aspiration. The needle is judged to be in the intercostal space as soon as air can be sucked up. (b) In order to prevent injury to the lung surface, the needle is held horizontally to the thoracic wall during aspiration (the beveled tip of the needle is directed to the pleural space). As soon as no more air can be aspirated, the needle is removed in this position.

Stress should be avoided at all costs. In animals with respiration difficulties, a thoracocentesis can be helpful both therapeutically and diagnostically (Fig. 12.1). All other patients with dyspnea benefit from rest, oxygen supplementation, and when necessary, analgesia.

Symptomatic therapy consists of oxygen supplementation (Fig. 12.2). Oxygen can initially be given by mask, or flow-by, at a rate of 5–15 l/min. During the subsequent treatment, it is more practical to place a nasal tube or to provide oxygen to the animal using a partially closed Elizabethan collar as an oxygen tent. The oxygen dosage is 100 ml/kg/min for the nasal tube and 200 ml/kg/min for the oxygen collar. Nasal oxygen tubes are contraindicated in patients with cranial trauma and/or brain edema as they can lead to sneezing and so to a detrimental increase in intracranial pressure.

Animals with cyanosis, oxygen saturation < 90% despite oxygen supplementation, hypoventilation (venous or end-expiratory CO_2 > 60 mmHg) or massively increased respiratory effort should be intubated and provided with manual artificial respiration using 100% oxygen. For the anesthetic protocol, anesthetics should be chosen that enable rapid intubation, e.g., propofol or etomidate to effect.

12.1.3 Circulation

Neurological emergency patients can be affected by shock, dehydration, hemorrhage or a combination of these conditions.

12.1.3.1 Shock
Shock can be elicited by a number of causes (hypovolemia, vasodilation, cardiac failure) and leads to a reduction in perfusion, with subsequent hypoxia and the accumulation of toxic metabolites which can lead to cell death. The reduced cardiac output per minute results in an activation of the sympathetic nervous system and a subsequent increase in heart rate and cardiac contractility. If these compensatory mechanisms are inadequate, peripheral vasoconstriction occurs, which is aimed at ensuring the perfusion of the vitally important organs such as the heart, brain and lungs. This occurs at the cost of all the other organs (skin, muscles, gastrointestinal tract, kidneys), which due to the aforementioned vasoconstriction are subjected to reduced perfusion or even no perfusion. This stage is designated as *decompensated* shock.

Clinically, compensated shock is associated with tachycardia, reddened mucous membranes, short capillary refill times (CRT), and a normal to increased blood pressure (Fig. 12.3a). With decompensated shock, tachycardia, pale to washed-out mucous membranes, prolonged CRT, cold extremities, and

12

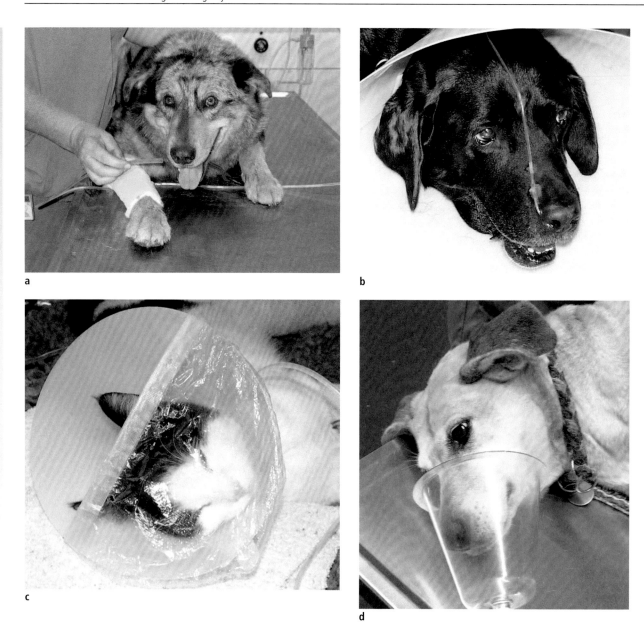

a

b

c

d

Fig. 12.2a–d
Methods of providing oxygen. (a) flow by, (b) nasal tube, (c) oxygen tent, (d) mask.

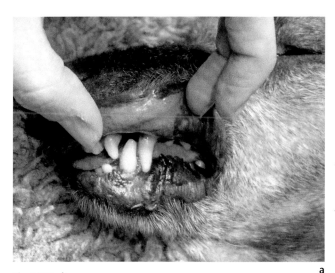
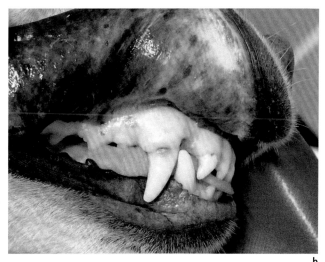

Fig. 12.3a, b
Different stages of shock. (a) Compensated shock with reddened mucous membranes and short capillary refill times. (b) Decompensated shock with pale mucous membranes and prolonged capillary refill times.

reduced consciousness are seen (Fig. 12.3b). The blood pressure can be normal, increased or reduced (Table 12.3).

The treatment of shock consists of oxygen supplementation and the normalization of perfusion. Apart from cardiogenic shock, the latter treatment is undertaken using fluid therapy. The type and amount of fluid infused depends on the basic problem and the degree of fluid deficit. Treatment is aimed at normalizing the intravascular volume. As the amount of infusion fluid required is dependent on the patient and the cause of the shock, fluid boluses are used (Table 12.4). Restoring the intravascular volume during shock should be done quickly. Fluid therapy involves the administration of repeated intravenous boli of 10–20 ml/kg of a crystalloid solution (over 5 to 20 minutes). The patient is re-evaluated after each bolus. Depending on the heart rate, mucous membrane color, and CRT, it can be decided whether another bolus is necessary or not. In this manner, over-infusion with deleterious or even fatal consequences can be prevented. As shock is associated with an intravascular fluid deficit, the most effective fluid therapy consists of a combination of crystalloid (e.g., Lactated Ringer's) and colloid (e.g., Voluven®, Haes®) solutions (Fig. 12.4). Colloids work oncotically and remain longer in the intravascular space, thereby reducing the risk of edema.

Cats are extremely sensitive to over-infusion; perfusion in this species should always be interpreted in connection with the body temperature. Hypothermic cats have pale mucous membranes with a prolonged CRT and so must be warmed before the perfusion can be correctly interpreted. We infuse cats carefully with small boli of combined fluid therapy (5–10 ml/kg crystalloid plus 3–5 ml/kg colloid), while **at the same time** increasing the cat's body temperature.

12

12.1.3.2 Dehydration

Dehydration can be assumed from the anamnesis (inappetence, fever, vomiting, or diarrhea) and the presence of dry mucous membranes, reduced skin turgor, or enophthalmos. The degree of dehydration is judged as % fluid deficit with respect to body weight (Table 12.5). The amount of fluid needed is calculated as follows:

Amount of infusion fluid needed = fluid deficit / 6–12 h + maintenance requirements

The fluid deficit (ml) = % dehydration × kg body weight × 10. This amount is given over 6 to 12 hours. If rehydration is undertaken over 10 hours, then the calculation of the hourly infusion rate is simple: % dehydration × kg body weight. In addition, 2 ml/kg/h is added as the maintenance requirement. In cases where there are other relevant causes of fluid loss (polyuria, vomiting, diarrhea), the estimated additional fluid loss / hour is added to the amount infused.

Dehydration means that there is an interstitial fluid deficit and is, therefore, most effectively treated with isotonic crystalloid solutions (e.g., Lactated Ringer's, 0.9% NaCl).

Table 12.3: Clinical signs of shock

Symptom	Compensated shock	Decompensated shock	Aims of therapy
Heart rate	Tachycardia	Tachycardia	Normal (breed dependent)
Colour of mucous membranes	Reddened	Pale	Pink, moist
Capillary refill time	< 1 s	> 2 s	1–2 s
Pulse	Throbbing	Weak	Strong, regular
Blood pressure	Normal to increased	Normal, increased, reduced	MAP > 60 mmHg
Urine production	Normal	Reduced	> 2 ml/kg/h

MAP = mean arterial blood pressure

Table 12.4: Examples of fluid therapy dosages

Cardiovascular problem	Dosage of isotonic crystalloids	Dosage of colloids
■ Hypovolemic shock		
Compensated	Dog: 10–30 ml/kg bolus** Dog: 15 ml/kg bolus** Cat: 10 ml/kg bolus**	– 5 ml/kg bolus** 5 ml/kg bolus**
Decompensated	Dog: 15–30 ml/kg bolus** Cat: 10 ml/kg bolus**	5 ml/kg bolus** 5 ml/kg bolus
Hemorrhage*	10 ml/kg bolus**	5 ml/kg bolus Whole blood / erythrocyte concentrate as required Dog: Oxyglobin® 5 ml/kg bolus (max. 30 ml/kg)
Additional heart sounds, Head trauma, lung problems	5–15 ml/kg bolus Dog: 5–10 ml/kg bolus**	1–3 ml/kg bolus 5 ml/kg bolus**
■ Coagulopathy	Cat: 3–5 ml/kg bolus** Plasma 8–15 ml/kg over 6 h	2–5 ml/kg bolus
■ Dehydration	% dehydration in ml over 6–24 h plus maintenance 2 ml/kg/h plus other losses/h	

* Aim: systolic blood pressure 100 mmHg, mean blood pressure > 60 mmHg.

** Repeat according to need.

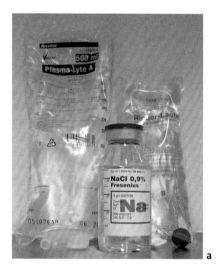 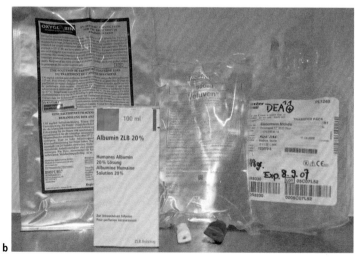

Fig. 12.4a, b
Infusion solutions. (a) Isotonic crystalloid solutions: Plasmalyte®, 0.9% NaCl, Lacteted Ringer's. (b) Colloids: Oxyglobin®, albumin 20%, Voluven®, plasma.

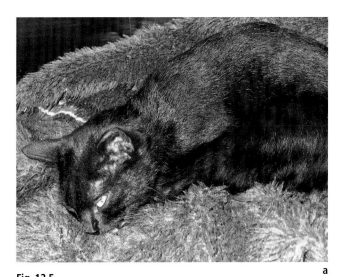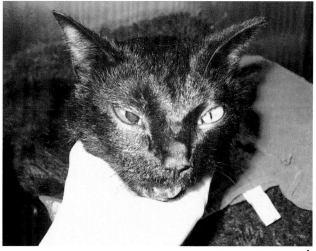

Fig. 12.5
Cat after craniocerebral trauma. The cat shows severe depression (a) as well as anisocoria with mydriasis on the right and miosis on the left (b).

12.1.4 Neurological status

The assessment of consciousness and concurrent neurological status is especially important in emergency patients. However, it can only be correctly assessed after the respiration and circulation have been stabilized. At this time, the animal's responsiveness, reaction and size of its pupils, menace response, and the muscle tone are tested (Fig. 12.5).

Plegic or paralyzed patients with a trauma anamnesis should be very carefully manipulated until vertebral trauma has been excluded. A reduced level of consciousness (stupor or coma) can be an indication of brain edema (see Chap. 12.2).

Muscle spasms lead to a massive increase in cell metabolism, oxygen utilization, and heat production. Oxygen should be substituted, perfusion ensured, and hyperthermic patients cooled (see Chap. 12.3).

Table 12.5: Clinical signs of dehydration

2–4%	Anamnesis of fluid loss (vomiting, anorexia)
5–7%	Dry mucous membranes, normal skin turgor
8–10%	Sticky mucous membranes, slight reduction in skin turgor
> 10%	In addition: sunken eyeballs, skin fold remains standing

12.1.5 Pain

Pain leads to tachycardia, tachypnea, hyper- or hypotension, reduced perfusion, and increased metabolism. Apart from the ethical reasons for giving animals analgesics, the interpretation of cardiovascular problems and tachypnea in patients with pain is difficult or even impossible. Suggestions for the implementation of analgesia are given in Chap. 9.3.

12

Further reading

RUDLOFF, E., KIRBY, R.: Colloid and cristalloid resuscitation. Vet Clin North Am. 2001; 31(6).

MOORE, K.E., MURTAUGH, J.R.: Pathophysiologic characteristics of hypovolemic shock. Vet Clin North Am. 2001; 31(6).

DAY, TK., BATEMAN, S.: Shock syndromes. In: DIBARTOLA S.P. (ed.), Fluid Therapy in Small Animal Practice, 3rd Edition. WB Saunders, Philadelphia, pp. 540–563.

CAMPS-PALAU, M.A., MARKS, S.L., CORNICK, J.L.: Small animal oxygen therapy. Comp Small Anim Pract. 1999; 21(7).

FORD, R.B., MAZZAFERRO, E.M.: Kirk and Bistners's Handbook of Veterinary Procedures and Emergency Treatment, 8th edition. Saunders Elsevier, Philadelphia.

12.2 Stabilization of selected neurological emergencies

12.2.1 Craniocerebral trauma

12.2.1.1 Introduction

Craniocerebral trauma can be caused in small animals by car accidents, by a fall from a great height, or injuries inflicted by other animals or humans. Trauma to the head can lead to primary and secondary lesions of the brain. Primary brain lesions include direct injury of the intracranial structures at the time of the initial trauma. Intracranial haemorrhage leading to a mass compression, direct neuronal and axonal contusion, and tearing injuries with cranial fractures are all possible. In comparison to humans, it appears that epidural and subdural haemorrhages are not so common in dogs and cats. These potentially surgically treatable lesions cannot be recognized without CT or MRI. In addition to the primary brain lesions that can be minimally influenced by the veterinarian, secondary brain lesions can arise due to the subsequent severe perfusion disturbances and metabolic dysregulation associated with such trauma. Such changes can be influenced by adequate treatment. The recognition and early treatment of secondary brain lesions is important and significantly influences the patient's prognosis.

12.2.1.2 Pathophysiology
Secondary traumatic brain lesions

Lesions which develop in addition to the injuries sustained during the initial trauma become apparent within minutes to days after the trauma. These secondary lesions can occur in the originally traumatized tissues or in healthy parts of the brain. Secondary brain lesions are the result of extracranial or intracranial processes.

Extracranial causes of secondary brain lesions

After craniocerebral trauma, the neuronal structures appear to be very sensitive to secondary lesions. Extracranial causes of neuronal lesions include a reduced oxygen supply (hypoxia and hypotension), changes in the electrolyte balance and glucose supply, as well as generalised inflammatory reactions.

Hypovolemic shock, anemia and respiratory dysfunction (e.g., lung contusions, pneumo- or hemothorax) are common changes in the polytraumatized patient, which can lead to a reduction in the oxygen supply to the brain.

As the brain, and especially the ATP production, is especially dependent on the supply of glucose, both hypoglycaemia and hyperglycemia in primary brain lesions can lead to a significant worsening of the animal's condition. Hypoglycaemia can also lead, in the short-term, to a critical reduction in ATP and therefore the energy supply of the neuronal tissues. Hyperglycaemia can potentiate the damage in traumatized, poorly oxygenated tissues as the resulting increased anaerobic glycolysis leads to a deleterious cellular acidosis.

A systemic inflammatory response (Systemic Inflammatory Response Syndrome, SIRS) with massive release of inflammation-potentiating cytokines (interleukins 1, 6, 8, and tumour necrosis factor) is possible in polytraumatized patients. Microvascular disturbances (e.g., increased endothelial per-

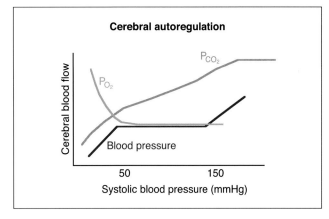

Fig. 12.6
Within the range of physiological blood pressure (50–150 mmHg systolic arterial blood pressure), the blood flow in the brain is maintained at a constant rate primarily by autoregulation. A regulatory increase in blood flow can occur secondary to a pathologically increased PCO_2 (hypoventilation) or pathologically low PO_2 (hypoxia).

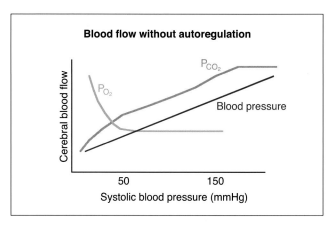

Fig. 12.7
After head injury, physiological autoregulation of blood flow within the normal blood pressure range is no longer possible. The blood flow in the unregulated regions of the brain rises or falls paralleling the systemic blood pressure. To ensure that constant adequate blood flow to the brain is guaranteed, fluid therapy should be instigated with the treatment of the head injury. This is achieved by monitoring systolic blood pressure (target: 100 mmHg).

meability) are the consequences of SIRS. In combination with the changes in the cerebral blood flow and the destruction of the blood-brain barrier, SIRS can lead to interstitial brain oedema with subsequently increased intracranial pressure.

Intracranial causes of secondary brain lesions

Craniocerebral trauma instigates a massive depolarization of the neurons. Glutamate, one of the most important neurotransmitters, is uncontrollably released into the extracellular space. Additional energy (ATP) is necessary for the K-ATPase pumps in the cell membranes to normalize the electrochemical gradients. Uncontrolled increases in intracellular calcium leads to cytotoxicity by activating enzymes such as phospholipases, proteases and nitrogen oxide synthases. The increased production of these enzymes leads in turn, for example via the formation of oxygen radicals, to irreversible cell lesions with the destruction of matrix proteins, DNA, RNA and membrane phospholipids.

The cerebral vasculature is normally regulated by pressure and metabolic autoregulation systems as well as the oxygen supply (Fig. 12.6). The normal perfusion pressure is defined as being the difference between the mean arterial blood pressure and the cerebral venous pressure. With a pathological increase in the ICP, the ICP itself becomes the limiting factor for the perfusion pressure (Fig. 12.7).

The cerebral blood vessels are autoregulated by a fine tuning between the nitrogen oxide production causing vasodilation and endothelin release causing vasoconstriction.

12.2.1.3 Emergency procedures in craniocerebral trauma

Due to the pathophysiological changes occurring with traumatic secondary brain lesions, the treatment of craniocerebral trauma is centered on the maintenance of an adequate perfusion and oxygen supply to the brain as well as measures for the control of the increased intracranial pressure (Fig. 12.8).

General treatment

The initial treatment of craniocerebral trauma has been the subject of controversy. The assumptions that high doses of methylprednisolone, hyperventilation, and high doses of mannitol can be helpful in the treatment of increased ICP has been refuted (Fig. 12.9).

High doses of steroids reduce the release of insulin, are glycolytic and gluconeogenic, and can therefore lead to a detrimental hyperglycemia. Numerous clinical studies have not been able to show any advantage in the administration of steroids for treating craniocerebral trauma and their use remains controversial.

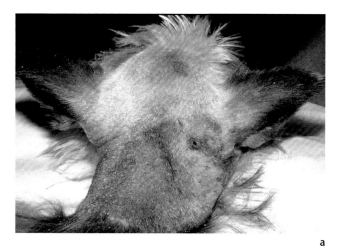

a

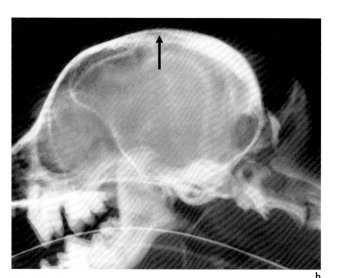

b

Fig. 12.8a, b
Injuries associated with a head injury caused by a bite. (a) External view and (b) x-ray view.

12

Although hyperventilation, by way of reducing the PCO_2, leads to a reduction in cerebral blood flow and so can induce a potential improvement in ICP, this therapy also has dangerous side-effects, namely, increased ischemia. The aim of ventilation as a therapy, therefore, is a normal or slightly reduced PCO_2.

In patients with a defective blood-brain barrier, high doses of mannitol can diffuse into the brain parenchyma and as it is osmotically active, it can lead to an even greater increase in ICP. Low to moderate doses (0.5–1.0 g/kg IV) are therefore suggested.

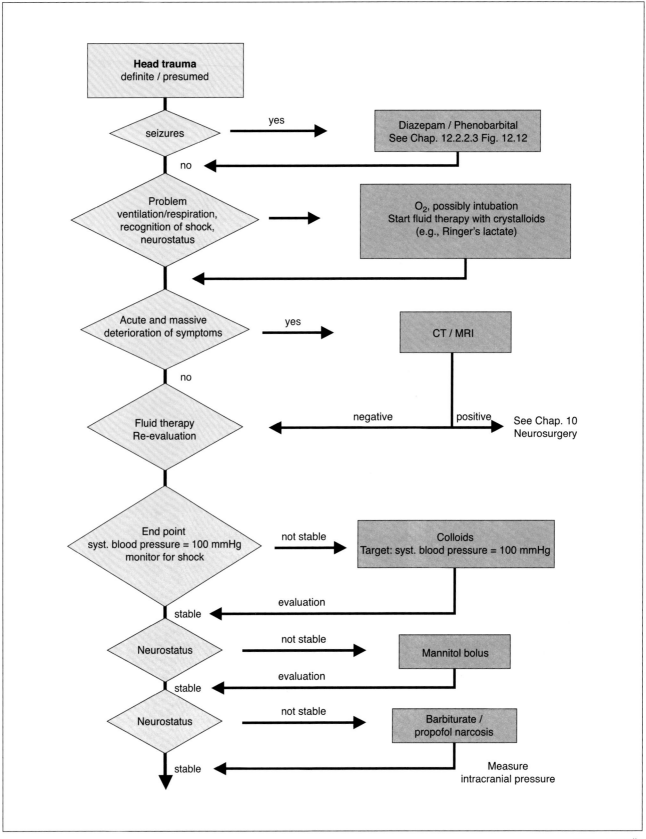

Fig. 12.9
Flow diagram of craniocerebral trauma management.

syst. = systolic

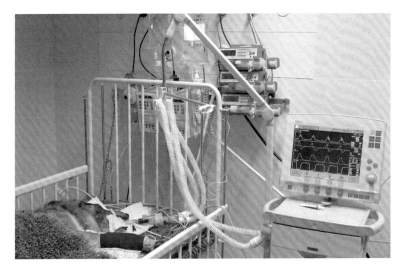

Fig. 12.10
Ventilated patient with brain oedema after trauma.

Fluid therapy
Lactated Ringer's / 0.9% NaCl
As with polytraumatized patients, fluid therapy should correct intravascular volume losses (hypovolemic shock) and ensure that the daily maintenance requirements are met. Hypovolemia or hypotensive situations should also be avoided, just like hypervolemia and hypertension. Early and rapid fluid therapy is necessary. To avoid over-dosing, fluid therapy should not be undertaken with the so-called "shock dosage" of 90 ml/kg; a number of small boli are used to attain an adequate volume. The infusion therapy can be done with either Lactated Ringer's or 0.9% NaCl. Normalized physiological parameters which give an indication of the perfusion and the intravascular volume should be used as the end point of the therapy (normal arterial and central venous blood pressure, normal heart rate and CRT, or pink mucous membranes).

Mannitol
Mannitol is an inert sugar molecule with a relatively small molecular weight. It remains virtually unmetabolized and is excreted unchanged via the kidneys. Mannitol is helpful in the treatment of increased ICP due to its osmotic and rheological effects (Table 12.6). Mannitol causes an increase in serum osmolarity, whereby free water is drawn out of the cerebral interstitium into the circulation, so that brain oedema is reduced. At the same time, these measures also improve the cerebral perfusion. Although the perfusion pressure is the most important factor for oxygen supply to the brain, both the vessel volume and the viscosity of the blood have an effect. Due to mannitol's plasma expansion effect, the blood viscosity is reduced, thereby increasing the blood flow.

High doses of mannitol can, however, lead to a deleterious diuresis. If the blood-brain barrier is injured, mannitol can flow into the cerebral interstitium and so increase the oedema present. Even if the blood-brain barrier is intact, mannitol can induce a reverse osmotic shift leading to microvascular damage. This is why a low-dose bolus therapy is preferable to a high-dose infusion therapy (0.5–1.0 g/kg q 4–6 h), and why this treatment should only be used in patients which have been volume expanded, have obvious deterioration of their neurological condition or have a poor prognosis despite other medical approaches.

Colloids
Colloids, due to their large molecular structure, have oncotic activity. Colloids are an interesting alternative to mannitol in head injuries as they theoretically pass less rapidly into the cerebral interstitium through a permeable blood-brain barrier (e.g., cerebral contusion) and so can reduce potential brain edema more effectively.

Additional therapies
Oxygen
The advantage of additional oxygen therapy (Fig. 12.10) is often ignored: a reduced oxygen supply is the main cause of secondary brain lesions.

12

Table 12.6: Effects of mannitol

Effect	Advantages	Disadvantages
Increase in serum osmolarity	■ Dehydration of the interstitium → reduction of ICP → increase in blood volume	■ Increased renal flow → diuresis
	■ Reduction in blood viscosity → improved perfusion	■ Osmotic diuresis ■ Emesis ■ Extravasation
Free radical scavenger		

ICP = intracranial pressure

The blood's oxygen concentration can be optimized by ensuring an adequate circulating hemoglobin concentration and a normal lung function, and by maximizing the inspiratory O_2 concentration (see Chap. 12.1.2).

Oxygen is best given by intubation and artificial respiration in an unconscious animal (Fig. 12.10). An improvised oxygen tent or cage can be used as an alternative to achieve inspiratory oxygen concentrations of up to 60%; however, the continual neurological monitoring necessary in the first 48 to 72 hours may make this approach impractical. The application of O_2 through nasal tubes is not advised as the irritation caused by the tubes can lead to sneezing or coughing, which in turn can raise the ICP. Flow-by oxygenation may be the safest and most effective manner to deliver oxygen in the conscious head trauma patient.

Barbiturate / Propofol anaesthesia

With severe, craniocerebral trauma, the patient can be placed in an artificial coma using a deep barbiturate anaesthesia (pentobarbital 2–15 mg/kg/IV followed by 0.2–4 mg/kg/h as continuous infusion) or propofol anaesthesia (2–6 mg/kg IV followed by 2–5 mg/kg/h as continuous infusion). The success of such treatment has not been documented in small animal medicine and is not widely accepted in human medicine; therefore, such anaesthesia should only be used as a last resort and in combination with an optimal fluid therapy and surveillance regimen.

Surgical treatment: see Chap. 10.2.2.

Further reading

PROULX, J., DHUPA N.: Severe brain injury. Part I. Pathophysiology. Comp Small Anim Pract. 1998; 20 (8) 897–905.

PROULX, J., DHUPA N.: Severe brain injury. Part II. Therapy. Comp Small Anim Pract. 1998; 20(9) 993–1005.

12.2.2 Status epilepticus

12.2.2.1 Introduction and definition

Status epilepticus is defined as an epileptic fit or seizure with generalized tonic-clonic activity lasting for more than 5 to 10 minutes, focal fits / seizures that last longer than 20 to 30 minutes, or a number of individual fits / seizures that occur within a short time period, between which the consciousness or EEG do not completely return to normal. Every type of focal or generalized seizure can lead to status epilepticus. The different causes of seizures and epilepsy are described fully in Chap. 18.5.

Status epilepticus is in itself a diagnosable, life-threatening, acute neurological emergency and requires immediate adequate management. This involves not only suitable and immediate treatment, but also subsequent intensive surveillance.

Status epilepticus with generalized tonic-clonic activity with or without loss of consciousness is the most common form seen. However, severe partial seizures can also be life threatening and should therefore be considered as emergencies.

12.2.2.2 Pathophysiology

Seizures are the result of a sudden and massive activation of neurons caused by an imbalance between the inhibitory and excitatory factors. Specifically, GABA-mediated inhibition and metabolic changes in the cell milieu (ions, energy substrates) play an important role in the initiation of epileptic seizures. Glutamate receptors and electrolyte changes in conjunction with other factors are responsible for the maintenance of an epileptic seizure.

Although the metabolic stress and the reduced oxygen supply to the brain which occur during a short epileptic fit can be compensated for, the massive cellular changes that occur during continual neuronal activation can potentially lead to cell death. The changes in the extracellular potassium and intracellular calcium concentrations, release of glutamate, and reduced oxygen tension all lead to a lack of ATP, hypotension, acidosis, and hyperthermia, which in turn can lead to secondary hypoxia and cell death.

Systematically, status epilepticus can lead to hyperthermia, hypotension, and endothelial damage with subsequent disseminated intravascular coagulation (DIC) and multiple organ failure.

12.2.2.3 Therapy

Cessation of the status epilepticus and the prevention of sequelae are the main therapeutic aims.

The emergency treatment follows the ABC principles. Due to their increased oxygen requirement, the patient is given **oxygen per mask or flow by** (Chap. 12.1.2). Further treatment often requires intravenous access. If this is not possible, 1 mg/kg diazepam can be given rectally (suppository formulation or the intravenous solution). After **venous access** has been set up, both fluid therapy and antiepileptic therapy with **diazepam 0.5–1 mg/kg IV** are initiated. Diazepam works quickly but only for a short time. In order to suppress further epileptic activity in the brain, patients that have already responded to diazepam should be treated with long-acting antiepileptics (phenobarbital 2–5 mg/kg IV, IM q4–6h or PO q 12 h). Diazepam can be repeated twice within a period of 10 minutes between each dose.

In the mean time, the metabolic causes of status epilepticus such as hypoglycemia, hypocalcemia, other electrolyte changes, azotemia, hypoxia, or massive acid-base changes should be excluded by blood analysis and where necessary treated. **Hypoglycemia** should especially be excluded in puppies. Glucose values < 3 mmol/l should be stabilized using a bolus infusion of glucose (0.5–1 ml/kg of a 50% solution, diluted to at least 25% IV). The infusion solution should be substituted, after the bolus therapy, with 5% glucose (a 5% solution is made by adding 50 ml 50% glucose to 500 ml Lactated Ringer's). Hypocalcemic animals should be treated with calcium. In the case of status epilepticus due to **hypocalcemia**, calcium should be administered intravenously with ECG monitoring over 15 to 20 minutes (e.g., with calcium gluconate 100 mg/kg).

Fluid therapy is performed according to need. Animals in status epilepticus are normally not in shock, but due to their increased metabolism have an increased need for fluid, and depending on the cause may be dehydrated. Normally, the maintenance requirement of such animals is at least 5 ml/kg/h of an isotonic crystalloid solution (e.g., Lactated Ringer's). If dehydration is present or fluid diuresis is desired (intoxications, renal failure), the fluid requirements are even higher.

If the status epilepticus cannot be suppressed with a maintenance dosage of diazepam and phenobarbital, then other treatments can be used. The patient can be put under **anaesthesia** using pentobarbital, propofol or gas anesthesia. The patient should be anaesthetised for at least 12 to 24 hours, which requires intensive surveillance. The patient should be intubated to prevent aspiration (Fig. 12.11). Artificial respiration may also be necessary; however, the majority of animals can breathe on their own and can be given oxygen supplementation via an oxygen catheter placed in the endotracheal tube without having to be placed on a respirator. The endotracheal tube should be aspirated or changed every couple of hours to prevent blockage or the ascension of bacteria. Anesthetized animals should also be given **phenobarbital 5 mg/kg** q 12 h, as the anaesthetic agents are not all antiepileptics and under certain circumstances only induce muscle relaxation.

An alternative to anaesthesia is the repeated treatment with phenobarbital. Phenobarbital can be given every 20 to 30 minutes to a maximum dosage of 24 mg/kg within 24 hours. As it can take hours before status epilepticus is suppressed in this way and the animal is subjected to massively increased metabolism during this time, the following therapy protocol is suggested: initially, diazepam 1 mg/kg IV and phenobarbital 5 mg/kg IV. If there is no reaction to this treatment, then repeat the diazepam after 10 minutes and give another dose of phenobarbital 5 mg/kg after 20 to 30 minutes. If this also does not show any effect (duration of the status epilepticus is already at least 30 minutes), phenobarbital is given again and the animal is placed at the same time under anaesthesia, intubated and monitored. Phenobarbital, 5 mg/kg, is repeated after 6 to 8 hours (see also Fig. 12.12).

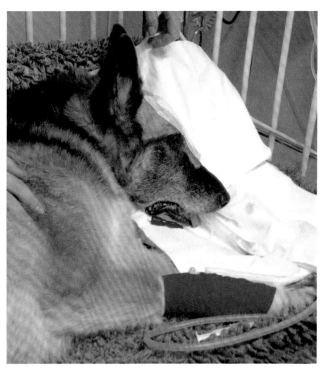

Fig. 12.11
Intubation without ventilation. Intubated patient under pentobarbital anaesthesia. If respiration is adequate, then the patient does not need to be artificially ventilated but can be left to breathe spontaneously through the endotracheal tube. The tube's cuff should be slightly inflated to protect the patient from aspiration. The cuff should be moved every 4–6 h and the endotracheal tube changed every 6–12 h. Oxygen can be supplemented via a tube placed in the endotracheal tube.

12

Animals in status epilepticus almost always present with hyperthermia. Active **cooling** with damp cloths, wetting of the fur, ice packs, cold infusions or if necessary bladder or abdominal lavage with cool infusion solutions can be undertaken to achieve a body temperature of 39.5°C. Although the normal body temperature range is 37.5–38.5°C, active cooling should be stopped at 39.5°C to prevent hypothermia from developing, especially if seizures avtivity abates.

Long-lasting status epilepticus can lead to brain oedema. If there are clinical signs of this condition, then the principles of treatment explained in Chap. 12.3.2.9 should be followed.

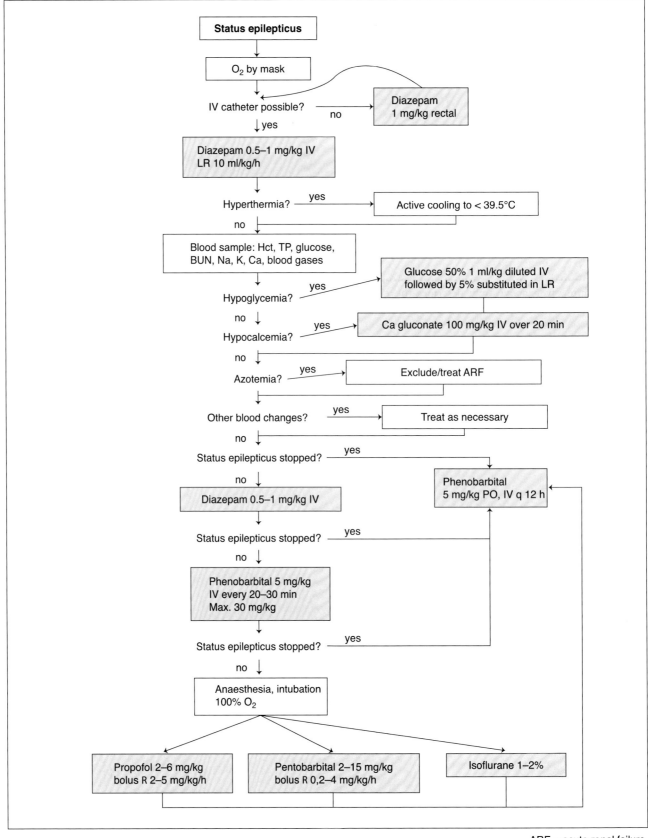

Fig. 12.12
Emergency stabilization of a patient with status epilepticus.

ARF = acute renal failure
LR = Lactated Ringer's

12.2.2.4 Monitoring

Monitoring of the vital parameters (respiration, circulation, temperature) is of crucial importance. Animals under anaesthesia should be intensively monitored: heart rate, heart rhythm, respiratory rate, temperature, colour of mucous membranes, CRT, SpO_2, blood pressure, and end-expiratory CO_2 should be controlled continuously. The nursing of a anaesthetised animal also includes the application of eye ointment, oral hygiene, adequate padding, and regular turning as well as control of urination.

The animals should not have any more seizures, neither generalized nor local. The recovery phase is controlled ideally with help of an EEG as excitation due to the side- or after-effects of the anaesthetics cannot always be differentiated from epileptic seizures.

12.2.2.5 Additional investigations and therapy

The procedure given above only describes the emergency treatment of a patient with status epilepticus. After the seizures have been suppressed, investigations into their cause and specific therapy are necessary. The diagnostic methods are described comprehensively in Chap. 18.5.

The specific therapies include, for example, measures taken for the suspicion of intoxication (see Chap. 12.2.3), treatment of brain oedema (see Chap. 12.3.2.9), brain surgery or the start of long-term treatment with anticonvulsive agents. The characteristics of the different anticonvulsants are described in Chap. 18.5.1.

Further reading

DRISLANE, F.W. (2005): Types of status epilepticus: Definitions and classification. In: Status Epilepticus. A Clinical Perspective. Humana Press, pp. 11–32.

PLATT, S.R. (2000): Status epilepticus: Patient management and pharmacologic therapy. Comp. Cont Educ. 22(8): 722–728.

JAGGY, A. (1998): Neurologische Notfälle beim Kleintier. Medizinverlage Stuttgart.

12.2.3 Intoxications

12.2.3.1 Introduction

Poisonings are often the cause of emergencies and can affect not only the gastrointestinal tract but frequently the nervous system. The causes of intoxications which lead to neurological symptoms are listed in Table 12.7.

An immediate diagnosis and therapy can considerably affect the progression of an intoxication (Table 12.8). The aim is to achieve early "detoxification" of the patient and prevent any further absorption of the toxin. If clinical signs of poisoning are already present, often symptomatic treatment is the only therapy possible due to the lack of a specific antidote or identification of the toxin.

In the following text, the general treatment of an intoxication is described, including "detoxification". A selection of toxins which can lead to neurological symptoms and their treatment are given in Table 12.8. Further information with respect to poisoning can be found in the relevant chapters (13.4.1, 13.4.2, 17.2.5.1, 18.4.5.5).

Table 12.7: Intoxications that can lead to neurological symptoms

Effect	Seizure / Tremor	Changes in consciousness	Tetany	Paralysis
Neuro-toxin	■ Bromethaline ■ Carbamates ■ Illicit human substances* ■ Ivermectin ■ Lead ■ Lidocaine ■ Metaldehyde ■ Mycotoxins ■ Opioids (high dosage) ■ Organo-phosphates ■ Pyrethroids ■ Zinc phosphide	■ Amitraz ■ Amphetamines ■ Barbiturates ■ Benzodiazepines ■ Bromethaline ■ Ethanol, methanol ■ Ethylene glycol ■ Illicit human substances* ■ Ivermectin ■ Methylxanthine / theobromine ■ Opioids ■ Phenothiazine	■ Botulinum toxin ■ Strychnine	■ Carbamates ■ Organo-phosphates

* (LSD, cocaine, marijuana)

12

Table 12.8: Clinical symptoms and treatment of selected neurotoxins

Neurotoxin	Mechanism	Clinical symptoms	Therapy
Amphetamines	CNS stimulation	Hyperactivity, tremor, ataxia, seizures, mydriasis, barking	Symptomatic
Barbiturates	Stimulation of GABA-mediated inhibition, glutamate inhibition	CNS depression	Symptomatic
Botulinum toxin	Inhibition of acetylcholine release	Weakness, paralysis	Antitoxin, atropine (0.2 mg/kg IV, SC, IM)
Bromethaline	Inhibition of oxidative phosphorylation	Ataxia, seizures, coma	Symptomatic
Carbamates	Reversible acetylcholine esterase inhibition	CNS: seizures PNS: tremor, tetany, miosis, salivation, diarrhea	Symptomatic, atropine (0.2 mg/kg IV)
Ethylene glycol	Osmotically active, metabolites are nephrotoxic	Stupor, ataxia, renal failure	Diuresis, vitamin B6 Antidote Dog: 4-methylpyrazole (20 mg/kg IV, then 15 mg/kg IV after 12/24 h and 5 mg/kg after 36 h) Cat: ethanol 20% (5 ml/kg IV 5 × q 6 h, then 4 × q 8 h)
Fungi	Various	Tremor, seizures, coma, diarrhea, vomiting, liver failure	Symptomatic
Illicite human substances*	Various	Disorientation, excitation, tremor, mydriasis, coma	Symptomatic
Ivermectin	GABA antagonist	Disorientation, hyperesthesia, tremor followed by weakness and paresis	Symptomatic, physostigmine (1 mg/kg IV), artificial respiration
Lead	Calcium inhibition	Tremor, seizures, weakness, blindness, hemorrhages, anemia	Symptomatic, chelation using DMSA or EDTA
Metaldehyde	Unknown	Tremor, seizures	Symptomatic, anticonvulsants
Methylxanthine	Inhibition of adenosine receptors, stimulation of catecholamines and release of Ca	Hyperexcitability, tremors, seizures, restlessness, tachycardia, arrhythmias	Symptomatic, diuresis, urinary catheter, β-blockers
Molds	Hepato- and neurotoxic	Tremor, seizures, salivation	Symptomatic
Opioids	Bind to opioid receptors	Excitation, stupor, coma	Naloxone
Organophosphates	Irreversible acetylcholine esterase inhibition	CNS: seizures PNS: weakness, paralysis, miosis, salivation, diarrhea	Pralidoxime (20 mg/kg IV, 3 × q 12 h) Atropine (0.2 mg/kg IV) for muscarinic symptoms
Pyrethroids	Inhibition of (Ca)ATPase and (CaMg)ATPase	Tremor, seizures, salivation, dyspnea	Symptomatic
Strychnine	Inhibition of Renshaw cells	Excitation, tetany, muscle paralysis	Symptomatic, (methocarbamol, phenobarbital)
Zinc phosphide	Inhibition of cytochrome oxidase	Seizures, vomiting	Symptomatic

* (LSD, cocaine, marijuana)

12.2.3.2 General therapy

Triage

If the first contact with the owner of an animal with definite or presumed intoxication occurs by telephone, the owner should be instructed on how to transport the animal to the veterinary practice. In certain cases, initial detoxification can be undertaken at home (washing the animal's fur in cases of topical intoxicity) especially where there are long driving times to the clinic. In the ideal situation, it is advisable for the animal to be brought immediately to a veterinarian. The owner should bring the packaging or the rest of the poison with them.

If the poison is known, information about the toxin can be obtained from the local toxicology centre by the veterinarian or the owner.

Immediate emergency procedures

The initial stabilization of each emergency patient consists of making the airway patent, assisting the breathing and stabilizing the circulation. Seizures should be immediately treated and measures for treating hyperthermia should be initiated.

Detoxification

Detoxification strategies include the removal of topical toxins, the induction of vomiting, gastric lavage, the application of activated charcoal and laxatives, and diuresis.

Topical toxins

Topical toxins should be removed using large amounts of lukewarm water. If necessary, a mild soap solution (washing-up liquid) can be used. The person washing the animal should protect themselves by wearing gloves. Afterwards, the animal must be dried and kept warm.

Gastrointestinal detoxification

The majority of toxins are ingested. If ingestion has taken place less than 2 to 4 hours previously, then it is possible that there is still toxin within the stomach and so it can be removed either by inducing vomiting or by gastric lavage.

Vomiting is induced in dogs using apomorphine (0.04 mg/kg IV, IM). Apomorphine can also be given at a higher dosage (0.25 mg/kg) over the conjunctiva. Apomorphine can lead to sedation and subsequent aspiration pneumonia, especially in patients that already have reduced consciousness. The effects of apomorphine can be antagonized by either naloxone or metoclopramide to effect.

Xylazine (0.4 mg/kg IV, IM) is the emetic of choice in cats and can, when necessary, be antagonized with yohimbine (0.5 mg/kg).

Hydrogen peroxide (1–2 ml/kg of a 3% solution) can be used as an alternative treatment for the induction of vomiting. Salt or soap solutions should not be used.

> Contraindications for the induction of vomiting include the ingestion of acid or alkali, altered consciousness (apathy, stupor, coma, hyperexcitability), seizures, tremor, bradycardia, respiratory distress, vomiting, laryngeal paralysis, and weakness. Vomiting should never be induced in rodents.

The induction of vomiting is especially contraindicated in intoxications with neurotoxins due to the changed consciousness or seizures as there is an increased danger of aspiration pneumonia.

Gastric lavage can be used if the toxin has been ingested within the previous 2 to 4 hours. Animals should be intubated before the procedure and the cuff inflated to prevent the aspiration of the lavage fluid. The prerequisite for this procedure is anaesthesia. The stomach is washed out using 5–10 ml/kg warm water until the lavage fluid remains clear. The contraindication for gastric lavage is the ingestion of acid or alkali.

The risks of a gastric lavage (e.g., anaesthetic risk and aspiration pneumonia) must be weighed against its use. In animals which need to be intubated because of other reasons (coma, seizures), the benefit of gastric lavage is usually greater than the risks and in addition it can also be undertaken when the intoxication has occurred more than 4 h previously.

Adsorption of toxins

After gastric detoxification, the most effective "decontamination" strategy is the application of active charcoal (1–4 g/kg PO) to bind the remaining toxin. Active charcoal can be given orally (Fig. 12.13) or by gastric tube. It is important to give **liquid medicinal active charcoal** as charcoal tablets have a much smaller adsorption surface. Active charcoal binds not only the majority of neurotoxins but also ingested medications. Laxatives such as sorbitol or lactulose can speed up toxin excretion.

Diuresis

Toxins absorbed from the gastrointestinal tract are metabolized in the liver and/or excreted via the kidneys. In certain circumstances, the degradation products can also be toxic (metaldehyde, ethylene glycol). Renal excretion can be accelerated by using fluid diuresis. Diuretics, such as furosemide or mannitol, are only indicated in acute renal failure. The excretion of ionic substances can be supported by changing the pH of the urine. This, however, requires the identification of the toxin and a regular blood gas analysis to control the acid-base balance. Hemodialysis or peritoneal dialysis are, (if they are available) very effective in the elimination of certain toxins from the blood.

12

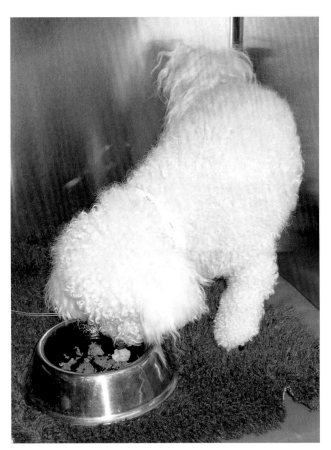

12

Fig. 12.13
Administration of activated charcoal. Liquid charcoal is tasteless and is tolerated by many dogs if it is mixed with a little meat or canned food.

Control of seizures

Seizures, hyperreactivity and tremors lead to a high metabolic use of substrates and oxygen, and should be suppressed. The therapy of seizures is described in detail in Chap. 12.2.2. Diazepam (0.5 mg/kg IV or rectal) is the first step in the therapy, followed by phenobarbital (5 mg/kg IV, IM every 20–30 min until the seizures have stopped or a total dosage of 24 mg/kg/ 24 hrs has been given; then 5 mg/kg every 12 h) and if necessary pentobarbital (0.2–4 mg/kg/h) or a continuous infusion with propofol.

If there is an indication that brain oedema is present (anisocoria, miosis or mydriasis, pathological nystagmus, bradycardia or bradypnea, absent pupillary or palpebral reflex in unanesthetized patients), then mannitol should be given (Chap. 12.2.1.3).

Monitoring

Monitoring of perfusion parameters, control of respiration, stabilization of body temperature as well as blood gas and electrolyte analyses are minimal requirements for patients with signs of intoxication.

Specific therapy
Antidotes

Specific antidotes are unfortunately only available for a few neurotoxins. They are, however, important in the treatment of medication overdosage as in many such cases the antidote is known (Table 12.8).

Metaldehyde

Metaldehyde is a tetramer of acetaldehyde. It is used in slug bait and, more rarely, in grill or oven lighters. Metaldehyde is hydrolyzed in the stomach to acetaldehyde. Both substances are quickly absorbed and lead within minutes to hours to tremors or seizures, tachycardia, panting, excitement, hypersalivation or vomiting. Death can occur due to respiratory and cardiac arrest if the animal is not treated.

There is no specific therapy for metaldehyde poisoning. Symptomatic therapy includes detoxification using gastric lavage and the administration of activated charcoal, fluid therapy, temperature control, and control of the seizures. Animals which mainly demonstrate tremors can be treated with methocarbamol (55–200 mg/kg slow IV) or diazepam (1–5 mg/kg IV) (Fig. 12.14). Animals in status epilepticus usually do not respond to diazepam and should be placed under propofol or isoflurane anaesthesia for 12 to 24 hours. In addition, the seizures should be stopped centrally and the animals should be given phenobarbital (5 mg/kg q 12 h) for a couple of days. Higher dosages of phenobarbital or the use of pentobarbital are controversial as both these drugs can prolong the denaturation of acetaldehyde in the liver.

The prognosis is normally good as long as secondary brain damage due to status epilepticus is prevented. Metaldehyde can, however, lead to a delayed liver failure.

Organophosphate / Carbamate intoxication

Organophosphates and carbamates are components of various insecticides. They are toxic in that they inhibit acetylcholine esterase, leading to prolonged activity of acetylcholine. The resulting muscarinic receptor stimulation leads to diarrhea, micturition, miosis, bronchospasm, vomiting, lacrimation, and salivation. Nicotinic stimulation leads to neuromuscular stimulation with tremors and tetany, followed by weakness and paralysis, while central stimulation leads to seizures, excitation, or coma.

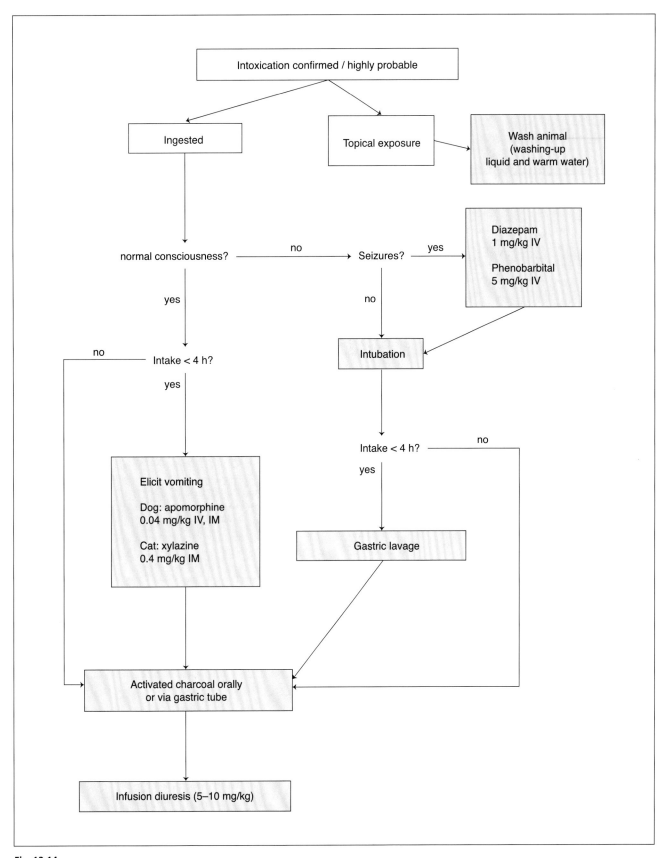

Fig. 12.14
Flow diagram: Decontamination for animals exposed to toxins.

The actual degree of toxicity of these compounds is dependent on the product. Organophosphates are more toxic than carbamates because they attach irreversibly to acetylcholine esterase and make the synthesis of new enzyme necessary.

The diagnosis is achieved by proving the presence of reduced plasma cholinesterase activity. The therapy is symptomatic and includes detoxification via gastric lavage and the administration of active charcoal. If the animal has had skin contact with the poison, it should be washed with a mild soap solution. In the initial stages of an organophosphate intoxication, 2-PAM / pralidoxime (20 mg/kg slow IV, 3 × q 12 h) can help to reactivate the acetylcholine esterase as it binds to the organophosphate. The complex is excreted in the urine and this can be hastened by using infusion diuresis. Anticholinergics (atropine 0.2 mg/kg IV), muscle relaxants, and anticonvulsants can be given depending on the clinical symptoms.

The prognosis is guarded. Amongst other complications, polyneuropathies can occur as late sequelae to this toxicity.

Pyrethroid intoxication

Pyrethroids are present in various products used against flea and tick infestations. They lead to an inhibition of (Ca)ATPase and (CaMg)ATPase in nervous tissue. The clinical symptoms are salivation, tremor, ataxia, seizures, vomiting and dyspnea. Progression can lead to death.

Therapy is symptomatic and includes the immediate washing off of any of the toxin on the fur, the initiation of vomiting or gastric lavage following oral ingestion, the administration of active charcoal, control of seizures, and the maintenance of respiration.

Chocolate

Chocolate contains the methylxanthines, theobromine and caffeine. The amount of these compounds present depends on the type of chocolate: the darker and more bitter it is, the more toxic it is. The lethal dose of milk chocolate is approx. 60 g/kg, while with plain or cooking chocolate as little as 6 g/kg can be lethal.

Methylxanthine inhibits adenosine receptors and stimulates the release of catecholamines as well as free calcium in the muscle cells, which can lead to CNS stimulation, tremors, tachycardia, cardiac arrhythmias, weakness, seizures and death.

In asymptomatic animals, vomiting should be elicited and activated charcoal administered. Due to the disturbances in consciousness seen in animals with symptoms, gastric lavage is often indicated. ECG monitoring of heart function is recommended and arrythmias or tachycardia should be treated as required. Seizures and tremors can be treated with diazepam or phenobarbital. Diazepam is not as effective as phenobarbital, which can inhibit benzodiazepine receptors in the CNS.

As methylxanthine is excreted via the kidneys, infusion diuresis is indicated. The bladder should be catheterized with an in dwelling catheter or kept empty by being regularly emptied because methylxanthine can be resorbed from the urine.

The prognosis is normally good when the treatment is started early enough.

Lead intoxication

Lead poisoning occurs after the ingestion of lead-containing paints, batteries or projectiles. Lead accumulates in the erythrocytes, bones and soft tissues. It interferes with intracellular calcium concentration and potassium-dependent processes such as nerve function, muscle contractility, platelet aggregation and renal function. This can lead to a multitude of different clinical symptoms: anemia, seizures, dementia, blindness, tremors, weakness, cardiac arrhythmias, hypotension, hemorrhage, renal failure, vomiting and diarrhea.

Patients should be treated symptomatically. If possible, the lead source should be removed. Lead can be chelated using either DMSA (2,3-dimercaptosuccinate; 10 mg/kg/day PO for 10 days) or EDTA (25 mg/kg of a 1% solution q 6 h SC for 4 to 5 days). The side-effects of these therapies include hypocalcemia, zinc deficiency and nephrotoxicity. Infusion diuresis encourages the excretion of chelated compounds and reduces the nephrotoxicity.

Ethylene glycol

Ethylene glycol is present in antifreeze, radiator fluids; more rarely, in cleaning fluids, varnishes and paints.

Ethylene glycol is very rapidly resorbed and is metabolized in the liver to a variety of metabolites. Ethylene glycol is itself osmotically active and increases osmolarity leading to stupor, ataxia, tremors, vomiting, and osmotic diuresis with subsequent dehydration. This *first stage* of intoxication occurs 30 min to 12 h after ingestion. In the *second stage,* the animal presents apathetic but otherwise normal. In the *third stage*, after 24 to 72 hours, the toxic metabolites lead to renal failure.

The diagnosis is attained from the anamnesis, clinical symptoms, the proof of an increased osmotic gap, metabolic acidosis, and by using commercial kits.

In the initial stage, the most important aspects are (1) the prevention of further uptake of the poison using gastric lavage and the administration of activated charcoal, and (2) rehydration and fluid diuresis. Either ethanol 20% can be given as an antidote (5.5 ml/kg 5 × q 4 h, then 4 × q 6 h) or 4-methyl-parasol, an alcohol dehydrogenase inhibitor (20 mg/kg IV followed by 15 mg/kg IV after 12 and 24 h, then 5 mg/kg after 36 h).

Peritoneal dialysis or haemodialysis are the only treatments recommended once acute anuric renal failure has developed.

The prognosis is guarded and is particularly dependent on early treatment with an antidote. The metabolism in cats is quicker and if they are not treated within 3 hours after intake of the poison, the intoxication is usually fatal.

Further reading

PETERSON, M.E., TALCOTT, P.A., (2001): Small Animal Toxicology, WB Saunders Co, Philadelphia.

GFELLER R.W., MESSONNIER S.P., (1998): Handbook of Small Animal Toxicology and Poisonings, Mosby, St. Louis.

KIRK R.W., BISTNER S.I., FORD R.B., (1995): Handbook of veterinary procedures and emergency treatments, 6th ed. WB Saunders, Philadelphia.

MILEWSKI L.M. et al., (2006): An overview of potentially life-threatening poisonous plants in dogs and cats JVECCS 16(1): 25–33.

HORNFELDT, C.S., MURPHY, M.J., (2001): Summary of small animal poison exposures. In: PETERSON M.E., TALCOTT P.A., (eds.) Small Animal Toxicology, WB Saunders Co, Philadelphia.

www.clinitox.ch

12.3 The neurological intensive-care patient

12.3.1 Introduction

The "Rule of 20" (according to Dr. KIRBY) helps make the monitoring of an intensive-care patient easier and ensures the early recognition of complications (Fig. 12.15).

The complex interrelationship of the body's physiological and pathophysiological mechanisms requires the inclusion of all the body's systems in the interpretation of an individual abnormality; for example, the heart rate. An increase in heart rate can be caused by a change in fluid balance, the oncotic pressure, the blood pressure, oxygenation, ventilation, heart function, acid-base balance, glucose concentration, consciousness, coagulation parameters, hematocrit, renal function, pain, temperature, and the psychological condition of the animal. Additionally, tachycardia can lead to changes in other body systems. The recognition, understanding, correct interpretation, and proper treatment of the interrelationships between the body's systems are the most important prerequisites for successful intensive-care therapy. The twenty-point rule should be undertaken at least once a day in the neurological patient, in addition to clinical investigation, interpre-

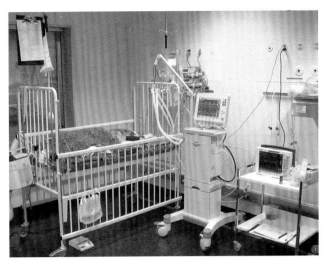

Fig. 12.15
An intensive-care patient after the removal of a brain tumor. Such animals are kept in an artificial coma for the first 24 hours. This requires intensive monitoring and nursing.

tation of results, and assessment of the diagnostic and therapeutic plans. The more critical the condition of the patient, the longer the time is needed for consideration of each of the respective points. If one considers the current situation of the patient, in addition to any changes, possible complications, and therapy with respect to each of the points on the list, then the interrelationship of the symptoms and their interpretation will be easier and complications can be prevented (Table 12.9).

12.3.2 The Rule of 20

The priority of the individual points is determined on an individual basis. However, it is easier if the points are always discussed in the same sequence so that none are forgotten.

12.3.2.1 Fluid replacement therapy

The hydration status and perfusion are determined as described in Chap. 12.1.3.

Monitoring of the fluid balance is performed by assessing the heart rate, pulse strength, colour and consistency of the mucous membranes, CRT, blood pressure, urine production, weight control, and the measurement of hematocrit / total protein.

12

Table 12.9: The "Rule of 20" for neurological intensive-care patients

"Rule of 20" parameter	Monitoring	Aims	Therapy	Comments
Fluid compensation	HR, pulse strength, MM, CRT, urine production, weight, ABP, Hct/TP, CVP	Normal perfusion and hydration	Crystalloids +/− colloids Blood products when needed	See Chap. 12.1.3
Blood pressure	Pulse strength, blood pressure	MAP > 60 mmHg Systolic 80–120 mmHg	Fluid therapy, vasopressors with restored blood volume	Prevent hypertension with hemorrhaging; vasopressors contraindicated with hypovolemia
Oncotic pressure	Albumin, COP	Albumin > 20 g/l COP > 15 mmHg	Colloids	
Albumin	Albumin	Albumin > 20 g/l	Human plasma albumin	Albumin important for wound healing, transport protein
Heart function and rhythm	HR, ECG, echocardiography, electrolytes, PaO_2	Maintenance of perfusion	Oxygen supplementation Depending on problem: antiarrythmics, dobutamine, pimobendan	
Oxygenation and ventilation	MM, respiratory rate, SpO_2, $PaCO_2$, PvO_2, PaO_2	SpO_2 > 90% $PaCO_2$ < 60 mmHg PaO_2 > 60 mmHg	Oxygen supplementation, ventilation, analgesia, bronchodilators	Hypoxia and hypercapnia reduce the cerebral blood flow
Glucose	Consciousness, glucose	Glucose 4–10 mmol/l	Hypoglycemia: 1 ml/kg 50% dextrose diluted IV followed by 5% dextrose CRI Hyperglycemia: short-acting crystalline insulin 0.05 IU/kg/h	The brain is glucose-dependent; however, hyperglycemia leads to an increased use of O_2
Electrolyte and acid-base balance	Blood gases (pH, CO_2, HCO_3), Na, K, Cl, Ca, P	Normal blood gas and electrolytes	See Chap. 12.3.2.8	Acute changes in the osmolarity (Na) or a too rapid correction of chronic changes can lead to neurological symptoms
Intracranial pressure and consciousness	Consciousness, cranial nerves, pupil position and reactivity, EEG	Normal reflexes, reactive symmetrical pupils, normal consciousness	Brain oedema: O_2, if needed with artificial respiration. Raising of upper body Mannitol	With raised ICP, the MAP must be > 80 mmHg to ensure adequate cerebral blood flow (CPP = MAP − ICP)

In critical neurological patients, a jugular or femoral catheter to measure central venous pressure (CVP) can be helpful (Fig. 12. 16). CVP is dependent on the venous return to the heart (volume), the intrathoracic pressure, the elasticity of the walls of the vena cava, and the cardiac function (reflux from the right heart chambers). Apart from the volume, the rest of these parameters do not change in the majority of intensive-care patients (NB: pneumothorax), so that CVP is proportional to the venous return to the heart. The CVP should be 2–6 cm H_2O. Values under 0 cm mean that the patient is suffering from hypovolemia, while there is danger of over-infusion with values in excess of 10 cm H_2O. An excessively low CVP can also be normalized with boli of crystalloid and/or colloid solutions. If there is normal or increased CVP with

signs of reduced perfusion, then a heart problem should be excluded.

Perfusion deficits result in tachycardia, reddened or pale mucous membranes, abnormal CRT, cold extremities, and in chronic stages, hypotension.

Treatment is with fluid boli (Chap. 12.1.3, Table 12.4).

Dehydration must be differentiated from perfusion deficits. There is a net extravascular fluid loss with dehydration (primarily from the interstitium). The signs of dehydration are dry mucous membranes and reduced skin turgor.

Table 12.9: The "Rule of 20" for neurological intensive-care patients (continued)

"Rule of 20" parameter	Monitoring	Aims	Therapy	Comments
Coagulation	MM (petechiae), PT, PTT, thrombocyte count, buccal mucosa bleeding time	Normal coagulation times, Thrombocytes > 100,000 /ml	Plasma 10 ml/kg q 8 h, thrombocyte concentrate, vitamin K	Treatment depends on cause
Erythrocytes and hemoglobin	Hct, regeneration, Hb	Hct 30–45%	Whole blood transfusion: 2 ml/kg/%Hct Erythrocyte concentrate: 1 ml/kg/%Hct	Aim is to have Hct lower as normal as better blood rheology
Immune status, leukocytes and antibiosis	Differential blood count (leucocyte count, left shift) bacterial culture and sensitivity CSF analysis	Specific antibiosis depending on culture and antibiotic sensitivity	Depends on infectious agent	Intracranial: antibiotic must be effective with intact blood-brain barrier.
Renal function	Urine production, serum creatinine, urinalysis	Urine production > 2ml/kg/h, concentratability, normal renal values, inactive sediment	Fluid diuresis, hemodialysis	Glucosuria; Cylinders: indication of tubule damage; Proteinuria: indication of glomerulopathy
Gastrointestinal tract	Intestinal movement, fecal consistency	Normal appetite and defecation	Depends on problem	
Nutrition	Body weight control	Calorie requirements Kcal/day: 30 × kg body weight + 70	Tube feeding (nasoesophageal, esophageal, gastric)	Enteral nutrition is preferable to parenteral
Medication metabolism and dosage	Renal function, liver function	Dosage is adapted to the kidney and liver function	If the metabolism or excretion is reduced, then increase the time interval between doses or reduce dosage	
Analgesia	Pain vocalization, HR, respiration	Pain-free condition	Opioids (fentanyl, morphine), possibly NSAIDs	NSAIDs contraindicated in many cases
Body temperature	Rectal temperature	Temperature 37.5–38.5°C	Warmth (hot water bottle, Bair-Hugger®, warm infusion solutions, blankets) or cooling (wet fur, ventilator, cool infusion solutions)	Hyperthermia increases the energy and oxygen requirements; cool only to 39.5°C to prevent hypothermia
Wounds and bandages	Control at least once daily (hygiene, pressure)		Clean wounds, keep bandages clean and dry	
General nursing		Avoid stress	Hygiene, physiotherapy, TLC	

ABP = arterial blood pressure, COP = colloid osmotic pressure, CPP = cerebral perfusion pressure, CRI = constant rate infusion, CRT = capillary refill time, CVP = central venous pressure, HR = heart rate, ICP = intracranial pressure, MAP = mean arterial blood pressure, MM = mucous membranes, PT = prothrombin time, PTT = partial thromboplastin time, TLC = tender loving care, TP = total protein.

Patients with increased fluid loss (diarrhea, vomiting, hyperthermia, seizures, sepsis, anorexia) are usually dehydrated. With severe chronic fluid loss, blood loss, or the transfer of fluid into third compartments (ascites, pleural effusion), an additional perfusion deficit can also arise. Extravascular fluid deficits can be replaced intravenously or subcutaneously. Intravenous fluid therapy enables more precise dosing, improved monitoring of the result and additionally, the speed of rehydration can be chosen. Basically, rehydration should be proportional to time of development of dehydration; this means that fluid losses in acute dehydration (e.g., massive vomiting with diarrhea) are replaced over 2 to 4 hours, while in more prolonged cases of dehydration the fluid deficit is replaced over 6 to 12 hours and in exceptional cases over 24 hours. Isotonic crystalloid solutions, such as Lactated Ringer's, are used in cases of dehydration because they are distributed effectively due to their normal osmotic pressure. The amount of fluid required depends on the degree of dehydration:

Rehydration volume (liter) = % dehydration × kg body weight / 100

The calculated amount of fluid required is administered over the time which the animal should be rehydrated. In addition to the fluid deficit, the maintenance requirements of the animal (2 ml/kg/h) should also be replaced.

12

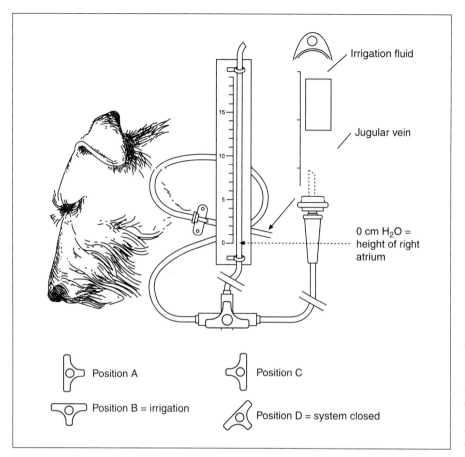

Fig. 12.16
The central venous pressure is measured using a jugular catheter which is connected via a fluid-filled tube to a manometer. The null point of the manometer is positioned at the height of the right atrium. Using a three-way tap in Position A, the manometer is filled. Afterwards, the three-way tap is turned to position C so that the manometer is connected to the jugular catheter and the height of the fluid column can adjust itself to the central venous pressure.

12.3.2.2 Blood pressure

Adequate perfusion is in part dependent on adequate blood pressure. The blood pressure can be measured directly using an arterial catheter or indirectly using oscillometry or Doppler methods (Fig. 12.17).

The mean arterial blood pressure (MAP) should be above 60 mmHg so that renal perfusion is ensured. The blood pressure is dependent on the intravascular volume, the heart function, and the vascular capacity. If the blood pressure is too low, then all three of these components must be optimized. When the blood pressure remains too low despite massive infusion therapy, then other causes must be investigated. Other causes of fluid loss (severe diarrhea, peritonitis), pain, hypoxia, hypothermia, cardiac dysfunction, electrolyte imbalance, brain stem lesions, or cardiac tamponade are all possible causes of hypotension and must be excluded. The measurement of CVP provides information about the intravascular volume. Heart problems must be excluded before either infusion therapy is maximized or vasopressor therapy is used.

Cardiac function can be increased by administering a continuous intravenous infusion of dobutamine (1–5 µg/kg/h in 5% dextrose). Dobutamine works as a positive inotropic agent increasing the cardiac output per minute. Due to the improved contractility, the oxygen requirements of the heart muscle is increased which is why good blood oxygenation needs to be ensured.

If hypotension persists despite normal intravascular volume and adequate contractility of the heart muscle, then vasopressors can be used. A continuous intravenous infusion of dopamine at a dosage of 5–10 µg/kg/h causes stimulation of the β_1-adrenergic receptors and results in increased contractility of the heart muscle and increased cardiac output. At a dosage of 10–20 µg/kg/h, dopamine mainly affects the α-receptors and leads to an increase in peripheral vascular resistance, which in turn raises the blood pressure. Regular control of the blood pressure is necessary and vasopressor therapy should be reduced as soon as the blood pressure is stable.

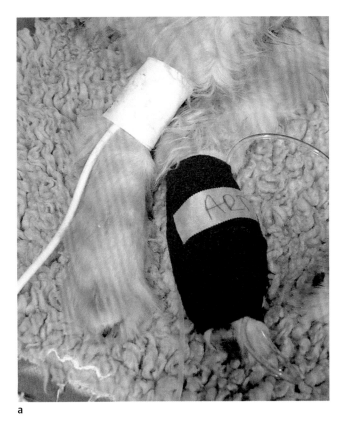

a

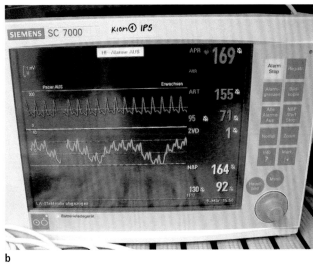

b

Fig. 12.17a, b
Blood pressure measurement via an arterial catheter (right foot) and a blood pressure cuff (a), which measures the systolic and diastolic blood pressure oscillometrically and calculates the mean blood pressure. (b) Continual presentation of the pressure curve (red curve).

12

Narcotics or sedatives / analgesics with a hypotensive effect (such as acepromazine or α_2-agonists) should not be used in hypotensive patients.

Severe hypertension needs to be restricted. Blood pressure persistently over 160 mmHg can lead to poor peripheral perfusion, retinal hemorrhage, myocardial hyperplasia, and renal damage. Basically, the underlying cause should be addressed. If this is not possible, vasodilators can be used, the choice of which depends on the cause of the hypertension.

12.3.2.3 Oncotic pressure

The intravascular volume is not only dependent on the osmotic pressure but also on oncotic or colloid osmotic pressure (COP). The COP is measured with an osmometer and should be between 20–25 mmHg.

Oncotically active infusion fluids include whole blood, plasma, dextran hydroxylethyl starch (Haes®, Volvuen®) and hemoglobin solution (Oxyglobin®).

Plasma contains relatively little albumin and is therefore not suitable for increasing the oncotic pressure. In patients with hypoproteinemia < 45 g/l or a hypoalbuminemia < 20 g/l, it can be assumed that the oncotic pressure is too low. After an initial intravenous bolus of 5–10 mg/kg of colloidal solution, maintenance of oncotic pressure is achieved by the continuous infusion of the colloid (e.g., hetastarch 1 ml/kg/h). In animals that eat and have an albumin concentration of > 20 g/l or a total protein > 50 g/l, it can be assumed that their own protein production is enough to maintain oncotic pressure.

12.3.2.4 Albumin

Albumin is not only important for the maintenance of oncotic pressure but is also responsible for the systemic transportation of hormones, cations and medications.

In association with systemic inflammation, a cytokine-induced suppression of albumin production can occur. Other possibilities leading to hypoalbuminemia are loss via the kidneys or gastrointestinal tract, liver insufficiency, and massive infusion therapy (dilution effect).

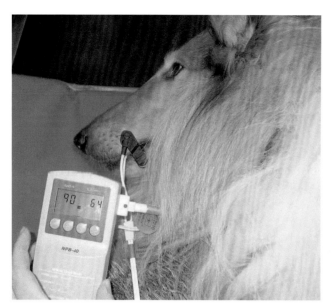

Fig. 12.18
Measurement of oxygen saturation using a pulse oximeter.

With decreasing blood albumin concentrations, the interstitial reserves of albumin are released. This albumin pool is also refilled when the blood albumin is replaced.

The albumin concentration in intensive-care patients should ideally be over 20 g/l. Animals with albumin concentrations below 15–20 g/l should be given albumin, plasma or whole blood to maintain albumin functions. However, 5 ml plasma/kg body weight is needed to increase the blood albumin by 1 g/l! The loss of albumin is also an indicator of the loss of other similar small proteins from the blood (e.g., antithrombin and coagulation factors), which cannot be measured using conventional laboratory methods. Some patients, therefore, will profit from plasma transfusions as plasma also contains these important molecules.

12.3.2.5 Heart function and rhythm

Arrhythmias and cardiac dysfunction can occur in neurological intensive-care patients in association with intracranial lesions or as a pre-existing problem.

Careful heart auscultation should be performed daily in the neurological intensive-care patient as abnormal heart sounds or arrhythmias can occur suddenly. Abnormal heart sounds are often only audible at a single position: in cats: often directly next to the sternum between ribs 4 and 7.

Cardiomyopathy can make cardiovascular stabilization very difficult, especially when the cardiac problem is secondary to other problems, such as sepsis or hypovolemia, which require intensive fluid therapy. Cats often have signs of hypertrophic cardiomyopathy without showing any clinical symptoms. Suddenly occurring abnormal heart sounds or "gallop" rhythms after fluid therapy are, therefore, not uncommon in this species. Cats with decompensating heart problems show at least one of the following symptoms: abnormal heart sounds or "gallop" rhythm, hypothermia, bradycardia, or increased to moist lung sounds. Cardiomyopathy must be excluded in cats that show any of these symptoms.

Cardiomyopathy can be dilated, hypertrophic or intermediary. Therapy depends on the type and degree of change as well as the clinical symptoms. Careful fluid therapy and continual monitoring are essential. A central venous catheter for measuring CVP makes the interpretation of perfusion and heart function easier.

A suddenly onset of abnormal heart sounds in the neurosurgical intensive-care patient can be associated with endocarditis or thrombosis. These complications should be excluded using echocardiography.

Patients with systemic inflammation often show arrhythmias secondary to hypovolemia and/or hypoxia. Inflammatory mediators (i.e., myocardial depressant factor) can, in addition to inducing arrhythmias, cause reduced myocardial contractility. In patients with arrhythmias, extracardiac causes such as hypoxia, hypovolemia, pain, and electrolyte imbalance should be excluded or counteracted before antiarrhythmic agents are used. Hypokalemia, hyperkalemia, hypocalcemia, hypercalcemia, and acidosis are common causes of arrhythmias.

Persistent arrhythmias are usually only treated with antiarrhythmics when they negatively affect perfusion (pulse deficit, reduced CRT, etc.). Antiarrhythmic therapy is directed at the type and frequency of the arrhythmia. An ECG is, therefore, necessary.

Patients with cardiac problems benefit from oxygen therapy. Ketamine should be avoided as it increases the oxygen requirement of the myocardium. For the same reason, hypotensive-acting medications should not be used.

12.3.2.6 Oxygenation and ventilation

Tachynpnea, dyspnea, cyanotic mucous membranes, increased lung sounds, "rattling", as well as inaudible lung sounds are all signs of respiratory problems and require further clarification. Measuring the blood oxygen saturation is a simple method for evaluating oxygenation and should be at least 95% (Fig. 12.18). Arterial blood gas analysis is a more invasive method; however, it allows the differentiation between an oxygenation and a ventilation problem.

Hypoxemic patients ($SpO_2 < 95\%$ or $PaCO_2 < 80$ mmHg) should be given oxygen therapy via a nasal catheter, oxygen tent or oxygen cage. Under certain circumstances, the animals must be intubated and given 100% oxygen with positive-pressure artificial respiration. Nasal tubes are contraindicated in patients with head injuries or increased ICP, as they can cause sneezing which leads to a massive increase in ICP.

Hypoventilation can be due to central or peripheral causes. The respiratory centre is in the medulla oblongata. Changes in its cell milieu or environment can lead to an altered respiratory pattern and hypoventilation. The peripheral causes of hypoventilation include neuromuscular disease affecting the thoracic musculature, paralysis of the phrenic nerve, or high cervical lesions of the spinal cord. An increase in the $PaCO_2$ leads to vasoconstriction, acidosis, and secondarily to disturbances in consciousness. Animals with hypoventilation ($PaCO_2 > 60$ mmHg) should be given artificial respiration.

Animals with a reduced degree of consciousness are liable to suffer from aspiration pneumonia. Comatose patients should therefore be intubated.

12.3.2.7 Glucose

The CNS is totally reliant on glucose as its energy source. The blood glucose value should lie between 5–8 mmol/l. Hyperglycemia leads to an increase in cellular metabolism and lactate production and can be just as damaging as hypoglycemia.

Hypoglycemia can lead to seizures and cell damage. The causes of hypoglycemia include trauma, sepsis, neoplasia, liver insufficiency, and starvation in puppies. The supplementation of glucose in hypoglycemia can be achieved by the administration of glucose in an isotonic crystalloid solution (5% glucose solution). When necessary, a bolus of 0.5–1 ml/kg diluted 50% glucose solution can be given, followed by a continuous 2.5% glucose infusion. Glucose-containing solutions should **not** be used for initial shock therapy, only as maintenance infusions and must be given intravenously.

12.3.2.8 Electrolyte and acid-base balance

In the neurological intensive-care patient, electrolyte changes can be secondary to or the primary causes of the neurological abnormalities. Both hypernatraemia and hyponatraemia can lead to CNS disturbances. The **sodium** concentration reflects the amount of intravascular free water. Hypernatraemia is an indication of a water deficit typically caused by dehydration, renal disease or diabetes insipidus (central or nephrogenic). Hypernatraemia leads to an increase in osmolarity. If the blood-brain barrier is intact, this then results in water movement out of the brain, causing neuronal dehydration. Accordingly, **acute hypernatraemia** must be corrected as quickly as possible. Once the intravascular volume has been corrected with isotonic crystalloid solutions, the water deficit is replaced with a hypotonic solution (dextrose mixture). The water deficit is calculated as follows:

Water deficit = 0.6 × kg body weight × [(serum sodium/145) − 1]

If hypernatremia occurs slowly, the brain can protect itself by producing so-called idiogenic osmoles, which increase the osmolarity of the brain tissue so that the same osmolarity is present on both sides of the blood-brain barrier. The production and degradation of idiogenic osmoles requires hours to days. Therefore, in the case of **chronic hypernatraemia**, serum sodium must be therapeutically reduced over hours to days so that brain oedema does not form. As a rule, the sodium concentration should be reduced by 1 mmol/l/h at the most. The infusion solution should have only a slightly reduced sodium concentration (e.g., NaCl 0.9% or a mixture with hypertonic NaCl). Regular monitoring of the serum sodium concentration (every 2–6 h) and subsequent adaption of the infusion solution are necessary.

Hyponatremia tends to be infrequent in neurological intensive-care patients with normal renal function. Pseudohyponatremia is seen with hyperproteinemia and hypertriglyceridemia, and reflects excessive binding of sodium molecules rather than an actual deficit. In such cases, the acute changes should be corrected quickly and the chronic changes more slowly.

Serum potassium should also be regularly monitored and where necessary administered, especially as serum potassium levels are often low in association with inappetence and the majority of commercial infusion solutions do not contain enough potassium, which causes a dilution effect. The amount of potassium administered depends on the deficit and should not be more than 0.5 mEq/kg/h (Table 12.10).

Hyperkalaemia is principally seen in association with renal or urinary tract problems and massive muscle trauma. Bradycardia and arrhythmia are typical symptoms of hyperkalaemia; however, in cats the heart rate is not a reliable sign of potassium changes. Immediate therapy must be started in cats with bradycardia due to hyperkalaemia as otherwise there is

12

Table 12.10: Potassium substitution

Serum potassium (mmol/l)	mEq potassium per 250 ml infusion solution	mEq potassium per liter infusion solution	Maximal infusion rate (ml/kg/h)
3.1–3.5	7	28	16
2.6–3.0	10	40	12
2.1–2.5	15	60	8
< 2.0	20	80	6

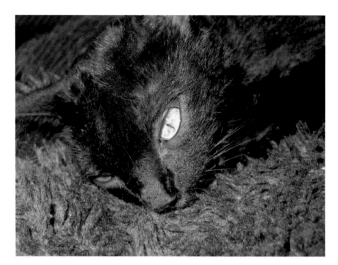

Fig. 12.19
A non-responsive miotic pupil can be a sign of raised intracranial pressure.

12

an acute danger of cardiac arrest. Immediate treatment is also necessary with arrhythmias or the typical ECG changes, such as a flat and prolonged P-wave and a high T peak, in order to prevent life-threatening disturbances from developing (Table 12.11).

Calcium is important for neuromuscular function. Hypocalcaemia can lead to trembling and/or seizures. Symptomatic hypocalcaemia is treated with a calcium bolus (calcium gluconate 100 mg/kg IV over 20 minutes). As hypercalcaemia can lead to cardiac arrhythmia, the calcium infusion should be performed under ECG control.

Potassium bromide is often incorrectly interpreted by many measuring instruments as chloride, which can lead to falsely increased chloride values.

Other electrolyte changes tend to be rare in the neurological intensive-care patient. However, electrolyte changes should be excluded in cases of inexplicable muscle weakness, seizures, massive infusion therapy, inappetence or arrhythmia.

Acid-base changes can be seen as either a primary or secondary problem in neurological intensive-care patients. Metabolic acidosis occurs with reduced perfusion, trauma, seizures and hyperthermia. It corrects itself if adequate fluid therapy is given and the underlying cause is removed. Hypoventilation caused by CNS or neuromuscular disease can lead to respiratory acidosis. The only treatment possible is intubation and artificial respiration. Bicarbonate is contraindicated in such cases as this leads to an increase in CO_2.

An increase in the anion gap (AG > 20 in the dog, AG > 27 in the cat) occurs in intoxications such as ethylene glycol, methanol, ethanol and aspirin as well as with severe rhabdomyolysis. The treatment consists of fluid therapy and the treatment of the primary cause.

12.3.2.9 Intracranial pressure and consciousness

A neurological investigation should be undertaken at least once daily. Monitoring of the consciousness is essential in neurological patients. Each degeneration of the state of consciousness and the neurological symptoms should be treated as potentially serious (Fig. 12.19). The causes of degeneration in consciousness are hypovolemia, hypoxia, hypoglycemia, electrolyte changes (sodium, potassium), hepatic encephalopathy, renal failure, sepsis, and changes in the intercranial pressure (ICP).

Hyperosmolarity or rapid changes in the osmolarity are frequent causes of changes in the degree of consciousness. The serum osmolarity should not be more than 320 mOsm/kg (see also Chap. 12.3.2.8). The exact serum osmolarity can only be measured using special methods, but it can be approximated quite simply:

Serum osmolarity (mOsm/kg) = 2 × Na^{2+} (mmol/l) + glucose (mmol/l) + BUN (mmol/l)

The ICP is not measurable under normal clinical conditions. The normal ICP in humans is 0–15 mmHg, and in dogs it is approximately 8–12 mmHg. The clinical symptoms of increased ICP are reduced pupillary reflex, stupor to coma, changes in the character of the respiration, bradycardia with concomitant hypertension, and cardiac arrhythmia. An increase in ICP leads to a reduction in the cerebral perfusion pressure (CPP). The maintenance of CPP is essential for life. From the following formula:

CPP = MAP – ICP

Table 12.11: Hyperkalemia therapy

Therapy	Dosage	Mechanism
Infusion with crystalloids	5–10 ml/kg/h	Diuresis
Glucose	1 ml/kg 50% glucose solution IV undiluted	Uptake of K$^+$ with glucose into the cells
Glucose and insulin	0.2 IU/kg insulin IV/IM + 1 g glucose per unit of insulin IV	Uptake of K$^+$ with glucose into the cells
Calcium gluconate	100 mg/kg IV over 20 min	Antagonism of K$^+$ effects on the heart
Sodium bicarbonate	1–2 mEq/kg over 30 min	Shift of K$^+$ out of the cells in exchange for H$^+$

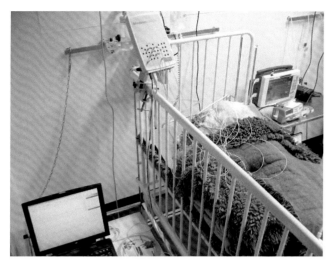

Fig. 12.20
Additional neurological investigations, for example, an electroencephalogram (EEG) can also be performed in comatose patients on the intensive station.

it can be seen that a cerebral perfusion pressure of 70–80 mmHg can be maintained by either having a mean arterial blood pressure (MAP) of at least 80–90 mmHg or by reducing the ICP. The maintenance of MAP can be achieved with adequate fluid therapy. Reducing the ICP can be achieved by placing the upper body above the lower (30° slope), giving mannitol (0.25–1 g/kg IV as bolus over 20 min; when necessary repeating after 2–4 h, 2 to 3 times), normalizing oxygenation and ventilation, inducing a slight hypothermia, or providing sedation. Hypoxia and hypercapnia lead to vasoconstriction and secondary ischemia, and must be avoided. Further details can be found in Chap. 12.2.1.

Other neurological investigations are indicated depending on the individual case and in certain circumstances in critical patients be undertaken in the intensive-care unit (Fig. 12.20).

12.3.2.10 Haemostasis
Hemostasis is an interplay between primary hemostasis, the coagulation cascade, antithrombosis, fibrinolysis and antifibrinolysis. All these systems are also closely connected to the different inflammatory systems.

Haemorrhage can occur due to thrombocytopaenia or thrombocytopathy, coagulation factor deficiency, or tissue damage. As the skull and the spine form a reasonably closed system, haemorrhage in the brain or spinal cord can lead to severe damage and classical symptoms of neuraxis compression.

The thrombocyte count can easily be judged on a blood smear. Each thrombocyte seen on a high-power field under the microscope is equivalent to approx. 15,000 thrombocytes.

Spontaneous bleeding first occurs, as a rule, when there are less than 40–50,000 thrombocytes. Thrombocytopathies can also lead to haemorrhage despite the presence of a correct number of thrombocytes. Thrombocyte function is tested using buccal mucosa bleeding time (BMBT). The treatment of thrombocytopaenia or thrombocytopathies is dependent on the cause (e.g., immune-mediated) and is often difficult. If available, thrombocyte infusions can be given.

Disturbances in the coagulation cascade can be caused by a reduced production (rodenticide intoxication, liver failure) or increased usage (massive bleeding, DIC). These can be diagnosed by the prothrombin time (PT), partial thromboplastin time (PTT) or the activated coagulation time (ACT). Normal values are dependent on the method used in the test. Treatment consists of administration of fresh frozen plasma and, if necessary, vitamin K.

Thromboses occur with DIC, antithrombin deficiency, vascular stasis, and tissue damage. They can also lead to neurological symptoms.

Every neurological patient can potentially develop hemorrhage or thromboemboli. Blood stasis, hypotension, tissue damage, systemic inflammation, haemolysis, or pansystemic diseases increase the risk of DIC. This condition can occur initially without any clinical symptoms. The aim is to recognize DIC as early as possible so that multiple organ failure due to microthrombi and bleeding can be prevented. Unfortunately, there are no definitive diagnostic tests for DIC. Thrombocytopaenia followed by prolonged coagulation times (initially shortened, but this phase is usually missed), reduced fibrin values, and increased fibrin degradation products are indications of DIC. The thrombocyte count and ACT should be controlled at least once daily in critical patients. If petechiae and haemorrhage occurs, then it must be assumed that a late stage of DIC is present. The prophylaxis and treatment of DIC are very similar: optimal perfusion and oxygenation must be ensured, and blood stasis must be prevented whenever possible.

The underlying cause should be treated (endotoxins, abscess, etc.). Lungs, kidneys, heart, brain and the gastrointestinal tract are susceptible to microthrombi and ischemia, and must be supported by treatment. Coagulation factors can be replaced by infusing freshly frozen plasma at a dosage of 6–10 ml/kg over 2 to 6 hours, repeated every 8 to 12 hours. It should be noted that coagulation factors are destroyed in plasma older than 6 h.

12.3.2.11 Erythrocytes and hemoglobin
The oxygen concentration of the blood (PaO_2) is mainly dependent on the haemoglobin concentration (Hb) and so indirectly on the haematocrit.

$$PaO_2 = (1.34 \times Hb \times SpO_2) + (0.003 \times PaO_2)$$

12

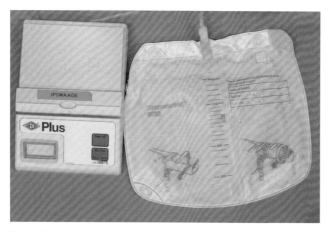

Fig. 12.21
The amount of urine produced is regularly calculated (*outs*) and compared with the amount of fluid infused (*ins*). Other fluid losses should also be included in the *outs* (vomiting, diarrhea).

12

A hematocrit value between 27 and 33% is optimal for oxygen transportation, and should be stabilized in anaemic patients to lie within this range. The haematocrit value can also be helpful in interpretation of the fluid balance: an increase in the haematocrit within hours is always an indication of fluid loss.

Compatibility must be ensured with the transfusion of whole blood or erythrocyte concentrates. In dogs, the first blood transfusion, as a rule, presents no problem as dogs do not naturally have any antibodies against other blood groups. A cross reaction test is, however, usually recommended. Such a cross reaction test is obligatory in dogs which have already received a blood transfusion, bitches which have had puppies, and in all cats.

Synthetic hemoglobin-containing products such as Oxyglobin® are new on the market. These infusion solutions contain polymerized bovine hemoglobin in a modified Lactated Ringer's solution. They massively increase the oxygen-carrying capacity of the blood due to the free hemoglobin. In addition, they act as plasma expanders and appear to improve the microcapillary perfusion and oxygenation as the molecules are smaller than erythrocytes. Oxyglobin® can be given to dogs as a single dose of 10–30 ml/kg infused over a number of hours (maximum 10 ml/kg/h). This product should be given in very small doses to cats as they are more susceptible to an overdose (initial bolus 2 ml/kg, afterwards 0.5–1 ml/kg/h). Oxyglobin® colors the serum orange and falsifies results of photometric enzyme activities (liver enzymes). The resulting icterus, however, does not interfere with measurement of oxygen saturation.

12.3.2.12 Immune status, leucocytes and antibiosis

The ability of the body to defend itself from infections can be monitored using the leucocyte count, left shifts, fever and immunoglobulin production. Increasing leucocyte count with a left shift and fever are signs of an uncontrolled infection. Bacterial infections are rare in neurological intensive-care patients. Intensive-care patients are, however, at risk of secondary bacterial infections due to aspiration pneumonia, intravenous catheters, and bacterial translocation in the gastrointestinal tract.

Immunosuppressed animals with neutropaenia require strict aseptic nursing and minimally invasive monitoring to prevent the occurrence of life-threatening secondary infections with or without hospital-acquired bacteria.

Antibiotic therapy should be undertaken based on the results of bacterial culture and sensitivity testing. Until the results of the bacterial culture are available, a Gram's stain of a cytological preparation can make the initial choice of antibiotic easier. Further information concerning antibiosis and therapy of specific infectious diseases can be found in Chap. 9.1.

12.3.2.13 Renal function and urine production

Urine production is dependant on the intravascular volume, the heart function, and the function of the kidneys and the urinary tract. All hypotensive patients are in danger of having renal failure. Urea, creatinine and electrolytes should, if possible, be measured before fluid therapy is initiated and monitored daily in risk patients. Initial prerenal azotemia should normalize after fluid therapy. Urine analysis provides further information with respect to renal function: a low specific gravity in connection with azotemia, proteinuria, glucosuria without hyperglycemia, and casts in the urine sediment are signs of kidney problems and should be further evaluated. With reduced urine production or azotemia, the intravascular volume should be determined first of all.

The MAP should be at least 60 mmHg. A sterile urethral catheter connected to a urine bag should be placed in cases of reduced urine production, disturbances in emptying of the bladder (associated with LMN or UMN dysfunction), or intensive fluid therapy (Fig. 12.21). This allows the amount of urine produced to be measured exactly and to be compared with the amount being infused (comparison of *ins* and *outs*).

Furosemide is a loop diuretic and can be given at a dosage of 2 mg/kg IV in acute renal failure and repeated when needed every hour. Mannitol can also be used (0.5 g/kg) except in cases of anuria.

12.3.2.14 Gastrointestinal tract

Intensive-care patients often suffer from secondary disturbances in their gastrointestinal motility; e.g., gastric paresis, paralytic ileus, or gastric ulceration. The causes of reduced gastrointestinal motility include abdominal surgery, anaesthesia, opioids, neuromuscular problems, and hypokalaemia. Reduced motility or a total lack of motility leads to vomiting, bacterial translocation, poor digestion and absorption, as well as potentiates gastric ulceration. Gastric ulceration can occur subclinically; however, it leads to an increased risk of bacterial translocation, blood loss and gastric paresis. The auscultation of intestinal sounds is a simple and helpful means of judging intestinal peristalsis. Sonography can confirm reduced or absent peristalsis and can provide additional information about its severity and possible cause. Once an obstructive cause of the reduced motility has been excluded, metoclopramide can be given as a continuous infusion (0.01–0.08 mg/kg/h). Additionally, the placement of a nasogastric tube is recommended to remove any accumulated gastric juices before vomiting and aspiration occurs. The tube also enables enteral feeding to be performed.

The prophylactic use of H_2-blockers is controversial as changes in the pH value of the stomach can enable gastric bacterial translocation and they can induce severe aspiration pneumonia when vomited or refluxed. Prophylactic gastric ulcer therapy with ranitidine (0.5–1 mg/kg IV, PO q 12 h) and sucralfate (0.5–1 g per animal PO q 8 h) are recommended when administering steroid therapy. Continuous vomiting should be suppressed using metoclopramide (0.1–0.5 mg/kg SC, IM, IV) or a phenothiazine such as thiethylperazine (dog: 0.1–0.4 mg/kg; cat: 0.1–0.2 mg/kg IM, IV). Both of these medications can cause sedation, making the assessment of disturbances in consciousness difficult. Intestinal obstructions must be excluded before metoclopramide is used as this medication leads to an increase in intestinal peristalsis.

Hypermotility can also be a pre- or postoperative complication. It can lead to abdominal pain, maldigestion / malabsorption, or intussusception. Metamizole at a dosage of 50 mg/kg slow IV q 6–8 h is an effective analgesic against abdominal pain associated with intestinal spasms.

12.3.2.15 Nutrition

Early feeding of a balanced diet is an important aspect of intensive care and is often neglected. Energy and protein deficiency quickly lead to reduced immune defense, muscle degeneration and weakness, as well as the collapse of the gastrointestinal barrier with the subsequent risk of sepsis and multiple organ failure. Early enteral nutrition with small amounts of high quality nutrients for the enterocytes is very important for maintenance of the intestinal mucosal barrier and the prevention of bacterial translocation followed by sepsis and organ failure. Oral glucose solutions (0.5–2 ml/kg PO q 1–2 h) also reduce the occurrence of gastric micro-ulcers.

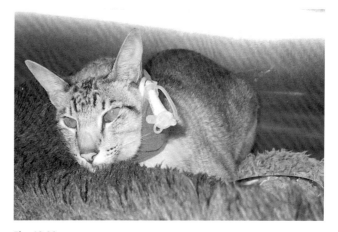

Fig. 12.22
Oesophageal feeding tube.

Enteral nutrition should therefore be started as soon as possible and can be easily given to anorectic animals using nasogastric, nasoesophageal, or oesophageal tubes (Fig. 12.22). The choice of tube depends on the basic disease affecting the patient, the functional nature of the larynx, oesophagus, and stomach as well as the assumed length of time needed for feeding by tube. The longer the animal has been anorexic, the slower the increase in calorie content and amount of feed given can be. In the first few hours, only water is given. Afterwards, a slow increase in volume and calorie concentration can be undertaken so that after 3 days the full amount of food required is fed.

The basal energy requirements at rest (RER: resting energy requirement) is the same for all patients:

RER (kcal) = (30 × kg body weight) + 70

Depending on the energy requirements of the disease (i.e., sepsis versus coma), the RER is multiplied by a factor of 1.2–1.5. This provides the IER (illness energy requirement). Partial parenteral nutrition with amino acid solutions or total parenteral nutrition is often necessary in completely inappetent intensive-care patients in order to cover their high energy requirements. Feeding after a long period of anorexia and parenteral nutrition can lead to a massive change in the electrolyte and glucose balance. As a result, these parameters should be monitored daily.

Anorexic cats are in danger of developing hepatic lipidosis and, in contrast to dogs, need arginine, vitamin A, niacin, arachidonic acid, and taurine added to their dietary formulations.

12

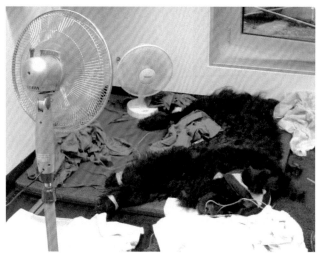

Fig. 12.23
Active cooling of a dog with hyperthermia using wet materials and electric fans.

12.3.2.16   Medication metabolism and dosage

Medication dosage should be adapted daily to the patient's body weight and underlying disease. Animals with renal and / or liver problems require reduced dosages, especially of those medications which are metabolized in the liver or excreted by the kidneys. The dosage of medications which have possible catastrophic effects when overdosed (e.g., insulin, aminoglycosides, dopamine or dobutamine) should be calculated anew each day in order to prevent fatal complications due to miscalculation or transcription mistakes.

The compatibility of medications in patients which receive a number of medications should also be ascertained. Cats often require lower dosages and the species-specific recommendations must be upheld.

12.3.2.17   Analgesia

Pain can be expressed in animals as tachycardia, tachypnea, hypertension, restlessness, depression to stupor, or aggression. The treatment of pain is not only important for ethical reasons, but it is also essential for the stabilization and interpretation of the circulation. Patients in pain show clinical signs similar to that of shock. Information about specific pain therapies as well as the advantages and disadvantages of the diverse groups of analgesics (including dosage) are to be found in Chap. 9.3.

12.3.2.18   Body temperature

The control of the body temperature is not only part of the initial therapy, but also an important aspect of monitoring the neurological intensive-care patient. Changes in body temperature in intensive-care patients can be due to extremes in ambient temperature or secondary to disease (hypothermia in shock patients; hyperthermia in status epilepticus). A prolonged abnormal body temperature can have serious consequences such as renal failure, muscle breakdown, acid-base disturbances or cardiac arrhythmia.

Hypothermia leads to a slower conduction in the heart, reduction of the metabolic processes, and reduces the body's oxygen requirements. This can be advantageous in certain circumstances (e.g., brain oedema). However, after the start of shivering due to cold, muscle contractions lead to a massive increase in metabolic processes and oxygen requirements. Hypothermia should be normalized using active warming (heating pads, warm infusions, blankets, Bair-Hugger®). When a drop in body temperature occurs in a previously stable patient, a reduction in cardiac function must be investigated.

The causes of hyperthermia include heat stroke (infra-red lamps), status epilepticus, inadequate ventilation of rooms, pyrogen release with inflammatory conditions, or a disturbance of the CNS thermoregulatory centre. The possible consequences include hyperventilation, dehydration, shock, acidosis, acute renal insufficiency, cerebrocortical necrosis, and DIC. Hyperthermia is treated primarily with infusion therapy and cooling (cold wet cloths, cold hairdryer) before NSAIDs are used (Fig. 12.23). Only when body temperatures cannot be reduced below 40°C should a single dose of an antipyretic be given. The cooling measures should be stopped once the body temperature has dropped below 39.5°C to prevent the development of hypothermia.

The choice of antibiotics used in patients with possible infections should be re-evaluated.

12.3.2.19   Bandages and wounds

Wounds should be inspected daily and the bandages changed at least once a day. Wet or dirty bandages must always be changed. Skin incisions should be checked for redness, excretion and integrity. Ecchymoses and haematomas around the surgical site should be marked with a waterproof marker so that a possible extension can readily be seen. The coagulation status of the patient should be monitored if ecchymoses are seen to enlarge, so that DIC or vasculitis can be excluded.

12.3.2.20 General nursing

Intravenous catheters, wounds, etc. should be controlled at least once a day. General hygiene is very important. If the animals cannot clean themselves, it must be ensured that they are dry and clean. Animals in lateral recumbency should be turned at least every 4 h or should be placed in sternal recumbency to reduce dependent congestion of the lungs. Passive physiotherapy and massage maintain the muscle tone and perfusion of the limbs and so reduces the risk of thromboemboli. Pressure weals and pressure necrosis should not develop with soft and dry bedding (Fig. 12.24); though once present they should be treated adequately.

In critically ill animals, surgical gloves should be used when dealing with all catheters, tubes and drains to prevent the development of nosocomial infections.

The recording of case history and the treatment protocols should also be performed during a period of intensive care. The use of the "Rule of 20" is an important part of this process.

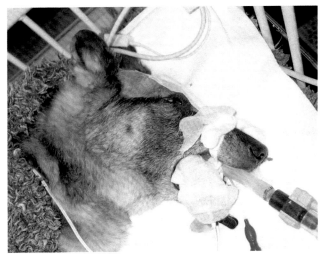

Fig. 12.24
A soft bed, regular turning, control of the body temperature, keeping the mucous membranes and cornea moist, and oral hygiene are all part of intensive care.

Further reading

BAGLEY, R.S., HARRINGTON, M.L., PLUHAR, G.E. et al. (1996): Effect of craniectomy / durotomy alone and in combination with hyperventilation, diuretics, and corticosteroids on intracranial pressure in clinically normal dogs. Am J Vet Res. **57**: 116–119.

HARRINGTON, M.L., BAGLEY, R.S., MOORE, M.P. et al. (1996): Effect of craniectomy, durotomy, and wound closure on intracranial pressure in healthy cats. Am J Vet Res. **57**: 1659–1661.

PURVIS, D., KIRBY, R. (1994): Systemic inflammatory response syndrom: Septic Shock. Vet Clin North Am. (Small Anim Pract.) **24** 1225–1248.

KIRBY, R. (1995): Current Veterinary Therapy XII. Saunders, Philadelphia, p. 139

SPRENG, D.E., SPRENG, R., KIRBY, R., SCHAWALDER, P. (1996): Überwachung des Notfall- und Intensivpatienten: Einfache diagnostische Hilfsmittel. Schweiz. Arch. Tierheilkunde 138: 11: 537–545

RUDLOFF, E., KIRBY R. (1998): Fluid Therapy. Vet Clin North Am. (Small Anim Pract.) **28** 297–328.

12

13 Peripheral Nervous System and Musculature

Dominik Faissler
Konrad Jurina
Laurent Cauzinille
Frédéric Gaschen
Fillipo Adama
André Jaggy

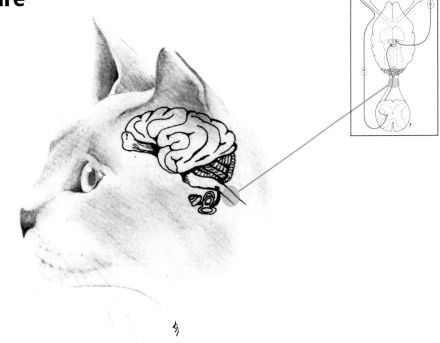

13.1 Introduction

The peripheral nervous system (PNS) exists as a connection between the brain stem or spinal cord and the musculature, glands and sensory receptors. In the dog and cat, the PNS consists of 12 pairs of cranial nerves and 36 paired spinal nerves. It can be divided into a somatomotor, a somatosensory and an autonomic part. Most peripheral nerves are mixed and contain motor, sensory and autonomic fibres. It is difficult to differentiate these three parts from each other under practical clinical conditions. Despite this, it makes sense for didactic purposes to consider each of these three parts separately. Strictly speaking, the musculature is not part of the PNS; however, there is a very close functional relationship between them. In the following, the terms PNS and lower motor neuron system (LMNS) are considered as being the same to make the terminology simpler and to help improve the understanding of this difficult chapter – although, as mentioned, this is not anatomically correct.

13.1.1. Classification of the changes in the PNS

Neuropathies and myopathies can be differentiated using various criteria. A system of classification is necessary because of the large number of different diseases affecting these structures, otherwise one may lose ones orientation and important diseases can be forgotten. The clinical picture of individual structures is very similar. Apart from primary disturbances of the autonomic and sensory nervous systems, motor symptoms usually predominate in LMNS diseases. For the diagnosis, therapy and prognosis, it is important to localise the segment of the LMNS which is predominantly affected. Different classifications are sensible and improve the understanding of disturbances of the PNS or LMNS.

13.1.1.1 Classification according to the differential diagnosis

The most useful and clinically helpful classification of LMNS disease is differentiation according to aetiology. The VITAMIN D principle can be used without any limitations for all forms of neuropathy, neuromuscular transmission disturbances and myopathies.

13

13.1.1.2 Classification according to anatomical localisation

An anatomical classification of disease is helpful in many cases. The clinically important structures are α-motor neuron, nerve root, nerve, synapse, sensory nerve fibres with their dorsal ganglia, and the autonomic nervous system.

The anatomical localisation provides an indication about the pathological mechanisms involved. Diseases of the α-motor neurons are often inherited and degenerative. Disturbances of the nerve roots and the proximal nerves in monoparesis are caused by trauma or neoplasia, while in polyneuropathies they are induced by inflammatory changes. The basic causes of distal neuropathies are commonly metabolic, idiopathic or degenerative diseases. Abnormal signal transmission in the synapse is often caused by an immunological or toxic agent.

The pathological mechanisms that adversely influence the function of muscle fibres are multiple. Reduced blood and energy supply compromises the function of the sodium-potassium pump, which limits the coupling and decoupling of actin and myosin. In severe cases, this can mean the death of the cell. Inflammatory infiltrates hinder the interaction between the contractile elements. In chronic cases, muscle fibres are destroyed and replaced by fibrous tissue. Electrolyte disturbances limit the transmission of the postsynaptic action potential that normally causes the release of calcium in the sarcolemma and so, the interaction between actin and myosin.

Many degenerative muscle diseases are caused by gene mutation. Due to an abnormal expression of dystrophin or other structural proteins, continual muscle fibre degeneration becomes programmed from birth. Dystrophin is a component of the sarcolemma and most probably plays a role in the interaction between the solid and the contractile elements of the striated muscle cell. Genetic defects in the chloride and sodium channels prevent rapid depolarisation of the membrane and lead to myotonia with muscle hypertrophy. Specific inherited enzyme defects can cause an exertion-dependent increase in lactate as well as muscle cell necrosis.

13.1.1.3 Classification according to pathological processes

The PNS can only show a limited number of pathological reaction mechanisms, none of which are specific for the primary cause of the disease. The reaction pattern of muscle to different noxious agents is relatively limited and their clinical manifestation is non-specific. Common pathological changes are:

Wallerian-like degeneration

Traumatic damage to a nerve leads to degeneration of the axon distal to the injury site with secondary demyelination and rapidly progressive neurogenic muscle atrophy. Chromatolysis occurs in the affected neurons. If the basal membrane of the nerve has not been severed, the axon can grow again. Complete transection of the nerve root with subsequent Wallerian-like degeneration is irreversible.

Degeneration of the axon

Swelling of the axon is most probably due to disturbance in the synthesis of neurofilaments and microtubuli. The accumulation of neurofilaments and microtubuli occurs mainly in the proximal part of the axon; the distal part of the axon degenerates. Secondary demyelination with muscle atrophy becomes visible, similar to that of Wallerian-like degeneration.

Another form of axon degeneration is distal axonopathy also known as dying-back neuropathy. The degeneration of the axon begins first of all at the nerve end and continues during the course of the disease to more proximal regions. This is mainly superseded by a slow secondary demyelination with neurogenic muscle atrophy.

Budding axons (a sign of regeneration) occur rarely. This syndrom is still not well understood. A disturbance of the rapid transport of metabolites in the distal nerve segments or disturbed return transport is presumed to occur. Metabolic, toxic, idiopathic and above all, degenerative causes are predominantly responsible for axon degeneration.

Demyelination

Primary loss of myelin occurs either due to damage to the Schwann cells or due to direct destruction of the myelin. The demyelination often affects the paranodal regions or certain specific segments of the nerve and is called either paranodal or segmental demyelination, respectively. Muscle atrophy usually does not occur in primary demyelination. Due to subsequent proliferation of Schwann cells, regeneration or remyelination is possible. Chronic demyelination and remyelination lead to "onion-bulb" proliferations around the nerve.

Transmission disturbances in the synapse

The causes of abnormal impulse transmission at the synapse are reduced neurotransmitter release from the presynaptic membrane, abnormal neurotransmitter metabolism in the synaptic space, or abnormal postsynaptic receptor function.

Abnormal contractility of the muscle fibres

Mechanical or electromechanical decoupling or the loss of muscle fibres leads to their dysfunction. The most common mechanisms have a degenerative, inflammatory or metabolic nature. Vascular disturbances are significant in cats (i.e. ischemic neuropathy).

13.1.2 Clinical symptoms

The most frequently occurring motor nerve deficits are paraparesis, tetraparesis, tetraplegia, reduced to absent spinal reflexes and reduced to absent muscle tone. Rapid progressive muscle atrophy can be another indicator of abnormal LMNS function. While motor deficits are at the forefront of diseases of the musculature, there are also sensory and autonomic deficits seen with neuropathies and disturbances of the synapses (e.g., Horner's syndrome, bradycardia or reduced tear production). The signs which indicate a disturbance of the sensory nervous system are ataxia, abnormal proprioception, dysaesthesia and the loss of nociception. The majority of diseases result in a mixed collection of clinical signs. Syndromes with predominantly sensory symptoms are rare. This also holds true for autonomic deficits, as primary autonomic nervous system disturbances only occur sporadically.

It should be noted that initially in many diseases of the LMNS, the hindlimbs are more obviously affected. It is also important to understand that abnormal cranial nerve function is frequently due to a generalised LMNS disease. The diagnosis of a megaoesophagus is potentially serious, so investigation for dysphagia is an important part of the clinical examination of the LMNS case.

Table 13.1 can aid in classifying motor, sensory or autonomic deficits which affect the α-motor neuron, nerve, synapse or muscle. In certain cases, the clinical examination alone can indicate a localisation to the LMNS. However, adjunct specialised investigations are necessary to confirm the diagnosis of PNS disease and to determine the affected part of this system.

13.1.3 Adjunct investigations

In monoparesis and monoplegia, the predominant pathologies include compressive, traumatic and neoplastic disease of the nerve, or focal inflammatory and idiopathic muscle disease. The key question in these patients is whether it is a neurological or an orthopaedic problem. Although the clinical results are important here too, other investigations must be done in many patients to answer this question. Flow diagram 13.1 describes one possible method of deciding which investigations need to be done. Resolution of the diagnosis can be very complex and time-consuming in patients with complicated case histories. The severity of the disease and the expectations of the owner are very important in such cases.

In generalised disturbances of the LMNS, the basic causes include inflammatory, metabolic, idiopathic, paraneoplastic and degenerative groups of diseases.

A systematic procedure is necessary in the search for all the possible causes. The clinical examination has a high degree of relative importance. A biochemistry profile (including

13

Table 13.1: Association of neurological deficits in the dog and cat to the different parts of the lower motor neuron system

	α-motor neuron	Nerve	Synapse	Muscle
■ **General weakness**	Possible	Possible	Often	Possible
■ **Paresis or paralysis**	Yes	Yes	Possible	Yes
■ **Proprioception**	Normal	Often abnormal, paresis	Abnormal with severe paresis	Abnormal with severe paresis
■ **Spinal reflexes**	Reduced to missing	Reduced to missing	Often normal, reduced to missing possible	Often reduced to missing, increased reflexes possible
■ **Muscle tone**	Reduced	Reduced	Normal to reduced	Reduced to increased
■ **Muscle mass**	Atrophy	Atrophy	Normal, rarely atrophy	Atrophy to hypertrophy
■ **Muscle pain**	No	Rare	No	Possible with myositis
■ **Other muscular abnormalities**	Fasciculation, tremor	–	–	Myotonic dimple, tremor, muscle spasm possible
■ **Nociception**	Normal to hyperaesthesia	Normal, hypoaesthesia, hyperaesthesia	Normal	Normal
■ **Cranial nerve abnormalities**	Possible	Loss of voice and other disturbances	Dysphagia, laryngeal paralysis, facial nerve paralysis	Possible
■ **Megaesophagus**	Possible	Possible	Often	Possible
■ **Autonomic disease**	–	Possible	Possible	–
■ **Distribution of the abnormalities**	Generalised, focal possible	Generalised, focal possible	Focal, only hindlegs, generalised	Focal, generalised

(This list describes only tendencies and does not replace further diagnostic clarification.)

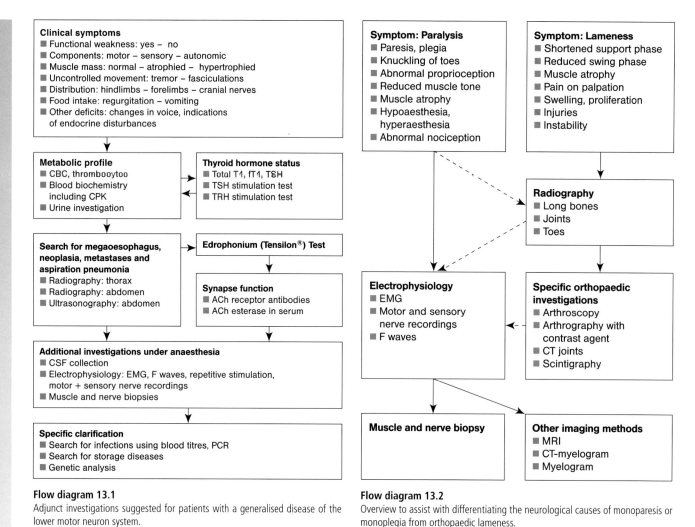

Clinical symptoms
- Functional weakness: yes – no
- Components: motor – sensory – autonomic
- Muscle mass: normal – atrophied – hypertrophied
- Uncontrolled movement: tremor – fasciculations
- Distribution: hindlimbs – forelimbs – cranial nerves
- Food intake: regurgitation – vomiting
- Other deficits: changes in voice, indications of endocrine disturbances

Metabolic profile
- CBC, thrombocytes
- Blood biochemistry including CPK
- Urine investigation

Thyroid hormone status
- Total T4, fT4, TSH
- TSH stimulation test
- TRH stimulation test

Search for megaoesophagus, neoplasia, metastases and aspiration pneumonia
- Radiography: thorax
- Radiography: abdomen
- Ultrasonography: abdomen

Edrophonium (Tensilon®) Test

Synapse function
- ACh receptor antibodies
- ACh esterase in serum

Additional investigations under anaesthesia
- CSF collection
- Electrophysiology: EMG, F waves, repetitive stimulation, motor + sensory nerve recordings
- Muscle and nerve biopsies

Specific clarification
- Search for infections using blood titres, PCR
- Search for storage diseases
- Genetic analysis

Symptom: Paralysis
- Paresis, plegia
- Knuckling of toes
- Abnormal proprioception
- Reduced muscle tone
- Muscle atrophy
- Hypoaesthesia, hyperaesthesia
- Abnormal nociception

Symptom: Lameness
- Shortened support phase
- Reduced swing phase
- Muscle atrophy
- Pain on palpation
- Swelling, proliferation
- Injuries
- Instability

Radiography
- Long bones
- Joints
- Toes

Electrophysiology
- EMG
- Motor and sensory nerve recordings
- F waves

Specific orthopaedic investigations
- Arthroscopy
- Arthrography with contrast agent
- CT joints
- Scintigraphy

Muscle and nerve biopsy

Other imaging methods
- MRI
- CT-myelogram
- Myelogram

Flow diagram 13.1
Adjunct investigations suggested for patients with a generalised disease of the lower motor neuron system.

Flow diagram 13.2
Overview to assist with differentiating the neurological causes of monoparesis or monoplegia from orthopaedic lameness.

13

creatine phosphokinase) CBC, urinalysis, serum antibodies against cholinergic receptors (see Chap. 4.3) and radiographs of the thorax and abdomen are helpful in the investigation of infections, metabolic abnormalities, myasthenia gravis, neoplasia and metastases or a megaoesophagus with possible aspiration pneumonia (see Chap. 6.2). Titres of infectious diseases that are borderline should be interpreted with care and only a four-fold increase should be deemed a significant indicator of an infection.

Anaesthesia in patients with a generalised LMNS disease carries with it a higher risk than normal as the function of the intercostal musculature and the diaphragm can be affected by such disease. The stress of anaesthesia can lead to decompensation in severely affected animals. Such patients often need intensive therapy, and artificial respiration with a ventilator can be vital for several days. Despite all the risks of anaesthesia, electrophysiology and muscle and nerve biopsies are

the most important investigations to confirm the diagnosis of LMNS disease, and may even provide the ultimate diagnosis. Flow diagram 13.2 describes the procedures recommended in the majority of neuropathies and myopathies to differentiate these diseases from orthopaedic causes of lameness. How far an individual patient can be diagnosed depends on the possible cause, the severity of the disease, the course of disease and the expectations of the owner.

Further reading

BLOT, S. (1995): Part 1. The skeletal striated muscle: structure, function and symptomatology. Part Med Chir Anim Comp. **30**: 11–25.

DUNCAN, I.D. (1991): Peripheral neuropathy in the dog and cat. Prog Vet Neurol. **2**: 111–128.

GANONG, W.F. (2001): Physiology of nerve and muscle cells. In: Review of medical physiology 20th ed. Lange Medical Books/ McGrath-Hill Medical Publishing Division, New York, pp. 49–80.

NIEDERHAUSER, U.B., HOLLIDAY, T.A. (1989): Electrodiagnostic studies of muscles and neuromuscular junctions. Sem Vet Med Surg. **4**: 116–125.

SUMMERS, B.A., CUMMINGS, J.F., DeLAHUNTA, A. (1995): Diseases of the peripheral nervous system: introduction and general pathology of the peripheral nervous system. In: Veterinary neurolopathology. Mosby, St. Louis, pp. 402–423.

13.2   Mononeuropathies

In this chapter, nerve diseases that cause deficits in a single limb will be discussed. Such deficits can affect individual nerves, a group of nerves or a whole plexus. Isolated cranial nerve deficits are also possible, but these will be considered with diseases of the brain stem (see Chap. 17.2).

All spinal nerves have a ventral and a dorsal nerve root. The ventral nerve root consists of two or more small fibres that are completely myelinated. Generally, nerve roots contain relatively little fibrous tissue and are, therefore, not as resistant to injury as the peripheral nerve. The ventral and dorsal nerve processes are bathed in CSF. After the ventral and dorsal parts have joined to form the nerve, the meninges switch over to perineurium and epineurium, which provide the peripheral nerves with a better degree of stability. As soon as the nerve has passed through the intervertebral foramen, it gives off motor, sensory and autonomic branches. The spinal nerves provide exactly defined muscle and cutaneous regions with motor, sensory and autonomic functions.

Table 13.2: Differential diagnosis of neuropathies as the cause of monoparesis or monoplegia in the dog and cat

V	■ Spinal cord infarct (dog/cat)
T	■ Peripheral nerve damage:
	– Radial nerve (dog/cat)
	– Femoral nerve (dog/cat)
	– Sciatic nerve (dog/cat)
	– Tibial nerve (dog/cat)
	– Peroneal nerve (dog/cat)
	■ Avulsion of the brachial plexus (dog/cat)
	■ Sacrococcygeal fractures and luxations (cat)
M	■ Local tetanus (cat)
N	■ Nerve sheath tumours (dog/cat)
	■ Lymphoma (cat)
	■ Meningioma (dog/cat)
	■ Paraganglioma (dog)
D	■ Foraminal disc prolapse (dog)
	■ Osteochondrosis dissecans of the lumbosacral joint (dog)
	■ Ventral spondylosis (dog)

The possible causes of mononeuropathies include damage to the ventral and dorsal roots, the proximal nerve segments and the plexus, or the distal nerve. As a consequence of the segmental innervation by individual nerves, characteristic clinical syndromes occur irrespective of whether one or more nerves are affected. The clinical deficits are somatomotor, somatosensory or autonomic in nature. The most important pathological mechanisms responsible for monoplegia are trauma and neoplasia. The differential diagnosis for these diseases in the dog and cat are given in Table 13.2.

13.2.1   Traumatic damage to individual nerves of the fore- and hindlimbs

Occurrence: Sometimes in the dog and cat

Aetiology: Traumatic nerve lesions can be caused by fractures, gun shot or pressure from plaster casts and other bandages, overextension during manipulation under anaesthesia and chronic damage due to implants. Surgical operations may be responsible for transection of nerve fibres. An injection of an irritating substance in or close to an important motor nerve can also lead to permanent damage.

Trauma to a nerve causes different degrees of tissue damage, which is divided into the following groups: neuropraxia, axonotmesis, neurotmesis and avulsion of the nerve root.

Neuropraxia is a functional disturbance of a nerve. The nerve's structure remains intact. The clinical deficits are caused due to compression, oedema and local demyelination. Obvious damage to the axon, such as Wallerian-like degeneration, does not occur. The recovery of nerve function usually takes 1 to 6 weeks depending on the degree of oedema and demyelination.

Axonotmesis describes traumatic damage to the axon with Wallerian-like degeneration and secondary demyelination distal to the trauma. Nerve conduction in the distal segment below the lesion is lost after 3 to 5 days. The fibrous structures and the basal membrane of the nerve fibres are retained. These basic structures enable the axon to regenerate. The regeneration process starts about 1 week after the damage and the axon grows 1–2 mm/day.

Neurotmesis is the most severe degree of peripheral nerve damage. The axon is severed and depending on the degree of damage, the endoneurium or perineurium is destroyed. If the outer tissue layer of the nerve, the epineural connective tissue, is torn, then both ends of the nerve will lie free in the limb. As soon as the basal membrane of the nerve fibre is damaged, the probability of regeneration deteriorates drastically; on the one hand, the nerve fibre can no longer find its way to its target

13

organ and on the other hand, the reactive connective tissue's response can block the fibre's path. The chance of spontaneous regeneration in completely severed nerves without surgical intervention is zero.

Avulsion of the ventral and dorsal nerve roots can lead to isolated dysfunction, especially of the radial nerve. Mechanical forces tear the ventral nerve root including the local neurons in the spinal cord or sever the ventral or dorsal roots close to the spinal cord. Either only a part (partial nerve root avulsion) or all of the small rootlets that form a nerve can be affected (complete nerve root avulsion). Injured nerve root fibres have a very limited capacity for regeneration. Any possible clinical improvement occurs mainly due to functional compensation of the intact parts of the nerve root. The diagnosis of nerve root avulsion is often associated with an unfavourable prognosis.

13.2.1.1 Radial nerve

Clinical: This is the most important nerve of the foreleg and includes both motor and sensory fibres. Its nerve roots originate from spinal cord segments C7, C8, T1 and T2. Traumatic damage to the peripheral part can arise with fractures of the humerus or damage to the lateral aspect of the elbow joint. Avulsion of the nerve roots which specifically contribute to the radial nerve can occur. Due to disturbed radial nerve function, the elbow can no longer be extended and the carpal joint is held in the knuckling position. The extensor carpi radialis reflex and the flexor reflex are reduced or absent. Rapid muscle atrophy is seen particularly affecting the triceps and the extensor carpi radialis muscles. Selective loss of sensitivity can be confirmed by testing the nociception on the dorsal distal limb approx. 1 cm proximal to the middle toe.

Diagnosis: Electrophysiology and radiography are the most important specialised investigatory techniques needed. EMG allows the pathological changes to be assigned to a specific region of the radial nerve. Improved localisation of the damage is possible using motor nerve conduction tests and F waves.

Therapy: Physiotherapy is essential for a positive end result independent of the severity of the lesion. Nerve anastomoses may result in functional improvement when there is complete transection of the nerve, as long as the lesion is distal enough to allow surgical access (see Chap. 10.5).

Prognosis: Recovery is possible with neuropraxia and axonotmesis. In severe cases with severance of the radial nerve at the level of the elbow and with mild avulsion, a carpal arthrodesis or tendon transplantation can be attempted as long as there is no self-mutilation.

13.2.1.2 Sciatic nerve

Clinical: The nerve fibres of this mixed nerve leave the spine through the foraminae caudal to the vertebrae L5, L6, L7 and S1. The sciatic nerve is subdivided into one tract that runs within the pelvis and another "extrapelvic" tract. The most important tracts leave the spinal cord at segments L6 and L7, and form the lumbosacral trunk, which runs medial and dorsal to the shaft of the ilium. After the lumbosacral trunk has joined with the nerve root S1, the nerve is called the sciatic nerve. Branches from this nerve supply the gluteus musculature while the rest of the sciatic nerve runs on around the acetabulum to the periphery. The sciatic nerve forks just above the stifle forming the tibial and peroneal nerves. The sciatic nerve contains nerve fibres for all the muscles of the hindlimb; only the adductors and the quadriceps-sartorius-iliopsoas group are innervated by other motor nerves.

The causes of a sciatic lesion are numerous. Pelvic and sacral fractures are important ones. Specifically, fractures of the shaft of the ilium, the acetabulum or the proximal femur are associated with an increased risk of trauma to the nerve. Iatrogenic lesions after surgery have been documented. The placement of intramedullary pins, surgical correction of hip dysplasia (triple pelvic osteotomy) and reduction of perianal hernias are associated with a danger of damaging the sciatic nerve. In addition, degenerative lumbosacral stenosis can lead to selective nerve root compression of the lumbosacral trunk, thereby causing a sciatic pain syndrome. Foraminal disc prolapse, bone fragments and in rare cases, spondylotic proliferation can all result in chronic compression (Figs. 13.1–13.5),

Depending on the degree of damage to the sciatic nerve, monoparesis to monoplegia of virtually the whole limb can occur. The affected hindlimb can still be drawn forward with the help of the quadriceps-sartorius-iliopsoas muscle group and be held in a medial position by the adductors. The tarsal joint collapses and the toes are held in a knuckling position. The patella reflex is normal to increased as the muscle antagonists are no longer functional. The flexor reflex and the muscle tone of almost the whole limb are often reduced.

Severe muscle atrophy that does not affect the quadriceps-sartorius-iliopsoas muscle group or the adductors makes itself quickly obvious. It is not uncommon for abnormal nociception to arise proximal to the third toe and plantar over the foot pads. Due to the massive loss of function, skin injuries are associated with persistent dragging of the leg and knuckling. Chronic self-mutilation can be a reason for amputation of the limb. In rare cases, lameness, retraction of the affected limb and pain can be seen.

Diagnosis: It can be difficult to separate orthopaedic from neurological symptoms in these cases, especially in the presence of pelvic fractures, (Fig. 13.6). The clinical picture is often very typical with neurological lesions, though some specialised investigations may be necessary. An EMG can re-

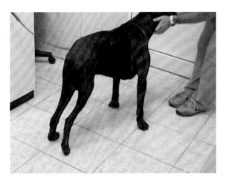

Fig. 13.1
A five-year-old Boxer was presented with lameness of the right hindlimb. The dog intermittently pulled the leg upwards. The neurological examination revealed a reduced flexor reflex, delayed proprioception of the right hindlimb and atrophy of the muscles innervated by the sciatic nerve. The lumbosacral region was tense and painful.

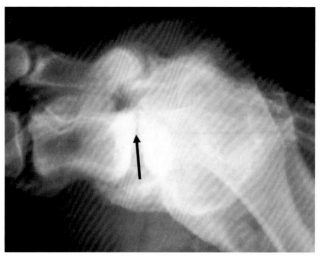

Fig. 13.2
Lateral radiograph of the five-year-old Boxer in Fig. 13.1 shows obvious changes in the lumbosacral region. Note the severe spondylosis, the sclerotic endplates of L7 and S1 as well as the conical intervertebral space between L7–S1 (arrow). However, an important indication of spinal canal stenosis is missing: an overshadowing of L7–S1.

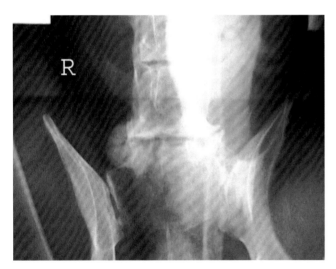

Fig. 13.3
The results of the ventrodorsal radiograph of the five-year-old Boxer show similar changes to Fig. 13.2. The spondylosis is more marked on the right side.

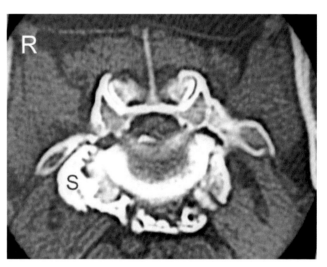

Fig. 13.4
The CT investigation of the same patient in Figs. 13.1–13.3 makes the compression of the right nerve root L7 due to osteoarthritic proliferation (S) more apparent.

13

late the abnormal cMAPs to the area innervated by the sciatic nerve (see Chap. 7.1.2).

The damaged site can be localised by studying the motor nerve conduction with respect to velocity and the amplitudes. F waves, sensory nerve conduction and cord dorsum poten-

tials provide important additional information. Radiography and in some cases CT or MRI can be very valuable.

Therapy: Exploration of the suspected section of the nerve, and decompression and stabilisation of fractures are important prerequisites for regeneration in cases with obvious neu-

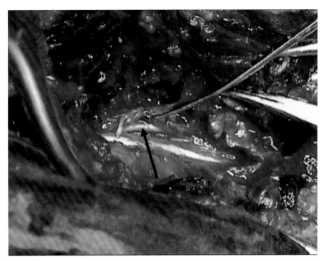

Fig. 13.5
Surgical decompression of the nerve roots in the five-year-old Boxer (Figs. 13.1–13.4) is shown in this picture. The approach was via a dorsal laminectomy, which was widened by a right-sided foramenectomy. The exposed right nerve root L7 can be seen underneath the nerve root retractor (arrow); the shiny white conus medullaris lies caudal to it.

rological deficits. Conservative therapy can be tried at first in all patients with mild deficits and without any fractures or luxations. If, however, surgical exploration is required because of the clinical symptoms and the adjunct investigations, then surgery should be done as early as possible (see Chap. 10.5). Prolonged damage to nerves can lead to Wallerian-like degeneration and fibrosis, which will hinder the regrowth of the nerve.

Prognosis: The prognosis depends on the degree and duration of nerve damage. An end-to-end anastomosis can be attempted if the nerve is completely severed. Due to the long regeneration time and the frequent complications such as muscle contraction, fibrosis, ankylosis of the joints, sensation disturbances and possible self-mutilation, the patient's prospects are very guarded, even with good physiotherapy. In neuropraxia and axonotmesis, recovery is possible with adequate physiotherapy.

13.2.1.3 Peroneal nerve

Aetiology: This nerve is one of the most important branches of the sciatic nerve. The peroneal nerve runs laterally over the proximal tibia where the risk of trauma is greatest. It provides motor innervation to the tarsal joint flexors and the carpal extensors on the distal hindlimb. Its sensory branches go to the palmar skin region distal to the tarsus. Causes of damage include trauma or injections of drugs.

Clinical: The neurological deficits include a lack of flexion of the tarsus and carpus. The patients can no longer lift up the distal part of their limb and the toes knuckle over spontaneously or are held in that position. The tibialis cranialis reflex is reduced or absent. Rapidly progressive muscle atrophy can be observed especially affecting the tibialis cranialis muscle.

Diagnosis: Electrophysiology and radiography are the primary adjunct investigations required. The pathological changes are restricted to the innervation area of the peroneal nerve with EMG (see Chap. 7.1.2).

Therapy: Complete severance is rare. Physiotherapy is essential (see Chap. 8.1).

Prognosis: Regeneration depends on the quality of the physiotherapy and the degree of nerve fibrosis.

13.2.1.4 Tibial nerve

Diagnosis: The tibial nerve innervates the important gastrocnemius muscle, which plays an important role in the extension of the tarsal joint. It also serves the flexors of the carpal joint and the toes. Its sensory branches innervate the plantar skin region distal to the tarsal joint. As the tibial nerve is protected within the musculature, isolated lesions rarely occur.

Clinical: The clinical signs of a lesion to the tibial nerve include a sunken tarsus, plantigrade positioning and collapse of the tarsal joint when the animal puts weight on it. The patella and flexor reflexes are normal. Nociception of the plantar skin zone distal to the tarsal joint may be abnormal.

Therapy: Complete severance is rare. Physiotherapy is essential (see Chap. 8.1).

Prognosis: Regeneration depends on the quality of the physiotherapy and the degree of nerve fibrosis.

13.2.1.5 Femoral nerve

Diagnosis: The femoral nerve originates from the spinal cord at the level of L4 and L5. The fibres run well protected within the musculature. This nerve provides motor innervation to the quadriceps, sartorius and iliopsoas muscles. Its sensory branch, the saphenous nerve, innervates the medial skin zone of the hindlimb. Isolated lesions of the femoral nerve are rarely seen in the dog, although gun shot wounds may damage the nerve both in the dog and cat and nerve sheath tumours can occasionally be documented (Figs. 13.7 and 13.8). Peripheral femoral nerve lesions can occur in cats that have been trapped somwhere (i.e. under a door or in a window) (see Chap. 13.5.1). Electrophysiological investigations are the most important aids necessary to confirm the diagnosis of damage to this nerve.

13

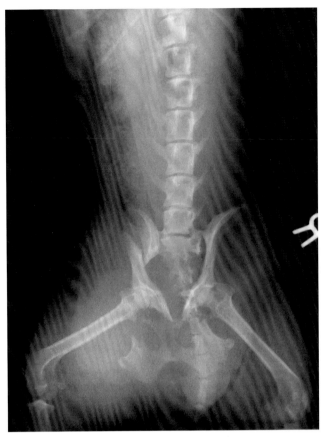

Fig. 13.6
A ten-year-old Terrier cross was hit by a car and presented with paraplegia. The results of the clinical examination indicated the presence of fractures in the pelvis. The multiple pelvic fractures could explain the pain and the instability; however, the loss of nociception in the plantar region of the left hindleg compared to the completely normal sensation in the right hindleg is an unequivocal indication of significant damage to the right sciatic trunk.

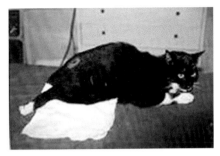

Fig. 13.7
A cat was hit by a pellet from an airgun and presented with right-sided focal paralysis of the femoral nerve. The weight-bearing function of the right hindleg was severely reduced: the affected leg collapsed and could not be drawn forward; it was held preferentially stretched backwards.

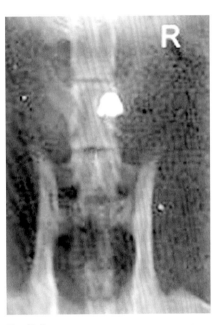

Fig. 13.8
Ventrodorsal radiograph of the cat in Fig. 13.7 shows the position of the pellet a few millimetres caudal to the right nerve root L6. The cat completely recovered within a few weeks with conservative therapy.

13

Clinical: The clinical symptoms are relatively typical. The patient collapses at the knee and cannot stand upright. If the lesion occurs bilaterally, then a frog-like stance of the hindlimbs can be observed. The patella reflex is reduced or lacking. The postural reflexes in the affected limb are usually normal. A reduced or absent reaction to noxious stimuli can be observed on the medial surface of the hindlimb.

Therapy: As lesions of the femoral nerves are rarely of the neurotmesis type, the treatment is concentrated on physiotherapy as well as other supportive measures (see Chap. 8.1).

Prognosis: Usually favourable.

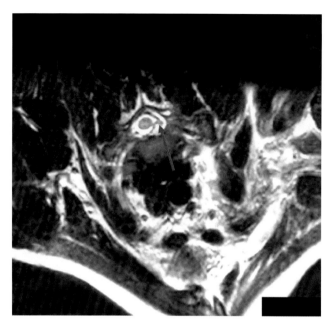

Fig. 13.9
A one-year-old male Labrador Retriever that had been hit by a car showed symptoms of brachial plexus avulsion. The neurological deficits such as monoplegia of the right foreleg, Horner's syndrome and the lack of pain perception under the elbow indicated that severe damage was present. MRI was done a few days after the accident. The figure demonstrates a T2w MRI cross-section through the C8 nerve root. On the right side, a filling defect is visible in the subarachnoid space, compatible with an avulsion (arrow). How many of the small nerve roots that form the root complex of C8 were affected remained unclear.

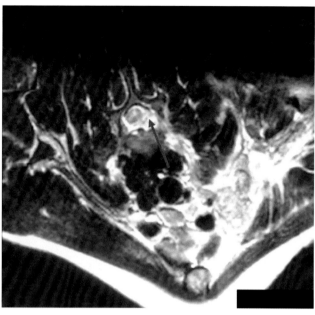

Fig. 13.10
This sequence is a T2w cross-section of the MRI investigation of the same Labrador Retriever as in Fig. 13.9. The figure shows a right-sided mass effect a few millimetres rostral to the avulsed C8 nerve root (arrow). The FLASH sequence identified this mass as haemorrhage and a haematoma. Resorption of the blood clots leads to a partial functional improvement in some of these types of patient.

13

13.2.2 Avulsion of the brachial plexus

Occurrence: This is a well-described problem. Male dogs and medium-sized breeds seem to be more commonly affected; cats that go outside may be sporadically affected, too.

Aetiology: Pulling on the nerves occurs due to traction of the limb during trauma and is usually responsible for this. Due to their high proportion of connective tissue, peripheral nerves can withstand a certain degree of stretching; however, if the strain limit is overstepped the nerve can tear at its weakest point. This is usually at the ventral nerve root close to the spinal cord, the dorsal nerve root proximal to the sensory ganglion, or the ventral and dorsal roots distal to the sensory ganglion. Nerve damage in the proximal nerve segments or within the plexus itself is rare. Injury to the nerve roots leads to Wallerian-like degeneration of all the affected nerves distal to the lesion.

Clinical: The extent of nerve damage (from cranial to caudal) as well as the severity of the root injury determines the clinical symptoms. The extent of injury can be divided into cranial plexus avulsion (C6, C7: suprascapularis, subscapularis, musculocutaneous and axillary nerves), caudal plexus avulsion (C8–T2: radial, median, ulnar, and lateral intercostal nerves), and complete avulsion (C6–T2). Knowledge about the severity of root damage is essential. For the understanding of this type of situation, it is important to know that the whole nerve root system is made up of numerous small rootlets. The question of whether all the small roots or only a certain proportion of them are affected has great prognostic value. If all the small roots are torn, then there is no hope of compensation and functional recovery. It is often difficult to judge the degree of root damage from the clinical picture, even with the help of specialised tests (Figs. 13.9 and 13.10). Although reliable prognostic factors are lacking, complete monoplegia, accompanied by abnormal skin sensation in the affected limb from the outset are, however, important indicators of a significant lesion and a poor prognosis. As the dorsal nerve roots are probably more mechanically resistant than the ventral ones, abnormal superficial sensation indicates the presence of a severe lesion.

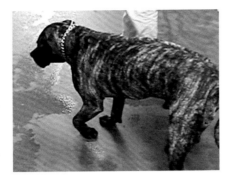

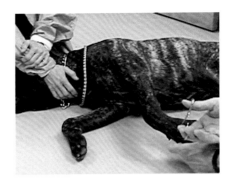

Fig. 13.11 (left)
A young Boxer with a plexus avulsion of the right foreleg was presented one week after a car accident. The posture of the foreleg in the knuckling position as well as the "hanging" elbow are typical of damage to the radial nerve, which is the most important neural structure in the forelimb.

Fig. 13.12 (right)
Careful testing of the sensation is essential when there is suspicion of a plexus avulsion or damage to a peripheral nerve. This picture shows the examination of the autonomic zone of the radial nerve in the Boxer described in Fig. 13.11. The loss of deep pain in this dog represents an unfavourable prognostic factor for a complete functional recovery.

If it remains uncertain as to whether the nerve roots are really affected in the patient vs. the proximal nerve segment or the plexus, the presence of an ipsilateral Horner's syndrome or proprioceptive dysfunction immediately after trauma can be of further use. When one or other of these symptoms are present, then the traumatised tissue must lie within the vertebral foramen. If these symptoms are not present, then it is possible that the lesion is more distal, which is prognostically more favourable. Histopathological investigations in dogs with monoparesis or monoplegia following trauma have, however, demonstrated the presence of damaged nerve roots in most cases.

Diagnosis: The anamnesis provides important information about a trauma. The clinical picture is often typical, though it can vary greatly (Figs. 13.11–13.13). Monoparesis or monoplegia with abnormal proprioception is usually present. Other clinical signs can include Horner's syndrome, abnormal panniculus reflex, abnormal proprioception in the ipsilateral hindleg, and abnormal superficial sensation. Investigation of autonomous skin zones is very valuable. It should be noted that the affected and the healthy sides must be compared with each other. Radiography of the long bones and the joints are necessary adjunct investigations. Electrophysiological evaluation of the limbs can quantify the extent and severity of the lesion, and repeated investigations can provide measurable information about the function of the nerves and musculature (Fig. 13.14).

Therapy: Specific therapy is not yet possible as surgical reimplantation of nerve roots has not as yet been completely successful in the dog. The only viable treatment is conservative therapy. Physiotherapy, hydrotherapy, electrostimulation and support or protective bandages / wraps are recommended approaches (see Chap. 8.1). Good physiotherapy is essential to keep muscle contraction and joint ankylosis down to a minimum. Adequate time should be given to the patient for nerve regeneration to occur. If self-mutilation, deep wounds or severe infections occur, amputation should be considered

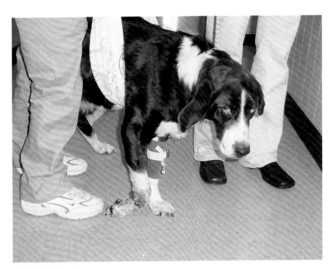

13

Fig. 13.13
A young, male Bernese Cattle Dog one month after a car accident. The clinical findings included knuckling, a hanging elbow, monoplegia, lack of deep pain perception below the elbow, Horner's syndrome in the right eye and a severe infection in the periphery of the right foreleg.

(Fig. 13.15). Carpal arthrodesis or tendon transposition should only be considered in the presence of mild deficits with some extensor function remaining.

Prognosis: Approximately 15% of dogs and cats with brachial plexus avulsion or lesions return to normal function of the affected limb. If obvious sensory deficits are present on the first examination, the chance for complete functional recovery is low.

Mild to moderate improvement of neurological status, however, occurs in many patients, so the abnormal limb does not have to be amputated as long as adequate physiotherapy is implemented.

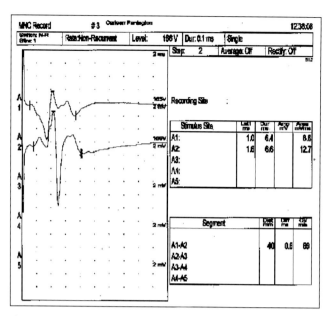

Fig. 13.14
This figure shows the results of a motor nerve conduction test of the radial nerve in a ten-year-old Labrador Retriever, which had been hit by a car four months previously. The patient had improved functionally from a severe monoparesis to a slight monoparesis with retained sensation in all autonomic zones. The electrophysiological investigation reveals a normal NCV and normal duration of the cMAPs, which indicate normal myelination of the radial nerve. The severely reduced amplitude, however, represents a reduced number of functional axons and nerve roots, and provides the diagnosis of a partial avulsion of the caudal plexus.

13

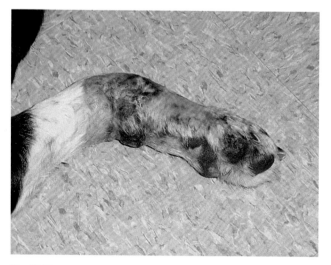

Fig. 13.15
The paw of a young male Bernese Cattle Dog one month after a car accident (same dog as in Fig. 13.13). The deeply penetrating infection was caused by self-mutilation and self-inflicted trauma. The predisposing factors were monoplegia, knuckling and lack of deep pain, as well as a lack of supportative measures such as protective bandaging and physiotherapy.

13.2.3 Sacrocaudal fractures and luxations

Occurrence: Occasional in outdoor cats

Aetiology: The main causes are related to vehicle accidents. The damage occurs due to an abrupt "pulling" on the tail, in a direction opposite to that in which the cat is moving or is being thrown/accelerated. Fractures and luxations of the proximal tail vertebrae, sacral vertebrae or more rarely, the caudal lumbar vertebrae occur due to this type of force. Damage to the sacral spinal cord, avulsion of the nerve roots and overstretching or compression of the nerves occur both because of excessive traction on the relatively short nerves or due to luxation fractures. The affected nerves and nerve roots include the coccygeal nerves, the pudendal nerve, the pelvic nerve and in rare cases, the L7 nerve root of the sciatic. Not uncommonly other injuries such as pneumothorax, limb fractures, pelvic fractures and skin injuries are present.

Clinical: The anamnesis and/or the presence of skin injuries in the tail region are often typical. The main symptom is paresis or plegia of the tail. Pain sensation is usually absent. A major concurrent problem is bladder function disturbance: a lesion of the pelvic nerve associated with this injury results in the detrusor reflex being reduced or totally absent. The brain is no longer informed about the degree of filling of the bladder because of pelvic nerve injury, and so conscious emptying of the bladder is no longer possible. A disturbance in the balance between the parasympathetic innervation of the bladder via the damaged pelvic nerve and the sympathetic supply through the intact hypogastric nerve most probably leads to an increased sympathetic tone, which could explain the increased tone of the bladder's internal sphincter. This high resistance also makes emptying of the bladder more difficult. Primary overflow incontinence occurs in very severe lesions of the pelvic nerve and the pudendal nerve. The urine flows continuously or at least with mild abdominal compression. Other indications of damage to the pudendal nerve are reduced perineal reflex, reduced tone of the anal sphincter, open anus, and reduced or missing perianal superficial sensation. In some patients, a mild paresis with abnormal proprioception occurs. Megacolon is often present.

Diagnosis: The important adjunct investigations in this condition include radiography of the pelvis, thorax and abdomen. Due to the high risk of urinary infection, urinalysis is also indicated. Electrophysiological investigations can be helpful in some cases.

Therapy: Specific treatment of the crushed nerves or nerve root avulsion is not possible. Therapy is symptomatic. The biggest problem is disturbance in bladder function. The medications bethanechol (0.5–1.0 mg/kg, PO, BID–TID), phenoxybenzamine (0.25–0.5 mg/kg, PO, BID–TID) or diazepam (0.25–0.5 mg/kg, PO, TID) support the spontaneous emptying of the bladder. Analgesics such as butorpha-

Table 13.3: Clinical symptoms and prognosis for cats with sacrocaudal fractures and luxations

Group	Clinical symptoms	Prognosis
1	Plegic and analgesic tail, normal reflexes, normal urination.	The motor function of the tail recovers in roughly 75% of cats within 3 months.
2	Plegic and analgesic tail, normal perineal reflex and anal sphincter tone, normal perineal sensation, no spontaneous urination but urination is attempted, large bladder, bladder can be emptied manually.	The tail function and spontaneous urination return in roughly 75% of cats; the time needed is approx. 1 month.
3	Plegic and analgesic tail, reduced perineal reflex and anal sphincter tone, urination not attempted, large bladder, it is difficult or impossible to empty the bladder manually.	Roughly half of these animals recover their motor function in the tail and achieve an improved bladder function, but the residual urine is greater than normal; recovery takes 1 to 2 months.
4	Plegic and analgesic tail, loss of perineal reflex, dilated and flaccid anus, primary overflow incontinence, urine can be easily expressed.	Improvement in the neurological status is observed, but only a few cats recover their normal tail and bladder function; possible recovery can be seen in 2 to 3 months.

nol are also valuable in many cases. If the detrusor reflex and continence are dysfunctional, the bladder should be emptied two to three times a day, either manually or using a catheter, which often cannot be done without sedation or anaesthesia (see Chap. 8.2.1) Administration of antibiotics is necessary to address subclinical or clinical infections. The ideal would be to choose the antibiotic according to bacteriological culture and sensitivity testing, but this is not always possible under practical conditions.

Prognosis: Healing of nerve damage requires time. Based on the clinical symptoms, the patients can be subdivided into four groups (Table 13.3), which facilitates an overview and improves the quality of the prognostic assessment. With the aid of this table, the trend of the degree and speed of neurological status recovery can be predicted.

13.2.4 Peripheral nerve sheath tumours

Occurrence: Sometimes in the dog; very rare in the cat.

Aetiology: The cause is unknown but may in part be associated with genetic predilections. The terms used for these tumours are neurinoma, neurolemoma, schwannoma, malignant schwannoma, neurofibroma, neurofibrosarcoma and nerve root tumour. This terminology can be very confusing and only schwannoma, neurolemoma and neurofibroma have been diagnosed in animals. Histologically, the tumours that develop from nerve roots and those from peripheral nerves are very heterogeneous. The name peripheral nerve sheath tumour has been accepted as these tumours predominantly arise from cell lines belonging to the nerve sheath and show similar biological behaviour to malignant schwannomas. Until advances have been made in the classification of these tumours in domestic animals, they are classified collectively as peripheral nerve sheath tumours.

Clinical: Peripheral nerve sheath tumours often affect the middle and caudal nerve roots of the cervical enlargement and the brachial plexus. They have also been seen in the lumbo-sacral trunk of the sciatic nerve. Thoracolumbar nerves can also become neoplastic. Nerve sheath tumours rarely produce metastases, but they can be very invasive locally. After their initial growth caudal and proximal along the periphery, invasion of the spinal cord is a devastating complication.

Mainly older dogs of medium and large breeds are affected. The clinical signs develop slowly and progressively, and at the beginning are often confused with an orthopaedic problem. The typical symptom is a progressive lameness with slow atrophy of the muscles. Pain is present in half of the patients. Depending on the nutritional status of the patient, nerve sheath tumours of the brachial plexus can occasionally be palpated. Horner's syndrome may occur when the caudal cervical nerve roots are affected. After tumour infiltration in the spinal cord, progressive paresis or tetraparesis occurs suddenly (Figs. 13.16–13.18).

Diagnosis: Adjunct specialised investigations are important. With a tumour in the nerve root area, it is not uncommon for enlarged intervertebral foraminae to be seen on plain radiographs. Myelography and CSF investigations can be helpful if the spinal cord or neighbouring nerve roots are affected, but a negative result does not exclude the presence of a nerve sheath tumour of the nerve roots (Figs. 13.19 and 13.20). A very important method of resolving the diagnosis is electrophysiology. The probability that a nerve sheath tumour causes an abnormal EMG is very high and it may occasionally be seen with the use of ultrasound. The best adjunct investigation is, however, MRI (Figs. 13.21–13.24). Localisation, extent and size of the neoplasia as well as possible spinal cord infiltration can be identified with MRI.

13

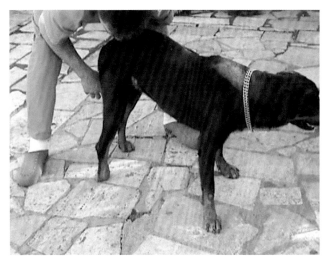

Fig. 13.16
A six-year-old Rottweiler was presented because of a chronic progressive lameness in the right foreleg that had developed into a hemiparesis. Proprioceptive deficits can be seen here in the right hindleg. A neurolemmal tumour of C7 was diagnosed in this patient.

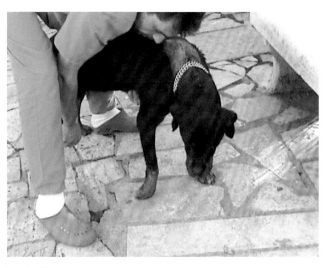

Fig. 13.17
The same Rottweiler as in Fig. 13.16. The proprioceptive deficits in the right forelimb can be seen with the wheelbarrow test.

13

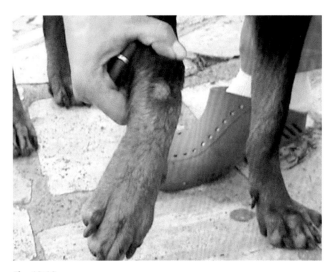

Fig. 13.18
The same Rottweiler as in Figs. 13.16 and 13.17. Repeated falling over due to proprioceptive dysfunction, weakness and muscle atrophy in the right forelimb as well as chronic licking have led to the development of a carpal granuloma.

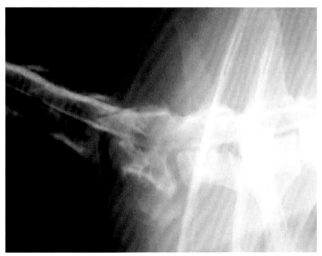

Fig. 13.19
The myelogram of the same Rottweiler as in Figs. 13.16–13.18 shows a dilated foramen at C6–C7 as well as blurred contours of the contrast columns in this region.

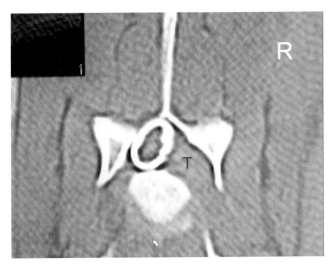

Fig. 13.20
The CT-myelogram of the same Rottweiler from Figs. 13.16–13.19 reveals a massively enlarged right nerve root C7 (T), which has grown through the dilated foramen and has started to compress the spinal cord.

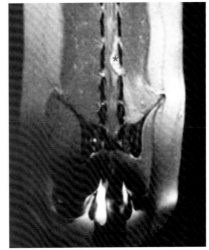

Fig. 13.21
A ten-year-old Shar Pei was presented with lameness in the left hindleg that had slowly developed over months. The dog had difficulties in moving its left hindleg forwards, knuckling, a loss of patella reflex and severe atrophy of the quadriceps and sartorius muscles. Audible fibrillation potentials were found on the EMG of these muscles. The T1w sequence from the MRI investigation revealed a pale mass (*) in the caudal area of L5.

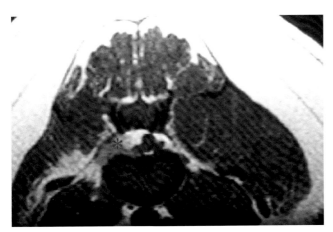

Fig. 13.22
A cross-section of the T1w image from the same Shar Pei in as Fig. 13.21 shows a longish, contrast-enhanced mass (*), which has started to grow into the spinal cord. The neoplasm has all the typical characteristics of a neurolemmal tumour.

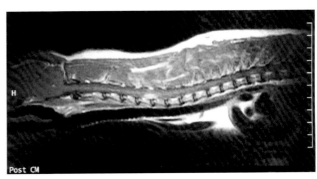

Fig. 13.23
A seven-year-old domestic cat was presented because of lameness of the right foreleg that had lasted for 10 weeks, with subsequent development of hemiparesis. The sagittal T1w MRI image after the administration of a contrast agent reveals a bright intramedullary mass in the caudal region of C5.

13

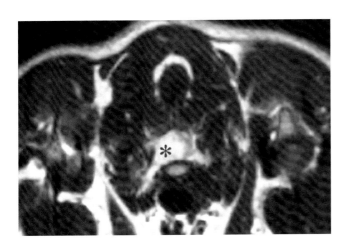

Fig. 13.24
A cross-section of the T1w MRI contrast study of the cat in Fig. 13.23 revealed a neoplasm (*) which was growing along the nerve roots and had severely infiltrated the spinal cord. This tumour shows all the typical characteristics of a neurolemmal tumour.

Therapy: The best form of treatment is the complete surgical resection of the tumour. This is difficult if the neoplasm has already infiltrated the spinal cord. Not uncommonly, amputation of the limb is undertaken given all of the oncological and functional aspects. Subsequent radiation therapy may be advantageous because peripheral nerve sheath tumours, as mentioned above, are locally very invasive and cannot be completely removed. However, investigations that confirm this therapeutic suggestion are lacking in veterinary medicine.

Prognosis: The patient's prognosis is usually unfavourable. Animals with nerve sheath tumours of the brachial plexus and peripheral nerves have a better prognosis than animals with the same tumours in the nerve root region. A study of 51 dogs determined a mean survival time of 2 years with surgically excised peripheral nerve sheath tumours, roughly 1 year with tumours in the brachial plexus area, and only half a year with tumours of the nerve roots.

13.2.5 Lymphoma

Occurrence: This tumour occurs infrequently in the nerve roots in cats.

Aetiology: Lymphoma is a common tumour of the cat. Feline leukaemia virus (FeLV) plays an important role in its pathogenesis.

Clinical: Feline lymphoma often has a multifocal organ localisation. Primary lymphatic tumours in the CNS are rare and usually the nervous system is secondarily affected, whereby extradural spinal cord compression is the most common lymphoma-associated presentation. A rapidly progressive tetraparesis or paraparesis is the logical consequence. Isolated involvement of the nerve roots is possible. The cervical enlargement is more frequently affected than the lumbosacral region. Usually more than one nerve root is infiltrated. Bilateral forms are also possible.

Diagnosis: CBC, biochemistry profile, urinalysis, radiography of the lungs and ultrasonography of the abdomen are the basic diagnostic methods used to determine the presence of a generalised form of feline lymphoma. The FeLV test can frequently be positive. CSF investigation is the first step in demonstrating that the nervous system is affected. Neoplastic lymphocytes can be seen, though non-specific mixed cell populations are possible. Imaging methods, such as myelography or MRI, provide further useful information for determining the localisation and extent of the disease. Biopsies are essential for confirming the diagnosis.

Therapy: Chemotherapy prolongs the survival time. The COP (vincristine, cyclophosphamide, prednisolone) and the COPA (vincristine, cyclophosphamide, doxorubicin, prednisolone) protocols induce clinical improvement. Other combinations such as vincristine, cyclophosphamide, methotrexate, L-asparginase and prednisolone have been described. Radiation therapy is useful in focal forms of the disease. Surgical therapy may be possible but is usually only diagnostic in its results.

Prognosis: The long-term results are poor. The majority of affected cats must be euthanised within 1 year despite chemotherapy.

Further reading

BAILEY, C. (1984): Patterns of cutaneous anesthesia associated with brachial plexus avulsion in the dog. J Am Vet Med Assoc. **185**: 889.

BREHM, D.M., VITE H.S., HAVILAND, J., Van WINKLE, T., (1985): A retrospective evaluation of 51 cases of peripheral nerve sheath tumors in the dog. J Am Anim Hosp Assoc. **31**: 349–359.

COCKHUTT, J.R., SMITH-MAXIE, L.L. (1993): Delayed onset sciatic impairment following triple pelvic osteotomy. Prog Vet Neurol. **4**: 60–63.

GRIFFITHS, I.R. (1974): Avulsion of the brachial plexus, 1: neuropathology of the spinal cord and peripheral nerves. J Small Anim Pract. **15**: 165–176.

GRIFFITHS, I.R., DUNCAN, I.D., LAWSON, D.D. (1974): Avulsion of the brachial plexus, 2: Clinical aspects. J Small Anim Pract. **15**: 177–182.

JACOBSON, A., SCHRADER, S.C., (1987): Peripheral nerve injury associated with fracture-dislocation of the pelvis in dogs and cats: 34 cases (1979–1982). J Am Vet Med Assoc. **190**: 569–572.

LANE, S.B., KORNEGAY, J.N., OLIVER, J.E. Jr, DUNCAN, J.R.: (1994): Feline spinal lymphosarcoma: A retrospective evaluation of 24 cases. J Vet Inter Med. **8**: 99–104.

OLIVER, E.O. Jr, LORENZ, M.D., KORNEGAY, J.N. (1997): Paresis of one limb. In: Handbook of Veterinary Neurology, 3rd ed. WB Saunders, Philadelphia, pp. 111–127.

SHARP, N.J.H. (1995): Neurological deficits in one limb. In: WHEELER S.J. (ed.) Manual of Small Animal Neurology, 2nd ed., BSAVA, Gloucestershire, pp. 159–178.

STANTON, M.E., WEIGEL, J.P., HENRY, R.E. (1988): Sciatic nerve paralysis associated with the biceps femoris sling: Case report and anatomical study. J Am Anim Hosp Assoc. **24**: 429–432.

STEINBERG, H.S. (1979): The use of electrodiagnostic techniques in evaluating traumatic brachial plexus root injuries, J Am Anim Hosp Assoc. **15**: 621–626.

STOICA, G., TASCA, S.I., KIM, H.T. (2001): Point mutation of neu oncogene in animal peripheral nerve sheath tumors. Vet Pathol. **38** (6): 679–688.

WHEELER, S., JONES, C., WRIGHT, J. (1986): The diagnosis of brachial plexus disorders in dogs. A review of twenty-two cases. J Small Anim Pract. **27**: 147–157.

13.3 Polyneuropathies

13.3.1 Inherited polyneuropathies

In this section, degenerative diseases which arise before the end of the first year of life and have a progressive course will mainly be considered. A genetic basis is often presumed or is already known. The exact pathological mechanisms have not been investigated in most cases and the causative biochemical defect has only been confirmed for some of the storage diseases.

This group of neurological diseases is not really very important in every-day clinical work. Inherited polyneuropathies occur very rarely in certain breeds. The symptomology can be very complex, but neurological deficits are the most notable. Extra-neural deficits occur in some storage diseases. As a rule, the first clinical signs are nonspecific: paraparesis, ataxia, tremor, lameness and even seizures have been described. In the later stages, motor dysfunction can affect all limbs. Additionally, megaoesophagus and laryngeal paresis/paralysis can also occur. Not uncommonly, more than one animal from the same litter is affected.

A tentative diagnosis can be made using the signalment, clinical picture, electrophysiology, muscle and nerve biopsies, and other complex biochemical methods. The following points indicate a degenerative inherited disease of the LMNS: (1) starts in puppy- or kittenhood; (2) more than one animal in the same litter is affected; and (3) chronic, progressive course with an initially good general health status. A comprehensive definitive diagnosis is sadly only usually attained with histopathology. Therapy can at best only be supportive. The long-term prognosis is unfavourable to grave.

13.3.1.1 Spinal muscular atrophy

Occurrence: Very rare.

Aetiology: Spinal muscular atrophies are caused by a premature degeneration of the motor neurons in the ventral horn of the spinal cord and brain stem. This form of neuronal degeneration mainly affects dogs but has been reported in cats. Chromatolysis of the neurons in the spinal cord, brain stem and peripheral ganglia is the most important histological abnormality. Additionally, a characteristic swelling of the proximal axons is seen in the Brittany Spaniel and the Rottweiler.

A dominant inheritance with variable penetrance has been described in the Brittany Spaniel.

Clinical: The breed-specific diseases are summarised in Table 13.4. Clinically, there is a chronically progressive, severe muscle atrophy and weakness with reduced spinal reflexes. Fasciculations or tremors can be important indicators of disease of the α-motor neurons. NB: Reflexes are normally difficult to evaluate in puppies.

Diagnosis: A tentative diagnosis can be based on the clinical picture. Important specialised investigations such as electrophysiology or nerve and muscle biopsies can be the next steps. A definitive diagnosis can often only be achieved with histopathology.

Therapy: Specific treatment is not possible; physiotherapy may be useful.

Prognosis: Usually unfavourable; certain mild forms can stabilise themselves clinically.

13.3.1.2 Motor axonopathy

Occurrence: Rare.

Aetiology: Medium-sized and large dog breeds are affected by this syndrome. Cats are rarely affected by axonopathies. Usually swelling of the axons is seen as an expression of the degenerative process. While an accumulation of neurofilaments in the proximal section of the nerve occurs in the progressive axonopathy found in the Boxer, the axon swelling in the Giant axon neuropathy of the German Shepherd (Fig. 14.10) lies in the peripheral segments. The pathological mechanism for these types of axonopathy is unclear. Abnormal protein synthesis, disturbances in the slow or rapid axonoplasmic transport, as well as retrograde flow of metabolites have been suggested. Genetic factors play a role but the mode of inheritance is largely unknown.

Clinical: Table 13.5 provides information about the affected breeds and the clinical disturbances seen. The clinical signs are manifested as chronic progressive paraparesis, increasing motor deficits in the forelimbs, sometimes megaoesophagus or laryngeal paralysis, and more rarely, tremors. Muscle atrophy is especially pronounced in the peripheral parts of the limbs.

Diagnosis: Signalment, clinical picture and electrophysiology as well as muscle and nerve biopsies are the most important factors which lead to a diagnosis.

Therapy: Supportive measures are possible.

Prognosis: Unfavourable.

13

Table 13.4: Overview of the acquired degenerative diseases of the α-motor neurons found in the dog

Disease	Species, breed	Age	Clinical symptoms
Progressive neuronopathy	Cairn Terrier	12 to 24 weeks	Chronic progressive paraparesis that develops into tetraparesis, head tremor is almost always present, head tilt and cataplexy occurs sporadically.
Focal spinal muscle atrophy	German Shepherd	4 weeks	Asymmetric paresis of the forelegs, valgus position, muscle fibrosis and muscle contraction.
Spinal muscular atrophy	Pointer	4 to 5 months	Weakness of the hindlegs that progresses to tetraparesis within 3 to 4 months
Spinal muscular atrophy	Rottweiler	4 weeks	Paraparesis which progresses to tetraparesis, stiff hindlimbs, in some cases megaoesophagus.
Spinal muscular atrophy	Brittany Spaniel	1. Acute form: 6 to 8 weeks	1. Tetraparesis, tetraplegia, head tremor, severe muscle atrophy.
		2. Intermediate form: 6 to 8 months	2. Tetraparesis, muscle atrophy is more pronounced in the proximal muscles.
		3. Chronic form: adults; seen in cats too	3. Very slow progressive weakness and muscle atrophy.
Neuronal abiotrophy	Swedish Lapland Hound	5 to 7 weeks	Paresis of the forelimbs; after a few weeks, progressive tetraparesis.

Table 13.5: Overview of the inherited degenerative axonopathies in the dog and cat

Disease	Species, breed	Age	Clinical symptoms
Canine giant axonal neuropathy	German Shepherd	14 to 15 months	Paraparesis, later tetraparesis; megaoesophagus and laryngeal paralysis are possible.
Progressive axonopathy	Boxer	1 to 3 weeks	Paraparesis, ataxia; after some months tetraparesis; head and eye tremors possible.
Inherited polyneuropathy	Alaskan Malamute	7 to 8 months	Paraparesis, later tetraparesis; megaoesophagus often present.
Idiopathic polyneuropathy	Alaskan Malamute	12 to 18 months	Progressive paraparesis progressing to tetraplegia, hyperaesthesia, muscle atrophy, hyporeflexia.
Distal sensory and motor polyneuropathy	Rottweiler	1.5 to 4 years	Paraparesis, which progresses to tetraparesis over a number of months.
Central and peripheral distal axonopathy	Burmese Cat	8 to 10 weeks	Paraparesis, hypermetria, plantigrade positioning of the hindlimbs

Table 13.6: Overview of the sensory axonopathies in the dog

Disease	Breed	Age	Clinical symptoms
Acral mutilation	English Pointer, German Short-haired Pointer	2 to 12 months	Reduced pain sensibility to complete loss of pain sensation; obvious automutilation, in some cases autoamputation.
Sensory neuropathy	Long-haired Dachshund	8 weeks	Very mild ataxia, abnormal proprioception, pain sensibility reduced, urinary and faecal incontinence, automutilation.
Sensory neuropathy	Boxer, Border Collie	2 months	Progressive ataxia, patella reflex and muscle tone reduced, proprioception abnormal, flexor reflex and muscle mass normal; in the final stages, there may be mild cerebellar symptoms.

13

Table 13.7: Overview of the acquired degenerative diseases of the Schwann cells and myelin

Disease	Species, breed	Age	Clinical symptoms
Congenital hypomyelinating polyneuropathy	Golden Retriever	7 weeks	Paraparesis, ataxia, bunny hopping, reduced reflexes, slight muscle atrophy, circumductive movements of the hindlimbs.
Feline hypertrophic polyneuropathy	Domestic cat	7 to 12 months	Plantigrade positioning of the hindlimbs, paraparesis, ataxia, abnormal proprioception, only slight muscle atrophy, generalised tremor.
Canine hypertrophic neuropathy	Tibetan Mastiff	7 to 10 weeks	Paraparesis, which quickly develops to tetraparesis; spinal reflexes and muscle tone are severely reduced, voice is changed. In some dogs, the neurological status can improve but these animals remain weak.

Table 13.8: Overview of the congenital metabolic diseases that can induce disturbances of the peripheral nervous system in the dog and cat

Disease	Species, breed	Age	Pathological changes	Clinical symptoms
Hyperchylomicronaemia	Domestic cat, Himalayan cat, Persian cat, Siamese cat	8 months	A deficiency of lipoprotein lipase leads to hyperlipidaemia and lipid granulomas in various organs with compression on the peripheral nerves.	Abdominal pain, pancreatitis, seizures, single or multiple peripheral neuropathies; radial and tibial nerve paralysis are the most common disturbances. Horner's syndrome is possible. Increase in chylomicrons, VLDH and LDH lipoproteins, cholesterol and triglycerides in the serum.
Hyperoxaluria	Domestic cat	5 to 9 months	A deficit of D-glycerate dehydrogenase, accumulation of oxalate crystals in the kidneys and in the proximal peripheral nerves, accumulation of neurofilaments.	Renal failure, kyphosis, pain in kidney region, spinal reflexes and proprioception reduced, reduced pain sensation. In serum: increased renal values, glucose, phosphate, and potassium; in urine: many oxalate and L-glycerate crystals.
Fucosidosis	English Springer Spaniel	6 to 12 months	A deficit of L-fucosidase causes an accumulation of fructose products in the lysosomes, vacuole formation in neurons and glial cells in the CNS, thickened peripheral nerves. Particularly, the cranial nerves and the brachial plexus are affected.	Changes in behaviour, ataxia, hypermetria, visual disturbances, thickened nerves can be palpated. Blood: lymphocytes with vacuoles. CSF: macrophages and lymphocytes with vacuoles. Nerve and muscle biopsies helpful.
Globoid cell leukodystrophy	Basset Hound, Beagle, Blue Tick Hound, Cairn Terrier, Pomeranian, Poodle, West Highland White Terrier; Domestic cat	3 to 5 months	A deficit of β-galactocerebrosidase leads to an accumulation of glactocerebrosides in the oligodendrocytes and Schwann cells. This causes destruction of the white matter in the CNS and leads to peripheral demyelination.	Ascending paralysis, patella reflex reduced, spastic forelegs, head tremor, possibly dementia and central blindness, slow nerve conduction velocities; nerve and muscle biopsies and MRI of the brain show abnormal results.
Niemann-Pick disease	Boxer, Miniature Poodle; Balinese cat, Domestic cat, Siamese cat	6 to 9 weeks	An unknown enzyme defect leads to an accumulation of sphingomyelin, cholesterol and glycosphingolipids in the lysosomes. This causes a swelling and vacuolation in many organs. Demyelination or hypomyelination is seen in the peripheral nerves. Macrophages and lymphocytes also contain vacuoles.	Two forms: (1) Central form (type C) with depression, head tremor, gait disturbances, blindness, positional nystagmus. (2) Peripheral form (type A) in Siamese cats with paresis, palmigrade and plantigrade positioning of the limbs, abnormal proprioception, reduced reflexes, fine whole body tremor. Electrophysiology and nerve and muscle biopsies are valuable for the diagnosis.
Glycogen storage disease type IV	Norwegian Forest Cat	5 to 8 months	A deficit of enzyme 1,4-D-glucan causes an accumulation of glycogen in the muscle and α-motor neurons.	Fever, generalised tremor, bunny-hopping gait, severe muscle atrophy. At a late stage, tetraplegia and muscle contracture. A muscle biopsy is valuable for the diagnosis.

13

13.3.1.3 Sensory axonopathies

Occurrence: Very rare.

Aetiology: The cause of this very rare degenerative disease is unknown. However, an autosomal recessive inheritance is presumed to be involved in all sensory neuropathies. The pathological changes affect the dorsal ganglia and the peripheral and central sensory axons. A primary degeneration of the neurons in the dorsal ganglia with Wallerian-like degeneration of the nerve fibres (Pointer), axon swelling (Boxer) and a distal axonopathy (Long-haired Dachshund, Border Collie) have been described.

Clinical: The clinical signs are shown in Table 13.6. Deficits in pain sensation and proprioception are predominant. Paresis, ataxia and reduced reflexes are less common but have been described in the Border Collie. The muscle mass is normal.

Diagnosis: Adjunct investigations: normal EMG, normal motor nerve conduction in most cases, abnormal values for sensory nerve conduction.

Therapy: No specific treatment is possible.

Prognosis: Unfavourable.

13.3.1.4 Abnormal Schwann cell function

Occurrence: Very rare.

Aetiology: Abnormal functioning of the Schwann cells leads to either a production of myelin with reduced density, demyelination and remyelination with primitive onion-bulb thickening of the nerves (Tibetan Mastiff); onion-bulb proliferations of the sensory and motor nerve roots (domestic cat); or reduced myelin production with peripheral hypomyelination (Golden Retriever).

Clinical: The clinical signs are listed in Table 13.7. Progressive gait disturbances are predominant. Some patients can recover to a certain degree but they do not reach normality.

Diagnosis: EMG is mostly unchanged; mild spontaneous activity is rarely present (see Fig. 7.1). The motor nerve conduction test shows a severely reduced conduction velocity with polyphasic action potentials. Investigations such as muscle and nerve biopsy are important.

Therapy: None.

Prognosis: Usually unfavourable; a certain degree of improvement can occur with hypomyelination.

13.3.1.5 Metabolic diseases

Occurrence: Very rare.

Etiology: These recessively inherited enzyme deficiencies all lead to a metabolic disease caused by self-intoxication due to toxic metabolites collecting in the lysosomes (see Chap. 3).

Clinical: The pathogenesis and clinical symptoms of the individual diseases are shown in Table 13.8. In the majority of cases, more than one organ system is affected. The function of the PNS and the CNS is disturbed in many cases. The neurological deficits are an important part of the syndrome. It must be noted that the multifocal nature of these diseases can cause a very complex clinical picture in which extraneural organs are also affected.

Diagnosis: The diagnosis of these syndromes has proven to be very laborious. The reasons for this lie, on the one hand, in the difficulty of determining the localization of the disease and on the other hand, specific tests for these diseases in the living animal are complicated. A systematic procedure is especially valuable in such cases. The basic tests which can indicate the presence of a metabolic disease are the red blood count, white blood count, blood chemistry profile, urine investigation, radiographic and ultrasonographic investigations, electrodiagnostics and CSF investigation as well as muscle and nerve biopsies. Further specific investigations should then be undertaken to substantiate the suspicion and to describe the enzyme defect. Looking at this list of tests, it becomes clear why so many of these diseases in animals are detected first by histopathology.

Therapy: No causal treatment is possible.

Prognosis: Very unfavorable.

13.3.2 Acquired polyneuropathies

In this group of polyneuropathies, diseases are discussed that occur in puppies and kittens though they are seen more commonly in young and old adult animals. These polyneuropathies are clinically relevant and are regularly found in practice. The pathological mechanisms responsible include inflammatory, metabolic-toxic, idiopathic, paraneoplastic or degenerative. In contrast to the inherited degenerative polyneuropathies, usually only individual animals are affected. The causes are also well described, particularly those of the acquired inflammatory, metabolic and paraneoplastic forms. A good comprehensive work-up of the patient leads to a diagnosis. The prognosis is definitely better than with the congenital polyneuropathies in most cases. Some of the patients with acquired inflammatory, metabolic, idiopathic or paraneoplastic polyneuropathies can at least be stabilised. With well-adjusted therapy, a good quality of life is possible. The potential causes are detailed in Table 13.9.

Table 13.9: Differential diagnoses of acquired polyneuropathies in the dog and cat

I	■ Toxoplasmosis (dog/cat) ■ Neosporosis (dog) ■ Acute polyradiculoneuritis (dog/cat) ■ Chronic polyradiculoneuritis (dog/cat) ■ Chronic inflammatory demyelinating polyneuropathy (dog/cat) ■ Sensory ganglioradiculoneuritis (dog)
M	■ Diabetic polyneuropathy (dog/cat) ■ Hypoglycaemic polyneuropathy (dog) ■ Hypothyroidism (dog) ■ Drug- and toxin-induced polyneuropathies (dog/cat)
I	■ Distal denervating polyneuropathy (dog)
N	■ Paraneoplastic polyneuropathy (dog/cat)
D	■ Spinal muscular atrophy (cat) ■ Distal symmetrical polyneuropathy (dog) ■ Dancing Doberman disease (dog) ■ Dysautonomia (dog/cat)

13.3.2.1 Toxoplasmosis
(See Chap. 20.3).

13.3.2.2 Neosporosis
(See Chap. 20.2).

13.3.2.3. Acute polyradiculoneuritis

Occurrence: Sporadic.

Aetiology: An acute form of polyradiculoneuritis, also known as Coonhound paralysis, has been observed in areas where racoons are endemic. The exact pathogenesis is unknown, but the occurrence of neurological disturbances is associated with a raccoon bite. The clinical changes have been reproduced by the experimental injection of raccoon saliva. Possibly, the saliva triggers an immune response against the peripheral nerves; however, this still remains unclear. A disease with an identical clinical picture is called acute idiopathic polyradiculoneuritis or acute idiopathic polyneuropathy. These comparable symptoms and pathological changes occur in areas where contact with a racoon is impossible. Its most probable pathogenesis is a disease affecting the immune system.

Pathological changes are mainly seen in the ventral nerve roots, and rarely in the dorsal ones or in the proximal nerves. The distal peripheral nerve sections are very rarely affected. An infiltration of macrophages, lymphocytes, plasma cells and sometimes neutrophils leads to demyelination and axon degeneration. Whether the demyelination is primarily a consequence of the inflammatory reaction or may be secondary to degeneration of the axon remains controversial. Histopathologically, the inflammatory reaction is obvious though most probably other mechanisms also play a role. As the nerve roots and the proximal nerves are mainly affected, the descriptive term acute idiopathic polyradiculoneuritis is applicable to this syndrome.

Clinical: Coonhound paralysis affects dogs of every age and every breed. Seven to eleven days after a racoon bite, rapidly progressive weakness of the hindlimbs and hyporeflexia occur. Acute polyradiculoneuritis is found world-wide, and dogs (rarely cats) of every age and breed can be affected.

Typical for this disease is the ascending nature of the paralysis. The first signs are paraparesis and hyporeflexia in the hindlimbs. Progressive dysfunction can affect the forelimbs and the head, depending on the severity of the disease. The neurological deficits can develop into tetraplegia, loss of spinal reflexes, facial nerve paralysis, loss of voice and respiratory disturbances (Figs. 13.25 and 13.26). Motor deficits are more pronounced than sensory ones. Food intake and appetite remain normal. The duration of the paralysis lasts from 2 weeks to 3 months.

Diagnosis: Electrophysiology provides an important adjunct investigation. The EMG reveals mild fibrillations, PSWs and in some cases, complex repetitive discharges (see Chap. 7.1.1). Signs of demyelination, such as slightly reduced mNCV, polyphasic action potentials and conduction blocks may be present.

13

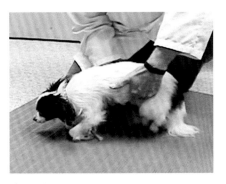

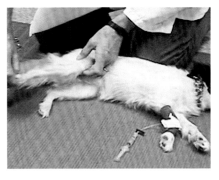

Fig. 13.26
The spinal reflexes in the Papillion in Fig. 13.25 were severely reduced as was the muscle tone. This photograph shows almost total lack of flexor reflex in the right hindleg. The problem could be localised to the LMNS.

Fig. 13.25
A two-year-old Papillion was presented with a rapidly progressive ascending paralysis and loss of voice. The neurological examination revealed a severe tetraparesis and loss of proprioceptive function in all four limbs.

13

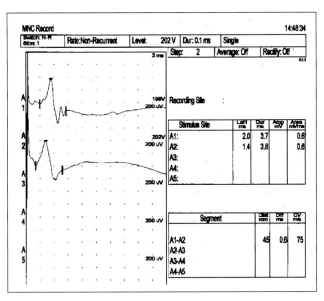

Fig. 13.27
Further investigations in the Papillion with an acute severe tetraparesis in Figs. 13.25 and 13.26 revealed a normal CBC, an increased protein concentration in the CSF taken by lumbar tap as well as a normal lung radiographs. The electrophysiological investigation was done five days after hospitalisation. Mild fibrillations, that tended to occur more often proximally, were recorded on EMG. The results shown in this figure of the peroneal nerve recording showed that the nerve conduction and the duration of the cMAPs are in the normal range. The amplitude of the cMAPs were massively reduced, which in addition to the clinical and other investigatory results, best fits with an acute polyradiculoneuritis. The patient recovered well within 1 month with the help of physiotherapy and without any other medication.

The most conspicuous changes are, however, the reduced or barely recordable action potential amplitudes (Fig. 13.27). Absent or reduced amplitudes of the F wave, prolonged F wave latencies and increased F wave ratios electrophysiologically indicate pathology in the proximal sections of the peripheral nerves. CSF taken by lumbar tap usually has a normal number of cells with increased protein content. Nerve biopsies in the distal sections are usually normal. Muscle pathology confirms neurogenic abnormalities.

Therapy: Corticosteroids may favourably affect the course of the disease, but this is unproven and controversial. More modern therapies such as plasmapheresis and intravenous immunoglobulin therapy may also be used in veterinary medicine in the future. Supportive measures, including physiotherapy and hydrotherapy remain the most important methods of treatment (see Chap. 8).

Prognosis: As long as severe respiratory paralysis requiring artificial respiration does not occur, the prognosis is favourable.

13.3.2.4 Chronic polyradiculoneuritis

Occurrence: Sporadic.

Aetiology: This abnormality is known as chronic idiopathic polyradiculoneuritis or chronic relapsing polyradiculoneuritis. The cause appears to be a disease of the immune system of unknown pathogenesis. The pathological changes are equivalent to those of acute polyradiculoneuritis. Round cell infiltrates consisting of plasma cells, macrophages and lymphocytes are seen in the ventral and dorsal nerve roots and are less pronounced in the peripheral nerve segments. An important histopathological characteristic is demyelination and remyelination which may lead to onion-bulb-like proliferations. Axonal necrosis with the budding of new axons is also present.

Fig. 13.28
A Staffordshire Terrier was presented because of a chronic ascending hemiparesis that had lasted for more than 3 months. Proprioception, reflexes, muscle tone and muscle mass in the right fore- and hindlimbs were significantly reduced. A right-sided facial nerve paralysis with atrophy of the temporalis muscle suggested a generalised disease of the LMNS. Chronic polyradiculoneuritis was presumed but neither administration of prednisolone over several months nor additional therapy with azathioprine led to clinical improvement. Histopathological investigation confirmed generalised infiltration of the nerve roots predominantly with macrophages and some lymphocytes. An immunological process was most likely.

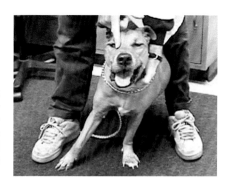

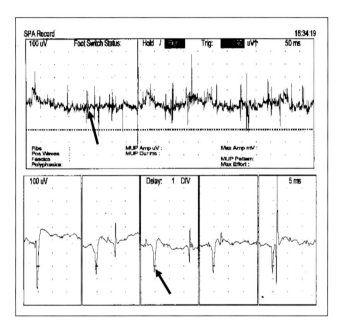

Fig. 13.29
This figure shows the fibrillations and the PSWs in the cranial tibial muscle in the Staffordshire Terrier from Fig. 13.28. Abnormal EMG results could be found in all four limbs as well as in the neck and head musculature.

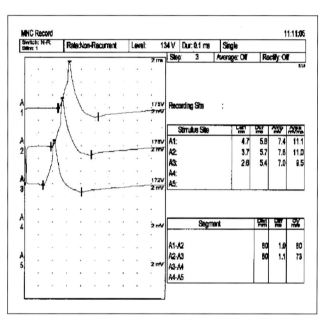

Fig. 13.30
Although the nerve conduction velocity of the peroneal nerve and the duration of the cMAPs in the Staffordshire Terrier from Figs. 13.28 and 13.29 remained in the normal range, the amplitudes of the cMAPs were moderately reduced. These results indicate that a disease of the axons is present.

13

Clinical: This disease has been described in both the dog and cat. The clinical signs are chronic and often intermittent. The paresis can be very slight at the beginning and may be confused with an orthopaedic lameness. In the later stages paraor tetraparesis may develop and the spinal reflexes are reduced; dysphonia and facial paralysis have also been described. Muscle atrophy is the logical consequence due to the disease's chronic course (Fig. 13.28). In one cat, fine tremor, disturbances of sensation and intense licking of the hindlimbs was observed.

Diagnosis: Important additional investigations include: electrophysiology with spontaneous activity on EMG (Fig 13.29), polyphasic and prolonged cMAPs, and reduced NCV (Figs. 13.30 and 13.31); CSF with a normal cell count and increased protein content; and muscle and nerve biopsies.

Therapy: Treatment with high doses of corticosteroids over many weeks may be successful (see Chap. 9.2).

Prognosis: Slow recurrence of the symptoms after stopping corticosteroid treatment is possible.

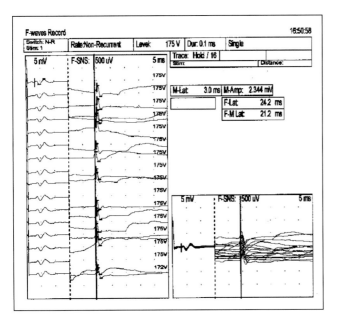

Fig. 13.31
This figure shows a study of the F waves in the Staffordshire Terrier from Figs. 13.28–13.30. The calculation of the F wave relationships can be useful in differentiating whether nerve disease affects the whole nerve equally, just the nerve roots or more obviously the distal part of the nerve. The results from the Staffordshire Terrier reveal an F wave relationship significantly above the normal value, which indicates severe disease of the nerve roots and the proximal segments of the nerve.

13.3.2.5 Chronic inflammatory demyelinating polyneuropathy

Occurrence: Rare.

Aetiology: This is also presumed to be an autoimmune disease. The predominant features are paranodal demyelination, remyelination and in some cases onion-bulb-like myelin proliferation. In contrast to chronic polyganglioradiculoneuritis, the inflammatory infiltrate is more moderate and consists mainly of macrophages. Axonal degeneration or necrosis is not present.

Clinical: This disease can affect dogs and cats of every age. The course is chronic progressive and is very often intermittent. The clinical signs include lameness, para- or tetraparesis, hyporeflexia and muscle atrophy. In the cat, plantigrade hindlimbs and ventroflexion of the neck may also occur. Changes in the voice, laryngeal paralysis, megaoesophagus and facial nerve paralysis can occur when the cranial nerves are affected.

Diagnosis: The results of the electrophysiological tests include: normal EMG, reduced NCV, polyphasic and prolonged action potentials.

Therapy: The administration of prednisolone 1–2mg/kg, PO, daily leads to a remission of the symptoms in the majority of cases. Afterwards the steroid dosage can be slowly reduced (see Chap. 9.2).

Prognosis: Some of the patients do not respond or respond unsatisfactorily to prednisolone. Relapses are not uncommon, but they can often be controlled with prednisolone.

13.3.2.6 Canine ganglioradiculitis

Occurrence: Rare.

Aetiology: The most conspicuous characteristics of this disease are degeneration and a nonpurulent inflammation of the dorsal nerve roots and the sensory ganglia. The ventral nerve roots are only marginally affected. These changes have been observed in both the spinal and cranial nerves. Lymphocytes and macrophages destroy the satellite cells and the myelin. Nerve fibres with large diameters, responsible for proprioceptive functions, appear to be more severely affected than the thinner fibres. The histological picture is reminiscent of an allergic neuritis. The cause of this disease is unknown. Mechanisms such as autoimmune disease, viral infections and toxins (e.g. mercury, pyridoxine and doxorubicin) have been considered. A paraneoplastic disease, HIV infection and borreliosis have been present in human beings with similar clinical and pathological changes.

Clinical: This disease has been described differently in various breeds, but the Siberian Husky is apparently most commonly affected. Young adult dogs are mainly affected. The changes are chronically progressive, but an acute form has also been described. The clinical signs include ataxia and hypermetria, abnormal proprioception in all four limbs and a reduced patella reflex. The flexor reflexes and muscle mass remain normal; atrophy of the masticatory muscles sometimes occurs. Other abnormal cranial nerve functions include hypalgesia of the face, difficulty prehending food, dysphagia and salivation, head tilt or a loss of hearing. In addition, megaoesophagus, dysphonia, Horner's syndrome and more rarely self-mutilation have been observed.

Diagnosis: The clinical picture is nonspecific and other diseases must be excluded. An important diagnostic aid is electrophysiology. EMG and mNCV are normal or are only minimally affected, while the sensory nerve conduction is usually not recordable or markedly reduced. The CSF remains unchanged, although a slight pleocytosis and increased protein content have been described. Atrophy of the sensory fibres has been seen in large cross-sections of a nerve biopsy from a mixed nerve.

Therapy: Specific treatment is not possible; corticosteroids appear not to be effective. Supportive measures are essential (see Chap. 8).

Prognosis: The prognosis is poor to guarded because of the limited therapeutic possibilities; however, cases of spontaneous recovery have been described.

13.3.2.7 Diabetic polyneuropathy

Occurrence: Sporadic.

Aetiology: Diabetic polyneuropathy is a common complication in human beings. The clinical signs predominantly include a loss of sensation in the distal limbs. Later, motor disturbances develop, too. Diabetic polyneuropathy in domestic animals is observed most commonly in the cat, though it does occur in the dog. Most probably, sensory abnormalities occur more commonly than has been assumed, but they are more difficult to diagnose in domestic animals than in human beings. Histological investigation of this disease in the dog and cat have revealed demyelination and remyelination in the long nerves. Degeneration of the distal axons is present, but it is only slight. The proximal segments of the nerves demonstrate virtually no changes.

Electron-microscopic investigations of the Schwann cells from diabetic cats indicate a primary injury of these myelin-building organs. One possible pathological mechanism for Schwann cell dysfunction is an abnormal myo-inositol metabolism, disturbed function of sodium / potassium ATPase or an abnormal phospholipid metabolism. Reduced protein synthesis in the neuron, reduced axonal transport in the periphery and interstitial hyperosmolarity, as well as ischemia due to abnormal blood vessels have all been mentioned as potential causes of the reduced diameter of the distal axons seen in this disease. In the subclinical stage in human beings, demyelination occurs first and only later does the distal axonopathy come to the fore. How much improved control of hyperglycaemia improves the nerve function is controversial in human beings. Reliable data on the course of diabetic polyneuropathy before and after therapy are not available for the dog and cat.

Clinical: In the dog, the clinical signs are either subclinical or mild. Paraparesis, slightly reduced reflexes and generalised muscle atrophy can occur. Cats show more prominent changes; paraparesis, plantigrade positioning of the hindlimbs, abnormal proprioception, reduced spinal reflexes and muscle atrophy have been seen. In severe cases, ventroflexion of the head can occur as well.

Diagnosis: The basic diagnostic abnormalities include increased blood glucose, glucosuria, ketonurea or an increased serum fructosamine concentration (see Chap. 4). EMG shows fibrillations, PSWs and complex repetitive discharges. Motor and sensory nerve conduction tests indicate a slightly reduced velocity and reduced amplitudes of the cMAPs. The abnormalities are more pronounced in the distal nerves.

Therapy: Insulin, diet, regular blood sugar profiles.

Prognosis: In the cat, an improvement of the polyneuropathy is often attained with adequate blood sugar control. Comprehensive studies are, however, lacking.

13.3.2.8 Hypoglycaemic polyneuropathy

Occurrence: Rare.

Aetiology: The cause for the hypoglycaemia is often an insulinoma. Due to malignant change of the B-cells in the pancreas, an intermittent or chronically low blood glucose concentration arises. Leiomyosarcoma is another tumour that can induce chronic hypoglycaemia. Seizures, syncope, behavioural changes and tremor are not uncommon, so generalised weakness, which is usually present, is often overlooked. In some cases, the dogs are presented primarily because of gait disturbances, which may be caused by a hypoglycaemic polyneuropathy.

The causative relationship between hypoglycaemia and neuropathy is not known. The question of whether chronic hypoglycaemia is the primary cause of the polyneuropathy or whether the nerve changes are associated with the tumour itself remains unclear. A correlation between the duration and degree of hypoglycaemia with the disease severity does not seem to be present. Histologically, the main characteristics are demyelination, remyelination and axonal degeneration. If paranodal or segmental demyelination progresses, then subclinical changes can become clinically apparent.

Clinical: Middle-aged or older dogs are affected. The possible clinical signs of the polyneuropathy include weakness, tetraparesis, abnormal proprioception, and slightly to moderately reduced spinal reflexes. An isolated case of facial paralysis has been described.

Diagnosis: Repeatedly abnormal blood glucose concentrations in association with the clinical symptoms: glucose values under 3.3.mmol/l after fasting; high insulin levels (> 20 mU/ml) with glucose values under 3.3 mmol/l and clinical symptoms; insulin-glucose ratio > 30 (plasma insulin [mU/ml] × 100): (plasma glucose [mmol/l] × 18–30); ultrasonography of the abdomen; MRI; exploratory laparotomy; EMG changes with fibrillations, PSW more pronounced in the distal limb musculature, reduced mNCV and reduced am-

13

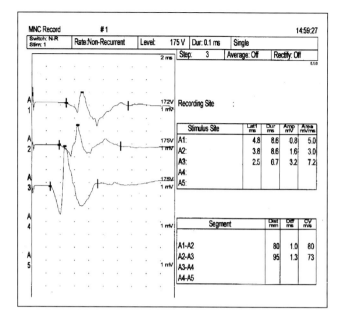

Fig. 13.32
An eight-year-old Golden Retriever was presented with an insulinoma and severe tetraparesis. The electrophysiological examination was very valuable in confirming and characterising the presence of a concomitant disease of the LMNS. The figure shows classical PSWs on an EMG investigation of the cranial tibial muscle.

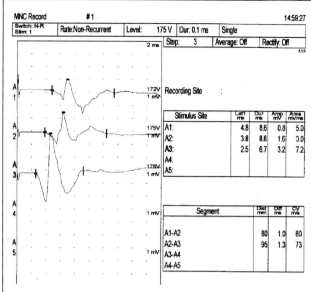

Fig. 13.33
Motor nerve conduction was also investigated in the Golden Retriever from Fig. 13.32. The most obvious finding was severe reduction in the amplitude of the cMAPs, which indicates primary degeneration of the axons. Although the nerve conduction velocity of the peroneal nerve was in the normal range, the increased duration of the cMAPs and the tendency for polyphasic amplitudes suggests a secondary concomitant disease of the myelin sheaths.

plitudes of the cMAPs; muscle and nerve biopsies are the keys to definitive diagnosis (Figs. 13.32 and 13.33).

Therapy: Stabilisation of the glucose values with intravenous infusions of dextrose, prednisolone administration, diet, and cage rest. Surgical removal of the primary tumour is associated with the best results, as long as metastasis to the surrounding organs, or more rarely to the lungs, has not taken place. For tumours that cannot be resected, chemotherapy with alloxan or streptozotocin can be attempted; however, comprehensive information about the success and use of these drugs is lacking in veterinary medicine. Strategies which are suitable for symptomatic therapy include: diet, prednisolone (0.25–3 mg/kg, PO, BID), diazoxide (5–30 mg/kg, PO, BID) or somatostatin octreoide acetate (10–20 mg, SC, BID–TID).

Prognosis: Often unfavourable. Roughly half of the patients already have metastases in the liver, lymph nodes or other sites at the time of diagnosis. In patients without metastases, surgical resection of the primary tumour can positively influence the polyneuropathy. Electrophysiological follow-up and repeated nerve and muscle biopsies have demonstrated functional and histological improvement of the peripheral nerves (Fig. 13.34).

13.3.2.9 Hypothyroidism
(See Chap. 15.4.3)

13.3.2.10 Drugs and toxins

Occurrence: Rare.

Aetiology: Some toxins, heavy metals and drugs damage the peripheral nerves and lead to demonstrable changes in their structure. The information available in the dog and cat are mainly derived from experimental studies. The cause of spontaneously occurring cases is usually speculative as the demonstration of a toxin is very costly and, therefore, rarely done.

Lead causes generalised demyelination as this heavy metal adversely affects the functioning of Schwann cells. The application of thallium or methylmecury silver diacyanide leads to swelling of the proximal axons with Wallerian-like degeneration of the distal nerve segments. Vincristine used in chemotherapy also causes axonal swelling and hinders axonal transport.

Necrosis of the distal nerve segments has been seen with the intake of triorthocresyl phosphate, acrylamide and salinomycin. The pathological mechanism of these distal axonopathies (or dying-back neuropathies) is not completely understood. Disturbances in the protein synthesis of the perikaryon, dysfunction of the rapid axonal metabolite transport and reduced retrograde axonoplasmic flow have been discussed. For some of the toxins listed in Tables 13.10 and 13.11, there is little information available about their pathophysiology and their clinical relevance should therefore be judged with care. The sensitivity of dogs and cats to these toxins can be different and even within a species there is not a strong correlation between exposure and symptoms. Questions about any possible toxins should, however, be asked in every case of peripheral polyneuropathy with an uncertain aetiology. Two lists of compounds that are possibly toxic to axons are given in Tables 13.10 and 13.11.

Clinical: The signs are very variable. The clinical signs can range from paraparesis to severe generalised disease of the LMNS that includes the cranial nerves.

Diagnosis: Anamnesis, possible exposure to a toxin or administered medications, and the exclusion of other diseases is essential. The determination of toxicity is only possible if the noxious agent is known or if there are hard and fast indications from the anamnesis. Electrophysiology, muscle and nerve biopsies as well as the removal of suspicious medications are the basis for describing the disturbances more fully.

Therapy: Toxic reactions to medications improve quickly when therapy is stopped. For most of the other intoxications there is no specific therapy. Supportive treatment is important.

Prognosis: The prognosis depends on the toxin or medication and the amount taken in by the animal.

13.3.2.11 Denervating distal axonopathy

Occurrence: Rare; dog.

Aetiology: The pathogenesis is unknown. A toxin or metabolic abnormality has not been proven so far. Spontaneous recovery seen in many patients is not typical of a purely degenerative disease. These idiopathic polyneuropathies have been predominantly seen in Great Britain. Histologically, the distal intramuscular axons are changed and degenerate. Budding of new axons is conspicuous, which most probably is the key to the clinical recovery. The proximal and middle segments of the nerves remain unchanged. The muscles show a typical neurogenic atrophy.

Clinical: There is no predisposition for age, gender or breed. The clinical symptoms occur within 1 to 4 weeks. Motor deficits are predominant. Muscle tone and reflexes are reduced. The neck muscles can also be affected. Cranial nerves: facial nerve paralysis is rare. The sensory functions remain unaffected. Respiratory paralysis has not been observed. The

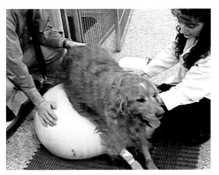

Fig. 13.34
The Golden Retriever from Figs. 13.32 and 13.33 one week after removal of the insulinoma. The dog's blood glucose values had normalised. Physiotherapy is essential as supportive treatment during reconvalescence of a hypoglycaemic polyneuropathy patient.

Table 13.10: Toxins and medications that have been associated with polyneuropathies in the dog and cat

Medications	Heavy metals	Other chemical compounds
Cisplatin (dog)	Lead (dog / cat)	Chlorpyriphos (cat)
Nitrofurantoin (dog)	Mercury (dog / cat)	Hexacarbon (cat)
Pyridoxine (dog)	Thallium (dog / cat)	Hexachlorophene (dog / cat)
Salinomycin (cat)		Trimethylphosphate (dog)
Vincristine (dog / cat)		Tri-ortho-cresyl phosphate

13

Table 13.11: Toxins and medications that have caused polyneuropathies in humans and other species and so may potentially be toxic for the dog and cat

Medications	Heavy metals	Other chemical compounds
Diphenylhydrantoin	Gold	Carbon disulphide
Doxorubicin		Carbon tetrachloride
Vinblastine		Lindane
		N-hexane
		Trichloroethylene

muscle atrophy is generalised, although the proximal extensor muscles are the ones most conspicuously affected.

Diagnosis: An important adjunct investigation is electrophysiology. EMG: spontaneous abnormal activity; motor nerve conduction: velocities in low normal range, and the action potentials are polyphasic, the amplitude of the cMAPs are reduced; sensory nerve conduction remains normal. Muscle and nerve biopsies provide important information for the diagnosis.

Therapy: No specific therapy is possible. Supportive measures are of paramount importance.

Prognosis: In the majority of cases, spontaneous recovery occurs within 1 month.

13.3.2.12 Paraneoplastic polyneuropathy

Occurrence: Sporadic.

Aetiology: The clinical significance of paraneoplastic neuropathies has been established in human beings, with several types of tumour causing subclinical or clinical neurological disturbances. Little has been published about the incidence of paraneoplastic polyneuropathies in the dog and cat. Despite this, there is an association between certain tumours and polyneuropathy. In a study on dogs with bronchial carcinoma, mammary gland adenocarcinoma, malignant melanoma, insulinoma, osteosarcoma, thyroid adenocarcinoma or mast cell tumour, nerve changes such as demyelination, remyelination and axon degeneration were more frequently seen in the affected animals than in control animals of the same age. Possible pathological mechanisms include the effects of biologically active substances produced by the tumour; tumour-induced antibodies against myelin or glycoproteins of the nerves; immunosuppression; opportunistic infections; or a deficit in essential compounds as a consequence of the tumour's competitive metabolism.

Clinical: The symptoms are variable and range from subtle subclinical deficits to severe, obvious disturbances. Para- or tetraparesis, abnormal proprioception, reduced spinal reflexes and muscle tone have been described in dogs with bronchial carcinoma, insulinoma, leiomyosarcoma, haemangiosarcoma and undifferentiated sarcoma.

Diagnosis: Confirmation of the neoplasm (radiography of the lungs, ultrasonography of the abdomen, CT, MRI, biopsy), exclusion of other concomitant metabolic disturbances, electrophysiology, muscle and nerve biopsies are essential.

Therapy: Surgery, radiation and chemotherapy are possible.

Prognosis: Depends on the type of tumour and the stage. Solitary operable tumours without metastases have the best prospects. Improvement of the neurological status has been described in a dog with bronchial carcinoma after successful tumour excision. In many patients, however, only palliative or symptomatic treatment is possible, which is hardly able to improve the polyneuropathy.

13.3.2.13 Spinal muscular atrophy in adulthood

Occurrence: Very rare; cat.

Aetiology: This disease of unknown aetiology has been described in several cats. The degeneration of α-motor neurons is limited to the spinal cord and the brain stem.

Clinical: The first signs occur in middle to older age. The course is slow and progressive. The neurological changes include generalised weakness, muscle fasciculations and atrophy. The fasciculations can even affect the tongue. In the later stages, ventroflexion of the neck, difficulty in ingesting food and severe tremor have been described. Reduced spinal reflexes occur in the advanced stages.

Diagnosis: A tentative diagnosis can be made on the basis of disease progression, clinical picture, electrophysiological results (fibrillations, reduced amplitude of the cMAPs), and muscle and nerve biopsies. A definitive diagnosis can only be achieved with histological investigation of the spinal cord.

Therapy: No specific therapy is possible; supportive measures are advised.

Prognosis: The disease is progressive. According to the available reports, the prognosis is very unfavourable.

13.3.2.14 Symmetrical distal polyneuropathy

Occurrence: Rare.

Aetiology: This disease is a distal sensorimotor polyneuropathy that particularly affects young adult dogs of medium-sized and large breeds. The cause is unknown. Pathologically, there is obvious degeneration of the distal motor neurons in the limbs and larynx. Different degrees of demyelination and remyelination can also be present. The sensory and autonomic nervous systems are only marginally affected. Neurogenic atrophy is prominent

Clinical: The clinical signs include chronic, progressive weakness of the hindlimbs, which then increasingly affects the forelimbs. The proprioceptive reactions are mildly to moderately altered. A prominant lameness in the forelimbs can occur. Muscle atrophy is obvious on the head and over the distal limbs. The sensory function remains normal.

Diagnosis: EMG: fibrillations and PSWs below the elbow and knee; nerve conduction: slight to moderate reduction in the NCV, slight polyphasic cMAPs with obviously reduced amplitudes. Muscle and nerve biopsy: distal axonopathy, demyelination, neurogenic muscle atrophy.

Therapy: No specific treatment is possible. The disease does not respond either to corticosteroids or thyroid hormone substitution.

Prognosis: Unfavourable. The course is similar to that of the majority of degenerative diseases: chronic progressive.

13.3.2.15 Dancing Doberman disease

Occurrence: Very rare.

Aetiology: Only Doberman Pinschers are known to be affected. A chronic progressive disturbance affects the gastrocnemius muscle and the distal part of the tibial nerve. Whether it is a primary myopathy or a distal axonopathy has not been clearly determined. The primary cause is also unknown, but Dancing Doberman disease shows some characteristics of a degenerative disease.

Clinical: The disease starts in young adult dogs and is chronic progressive in nature. The clinical picture is dominated by flexion of the hock. Initially, only one limb is affected, but it often progresses to become apparent in both hindlimbs. Paraparesis and proprioceptive deficits in the hindlimbs are often present in addition to an increased patella reflex. Atrophy of the gastrocnemius muscle is usually obvious. Weakness of the hindlimbs leads to a restless, stepping and "dancing" movement, which gives the disease its name.

Diagnosis: Signalment, clinical picture, course of disease and selective atrophy of the gastrocnemius muscle are important diagnostic indicators. Adjunct investigations include (i) electrophysiology with fibrillations, PSWs and complex repetitive discharges on the EMG, (ii) muscle and nerve biopsy with axonal necrosis and muscle changes similar to those of a myotonic myopathy.

Therapy: None known as yet.

Prognosis: The disease is very slowly progressive. Usually the quality of life can be retained over a number of months up to 6 years.

13.3.2.16 Dysautonomia

Occurrence: Rare.

Aetiology: The first cases of dysautonomia in the cat occurred in the UK. Since then, feline dysautonomia has been observed in Scandinavia, sporadically in other European countries and the USA. The main pathological change is degeneration of the neurons of the autonomic nervous system. The most obviously affected ones include those of the pelvic, mesenteric and ciliary ganglia. Degenerative changes can also occur in the CNS of dogs and cats. The intermediolateral grey matter of the spinal cord, the motor neurons of the ventral spinal cord and the nuclei of the cranial nerves are abnormal in some patients. Electron-microscopic investigations of the degenerating neurons demonstrate disturbed protein synthesis. The basic cause remains unknown; neither a neurotoxin, an environmental factor nor infections have been found. Epidemiological studies in dogs have shown that young adult dogs have a higher risk of becoming affected during the months February to April. Another risk group are dogs which spend most of their time outside in rural areas. Additionally, it appears that certain regions in the USA have distinctly more cases of canine dysautonomia than others.

Clinical: Dysautonomia can occur in dogs and cats of every age, but animals in the second or third year of life are more commonly affected. The course is acute, but also chronic progressive forms are presumed to occur. The most common clinical signs in the dog include dysuria, enlarged bladder, mydriasis, loss of pupillary reflex, dry mucous membranes and reduced tear production. Other important symptoms include protrusion of the nictitating membrane, loss of weight, apathy, reduced appetite, regurgitation / vomiting, constipation and diarrhoea. In the cat, depression, anorexia, constipation, regurgitation, dry nose, reduced tear production and dilated pupils with prolapse of the nictitating membrane are frequent. Bradycardia, reduced anal reflex, faecal and urinary incontinence, and paraparesis are other clinical signs which have been documented.

Diagnosis: Adjunct investigations are helpful. Evaluation of tear production is performed with a Schirmer tear test (normal values: cat $>$ 20 mm/min; dog $>$ 25 mm/min). After parasympathetic denervation, 1–2 drops of 0.05% pilocarpine solution in the eye lead to a rapid constriction within 15 minutes. A low mean arterial blood pressure which does not increase after orthostatic manipulation and significant bradycardia are other clinical signs reported in the cat. A lack of cardiac response to the administration of atropine (0.02–0.04 mg/kg, IM or IV), is part of the autonomic dysfunction noted.

A new test described in the dog is the intradermal histamine injection. Local oedema and erythema occur in healthy animals within 30 minutes after the application of 0.05–0.1 ml histamine (1:1000–1:10000). In dogs with dysautonomia, roughly half of the patients respond with local oedema, but no erythema is observed in the majority of them. Radiography: megaoesophagus with an air-filled stomach and intestines; the bladder can be greatly dilated and filled with urine. Secondary haemoconcentration and urinary tract infections are not uncommon. A definitive diagnosis can only be achieved with histopathology.

13

Therapy: Symptomatic therapy includes the following possibilities: isotonic electrolyte solutions; parenteral feeding via stomach tube; 1% pilocarpine eye drops BID to constrict the pupils; tear replacement therapy in both eyes QID; bethanechol to support bladder contraction 0.5–1.0 mg/kg, PO, TID; metoclopramide 0.2–0.5 mg/kg, PO, SC, IV, TID to improve the gastrointestinal motility; lactulose for severe constipation.

Prognosis: In general, unfavourable: roughly 70% of cats and dogs must be euthanised. There is a high risk of aspiration pneumonia with megaoesophagus. In certain cases, the condition can stabilise and the animal's quality of life is good with adequate symptomatic therapy.

Further reading

CUDDON, P. (2002): Acquired canine peripheral neuropathies. In: Neuromuscular diseases. Vet Clin North Am Small Anim Pract. **1**: 207–250.

CUDDON, P. (1998): Electrophysiologic assessment of acute polyradiculoneuropathy in dogs: Comparison with Guillan-Barré syndrome in people. J Vet Intern Med. **12**: 294–303.

DYER INZANA, K. (2000): Peripheral nerve disorders. In: ETTINGER S.J., FELDMANN E.C. (eds.) Textbook of Veterinary Medicine, 5th ed., W.B. Saunders Company, Philadelphia, pp. 662–683.

HARKIN, K.R., CASH, W.C., SHELTON, G.D. (2005): Sensory and motor neuropathy in a Border Collie. J Am Vet Med Assoc. **227** (8): 1263–1265.

O'BRIEN, D.P., JOHNSON, G.C., (2002): Dysautonomia and autonomic neuropathies. In: Neuromuscular diseases. Vet Clin North Am Small Anim Pract. **1**: 251–266.

PLATT, S.R. (2002): Neuromuscular complications in endocrine and metabolic disorders. In: Neuromuscular diseases. Vet Clin North Am. Small Anim Pract. **1**: 125–146.

TOWELL, T.L., SHELL, L.C. (1994): Endocrinopathies that affect peripheral nerves of cats and dogs. Compend Contin Educat. **16**: 157–161.

VERMEERSCH, K., VAN HAM, L., BRAUND, K.G., BHATTI, S., TSHAMALA, M., CHIERS, K., SCHRAUWEN, E. (2005): Sensory neuropathy in two Border Collie puppies. J Small Anim Pract. **46** (6): 295–299.

13.4 Neuromuscular transmission abnormalities

In the synapse, the action potentials are transmitted from the nerve to the effector organ, which is a complicated process. The electrical impulse develops in the hilus region of the neuron, moves along the nerve into the distal branch and elicits different chemical reactions in the presynaptic zone of the nerve ending. The action potential causes an influx of cal-

Table 13.12: Differential diagnoses of neuromuscular synapse diseases in the dog and cat

I	■ Myasthenia gravis (dog/cat)
T	■ Tetanus (dog/cat)
	■ Botulism (dog)
	■ Organophosphate poisoning (dog/cat)
	■ Tick paralysis (dog)
	■ Snake bite (dog/cat)

cium into the axon, which is an important prerequisite for the secretion of acetylcholine, contained within vesicles, in the synaptic space. After the diffusion of acetylcholine through the synaptic space, this neurotransmitter causes the sodium and potassium channels in the postsynaptic receptor membrane of the musculature to open. An avalanche-like influx of sodium generates an electrical impulse. The action potential distributes itself rapidly over the whole muscle cell, and the electrical activity increases the calcium permeability of the longitudinal tubuli of the sarcoplasmic reticulum. Due to the resulting massive influx of calcium in the muscle fibrils, the calcium molecule can bind to troponin, which facilitates the interaction between actin and myosin and so, makes muscle contraction possible.

In general, diseases of the synapse cause symptoms of the LMNS, such as hypotonia or atony, flaccid paralysis, and hypo- or areflexia. In chronic cases, muscle atrophy may occur but this is not common. Inflammation toxic reactions, and in rare cases anomalous diseases are the most frequent responsible pathological mechanisms in veterinary medicine. For didactic reasons, the list of possible causative diseases is classified according to the localisation of the disturbance in presynaptic, synaptic and postsynaptic diseases. The differential diagnoses are listed in Table 13.12.

13.4.1 Presynaptic disturbances

13.4.1.1 Tetanus

Occurrence: Rare in dogs and cats.

Aetiology: Tetanus is a presynaptic disturbance that is caused by the neurotoxic polypeptide tetanospamin.

A few hours after anaerobic contamination of a wound with the spores of *Clostridium tetani*, this substance is synthesised *in situ*. The neurotoxin blocks the presynaptic release of the inhibitory neurotransmitters glycine and GABA from the Renshaw cells, by hindering the coupling of the neurotransmitter vesicles to the presynaptic membrane. These Renshaw interneurons normally reduce the activity of the LMNS, and especially that of the extensor muscles. Due to this dysinhibi-

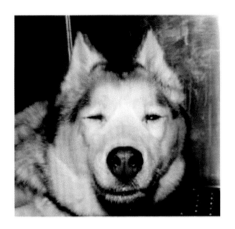

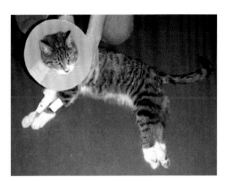

Fig. 13.35 (left)
Risus sardonicus in a Husky with tetanus. The ears are notably turned backwards and the orbicularis oculi muscles are contracted making the eyelids appear to be half-closed.

Fig. 13.36 (right)
This photograph shows a domestic cat with focal tetanus of the hindlimbs. Both hindlegs are extremely stiff and extended backwards with the paws held in flexion. The animal was presented one week after castration with a scrotal infection and progressive ascending weakness of the hindlimbs.

tion of the LMNS, a characteristic condition of continual and increased muscle tone is induced. Two possible pathways for the transport of the toxin are possible. The neurotoxin can travel to higher CNS centres via retrograde axonal transport of the peripheral nerves, ultimately reaching the interneuron pool. This mechanism leads first of all to localised tetanus. Subsequently, generalisation of the disease occurs as the toxin diffuses through the CNS. Additionally, haematogenous dissemination can directly result in the generalised form. Young dogs, undergoing tooth replacement or dogs and cats with skin injuries can become affected with tetanus if the environment is contaminated with *C. tetani* spores.

Clinical: The typical clinical signs do not involve a flaccid paralysis as is usual with diseases of the LMNS. In contrast, spasticity and increased muscle tone are the predominant symptoms.

In the generalised form, spasm of the extensor muscles leads to a stiff gait; upright tail; upright, almost parallel ear posture; drawn back lips (risus sardonicus; Fig. 13.35); increase jaw tone (lockjaw / trismus); wide-opened eyes and sometimes prolapse of the third eyelid. The autonomic symptoms of dysuria, urine retention and constipation may also be present. The clinical signs become more pronounced with excitement. Lateral recumbency with extensor spasm, opisthotonus, and cyanosis due to spasm of the diaphragm are possible. Death can arise due to starvation and dehydration because of trismus or be due to respiratory failure.

In the focal form in the cat, often only one limb is affected (Fig. 13.36). The affected fore- or hindlimb has increased muscle tone, is stiff, rigid and is "held" almost horizontally backwards. Carpal flexion in the forelimbs and flexion of the toes in the fore- or hindlimbs is typical for this disease. The spinal reflexes are increased if they can be elicited at all. Due to the chronic course of the disease, muscle atrophy often occurs.

Diagnosis: The clinical picture provides obvious indications of this disease. Definitive proof is not easy. Culture of *C. tetani* is very difficult and time-consuming. EMG can provide important adjunctive information. Even under anaesthesia, spontaneous motor cMAPs can be observed. The velocity and amplitude of the cMAPs are normal based on nerve conduction studies.

Therapy: If there is an infection, the wound should be cleansed. Tetanus antitoxin (25–110 iu/kg, IV, IM) is only effective against the free or unbound neurotoxin in the wound, blood and synaptic space. As soon as the neurotoxin enters the nerve or presynaptic nerve ending, antitoxin is no longer effective. Anaphylactic shock immediately following an intravenous injection of antitoxin is possible. Penicillin G (40000–100000 iu/kg, IV, IM, initially QID; thereafter 20000 iu/kg IV, IM, BID) is used to treat the *C. tetani* that are still active in the wound. An effective alternative is metronidazole 10–15 mg/kg IV, PO, TID. GABA antagonists such as diazepam 0.5 mg/kg, IV, TID or clonazepam 0.5–2 mg/kg, PO, BID–TID can be used to induce muscle relaxation. An alternative, chlorpromazine 0.5–2 mg/kg, BID PO, can produce a very pleasant sedative effect in addition to muscle relaxation. Feeding via stomach tube may be needed. If there is urinary incontinence, the bladder should be regularly catheterised. A quiet and protected bed and supportative measures such as physiotherapy are also important for the success of the treatment, especially in the local form affecting the limbs.

Prognosis: The tetanus toxin is active for 2 to 3 weeks. In the generalised form, the symptoms regress after this period of time. The local form affecting the limbs in the cat can last for 2 to 3 months.

13

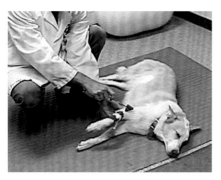

Fig. 13.37
A ten-year-old Collie Crossbreed was brought to the hospital with tetraplegia, loss of voice and abdominal respiration ten hours after having eaten rotten meat. The dog was too weak to raise its head.

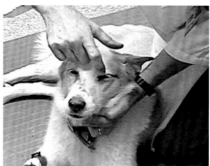

Fig. 13.38
The palpebral reflex, jaw tone and swallowing reflex were all severely reduced in the dog from Fig. 13.37.

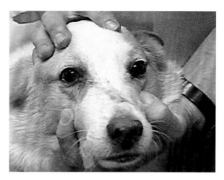

Fig. 13.39
A physiological nystagmus could not be stimulated in the Collie Cross from Figs. 13.37 and 13.38. The cause of the animal's severe and very generalised deficits in the LMNS proved to be botulinum toxin.

13.4.1.2 Botulism

Occurrence: Infrequent in the dog; very rare in cats.

Aetiology: The botulinum toxin is a neurotoxin which is formed by the bacterium *Clostridium botulinum*. Dogs, and cats, have been reported to be affected by botulinum toxin type C. The intake of the toxin results from the ingestion of dead, rotting animal or bird flesh, excreta from affected animals or contaminated foods. The toxin can also be produced in wounds under anaerobic conditions. The neurotoxin blocks the presynaptic release of acetylcholine as it prevents the coupling of the acetylcholine vesicle on the presynaptic membrane, so that the calcium influx can no longer induce a release of this neurotransmitter. The toxin binds irreversibly to the presynaptic membrane. For clinical recovery, the axon must bud anew.

Clinical: The clinical signs occur within 24 to 48 hours of ingestion. The main symptom is a generalised flaccid paralysis which can initially start as a mild pelvic limb gait abnormality (Fig. 13.37). The clinical signs include progressive tetraparesis to tetraplegia, and paralysis of the cranial musculature. Facial nerve paralysis, ophthalmoplegia, dysphagia, disturbances in swallowing, megaoesophagus and dysphonia can occur. Symptoms of autonomic nervous system dysfunction, such as bradycardia, reduced tear production, ileus, mydriasis and a dilated bladder, may also become apparent (Figs. 13.38 and 13.39). Sensation and nociception remain normal. The risk of aspiration pneumonia is high in the recumbent dog and respiratory paralysis is possible.

Diagnosis: Electrophysiological investigations provide the most important diagnostic indication of disease. The EMG is initially normal; fibrillations and PSWs are seen in the recovery phase. Nerve conduction reveals reduced cMAPs, and a slightly reduced NCV. Reduction in the cMAP amplitudes of 7% or more with 3 Hz repetitive nerve stimulation has been described in several dogs. In how far this decrement is a reliable result for the diagnosis of botulism remains unclear. The definitive diagnosis of this disease is difficult and it relies on the detection of toxin. The neurotoxin can be found in the serum, faeces or vomit.

Therapy: Neutralisation of the botulinum toxin in the initial phase is possible, prior to the irreversible binding. In the dog, an antitoxin against type C should be given within the first five days from the start of symptoms. The use of penicillin is controversial. The most important part of treatment is the supportive measures. Feeding via stomach tube is essential.

Prognosis: The prognosis is guarded. The disease can last for 3 to 4 weeks before improvement occurs.

13.4.1.3 Tick paralysis

Occurrence: Rare in dogs.

Aetiology: Paralysis after a tick bite has been described in North America and Australia. The paralysis is due to a neurotoxin which can be found in the saliva of female *Dermacentor variabilis*, *Dermacentor andersoni* or *Ixodes holocyclus*.

These tick species are not found in Europe. The toxin blocks neuromuscular transmission within a few days by inhibiting the depolarisation of the nerve ending's presynaptic membrane necessary for the release of acetylcholine.

Clinical: An ascending flaccid paralysis occurs within a few days and can cause death through respiratory paralysis.

Diagnosis: Symptomatic; the detection of attached ticks as well as a rapid improvement after they have been removed are important indicators. Electrophysiological investigations can also be useful.

Therapy: Clinical improvement can be attained within 24 hours after removing the ticks.

Prognosis: Usually favourable.

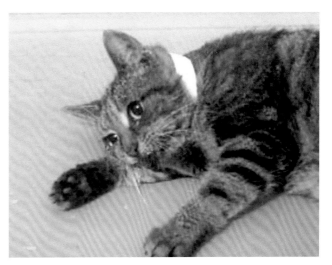

Fig. 13.40
A cat sprayed with organophosphates manifested notable tetraparesis and dilated pupils.

13.4.2 Synaptic disturbances

13.4.2.1 Organophosphates

Occurrence: Rare.

Aetiology: Intoxication with organophosphate- or carbamate-containing insecticides is seen every now and then. While organophosphates bind irreversibly with acetylcholine esterase, carbamate forms a reversible bond. Both substances inhibit the activity of acetylcholine esterase in the synaptic space. Acetylcholine accumulates and so causes over-stimulation and "tiring" of the central and peripheral receptors. The increased acetylcholine concentration over-stimulates the somatic nicotinic, nicotinic preganglionic parasympathetic and sympathetic, and the muscarinic postganglionic parasympathetic receptors.

Clinical: The clinical signs are somatic (muscle tremor, fasciculations, stiff gait, paralysis) and autonomic (miosis, mydriasis, hypersalivation, bradycardia, tachycardia, abnormal respiration, vomiting, diarrhoea, anorexia, continual micturition). Central disturbances such as seizures can occur, too. The distribution pattern and the degree of deficits depend on the causative agent, the dosage and other factors. As far as it is known, carbamates do not cause weakness in cats. Intoxication with fenthion in the dog predominantly induces somatic symptoms, while autonomic dysfunction remains minimal. The clinical signs include muscle tremor, para- or tetraparesis and exertional weakness. Ventroflexion, paraparesis, generalised hyperaesthesia and dilated pupils have been reported in a cat treated with chlorpyrifos (Fig. 13.40).

Diagnosis: Occasionally the owner can attest to proven toxin exposure which is extremely useful. A serum acetylcholine esterase activity < 25% of the normal value is another helpful indicator. These values should be interpreted with care in the cat, as cats with acetylcholine esterase values that are only 10% of the normal do not necessarily show any clinical symptoms. Electrophysiological investigations do not appear to be very helpful. A reduction in the amplitudes after repetitive stimulation has been reported in dogs with fenthion poisoning. Prolonged insertion potentials, fibrillations and PSWs were seen in two cats exposed to chlorpyrifos.

Therapy: Detoxification is the most important therapeutic measure. Possible treatments include emptying of the stomach, oral administration of activated charcoal and washing of the fur, or repeated bathing of the patient. Atropine should be given but with great care. This substance only blocks acetylcholine at the muscarinic postganglionic parasympathetic synapses; the nicotinic receptors are barely influenced at all. Atropine should only be used for life-threatening respiratory complications and bradycardia. In all other cases, the unpleasant side-effects such as tachycardia and possible stimulation of the CNS can be considerable. Pralidoxime is a medication that can cause release of organophosphate from acetylcholine esterase. As organophosphates are irreversibly bound, this process is very slow and often incomplete. The best results are achieved when pralidoxime is given within 24 hours of the toxin exposure.

Treatment with pralidoxime (10–15 mg/kg, IM, SC, BID–TID) should last for at least 2 days before its success can be judged. The clinical signs induced by overstimulation of the nicotinic muscle receptors such as tremor and weakness can be treated with diphenhydramine 1–4 mg/kg, PO, TID. Supportative measures are also very important and increase the success of treatment.

Prognosis: The disease can last for many weeks and the prognosis depends on the causative agent and its dosage.

13

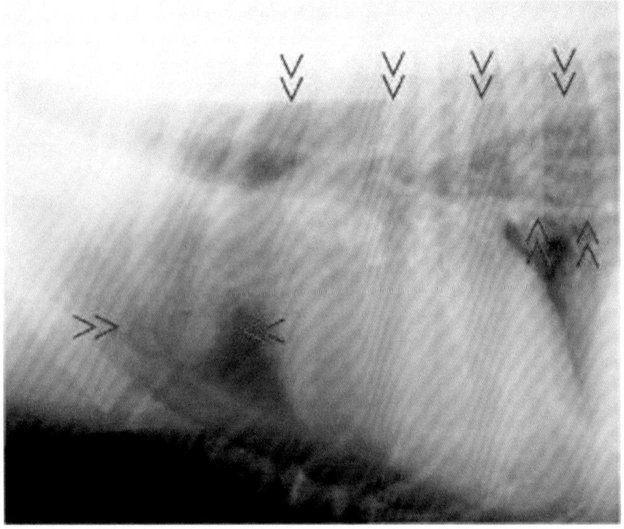

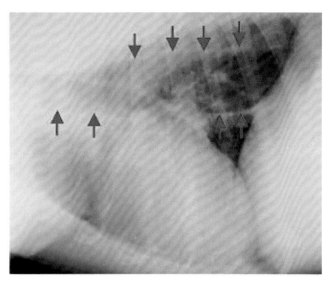

Fig. 13.41
A radiograph of the lungs in an adult Golden Retriever reveals megaoesophagus and a mass cranial to the heart (arrows; thymoma). The patient was presented because of chronic regurgitation and generalised weakness. The animal's acetylcholine receptor antibody titre was significantly increased compatible with myasthenia gravis.

Fig. 13.42
Regurgitation and a radiographically conspicuous megaoesophags (arrows) were the main signs in an adult Collie. The dog's raised acetylcholine receptor antibody titre pointed to myasthenia gravis.

13.4.3 Postsynaptic disturbances

13.4.3.1 Myasthenia gravis

Congenital myasthenia gravis

Occurrence: A rare, autosomal recessive inherited form of myasthenia gravis occurs in the Jack Russell Terrier, Springer Spaniel, the Smooth Fox Terrier, the Gammel Dansk Honsehund and the Smooth-Haired Miniature Dachshund. This disease has been sporadically described in other dog breeds and cats.

Aetiology: An inadequate number of postsynaptic nicotinic acetylcholine receptors are formed due to a genetic defect. Increased antibody titres against acetylcholine receptors have not been found.

Clinical: The clinical signs are similar to those of the acquired form and occur at an age of 2 to 5 months. Megaoesophagus is rare. The main symptoms are progressive generalised weakness and muscle atrophy. The disturbances can progress to tetraplegia.

Diagnosis: Important diagnostic aids include the Tensilon® (edrophonium) test and repetitive nerve stimulation at a frequency of 2–3 Hz. Significant reduction of the action potential amplitude following reflective stimulation is an important indicator of myasthenia gravis.

Therapy: Pyridostigmine bromide (Mestinon®) 0.2–2 mg/kg, PO, BID–TID, is suitable for the treatment of congenital myasthenia gravis in the dog.

Prognosis: The prognosis in the dog is poor except for the Smooth-Haired Miniature Dachshund, in which it is good, due to the spontaneous resolution seen by 6 months of age. It is difficult to determine a prognosis for affected cats as only individual cases have been described.

Acquired myasthenia gravis

Occurrence: Sporadically in the dog; rare in the cat.

Aetiology: Acquired myasthenia gravis is a disease of the immune system in which antibodies limit the function of the postsynaptic nicotinic acetylcholine receptors of the striated musculature. The acetylcholine receptors are found on protein subunits that form the sodium channels in the post-synaptic membrane. The main function of these sodium channels is the transformation of a chemical reaction into an electrical excitatory signal. This function is adversely affected due to the coupling of the antibodies with the acetylcholine receptors; the receptors may even be destroyed. Sodium influx with subsequent depolarisation of the muscle fibres is made more difficult or is impossible.

The group of acetylcholine antibodies is very heterogeneous and every animal has its own specific distribution.

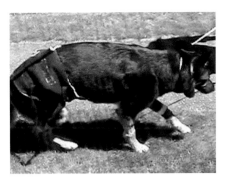

Fig. 13.43

A six-year-old German Shepherd was presented with severe tetraparesis and lack of endurance. The dog could not walk for more than two to three paces before all four limbs stiffened. The animal's first acetylcholine receptor antibody titre was in the normal range, while the second one taken a week later showed an increased titre. This led to a tentative diagnosis of myasthenia gravis.

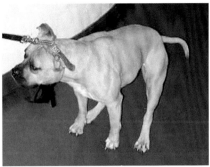

Fig. 13.44

An American Staffordshire Terrier was presented due to weakness. The dog became very stiff in the hindlimbs after a few metres and could hardly move. Other diagnostic investigations provided a clear diagnosis of acquired myasthenia gravis.

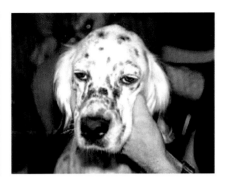

Fig. 13.45

This Brittany Spaniel was presented because of regurgitation and poor endurance. After a few metres the dog was unable to stand or to walk. The neurological examination of the cranial nerves revealed a palpebral reflex which very quickly tired: after being elicited two to three times it could not be stimulated again. The dog's increased acetylcholine receptor antibody titre indicated myasthenia gravis.

The majority of these antibodies belong to the IgG class. Recent investigations indicate that the antibodies can also be directed against the striated musculature and the sodium channels, which would directly hinder muscle contraction. The origin of the antibodies is still not clear. The T-helper cells, which have a modulating effect on the immune system, play an important role. The question as to which antigen(s) causes the production of the antibodies also remains unsolved. In human beings, diseases of the thymus such as hyperplasia or thymoma have been often observed in association with acquired myasthenia gravis. Probably, newly evolved epitopes trigger the antibody production. In the dog, a correlation between thymoma and myasthenia gravis has been reported (Fig. 13.41). In individual cases, other neoplasms such as osteosarcoma, cholangio-cellular adenocarcinoma, adenocarcinoma, cutaneous lymphoma and anal gland carcinoma have been associated with acquired myasthenia gravis, as have hypoadrenocorticism, hypothyroidism and polymyositis.

Clinical: Dogs of every breed and age can develop myasthenia gravis, although a biphasic age distribution has been described, with young adult and middle-aged dogs being more frequently affected. German Shepherds, Golden and Labrador Retrievers and mixed-breed dogs are most commonly presented. If the number of myasthenic patients is compared with the size of the population of the individual breeds, then the Akita Inu, Terriers, German Short-haired Pointer and the Chihuahua have a higher risk of developing this disease than other breeds. An inherited predisposition has been reported in Newfoundlands and Great Danes.

For didactic reasons, it is advantageous to subdivide the clinical symptoms into three groups:

1. **Focal form:** In this form, megaoesophagus is the predominant symptom (Fig. 13.42). A reduced swallowing reflex, facial muscle weakness and laryngeal paralysis may also be present.

2. **Generalised form:** The anamnesis describes acute onset of exercise intolerance. The main symptom is a para- or tetraparesis, which occurs in many dogs after exertion or is obviously increased after an exercise test. During an exercise test, the limbs start to tremble, the musculature becomes increasingly stiff and the stride length shorter. After a short recovery phase, the motor functions improve (Fig. 13.43). In roughly two thirds of the dogs, only the hindlimbs are affected or are more obviously affected (Fig. 13.44). An exercise test can in some patients induce weakness in all limbs or increase its severity. The neurological examination reveals normal proprioception as long as the patient is able to carry its own weight. The spinal reflexes are unchanged. The majority of dogs with a generalised form have megaoesophagus, too. Facial muscle weakness, swallowing problems and laryngeal paralysis appear to be rare in this group. Repetitive stimulation of the palpebral reflex can reveal signs of tiring (Fig. 13.45).

3. **Myasthenic crisis:** An acute para- or tetraparesis occurs. Megaoesophagus is almost always present. This form progresses rapidly and after a few days respiratory dysfunction can arise, too.

13

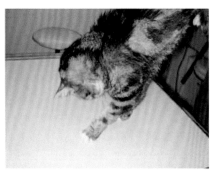

Fig. 13.46
This European domestic cat shows a severe generalised weakness. It has no proprioceptive functions in its forelegs nor can it raise its head. Further tests confirmed the diagnosis of an acquired myasthenia gravis.

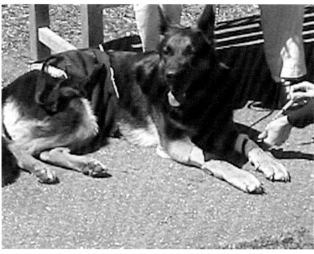

Fig. 13.47
A positive Tensilon test can be very helpful, though negative results do not exclude myasthenia gravis. This six-year-old German Shepherd was given 0.15 mg/kg edrophonium chloride intravenously, 30 seconds later the dog could walk almost normally for about 3 minutes before the symptoms of myasthenia gravis returned.

Cats can also be affected with myasthenia gravis, though rarely. Abyssinians are the most commonly affected breed. The clinical symptoms in the cat can also be subdivided into focal, generalised and myasthenic crisis forms.

1. **Focal form:** Very rare in cats. Megaoesophagus is less common than in the dog as cats have a high proportion of smooth muscle fibres in their oesophagus.
2. **Generalised form:** This is the most common form in cats. Ventroflexion of the neck is a symptom specific to cats but not specific for this disease (Fig. 13.46).
3. **Myasthenic crisis:** Occurs rarely in the cat.

Diagnosis: Adjunct investigations are important to confirm the tentative diagnosis. The CBC, biochemical profile and urinalysis should be used to exclude other metabolic, endocrine or inflammatory causes of weakness. Radiography of the thorax must be done to search for megaoesophagus, thymoma, other tumours and metastases. Small mediastinal thymomas are often not visible on radiographs and a CT of the lungs can be very important in individual cases. A thyroid hormone profile is recommended.

A quick and practical method of confirming acquired myasthenia gravis is the Tensilon test. Intravenous or intramuscular administration of the short-acting acetylcholine esterase inhibitor endrophonium chloride (Tensilon®) induces a marked improvement of the gait disturbances within one minute in many, but not all, cases (dog: 0.1–0.2 mg/kg, IV; cat 0.25–0.5 mg/cat, IV; Fig. 13.47). The risk of the use of this drug is a cholinergic crisis (respiratory disturbances, ptyalism, vomiting, miosis, tachycardia, hypotension, muscle spasms, weakness) which can be effectively treated if atropine is given immediately.

A positive response to the Tensilon test is not specific for myasthenia gravis. False positive results occur in other myopathies or neuropathies. EMG and the motor and sensory nerve conductions are normal. The repetitive stimulation of a smaller distal muscle (palmar or plantar interosseus muscle, tibialis cranialis muscle, mastication muscles) at 3–5 Hz reduces the amplitude with increasing duration of stimulation. If the amplitude of the third, fourth or fifth action potential is at least 10% smaller than the initial value, the patient has a high probability of being affected by myasthenia gravis (Fig. 13.48). Another reliable electrophysiological method is single fibre EMG. This test is complicated and therefore is not commonly used.

The "gold standard" for the diagnosis of myasthenia gravis is the presence of circulating antibodies against postsynaptic acetylcholine receptors. A titre of > 0.6 nmol/l is indicative this disease. The titre can be negative in the early stages or after treatment with glucocorticoids, and the test should be repeated if the clinical picture remains convincing for this disease. Increasing titres are also a clear indication of myasthenia gravis. Although the correlation between severity of disease and the concentration of acetylcholine receptor antibodies is not significant, there is a tendency for patients with higher titres to be affected more severely.

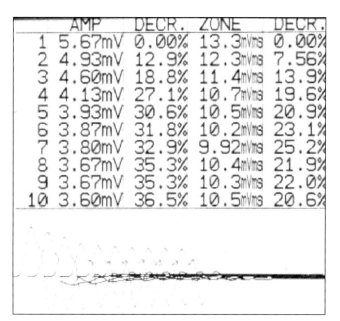

Fig. 13.48
Repetitive nerve stimulation tests the fatigability of the synaptic transmission. Here are the results of the Staffordshire Terrier from Fig. 13.44. There is a conspicuous 18.8% reduction in the amplitudes of the third cMAP compared to the first cMAP. A loss in amplitude of 6–10% is a significant diagnostic result suggestive of disturbance in neuromuscular transmission.

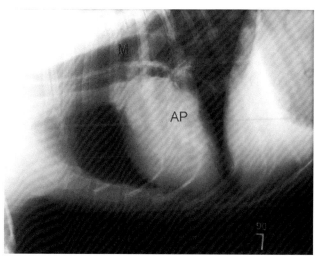

Fig. 13.49
This radiograph of the lungs was taken from a four-year-old German Shepherd with a significantly increased acetylcholine receptor antibody titre. In addition to poor endurance and regurgitation, the patient also showed coughing and an increased body temperature. Note the megaoesophagus (M). There are also signs of aspiration pneumonia (AP) in the right middle lobe of the lungs.

13

Therapy: Symptomatic treatment consists of giving cholineesterase inhibitors. Due to inhibition of the rapid hydrolysis of acetylcholine in the synaptic space, these medications serve to increase the concentration of the neurotransmitter. The resulting improved activation of free receptors leads to a better muscular response. The dosage must be adjusted to the individual animal. Pyridostigmine bromide (Mestinon®), 0.2–2 mg/kg, PO, BID–TID has proven to be successful in the treatment of acquired myasthenia gravis. Injectable neostigmine bromide 0.05 mg/kg, IM, QID can be used to avoid oral medication in the presence of megaoesophagus. The disadvantage of neostigmine is, however, its somewhat stronger muscarinic effect.

To prevent aspiration pneumonia, the animal should be fed by hand in an upright position and made to stay this way for 15 minutes after the meal to encourage emptying of the oesophagus into the stomach. A stomach tube is another alternative feeding mechanism for a short time.

The use of glucocorticoids is controversial, especially when aspiration pneumonia has been diagnosed. However, glucocorticoids may be very advantageous. In human beings, the clinical signs of myasthenia gravis can be exacerbated when the initial corticosteroid dosage is too high. The rule of thumb is, therefore, the more obvious the symptoms of weakness, the lower the starting dose of glucocorticoids. The recommended initial dosage of prednisolone is 0.5 mg/kg/day

and this should be gradually increased to 4 mg/kg/day. If the side-effects of the glucocorticoids are too severe or the treatment's success is not as expected, then another glucocorticoid can be used. Good success has been attained with azathioprine 2 mg/kg/day either alone or in combination with prednisolone. The use of mycophenolate and cyclosporine has also been reported in dogs with this disease. If a thymoma or other tumour is present, then surgical intervention can be very advantageous.

Other therapeutic possibilities, especially for a myasthenic crisis include intravenous globulin therapy or plasmapheresis; however, experience with these methods in dogs is limited.

Prognosis: In very rare cases, spontaneous resolution of acquired myasthenia gravis is possible in the dog. The prognosis can be favourable if the treatment is specific, strict and started early enough. Quick recovery of gait disturbances can occur and the function of the pharynx and oesophagus can be improved. A guarded to poor prognosis must be given if aspiration pneumonia secondary to swallowing difficulties and dysphagia is documented (Fig. 13.49). A myasthenic crisis has a very poor prognosis.

The prognosis in the cat is often favourable as megaoesophagus is rare in this species.

Further reading

COLEMAN, E.S. (1998): Clostridial neurotoxins: Tetanus and botulism. J Cont Educ. **20**: 1089–1096.

MALIK, R., FARROW, B.R.H. (1991): Tick paralysis in North America and Australia. Vet Clin North Am Small Anim Pract. **21**: 157–171.

DEWEY, C.W., BAILEY, C.S., SHELTON, G.D., KASS, P.H., CARDINET III, G.H. (1997): Clinical forms of acquired Myasthenia Gravis. J Vet Intern Med. **11**: 50–57.

DICKINSON, P.J., STURGES, B.K., SHELTON, G.D., LECOUTEUR, R.A. (2005): Congenital myasthenia gravis in Smooth-Haired Miniature Dachshund dogs. J Vet Intern Med. **19** (6): 920–923.

DUCOTE, J.M., DEWEY, C.W., COATES, J.R. (1999): Clinical forms of acquired Myasthenia Gravis in cats. J Contin Educ. **21**: 440–447.

KING, L.G., VITE, C.H. (1998): Acute fulminating myasthenia gravis in five dogs. J Am Vet Med Assoc. **212**: 830–834.

SHELTON, G.D., SCHULE, A., KASS, P.H. (1997): Risk factors for acquired myasthenia gravis in dogs: 1154 cases (1991–1995). J Am Vet Med Assoc. **211**: 1428–1431.

SHELTON, G.D. (1998): Myasthenia Gravis: lessons from the past 10 years. J Small Anim Pract. **39**: 368–372.

SHELTON, G.D., HO, M., KASS, P.H. (2000): Risk factors for acquired myasthenia gravis in cats: 105 cases (1986–1998). J Am Vet Med Assoc. **216**: 55–57.

13.5 Monomyopathies

Monomyopathies are diseases of individual muscles or muscle groups. In the majority of cases, the animals show reduced movement of the affected limb or joint, and paresis / paralysis and / or atrophy of individual muscles. The neurological examination is usually unremarkable. The monomyopathies are a heterogeneous group of diseases. The cause of many of these disturbances is often unknown at the moment. Inflammatory or immune-related changes and the consequences of (micro-)traumatic influences are the main purported causes. Possible differential diagnoses are shown in Table 13.13.

13.5.1 Ischemic myopathies

Occurrence: Frequent.

Aetiology: Ischemic neuromyopathy occurs almost exclusively in cats. The most common cause is arterial thromboemboli which lead to partial or complete blockage of the abdominal aorta or its branches. Different parts of the body

Table 13.13: Differential diagnoses of monomyopathies in the dog and cat

V	■ Ischemic (neuro)myopathy (cat)
I	■ Myositis of the mastication muscles (dog) ■ Extra-ocular myositis (dog) ■ Focal myositis: *Clostridium* spp., *Staphylococcus* spp., and other bacteria (dog / cat)
T	■ Myopathy of the gracilis muscle (dog) and the semitendinosus muscle (dog / cat) ■ Myopathy of the infraspinatus muscle (dog) ■ Myopathy of the teres minor muscle (dog)
I	■ Coccygeal myopathy (limber tail) (dog / cat)
D	■ Myositis ossificans (dog / cat) ■ Von Willebrand heterotopic osteochondrofibrosis in the Doberman (dog)

are affected depending on the location of the thrombus. Arterial thromboemboli are a frequent complication of cardiomyopathy. It is presumed that vasoactive substances, especially serotonin, play a key role in the pathogenesis. Due to the release of serotonin from the aggregated thrombocytes, vasoconstriction of the remaining, non-thrombosed blood vessels occurs causing ischemia.

Ischemic myopathies can also occur if the animal gets trapped somewhere (i.e., under a garage door or in a ventilation system); this can lead to obstruction of the blood supply, as with an arterial thrombo-emboli, in the area caudal to the entrapment. Inadequate arterial blood supply can lead to ischemic damage to the spinal cord, nervous tissues and musculature.

Clinical: The clinical signs usually occur peracutely. They are typified by a paraparesis to paraplegia of the LMNS type (Fig. 13.50). Monoparesis is rarely seen. The abnormalities are usually more severe distally than proximally. Additional deficits of superficial sensation and proprioception are possible if there is massive involvement of the spinal cord and / or the nerves. Absent or weak femoral pulses are palpated in cats with a thrombus in the abdominal aorta or its branches. In addition, a holosystolic heart sound can be heard. The distal limbs are cold and cyanotic, especially in the area of the claws (Fig. 13.51). Often the limb muscles are swollen and very hard. The majority of affected animals are in severe pain.

Cats which have been trapped somewhere can often still make crawling movements with their hindlimbs. Very frequently, a bilateral areflexia of the patella reflex is present; more rarely the flexor reflex is affected. In comparison to aortic thromboemboli, the femoral pulse is still present, there are no signs of severe pain and digital cyanosis is not visible. Depending on the duration of the entrapment, the skin at the site of compression may be damaged, too.

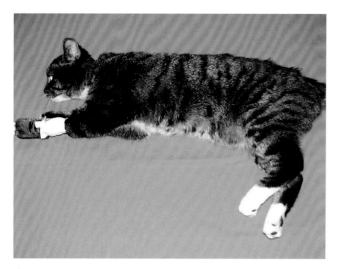

Fig. 13.50
European domestic cat, male, castrated, five years old, with arterial thromboembolism of the abdominal aorta in connection with hypertrophic cardiomyopathy. The cat showed a lower motor neuron type of flaccid paralysis of both hindlimbs with a bilateral lack of femoral pulse and cold distal limbs.

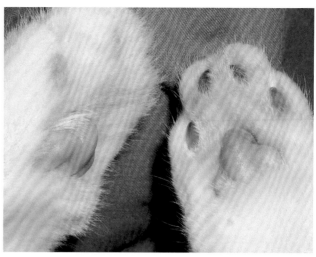

Fig. 13.51
European domestic cat, female, castrated, nine years old, with one-sided arterial thromboembolism of the abdominal aorta in connection with a hypertrophic cardiomyopathy. The cyanotic pads of the foot are conspicuous on the affected hindlimb.

13

Diagnosis: The diagnosis can be made with the aid of the anamnesis (i.e., known cardiomyopathy, entrapment) and the clinical results. Laboratory diagnostic tests reveal a massive increase in creatine kinase as an expression of the muscle damage. Radiographs of the spine are unremarkable. Radiographs of the thorax and echocardiography can confirm the diagnosis of cardiomyopathy. Ultrasonography can often demonstrate the aortic thrombus, so that angiography is not necessary.

Electromyography of the affected muscles can reveal absent or reduced insertion potentials.

The differential diagnosis should primarily exclude spinal or spinal cord trauma and neoplasia of the vertebral canal or spinal cord.

Therapy: In cases of thromboemboli, fibrinolysis can be attempted using streptokinase or tissue plasmogen activator (tPA); however, there have not been studies which confirm the utility of this approach. Heparin or acetylsalicylic acid can be given to prevent expansion of the thrombus due to their ability to inhibit thrombocyte aggregation. Analgesic treatment (buprenorphine, carprofen, opioids) and sedation (acepromazine) should be given, as should a diuretic (furosemide) after rehydration. A serotonin antagonist (cyproheptadine) can be given to reduce the vasoconstriction of the collateral vessels. Nursing care is essential. Surgical removal of the thrombus is associated with multiple risks and is not generally recommended. The risk of re-embolisation is very high. For more detailed information about treating aortic thromboemboli in the cat please refer to specialist cardiological literature.

Cats which have been trapped somewhere and have concurrent spinal injury can be treated with a neuroprotective regimen of methylprednisolone sodium succinate (MPSS); however, there are no clinical studies proving the efficacy of this treatment. Initially, within 8 hours after the insult, 30 mg prednisolone/kg is given intravenously. After another 2 and then 6 hours, 15 mg/kg IV is given; thereafter 2.5 mg/kg/h is given as a continual intravenous infusion over 24 to 48 hours. The use of MPSS after 8 hours is not recommended as there are no beneficial effects expected and the risk of side-effects increases. Intensive physiotherapy should be started as early as possible.

During the reperfusion of previously ischemic areas, there is massive release of toxins, including potassium. Close monitoring of the patient and determination of the animal's serum potassium and urea concentrations, is of great significance.

Prognosis: For arterial thromboemboli: guarded to hopeless for the long term; for injury related to being trapped: guarded to good.

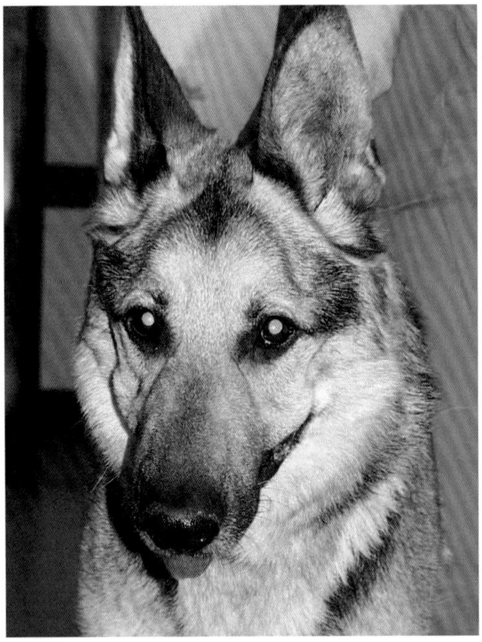

Fig. 13.52
German Shepherd, male, six years old with chronic myositis of the mastication muscles. The dog showed severe bilateral muscle atrophy of its mastication muscles and trismus.

13

13.5.2 Myositis of the masticatory muscles

Occurrence: Sporadic.

Aetiology: The mastication muscles (masseter, temporalis and pterygoid muscles) develop embryologically from the mesoderm of the first pair of branchial arches. These muscles have a high proportion of type 2 fibres and their own form of myosin. Accordingly, they differ histologically and biochemically from the other striated muscles. Due to an autoimmune reaction that is selectively aimed at these fibres, there are inflammatory changes that induce haemorrhage, oedema and myonecrosis. Muscle biopsy allows the presence of macrophages, lymphocytes, plasma cells, and individual neutrophils and eosinophilic granulocytes to be identified. With a more chronic course, the muscle fibres are replaced by connective tissue and are infiltrated with lymphocytes and plasma cells. The muscle damage is irreversible at this stage. Breed predisposition for the German Shepherd and the Doberman has been described.

Clinical: The affected animals show extreme swelling of the masticatory muscles during the acute phase. In some animals, this is associated with pain on palpation or movement of the mouth; other animals give no indication of pain. Food and water intake is reduced. In this initial phase, the body temperature may be raised. At the beginning, serum creatine kinase and the gamma globulin fraction may be moderately increased. Sometimes an eosinophilia is present in the peripheral blood. EMG reveals fibrillations, PSWs and complex repetitive discharges in the masticatory muscles, while the other skeletal muscles demonstrate no changes. This can be useful in questionable cases to differentiate the disease from polymyositis.

In the final stages of chronic disease, extreme atrophy of the masticatory muscles develops (Fig. 13.52). Often a progressive trismus occurs which is called pseudo-trismus. The mouth can neither be opened nor closed completely. This can, in extreme cases, make the intake of food or water impossible. In some patients, the acute phase is inapparent, so that the animals are initially presented with atrophy of the masticatory muscles and the problems associated with this. Polymyositis, neurogenic muscle atrophy after idiopathic trigeminal neuritis and abnormalities of the temporomandibular joint should be excluded from the differential diagnosis.

Diagnosis: This can be based on the clinical results. A muscle biopsy and the serological findings of antibodies against type 2M fibres are the most important adjunct investigations.

Therapy: The therapy in the acute phase consists of corticosteroids at an immunosuppressive dosage: prednisolone 2–4 mg/kg/day divided into two doses for 3 to 7 days, thereafter 1 mg/kg/day as a single dose for 1 week, followed by 0.5 mg/kg/day for approx. 1 month, then a slow tapering off. The prednisolone dose must be individually calculated during relapses. Azathioprine is also very effective at a dose of 2 mg/kg and can be combined with prednisolone (Fig. 13.53). Relapses are frequent and can result in severe muscle fibrosis and atrophy.

It has been advised that mechanical "opening" of the mouth can be undertaken carefully under anaesthesia to improve the mobility of the jaw if it is compromised by the disease; however, this risks serious temporomandibular joint damage and its beneficial effect is short-lived due to further fibrosis (Fig. 13.54). Animals with this disease must be stimulated to move their mouths as actively as possible (e.g. chewing on rubber balls or a chewing bone), so that a physiotherapeutic effect is achieved. Despite these measures and medication, it can often be difficult to achieve permanent improvement. The best parameter for the assessment of the treatment's success is the degree of lower jaw mobility.

Prognosis: Guarded to good if treatment is given in time and during the acute phase; poor to hopeless in the presence of severe muscle atrophy, fibrosis and therapy-resistant pseudo-trismus.

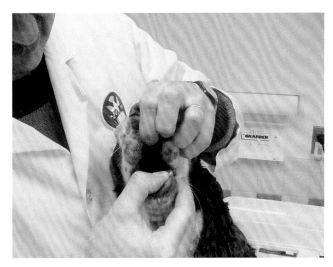

Fig. 13.53
A two-year-old Spaniel with histologically proven myositis of the mastication muscles. The biopsy showed an inflammatory infiltrate, a moderate fibrosis and positive 2M antibodies. The patient could open its mouth roughly 3 cm before the start of therapy. This photograph shows the dog after one month on prednisolone and azathioprine. The mouth can now be opened twice as wide as before. The lower jaw is a good control for determining the success of a drug therapy.

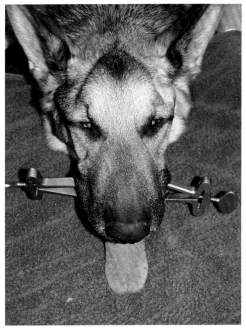

Fig. 13.54
The same dog as in Fig. 13.52. Treatment of the trismus under anaesthesia using a Heister's mouth gag is shown here; great caution should be used if pusuing this contentious treatment as injury can occur to the temporomandibular joints. The long-term success of this treatment is debatable.

13

13.5.3 Extraocular myositis

Occurrence: Rare.

Aetiology: A breed predisposition occurs in the Golden and Labrador Retriever, though the exact cause is unknown. It is presumed that this disease is an immune myositis of the extra-ocular musculature. Analogous to masticatory myositis, the presence of unique fibre types in these muscles as compared to the rest of the striated musculature is thought in part to be a factor responsible for the disease. Histologically, areas with a dense infiltration of lymphocytes, histiocytes and plasma cells including a few eosinophils and neutrophilic granulocytes are interspersed with areas of necrosis or fibrosis in the muscle bodies. The eye, the retrobulbar fat, the blood vessels and the nerves are unchanged.

Clinical: Usually young to young adult dogs from different breeds are affected. In the acute form, the main clinical symptom is bilateral exophthalmos. The conjunctiva and sclera are inflamed and show evident chemosis. In addition, there is partial prolapse of the nictitating membrane. The animals often have a staring look as they only have limited movement of their eyeballs. Sight is not affected. The direct and indirect pupillary reflexes are normal. Palpation does not elicit pain. The general clinical and neurological examinations are otherwise unremarkable. The same holds true for the laboratory tests. In some dogs, a unilateral or bilateral restrictive ventral or ventromedial strabismus with endophthalmus without any previous clinical evidence of exophthalamus has been described. This is considered as being the chronic form of extra-ocular myositis. Sometimes these animals have limited visual acuity because of the extreme displacement of the eyeball.

Diagnosis: The use of ultrasonography or MRI allows inflammatory changes in the extra-ocular muscles to be identified excluding some of the differential diagnoses.

With unilateral exophthalmus, retrobulbar processes (abscess, neoplasia, haematoma) or a mucocele of the zygomatic gland should be considered. In bilateral exophthalmus, myositis of the masticatory muscles should be excluded.

Therapy: The therapy of choice is administration of corticosteroids at an immunosuppressive dosage: prednisolone 2–4 mg/kg/day divided into two doses for 3 to 7 days, thereafter 1 mg/kg/day for 1 week, followed by 0.5 mg/kg/day for approx. 1 month, then a slow tapering off. The prednisolone dose must be calculated individually during relapses. Azathioprine can be given additionally at a dose of 2 mg/kg PO, if the side-effects of the corticosteroids are excessive or if there are other reasons necessitating reduction in the dosage of prednisolone. A topical eye ointment may help treat the local ocular inflammatory changes.

Surgical correction of a restrictive strabismus can be successful, especially if it affects the visual acuity.

Prognosis: Guarded to good if the therapy is initiated early enough.

13.5.4 Myopathy of the gracilis and semitendinosus muscles

Occurrence: Sporadic.

Aetiology: Various theories about the cause of this disease exist, though none of them have been confirmed as yet. The effects of trauma, repeated microtraumas, an autoimmune reaction, a primary neuropathy or vascular change are being discussed. Young adult male German and Belgian Shepherd dogs are most frequently presented with this disease. In the majority of cases, there is a unilateral lesion which either affects the gracilis or semitendinosus muscles individually or together. However, 26 of affected dogs have shown a bilateral lesion. Depending on the extent of the lesion there is partial or complete replacement of the muscle fibres by collagenous connective tissue especially in the region of the musculotendinous junction. Inflammatory reactions are mild. The caudolateral part of the gracilis muscle may become a fibrous cord, while the cranial part of the muscle only exhibits mild changes. As a consequence of the muscle fibrosis, there is mechanical impedance to hip joint abduction and in the extension of the knee and tarsal joints. The histopathological changes are similar to the results of the deep (musculoaponeurotic) form of aggressive fibromatosis in human beings. Similar changes have also been described in a Himalayan Cat.

Clinical: The animals have a chronic progressive lameness of the affected limbs. Their gait is very typical and is more pronounced with quick movements. The stride length is shortened. During the forwards movement of the leg, the paw is moved inwards with a sudden and elastic hypermetric movement, and the tarsal joint is rotated outwards ("chicken stepping"). During the later phase of the swing, there is also inwards rotation of the knee. Due to the anatomical course and function of the gracilis and semitendinosus muscles, the clinical picture is the same independent of which muscle is affected. The severity of the gait disturbance may be different in each leg, even when there is bilateral change. Palpation reveals a hard thickening of the affected muscle, which is particularly obvious in the region of the musculotendinous junction. In

dorsal recumbency, abduction of the limbs at the hip joint and extension of the knee and tarsal joint is limited – even in anaesthetised animals (Fig. 13.55).

Diagnosis: With the aid of EMG, fibrillations, PSWs and myotonic discharges are detected in the initial stages of the disease. In animals with an advanced degree of fibrosis, the lack of insertion potentials is obvious. The abnormal architecture of the muscle can be well visualised using ultrasonography.

Therapy: Any attempts at influencing the lameness with anti-inflammatory drugs or glucocorticoids have been without success. Surgical intervention can be attempted but this is associated with a high rate of relapse. A complete myotenectomy is favoured to prevent fibroplasia with renewed unification of the muscle stumps in the area of the operation. Reunification still represents the main postoperative complication despite the use of different techniques to prevent it (invagination of the edges of the resection; interposition of autologous fat tissue between the ends of the resected muscle; application of glucocorticoids, NSAIDs, colchicines or D-penicillamine). Once the wound has healed, physiotherapy should be initiated (see Chap. 8). In many of these dogs, renewed fibrosis of the resected muscle occurs within 3 to 5 months.

Prognosis: Guarded.

13.5.5 Myopathy of the infraspinatus muscle

Occurrence: Rare.

Aetiology: The exact cause is unknown. A breed predisposition has been described for hunting (German Short-haired and Wire-haired Pointers) and working dogs. Trauma to the muscle body and/or the tendon of the infraspinatus muscle, or severe overuse have been discussed as possible causes, while damage to the suprascapularis nerve or ischemic contraction is thought to be less likely. Histologically, scarring of the transitional zone between the muscle and tendon is often seen. The tendon itself remains unchanged.

Clinical: The animals show a typical, usually unilateral chronic lameness of the affected limb. In the early stages, the muscle body of the infraspinatus swells and pain can be elicited by palpation of the shoulder joint. In the later stages, an obvious muscle atrophy of the infraspinatus, and possibly the supraspinatus and deltoid muscles, becomes apparent. The limbs are permanently held in an outward rotation with adduction of the elbow and abduction of the distal limb. The shoulder joint is continuously extended and the carpal joint is bent and abducted. In the swing phase, the animals exhibit a throwing forward of the affected limb (carpal flip). There is a severe inhibition of shoulder joint flexion.

Diagnosis: Radiographs of the shoulder joint may reveal sclerosis of the insertion site of the infraspinatus muscle and periosteal reactions on the spine of the scapular. The best views for showing this are taken with the animal lying down or standing, at an angle of 20–25° to the median plane so that the insertion site (infraspinatus fascia) is depicted tangentially. These views can also be used to exclude other causes of lameness that can be found in the shoulder joint. Ultrasonography is better than radiography for the diagnosis of this condition as the altered architecture of the muscle can be shown. These changes are particularly obvious in the transitional zone between the muscle and the tendon. EMG can reveal fibrillations, PSWs, myotonic discharges of high frequency and amplitude, or a lack of insertion potentials, depending on the stage of the disease.

Therapy: The therapy of choice is tenotomy or partial tenectomy of the infraspinatus tendon in the region over the major tubercle. The restriction of shoulder joint movement can be improved by doing this. The characteristic abnormal gait disappears immediately postoperatively. Instability in the shoulder joint is not a post-operative factor. The animal's exercise should be limited to leash walking for roughly 2 to 3 weeks. Physiotherapy does not seem to be necessary. Reformation of the tendon does not occur in this disease.

Prognosis: Good.

13.5.6 Myositis ossificans

Occurrence: Rare.

Aetiology: Myositis ossificans is a heterotropic osteogenesis in the striated muscle of unknown origin. In human beings, a generalised form (progressive) is differentiated from a focal form. There are cases studies describing the generalised form in dogs and cats. In some of these studies, the disease is referred to as fibrodysplasia ossificans. This is considered to be a primary disease of the connective tissue of unknown cause. There is proliferation of connective tissue, which results in degeneration of the muscle fibres and their replacement with connective tissue, cartilage or bone. In the majority of cases, this is focal. The changes are initiated by traumatic damage to a muscle. The resulting haematoma is not resorbed but undergoes conversion into connective and bony tissues. Cartilage is formed and endochondral ossification occurs, resulting in the formation of large islands of bone in the musculature. These islands contain zones of bone marrow, osetoid, trabeculae and compact bone. The muscles of the thigh were affected in the majority of the cases described. In contrast to human beings, myositis ossificans, as a consequence of neuromuscular dis-

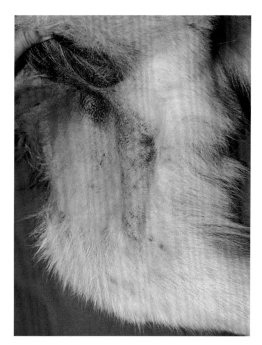

Fig. 13.55
German Shepherd, male, four years old with fibrotic myopathy of the gracilis muscle. Hard, cord-like gracilis muscles could be palpated on both hindlegs.

ease, chronic disease or a pseudo-malignant form has not been seen in the dog or cat. New experimental investigations have shown that certain proteins (e.g. BMP = bone morphogenic protein) and growth factors in bone tissue have a significant role in heterotropic osteogenesis.

Many authors consider that the von Willebrand heterotropic osteochondrofibrosis in the Doberman Pinscher is possibly a disease in its own right and not one that belongs to focal myositis ossificans. In this disease, microvascular haemorrhage within the musculature occurs as a consequence of a deficit of the von Willebrand factor. Heterotropic bone formation then occurs at these sites.

Clinical: The generalised form primarily affects young animals. They demonstrate progressive weakness of their limbs and a stiff gait. The individual muscles may be thickened and painful. There is an obvious limited movement of the joints. The disease disseminates to all of the muscles in the body, apart from the heart, diaphragm and the smooth muscles. Death occurs in the final stages due to damage to the respiratory muscles.

13

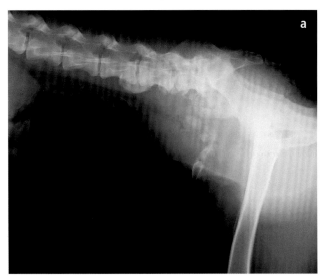

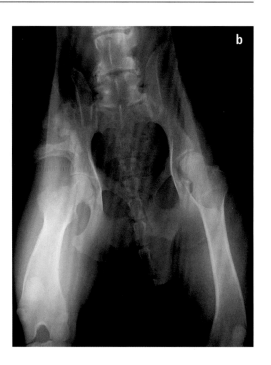

Fig. 13.56a, b
Doberman, female, three years old. Lateral radiograph of the abdomen (a) and ventrodorsal radiograph of the pelvis (b). The dog was presented because of a chronic lameness of the right hindleg. Clinically, reduced extension of the hip joint was conspicuous in addition to atrophy of the quadriceps muscle. In addition to the obvious degenerative changes seen in the caudal lumbar spine on the radiographs, numerous calcified shadows can be observed in the thigh muscles.

In the focal form, the animals primarily show chronic lameness and limited movement of the affected limb. One of the signs is a firm thickening of the muscles which can be palpated. Depending on the duration, an obvious disuse atrophy of the musculature can be observed.

Diagnosis: Radiographically, areas with obvious soft tissue "shadows" or calcifications within the muscle can be seen. Often there is no connection to the periosteum of the neighbouring bones. In some cases, however, a periosteal reaction is present. In some cases, the diagnosis must be confirmed with a muscle biopsy (Fig. 13.56).

Therapy: There is no therapy available for the generalised form. Glucocorticoids can slow down the progression of the disease. The use of diphosphonates (etidronate diphosphonate dinatrium, EHDP) is not successful. The focal form can be influenced by surgical measures with as much affected tissue as possible being resected. Sometimes it may be necessary to remove large parts of more than one muscle. If complete removal is not possible, then partial resection should be done to retain as much mobility as possible of the affected limb. A histological investigation of the excised tissue is absolutely necessary to exclude the possibility of neoplasia. Intensive physiotherapy should be used as a supportive measure.

Prognosis: The prognosis in the generalised form is poor; in the focal form the prognosis is good to guarded depending on the extent of the disease when diagnosed.

13.5.7 Coccygeal myopathy (limber tail, cold tail)

Occurrence: Rare.

Aetiology: The actual cause of this disease is unknown. The predisposing factors are thought to include prolonged transport in a cage, poor physical condition, over-activity, cold and damp weather or swimming in cold water. This problem occurs relatively frequently in Pointers and Retrievers used for hunting. Most probably there are perfusion disturbances of the coccygeal muscles, which lead to injury of this muscle group.

Histopathologically, there is bilateral damage to the muscle fibres, especially in the area of the ventrocaudal intertransversus muscle. The tendons, blood vessels and intramuscular nerves are unchanged.

Clinical: Usually young to young adult dogs are affected. The anamnesis provides an indication of possible predisposing factors. On clinical examination, the animals can initially have ruffled fur and sensitivity to touch in the dorsal area of the proximal part of the tail. The main symptoms include an acute, flaccid paralysis of the tail either directly at its root or a few centimetres distal to it. The dog often moves with its head sunken down and its tail pulled in. Some dogs are agitated and run around without sitting down. The hindlegs are clinically unaffected.

Diagnosis: There may be a slight increase in serum creatine kinase levels. After a few days, EMG can be used to demonstrate changes in the coccygeal muscles.

The differential diagnosis should include sacrococcygeal fractures, diseases of the sacral spinal cord and the cauda equina, as well as diseases of the prostate or anal glands.

Therapy: In the majority of cases, spontaneous resolution occurs within a few days. The application of anti-inflammatory drugs can speed up this process.

Prognosis: Good; relapses are rare.

Further reading

ALLGÖWER, I., BLAIR, M., BASHER, T., DAVIDSON, M., HAMILTON, H., JANDECK, C., WARD, D., WOLFER, J., SHELTON, G.D. (2000): Extraocular myositis and restrictive strabismus in 10 dogs. Vet Ophthalmol. **3**: 21–26.

BENETT, R.A. (1986): Contracture of the infraspinatus muscle in dogs. A review of 12 cases. J Am Anim Hosp Assoc. **22**: 481–487.

DÜLAND, R.T., WAGNER, S.D., PARKER, R.B. (1990): von Willebrand heterotopic osteochondrofibrosis in Doberman Pinschers: Five cases (1980–1987). J Am Vet Med Assoc. **197**: 383–388.

FISCHER, I., WEISS, R., CISINAUSKAS, S., VANNINI, R., JAGGY, A. (2002): Akute traumatische Nachhandlähmung bei 30 Katzen. Tierärztl Prax. 30: 361–366.

LASTE, N.J., HARPSTER, N.K. (1995): A retrospective study of 100 cases of feline distal aortic thromboembolism: 1977–1993. J Am Anim Hosp Assoc. **31**: 492–500.

LEWIS, D.D. (2000): Gracilis – Semitendinosus Myopathy. In: BONAGURA, J.D. (ed.): Kirk's Current Veterinary Therapy XIII. Small Animal Practice. W.B. Saunders Company, Philadelphia. pp. 989–992.

LEWIS, D.D. (1988): Fibrotic myopathy of the semitendinosus muscle in a cat. J Am Vet Med Assoc. **193**: 240–241.

GILMOUR, M.A., MORGAN, R.V., MOORE, F.M. (1992): Masticatory myopathy in the dog: A retrospective study of 18 cases. J Am Anim Hosp Assoc. **28**: 300–305.

SCHOEMAN, J.P. (1999): Feline distal aortic thromboembolism: areview of 44 cases (1990–1998). J Fel Med & Surg, **1**: 221–231.

SHELTON, G.D., BANDMAN, E., CARDINET, G.H. 3rd (1985): Electrophoretic comparison of myosins from masticatory muscles and selected limb muscles in the dog. Am J Vet Res. **46**: 493–498.

SHELTON, G.D., CARDINET, G.H. 3rd, BANDMAN, E., CUDDON, P. (1985): Fiber type specific autoantibodies in a dog with eosinophilic myositis. Muscle Nerv. **8**: 783–784.

STEISS, J., BRAUND, K., WRIGHT, J., LENZ, S., HUDSON, J., BRAWNER, W., HATHCOCK, J., PUROHIT, R., BELL, L., HORNE, R. (1999): Coccygeal muscle injury in English Pointers (Limber Tail). J Vet Intern Med. **13**: 540–548.

VAN WINKLE, T.J., HACKNER, S.G., LIU, S.M. (1993): Clinical and pathological features of aortic thromboembolism in 36 dogs. J Vet Emerg Crit Care. **3**: 13–21.

WALDRON, D., PETTIGREW, V., TURK, M., GIBSON, R. (1985): Progressive ossifying myositis in a cat. J Am Vet Med Assoc. **187**: 64–68.

WARREN, H.B., CARPENTER, J.L. (1984): Fibrodysplasia ossificans in three cats. Vet Pathol. **21**: 495–499.

WATT, P.R. (1992): Posttraumatic myositis ossificans and fibrotic myopathy in the rectus femoris muscle in a dog: A case report and literature review. J Am Anim Hosp Assoc. **28**: 560–564.

13.6   Polymyopathies

The musculature is not only the largest and heaviest organ in the dog and cat, but its functions are also complex. Muscles can only work correctly when they are optimally supported by all the other components of the body, especially the cardiovascular function; carbohydrate, lipid and protein metabolism; PNS function and CNS function.

An axon supplies more than one muscle fibre and so forms a motor unit. Gradation of the muscle activity is possible because a variable amount of motor units can be recruited. The more axons responsible for a specific number of muscle fibres, the better the muscle is suitable for fine and exact movements. The different axons also determine the metabolic characteristics of the individual muscle fibres, meaning that the rapid and the slow contracting fibres are supplied by different types of α-motor neurons and axons. The rapidly contracting type 2 fibres specifically require glycogen. The slow contracting type 1 fibres have a predominantly oxidative metabolism and are rich in mitochondria. Under stressful situations, the musculature is the organ with the highest blood perfusion, which indicates a central role for an intact energy metabolism.

In the past few years, a wide spectrum of new muscle diseases has been described. Sadly, the pathophysiology of many of these disturbances is not currently understood. The most important pathological mechanisms responsible for muscle disease include inflammatory, metabolic and degenerative. The differential diagnoses of polymyopathies are summarised in Table 13.14. It must, however, be emphasized that systemic and cardiovascular diseases and abnormalities of the nervous system can induce secondary muscle dysfunction. Pathognomonic symptoms do not exist for the primary or secondary muscle diseases. The main symptom is weakness, which often increases with exercise. Muscle atrophy, in rare cases hyper-

13

trophy, abnormal reflexes and muscle tone, tremor and spasms are other signs of muscle disease. Without further investigation, specific diagnosis and treatment are impossible. The most important muscle diseases are discussed in this chapter.

The diagnostic investigation of muscle disease begins with a detailed anamnesis. Specifically, the course of the disease, similar problems identified with related dogs or cats, and evidence of other organ system disease, are all important. Targeted laboratory investigations can help with identification of muscle abnormalities. An increased serum creatine kinase (CK) is observed with muscle disease as a consequence of muscle fibre necrosis, and also increased permeability of the sarcolemma in degenerative diseases. Prolonged anorexia in the cat can lead to a significant increase in serum CK due to muscle loss, and this should be included in the differential diagnosis.

Other specific methods for the investigation of muscles include EMG and nerve function tests, in addition to histology, histochemistry and immunohistochemistry of a muscle biopsy (see Chap 7). Imaging methods such as ultrasonography or MRI can also be useful in certain conditions (Flow diagram 13.2, Chap. 13.1.3).

13.6.1 Acquired polymyopathies

13.6.1.1 Toxoplasmosis
(See Chap. 20.3)

13.6.1.2 Neosporosis
(See Chap. 20.2)

13.6.1.3 Hepatozoon canis

Occurrence: Rare in the dog; worldwide in warm areas (see Chap 20.8).

Aetiology: The protozoa *Hepatozoon canis* is transmitted by infected ticks of the species *Rhipicephalus sanguineus*. The infection is a problem in southern regions of the USA, Europe and Africa. Young dogs are most commonly affected. Immunosuppression promotes the development of this infection.

Clinical: Many animals are infected subclinically. Possible clinical signs include fever, apathy, anorexia, weight loss, muscle pain as well as purulent ocular and nasal discharge. The muscle pain leads to a stiff gait and the animal adopts abnormal postures.

Table 13.14: Differential diagnosis of polymyopathies in the dog and cat

I	■ *Toxoplasma gondii* (dog / cat)
	■ *Neospora canis* (dog)
	■ *Hepatozoon canis* (dog)
	■ *Leptospira icterohaemorrhagica* (dog)
	■ Microfilaria (dog)
	■ *Trichinella spiralis* (dog)
	■ Polymyositis (dog / cat)
	■ Dermatomyositis (dog)
M	■ Hypothyroidism (dog)
	■ Hyperthyroidism (cat)
	■ Hyperadrenocorticism (dog)
	■ Hypokalaemic polymyopathy (cat)
	■ Hypernatraemic polymyopathy (cat)
	■ Hypercalcaemia (dog / cat)
	■ Hypocalcaemia (dog / cat)
D	■ Muscular dystrophy (dog)
	■ Hypertrophic polymyopathy (cat)
	■ Merosin deficiency (cat)
	■ Labrador Retriever myopathy
	■ Myopathy of the Devon Rex Cat
	■ Degenerative myopathy in the Bouvier des Flandres
	■ Nemaline rod myopathy (dog / cat)
	■ Juvenile distal myopathy in the Rottweiler
	■ Lipid storage myopathies (dog)
	■ Mitochondrial myopathy (Clumber Spaniel, Sussex Spaniel, Old English Sheepdog)
	■ Glycogen storage disease type II in the Swedish Lapland Hound
	■ Glycogen storage disease type III in the German Shepherd and Akita Inu
	■ Glycogen storage disease type IV in the Norwegian Forest Cat
	■ Malignant hyperthermia (dog / cat)
	■ Exertion-dependent rhabdomyolysis (dog)
	■ Exertion-dependent muscle spasms in Terriers, Dalmatians and Cavalier King Charles Spaniel
	■ Exertion-dependent collapse in the Labrador Retriever
	■ Intermittent hyperkalaemia (American Pit Bull)
	■ Hypokalaemic polymyopathy in the Burmese Cat
	■ Myotonia (dog / cat)

Diagnosis: The CBC provides an indication of chronic infection. The blood biochemistry is usually compatible with a cholangiohepatitis. Radiographs of the long bones demonstrate a massive periosteal reaction. The CSF may reveal neutrophilic pleocytosis. EMG provides obvious indications of muscle abnormalities, but the definitive diagnosis is attained with a muscle biopsy.

Therapy: As yet no curative treatment has been established. Diminazene, imidocarb, tetracyclines, primaquine, toltrazuril and clarithromycin have been tested as specific therapies, but the results are difficult to interpret due to the small number of patients treated with each of these drugs. Anti-inflammatory drugs can also be used. Corticosteroids, however, often make the clinical symptoms worse.

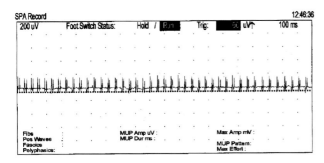

Fig. 13.57
A six-year-old Labrador retriever was presented because of an acute severe lack of endurance, tetraparesis and generalised reduction in reflexes. The EMG investigation showed intense spontaneous activity composed of complex repetitive discharges (shown here) and fibrillations in the right temporalis muscle, right shoulder area and left thigh.

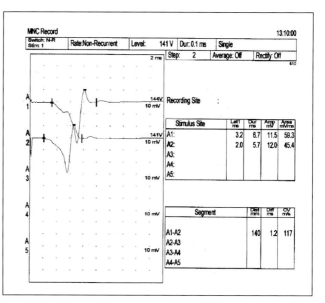

Fig. 13.58
The normal motor conduction study of the peroneal nerve in the left hindlimb of the dog in Fig. 13.57 indicates a primary muscle disease as the cause of the weakness. The results of the muscle biopsy indicated an autoimmune aetiology. The clinical symptoms improved quickly with a combination of prednisolone and azathioprine.

Prognosis: The long-term prognosis is poor. The course of the disease is intermittent with episodes of fever and muscle pain. Spontaneous remission is possible.

13.6.1.4 Idiopathic polymyositis

Occurrence: Infrequent in the dog; rare in the cat.

Aetiology: Polymyositis has been observed in association with many diseases. In the dog, idiopathic, immune-mediated inflammatory destruction of the muscle is described. New studies have shown that a T-cell-induced immune reaction is responsible. The same inflammatory muscle changes have also been seen in association with systemic lupus erythematosus, myasthenia gravis, thymoma and some immune-mediated skin diseases. A so-called dermatomyositis exists in the Collie, Sheltie and related breeds. Adult cats infected experimentally with feline immunodeficiency virus (FIV) demonstrate similar histological and sometimes electromyographic changes, though these had a subclinical course. Certain cats with thymoma can develop a paraneoplastic polymyositis, which sometimes results in dysphagia. Idiopathic polymyositis rarely occurs in the cat.

Clinical: Mainly middle-aged and older animals are affected. The clinical picture is that of a generalised muscle weakness of differing degrees. In some patients, the predominant symptom is a stiff gait. Ventroflexion of the neck has been sporadically observed in cats, but even dogs may have difficulty in raising their heads. Affected cats can also have dysphagia, especially with paraneoplastic and idiopathic forms. Laryngeal paralysis and changes in the voice can occur. Muscle pain or swelling is possible. Aspiration pneumonia is a serious complication.

Diagnosis: The serum CK is often increased. Non specific EMG changes such as fibrillations, PSWs, complex repetitive or pseudo-myotonic discharges with normal NCV are possible (Figs. 13.57 and 13.58). Histological investigation reveals a multifocal inflammatory infiltrate with lymphocytes and plasma cells. Disseminated necrosis and regenerating muscle fibres are also visible. In certain cases, a degenerative pattern with necrosis and fibrosis is present. Serum anti-nuclear antibody presence may be further supportive of an immune mediated process

13

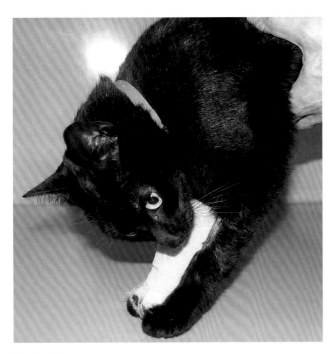

Fig. 13.59
A two-year-old castrated male cat with ventroflexion of the neck and hypokalaemia (serum K+ concentration 2.86 mmol/l; reference range: 3.50–5.00 mmol/l) due to chronic renal failure.

13

The criteria for a definitive diagnosis of idiopathic polymyositis are poorly defined in veterinary medicine. A definitive diagnosis should be based on the clinical signs of muscle weakness, the exclusion of infectious causes or neoplasia, increased CK levels, EMG changes and histological proof of inflammatory muscle changes.

Therapy: Immunosuppressive dosages of glucocorticoids (prednisolone 2 mg/kg, PO, BID) are initially used to treat idiopathic polymyositis. A tapering dose regimen is then advised to effect. Treatment with azathioprine (2mg/kg PO daily until remission, then 0.5–2.0 mg/kg PO every other day) in addition to prednisolone or azathioprine alone has been an effective in some patients.

Prognosis: The prognosis depends on the primary disease. Idiopathic polymyositis can at times respond well to therapy, but relapses are not uncommon. The presence of dysphagia and/or megaoesophagus is an unfavourable sign.

13.6.1.5 Hypokalaemic polymyopathy

Occurrence: Frequent in the cat.

Aetiology: This acquired disease is mainly associated with chronic renal failure. Between 10 and 30% of cats with renal disease suffer from hypokalaemia. Even though hypokalaemia only causes clinical symptoms in a few cases, minor reduction of the potassium concentration in the serum of cats with chronic nephropathies should not be ignored as it can play a role in the progression of renal disease.

Hypokalaemia is the result of a series of different causes. Predisposing factors include reduced intake (potassium-poor foods), ingestion of urine-acidifying substances (DL-methionine or ammonium chloride) or a low magnesium or high protein content of the diet. In chronic renal failure, potassium is eliminated more readily in the urine due to various mechanisms. Affected cats have a markedly higher potassium excretion factor of 35.8 compared to 1.8–15.1 in healthy cats. Other rare causes of hypokalaemia include chronic enteropathies, diabetes mellitus at the initiation of insulin therapy, post-obstructive diuresis and hyperaldosteronism.

As potassium is mainly stored in the intracellular compartment, the serum potassium concentration is not necessarily a true representation of the total amount of potassium in the body. A change in the transmembranous potassium concentration gradients influences the membrane excitability of the muscle cells. Hypokalaemia initially causes hyperpolarisation of the cells which makes the initiation of action potentials difficult. Later, there is increased sodium permeability of the cell membrane, which is accompanied by hypopolarisation and profound muscle weakness.

The prevalence of hypokalaemia in cats with chronic nephropathies is often underestimated. In the presence of metabolic acidosis, potassium is additionally transferred from the intracellular space into the extracellular compartment leading to increased loss through the kidneys. When the metabolic acidosis is corrected, extracellular potassium is pushed back into the cells and hypokalaemia gets worse. In rats, hypokalaemia causes a reduction in renal blood perfusion and glomerular filtration rate. The synthesis of ammonia in the distal tubuli is increased. These factors can cause further progression of renal failure. However, similar mechanisms have not been definitely proven in the cat.

Clinical: The typical clinical sign is that of a generalised muscle weakness with profound weakness at activity. The gait is stiff and the forelegs are often positioned far forwards cranially. In severe cases, weakness of the neck is dramatic (Fig. 13.59). In contrast to dogs, cats do not have a nuchal ligament and therefore muscle weakness in this species is associated with obvious ventroflexion of the neck.

Table 13.15: Guide to the determination of the dosage of intravenous potassium substitution in cats with hypokalaemia

Potassium concentration in serum (mmol/l)	KCl per 250 ml infusion bag	KCl per 500 ml infusion bag	KCl per 1000 ml infusion bag	Maximum infusion rate (ml/kg/h)
≤ 2	20	40	80	6
2.01–2.50	15	30	60	8
2.51–3.00	10	20	40	12
3.01–3.50	7.5	15	30	16

Diagnosis: The causes of a ventroflexion of the neck must be differentiated: hyperthyroidism, polymyositis, organophosphate poisoning, myasthenia gravis, or in the Devon Rex, the inherited myopathy typical of this breed. In addition, thiamine deficiency can lead to a similar clinical picture, whereby flexion of the neck is due to uncontrolled muscle contraction.

Serum biochemistry reveals a low or low normal serum potassium concentration. Azotaemia indicates, when present with other renal biochemical abnormalities, the presence of chronic renal failure. The serum concentration of the muscle enzyme CK may be significantly increased.

Therapy: Initially, potassium is given by infusion (Table 13.15). The dosage of potassium chloride may not exceed 0.5 mmol/kg/h otherwise cardiac arrhythmias may occur as a complication. When the cat is stable and eats, then potassium gluconate in the form of a powder or syrup is given at an initial dose of 5–8 mmol/ day, PO. The daily maintenance dosage is approx. 2–4 mmol/cat. The dosage is adapted to the individual using regular serum potassium measurements. This treatment can also lead to improvement in the general condition of a cat with chronic renal failure. In addition, specific treatment for uraemic syndrome and the progression of renal disease should be considered. In rare cases, serum potassium may be reduced with infusion therapy, most probably due to a dilution effect. This can then lead to dramatic worsening of the polymyopathy, so that the respiratory muscles are affected, too.

Prognosis: The prognosis is dictated by the severity of chronic renal disease; with adequate treatment many cats may live for months or even years.

13.6.1.6 Hypercalcaemia

Occurrence: Rare in the cat and dog.

Aetiology: The most important causes of increased calcium concentration in the blood include benign tumours of the parathyroid, lymphoma, multiple myeloma, anal gland carcinoma, squamous cell carcinoma and mammary gland tumours. Calcium values over 3.5 mmol/l lead to functional disturbances of the kidneys, gastrointestinal tract, the nervous system, the limbs and the heart muscle. If the calcium concentration × the phosphorus concentration (Ca mmol/l × phosphorus mmol/l) is > 5.6, then calcium deposition in the organs is possible. The cause of muscle dysfunction is most probably an inhibition of the sodium / potassium pumps as well as a reduced potassium permeability of the cell membranes.

Clinical: The possible symptoms include PU / PD, inappetence, anorexia, vomiting, diarrhoea, severe weakness and muscle atrophy. Tremor and muscle spasms are frequent concurrent symptoms.

Diagnosis: Investigation of the disease includes a search for neoplasia, the measurement of total and ionised calcium (normal values: 1.25–1.45 mmol/l), analysis of the parathyroid hormone, and ultrasonography or scintigraphy of the parathyroids.

Therapy: Treatment is aimed at the underlying cause. If necessary, surgical removal of abnormal parathyroid tissue may be recommended.

Possible symptomatic measures for initial stabilisation of the calcium concentration include infusion with sodium chloride, furosemide, prednisolone, biphosphonate, mithramycin or sodium EDTA. Prednisolone and furosemide are suitable for long-term therapy.

Prognosis: The management of these patients is time-consuming, depending on the basic cause.

13

13.6.1.7 Hypocalcaemia

Occurrence: Rare.

Aetiology: Lactation, or atrophy of the parathyroids, as well as intended or accidental removal of these organs can all lead to a decreased production of parathormone. The subsequently reduced calcium concentration destabilises the resting potentials of the neurons, peripheral nerves and muscle cells. The resulting over excitability determines the clinical picture.

Clinical: The typical clinical signs in the dog include nervousness and seizures. Disturbances of the LMNS causing spasms of limb muscles, pain, focal muscle fasciculations, stiff gait, and or weakness also occur frequently. Another important clinical indication of hypocalcaemia is intense rubbing of the face on firm surfaces or the floor. Repeated licking of the limbs may also been seen.

Diagnosis: In the assessment of serum calcium concentration, the albumin level must also be taken into consideration. Correction of the calcium level for deficits in albumin can be done and the reader is referred to internal medicine texts for the methodology. A corrected total calcium concentration < 1.6 mmol/l indicates that there is a severe deficit. The clinical symptoms depend on the concentration of ionised calcium that can be easily measured in a clinic or a larger laboratory (normal value 1.25–1.45 mmol/l).

Therapy: Treatment is symptomatic. Calcium gluconate intravenously or subcutaneously; oral calcium and oral vitamin D metabolites (dihydrotachysterol, calicitriol) improve the clinical condition; internal medicine texts should be consulted for further information.

Prognosis: Life-long therapy is necessary.

13.6.1.8 Hypothyroidism
(See Chap. 15.4.3)

13.6.1.9 Hyperthyroidism

Occurrence: Frequent in the cat.

Aetiology: Hyperthyroidism is one of the most frequent endocrinopathies of older cats. Although mild muscle weakness occurs relatively often, cases with obvious muscle signs are rare, and only affect a few hyperthyroid cats. In human beings, in addition to other clinical signs, there is reduction in the reserves of energy-rich compounds in the skeletal muscles and displacement of calcium into the muscle cells. With successful treatment of hyperthyroidism, calcium retention disappears and renal loss of potassium due to subclinical renal dysfunction becomes apparent. This can then lead to a hypokalaemic polymyopathy.

Clinical: There is often generalised muscle weakness and the animal shows rapid exhaustion on minimal exertion. In some cases, ventroflexion of the neck becomes apparent before the hyperthyroidism is diagnosed.

Diagnosis: Along with the typical laboratory investigations for hyperthyroidism, the serum concentration of CK can be increased. Hyperthyroidism is diagnosed with determination of the serum thyroxine concentration. Total T4 and free T4 are also useful parameters. In uncertain cases, a T3 suppression test is indicated.

Therapy: Possible alternatives include medication, surgery or radiation therapy. In addition, the replacement of possible potassium deficits is important. The risk of hypokalaemia immediately postoperatively occurs in thyroidectomised animals given intraoperative potassium therapy.

Prognosis: The prognosis of feline hyperthyroidism depends on the chosen therapy and the experience of the surgeon. The myopathy disappears shortly after the start of therapy. In cats with clinical chronic renal failure, long-term potassium replacement therapy must be planned.

13.6.1.10 Spontaneous hyperadrenocorticism

Occurrence: Frequent in the dog; very rare in the cat.

Aetiology: Loss of muscle mass is induced by the catabolic effects of cortisol. Weakness as a sign of muscle dysfunction has been described in roughly three quarters of all Cushing's patients. Cushing's myopathy is a so-called pseudomyotonia. Stiff hindlimbs, muscle atrophy and in severe cases even muscle contractions are apparent in affected dogs. The cause of this phenomenon is unknown. Histological and ultrastructural investigations in dogs with Cushing's myopathy have shown atrophy of both type 1 and type 2 muscle fibres, variation in the diameter of the muscle fibres, focal necrosis, fat deposits, abnormal mitochondria and intrafibrillar glycogen deposits. The deposition of nemaline rods in type 1 muscle fibres and the presence of so-called "ragged" red fibres have also been described. The grouping of affected muscle fibres indicates that nerve fibres are also involved in the disease process. Most probably, a disturbance of the chloride or sodium channels is responsible for the pseudomyotonia.

Clinical: Dachshund, German Shepherd, Labrador Retriever and Poodle are the most commonly affected breeds. Muscle changes accompany the Cushing's syndrome. Even though PU/PD, polyphagia, pendulous abdomen, overweight, alopecia, thin skin, exophthalmus and abnormal function of the sex hormones are the main symptoms; many dogs suffer from exercise intolerance, weakness, lameness and muscle atrophy.

Diagnosis: In addition to weakness and other signs typical for hyperadrenocorticism, laboratory investigations are essential. ACTH stimulation test, dexamethasone suppression test with a high or low dose of dexamethasone and endogenous ACTH are the most important hormonal methods of clarifying the diagnosis. Imaging techniques such as ultrasonography of the abdomen or in some cases MRI of the brain can be valuable. Serum CK may be slightly increased. The changes in EMG provide indications about the pathological mechanism of the weakness. Mild fibrillations or PSWs can indicate the presence of a Cushing's myopathy, although complex repetitive or pseudo-myotonic discharges can also be present.

Therapy: Depending on the cause, medical or surgical treatment of Cushing's may be warranted; radiation therapy may even be indicated.

Prognosis: The muscle weakness improves with normalisation of the serum cortisol concentration.

13.6.1.11 Iatrogenic steroid-induced myopathy

Occurrence: Frequent in the dog; rare in the cat.

Aetiology: Glucocorticoids are frequently used in veterinary medicine, however, the frequency of this steroid-induced myopathy in domestic animals is unknown. With a prednisolone dosage of 4 mg/kg/day, muscle changes can be observed in the dog after 2 weeks; after 4 weeks, reduced diameter of the muscle fibers can be seen. Similar but milder indications of a myopathy were found in cats that had been given triamcinolone 3–4 mg/kg/day. Some observations indicate that long-term glucocorticoid therapy, even at low doses, leads to weakness and visible muscle atrophy. Cortisone given for therapeutic purposes increases muscle protein catabolism and reduces the synthesis of muscle fibres. These side-effects are more pronounced in patients with low protein reserves.

Clinical: In addition to the typical corticosteroid side-effects, there is progressive, generalised muscle atrophy and weakness. Temporalis muscle atrophy is often the first sign noticed by the owner.

Diagnosis: Anamnesis, clinical results and ACTH stimulation test.

Therapy: Reduction of the cortisone dosage, oral administration of high-quality protein supplements, physiotherapy.

Prognosis: Depends on the cause necessitating administration of cortisone.

13.6.2 Congenital myopathies

Congenital myopathies are rare. Early recognition of these diseases is extremely important for breeders and breeding advisors. While polymyopathies of other aetiologies are not breed-specific, the congenital diseases have only been described in certain breeds. Genetic transmission has been proven or suggested in these diseases. An important characteristic is their occurrence in the first year of life. Important differential diagnoses are given in Table 13.14.

13.6.2.1 Muscular dystrophy in the dog

Occurrence: Rare; described in specific dog breeds.

Aetiology: Muscular dystrophy in the dog is a heterogeneous group of progressive diseases in which the main symptoms are muscle atrophy and weakness. The abnormalities are caused by the lack or dysfunction of dystrophin, which is an important stabiliser of the muscle fibre membrane. Its inheritance is recessive and is linked to the X-chromosome. Female animals are the carriers and they either remain asymptomatic or are only affected mildly. Male dogs show the full clinical picture. The high mutation rate of the large dystrophin gene causes sporadic individual cases or outbreaks within a family. Muscular dystrophy with dystrophin deficiency has been proven as occurring or is thought to be highly probable in the following breeds: Brittany Spaniel, German Short-haired Pointer, Golden Retriever, Groenendaler, Irish Setter, Labrador Retriever, Miniature Schnauzer, Pembroke Welsh Corgi, Rat Terrier, Rottweiler and Samoyed.

Clinical: The first signs often occur at 2 months of age. The typical symptoms include exercise intolerance, tetraplegia, stiff gait, inability to open the mouth and muscle atrophy in all four limbs. Many patients have difficulty in swallowing as the oesophageal musculature is hypertrophic. Later on, adduction of the elbow joints and lordosis of the spine can also develop. In mild cases, the disease can stabilise after a number of months but due to the connective tissue deposits within the muscle, the animal's movements remain constrained.

Diagnosis: Serum CK levels increase to a value between 10,000–30,000 U/l or even higher. On EMG, severe abnormal spontaneous activity with fibrillations, PSWs, complex repetitive and pseudo-myotonic discharges can be seen. The definitive diagnosis is obtained by muscle biopsy which demonstrates the lack of dystrophin. Histopathological investigations of the skeletal musculature in the Golden Retriever revealed a severe variation in the diameter of muscle fibres, dominance of the type 1 fibres, focal or segmental necrosis, phagocytosis, fibrosis and intra-cytoplasmic calcium deposits.

13

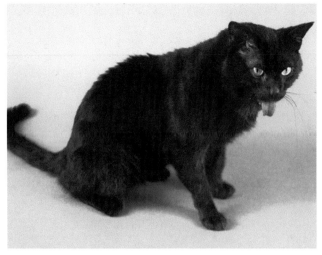

Fig. 13.60
A two-year-old cat with hypertrophic polymyopathy as a result of dystrophin deficiency. Hypertrophy of the limb musculature is especially noticeable in the proximal parts of the limbs (thigh, brachium). The neck musculature is also very prominent. The tongue is enlarged in this animal and hangs out of the mouth as the hypertrophic pharyngeal and laryngeal muscles make its retraction difficult.

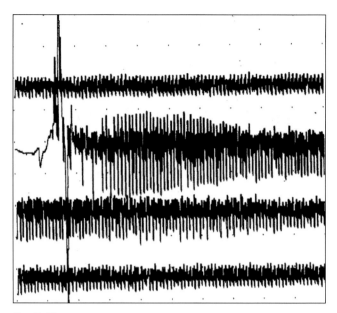

Fig. 13.61
Spontaneous myotonic discharges with typical crescendo-descendo course are depicted in this EMG. The corresponding acoustic signal sounds like a dive bomber out of World War II. In dystrophin deficiency, these discharges as accompanied by various other EMG changes.

Therapy: Supportive measures and physiotherapy in mildly affected animals (see Chap. 8.1).

Prognosis: The patient's life expectancy depends on the severity of the clinical signs. Due to involvement of the diaphramatic muscles, severe respiratory disturbances can occur. A chronic progressive cardiomyopathy can occur which is a further reason for a reduced life expectancy.

13.6.2.2 Hypertrophic polymyopathy (muscular dystrophy) in the cat

Occurrence: Rare.

Aetiology: Case studies from Europe (the Netherlands, Switzerland) and North America are described in the literature. This muscle disease serves as one of the three animal models for Duchenne myopathy in human beings. The responsible gene is also found on the X-chromosome, and so the myopathy is transmitted by clinically healthy female cats and only some of their male progeny are affected. The missing protein dystrophin has a critical function in the subsarcolemmal space in the muscle cell as a connection between the intracellular cytoskeleton and the extracellular matrix. Presumably, dystrophin fulfils a number of important tasks in maintaining the integrity of the cell.

Clinical: The clinical signs of dystrophin deficiency in the cat are rather characteristic. In comparison to the dog, a hypertrophic myopathy is present in affected male cats, which is recognisable both in the axial and in the proximal part of the appendicular skeletal musculature (Fig. 13.60). Due to generalised skeletal muscle hypertrophy, many males with dystrophin deficiency develop different complications. The extreme hypertrophy of the diaphragmatic muscles with obstruction of the oesophagus at the hiatus leads to megaoesophagus. The hypertrophy of the tongue muscles makes the uptake of water difficult and leads to dehydration and hyperosmolarity. Subclinical involvement of the heart muscle has been proven. These cats are oversensitive to stress and certain anaesthetics, so that rhabdomyolysis can quickly develop.

Diagnosis: The muscle enzymes are evidently increased. EMG investigations show a multitude of changes, though the myotonic discharges are the most impressive (Fig. 13.61). Histological investigations of the affected muscles show a nonspecific picture of multifocal muscle degeneration and regeneration but without an increase of connective tissue and muscle fibre hypertrophy (Fig. 13.62). Immunohistochemical investigation for subsarcolemmal dystrophin is essential for a definitive diagnosis.

13

Therapy: Specific therapy is impossible. Dystrophic male cats need supportive care including rest and regular subcutaneous fluid infusions.

Prognosis: The prognosis in cats depends on the severity of the complications. Affected male cats have been able to reach an age of 5 to 10 years with a good quality of life.

13.6.2.3 Merosin deficiency myopathy

Occurrence: Very rare in cats: only two cases from North America have been described so far.

Aetiology: Merosin (laminin a2) is a component of the basal membrane of muscle fibres, Schwann cells and endothelial cells in the brain. Merosin deficiency is the cause of congenital muscular dystrophy in human beings.

Clinical: The main clinical signs include progressive muscle weakness with muscle atrophy and contraction of the extensors of the hindlimbs and hypotonia of the forelimbs.

Diagnosis: The first abnormalities occur at approximately 6 months of age. The serum concentration of CK is increased. Electrophysiological results include a reduced NCV with normal spontaneous muscle activity. Histological investigations reveal endomysial fibrosis and muscle fibre necrosis. The neural abnormalities include axons with thin or absent myelin sheaths, periaxonal swelling and degeneration of the Schwann cells. Immunohistochemical staining for merosin is negative.

Therapy: None.

Prognosis: Hopeless. Both cats reported had to be euthanised.

13.6.2.4 Labrador myopathy

Occurrence: Rare.

Aetiology: A degenerative muscle disease in the Labrador Retriever was first described in 1976. Since then individual cases have occurred in the USA, Australia and Europe. An autosomal recessive inheritance was confirmed. The actual cause for the muscular degenerative changes is still unknown. Histological signs of secondary neurogenic disease have also been observed with this disease.

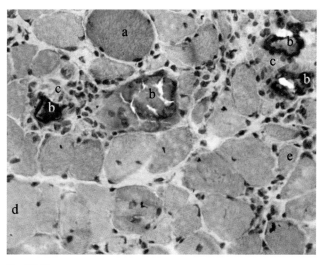

Fig. 13.62
Lateral vastus muscle of a six-month-old male cat with hypertrophic polymyopathy (HE stain). The following abnormalities can be seen: (a) contracted, hypereosinophilic muscle fibres; (b) dystrophic calcification of degenerate muscle fibres; (c) area of regeneration with proliferation of small cells with a high nucleus:cytoplasm ratio; (d) a wide variation in the diameter of the muscle fibres with large hypertrophic and small muscle fibres. No dystrophin could be found in the subsarcolemmal space using immunohistochemistry.

Clinical: The first clinical signs are visible at an age of 2 to 7 months with most puppies affected 3 to 4 months after birth. The clinical signs include exercise intolerance, uncoordinated gait and frequent collapse of the forelimbs. In severe cases, lordosis of the spine with cervical ventroflexion, a bunny-hopping gait and swallowing problems also develop. Often cold intolerance is seen with deterioration of the clinical signs in cold surroundings.

The neurological examination reveals a general reduction in the spinal reflexes. The proximal limb muscles and sometimes the mastication muscles are particularly affected by muscle atrophy. In rare cases, dysphagia and megaoesophagus have been observed. Other complications in adult dogs include patella luxation and degenerative joint disease.

Diagnosis: The presence of the disease is proven by the clinical picture, the electrophysiological investigation and muscle and nerve biopsies.

EMG often reveals fibrillations, PSWs and complex repetitive discharge patterns. This abnormal spontaneous activity is found predominantly in the proximal limb muscles, and in the head. The mNCV of the diseased dogs are in the normal range.

13

Histologically, a great variety of muscle changes can be found with primary degenerative muscle changes being most conspicuous. Sometimes histological reactions are seen which indicate the presence of secondary neurogenic influences.

Therapy: No specific therapy available; supportive measures and physiotherapy are helpful in some cases.

Prognosis: The disease course can be very variable. Mildly affected dogs can stabilise at 1 year of age and lead a good life as a family dog, although muscle atrophy remains. Dogs with severe gait disturbances or problems with swallowing have an unfavourable prognosis.

13.6.2.5 Myopathy of the Devon Rex Cat

Occurrence: Reports from Great Britain and Australia about this breed-specific myopathy are available, which is also known as Devon Rex spasticity. The disease apparently occurs more frequently in certain breeding lines.

Aetiology: Unknown. This is an autosomal recessive inheritable disease.

Clinical: The clinical signs are typical. The first clinical signs appear at a few weeks or months of age. Characteristic signs include ventroflexion of the neck and generalised muscle weakness, especially after exertion, stress or excitement. The animals have a hypermetric gait in the forelimbs, synchronised pendulous head movements and dorsal hunching of the shoulders as a consequence of the weakness of the shoulder "girdle" muscles. Finally, the animals collapse in sternal recumbency (chin on sternum phenomenon). Often the affected cats take on a classical "begging" position. Individual cats have problems with eating and swallowing.

Diagnosis: There is no increase in the serum muscle enzymes. Enlargement of the oesophagus is often seen on radiographs of the thorax. EMG demonstrates moderate abnormalities (few fibrillations and PSWs). The following abnormalities have been observed histologically: large variation in the diameter of the muscle fibres, increased number of nuclei with a tendency for central migration, necrotic and regenerative muscle fibres.

Therapy: None.

Prognosis: The course of this myopathy is progressive until the age of approx. 6 to 9 months. The disease then stabilises or it continues to progress slowly. The least favourable prognosis is for cats with severe dysphagia. Affected cats and their parents or siblings should not be used for breeding.

13.6.2.6 Degenerative polymyopathy in the Bouvier des Flandres

Occurrence: Very rare.

Aetiology: The exact cause is not known. Metabolic causes have been excluded. Atypical for a degenerative disease is the onset at 2 to 7 years of age. Female animals are affected more commonly.

Clinical: The clinical picture is typified by exercise intolerance, muscle atrophy, reduced muscle tone, regurgitation and megaoesophagus.

Diagnosis: Serum CK is normal to moderately increased. Complex repetitive discharges can be seen on EMG. Histological investigation shows a degenerative muscle disease which is partially reminiscent of Labrador myopathy and also partially reminiscent of the muscular dystrophy found in Golden Retrievers.

Therapy: None possible.

Prognosis: The course is progressive.

13.6.2.7 Nemaline-rod myopathy

Occurrence: Very rare.

Aetiology: Unknown. This myopathy has been described in various dog breeds and in five related cats from the USA.

Clinical: The age of affected dogs varies from 10 months to 13 years. The most noticeable clinical symptoms include palmi- and plantigrade positioning of the limbs, exercise intolerance, generalised muscle atrophy, reduced spinal reflexes and generalised tremor.

The affected cats were 0.5 to 1.5 years of age and exhibited weakness, swaying gait, loss of weight and listlessness, progressing to exercise intolerance, a hypermetric gait with a kyphotic back, generalised tremor and very severe muscle atrophy. The clinical signs gradually increased in severity.

Diagnosis: Laboratory investigations reveal a moderately increased CK. EMG reveals hardly any abnormalities. The histology of the muscles demonstrates wide variation in the size of muscle fibres with many atrophic fibres, centralisation of the nuclei, and the accumulation of so-called nemaline rods in some muscle fibres.

Therapy: None.

Prognosis: Poor.

13.6.2.8 Juvenile distal myopathy in the Rottweiler

Occurrence: Rare.

Aetiology: The cause is unknown therefore an exact aetiological classification is impossible. Histochemical investigation does not reveal any dystrophin abnormalities. Some animals have reduced plasma and muscle carnitine concentrations.

Clinical: The clinical signs start in puppyhood. Weakness of the distal muscle groups is conspicuous. The affected dogs exhibit typical palmigrade or plantigrade positioning of the limbs. The toes of all four feet are spread out and the tarsal joint can only be held flexed. Depression and exercise intolerance are additional symptoms.

Diagnosis: The CK is normal or is only slightly increased. Electrophysiological investigations are unremarkable. Histological investigation reveals that the muscle tissue is replaced by fat. Dystrophin staining is normal.

Therapy: Oral therapy with carnitine 50 mg/kg BID, coenzyme Q_{10} 4 mg/kg SID and standard human adult doses of vitamin B complex can be attempted.

Prognosis: Due to limited experience with this disease, it is difficult to formulate a prognosis.

13.6.2.9 Lipid storage myopathy

Occurrence: Very rare.

Aetiology: Muscle disease due to intramuscular lipid accumulation has recently been documented in dogs. The exact cause is not known. An accumulation of predominantly triglycerides has been found in type 1 muscle fibres. This buildup of long-chain fatty acids is most probably due to a defect in the oxidative cycle. Carnitine appears to be an important building block for enzymes helpful in the transport of acetyl CoA into the mitochondria. A deficit of carnitine is associated with lipid storage myopathies and is due to a primary disease or secondary to abnormal β-oxidation, both resulting in low plasma and muscle carnitine concentrations. Carnitine also plays a role in the use of glucose in the Krebs cycle and in the metabolism of branched amino acids. In addition to the intramuscular fat deposits, lactate or pyruvate acidosis and a raised plasma concentration of alanine, glutamine, valine and leucine may occur. In affected animals organic acids are excreted in high concentrations in the urine. In addition to carnitine, Coenzyme Q_{10} has been described as being an important catalyst for mitochondrial β-oxidation.

Clinical: The signs include diffuse and obvious muscle pain as well as weakness with the head held low. Other nonspecific symptoms such as stiff gait, lameness, muscle spasms, exercise intolerance and tremor have been described.

Diagnosis: Serum CK can be normal. Muscle biopsy is an essential step for definitive diagnosis. The most conspicuous abnormalities are the numerous fat droplets in type 1 fibres and sometimes in type 2 fibres. Other diagnostic tests include the measurement of lactate and pyruvate concentrations before and after exercise, determination of amino acid concentrations in the serum, quantitative analysis of organic acids in the urine and the determination of carnitine concentration in the plasma, urine and muscle.

Therapy: Oral therapy with L-carnitine 50 mg/kg BID, coenzyme Q_{10} 4 mg/kg SID; Vitamin C 50 mg/kg SID as well as standard daily doses of vitamin B complex leads to a significant clinical improvement in some patients.

Prognosis: Due to limited experience with this disease, prognosis is difficult to determine.

13.6.2.10 Mitochondrial myopathies

Occurrence: Very rare.

Aetiology: A few Clumber Spaniels and Sussex Spaniels in the UK, Finland and the USA have been shown to suffer from a deficit of the mitochondrial enzyme pyruvate dehydrogenase, which is responsible for the metabolism of glucose in the Krebs cycle. Lactate acidosis occurs with exertion and excessive glucose use. A mitochondrial myopathy has also been described in an English Sheepdog puppy and has been presumed in a Jack Russell Terrier.

Clinical: The most important clinical signs are exercise intolerance and muscle spasms.

Diagnosis: The classical diagnostic methods such as serum CK levels, metabolic investigations, EMG, nerve conduction tests or repetitive nerve stimulation are not of specific use in this disease, but are important for the exclusion of other diseases. In the muscle biopsy, the presence of ragged red fibres is the first indication of an abnormality. Measurement of the lactate and pyruvate concentrations whilst resting and after exercise is an important screening test. An excessive increase in lactate after movement, and a lactate: pyruvate ratio of > 10 are diagnostic features compatible with a pyruvate dehydrogenase deficiency. Pyruvate dehydrogenase activity can be measured in fibroblast cultures.

Therapy: Supplementation of riboflavin and L-carnitine (50 mg/kg BID) to the diet has been suggested. Feeding a diet low in carbohydrates and rich in fats (50% or more fat, maximal 20% carbohydrates) has also been recommended.

Prognosis: With no cure, the prognosis is poor.

13

13.6.2.11 Glycogen storage disease type II in the Lapland Hound

Occurrence: Very rare.

Aetiology: A deficiency of α–1,4-glucosidase has been described in the Lapland Hound. This enzyme deficit leads to a massive accumulation of glycogen in the majority of the organs, including the muscles.

Clinical: The clinical signs start in puppyhood. The signs are generalised weakness, dysphagia, vomiting and dyspnoea.

Diagnosis: The definitive investigations include muscle biopsy and the investigation of tissue samples from other organs. The biochemical defect can be analysed in connective tissue cultures.

Therapy: None.

Prognosis: The majority of these dogs do not reach the second year of life.

13.6.2.12 Glycogen storage disease type III in the German Shepherd and Akita Inu

Occurrence: Very rare.

Aetiology: A defect in the enzyme amylo-1,6-glucosidase leads to the deposition of a glycogen-like compound in various organs.

Clinical: Weakness and increase in the size of the abdomen due to hepatomegaly occur in early puppyhood.

Diagnosis: Important investigations include muscle and liver biopsy.

Therapy: None.

Prognosis: Very poor.

13.6.2.13 Glycogen storage disease type IV in the Norwegian Forest Cat

Occurrence: Very rare.

Aetiology: An enzyme defect is presumed which inhibits the synthesis of the branched form of glycogen. Abnormal glycogen is stored in muscle and nerve tissue. The disease is inherited by a simple autosomal recessive gene.

In North America, the disease is a problem in the Norwegian Forest Cat, while in Europe this disease has not been diagnosed. However, it appears that cats subsequently identified as being carriers had been exported from Norway and Germany to the USA. Possibly, the disease is so rare in Europe that it is not recognised. Another possible cause for this lack of recognition could be the fulminant nature of disease found in kittens.

Clinical: The clinical signs start at an age of approx. 5 months and consist initially of intermittent depression, increased body temperature, generalised muscle tremor and abnormal gait. Progressive, severe, generalised muscle atrophy with contracture of the limbs develops over weeks to months. Some cats can not move because of this and remain in lateral recumbency. Chewing and swallowing difficulties have also been observed. Serum CK and ALT are significantly increased. In addition, a fulminant form has been documented in which kittens are affected by collapse of the lungs and circulation followed by death within a few hours after birth.

Diagnosis: Spontaneous fibrillations and pseudo-myotonic discharges can be found with EMG in many muscles. A concentric hypertrophic cardiomyopathy has also been found associated with these cases.

The histological changes consist of cytoplasmic inclusion bodies in many different types of tissue. The most conspicuous changes are found in the skeletal and heart muscles, and the neurons. A molecular genetic test has been developed and is available in North America.

Therapy: None.

Prognosis: Hopeless. The cats die before 10 months of age. This is why early identification of carriers is desirable in affected breeding lines.

13.6.2.14 Malignant hyperthermia

Occurrence: Very rare.

Aetiology: Malignant hyperthermia with a body temperature of more than 42°C represents a hypermetabolic syndrome of the skeletal musculature. There is an inherited predisposition. Gaseous anaesthesia (halothane, enflurane), medications such as lidocaine or succinyl choline, stress, exertion, and an already elevated body temperature have been purported as trigger factors. Individual or combined trigger factors stimulate abnormal regulation of the myoplasmic calcium. The defect lies in the sarcoplasmic reticulum, which releases calcium after stimulation but afterwards cannot transport it back. Excessive glycogenolysis induces hypoxia, an accumulation of CO_2 and lactic acidosis. Males and heavily muscled dogs are more commonly affected. In cats with rhabdomyolysis, the animals usually have dystrophin deficiency and hypertrophic myopathy. All such cats die during or immediately after anaesthesia.

Clinical: The clinical signs include pyrexia, tachycardia and generalised or focal muscle rigidity of the mastication muscles. Cardiac or renal failure, pulmonary oedema or disseminated intravascular coagulopathy are possible, and are severe complications.

Diagnosis: An unexpected increase in body temperature; exclusion of fever (infections, immune-mediated inflammation, neoplasia) and other causes of hyperthermia (seizures, heat stress, bodily exertion). Laboratory investigation to determine secondary complications is often needed.

Therapy: Stop the anaesthesia; correction of the electrolyte disturbance and the acid-base imbalance; fluid therapy, possibly with the addition of bicarbonates; control of body temperature; muscle relaxation (dantrolene 2–5 mg/kg IV) and rest are the most important therapeutic measures.

Prognosis: Frequently very poor.

13.6.2.15 Exertion-dependent rhabdomyolysis

Occurrence: Rare.

Aetiology: This disease is particularly seen in Greyhounds that have been used in races. However, it can also be seen in captured wild animals and after prolonged grand mal epileptic seizures. The pathogenesis is unclear. In the Greyhound, lactic acidosis, swelling of the muscle fibres and local muscle cell necrosis have been described. Metabolic defects and immune-mediated abnormalities cannot be completely excluded.

Clinical: The first signs of the disease occur within 24 to 72 hours after exertion. The most common clinical signs include depression, dehydration, stiff gait, increased muscle tone and/or swollen and painful muscles in the limbs. The hindlegs are most obviously affected. In severe cases, the patients remain in lateral recumbency and are incapable of moving. Sometimes severe myoglobinuria is associated with a risk of renal failure. In the serum, potassium and phosphorus are often significantly increased. Abnormal kidney values and urine results with myoglobinuria are not unusual.

Diagnosis: Anamnesis, clinical signs, laboratory investigation such as biochemical profile including serum CK, lactate and urinalysis.

Therapy: Correction of the electrolyte disturbance and the acid-base imbalance; fluid therapy, possibly with the inclusion of bicarbonates; control of the body temperature; muscle relaxation and rest are the most important therapeutic measures.

Prognosis: The prognosis depends on the degree of muscle damage and renal failure. Particular attention should be paid to monitoring the kidney function.

13.6.2.16 Episodic muscle hypertonia in Terriers, Dalmatians and Cavalier King Charles Spaniels

Occurrence: Very rare.

Aetiology: This paroxysmal disease with hyperkinetic episodes is particularly well described in the Scottish Terrier (Scotty cramp), but individual cases have also been described in the Dalmatian, Jack Russell Terrier and Norwich Terrier. The defect is presumably inherited by a recessive gene. The disease appears not to be a primary muscle disease, but is described in this chapter as the clinical signs may indicate that it is one. It is thought that a serotonin imbalance occurs in the part of the nervous system that controls muscle tone. Neither muscle abnormalities nor structural changes in the nervous system have been found. A clinically similar syndrome has been observed in the Cavalier King Charles Spaniel.

Clinical: The problem occurs in animals as young as 6 weeks to 18 months. The episodes can be elicited by work, excitation or stress. The typical clinical signs include an increasingly stiff gait, hunching of the back, spasms of the cervical and facial muscles, and hyperextension of the hindlimbs. Certain animals are unable to stand and remain in lateral recumbency. This spastic condition improves usually after a period of rest. The animal remains conscious throughout the whole episode which can last for several minutes.

13

Diagnosis: Signalment, clinical presentation and the lack of structural abnormalities support a tentative diagnosis. Methysergide 0.3 mg/kg PO can elicit an episode within approx. 2 hours.

Therapy: Diazepam, chlorpromazine and acepromazine can stop an episode. Preventative medical therapy may be effective in the long term. Clonazepam treatment appears to be effective in some Cavalier King Charles Spaniels. Supportive measures such as rest and limited exertion are the most important therapies. Phenotypic carriers should not be used for breeding purposes.

Prognosis: Favourable.

13.6.2.17 Intermittent hyperkalaemia

Occurrence: Very rare.

Aetiology: Periodic hyperkalaemia is caused by a mutation of the sodium channels in human beings. After an action potential, these channels cannot be closed and the membrane potential is significantly prolonged. A measurable change associated with this congenital sodium channel dysfunction is that increased concentrations of potassium remain in the extracellular compartment, which depending on the degree of exertion, leads to weakness, paralysis or myotonia and increased muscle tone.

A similar syndrome, predominantly causing paralysis, has been described in an American Pit Bull Terrier. Although the molecular basis has not been investigated in this breed, the presence of a dysfunction of the sodium channels appears likely.

Clinical: A seven-month-old American Pit Bull Terrier has been described with exertion-dependent collapse. The 10- to 15-second episodes were characterised by a loss of muscle tone in the limbs and neck, protruding tongue and normal consciousness.

Diagnosis: CBC, biochemistry profile, electrophysiological tests and endocrine investigations were unremarkable. The serum CK was slightly raised. The potassium concentration increased after exercise and only returned to normal over a number of hours. Other causes of hyperkalaemia such as hypo- and hyperadrenocorticism, aldosterone deficiency and rhabdomyolysis could be excluded. Treatment with acetazolamide and fludrocortisone at standard doses reduced the frequency of collapse, which confirmed the diagnosis.

Therapy: Acetazolamide, fludrocortisone, low potassium diet, prevention of hypothermia.

Prognosis: Difficult as virtually no experience of this condition exists in dogs.

13.6.2.18 Hypokalaemic polymyopathy in the Burmese Cat

Occurrence: Very rare.

Aetiology: It is thought that the inheritance is autosomal recessive; however, the exact aetiology in the Burmese cat is unknown. In human beings, this disease is caused by a disturbance of the calcium channels.

Clinical: Burmese cats with this congenital muscle disease have been reported in Great Britain, New Zealand, Australia and the Netherlands. The syndrome is similar to periodic hypokalaemic paralysis in human beings. Periodic muscle weakness has been observed in young Burmese kittens (starting at an age of 4–12 months). Episodes with generalised muscle weakness and ventroflexion of the neck occur acutely. Activity related weakness is prominent. Hypermetria in the forelegs with pendulous head movements has been described. Head tremor is possible.

Diagnosis: There is a significant increase in serum CK. The EMG reveals mild changes such as excessive insertion activity and PSWs. Histologically, there is mild, diffuse necrosis of the muscle fibres.

Therapy: Potassium supplementation as in acquired hypokalaemic polymyopathy is indicated (see Chap. 13.6.1.5).

Prognosis: Favourable with potassium supplementation. However, neither affected animals nor their parents or siblings should be used for breeding purposes.

13.6.2.19 Central core-like myopathy

Occurrence: Rare in the Great Dane.

Etiology: Specific for this disease is damage of the central area of the muscle fibers. The associated central ring-like area of lucency (core) can be made visible with a number of staining techniques. Electron microscopic investigations have shown an accumulation of mitochondria, glycogen, and destroyed muscle fibrils in the lucent area. These central changes are mainly seen in Type I muscle fibers, although they can also affect Type II fibers. The cause of this disease is unknown. Though a genetic background is thought to be present in the Great Dane, an extensive clarification of the disease is lacking.

Clinical: In the majority of cases, the first indications of the disease are seen before the dogs are one year old. Male and female dogs are affected equally. The main neurological finding is weakness, which is more pronounced when affected dogs

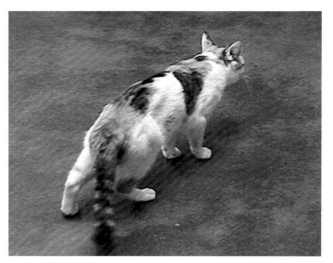

Fig. 13.63

An eighteen-month-old domestic cat was presented because of syncope that could be elicited by excitement or stress. The clinical examination showed a generalised, over-proportioned muscling of the limbs, torso and head.

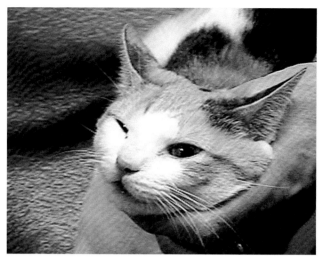

Fig. 13.64

A spastic palpebral reflex was evident in the cat from Fig. 13.63. After stimulation of the edge of the right eyelid, the cat needed 2–3 minutes before it could open its eye again.

are worked and which can lead to collapse. The animals have a slight to moderate loss of muscle mass, shortened step length, and in some dogs, tremor and reduced spinal reflexes (especially the patella reflex).

Diagnosis: The serum creatinine kinase may be raised. The EMG shows nonspecific changes such as fibrillation potentials or positive sharp waves (PSW). The most important additional investigation is a muscle biopsy, which will confirm the diagnosis.

Therapy: No specific treatment is available, though supportive measures can be useful for a while.

Prognosis: The long-term prognosis is unfavorable; however, a life expectancy of 1–2 years is possible with this disease.

13.6.2.20 Myotonia

Occurrence: Very rare.

Aetiology: Myotonia is a disease of the skeletal muscles in which a mechanical, electrical or arbitrary stimulation of the muscles results in a prolonged or continual contraction. An inheritable form is known to occur in the Chow Chow and Miniature Schnauzer. An autosomal recessive inherited defect in the sarcolemmal chloride channel has been proven in the

Schnauzer. A similar situation has been presumed in the Chow Chow and the cat.

Clinical: The first indications of this disease become apparent whilst the animal is a puppy / kitten. The typical clinical signs include good muscle development on the head and limbs, stiff gait and short stride length, especially in the hindlimbs (Fig. 13.63). The stiff gait is more prominent after rest or during cold weather. Climbing stairs can be difficult for these animals. Flight reactions lead to massive muscle spasms, during which the animals lose control of themselves and remain lying in lateral recumbency for a few seconds with normal consciousness. Such spasms may only affect local muscle groups such as the muscles around the eyes (Fig. 13.64), the muscles for moving the earlobe or the laryngeal muscles. The palpebral reflex is prolonged because the orbicularis oculi muscle needs time to recover from the spasms. Dysphonia is also caused by contraction of hypertrophic muscles. Respiratory disturbances due to stenosis of the upper airways as a consequence of the generalised muscle hypertrophy may also occur. A myotonic dimple can be induced by percussing the tongue under anaesthesia.

13

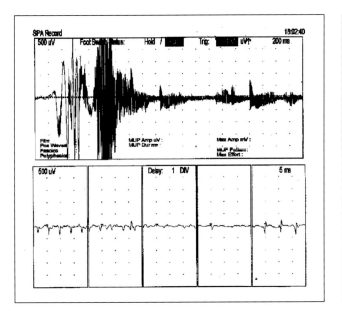

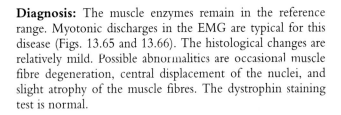

Fig. 13.65
The EMG from the cat in Figs. 13.63 and 13.64 showed an obviously increased insertional activity which progressed to crescendo-decrescendo spontaneous activity.

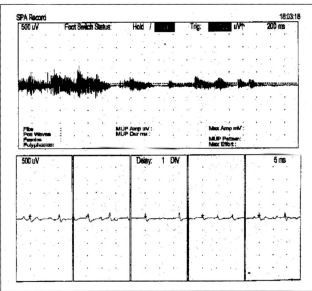

Fig. 13.66
Although the continual crescendo-decrescendo spontaneous activity in Fig. 13.65 could be classified as a myotonic discharge pattern, the acoustic signal sounded more like a racing car than a dive bomber. The clinical and electrophysiological results, muscle biopsy and positive dystrophin test were the bases for a diagnosis of congenital myotonia.

Diagnosis: The muscle enzymes remain in the reference range. Myotonic discharges in the EMG are typical for this disease (Figs. 13.65 and 13.66). The histological changes are relatively mild. Possible abnormalities are occasional muscle fibre degeneration, central displacement of the nuclei, and slight atrophy of the muscle fibres. The dystrophin staining test is normal.

Therapy: Slow-release procainamide (40 mg/kg, PO, BID-TID) can be used in the dog. An alternative in the dog is mexiletine 8.3 mg/kg, PO, TID. Potassium bromide is contraindicated. Our own experience in cats has shown that slow-release procainamide 40–50 mg/kg, PO, TID leads to obvious improvement in clinical signs.

Prognosis: Successful therapy improves the situation but it does not completely stop the muscle spasms.

13

Further reading

BELLAH, J.R., ROBERTSON S.A., BÜRGELT, C.D. McGAVIN, D. (1989): Suspected malignant hyperthermia after halothane anesthesia in a cat. Vet Surg. **18**: 483–488.

BLAXTER, A., LIEVESLEY, P., GRUFFYD-JONES, T., WOTTON, P. (1986): Periodic muscle weakness in Burmese kittens. Vet Rec. **118**: 619–620.

BRAUND, K.G., DILLON A.R., MIKEAL, R.L., AUGUST J.R. (1980): Subclinical myopathy associated with hyperadrenocorticism in the dog. Vet Pathol. **17**: 134–148.

BRAUND, K.G., STEINBERG, H.S., MENTHA, J.R., AMLING, K.A. (1990): Investigating a degegerative polymyopathy in four related Bouvier des Falndres dogs. Vet Med. **85**: 558–570.

CARPENTER, J., HOLZWORTH, J. (1982): Thymoma in 11 cats. J Am Vet Med Assoc. **181**: 248–251.

DOW, S.W., FETTMAN, M.J., LECOUTEUR, R.A., HAMAR, D.W. (1987): Potassium depletion in cats: renal and dietary influences. J Am Vet Med Assoc. **191**: 1569–1575

DOW, S.W., LECOUTEUR, R.A., FETTMAN, M.J., SPURGEON, T.L. (1987): Potassium depletion in cats: hypokalemic myopathy. J Am Vet Med Assoc. **191**: 1563–1568.

DUBEY, J.P., LAPPIN, M.R. (1998): Toxoplasmosis and neosporosis. In GREENE, C.E. (ed.): Infectious Diseases of the Dog and Cat. W.B. Saunders, Philadelphia 1998, pp. 493–509.

DUBEY, J.P., CARPENTER, J.L. (1993): Histologically confirmed clinical toxoplasmosis in cats: 100 cases (1952–1990). J Am Vet Med Assoc. **203**: 1556–1566.

GASCHEN, F.P., HAUGH, P.G., SWENDROWSKI, M.A. (1994): Hypertrophic feline muscular dystrophy – A unique clinical expression of dystrophin deficiency. Fel Pract. **22**: 23–27.

GASCHEN, F.P., ADÉ-DAMILANO, M., GASCHEN, L., SEILER, G., WELLE, M., BORNAND-JAUNIN, V., GONIN-JMAA, D., NEIGER-AESCHBACHER, G. (1998b): Lethal peracute rhabdomyolysis associated with stress and general anesthesia in three dystrophin-deficient cats. Vet Pathol. **35**: 117–123.

HANSON, S.M., SMITH, M.O., WALKER, T.L., SHELTON, G.D. (1998): Juvenile-onset distal myopathy in Rottweiler dogs. J Vet Med. **12**: 103–108.

HICKFORD, F.H., JONES, B.R., GETHING, M.A., PACK, R., ALLEY, M.R. (1998): Congenital myotonia in related kittens. J Small Anim Pract. **39**, 281–285.

JEZYK, P.F. (1982): Hyperkalemic periodic paralysis in a dog. J Am Anim Hosp Assoc. **18**: 977–980.

JONES, B. (2000): Hypokalemic myopathy in cats. In BONAGURA, J.D. (ed): Kirk's Current Veterinary Therapy XIII. W.B. Saunders, Philadelphia, pp. 985–987.

MALIK, R., MEPSTEAD, K., YANG, F., HARPER, C. (1993): Hereditary myopathy of Devon Rex cats. J Small Anim Pract. **34**: 539–546.

MASON, K. (1987): A hereditary disease in Burmese cats manifested as an episodic weakness with head nodding and neck ventroflexion. J Am Anim Hosp Assoc. **24**: 147–151.

O'BRIEN, D.P., JOHNSON, G.C., LIU, L.A., GUO, L.T., ENGVALL, E., POWELL, H.C., SHELTON, G.D. (2001): Laminin alpha-2 (merosin)-deficient muscular dystrophy and demyelinating neuropathy in two cats. J Neurol Sci. **189**: 37–43.

PLATT, S.R. (2002): Neuromuscular complications in endocrine and metabolic disorders. Vet Clin North Am Small Anim Pract. **32**: 147–167.

PODELL, M., CHEN, E., SHELTON, G.D. (1998): Feline immunodeficiency virus associated myopathy in the adult cat. Muscle Nerve **21**: 1680–1685.

PODELL, M. (2002): Inflammatory Myopathies. Vet Clin North Am Small Anim Pract. **32**: 147–167.

RAND, J.S., EBERLE, B., SUTER, P.F. (1990): Hypokaliämische Myopathie bei drei Katzen. Kleintierpraxis. **35**: 265–272.

ROBINSON, R. (1992): "Spasticity" in the Devon Rex cat. Vet Rec. **130**: 302.

SHELTON, G.D., ENGVALL, E. (2002): Muscular dystrophies and other inherited myopathies. Vet Clin North Am Small Anim Pract. **32**: 147–167.

TOLL, J., COOPER, B., ALTSCHUL, M. (1998): Congenital myotonia in two domestic cats. J Vet Intern Med. **12**: 116–119.

VITE, C.H. (2002): Myotonia and disorders of altered muscle cell membrane excitability. Vet Clin North Am Small Anim Pract. **32**: 169–187.

13

14   Spinal Cord

Andrea Tipold
Marco Bernardini
Marion Kornberg

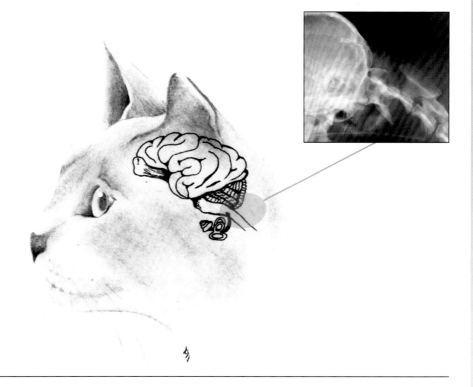

14

The spinal cord lies in the vertebral canal and extends from the medulla oblongata to the cauda equina (see Fig. 18.1). It consists of both grey matter which contains the different nerve cells and the centres of reflex activity, and white matter in which the long ascending and descending tracts run. These tracts form the connection between the periphery and the brain, and are made up of fibres which join the individual segments of the spinal cord together.

The clinical signs of diseases of the spinal cord depend on the localisation of the lesion (see Chap. 1.4.8). In lesions of the cervical spinal cord, gait disturbances which affect all four limbs can be seen (generalised ataxia, tetraparesis, tetraplegia, hemiparesis, hemiplegia). In lesions caudal to the cervical enlargement, the gait disturbances are often limited to the hindlegs (ataxia, paraparesis, paraplegia). In addition, diseases of the spinal cord are subdivided into compressive and non compressive diseases.

The determination of prognosis in spinal disease is done not only according to the cause of the lesion, but also the clinical symptoms (localisation and extent of tissue damage). Generally, it can be said that a lesion in the area of the grey matter in either spinal cord enlargement (cervical [C6–T2] or lumbar [L4–S3]) has a worse prognosis than a lesion that lies outside of these areas. This means that the prognosis tends to be more guarded with paralysis and loss of reflexes than with par-alysis and intact reflexes. Pain sensation is also used for determining the prognosis: if no pain sensation (nociception) is present then the prognosis is guarded to poor. Exceptions include acute compressive lesions that are associated with a high degree of oedema. After suitable therapeutic measures and treatment of the oedema, the pain sensation may return.

Individual spinal cord diseases are listed in Tables 14.1 and 14.2 according to their main symptoms (paraparesis / tetraparesis or paraplegia / tetraplegia) and according to the type of lesion (compressive or non-compressive).

Diseases of the spinal cord are, in principle, classified according to the scheme given in Fig. 14.1. After localisation of the lesion to the spine and / or spinal cord, special diagnostic investigations are necessary to characterise the nature of the lesion more accurately. These initially include imaging techniques. Some changes can be seen on a plain radiograph (e.g. fractures / luxations, changes in vertebral structure, malformations; see also Chap 6). If the diagnosis cannot be attained with this technique or the extent of the spinal cord disease must be evaluated in more detail, then the diagnostic investigation can be expanded.

Table 14.1: Diseases of the spinal cord: main symptom paraparesis

		Compressive lesions	Non-compressive lesions		Compressive lesions	Non-compressive lesions
V		■ Haemorrhage (dog/cat)	■ Spinal cord infarct (dog/cat) (fibrocartilaginous emboli) ■ Arteritis (dog) ■ Haematomyelia (dog) ■ Ischemic myopathy (dog/cat) (aortic thrombus)	**A**	■ Malformation of the vertebrae – hemivertebrae, wedge-shaped and fused vertebrae (dog/cat) ■ Congenital exostoses/osteo-chondromatosis (dog/cat) ■ Meningeal cysts/arachnoid cysts (dog) ■ Sacrococcygeal dysgenesis (cat)	■ Hydromyelia/syringomyelia/myelodysplasia (dog/cat) ■ Dermoid sinus (dog) ■ Spina bifida (dog/cat)
I		■ Discospondylitis (dog/cat)	■ Distemper (dog) ■ Central European tick encephalitis (dog) ■ Rabies (dog/cat) ■ Feline infectious peritonitis (cat) ■ Borna disease (cat) ■ Bacterial myelitis/abscess (dog/cat) ■ Ehrlichiosis (dog) ■ Protozoal myelitis (dog/cat) ■ Larva migrans/filaria (dog/cat) ■ Mycotic myelitis (dog/cat) ■ Prototothecosis (dog/cat) ■ Sterile purulent meningitis-arteritis (dog) ■ Granulomatous meningoence-phalomyelitis (dog) ■ Feline poliomyelitis (cat)	**M** **N**	■ Hypervitaminosis A (cat) ■ Intramedullary (dog/cat): glioma, ependymoma ■ Intradural-extramedullary (dog/cat): meningioma, nerve root tumour (schwannoma, neuro-fibroma), nephroblastoma ■ Extradural (dog/cat): osteosarcoma, fibro-sarcoma, chondrosarcoma, haemangiosarcoma, metastases ■ Multiple localisations (dog/cat): metastases, lymphoma, histiocytosis, myeloma	 ■ Intramedullary (dog/cat): lymphoma
T		■ Fracture (dog/cat) ■ Luxation/subluxation (dog/cat) ■ Traumatic intervertebral disc herniation (dog/cat) ■ Haemorrhage (dog/cat)	■ Contusion (dog/cat) ■ Laceration (dog/cat) ■ Haemorrhagic myelomalacia (dog/cat)	**D**	■ Disc disease (dog/cat) ■ Spondylosis deformans (dog) ■ Dural ossification (dog) ■ Multiple cartilaginous exostoses (dog)	■ Degenerative myelopathy (dog) ■ Afghan myelopathy (dog) ■ Neuronopathy (dog) ■ Stockard's paralysis (dog)

14

Investigation of CSF helps to determine whether there is a primary inflammatory disease or a secondary inflammatory reaction (tumour, acute disc disease). With the aid of CT, MRI and myelography or myelo-CT, the lesion can be characterised in the majority of cases. Should this not be the case or if the results are equivocal, a biopsy can provide further information. In addition, by using a process of elimination to exclude other diseases, the diagnosis may have to be left as tentative (e.g., spinal cord infarct, degenerative spinal cord diseases).

14.1 Spinal cord diseases

In the following sections, the most common diseases of the spinal cord are described. To prevent repetition, the resulting clinical signs of paraparesis/tetraparesis and paraplegia/tetraplegia are considered together.

14.1.1 Vascular diseases

14.1.1.1 Spinal cord infarcts (fibrocartilaginous emboli)

Occurrence: Common.

Table 14.2: Diseases of the spinal cord: main symptom tetraparesis

	Compressive lesions	Non-compressive lesions		Compressive lesions	Non-compressive lesions
V	■ Haemorrhage (dog/cat)	■ Spinal cord infarct (dog/cat) (fibrocartilaginous emboli) ■ Arteritis (dog) ■ Haematomyelia (dog)	**M** **N**	■ Hypervitaminosis A (cat) ■ Intradural-extramedullary (dog/cat): meningioma, nerve root tumour (schwannoma, neuro-fibroma), nephroblastoma ■ Extradural (dog/cat): osteosarcoma, fibrosarcoma, chondrosarcoma, haemangiosarcoma, metastases ■ Multiple localisations (dog/cat): metastases, lymphoma, histiocytosis, myeloma	
I	■ Discospondylitis (dog/cat)	■ Distemper (dog) ■ Central European tick encephalitis (dog) ■ Rabies (dog/cat) ■ Feline infectious peritonitis (cat) ■ Borna disease (cat) ■ Bacterial myelitis/abscess (dog/cat) ■ Ehrlichiosis (dog) ■ Protozoal myelitis (dog/cat) ■ Larva migrans/filaria (dog/cat) ■ Mycotic myelitis (dog/cat) ■ Prototheocis (dog/cat) ■ Granulomatous meningoence-phalomyelitis (dog) ■ Feline poliomyelitis (cat)			
			D	■ Disc disease (dog/cat) ■ Cervical malformation/malarticulation (dog) ■ Spondylosis deformans (dog) ■ Calcinosis circumscripta (dog)	■ Hereditary ataxia (Fox Terrier, Jack Russell Terrier) ■ Afghan myelopathy (dog) ■ Hound ataxia (dog) ■ Demyelinating myelopathy (dog) ■ Leukoencephalomyelopathy (Rottweiler) ■ Necrotising myelopathy (Kooiker) ■ Axonopathy (dog) ■ Progressive degeneration (Ibizan Hound) ■ Globoid cell leukodystrophy (dog/cat) ■ Mucopolysaccharidosis (dog/cat) ■ Spinal muscular dystrophy (dog)
T	■ Fracture (dog/cat) ■ Luxation/subluxation (dog/cat) ■ Traumatic intervertebral disc herniation (dog/cat) ■ Haemorrhage (dog/cat)	■ Contusion (dog/cat) ■ Laceration (dog/cat) ■ Haemorrhagic myelomalacia (dog/cat)			■ Dalmatian leukodystrophy (dog) ■ Alexander's disease (dog) ■ Hypomyelogenesis (dog/cat) ■ Primary spinal cord degeneration (cat) ■ Spongiform degeneration (dog/cat) ■ Motor neuron disease (dog/cat)
A	■ Cervical malformation/malarticulation (dog) ■ Atlanto-axial subluxation (dog/cat) ■ Occipital dysplasia (dog) ■ Malformation of the vertebrae (dog/cat) ■ Meningeal cysts/arachnoid cysts (dog)	■ Hydromyelia/syringomyelia/myelodysplasia (dog/cat) ■ Dermoid sinus (dog) ■ Spina bifida (dog/cat)			

14

Aetiology: Nucleus pulposus material from the disc leads to obstruction of the spinal vessels and subsequent anaemic infarction of the grey and white matter in the affected spinal cord segment(s). The mechanism by which disc material enters the vessels has not been fully elucidated.

Clinical: Every dog breed and every age group can be affected. Most commonly, however, fibrocartilaginous emboli occur in adult dogs (5, 35). Cats can also be affected, but more rarely than dogs. The clinical signs develop acutely or peracutely. The infarcts are often in the lumbar or cervical enlargement but can occur at any point within the spinal cord (Fig. 14.2). The clinical signs are often lateralised but can be bilateral.

Diagnosis: The diagnosis is made by a process of elimination and diagnostic imaging. With the aid of myelography, compressive lesions can be excluded. Swelling of the spinal cord may be seen in acute cases of infarction. In some cases, oedema can be seen on MRI images (see Fig. 6.32).

Therapy: Glucocorticoids such as methylprednisolone (30 mg/kg) or dexamethasone (2 mg/kg) can be given in the first hours of the disease but there is no proof that this therapy is effective. Long-term therapy with glucocorticoids is definitely not indicated. The most important adjunct therapies include control of the bladder and its emptying, and physiotherapy.

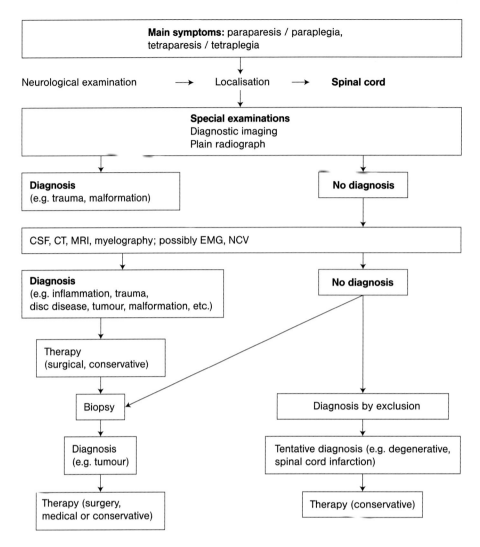

Fig. 14.1
Outline of the approach to patients with spinal lesions.

Prognosis: The prognosis depends on the clinical signs. If localisation is in the thoracolumbar region and if pain sensation is retained, then the prognosis is good to guarded. If the infarct affects an intumescence and pain sensation is absent, the prognosis is poor. Usually in these latter cases, the affected limb remains paralysed.

14.1.1.2 Spinal cord haemorrhage

Occurrence: Rare.

Aetiology: Haemorrhage is usually secondary to a primary disease process (malformation of blood vessels, intoxication, disseminated intravascular coagulopathies, trauma, arteriitis, explosive disc prolapse).

Clinical: The clinical signs start acutely. A progression of the symptoms cranially and caudally is possible.

Diagnosis: Determination of the primary disease using blood tests (clotting, thrombocytes), investigation of the CSF (possibly xanthochromia, pleocytosis with an arteriitis), and imaging techniques.

Therapy: Therapy of the primary disease.

Prognosis: The prognosis depends on the clinical deficits, the extent of haemorrhage, and the primary disease. It is poor with explosive disc prolapse and ascending haemorrhagic myelomalacia; good to guarded with trauma and arteriitis.

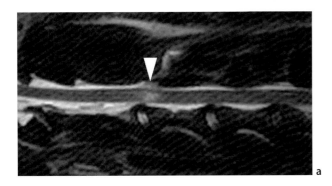
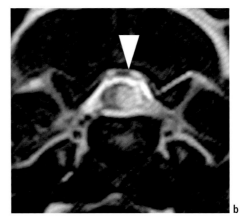

Fig. 14.2a, b
Spinal cord infarct in a ten-year-old Appenzeller Cattle Dog with severe hemiparesis. (a) Sagittal T2w sequence: hyperintense intramedullary lesion in the spinal cord segment dorsal to the cranial endplate of C3. (b) In the transverse T2w section, there is mild asymmetrical swelling with a focal, sharply demarcated zone of increased signal intensity on the left side of the spinal cord. The area dorsal to the affected segment is most probably a vein (interarcualis vein; arrowhead). (Pictures: Johann Lang, Berne.)

14.1.2 Inflammatory changes

14.1.2.1 Discospondylitis

Occurrence: Rare.

Aetiology: Discospondylitis usually develops due to bacterial infection after iatrogenic trauma (e.g. curettage of a disc), a migrating foreign body, penetrating trauma, paravertebral injection and septic emboli that originate from a primary focus. The primary focus of infection often cannot be found; it can reside in the urogenital or respiratory tract, skin, gingiva or heart valves. The following bacteria have been more frequently reported: *Staphylococcus aureus* or *intermedius*, *Brucella canis*, *Nocardia* and *Streptococcus canis*. Fungi can be responsible for discospondylitis (e.g. *Aspergillus* spp.).

Clinical: This disease occurs in young to adult animals in larger breeds of dog; it very rarely affects cats. In principle every intervertebral disc can be affected. The clinical symptoms are variable and range from mild discomfort over the spine to stiffness and severe pain, to severe paresis or even paralysis – depending on the extent of the concurrent compression of the spinal cord. In some animals, depression, anorexia and increased body temperature are evident.

Diagnosis: Radiography: initially concentric lysis can be seen on the neighbouring endplates of the vertebrae. Chronic forms are characterised by varying degrees of osteolysis, osteogenesis, sclerosis, shortened vertebral bodies and narrowed intervertebral spaces (see Fig. 6.33). Bone proliferation in the ventral area of the vertebral body can lead to the formation of "bridges". Discospondylitis can affect more than one disc space. The most commonly affected sites include the caudal cervical, thoracolumbar and lumbosacral segments of the spine. Radiological changes are not always evident at the start of clinical signs; it may be 7 to 10 days for these to become apparent. In order to ensure that the therapy is suitable, an attempt should be made to isolate the causative bacteria. Blood and urine cultures can be positive in 40–45% of all cases. Percutaneous aspiration of the infected disc can be attempted in the presence of fluoroscopy.

Therapy: Antibiotics should be given for at least 2 to 4 months. Until it is proven otherwise, the discospondylitis is treated as if it is due to a staphylococcal infection. Cephalosporins have been successfully used in the therapy of small animals (e.g. cephalexin 22 mg/kg, PO, BID). If bacterial culture and sensitivity reveals a different bacterial cause then the antibiotic should be changed. Analgesics are sensible if there is severe pain. In some cases – with a lack of response to conservative therapy – surgical curettage of the disc is recommended. If there are severe neurological deficits (paresis, paralysis) and spinal cord compression, then surgical decompression and stabilisation is indicated. With improvement and regular clinical and radiological monitoring, stabilisation and then improvement of the osteolysis is seen. The step-wise replacement of the disc by new bone tissue can lead to vertebral fusion.

Prognosis: The prognosis in the majority of cases is favourable when early and aggressive therapy is used. The prognosis is guarded in chronic disease and where there is severe involvement of the spinal cord.

14

14.1.2.2 Myelitis

Occurrence: Common.

Aetiology: Inflammatory processes of the CNS are predominantly multifocal, though they may be limited to the spinal cord. As with intracranial diseases, inflammation of the spinal cord can be induced by viral, bacterial and parasitic infections. Fungal infections are rare. Bacterial infections are usually a consequence of bite injuries or other types of perforating trauma. In addition to the inflammatory diseases of known aetiology in the spinal canal, there are many with unknown causes. These latter diseases include steroid-responsive meningitis-arteritis (8), which may be one of the most commonly seen inflammatory diseases of the CNS, and granulomatous meningoencephalitis (12, 69).

Diagnosis: General clinical examination: extraneural symptoms can be found in approx. 50% of the cases. CBC: e.g. lymphopaenia with distemper; leukocytosis with sterile purulent meningitis-arteritis. CSF: this often reveals the presence of an inflammatory reaction (pleocytosis, increased protein, increased IgG).

Therapy: There is at present no specific therapy available for viral infections; these are treated purely symptomatically. Bacterial infections are treated with antibiotics. Protozoal infections are treated with a combination of trimethoprim / sulfadiazine (dog and cat: 15–30 mg/kg BID) and/or clindamycin (dog and cat: 10–20 mg/kg BID) for at least 14 days. To prevent bone marrow suppression, folic acid (5 mg, PO, SID) or brewer's yeast (100 mg/kg, PO, SID) should be given. The treatment of inflammatory diseases of unknown aetiology consists of anti-inflammatory (glucocorticosteroid) or immunosuppressive (e.g. azathioprine, cytosine) drugs.

Prognosis: Dependent on the primary disease (favourable to poor).

14.1.2.3 Feline poliomyelitis

Occurrence: Rare.

Aetiology: This disease occurs sporadically in Europe and North America without any breed, age or sex predisposition. It can occur in combination with encephalitis or purely as a disease of the spinal cord. The aetiology is unknown; a virus is most likely. Whether it is caused by the Borna virus and is equivalent to Staggering disease or it is a disease in its own right, remains to be elucidated.

Clinical: The clinical signs begin insidiously and progress slowly over weeks to months. In many cases, the animals stabilise and some cats can recover. The main symptoms can be explained by the poliomyelitis and manifest as spinal cord lesions affecting the LMNS. Muscle atrophy can be observed fairly early on in the disease. Less commonly, the inflammation spreads throughout the brain leading to seizures, cerebellar signs and abnormalities of the pupils.

Diagnosis: The diagnosis is based on the clinical symptoms, its insidious progressive course, and the obvious muscle atrophy. A monocytic pleocytosis has been observed in the CSF. Other common cat diseases such as FeLV, FIV or FIP must be excluded. Radiography of the spine including myelography is unremarkable (see Fig. 6.35). With the aid of this type of information, a tentative diagnosis can be made.

Therapy: Supportive care; physiotherapy.

Prognosis: Guarded. The disease process stabilises in some cats, while others can recover.

14.1.2.4 Steroid-responsive meningitis-arteriitis (SRMA)

Occurrence: Common in dogs; very rare in cats

Aetiology: Unknown. An exogenous stimulus has been presumed due to the results of epidemiological studies (infectious agents, toxins, etc.). Pathogenetically, immune-mediated changes are most probable as an excessive intrathecal and systemic IgA production appears to play a key role (8).

Clinical: The dogs are presented mainly because of relapsing pain and fever attacks. Two forms can be differentiated because of their differing clinical examination results and changes in the CSF. The classical form is characterised by stiffness of the head and neck, pain and increased body temperature. In the second, more protracted atypical form, the neurological examination reveals deficits indicative of a spinal cord disease or a multifocal lesion (74).

Diagnosis: Blood tests: in the acute form, leukocytosis, neutrophilia with a left shift and increased sedimentation rate have been seen. In the chronic form, blood tests are unremarkable. In the acute form, the CSF reveals a mild to moderate increase in protein and a severe neutrophilic pleocytosis with many thousands of cells/μl. In the chronic form, CSF can be normal or exhibit a mild pleocytosis with a mixed or monocytic population. As there are no clearly interpretable results to be found in the CSF in the chronic form, a process of elimination must be used to exclude other spinal cord diseases (radiography, possibly myelography, CT, MRI). Diagnostic for this form of the disease is the investigation of serum and CSF for IgA: an increase in IgA in both is characteristic for SMRA. An increase in intrathecal IgA alone, without systemic increase, is uncharacteristic and occurs with other types of inflammatory disease in the CNS (encephalomyelitis, reaction to tumour tissue).

Therapy: Prednisolone: long-term therapy for approx. 6 months. The dosage must be individually adjusted via continual monitoring. When the clinical examination is unremarkable and if repeated, the CSF normal, the dosage can be halved. With a pathological CSF result, the prednisolone dose must be continued or even increased as there is danger of a relapse; however, interpretation of the CSF to determine active disease vs. residual or "healing" phase inflammation can be difficult. The oral prednisolone dosage starts at 4 mg/kg SID for 1 to 2 days and is reduced step-wise by half each time (approx. 1 week of 2 mg/kg SID; then 1 mg/kg SID for 2 to 4 weeks). Combination with an immunosuppressive drug is possible if there are frequent relapses or the patient responds poorly to prednisolone alone. Antibiotics can be given at the start until a negative bacteriological investigation of the CSF is confirmed. Bacterial meningitis is, however, very rare in the dog. With prolonged glucocorticosteroid therapy, prophylactic treatment to prevent gastrointestinal ulceration should be given, too.

Prognosis: The prognosis can be good to guarded. With frequent relapses, therapy is more complicated and lengthy. The prognosis is favourable, when the animal is young and the treatment is started early enough.

14.1.3 Traumatic diseases

Occurrence: Common in dogs and cats.

Aetiology: Usually, trauma in the region of the spine and/or spinal cord is due to traffic accidents, falls, and fights with other animals. The clinical picture depends not only on the initial trauma, but also on secondary damage which may develop while the body tries to compensate for the deficit (29, 32). The spinal cord is surrounded and protected by a stable bony canal; therefore, a strong force is required to damage it. In severe accidents, multiple areas of the spinal column can be traumatised as can other parts of the body. Even with clear neurological symptoms, a thorough clinical examination of the other organs systems must be done in conjunction with the neurological examination. The reasons for spinal cord injury can include the following: vertebral fracture, luxation or prolapsed disc. These abnormalities may lead to spinal cord oedema and/or intramedullary, epidural or subdural haemorrhage.

The degree of cord damage depends on three factors:
1. Duration of compression
2. Degree of compression and
3. Speed and force of cord concussion.

Damage to the spinal cord can be structural or functional. In the former case, the lesion is irreversible. In the latter, there are often microcirculation changes resulting in haemorrhage or ischemia. The neurological signs may improve after a few hours, or there may be permanent functional damage to the nervous tissue. Injury to the grey matter is always more serious than that to the white matter (an axon can recover). There is a larger vascular network in the grey matter, so haemorrhage tends to be more likely.

Clinical: The first therapeutic measure is focussed on immobilisation of the patient. This can be done mechanically, in that the animal is fixed on a table or flat board, or by using medication (for example, butorphanol or opioids; see Chap. 9.3). The integrity of the bladder, the haematocrit and the function of the other organs such as liver, spleen and kidneys should be assessed. Before providing sedation, a short neurological examination should be performed, but further spinal damage must be avoided whilst undertaking this.

If the trauma is purely spinal, then the animal's consciousness will remain normal. The body posture can be normal or abnormal. A luxation or fracture can be manifested by kyphosis. Gait abnormalities can range from a slight ataxia and/or paresis to complete inability to move.

A so-called **Schiff-Sherrington phenomenon** may be observed with injuries which involve acute concussion of the spinal cord between the two spinal cord enlargements (i.e., T3–L3 injury) (Fig. 14.3). This phenomenon is an exception in neurology as the clinical symptoms, which include hyperextension of the forelimbs or opisthotonus, occur with a lesion which lies caudal to the forelimbs. In addition to hyperextension of the forelimbs, there is paralysis of the hindlimbs. A Schiff-Sherrington phenomenon indicates the presence of a very severe lesion, though prognostically this is not always unfavourable. It should not be confused with other rigid body positions due to pain, cervical spinal cord disease or cerebral/cerebellar injury. The anatomical functional basis of this phenomenon lies with the so-called border cells, whose axons are atypical ascending tracts of the UMNS. The cell bodies of these cells reside laterally in the grey matter of the lumbar cord (L1–L7) between the ventral and intermediate horns. Their axons cross over and ascend up the spinal cord in the contralateral fasciculus proprius and form synapses with the LMNs of the extensors in the forelimbs. This mechanism is important in regulating the gait. As the effect of the border cells is inhibitory, a lesion in this system causes increased activity of the extensors. Although an investigation is difficult in a patient exhibiting this phenomenon, the positioning and placement reactions of the forelimbs are not changed as the proprioceptive tracts are not involved.

14

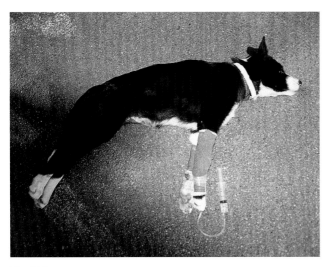

Fig. 14.3
Two-year-old female dog after a car accident. Schiff-Sherington characterised by increased extensor tone in all four limbs as well as lateral recumbency. The dog had massive compression of the thoracolumbar spinal cord with luxation of two neighbouring vertebrae, T12 and T13.

14

The existence of "**spinal shock**" in dogs and cat is controversial. It is characterised by a flaccid paresis of the limbs subsequent to spinal cord trauma that involves the UMNS. This shock is normally only transient, though it may have a variable duration.

Diagnosis: The diagnosis is achieved radiographically. It is sensible to take lateral views of the whole spine and not just focus on the site of a known lesion. Ventrodorsal views are useful, but the value of an additional view needs to be considered in terms of whether it will provide more information or induce more damage due to the manipulation of the animal necessary for this view. Anaesthetised animals should be moved very carefully indeed, so that further damage does not occur due to a drug-induced reduction of muscle tone which can make lesions more unstable. These animals must be additionally physically stabilised before being manipulated. The extent of spinal cord compression can be judged using myelography. However, excessive flexion of the spine during lumbar injection of contrast agent should be avoided. Other investigation methods include CT and MRI. A CT investigation following injection of contrast in the subarachnoid space (myelo-CT) is useful.

Therapy: Immediate treatment with methylprednisolone sodium succinate (MPSS) has been described but as yet is unproven in veterinary medicine and is controversial (see Chap. 9.2.4.3). Its effect may depend on the time between the injury and its administration. An initial dosage of 30 mg/kg, IV, should be given (at time zero), followed by a bolus of 15 mg/kg, IV, two hours later. Another bolus of

15 mg/kg, IV, is given four hours later (six hours after time zero). This treatment can be continued over the next 24 to 48 hours with 15mg/kg IV q 6 hrs. A better alternative, which requires hospitalisation of the patient, is constant infusion of 5.4 mg/kg/h, IV, over 12 to 24 hours. If more than 8 hours have passed since the trauma, therapy with MPSS is contraindicated. The most frequent side-effects with MPSS are melaena, diarrhoea, vomiting and haematemesis. Usually these side-effects are not severe and but may cause prolongation of the convalescence period. The prophylactic use of ranitidine or cimetidine and/or sucralfate has been recommended for the prevention of gastrointestinal ulceration but the benefits remain unsubstantiated. The use of omeprazole and misoprostol, both of which are extremely expensive, has also been described (49, 51, 52, 59, 60).

In the majority of cases of spinal cord injury, the spinal column needs to be surgically stabilised (see Chap. 10.3). Two types of operation are possible: internal or external stabilisation. With internal fixation, screws, Kirschner pins, plates and cement (polymethylacrylate) are used to stabilise the vertebral bodies. Decompression of the spinal cord via hemilaminectomy is obligatory. The disadvantages of surgery include the risks which are associated with an operation on the spine and the cost. External fixation is based on restraint using bandaging and cast materials. Aluminium, wood or plastic are moulded along the back, padded and fixed with bandaging material. The immobilisation achieved is relative and can be considered most effective in small dogs and cats with mild damage. The advantages of this method are its low cost and the lack of risks due to surgical manipulation.

Strict cage rest must be maintained following both of these treatment methods, though especially with external fixation. This is achieved by placing the animal in a small cage, although the patient should be carried out to defecate and urinate. The cage rest should last between 2 and 8 weeks, depending on the weight of the patient, the type of lesion and the method of stabilisation. Physiotherapy and other necessary adjunct treatments are considered in Chaps. 8 and 14.2.2.

Prognosis: The prognosis depends on the initial injury and the response of the patient to therapy. From a prognostic point of view, the presence of sensation caudal to the lesion is a favourable sign. The majority of animals which retain superficial sensation after a trauma have the potential for a good recovery. Lack of superficial sensation but intact nociception (deep pain) can infer a good prognosis, though a prolonged healing time should be expected. Lack of nociception for 24 to 48 hours after the trauma is associated with a poor prognosis.

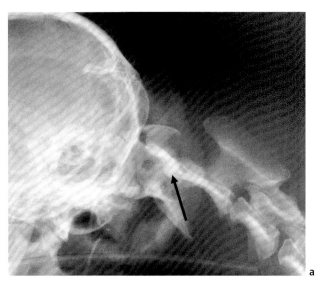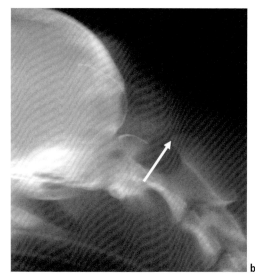

Fig. 14.4a, b
(a) Lateral view with rotated skull in a Yorkshire Terrier with atlanto-axial subluxation and (b) slice view of the same animal. C2 is subluxated cau-dodorsally; the space between the dorsal arch of C1 and the spinous process of C2 is enlarged. The stump-like dens of the axis points obliquely and dorsally into the middle of the vertebral canal (black arrow). Take note of the very thin and convex dorsal arch (white arrow). (Pictures: Johann Lang, Berne.)

14.1.4 Anomalies

14.1.4.1 Atlanto-axial subluxation (AASL)

Occurrence: Rare in dog. Extremely rare in cat.

Aetiology: There is no intervertebral disc between the atlas and the axis. The dens of the axis is connected to the occiput and the atlas by ligaments (transverse, apical, alar and atlanto-axial ligaments). The atlanto-axial joint can be congenitally malformed. The most common abnormality is an agenesis or hypoplasia of the dens, while the lack of one or more ligaments tends to be rare. In addition, the dens can be badly deformed. Of the acquired diseases affecting this area, a fracture of the dens is the most common; rupture of the transverse ligament is less frequent. In all these diseases, there is an AASL with secondary compression of the cervical spinal cord (75).

Clinical: The congenital disease usually occurs in toy breeds in the first year of life; rarely are large dog breeds and cats affected. The clinical symptoms are chronic progressive. The animal exhibits pain in the cervical region especially when it flexes its neck, and can demonstrate tetraparesis, ataxia and proprioceptive deficits in all limbs. Traumatically acquired disease has an acute start, and affects all breeds and ages. The clinical symptoms are much more dramatic: these patients are usually tetraplegic (1, 31).

Diagnosis: If there is a suspicion of AASL, then the examination should be done with great care to prevent further injury, which may even be fatal. Diagnostic radiographs of the cervical vertebrae are performed in the lateral view, and when possible in the conscious animal. The presence of a large distance between the lamina of the atlas and the cranial part of the spinous process of the axis or the lack of an angle between C1 and C2 may be recognised. To identify the absence of or a fracture of the dens, it is necessary to take a VD radiograph with the animal's mouth held open. However, putting the animal in this position is dangerous; therefore a slightly oblique lateral view is preferable (Figs. 6.11 and 14.4).

Therapy: Treatment is surgical as medication can only result in partial and temporary improvement. In the case of traumatic AASL, the standard surgical methods of treating spinal cord trauma can be recommended. The animal should be externally fixated until the time of surgery. There are different techniques available for surgical stabilisation. The one most commonly used is the transarticular implantation of screws or Kirschner pins via a ventral approach (see Chap. 10.3). An alternative is dorsal cerclage between the lamina of the atlas and the spinous process of the axis (33, 47, 70, 73).

Prognosis: The prognosis is favourable if the operation is undertaken early with genetic malformations causing only mild clinical signs. The prognosis of traumatic AASL tends to be more guarded, depending on the extent of spinal cord damage.

14

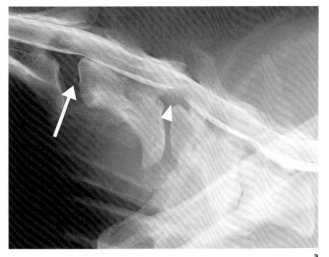 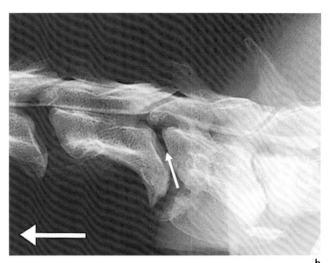

a
b

Fig. 14.5a, b
Disc herniation and cervical spondylomyelopathy in a ten-year-old Borzoi. Myelography (a) without and (b) with traction of the cervical spine (lower arrow shows direction of traction placed on spine). Collapsed intervertebral space C6–C7 with sclerosis of the endplates and the spongiosa of the vertebral bodies, in addition to spondylosis. The intervertebral space C5–C6 is narrowed and shows ventral spondylosis. The disc C4–C5 has a focus of mineralisation (arrow). The spinal cord compression in this dog was due to mineralised and extruded disc material from C5–C6. Note the forking of the ventral contrast column (arrowhead). There is practically no reduction of the compression under traction and only minimal widening of the collapsed intervertebral space C6–C7.

14.1.4.2 Cervical malformation/malarticulation: Caudal cervical spondylomyelopathy

Occurrence: Common.

Aetiology: Caudal cervical spondylomyelopathy (CCSM) is a disease which occurs due to an anomaly of the cervical vertebrae (C3–C7) and/or their joint structures (intervertebral discs or ligaments). Progressive stenosis of the vertebral canal develops with an associated progressive compressive myelopathy. This disease has been described for many years and has been given different names such as cervical spondylopathy, caudal cervical spondylopathy, malformation/malarticulation of the cervical vertebrae, cervical vertebral instability, cervical vertebral stenotic myelopathy, etc.

Its most well-known name is "Wobbler" due to the typical swaying gait of the affected animals (31, 45, 66).

The following problems are present with this disease:
- Changes in the shape or size of the vertebral canal (C4–C7)
- Changes in the dimensions, size and/or position of the articular processes
- Hyperostosis of the joint surfaces
- Prolapse of the intervertebral disc
- Hypertrophy of the dorsal longitudinal ligament
- Hypertrophy of the yellow ligament

CCSM has a multifactoral aetiology which probably includes rapid growth due to qualitatively and quantitatively excessive nutrition, genetic predisposition and/or trauma.

Clinical: CCSM has been described in a relatively large number of breeds: Basset, Bernese Mountain Dog, Bobtail, Borzoi, Chow Chow, English Setter, Fox Terrier, German Shepherd, Giant Schnauzer, Golden Retriever, Pyrenean Mountain Dog, Rhodesian Ridgeback, Rottweiler, Weimaraner, etc. The most commonly affected breeds are, however, the Great Dane and the Doberman. The first signs are seen within the first and second year of life in the Great Dane and after about 3 years in the Doberman. It appears that males are more commonly affected than females. The first clinical symptom is ataxia of the hindlimbs: the animal walks with excessively broad strides and tends to trot. Shortly afterwards, a spastic paresis develops that makes the ataxia appear more pronounced. At the same time, proprioceptive deficits are noted. The clinical signs become worse with time and the forelimbs become involved in the gait disturbance. The dog exhibits dragging of the toes with abnormal wearing of the claws. Spastic paresis of the forelimbs is often observed in the Great Dane, as the compression is due to changes in the shape of the vertebral canal at the level of C4. Hypermetria has been seen in the Doberman: the dog only makes short strides with the forelimbs that are not in unison with the long strides of the hindlegs as the compression is in the caudal region of the cervical spine.

14

With worsening of the disease, the cervical muscles become stiff as the animal tries to stabilise this region. The head is held down, the neck is bent and the animal refuses to move its neck. The dog has difficulty in standing up and falls over if it tries to lift its leg. Mating is impossible and disturbances in micturition can occur. Pain can be present, but not necessarily so. The spinal reflexes are normal in the forelimbs or reduced; in the hindlimbs they are normal or increased. The more caudal the compression, the more severe the muscle atrophy in the forelimbs, especially around the shoulder (supraspinatus and infraspinatus muscles). Horner's syndrome may be present but is rare.

Diagnosis: The diagnosis is obtained using imaging techniques (radiography, myelography, CT, MRI) (Fig. 14.5).

Plain radiograph:
- Changes in the dimensions and shape of the vertebral body and intervertebral space.
- Changes in the shape of the joint surfaces.
- Stenosis of the vertebral canal.
- Dislocation of a vertebra (subluxation).

Many variations found on a plain radiograph have no clinical relevance. For an exact interpretation, one should always perform myelography (Fig. 14.6). The standard views can reveal ventral compression caused by disc prolapse (single or multiple) or by hypertrophy of the dorsal longitudinal ligament. They can also reveal dorsal compression due to hypertrophy of the yellow ligament or a dorsolateral compression due to hyperostosis of the facet joints. The degree of compression also depends on the posture of the neck. Traction worsens the situation, while bending makes the compression less pronounced. The ventroflexion which the patients spontaneously adopt is an instinctive change in posture, so that the most comfortable position is attained. The spinal cord compression can be static (unchanged with changes in position of the neck) or dynamic. This can be determined by using stress views in which lateral radiographs are obtained with the neck extended, flexed and under traction.

Therapy: It is difficult to offer a definitive treatment for CCSM as it involves an inherited factor. The earlier the disease is recognised, the quicker one can react and try to slow down its evolution. In dogs with mild clinical deficits, cage rest and analgesics can be associated with an improvement. With normal activity, however, there is usually a worsening of the clinical signs which is why every movement that puts a strain on the cervical spine should be avoided. The Doberman is often trained as a guard dog which may be associated with unsuitable movements. Traction on a collar can be damaging and so a chest harness should be used. The dog should be prevented, as far as possible, from jumping too much or making abrupt movements. With dynamic compressions, adherence to these rules with early recognition of the disease significantly reduces its development.

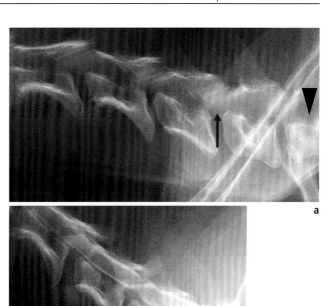

a

b

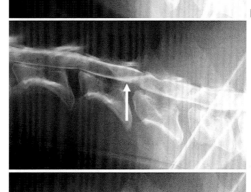

c

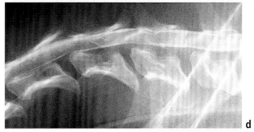

d

Fig. 14.6a–d
Myelography. Cervical spondylomyelopathy in a Doberman with ataxia and tetraparesis. The vertebrae C5–C7 are deformed and slightly subluxated dorsally; the vertebral canal is stenosed. (a) The intervertebral space C5–C6 is obviously narrowed; the one between C6–C7 is widened dorsally, giving it a wedge-like shape (arrow). Dural mineralisation in the cervicothoracic area (arrowhead). (b–d) The myelograms reveal a dynamic ventral compression of the spinal cord (arrow), which was almost completely reduced by ventroflexion (d) and traction (not shown). (Pictures: Johann Lang, Berne.)

14

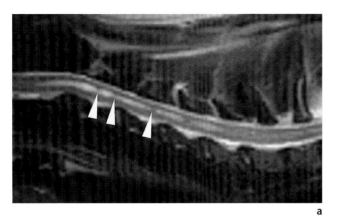

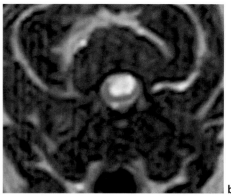

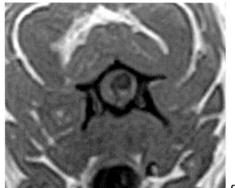

Fig. 14.7a–c
Sagittal T2w (a) and transverse T2w (b) and T1w (c) sequences of extensive syringohydromyelia in a Cavalier King Charles Spaniel. On the T2w sequences, the syringohydromyelia is shown as a hyperintense area in the central canal which is septated in the neck region (arrowheads). On the T1w sequence, by comparison, it is hypointense, enabling differentiated imaging of the central canal and the syrinx. (Pictures: Johann Lang, Berne.)

Often the clinical signs are so obvious and severe that surgery cannot be avoided. Surgery consists of removing a static compression and stabilising a dynamic compression. The choice of technique depends on the type of compression (static or dynamic), its localisation (dorsal or ventral), and the extent (one or more sites) of the lesion. Ventral decompression, stabilisation using transvertebral screws, distraction and fusion, the use of screws and polymethylacrylate and continuous dorsal laminectomy have all been described (see Chap. 10.3). The postoperative period is very difficult especially for animals which cannot stand. All the problems that can occur in a tetraplegic animal are exacerbated with increasing size of the patient. They can be so severe that they negate the benefit of an operation. The owner must be informed of this at the time of diagnosis (14).

Prognosis: The prognosis is guarded. It depends on the degree and reversibility of the spinal changes, their distribution, the severity of the anatomical changes, the duration of the compression, and the success of the decompression and/or stabilisation. A typical complication is the so-called domino effect: this is compression of the neighbouring intervertebral spaces secondary to the operation. Other complications are induced by postoperative mistakes in handling, which usually are due to the size of the animal.

14.1.4.3 Dermoid sinus

Occurrence: Rare: inherited in Rhodesian Ridgeback and crosses of this breed; reported in Boxer, Shi Tzu, Springer Spaniel and Yorkshire Terrier (19, 57, 67). Very rare in the cat.

Aetiology: A disturbance in neural crest development; longitudinal sinus lined with hair and glands in the region of the dorsal midline extending cranially or caudally from the vertebra to the spinous process; there can be communication with the dura.

Clinical: The sinus can be palpable in the skin. Neurological symptoms are possible, may be complicated by infections, and depend on the localisation.

Diagnosis: Clinical symptoms, fistulography, myelography, CT, MRI.

Therapy: Surgery; antibiotics.

Prognosis: Guarded.

14

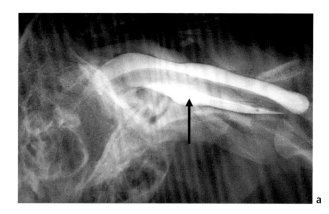
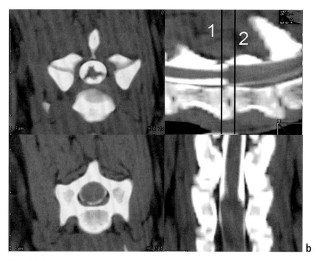
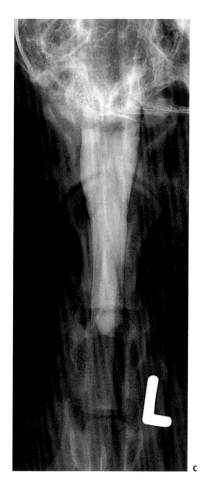

Fig. 14.8a–c

Myelography and CT of a sub-(intra-)arachnoid cyst in a Labrador Retriever. (a, c) The myelograms reveal a severely dilated subarachnoid space and compression of the spinal cord at the transition between C2 and C3 (arrow). (b) CT of an intra-arachnoid cyst at the level of C5: massive dilatation of the subarachnoid space with compression of the spinal cord from all sides, and a deformed spinal cord (top left) at the level of Section 1 in the sagittal reconstruction. Immediately caudal to the cyst at the level of Section 2, the spinal cord is very broad with a narrow subarachnoid space (bottom left). The ventrolateral filling defects are caused by the nerve roots. Both reconstruction levels show identical conditions. (Pictures: Johann Lang, Berne.)

14

14.1.4.4 Myelodysplasia / Spinal dysplasia / Spinal dysraphism

Occurrence: Rare; described in Cavalier King Charles Spaniel, Dalmatian, Rottweiler, Weimaraner, and in most cat breeds.

Aetiology: Myelodysplasia is a general term for a number of malformations of the spinal cord. Disturbances of neural crest development can occur as **hydromyelia** (local dilatation of the central canal in the spinal cord), **syringomyelia** (cavity formation in the grey matter of the spinal cord), or in the form of other malformations such as doubling of or lack of the central canal. This disease is called "spinal dysraphism" in the Weimaraner and is presumably inheritable. It occurs particularly in the thoracic or lumbar spine, rarely in the cervical (7, 68).

Clinical: Animals with this disease become clinical between the sixth and eighth week of life due to their broad-legged stance and bunny hopping – the hindlimbs always move at the same time; the spinal reflexes are normal. This form of malformation is often combined with others, such as scoliosis, hemivertebrae or hydrocephalus. There is also a possible abnormal hair tuft on the animal's nape and abnormalities of the sternum.

Diagnosis: Age, breed and clinical signs provide an indication of the disease. Myelography may be needed for further clarification. A swelling of the spinal cord may be evident. The use of CT or MRI is also indicated (Fig. 14.7).

Therapy: None. A laminectomy may give relief but not resolution. However, a normal life may be possible.

Prognosis: Guarded to poor.

14.1.4.5 Meningeal cysts/Intra-arachnoid cysts

Occurrence: Rare.

Aetiology: The aetiology is unclear. It is possibly a dysraphic disturbance as it mainly affects young animals. It is especially seen in the Boston Terrier, Chow Chow, Doberman, Rhodesian Ridgeback, Rottweiler, Shi Tzu, Weimaraner or cats; though principally every breed can be affected. In older animals, it is thought to be associated with trauma. Typical for this disease are intradural, extramedullary fluid-filled cysts located dorsally on the midline (21, 22, 55).

Clinical: The clinical signs vary according to the localisation of the cysts. Usually they are present in the cervical or thoracolumbar regions.

Diagnosis: A myelogram, CT or MRI is necessary for ensuring a diagnosis. Sometimes such cysts can be found incidentally (Fig. 14.8).

Therapy: A dorsal laminectomy as well as a durotomy +/− durectomy or marsupialisation of the dura may be necessary. Conservative therapy with glucocorticosteroids may sometimes help.

Prognosis: Guarded to good.

14.1.4.6 Spina bifida

Occurrence: Rare. Dogs: English Bulldog; cats: Manx Cat; other breeds may be affected.

Aetiology: This disease is due to the lack of closure of the spinous processes; it may be accompanied by a meningomyelocele.

It mainly affects the lumbar region. Other malformations such as hydromyelia/syringomyelia or hydrocephalus are also possible in conjunction with the spina bifida (11).

Clinical: Mild to severe paresis, urinary and faecal incontinence as well as anal analgesia may be apparent.

Diagnosis: The diagnosis can in some cases be suspected based on palpation; however, the majority of cases require radiography, myelography, CT or MRI (Fig. 14.9).

Therapy: Surgical correction is possible but with questionable success.

Prognosis: Guarded to poor.

14.1.4.7 Sacrococcygeal dysplasia/Dysgenesis/ Sacrocaudal hypoplasia

Occurrence: Manx Cat; rare in other breeds.

Aetiology: This is a malformation which has been described in the tailless Manx Cat and has been found to have an autosomal-dominant inheritance. The following anomalies can occur due to incomplete penetrance of the dominant gene for taillessness: subcutaneous cysts, myelocele, meningomyelocele, syringomyelia in the caudal lumbar to sacral region; the cauda equina may be truncated or completely missing.

Clinical: Depending on the extent of disease, clinical signs can be seen just after birth or later in life: plantigrade positioning of the feet to paresis and paraplegia, urinary and/or faecal incontinence, and sensation disturbances of the perianal region. Bunny hopping is considered "normal" in this breed. The pelvic limb spinal reflexes are reduced. The clinical signs are not progressive.

Diagnosis: Typical changes in the Manx Cat. Imaging techniques such as radiography, myelography, CT and MRI are used to confirm the diagnosis.

Therapy: None.

Prognosis: Guarded to poor.

14.1.4.8 Occipital dysplasia

Occurrence: Rare. Dogs: toy breeds such as Chihuahua, Maltese and Yorkshire Terrier.

Aetiology: Congenital widening of the foramen magnum and a shortening of C1 can occur in toy dog breeds. This disease is often combined with hydrocephalus (56).

Clinical: Cerebellar ataxia and cervical pain can occur, but often the animal does not show any clinical signs.

Diagnosis: Radiographs through the open mouth in the sedated animal reveal a keyhole-like foreman magnum (see Fig. 6.43b). Usually other causes are responsible for the neurological disturbances, so further diagnostic investigations must be done carefully as there is marked individual variation in the size of the foramen magnum, which is not associated with the clinical symptoms.

Therapy: None.

Prognosis: Good to guarded.

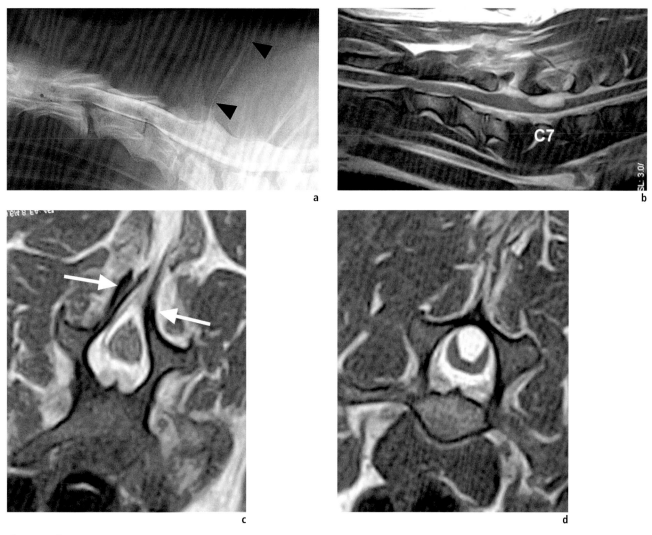

a

b

c

d

14

Fig. 14.9a–d
(a) Myelography with sagittal (b) and transverse (c, d) MRI images (CBASS fluid-sensitive, high resolution sequence) of a complex malformation of the cervical spine with spina bifida in a five-month-old Flat-coated Retriever (same dog as in Fig. 6.12). The myelogram shows a continual contrast line from the subarachnoid space over C6 in the subcutis of the nape (dermoid sinus; arrowheads). Note the apparent widening of the spinal cord over C7. Deformation of the cervical spine with shortened and partially fused vertebrae. Malformed discs, highly reduced signal intensity of disc C6–C7. (b) Cyst-like cavity in the bone marrow over C7. (c) The spinous process of C6 is duplicated from lack of fusion (spina bifida). Hyperintense CSF is present in the dermoid sinus, which extends dorsally. The spinal cord is pulled out dorsally forming drop-like extensions. (d) Large cyst lying dorsally in the spinal cord with high signal intensity (syringomyelia) at the level of C7. (Pictures: Johann Lang, Berne.)

14.1.4.9 Vertebral malformations/Hemivertebrae

Occurrence: Common. Dogs: English and French Bulldogs, German Short-haired Pointer, Pekingese, Pug, Rottweiler, Boston, West Highland White and Yorkshire Terriers.

Aetiology: Vertebral malformations are due to abnormal closure of the neural crest during embryonal development. The breeds with abnormal tails such as the ones mentioned above often have malformations in the thoracic region (T2–L1) (16).

The possible vertebral abnormalities include:
- Fused vertebrae: the vertebrae are not separated.
- Wedge-shaped vertebrae: the vertebra is deformed into a "wedge".
- Butterfly vertebrae: the vertebra has a sagittal cleft; usually found in the thoracic spine without any clinical symptoms.
- Transitional vertebrae (see Fig. 6.13): vertebrae at the junctions of the different spinal segments (cervical/thoracic/lumbar) have transitional characteristics such as:
  - Sacralisation: fusion between the last lumbar vertebra and the sacrum.
  - Lumbarisation: congenital isolation of the first sacral vertebra.
- Scoliosis: lateral deviation of the spine; can be due to unilateral hemivertebrae (see Fig. 1.3).
- Kyphosis: dorsal convex deviation of the spine; can be due to dorsal hemivertebra (see Fig. 1.3).
- Lordosis: ventral convex deviation of the spine; can be due to ventral hemivertebrae (see Fig. 1.3).

Clinical: The animals often do not show any clinical signs. Paresis, paraplegia, pain, faecal and urinary incontinence may occur in affected animals within the first year of life as the consequence of chronic compression. The occurrence of scoliosis, kyphosis, lordosis or fractures of the abnormal vertebrae has been described.

Diagnosis: Age, breed and clinical signs form the basis of a tentative diagnosis. The diagnosis can often be confirmed with plain radiography. Myelography can be used to visualise the degree of spinal cord compression but MRI is most useful for this purpose.

Therapy: Surgical stabilisation or decompression can result in improvement in many cases. However, surgical correction may be very difficult.

Prognosis: Guarded.

14.1.4.10 Congenital exostoses/ Multiple cartilaginous exostoses/ Osteochromatosis

Occurrence: Rare. Dogs: Alaskan Malamute, German Shepherd, Yorkshire Terrier, Terrier Crosses. Cats.

Aetiology: This is a benign proliferation of cartilage at the growth zones of the bones, vertebral bodies, spinous processes or ribs. Growth of the exostoses may stop at the time of the closure of the epiphyses. It is thought to be inheritable in the dog (15, 30).

Clinical: Pain in young animals in the affected region of the body – mainly thoracic or lumbar spine – during the growth phase in the first year of life is the most obvious symptom. Neurological deficits such as progressive paraparesis or tetraparesis are possible, depending on the severity and localisation of the spinal cord compression.

Diagnosis: The clinical signs occur during the growth phase. Radiologically, these abnormalities can be seen as radiodense well-demarcated areas of differing sizes (see Fig. 6.15). They are often round with radiopaque centres. A biopsy can confirm the suspicion. Myelography can demonstrate the degree of spinal cord compression, but CT or MRI gives a better 3D impression of the lesion

Therapy: Surgical removal may be necessary (2).

Prognosis: Guarded. The exostoses may stop growing when the epiphyses close, but there is also a possibility of transformation to a chondrosarcoma.

14.1.5 Metabolic diseases

14.1.5.1 Hypervitaminosis A

Occurrence: Rare. Cats.

Aetiology: Hypervitaminosis A can be induced in cats by excessive intake of foods such as raw liver. The consequences include hypertrophic changes in the bones with ankylosis, primarily in the cervical spine and joints.

Clinical: The clinical signs arise due to the immobility of the spine and the compression of nerves. Depression and a "rabbit-like" sitting position are conspicuous in adult animals. The coat is uncared for as the cats can hardly clean themselves. Other conspicuous signs include pain and hyperaesthesia (especially when the neck is manipulated), muscle atrophy, ventroflexion of the neck and lameness in the forelimbs (27).

14

Diagnosis: Hypertrophic and ankylotic changes are present on radiographs, especially in the cervical spine and its joints.

Therapy: None. An immediate change in nutrition and analgesics can only prevent the development of further clinical symptoms rather than cure the disease.

Prognosis: Poor.

14.1.6 Neoplastic diseases

Occurrence: Relatively common.

Aetiology: Primary tumours of or metastases to the spine and the vertebral column are well documented in dogs and cats. The tumours which affect the spine are divided into intramedullary, intradural-extramedullary and extradural depending on their location; extradural tumours are most common (Fig. 14.10). Gliomas are less common in this region than in the brain. Tumours of the spine often originate from the meninges (meningiomas; see Fig. 6.31) of the spinal cord or the nerve roots. Neoplasms of the spinal cord, the spinal meninges and the spinal column primarily cause neurological dysfunction through spinal cord compression. Some tumours may infiltrate the spinal cord; however, even primarily invasive tumours compress the surrounding tissue. Lymphosarcoma affecting the spinal cord is commonly seen in cats.

Clinical: Any age group can be affected. In young animals, for example, lymphoma in the cat and the so-called nephroblastoma of the dog are considerations (Fig. 14.11). Tumour-related neurological deficits can develop chronically or acutely; though the majority are progressive. Pain is often seen with extradural tumours prior to other neurological symptoms. The clinical signs are dependent on the localisation and correspond to a focal lesion (24, 44).

Diagnosis: Advanced imaging techniques are essential. Metastases can be identified with the aid of radiography of the thorax. Aggressive bone tumours may be directly visualised using survey radiography or CT of the spine. However, primary spinal cord tumours require myelography, myelo-CT or MRI to be assessed. At least two views should be taken and assessed with myelography (lateral, VD, possibly oblique). The pattern formed by the contrast column depends on the type of tumour and its location (intramedullary, intradural-extramedullary, extradural; see Chap. 6.3.2.4). With equivocal or negative myelography results, CT or MRI should be undertaken. CSF analysis can reveal abnormalities (increase in protein and cell counts, due to secondary inflammation).

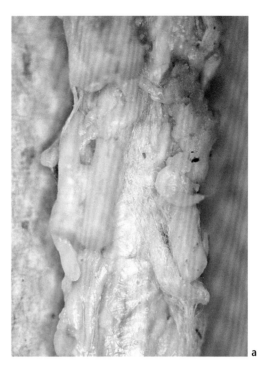

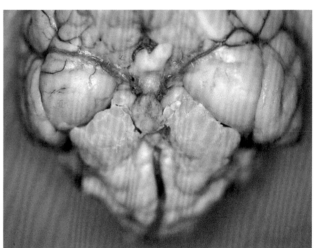

Fig. 14.10a, b
German Shepherd, seven years old, male, with extensive giant onion bulb formation (GOBF) polyneuropathy which has resulted in secondary compression of the spinal cord and brain stem. (a) Ventral view of the spinal cord showing massively thickened spinal roots and nerves. (b) Ventral view of the brain with massively thickened cranial nerves.

14

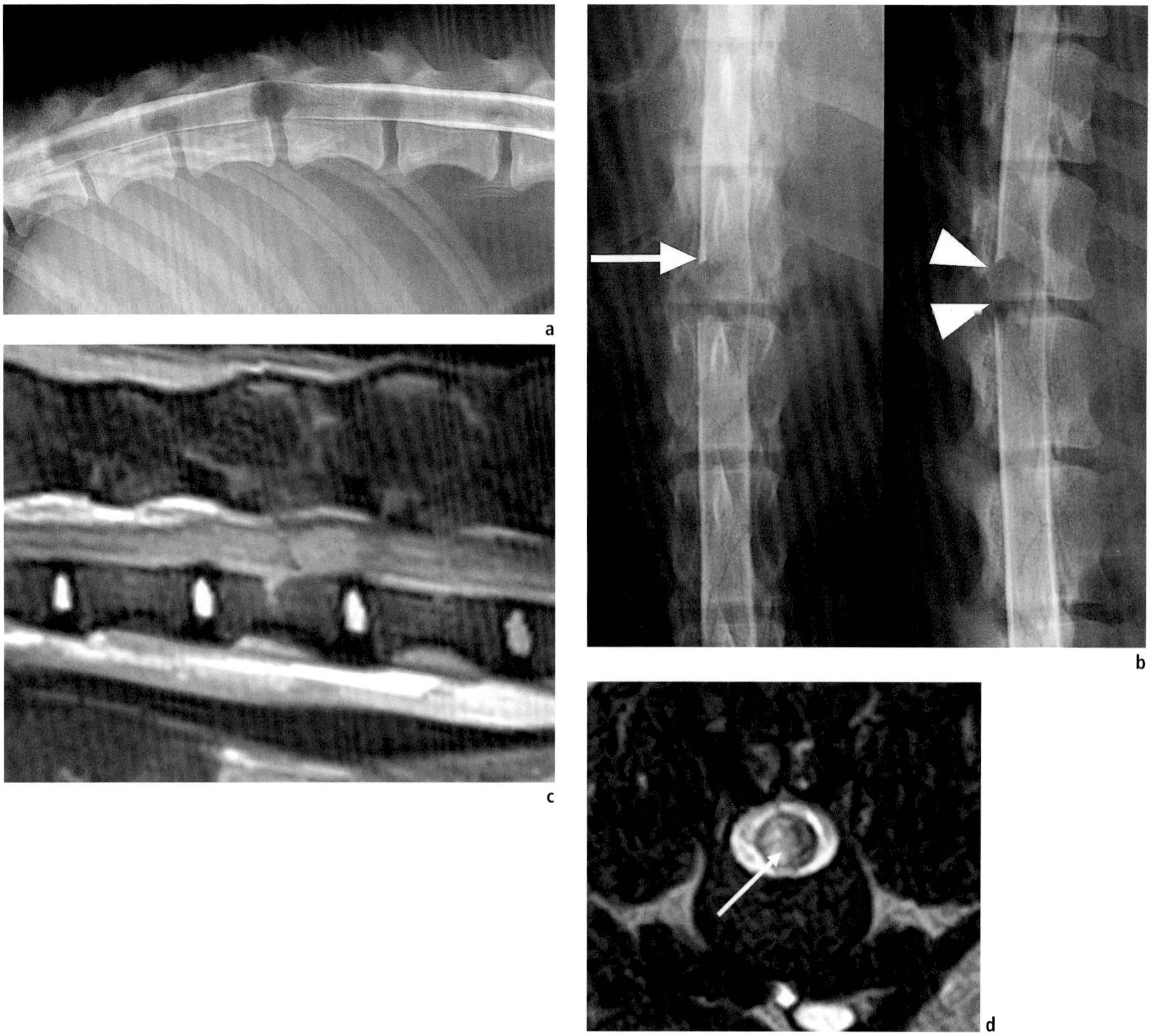

Fig. 14.11a–d
Nephroblastoma in a two-year-old Barbet with progressive paraparesis. (a, b) Myelography of the region T13–L1. (a) The lateral view shows a focal swelling of the spinal cord at T13–L1 with a filling defect. (b) The ventrodorsal projection additionally reveals a "golf tee", that reveals the intradural-extramedullary nature of the tumour (arrow). The oblique view very clearly reveals a local swelling of the spinal cord in the area of the adhesion with the meninges (arrowheads). (c, d) In the T2w sagittal and transverse MRI sequences, the tumour appears hyperintense and moderately well demarcated (arrow). The spinal cord is compressed by two thirds. (Pictures: Johann Lang, Berne.)

14

A severe neutrophilic pleocytosis can be seen in association with meningiomas. Tumour cells are rarely identified in CSF. However, large, lymphoblast-like cells or atypical lymphocytes can be seen in cytospin preparations of the CSF of CNS lymphoma cases. These are often accompanied by smaller "normal" inflammatory lymphocytes. With a suspicion of myeloma, investigation of the bone marrow can be useful in determining the diagnosis. The final diagnosis and histological classification of the tumour is only possible after surgical biopsy in the majority of cases (36, 40, 61).

Therapy: The therapeutic options for a tumour of the spinal column or spinal cord are surgical resection and/or radiation/chemotherapy. Some extradural tumours that do not involve bony structures and some intradural-extramedullary tumours can be successfully removed surgically. This is particularly true of meningiomas, extradural lymphosarcomas and some nerve root tumours. If a therapy is decided upon, then it should be undertaken as aggressively as possible. After surgical removal of a tumour, it is recommended that adjunct chemotherapy and/or radiation therapy should be initiated. As a rule, radiation therapy dosages of between 45.6 and 48.0 Gy are used, divided over at least 12 fractions given as 3.8–4.0 Gy three times a week. Lower doses (30–36 Gy divided into 5–6 fractions) have also been described. Chemotherapeutics can be used for treating gliomas; e.g., lomustine (CCNU).

This medication is lipid soluble and can therefore penetrate the blood-brain barrier. The dose of CCNU in the dog is 50–80 mg/m^2 body surface area every 5 to 8 weeks. Therapy with glucocorticoids usually only provides temporary improvement.

With the aid of surgery, two problems at the same time are addressed: a biopsy for histological investigation and the removal of the tumour with decompression. The surgical method of choice is usually a dorsal laminectomy; but a a hemilaminectomy can be performed if this makes the tumour more accessible. This is determined with the aid of imaging. Only occasionally can the whole grossly visible tumour be removed without damaging the adjacent spinal cord. Instrumental aids such as magnifying lenses or operating microscopes assist with visualisation of the edges of the tumour. Patients may have a worse neurological status immediately after the operation. In addition to possible mechanical trauma, the cause of this phenomenon is related to reperfusion injury which can potentially occur with every cause of chronic spinal cord compression. The preoperative administration of potent anti-inflammatories is recommended (methylprednisolone, dexamethasone). In the literature, there is relatively little data documenting survival times for spinal cord tumours following specific therapies. Combination therapies probably provide the best results (41).

Prognosis: The prognosis can be guarded to hopeless, depending on the therapeutic options available and on the neoplastic process itself (well demarcated or infiltrative). The prognosis is especially poor with intramedullary or infiltrative tumours. Cats with operable tumours affecting the cord have a distinctly better prognosis than cats with lymphosarcoma of the cord itself. The progression appears to be most rapid with intramedullary tumours; intradural-extramedullary tumours have the slowest rate of growth, with extradural tumours having intermediate growth rates. According to published data, the mean survival rate with tumours affecting the spinal cord is 135 days (15 to 600 days). The median survival time for dogs with intraspinal meningiomas is 15 to 19 months following surgical and radiation treatment.

14.1.7 Degenerative diseases of the spine and spinal cord

14.1.7.1 Disease of the intervertebral discs

Degenerative disease of the intervertebral discs does not necessarily result in neurological signs because the nervous tissue is not primarily affected unless there is concurrent herniation of disc material. However, as the clinical signs of disc degeneration are associated with secondary compression of the spinal cord, these diseases are discussed within this section.

Anatomical and physiological principles

Intervertebral discs are situated between the vertebral bodies throughout the whole spine, apart from between the atlas and axis, and in the sacral region. The disc consists of two structures: the nucleus pulposus and the annulus fibrosus, which is thinner dorsally. The nucleus is made up of a gelatine-like substance. The proteogylcans contained in this substance help store enormous amounts of water and so provide the disc with its tremendous elasticity. The composition of the nucleus pulposus varies greatly between chondrodystrophic breeds and nonchondrodystrophic ones. The annulus fibrosus consists of concentric lamellae of fibrous cartilage and elastic fibres. The outer two to four layers are vascularised directly while the others are supplied via indirect perfusion. The situation is similar for the disc's innervation.

Disc herniation implies a complete or partial displacement of the disc, which is predominantly caused by disc degeneration, and more rarely by trauma. Disc disease is divided into two groups: Hansen type I and Hansen type II, named after Hansen who first made this distinction.

14.1.7.2 Intervertebral disc extrusion

Occurrence: Common. This is a typical phenomenon in chondrodystrophic breeds such as Cocker Spaniel, Dachshund, Pekingese, Shih Tzu, etc. It can also affect medium-sized to large breeds, such as the German Shepherd. It is rare in cats.

14

Aetiology: The extrusion of an intervertebral disc in chondrodystrophoid dog breeds is due to chondroid degeneration of the nucleus pulposus, which can start in the sixth to eighth month of life. The nucleus is replaced by hyaline cartilage and its water content therefore reduces. The nucleus material can extrude dorsally or dorsolaterally through a tear in the connective tissue annulus. A genetic predisposition is thought to be part of the underlying cause, but whether or not physical stress plays a role is difficult to judge. Usually, extrusion occurs suddenly when the dog jumps or makes a sudden or awkward movement during play. The clinical symptoms are caused acutely by concussion and compression of the spinal cord. The causative, slowly progressive degenerative process, however, has been present for months or even years. Normally, clinical problems occur after the second year of life. Between the second and sixth years of life, extrusions occur most commonly in the thoracolumbar region; extrusions in the cervical spine, mainly occur between C2 and C3. The frequency of cervical cord extrusion reduces with each disc space caudal to this site. Haemorrhage, secondary to rupture of the ventrally situated venous sinus, exacerbates the degree of spinal cord compression.

Pain always occurs with disc extrusion and is secondary to compression of the meninges or the nerve roots. It is unclear whether the pain can also be due to the irritation of receptors in the annulus or the dorsal longitudinal ligament.

Concussion and compression of the spinal cord leads to perfusion disturbances and hypoxia. The reversibility of the spinal cord damage may be indirectly proportional to the duration of the compression. Nerve cell necrosis can develop relatively quickly and is not reversible. The clinical picture is more severe when the lesion is at the level of an intumescence. When there is damage to the spinal cord between the intumescences, demyelination of the tracts in the white matter can be compensated for by remyelination. The cytotoxic effects of glutamate in the area of the compression may be responsible for the secondary damage to the spinal cord as its concentration in the CSF has been found to be proportional to the severity of the clinical symptoms (26, 50).

Clinical: The clinical symptoms depend on various factors:
- The amount of extruded disc material.
- The force with which the disc material extrudes. The nucleus is contained within a firm connective tissue ring; as soon as a small opening occurs in the ring, the nucleus can extrude out. Extrusion in the direction of the spinal cord leads to severe trauma.
- The relationship between the diameter of the spinal cord and the diameter of the vertebral canal. If there is enough room in the vertebral canal, the extruded material may not necessarily cause compressive damage to the spinal cord. In the cervical region, the epidural space is relatively large, while that in the lumbar region tends to be small. The most unfavourable ratio is found in the thoracic and cranial lumbar regions of the spine as the spinal cord prac-

tically fills the whole of the vertebral canal. Between T1–T11, there are intercapital ligaments that extend from one rib head to another, and these can prevent dorsal disc extrusion. Most commonly, disc extrusion is observed between T11 and L3.

The following clinical subdivision has been documented for disc herniation in the thoracolumbar region:

Grade I. The animal has acute back pain without neurological deficits. The patient may have kyphosis. Using palpation from the cranial part of the spine caudally, attempts can be made to localise the compression according to the pain response of the patient, which can vary greatly according to the nature of the animal. The abdominal musculature becomes tense in response to pain. Despite the presence of pain alone, massive compressive disease cannot be excluded.

Grade II. In addition to the pain described in Grade I, paraparesis (mainly spastic) and ataxia of the hindlimbs can be observed in Grade II patients. The neurological symptoms can vary in degree. The animal can walk. Proprioception deficits are present during the neurological examination.

Grade III. Severe paraparesis. The animal can no longer stand up and walk. Voluntary movements can be made with support.

Grade IV. The animal is paraplegic. Even with support, it can no longer make voluntary movements. The clinical picture is, however, very similar to Grade III. Differentiation between these grades is important for the prognosis.

Grade V. In addition to paraplegia, problems with urination also occur. Overflow incontinence is recognisable by the dribbling of urine. This should not be confused with normal urination or incontinence.

Grade VI. An additional symptom to those present in Grade V, is the loss of nociception.

Extrusion in the cervical spine leads to tetraparesis or less commonly tetraplegia; only rarely is there loss of nociception or uncontrolled micturition. The spinal canal is relatively wide in the cervical region and so the spinal cord is rarely severely compressed. The most important symptom is pain. The animals contract their cervical muscles, resist examination, and may vocalise in pain. The patients sometimes do not get up because of the pain and try to avoid all unnecessary movements. This should not be confused with paresis. Other patients, in comparison, remain standing with their heads flexed downwards almost touching the floor.

Diagnosis: The diagnosis is confirmed using different advanced imaging techniques. These investigations are performed under anaesthesia enabling the spine to be placed in the correct position, and so that contrast agents can be injected into the subarachnoid space.

14

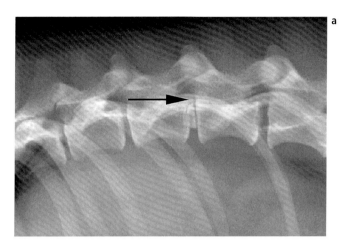

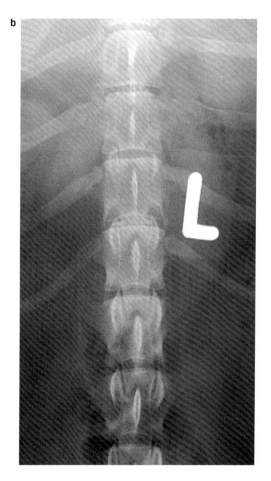

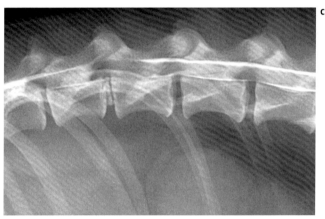

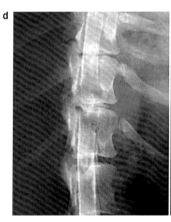
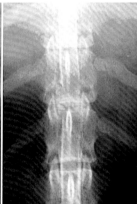
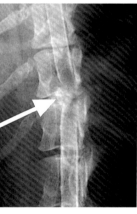

Fig. 14.12a–d
Disc herniation. (a) The plain radiograph shows a mineralised disc at T12–T13 with a protruding dorsal edge and a fine focus of mineralisation lying above it (arrow). The intervertebral space and the intervertebral foramenae are narrow. (b) T10–T11 is normally narrower than the neighbouring spaces. (c, d) Myelography. (c) On the lateral view, the widened spinal cord is displaced ventrodorsally and the contrast columns are compressed. (d) The mineralised and extruded disc material lying ventral to the right in the vertebral canal and the spinal cord compression first becomes visible in the view where the dog has been turned around its longitudinal body axis (arrow). (Pictures: Johann Lang, Berne.)

14

The following phenomena may be seen on plain radiographs:
- The presence of a calcified disc (Fig. 14.12): though this should not be over evaluated diagnostically. A calcified disc is a degenerative phenomenon, which has been present for some time. If the calcified disc remains in situ, then no clinical symptoms will arise. It has lost its function as a shock-absorber, but it still provides a certain degree of stability between the neighbouring vertebrae. Sometimes a prolapsed calcified disc is visible within the vertebral canal.
- Narrowing of the intervertebral disc space.
- Narrowing of the intervertebral foramen.

Localisation of a disc herniation can be presumed from a radiograph, though some type of advanced imaging is necessary in order to prove the presence of spinal cord compression. Myelography is performed when the neurological examination indicates that surgery may be necessary. If it is foreseeable that the patient can be helped with conservative treatment, then this adjunct investigation may at first be wavered due to the increased risk for the patient with the anaesthesia or the increased costs associated with the procedure (17).

The injection of contrast agent into the vertebral canal can provide the following information:
- The diagnosis may be confirmed.
- The site of the compression can be precisely localised. Extradural compression is usually ventral or ventro-lateral. The disc material can also accumulate to one side compressing the spinal cord laterally. In many patients, the prolapsed material does not lie on the side of the more severe clinical symptoms. In rare cases, the extruded material is wrapped around the spinal cord, whereby it is compressed dorsally, too.
- The actual extent of the compression can sometimes be seen.

Correct interpretation of the myelogram requires experience. In some cases, myelography is not diagnostic: narrowing of the subarachnoid space can prevent uniform dissemination of the contrast agent. Such impairment can occur with herniation of large amounts of disc material over a long segment of the spinal cord or when myelography is performed within hours of the occurrence of the first clinical symptoms. Changes in the blood supply to the spinal cord due to disc extrusion can lead to oedema. This oedema often extends over more than one segment of the spinal cord which increases its diameter. This latter change can also be associated with intramedullary lesions. Despite these problems, myelography can be an important diagnostic tool for diseases of the spine and spinal cord in the dog and cat. A more precise investigation of specific spinal cord segments can be done using CT or MRI. Both of these techniques can visualise prolapsed disc material and haemorrhage. With CT, the recognition of disc material is proportional to the degree of mineralisation and the chronicity of the process. CT is also performed after myelography, as long as there is contrast agent in the subarachnoid space (myelo-CT). Other investigations such somatosensory-evoked or magnetic-evoked potentials have not been used in routine diagnostics (6, 9, 34, 39, 42, 53, 63, 72).

Therapy: Treatment can be conservative or surgical. The former is appropriate in dogs with clinical signs of Grades I and II. With absolute box rest, it is hoped that fibrosis and scarring will develop. In conservative therapy, the animal is placed in a small cage, so that it lies down as much as possible. This restriction of movement should last for at least 3 to 4 weeks; afterwards, exercise should be slowly reintroduced. Ideally one could consider, hospitalisation, but this is often not possible due to the cost or lack of facilities. Due to the difficulties in restraining dogs, conservative treatment often results in failure. During the period of immobilisation, it is recommended to give the patient anti-inflammatory drugs (prednisolone 0.5–1 mg/kg SID). This medication is only of use when the animal is kept completely quiet as with pain reduction, the dog may move around too much, leading to a drastic deterioration of the neurological status. Other complications of glucocorticoids such as intestinal bleeding or haematemesis can also occur. To reduce these side-effects, different drugs such as sucralfate, cimetidine or ranitidine have been used, though their prophylactic effects have been questioned. Omeprazole and misoprostol seem not to be very effective, and they are also very expensive. Other side-effects of steroids include pancreatitis and intestinal perforation.

Surgery is recommended in animals with Grades III, IV and V clinical signs, as well as those animals in Grade VI which have been affected for less than 48 hours. In dogs with clinical signs of Grade VI, surgery is not recommended when there has been no pain response for more than 48 hours based on the poor prognosis. Different techniques have been described; the most common is hemilaminectomy (see Chap. 10.3). This method allows the site of compression to be reached with only minimal destabilisation of the spine, so that the herniated disc material can be removed from the vertebral canal. With a minihemilaminectomy, the articular process is preserved; however, it only allows a minimal view of the spinal cord and so makes the complete removal of the herniated material more difficult. With a dorsal laminectomy, the view of the spinal cord is good but disc material lying ventrally either cannot be removed at all or can only partially be retrieved. In the case of oedema or haemorrhage of the spinal cord, durotomy can be performed if it is assumed that the inelastic dura is causing restriction of blood circulation. Myelotomy is not recommended. Fenestration is not a method used for achieving decompression.

A lateral approach can be chosen in the cervical region when the herniated disc material is situated laterally with respect to the cord. The classical approach to the cervical spine is, however, the so-called ventral slot: a ventral window is drilled in the neighbouring vertebral bodies at the level of the disc herniation to remove the extruded material.

The window should never be more than a third of the width of the vertebral body, otherwise subluxation of the vertebrae could occur. During the healing process, the space made by curettage is replaced with fibrocartilaginous material. Another possibility for spinal decompression – especially with multiple disc herniations – is a dorsal laminectomy. Other methods such as chemonucleolysis have been described but should not be considered for the treatment of herniated discs (13, 20, 25, 38, 48, 65).

Postsurgical measures:
1. The patient should be kept quiet for 3 to 4 weeks. It may not jump or climb stairs. Animals that cannot move themselves should be placed on a soft mattress to prevent decubitus ulcers. A heated environment may be necessary. Dogs must be turned three to four times a day. Afterwards, an attempt to rebuild the muscles can be undertaken by taking the animal on longer and longer walks. However, the dog should be kept on the lead during this time to prevent abrupt movements. It should be made clear to the owner that the dog will not be able to achieve the same degree of physical prowess as before in many cases and that the occurrence of other disc herniations is possible. The discs cranial and caudal to the operation site are at most risk as they have altered dynamic forces to deal with due to the neighbouring missing disc.
2. Physiotherapy should be started immediately during the convalescence period to prevent muscle atrophy (see Chap. 8.1). The owner should extend and flex the affected limb for 5 to 10 minutes, three to four times a day. Exercises while standing with support are important. Electrotherapeutic devices for muscle stimulation are available. They are more effective than passive movement therapy. If they are used incorrectly, however, they tend to be unpleasant for the animal and cause more damage than good. Swimming or using an underwater treadmill is highly recommended for animals that cannot stand but are capable of conscious movement.
3. The biggest problem in animals with a lesion of the spinal cord is a disturbance of micturition, which may be due to the original injury or due to the operation. The bladder should be emptied at least three times a day as urine retention can lead to bladder inflammation and result in septicaemia. In addition, the detrusor muscle can lose its ability to contract because of overstretching. Pharmacological support of bladder emptying is possible (see Chaps. 8.2.1 and 14.2, Table 14.3).
4. Other possible postoperative complications include decubitus ulcers, wounds due to lying on hard surfaces without physiotherapy and uncontrolled urinary loss. The urine can additionally scald the skin. Seroma formation in the area of the surgical wound can develop due to excessive movement. Small seromas can be treated with warm compresses to stimulate their resorption; larger ones can be aspirated under aseptic conditions or by the introduction of a drain.
5. The daily calorie intake should be reduced to prevent an increase in weight. Excessive weight hinders the patient's mobility. Overweight animals must be put on a diet.
6. Individually-made carts can support the movements of the hindlimbs or be used for locomotion if paralysis remains.

14.1.7.3 Intervertebral disc protrusion

Occurrence: Common. Occurs mainly in medium-sized and large breeds such as the German Shepherd and especially in animals that are subjected to hard physical work.

Aetiology: These Hansen type II herniations are characterised by a fibroid degeneration of the disc. The whole of the disc pushes itself out from its usual position and compresses the spinal cord.

Clinical: The disc protrusion is mainly chronic and is usually subclinical. The animals are first brought for examination when the process has been in existence for some time. Clinical symptoms are usually not observed before the fifth or sixth year of life. The average age of the animals at the time of first presentation to a veterinarian is much later. Cervical protrusions are infrequently seen, though in some breeds they occur as part of CCSM (Chap. 14.1.4.2). Protrusion of the lumbosacral discs is more common (see Fig. 6.19). Due to the compression in the thoracolumbar region, there is secondary demyelination of the white matter leading to ataxia and paraparesis. The animal is usually not painful even on palpation of the spine.

Diagnosis: The diagnosis is made with the help of radiography and advanced imaging. Osteoarticular degeneration can be seen on plain radiographs, e.g. arthrosis of the joint surfaces, sclerosis of the epiphyses and spondylosis, which can be so progressive that various vertebrae are fused into a single bony structure. Other possible forms include narrowing of the intervertebral spaces and the foraminae. These changes are, however, not pathognomonic for compression of the spinal cord as they can represent normal age-related degeneration without any neurological deficits. Myelography should also be used for a definitive diagnosis. More than one neighbouring disc may be affected.

The contrast agent flows around the protruded tissue and the spinal cord may appear narrowed at the site. The presence of contrast in the subarachnoid space close to the area where the maximal spinal cord compression is found indicates that the process is slowly degenerative without concurrent oedema and cord swelling. Naturally, CT and MRI are more sensitive and specific imaging modalities for this disease.

Therapy: Treatment is either medical or surgical. The success of either depends on an early recognition of the disease. The use of anti-inflammatory drugs can provide temporary relief. A limitation on the physical activity of the dog can

14

substantially slow down the degeneration. If the animal has obvious pain and the diagnosis is made during an acute or subacute phase before the degenerative process is clinically relevant, then surgery is appropriate. With the onset of ataxia and paraparesis, the success of decompression surgery starts to decrease.

Prognosis: Guarded. NB: surgical decompression may lead to reperfusion damage and hence more severe neurological dysfunction than that seen prior to surgery.

14.1.7.4 Degenerative myelopathy of large dog breeds

Occurrence: Common. Dogs: German Shepherd and its crosses, Boxers, Corgis, Chesapeake Bay Retrievers, Collies Siberian Husky, and other large breeds of dog. Rare in cats.

Aetiology: In this disease, there is myelin degeneration particularly affecting the thoracolumbar spinal cord and the dorsal nerve roots. Different causes such as vitamin B or E deficiency, autoimmune or vascular diseases have been discussed. Recently, a genetic predisposition for the disease has been confirmed.

Clinical: Slowly progressive non-painful ataxia of the hindlimbs in middle-aged animals is typical for this disease. The proprioceptive reactions are abnormal in one or both hindlinbs. The intact spinal reflexes indicate a lesion between T3 and L3, although the patella reflex may be reduced (43).

Diagnosis: The diagnosis can only be made from the clinical signs and by a process of elimination. Blood tests are now available which can confirm whether a certain case has a genetic predisposition for the disease, but does not confirm the presence or absence of the disease. Radiographs, myelography and MRI are normal. Evoked potentials may be abnormal. CSF taken from a lumbar tap may show a slight increase in protein.

Therapy: None at this time. According to the literature, oral aminocaproic acid (Amicar®) 500 mg TID, vitamin E (2000 IU, SID) and vitamin B12 are useful but this regime has not been proven to be effective. Physiotherapy is important for the progressive muscle loss. Glucocorticoids should only be given on a short-term basis when acute deterioration of the clinical signs occurs, which is rare.

Prognosis: Poor; patients are usually recumbent within 12 to 18 months.

14.1.7.5 Ataxia and myelopathy of the Terrier/ Hereditary ataxia

Occurrence: Rare. Dogs: Fox Terrier, Jack Russell Terrier.

Aetiology: An autosomal recessive inheritance is thought to occur in the Fox Terrier. There is degeneration of the cervical and thoracic white matter (axonopathy). In the Jack Russell Terrier, the auditory nerves and sometimes the peripheral nerves are also affected (28).

Clinical: Between the second and sixth month of life, the animals exhibit a generalised ataxia with hypermetria of the forelimbs, a broad-based stance of the hindlimbs, and focal muscle tremor. The clinical signs worsen so that the animals tend to fall over and can no longer stand upright. After a while, stabilisation of the clinical signs may occur.

Diagnosis: Breed and clinical picture enable a tentative diagnosis to be made. Changes may be seen in auditory evoked potentials. Other diseases of the cervical spinal cord must be excluded.

Therapy: None.

Prognosis: Guarded. The disease is not lethal and it can even stabilise. Breeding affected dogs is not recommended.

14.1.7.6 Hound ataxia

Occurrence: Rare. Dogs: Beagle, Foxhound.

Aetiology: The aetiology is unclear. It is thought that this disease is a nutritional disturbance associated with the feeding of mainly tripe diets. There is degeneration of the spinal cord especially in the thoracic white matter, though the grey matter of the brain stem, cerebellum and sciatic nerve may also be affected.

Clinical: The animals show a progressive spastic paralysis between the second and seventh year of life. The panniculus reflex caudal to T13 is absent in many animals, even though the spinal reflexes are normal (54).

Diagnosis: Diagnosis in dogs of these breeds with a compatible clinical picture can only be made by a process of elimination. The serum methionine concentration is low in affected patients but is not specific.

Therapy: A change in the feeding regimes may possibly help. Supportive care and physiotherapy should be advised.

Prognosis: Guarded.

14.1.7.7 Afghan myelopathy

Occurrence: Rare. Dogs: Afghans.

Aetiology: This disease was first described in 1973, but its cause has not as yet been elucidated. It may have an inheritable aetiology, with it possibly being an autosomal recessive without sex predisposition. Only the CNS is affected. There is predominantly degeneration of the cervical and thoracolumbar white matter (leukodystrophy). The changes are bilateral and most notable between C5–L3 (10).

Clinical: The animals exhibit paresis and bunny hopping in the first year of life. The clinical signs are progressive and deterioration occurs within 4 to 6 weeks with the development of tetraplegia. The spinal reflexes may be normal or increased. Dyspnoea and death result from the massive myelin destruction.

Diagnosis: Breed, age and clinical signs are typical. The Pandy reaction in the CSF may be slightly positive but is none specific.

Therapy: None.

Prognosis: Hopeless.

14.1.7.8 Degenerative myelopathy of the Toy Poodle

Occurrence: Very rare. Dog: Toy Poodle.

Aetiology: Unknown. A diffuse, presumably congenital demyelination of the spinal cord and the brain stem is responsible for the clinical signs (58).

Clinical: The animals show a progressive spastic paresis leading to tetraplegia between the second to fourth month of life.

Diagnosis: Breed and clinical signs are typical. The CSF is unchanged.

Therapy: None.

Prognosis: Poor.

14.1.7.9 Leukoencephalomyelopathy of the Rottweiler

Occurrence: Rare. Dog: Rottweiler (23, 76).

Aetiology: There is demyelination throughout the whole CNS, though the dorsal and lateral cervical spinal cord and brain stem are affected in particular. The cause is thought to be an autosomal recessive genetic factor.

Clinical: A progressive ataxia of all the limbs develops between the first and third year of life, while the spinal reflexes remain intact. The clinical signs usually begin in the thoracic spine. Within 6 to 12 months, affected animals have problems standing up or remaining standing.

Diagnosis: Diagnosis is by process of elimination. Neuroaxonal dystrophy and cervical malformation / malarticulation are important differential diagnoses.

Therapy: None.

Prognosis: Poor.

14.1.7.10 Dalmatian leukodystrophy

Occurrence: Very rare. Dogs: Dalmatian.

Aetiology: An inheritable autosomal recessive aetiology is presumed. The changes affect the spinal cord and also the cerebrum (atrophy with dilatation of the lateral ventricles). Diffuse myelin loss in the white matter, vacuolisation, oedema and many lipid-filled macrophages are seen on histopathology.

Clinical: The disease becomes apparent between the third and sixth month of life with visual disturbances, ataxia of the hindlimbs and later the forelimbs. In many cases, the animals cannot get up after a short period of time (4).

Diagnosis: Based on the symptoms and a process of elimination.

Therapy: None.

Prognosis: Poor.

14.1.7.11 Fibrinoid leukodystrophy / Encephalomyelopathy / Alexander's disease

Occurrence: Very rare. Dogs: Black Labrador Retrievers, Scottish Terrier and Toy Poodle.

Aetiology: The cause is unknown. Histologically, there is a fibrinoid degeneration of the astrocytes (= Rosenthal fibres) throughout the CNS, which is presumably inherited.

14

Clinical: The affected animals develop paresis of the hindlimbs in the third to sixth month of life, with subsequent development of ataxia and generalised weakness; sometimes tremor, behavioural changes and seizures (Scottish Terrier) are seen.

Diagnosis: Possible via biopsy (histology).

Therapy: None.

Prognosis: Poor.

14.1.7.12 Necrotising myelopathy of the Kooiker Hound

Occurrence: Rare. Dogs: Kooiker Hound.

Aetiology: It is presumed that the aetiology is an autosomal recessive gene without sex predisposition. There is diffuse degeneration of the white matter in the spinal cord especially in the cervical region, similar to the changes seen in the Afghan and Rottweiler (see Chaps. 14.1.7.7 and 14.1.7.9, resp.).

Clinical: Affected animals show a progressive hindlimb paresis from the third month of life onwards, which later affects the forelegs, too. The reflexes are increased.

Diagnosis: Breed, clinical signs.

Therapy: None; usually euthanasia at about 12 months old.

Prognosis: Poor.

14.1.7.13 Axonopathy in the Labrador

Occurrence: Very rare; disease in Labrador Retriever first described in 1988.

Aetiology: Possibly genetic, autosomal recessive inheritance leading to degeneration of the white matter and axons, particularly in the thoracic to medullary region and the cerebellum, with aplasia or hypoplasia of the corpus callosum.

Clinical: The puppies develop weakness of the hindlimbs, while the forelimbs appear stiff and broad-based. The signs become progressive leading to hypermetria of both the fore- and hindlimbs. The animals tend to fall over. Later, tremor of the head may develop.

Diagnosis: Clinical signs and breed are typical.

Therapy: None.

Prognosis: Poor.

14.1.7.14 Progressive degeneration in the Ibiza Hound

Occurrence: Very rare. Dogs: Ibiza Hound.

Aetiology: First described in 1981, diffuse degeneration of the axons with encephalopathy and neuropathy. An autosomal recessive inheritance is suspected.

Clinical: As soon as the puppies try to walk, they show a progressive gait disturbance affecting the hindlimbs and then later the forelimbs. The gait disturbances are notable as spasticity and hypermetria. The animal's movements are awkward, causing it to fall over. The patella reflex is absent. There is no muscle atrophy. Seizures have been observed in some animals. The functions of the cranial nerves are normal.

Diagnosis: Clinical signs and breed.

Therapy: None.

Prognosis: Poor.

14.1.7.15 Calcinosis circumscripta / Tumoural calcinosis

Occurrence: Rare. Dogs: Bernese Cattle Dog, German Shepherd, Great Dane, Rottweiler, St. Bernard, Springer Spaniel and Hungarian Viszla. Rare in cats.

Aetiology: This is a focal or multifocal mineralisation of the tissues, which is often observed around the joints on the extremities, on the paws or in the mouth and dorsal to C1–C2 or T2–T3. Especially affects large breeds and male animals. The aetiology is unknown, though it is presumed to have an inheritable component. Renal disease is often additionally observed (3).

Clinical: The animals show a progressive spastic paralysis between the fifth to seventh month of life that progresses to tetraparesis and ataxia.

Diagnosis: Clinically a firm, nonpainful mass can be palpated. Radiologically, this mass can be seen as an easily visible calcification between the atlas and axis or less commonly at other sites. Compression of the spinal cord can be confirmed with myelography, CT or MRI. Biopsy verifies the tentative diagnosis.

Therapy: Surgical removal of the compressive calcification usually leads to an immediate improvement in the clinical signs and resolution of a normal gait.

Prognosis: Guarded to good.

14.1.7.16   Spinal muscular atrophy

Occurrence: Rare. Dogs: Brittany Spaniel, English Pointer, Doberman, German Shepherd, Great Dane / Bloodhound crosses, Great Dane / St. Bernard crosses, Rottweiler and Swedish Lapland Hound. Rarely in cats.

Aetiology: Chronic progressive degeneration of the motor neurons in the grey matter of the spine and the brain stem nuclei occurs in this disease. The disease in the Great Dane / St. Bernard or Great Dane / Bloodhound crosses is also known as Stockard's disease, though this only has historical significance. The disease is inheritable in the Brittany Spaniel with an autosomal dominant pattern; a similar aetiology is presumed to be present in the other breeds.

Clinical: Subsequent to the motor neuron degeneration, there is massive atrophy of the paraspinal and pelvic muscles. The animals develop weakness, paresis, and from the fifth to seventh week of life, paralysis. The cranial nerves are more rarely affected (Brittany Spaniel). Megaoesophagus may occur (Rottweiler).

Diagnosis: Clinical signs, breed and age support the presence of this disease. The spinal reflexes are reduced. Spontaneous activity can occur on the EMG (Fibrillations, PSWs).

Therapy: None.

Prognosis: Guarded. Some animals die due to respiratory problems, while others can live an almost normal life.

14.1.7.17 Gangliosidosis

Gangliosidosis, Globoid cell leukodystrophy (Chap. 14.1.7.18) and **mucopolysaccharidosis** (Chap. 14.1.7.19) are so-called storage diseases. Due to a genetic defect, the catabolic degradation of a substance is stopped and the respective substrate accumulates.

Occurrence: Rare, although gangliosidosis is one of the most common forms of storage disease found in animals.

Gangliosidosis 1 (GM1) – Dogs: Beagle crosses, Portuguese water dog, Springer Spaniel. Cats: domestic, Korat and Siamese.

Gangliosidosis 2 (GM2) – Dogs: German Short-haired Pointer and Japanese pointer. Cats: domestic and Korat.

Aetiology: Gangliosidosis is a lipid storage disease belonging to the group of sphingolipidoses. Due to a defect in a lysosomal enzyme, gangliosides and glycolipids accumulate in the nervous system and sometimes in the viscera. The consequence is a massive neuronal degeneration with chromatolysis, vacuolisation and displacement of the cell nuclei to the periphery. Two forms have been proven in animals: GM1 with a defect of β-galactosidase and GM2 with a defect of β-hexosaminidase. An autosomal recessive inheritance has been presumed (18).

Clinical: Clinical symptoms occur at 2 to 18 months of age. First of all a discrete head tremor is visible, with ataxia and dysmetria. Vision disturbances and nystagmus then follow. In the cat, corneal clouding has been seen. The gait is characterised by hypermetria and spastic para- to tetraplegia. Changes in behaviour such as dementia, aggression and seizures can be observed. Sudden death is possible.

Diagnosis: Biochemical analysis identifying the storage substance is necessary. This is possible with urinalysis in a specialized laboratory. In addition, enzyme assays in the leukocytes, liver or skin can be performed. In the Springer Spaniel and Portuguese water dog, abnormally large intervertebral disc spaces have been seen radiographically. In some cases, there is hepatomegaly.

Therapy: None.

Prognosis: Hopeless.

14.1.7.18   Globoid cell leukodystrophy (Krabbe's disease)

Occurrence: Rare. Dogs: Cairn and West Highland White Terriers, Bassett, Beagle, Pomeranian, Poodle, Kelpie. Rare in the domestic cat.

Aetiology: This is also a storage disease but the enzyme defect affects β-galactosidase. Galactocerebrosides accumulate in the oligodendrocytes and Schwann cells leading to a destruction of the white matter in the whole of the nervous system (PNS and CNS). The mode of inheritance of this leukodystrophy is autosomal recessive.

Clinical: The animals become clinical between the third and fifth month of life due to spinal and / or cerebral or cerebellar symptoms. Ataxia, paresis and reduced spinal reflexes as well as muscle atrophy and / or tremor, hypermetria and visual disturbances are the most common signs.

Diagnosis: There is an increase in CSF protein, though the cell count remains normal. Changes are present in EEG and other electrophysiological investigations (PSWs, fibrillations, prolonged NCV). Suspicion of this disease can be confirmed with a nerve biopsy, demonstration of reduced enzyme activity in the leukocytes or by a PCR test.

Therapy: None.

Prognosis: Poor to guarded.

14

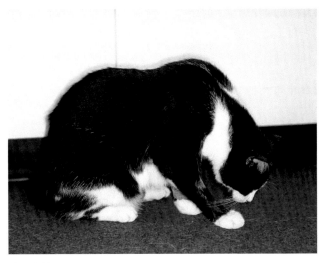

Fig. 14.13
Ventroflexion in a five-year-old European domestic cat (female, neutered) with hypomyelinogenesis.

14.1.7.19 Mucopolysaccharidosis (MPS)

Occurrence: Rare.

MPS I – Dogs: Miniature Pinscher, mixed-breed dogs, Plott Hound and domestic cat.

MPS VI: Siamese and domestic cats at an age of 3 to 10 months.

Aetiology: In MPS I, there is a deficiency of iduronidase and mucopolysaccharides accumulate. The disease is inherited as an autosomal recessive. In MPS VI, a deficit of arysulfatase B also leads to accumulation of mucopolysaccharides.

Clinical: MPS I: the animals are younger than 6 months. They are presented because of lameness, broad face, flat nose, short ears, corneal clouding, and rarely due to neurological disturbances such as progressive paresis. Vertebral fusion, bone dysplasia, funnel chest, luxation of the femoral head and/or hepatosplenomegaly can be shown radiographically. It is thought that there is an association with meningiomas.

MPS VI: Siamese cats are presented at an age of 2 to 3 months with similar clinical signs as in MPS I. Due to compression of the spinal cord, paraplegia and micturition disturbances can occur. Seizures have been described. Radiological osseous changes are visible with this disease: bone dysplasia, exostoses, spondylosis, osteoarthrosis of the vertebral joints and hypoplasia of the dens.

Diagnosis: Affected animals excrete more glycosaminoglycans (dermatan and heparin sulphates) than normal in their urine. Measurement of activity of both the affected enzymes is possible.

Therapy: Surgical decompression of the spinal cord and depending on the case, a bone marrow transplant may be necessary.

Prognosis: Guarded.

14.1.7.20 Hypomyelinogenesis

Occurrence: Rare. Dogs: Bernese Cattle Dog, Chow Chow, Dalmatian, Lurcher, Springer Spaniel, Samoyed and Weimaraner. Cats: Siamese (71).

Aetiology: Due to a reduced number of oligodendrocytes or a disturbance in their function, there is a myelin deficit in the whole of the CNS, though the peripheral nerves remain unchanged. Inherited factors (X-linked), toxins or *in utero* infections are thought to be possible causes of this disease.

Clinical: Wide-based stance, hypermetria. A generalised tremor obvious in stressful situations and excitement, but which disappears when the animal is at rest or sleeps is typical for this disease. In comparison to the tremor of cerebellar disease, hypomyelinogenesis affects the whole body and the tremor is more pronounced. Seizures have been described in the Springer Spaniel. Nystagmus is possible.

Diagnosis: Age, breed, clinical signs, normal results of all investigations apart from pathology (Fig. 14.13).

Therapy: None. It is possible that the clinical signs may plateau with time, but many animals die in the first 3 to 4 months of life.

Prognosis: Guarded.

14.1.7.21 Degenerative lumbosacral stenosis (DLSS)

The most common osteoarticular disease to be found in aged medium-sized and large dogs is DLSS. It is more commonly known as **cauda equina syndrome** (37, 62, 64).

Anatomy: The intervertebral disc space of L7 and S1, including the associated ligaments, is affected in this disease.

Each vertebra has dorsal and lateral bone laminae that form the boundaries of the vertebral canal. The dorsal longitudinal ligament lies within the vertebral canal and adheres to the dorsal surface of the vertebral bodies and the intervertebral discs. The ventral longitudinal ligament lies on the ventral surface of the vertebral bodies and intervertebral discs. Cranial and caudal to the vertebrae lie the joint surfaces, underneath which lies the intervertebral foramen. The laminae are joined together dorsally by the interarcuate ligaments. Between L7 and S1, the interarcuate ligament is particularly long as the space between these vertebrae is relatively wide. Other ligaments that provide stability to this region include the supraspinal and interspinal ligaments. Because the spinal cord segments are shorter than their respective vertebral segments, it ends at the level of L6 in dogs, as the conus medullaris. The meninges, arachnoidea and the dura mater continue on more caudally to the level of S1 (more rarely at L7). This is the site of the so-called cauda equina.

The cauda equina is made up of different nerve roots which form the following nerves:
1. The sciatic nerve originates in segments L6–L7–S1. It provides motor innervation to the semimembranosus, semitendinosus and biceps femoris muscles. More distally, it branches into the tibial nerve (which controls the gastrocnemius, popliteal, and the superficial and deep digital flexor muscles) and the peroneal nerve (which innervates the tibialis cranialis, fibularis longus and the long digital extensor muscles). This nerve complex is also responsible for the sensory innervation of the whole of the hindlimbs distal to the knee with exception of a small medial strip innervated by the saphenous branch of the femoral nerve.
2. The pudendal nerve originates in the spinal cord segments S1–S2–S3. It provides motor innervation to the external anal sphincter and the caudal rectus muscle. It provides sensory innervation to the prepuce, peritoneum, vulva and scrotum.
3. The pelvic nerve originates from the spinal cord segments S1–S2–S3. It innervates the smooth muscles of the bladder and rectum.
3. The caudal nerves arise from Cd1–Cd5; they are responsible for the motor and sensory innervation of the tail.

Occurrence: Common.

Aetiology: DLSS occurs due to stenosis of the lumbosacral vertebral canal leading to compression of the blood vessels and nerves which form the cauda equina. DLSS can start between L6 and L7, but it occurs more commonly between L7 and S1. The hindlimbs are responsible for moving the body forwards and so the joint between L7–S1 is particularly subjected to strain during running or jumping, i.e. physical activity. Arthrosis can develop relatively easily in this joint. The degenerative changes are progressive and occur in older animals.

The following factors can accelerate the process and make it worse:
1. Breed: Boxer, Doberman, German Shepherd, Rottweiler, Schnauzer, and Siberian Husky are particularly affected; the Poodle is one of the small breeds affected.
2. Body weight: animals under 20 kg are rarely affected.
3. Strain.

4. Genetic malformations: every abnormal structure puts the region under a greater or unbalanced strain. The most common associated defect is a so-called transitional vertebra, i.e. sacralisation of the last lumbar vertebra or lumbarisation of S1. The clinical picture worsens when this problem leads to unilateral or bilateral changes in the sacroiliac joint.

Excessive strain at the level of L7–S1 can induce the following problems:

Intervertebral disc herniation (Hansen type II).
- Hypertrophy of the interarcuate ligaments or the dorsal longitudinal ligament.
- Subluxation.
- Hypertrophy of the joint surfaces.

Clinical: A constant factor is pain. At the beginning, it is not recognised by the owner and it is often interpreted by them as their animal "becoming lazy" or "aging". The dog does not want to walk upstairs or jump into the car, etc.

Manifestations of pain can be elicited during the neurological examination with the following manipulations:
- Overextension of the tail with or without concomitant pressure on the lumbosacral region.
- Energetic pressing down on the L7–S1 joint, resulting in the animal sitting down or showing pain in other ways.
- Overextension of the hindlegs (both together and individually). The expression of pain with this manipulation occurs not only with DLSS, but it may also be due to orthopaedic disease.

The pain is reduced by cage rest and increased with physical activity. Despite this, it should not be forgotten that an arthrosis forms the basis of this syndrome, which in general causes less problems after a "warming-up" period of exercise. Weakness is another clinical sign seen during the course of DLSS. The hindlimbs are "dropped" in their posture as the joints are more flexed than normal and it is difficult for the animal to stand up. The paresis can also manifest in the tail muscles. Pain and weakness are early signs of DLSS and may be the only ones present.

In the later stages of this disease, the following clinical signs can be seen:
- Atrophy of the muscle groups innervated by the sciatic nerve. The whole of the hindlimb musculature can be affected with the exception of the quadriceps muscles which are innervated by the femoral nerve.
- Proprioception deficits.
- The flexor reflex is reduced, but only rarely is it completely absent. In the majority of cases, it appears normal when examined superficially.
- A normal response to this reflex is a strong retraction of the hindlimbs. In cases of DLSS, the flexion of the coxofemoral joint is not affected as the femoral nerve is not in-

14

volved in the disease process. In contrast, flexion of the knee and the tarsal joints is reduced or lacking. Another abnormal response to this reflex is repeated flexion and extension of the limbs as if the dog is trying to kick the investigator. This is interpreted as weakness.

- The tibialis cranialis reflex is often normal or reduced; it is rarely absent (stenosis L6–L7).
- The patella reflex is normal or appears to be increased (pseudohyperreflexia).
- The perineal reflex is often reduced and the anus can be dilated, although not always.

Sensation is often normal. The nails may be more worn than those of the normal limbs due to the weak "dragging" gait; this may affect one side more than the other. Incontinence occurs more in the later stages. Other differential diagnoses causing pain in the pelvic area must be excluded (e.g. prostate disease or arthrosis of the hips). Trauma can lead to fractures, luxation, haematoma and/or oedema at the level of the cauda equina. The acute onset and anamnesis allow for an easy differentiation. Discospondylitis can cause acute clinical signs and must be taken into consideration, especially in young animals. Neoplasia (primary or metastases) of the surrounding tissues (prostate or anal glands) and especially of the bone can have similar clinical signs.

Diagnosis: Plain radiography can reveal degenerative changes in the bone, subluxation, hypertrophy of the joint surfaces, sclerosis of the epiphyses, discospondylitis, narrowing of the intervertebral spaces and spondylosis. A definitive diagnosis can only be attained with contrast investigations to show compression of the nervous structures. In myelography, the contrast agent is poorly disseminated and collects in the dural sac (see Fig. 6.27). The limitation of this investigation is that lateral compression may not necessarily be seen as the dural sac can terminate at the level of L7 in approx. 20% of dogs. The results can be improved if myelography is performed with flexion and extension of the spine. Epidurography allows visualization of lesions if the lumbosacral region can be outlined with contrast. CT and MRI are the most precise methods for revealing significant changes, especially in combination with EMG testing.

Therapy: The first stage of therapy is cage rest. Through rest, the inflammation that is at least partially responsible for the clinical symptoms can resolve. The use of steroidal anti-inflammatory drugs can support the healing process but they are contraindicated if the animal is able to move around too much. Conservative treatment is recommended for those cases in which the only symptom is pain or when more than one intervertebral disc space is affected. The long-term success of the therapy depends also on radical changes being made in the animal's habits. The changes must be directed to ensure that the lumbosacral joint is protected. An increase in body weight is unwanted with this disease. In relapsing or clinically severely affected cases, decompression of the nerve fibres must be performed. A dorsal laminectomy at the level of L7–S1, removal of the yellow ligament or the disc, foramenectomy, facetectomy and stabilisation of the joint are all different techniques that can be used depending on the degree of change.

Prognosis: The prognosis is usually good as the cauda equina, in contrast to the spinal cord, is able to recover quite well. In some cases, the main problem is management of large, heavy animals over a very long period of convalescence. The animals must be rested for 2 to 3 months post-surgery due to the risk of post operative scarring

Literature

1 BAILEY, C.S., MORGAN J.P. (1992): Congenital spinal malformations. Vet Clin North Am Small Anim Pract. **22**: 985–1015.

2 BECK, J.A., SIMPSON, D.J., TISDALL, P.L.(1999): Surgical management of osteochondromatosis affecting the vertebrae and trachea in an Alaskan Malamute. Aust Vet J. **77**: 21–23.

3 BERROCAL, A., TJALSMA, E.J., KOEMAN, J.P. (1992): Calcinosis circumscripta in two cats, Feline Pract. **20**: 9–2.

4 BJERKAS, I., (1977): Hereditary cavitating leukodstrophie in Dalmatian dogs. Acta Neuropathol. **40**:163–169.

5 CAUZINILLE, L., KORNEGAY, J.N. (1996): Fibrocartilaginous embolism of the spinal cord in dogs: review of 36 histologically confirmed cases and retrospective study of 26 suspected cases. J Vet Intern Med. **10**: 241–245.

6 CHAMBERS, J.N., SELCER, B.A., SULLIVAN, S.A., COATES, J.R. (1997): Diagnosis of lateralized lumbosacral disk herniation with magnetic resonance imaging. J Am Anim Hosp Assoc. **33**: 296–299.

7 CHILD, G., HIGGINS, R.J., CUDDON, P.A. (1986): Acquired skoliosis associated with hydromyelia and syringomyelia in two dogs. J Am Vet Med Assoc. **189**: 909–912.

8 CIZINAUSKAS, S., JAGGY, A., TIPOLD, A. (2000): Long-term treatment of dogs with steroid-responsive meningitis-arteriitis: clinical, laboratory and therapeutic results. J Small Animal Pract. **41**: 295–301.

9 COATES, J.R. (2000): Intervertebral disk disease. Vet Clin North Am Small Anim Pract. **30**: 77–110.

10 CUMMINGS, J.F., deLAHUNTA, A. (1978): Heriditary myelopathy of Afghan hounds, a myelinolytic disease. Acta Neuropathol. **42**: 173–181.

11 DEFORSTER, M.E., BASKUR, P.K., (1979): Malformations and the Manx-syndrome in cats. Can Vet J. **20**: 304–314.

12 DEMIERRE, S., TIPOLD, A., GRIOT-WENK, M.E., WELLE, M., VANDEVELDE, M., JAGGY, A. (2001): Correlation between the clinical course of granulomatous meningoencephalomyelitis in dogs and the extent of mast cell infiltration. Vet Rec. **148**: 467–472.

14

13 DHUPA, S., GLICKMAN, N.W., WATERS D.J. (1999): Functional outcome in dogs after surgical treatment of caudal lumbar intervertebral disk herniation. J Am Anim Hosp Assoc. **35**: 323–331.

14 DIXON, B.C., TOMLINSON, J.L., KRAUS, K.H. (1996): Modified distraction-stabilisation technique using an interbody polymethyl methylacrylate plug in dogs with caudal cervical spondylopathy. J Am Vet Assoc. **208**: 61–68.

15 DOIGE, C. (1987): Multiple cartilaginous exostoses in dogs. Vet Path. **24**: 276–278.

16 DONE, S.H. (1975): Hemivertebra in the dog: clinical and pathological observations. Vet Rec. **96**: 313–317.

17 DUVAL, J., DEWEY, C., ROBERTS, R., ARON, D. (1996): Spinal cord swelling as a myelographic indicator of prognosis: a retrospective study in dogs with intervertebral disc disease and loss of deep pain perception. Vet Surg. **25**: 6–12.

18 EWANS, R.J. (1989): Lysosomal storage diseases in dogs and cats. J Small Animal Pract. **30**: 144–150.

19 FATONE, G., BRUNETTI, A., LAMAGNA, F., POTENTA, A. (1995): Dermoid sinus and spinal malformations in a Yorkshire terrier: diagnosis and follow – up. J Small Anim Pract. **36**:178–180.

20 FITCH, R.B., KERWIN, S.C., HOSGOOD, G. (2000): Caudal cervical intervertebral disk disease in the small dog: role of distraction and stabilization in ventral slot decompression. J Am Anim Hosp Assoc. **36**: 68–74.

21 FRYKMANN, O.F. (1999): Spinal arachnoidal cyst in four dogs: diagnosis, surgical treatment and follow-up results. J Small Anim Pract. **40**: 544–549.

22 GALLOWA, A.M., CURTIS, N.C., SOMMERLAD, S.F., WATT, P.R. (1999): Correlative imaging findings in seven dogs and one cat with spinal arachnoidal cysts. Vet Radiol Ultrasound. **40**: 445–452.

23 GAMBLE, D.A., CHRISMAN, C.L. (1984): A leukoencephalomyelopathy of Rottweiler dogs. Vet Pathol. **21**: 274–280.

24 GAVIN, P.R., FIKE, J.R., HOOPES, P.J. (1995): Central nervous system tumors. Semin Vet Med Surg. **10**: 180–189.

25 GILL, P.J., LIPPINCOTT, C.L., ANDERSON, S.M. (1996): Dorsal laminectomy in the treatment of cervical intervertebral disk disease in small dogs: a retrospective study of 30 cases. J Am Anim Hosp Assoc. **32**: 77–80.

26 GHOSH, P., TAYLOR, T.K., BRAUND, K.G., LARSEN, L.H. (1976): A comparative chemical and histochemical study of the chondrodystrophoid and nonchondrodystrophoid canine intervertebral disc. Vet Pathol. **13**: 414–427.

27 GOLDMAN, A.L. (1992): Hypervitaminosis A in a cat. J Am Vet Med Assoc. **200**: 1970–1972.

28 HARTLEY, W.J., PALMER, A.C. (1973): Ataxie in Jack Russell terriers. Acta Neuropathol (Berl). **26**: 71–74.

29 HAWTHORNE, J.C., BLEVINS, W.E., WALLACE, L.J., GLICKMAN, N., WATERS, D.J. (1999): Cervical vertebral fractures in 56 dogs: a retrospective study. J Am Anim Hosp Assoc. **35**:135–146.

30 JACOBSON, L.S., KIRBERGER, R.M. (1996): Canine multiple cartilaginous exostoses: unusual manifestation and review of the literature. J Am Anim Hosp Assoc. **32**: 45–51.

31 JAGGY, A., LANG, J. (1986): Zervikale Spondylopathie ("Wobbler-Syndrom") beim Hund. Schweiz Arch Tierheilk. **128**: 385–399.

32 JANSSENS, L.A.A. (1991): Mechanical and pathophysiological aspects of acute spinal cord trauma. J Small Animal Pract. **32**: 572–578.

33 JEFFERY, N.D. (1996): Dorsal cross pinning of atlantoaxial joint: new surgical technique for atlantoaxial subluxation. J Small Animal Pract. **37**: 26–29.

34 JENSEN, V.F., ARNBJERG, J. (2001): Development of intervertebral disk calcification in the Dachshund: a prospective longitudinal radiographic study. J Am Anim Hosp Assoc, **37**: 274–282.

35 JUNKER, K., VAN DEN INGH, T.S., BOSSARD, M.M., VAN NES, J.J. (2000): Fibrocartilaginous embolism of the spinal cord (FCE) in juvenile Irish Wolfshounds. Vet Q. **22**:154–156.

36 KIPPENES, H., GAVIN, P.R., BAGLEY, R.S. SILVER, G.M., TUCKER, R.L., SANDE, R.D. (1999): Magnetic resonance imaging features of tumors of the spine and spinal cord in dogs. Vet Radiol Ultrasound **40**: 627–633.

37 LANG, J. (1988): Flexion-extension myelography of the canine cauda equina. Vet Radiol Ultrasound **29**: 242–257.

38 LEMARIE, R.J., KERWIN, S.C., PARTINGTON, B.P., HOSGOOD, G. (2000): Vertebral subluxation following ventral cervical decompression in the dog. J Am Anim Hosp Assoc. **36**: 348–358.

39 LEVITSKI, R.E., LIPSITZ, D., CHAUVET, A.E. (1999): Magnetic resonance imaging of the cervical spine in 27 dogs. Vet Radiol Ultrasound **40**: 332–341.

40 LEVY, M.S., MAULDIN, G., KAPATKIN, A.S., PATNAIK, A.K. (1997): Nonlymphoid vertebral canal tumors in cats: 11 cases (1987–1995). J Am Vet Med Assoc. **210**: 663–664.

41 LEVY, M.S., KAPATKIN, A.S., PATNAIK, A.K. MAULDIN, G.N., MAULDIN, G.E. (1997): Spinal tumors in 37 dogs: clinical outcome and long-term survival (1987–1994). J Am Anim Hosp Assoc. **33**: 307–312.

41a PETERSEN, S.A., STURGES, B.K., DICKINSON, P.J., POLLARD, R.E., KASS, P.H., KENT, M., VERNAU, K.M., LECOUTEUR, R.A., HIGGINS, R.J. (2008): Canine intraspinal meningiomas: imaging features, histopathologic classification, and long-term outcome in 34 dogs. J Vet Intern Med. **22** (4): 946–953.

41b DERNELL, W.S., VAN VECHTEN, B.J., STRAW, R.C., LARUE, S.M., POWERS, B.E., WITHROW, S.J. (2000): Outcome following treatment of vertebral tumors in 20 dogs (1986–1995). J Am Anim Hosp Assoc. **36** (3): 245–251.

42 LIPSITZ, D., LEVITSKI, R.E., CHAUVET, A.E., BERRY, W.L. (2001): Magnetic resonance imaging features of cervical stenotic myelopathy in 21 dogs. Vet Radiol Ultrasound **42**: 20–27.

43 LONGHOFER, S.L., DUNCAN, I.D., MESSING, A. (1990): A degenerative myelopathy in young German shepard dogs, J Small Anim Pract. **31**:199–203.

14

14

44 LUTTGEN, P.J. (1992): Neoplasms of the Spine. Vet. Clin. North Amer Small Anim Pract. **22**: 973–984.

45 LYMAN, R.L., SEIM, H.B. (1991): Viewpoint: Wobbler syndrome. Prog Vet Neurol. **2**: 143–150.

46 MANDIGERS, P.J., VAN NES, J.J., KNOL, B.W., UBBINK, G.J., GRUYS, E. (1993): Hereditary necrotising myelopathy in Kooiker dogs. Res Vet Sci. **54**: 118–123.

47 MCCARTHY, R.J., LEWIS, D.D., HOSGOOD G. (1995): Atlantoaxial subluxation in dogs. Comp Cont Ed. **17**: 215–226.

48 MCKEE, W.M. (1992): A comparison of hemilaminectomy (with concomitant disc fenestration) and dorsal laminectomy for the treatment of thoracolumbar disc protrusion in dogs. Vet Rec. **130**: 296–300.

49 MEINTJES, E., HOSGOOD, G., DANILOFF, J. (1996): Pharmaceutic treatment of acute spinal cord trauma. Comp Contin Ed. **18**: 625–635.

50 MORGAN, J.P., PARENT, J.M., HOLMBERG, D.L. (1993): Cervical pain secondary to intervertebral disc disease in dogs; Radiographic findings and surgical implications. Progr Vet Neurol. **4**: 76–80.

51 NEIGER, R., GASCHEN, F., JAGGY, A. (2000): Gastric mucosal lesions in dogs with acute intervertebral disc disease: characterization and effects of omeprazole or misoprostol. J Vet Intern Med. **14**: 33–36.

52 OLBY, N. (1999): Current concepts in the management of acute spinal cord injury. J Vet Intern Med. **13**: 399–407.

53 OLBY, N.J., MUNANA, K.R., SHARP, N.J., THRALL, D.E. (2000): The computed tomographic appearance of acute thoracolumbar intervertebral disc herniations in dogs. Vet Radiol Ultrasound **41**: 396–402.

54 PALMER, A.C. (1988): Hound ataxie. Vet Rec. **122**: 263–265.

55 PARKER, A.J., ADAMS, W.M., ZACHARY, J.F. (1983): Spinal arachnoid cysts in the dog. J Am Anim Hosp Assoc. **19**: 1001–1008.

56 PARKER, A.J., PARK, R.D. (1974): Occipital dysplasia in the dog. J Am Anim Hosp Assoc. **10**: 520–525.

57 PRATT, J.N., KNOTTENBELT, C.M., WESH E.M. (2000): Dermoid sinus at the lumbosacral junction in an English Springer Spaniel. J Small Anim Pract. **41**: 24–26.

58 RICHARDSON, J.A., TANG, K., BURNS, D.K. (1991): Myeloencephalopathy with Rosenthal fiber formation in a miniature Poodle. Vet Pathol. **28**: 536–538.

59 ROHRER, C.R., HILL, R.C., FISCHER, A., FOX, L.E., SCHAER, M., GINN, P.E., PREAST, V.A., BURROWS, C.F. (1999) Efficacy of misoprostol in prevention of gastric hemorrhage in dogs treated with high doses of methylprednisolone sodium succinate. Am J Vet Res. **60**: 982–985.

60 RUCKER, N.C. (1990): Management of spinal cord trauma. Progr Vet Neurol. **1**: 397–412.

61 RUSBRIDGE, C., WHEELER, S.J., LAMB, C.R., PAGE, R.L., CARMICHAEL, S., BREARLY, M.J., BJORNSON, A.P. (1999): Vertebral plasma cell tumors in 8 dogs. J Vet Intern Med. **13**: 126–133.

62 SCHMID, V., LANG, J. (1993): Measurements on the lumbosacral junction in normal dogs and those with cauda equina compression. J Small Anim Pract. **34**: 437–442.

63 SCHULZ, K.S., WALKER, M., MOON, M., WALDRON, D., SLATER, M., MCDONALD, D.E. (1998): Correlation of clinical, radiographic, and surgical localization of intervertebral disc extrusion in small-breed dogs: a prospective study of 50 cases. Vet Surg. **27**: 105–111.

64 SCHWARZ, T., OWEN, M.R., LONG, S., SULLIVAN M. (2000): Vacuum disk and facet phenomenon in a dog with cauda equina syndrome. J Am Vet Med Assoc. **217**: 862–864.

65 SCOTT, H.W., MCKEE, W.M. (1999): Laminectomy for 34 dogs with thoracolumbar intervertebral disc disease and loss of deep pain perception. J Small Anim Pract. **40**: 417–422.

66 SEIM, H.B. (2000): Diagnosis and treatment of cervical vertebral instability-malformation syndromes. In Kirk's Current Veterinary Therapy XIII, 992–1000.

67 SELCER, E.A., HELLMANN, R.G., SELCER, R.R. (1984): Dermoid sinus in a Shi-Tzu and a Boxer. J. Am Anim Hosp Assoc. **20**: 634–636.

68 SHELL, L.G. (1988): Spinal dysraphism, hemivertebra and stenosis of the spinal canal in a Rottweiler puppy. J Am Anim Hosp Assoc. **24**: 341–344.

69 SORJONEN, D.C. (1992): Myelitis and meningitis. Vet Clin North Am Small Anim Pract. **22**: 951–964.

70 STEAD, A.C., ANDERSON, A.A., COUGHLAN A.R. (1993): Bone plating to stabilise atlantoaxial subluxation in four dogs. J Small Anim Pract. **34**: 462–465.

71 STOFFREGEN, D.A., HUXTABLE, C.R., CUMMINGS, J.F. (1993): Hypomyelination of the central nervous system of two Siamese kitten littermates. Vet Pathol. **30**: 388–391.

72 SUKHIANI, H.R., PARENT, J.M., ATILOLA, M.A., HOLMBERG, D.L. (1996): Intervertebral disk disease in dogs with signs of back pain alone: 25 cases (1986–1993). J Am Vet Med Assoc. **209**: 1275–1279.

73 THOMAS, W.B., SORJENEN, D.C., SIMPSON, S.T. (1991): Surgical management of atlantoaxiale subluxation in 23 dogs. Vet Surg. **20**: 409–412.

74 TIPOLD, A., JAGGY, A (1994): Steroid-responsive meningitis-arteritis in dogs – long-term study of 32 cases. J Small Animal Pract. **35**: 311–316.

75 WATSON, A.G., DE LAHUNTA A. (1989): Atlantoaxial subluxation and absence of transverse ligament of the atlas in a dog. J Am Vet Med Assoc. **195**: 235–237.

76 WOUDA, W., VAN NES J.J. (1986): Progressive ataxia due to central demyelination in Rottweiler dogs. Vet Q. **8**: 89–97.

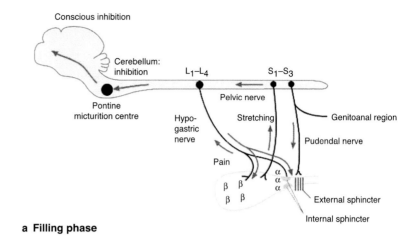

a Filling phase

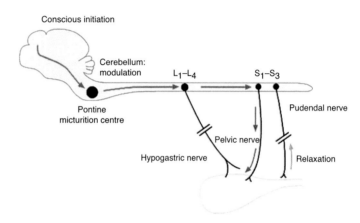

b Emptying phase

Fig. 14.14
Physiological depiction of the micturition reflex. (a) Filling phase (α: α-adrenergic receptors; β: β-adrenergic receptors) and (b) emptying phase.

14

14.2 Bladder disturbances
Susi Arnold, Frank Steffen, André Jaggy

During the filling phase, the bladder serves as a reservoir for the urine, whereby the urethra functions as an external seal. As soon as the urinary bladder has reached a critical degree of filling, micturition takes place reflexively. The bladder serves as an ejection organ and the urethra as an outflow organ.

The filling phase of the bladder and the release of urine are subjected to complex neuronal control. A functional abnormality of the responsible nerve pathways leads to a concomitant disturbance in bladder function.

14.2.1 Micturition reflex

With increasing bladder filling, the pressure rises (negligibly at first) until the elasticity limit of the detrusor smooth muscle fibres is reached. At this point, the stretch receptors are activated and send sensory signals, which run in the pelvic nerves arising from the sacral spinal cord S1–S3, to the spinal cord and then on to the brain stem. At this level, motor nerve cells are stimulated, which then send a signal back to the sacral spinal cord where preganglionic parasympathetic nerves stimulate postganglionic parasympathetic fibres, (which also run in the pelvic nerves), and initiate contraction of the bladder (Fig. 14.14).

In addition to the sensory fibres within the pelvic nerves which form part of the detrusor reflex arc, sensory fibres also run from the bladder via the hypogastric nerves to the spinal cord at the level of L1–L4 in the dog and L2–L5 in the cat. Spinal cord lesions localised caudally in the lumbar or sacral spinal cord, result in loss of the detrusor reflex; however, distension of the bladder is still appreciated as being painful.

The brain stem coordinates the sequence of the micturition reflex and makes certain that this lasts until there is complete emptying of the bladder. Sectioning of the spinal cord at any level between the sacral spinal cord and the brain stem turns off the micturition reflex.

14.2.1.1   Arbitrary control of micturition

The sensory fibres that transmit information about bladder wall stretching to the brain stem also have connections with the cerebrum and cerebellum. The cerebrum is responsible for behavioural control of the micturition reflex which can stop urine flow for a short period (marking behaviour) or for a longer term (house-training). Lesions in the cerebrum can, depending on the circumstances, result in loss of house-training. The frequency of micturition is controlled by connections from the cerebellum to the myelencephalon or medulla. Lesions in the respective cerebellar region lead to an increase in micturition frequency (8).

14.2.1.2   Closure function of the urethra

Closure of the urethra is based on the coordination of different physiological mechanisms. These can be subdivided into two main components: a neuromuscular component (smooth and striated muscles) and a non-neuromuscular component (submucosal vessel plexus and connective tissue). The neuromuscular component forms a total of 60% of the urethral wall pressure, whereby 50% is due to the sympathetic nervous system and 10% to the parasympathetic. The somatic nervous system with its effects on the striated muscle appears not to have any significance for the maintenance of continence. Half of the remaining 40% of the urethral resting pressure is due to the urethral and periurethral connective tissue, and half is due to the submucosal vessel complex (1, 2, 3, 10, 11).

14.2.1.3   Internal and external urethral sphincters

Only smooth muscle fibres are present in the proximal half of the urethra in the female dog. All of these muscle cells are collected together under the term "internal urethral sphincter". The internal urethral sphincter ensures the closure of the urethra during the filling phase of the bladder and is therefore responsible for continence. In the distal half of the female urethra, striated muscles called the external urethral sphincter can be found. The external urethral sphincter contracts in the presence of high abdominal pressure and thereby supports the closure function of the internal sphincter. In comparison, the striated muscles do not make a significant contribution to continence under normal pressure conditions.

In male dogs, the pars membranica and the pars prostatica of the urethra are both histologically and functionally equivalent to the whole of the urethra in the female. Both parts form the proximal 15% of the urethral length and are responsible for continence. In the distal urethra, the striated muscles are the most prominent; they are used to stop the flow of urine during marking.

When there is an abrupt increase in abdominal pressure (coughing, barking), the muscle fibres of the external sphincter are stretched and the sensory nerve fibres transmit the signal via the pudendal nerve to the sacral spinal cord. In both the dog and cat, the motor neurons are located between L7–S3, though mainly in S1 and S2. The response is transmitted via the motor neurons in the pudendal nerve to the external urethral sphincter, which contracts for a short time and so hinders the release of urine. The external sphincter can also be arbitrarily influenced by the nerve tracts that run from the cerebrum to the sacral spinal cord. Lesions in the cerebrum and spinal cord can lead to an increase in tone of the external sphincter and so hamper the urine flow during micturition. Lesions in T3–L3 can interfere with the detrusor reflex and increase the sphincter tone. If the detrusor reflex is elicited without relaxation of the external sphincter, this is termed reflex dyssynergia (8).

The internal urethral sphincter is controlled by the sympathetic nervous system and is imperative in the maintenance of continence. The bladder is also innervated by sympathetic nerves, which run in the hypogastric nerve and whose preganglionic neurons lie in the L1–L4 spinal segments in the dog and L2–L5 in the cat (7, 9). Alpha-adrenergic receptors are specifically located in the trigone and neck of the bladder. They cause contraction of the smooth muscles, which is most probably of significance in the prevention of retrograde ejaculation. Beta-adrenergic receptors are predominantly located in the bladder wall and result in relaxation of the detrusor.

14.2.1.4   Innervation of the detrusor

Although every motor nerve fibre innervates a number of smooth muscle cells, not every smooth muscle cell is directly innervated. When a stimulus arrives, the directly innervated cells contract first and transmit the signal over tight junctions to their neighbouring cells, with the result that the whole of the detrusor contracts within a short time.

14.2.2 Patients with micturition disturbances

An accurate anamnesis can make the diagnostic work-up much easier in patients with micturition disturbances. Often the type of questioning determines whether the information is significant or not. Owners may readily say that their pet has started to urinate in the home; it is important here to differentiate between loss of house-training and urinary incontinence. With loss of house-training, the dog or cat takes on the correct posture for micturition and urinates outside of its sleeping area. In urinary incontinence, by comparison, urine is released spontaneously and often within the dog's sleeping area. The question of whether the dog shows normal micturition behaviour whilst awake is always important. A change in the strength of the urine flow may recently have been observed or the frequency of micturition may have increased. In the latter case, it is significant as to whether the dog has sniffed around prior to micturition; and/or that the increased micturition frequency is compatible with normal marking behaviour or whether the dog abruptly urinates as if in an urgent need, which would be considered pathological.

The clinician should take enough time to gain a complete picture of the patient's micturition behaviour. Before uri-

nation, the bladder should have a certain degree of tone and be palpable. A flaccid bladder is usually pathological. After urination, the bladder should be almost completely empty. It is then maximally contracted and only contains residual urine, which in the dog is normally less than 10 ml. In this case, it can be assumed that the detrusor reflex is functioning normally. Spontaneous bladder contraction can occur in cases which have lost the detrusor reflex due to neurological disease; however, in such cases the residual urine volume is abnormally high (Table 14.3).

Many diseases of the lower urinary tract such as bacterial cystitis, urolithiasis, malformation or neoplasia may manifest themselves clinically similar to a neurological disturbance of micturition. One should always check the anatomical integrity of the lower urinary tract and especially exclude bacterial infections before trying to localise a neurological disturbance.

14.2.2.1 Overstretching of the bladder

Massive overstretching of the bladder wall can damage the tight junctions and the detrusor may no longer contract. The bladder of affected patients is flaccid after emptying and is difficult to express manually because the sphincter function is normal. The patient may be able to partially empty its bladder

Table 14.3: Diagnosis, prognosis and treatment of micturition disorders in small animals

	Diagnosis	Prognosis, treatment
Incontinence	■ Reduced urethral sphincter tone Castration (females) ■ Paralysis of the pudendal nerve ■ Reduced urethral sphincter tone ■ with additional bladder paralysis	■ Hormone treatment, adrenergic stimulation (e.g. phenylpropanolamine 15–20 mg, PO, SID) ■ Renervation possible (depending on the type of lesion) ■ Empty bladder (three times a day); cystitis treatment, cholinergic detrusor stimulation (bethanechol 2.5–25 mg SID to TID, PO or SC) Prognosis with cauda equina lesions: good to guarded. Prognosis with lesions of the sacral spinal cord: poor.
Retention	■ Spasm of the urethral sphincter ■ Spinal cord lesions above S1–S3 ■ Normal sphincter tone ■ Bladder atony (with chronic obstruction) ■ Normal sphincter tone ■ Paralysis of pelvic nerve	■ Empty bladder (three times a day): cystitis treatment; relaxation of sphincter with α-blockers (phenoxybenzamine 0.25–0.5 mg/kg PO, SID to TID) and diazepam 0.25–1.0 mg/kg PO. Prognosis depends on the primary spinal lesion. ■ Treat primary cause; empty bladder frequently (possibly permanent catheter); cystitis treatment; detrusor stimulation (bethanechol 2.5–25 mg, PO or SC, SID to TID). Prognosis of chronic dilatation: guarded. ■ Renervation of pelvic nerve possible (depending on the type of lesion).
Anomalous micturition (reflex dyssynergy)	■ Brain lesion ■ Partial spinal cord lesion	■ Possible sphincter relaxation with α-blockers (phenoxybenzamine 0.25–0.5 mg/kg PO, SID to TID) and diazepam. 0.25–1.0 mg/kg PO. Prognosis depends on primary lesion.
Loss of house training (without incontinence)	■ Brain lesion ■ Polyuria/polydipsia ■ Purely behavioural disturbances	■ Treatment of the primary lesion (see Chap. 18). Prognosis depends on primary lesion.

14

using its abdominal muscles. Such attempts at micturition indicate that the sensory connections are intact and are indicative of a primary detrusor problem. One of the most common causes of overstretching of the bladder is an obstructive urinary stone.

Overextension of the bladder can also result secondary to increased sphincter activity (UMNS / pudendal nerve). This complication occurs in patients with damage to the thoracolumbar spinal cord if regular emptying of the bladder is not ensured. With reversible damage, the bladder usually recovers within 2 weeks; if there is a more prolonged loss of function, then it undergoes fibrosis and recovery may be permanently compromised.

14.2.2.2 The patient does not urinate, the bladder can be manually expressed

Rarely, lesions in the region between the myelencephalon and spinal cord segment L7 lead to a loss of detrusor reflex without an increase in the tone of the external urethral sphincter. Traumatic damage to the pelvis can lead to injury of the pelvic plexus without injury to the pudendal nerve. The patient cannot urinate, but the bladder can be relatively easily expressed by hand. The perineal reflex is intact. Certain pharmacological compounds can also lead to urinary retention; e.g. calcium channel blockers, anticholinergics, opioids and tricyclic antidepressants such as clomipramine.

Hospitalisation, pain or disease which lead to the animal remaining recumbent and so hinder it urinating, are possible causes of urinary retention with an expressible bladder.

14.2.2.3 The patient does not urinate, the bladder can be easily expressed or the urine is spontaneously released

Lesions of the sacral spinal cord or the nerve roots lead to a loss of both the reflexes of the detrusor and the urethral sphincter. The bladder can be easily expressed and there is a possible continual loss of urine. The perineal reflex is weak or missing. Neurological diseases that are the cause of this common form of urinary incontinence are listed in Table 14.3.

14.2.2.4 Increased micturition frequency

The frequent, spontaneous release of small amounts of urine is suspicious for a partial lesion of the spinal cord (UMNS) or the cerebellum. Bacterial cystitis can also induce similar clinical signs. The bladder is always completely emptied. The bladder capacity slowly reduces due to the high frequency of micturition. The perineal reflex is normal.

14.2.2.5 Sudden cessation of urine flow during micturition

After normal initiation of micturition, the urine flow suddenly and spontaneously stops due to contraction of the external urethral sphincter. Often the patient remains in the micturition stance although no urine is released. This is the typical picture of reflex dyssynergia. The detrusor reflex is normal while the perineal reflex is often increased.

The term dyssynergia in this situation means simultaneous contraction of muscles which have opposite effects. The cause of the dyssynergia between the detrusor and the internal and external urethral sphincters lies in the suppression of the normal inhibitory pontospinal signals from the micturition centre to the sympathetic and somatic reflex centres in the spinal and sacral cord; these inhibitory signals normally lead to flaccidity of the urethral muscles. An idiopathic form of this disease is known as detrusor-sphincter dyssyneria (urethrospasm, functional bladder neck obstruction, reflex dyssynergia) and usually affects male dogs of large and medium-sized breeds (young to middle age). The syndrome is seen both in neutered and intact animals. Sexual excitement can potentially increase the problem, so neutering may help but rarely completely. Excessive water intake or excessive physical activity are further predisposing factors seen in individual dogs.

Other causes of dyssynergia or incoordinated micturition with cessation of urine flow include partial lesions of the UMNS or diseases of the cauda equina.

14.2.2.6 Urinary incontinence as a consequence of urethral incompetence

Reduction of the sphincter function leads to urinary incontinence. The patient can completely empty the bladder during micturition (normal detrusor function), but the urine is spontaneously / involuntarily released in small amounts. This type of incontinence occurs mainly in female dogs and is the most serious side-effect of neutering. The dogs usually lose urine whilst sleeping and only in severe cases is urine lost whilst the animal is awake. This type of incontinence occurs most frequently in connection with increased abdominal pressure (barking, jumping, coughing, etc.).

Reduced urethral closure can be seen as a consequence of a urethral lesion after prostate operations, perineal urethrostomy or improper catheterisation.

14

Literature

1 AWAD, S.A., DOWNIE, J.W. (1976): Relative contributions of smooth and striated muscles to the canine urethral pressure profile. Brit J Urol. **48**: 347–354.

2 BUMP, R.C., FRIEDMAN, C.I., COPELAND, W.E. (1988): Non-neuromuscular determinants of intraluminal urethral pressure in the female baboon: Relative importance of vascular and nonvascular factors. J Urol. **139**: 162–164.

3 DOWNIE, J.W., AWAD, S.A. (1976): Role of neurogenic factors in canine urethral wall tension and urinary continence. Invest Urol. **14**: 143–147.

4 ESPINEIRA, M.M.D., VIEHOFF, F.W, NICKEL, R.F. (1998): Idiopathic detrusor-urethral dyssynergia in dogs: A retrospective analysis of 22 cases. J Small Anim Pract. **39**: 264–270.

5 LANE, I.F. (2000): Diagnosis and management of urinary retention. Vet Clin North Am Small Anim Pract. **30**: 25–57.

6 MOREAU, P.M. (1989): Pharmacologic management of urinary incontinence. Proceedings of the 4th Annual Symposium of the ESVNU, October 11th, D-Giessen. pp. 112–143.

7 OLIVER, J.E. Jr., BRADLEY, W.E., FLETCHER, T.F. (1969): Spinal cord representation of the micturition reflex. J Comp Neurol. **137**: 329–346.

8 OLIVER, J.E., LORENZ, M.D. (eds.) (1983): Visceral dysfunction. In: Handbook of veterinary neurologic diagnosis. W.B. Saunders Company, Philadelphia, pp. 90–106.

9 PURINTON, P.T., OLIVER, J.E., Jr. (1979): Spinal cord origin of innervation to the bladder and urethra of the dog. Exp. Neurol. **65**: 422–434.

10 RAZ, S., CAINE, M., ZEIGLER, M. (1972): The vascular component in the production of intraurethral pressure. J Urol. **108**: 93–96.

11 RUD, T. (1980): Urethral pressure profile in continent women from childhood to old age. Acte Obstet Gynecol Scand. **59**: 331–335.

14

15 Vestibular Apparatus

Massimo Baroni
Massimo Mariscoli
André Jaggy

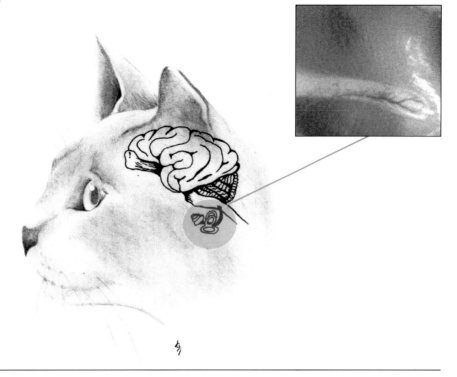

The position of the body in space generates a multitude of information which is transferred to the brain for processing. It is the brain's function to organise the apparent cacophony of information that arises from three different systems: the visual, proprioceptive and vestibular systems. The vestibular system is essential for the maintenance of normal body positioning and balance, whereby information about gravity, body rotation and its acceleration/deceleration is processed. The vestibular system is not important in the initiation of movement, but it needs to function efficiently to coordinate head position, eye movements and the extensor muscle tone – all of which depend on the position of the body in space and its movement.

15.1 Functional anatomy

The vestibular system consists of a peripheral (labyrinth with sensory receptors and the vestibular nerve) and a central part (vestibular nucleus in the brain stem; see Fig. 1.26).

The sensory vestibular receptors lie in the membranous labyrinth, within the bony labyrinth, located in the petrous bone. Three different regions that all belong to the vestibular system can be differentiated in the labyrinth: the utricle, the saccule and the semi-circular canals. The utricle is a widening of the membranous labyrinth at the base of the semi-circular canals. The saccule is a ball-shaped structure that lies between the utricle and the cochlea. Both the utricle and saccule contain a vestibular sensory receptor, the macula. This consists of a connective tissue layer that is covered with neurosensory epithelium, which is itself made up of special cells with hair-like processes on their apical surfaces (hair cells). There are two types of hairs on the hair cells: a large number of stereocilia and a single kinocilium. The surface of the macula is covered with a gelatinous substance, the otolithic membrane that contains a certain number of calcium carbonate crystals, the otoliths or otoconia. Bending of the stereocilia in the direction of the kinocilium causes depolarisation of the cell membrane and induction of an action potential. In contrast, movement of the stereocilia away from the kinocilium causes hyperpolarisation of the cell.

Stimulus of the macula occurs through linear acceleration (1).

The three semi-circular canals, which arise from the utricle, run orthogonally and they are differentiated into the rostral, caudal and lateral ducts.

15

At the origin of each duct, there is an ampulla, which contains the sensory receptors and is called the crista ampullaris. It consists of a connective tissue base that supports the neurosensory epithelium. As in the macula, this epithelium develops hair cells (stereocilia and a kinocilium). These cilia are also embedded in a gelatinous membrane, the cupula, which extends throughout the whole duct. The whole of the membranous labyrinth, including the semi-circular canals, is filled with endolymph, a fluid which is similar to intracellular cytoplasm. Movement of the head causes the endolymph in the canal, lying in the plane of the movement, to flow. The flow of endolymph then causes bending of the cupula and the stereocilia. The bending of the stereocilia stimulates the cell membrane either to depolarise or hyperpolarise, depending on the direction of the movement. Every semi-circular canal on one side of the head has its opposite on the other side, which also lies in the same plane (left and right lateral, left rostral and right caudal, left caudal and right rostral). Each of the semi-circular canals in a pair is oriented in a diametrically opposite direction, so that depolarisation of one is accompanied by hyperpolarisation of the other. Accordingly, one vestibular apparatus will be more strongly stimulated by a movement than the contralateral side. The crista ampullaris is influenced by movements that have an angular acceleration.

The stimulus from the sensory receptors is transferred to the brain via the vestibular part of CN VIII. The bodies of the bipolar neurons, which form the vestibular nerve, lie in a ganglion located in the inner auditory canal in the petrous bone. Peripheral axons of these neurons extend to the hair cells, while their central axon synapses with the vestibular nuclei. Some fibres, however, do not have such synapses, and ascend directly to the cerebellum.

There are four vestibular nuclei on each side: medial, lateral, rostral and caudal. They lie in the dorsal part of the medulla, in the area bordering the lateral wall of the fourth ventricle and directly in the neighbourhood of other important structures, such as the caudal cerebellar peduncle and the ascending system of consciously appreciated proprioception. The vestibular nuclei have anatomical and functional connections with different parts of the CNS. They are connected to the nuclei of the nerves responsible for eye movements (CN III, IV and VI) in the brain stem via the medial longitudinal fasciculus (see Fig. 1.26). Some of the axons extend into the vomiting centre in the reticular formation of the medulla. An important transmission line, the vestibulospinal tract (lying predominantly in the ventral funiculus of the spinal cord) connects the vestibular nuclei with the interneurons of the ventral grey matter of the cord. A vestibular stimulus which travels through this tract stimulates the ipsilateral extensor muscles and at the same time, inhibits the ipsilateral flexor muscles. Some fibres cross over the middle and inhibit the tone of the contralateral extensors. The fibres which ascend via the caudal cerebellar peduncle to the cerebellum (flocculonodular lobe and fastigeus nucleus) come from the nuclei or directly from the vestibular nerve These connections are es-

sential for maintaining balance during gait and for body posture. Finally, it appears that the vestibular system is functionally connected, via the medial geniculate body and the internal capsule, with the temporal cortex for conscious awareness of equilibrium.

15.2 Disturbances of vestibular function

Posture

Head tilt is the cardinal symptom of a vestibular syndrome. The head posture in a healthy animal is checked by a coordinated stimulus of both inner ears (vestibuli), which then provide the brain periodically with all the necessary information for the maintenance of correct head posture. If, for example, a dog has a head tilt to the right, the right vestibuli are excited and the left inhibited. In the case of a unilateral vestibular disease, the rate of excitation of the affected side is reduced which leads to false information with respect to the position of the head reaching the brain. As a consequence, one can observe a tilting of the head in the direction of the affected side (head tilt).

Gait

The term vestibular ataxia contains all the pathological changes that can be observed in the gait of an animal with vestibular syndrome. Depending on the severity of the disease, the animal shows a lateral twist, falling or rolling movements in the direction of the side of the lesion. Sometimes tight circling in this direction can also be observed.

All these clinical signs are associated with a loss of control of the vestibular system on the muscle tone. As the reduced extensor tone on the affected side is coupled with an increased extensor tone on the contralateral side, the animal cannot maintain its balance in the direction of the hypotonic side of the body; consequently, the more acute the disease, the more severe the ataxia. In a peracute syndrome, the animal is no longer capable of standing, at least in the first hours after the start of the clinical signs. In chronic cases, and even severe ones, the ataxia is milder. A lateral twist is the most common symptom.

Nystagmus

Spontaneous nystagmus is a typical concomitant symptom of vestibular disease, especially in the acute stage. In healthy animals, the eye movements are controlled by the vestibular system as an answer to the head or body movements. The vestibular apparatus sends the information via the medial longitudinal fasciculus to the nuclei of CN III, IV and VI; thereby controlling the contractions of the extraocular muscles. If one inner ear (vestibule) is damaged, the incoming information from both sides is no longer balanced, and this imbalanced influence is interpreted by the brain as a head movement. Its answer is the induction of a spontaneous nystagmus (see Table 1.2). Nystagmus is often not present in chronic diseases of the vestibular system because a central compensation for the vestibular deficit occurs. One can differentiate between a rapid and a slow phase in nystagmus, whereby the rapid phase shows the direction of the nystagmus.

Nystagmus can be horizontal, vertical, rotatory ± positional (the direction changes with passive movement of the head or the nystagmus is induced by manipulating the head). In horizontal or rotatory nystagmus, the rapid phase indicates the side of the lesion. In diseases, which affect the central part of the vestibular system all the different forms of nystagmus can be seen; in peripheral lesions, however, horizontal or rotatory forms are present in the majority of cases. In other words, vertical or positional nystagmus are typical for central vestibular disease.

Pendular nystagmus must be differentiated from the previously described forms. In this type of nystagmus, the rapid and slow phases cannot be differentiated from each other. Pendular nystagmus is a type of tremor and can be observed with cerebellar disease.

Strabismus

Ventral strabismus can be visible on the side of the vestibular lesion – sometimes it is more pronounced when the animal's neck is overextended.

Associated clinical symptoms

Facial nerve paralysis is often associated with a peripheral disease of the vestibular system (see Fig. 1.25). The facial nerve originates from the brain stem close to the vestibulocochlear nucleus, enters the internal auditory meatus and then runs through the facial channel in the petrous bone. It exits the petrous portion of the temporal bone, and so the cranium, through the stylomastoid foramen. Bearing this anatomical relationship in mind, it is easy to understand why a lesion located in the petrous bone can affect both the vestibular system and the facial nerve. A central vestibular lesion may even impair the facial nerve and in such cases, other structures in the brain stem are also affected; tetraparesis and multiple cranial nerve deficits can be the consequence.

Horner's syndrome can also be observed in peripheral disease of the vestibular system. Indeed, the sympathetic nerve fibres to the eye cross through the tympanic bulla and are often damaged in diseases of the middle ear.

A unilateral loss of hearing occurs often due to the anatomical connection between the auditory and vestibular systems in association with a peripheral vestibular disease. In addition, a central disease of the vestibular system may often extend to the brain stem and so to the vestibular nuclei. In addition, the descending motor tracts (paresis), ascending proprioceptive tracts (ataxia), other cranial nerve nuclei (multiple cranial

nerve deficits), and the reticular system (reduced consciousness) may be included in the disease process.

The clinical symptom of vomiting tends to be rare in animals in association with vestibular disease; despite this, it may occur with peracute disease.

Postural and placement reactions

The testing of postural and placement reactions is essential for the differentiation of central and peripheral vestibular syndromes. An examination of the patient's proprioception is most useful for testing whether the lesion is in the central structures of the vestibular system (the brain stem) or not. Ascending proprioceptive nerve fibres run very close to the vestibular nuclei at the level of the caudal brain stem. Usually because of this, they are mutually damaged by lesions in this area, even focal ones. Due to the position of the vestibular nuclei in the caudal brain stem, the proprioceptive deficit is observed on the side of the lesion. In peracute syndromes, independent of whether they are peripheral or central, the assessment of proprioception can be difficult or even impossible as the animal cannot stand. In such cases, it is useful to examine the animal again after a few hours or on the next day, when the vestibular ataxia has been better compensated for (see Fig. 1.41).

15.2.1 Paradoxical vestibular syndrome

As already described above, both the central and peripheral vestibular syndromes are associated with head tilt to the side of the lesion. In diseases with a central location that affects the cerebellar peduncles and flocculonodular lobe (archicerebellum), a head tilt in the direction of the contralateral side can be observed. The other clinical symptoms (ventral strabismus, hypotonus of the extensor muscles with sinking down or falling over), which are caused by the lesion also all affect the contralateral side (Fig. 15.1). In such cases, the correct neuroanatomical localisation is confirmed by testing the proprioception, which indicates a deficit on the side of the lesion, i.e. contralateral to the head tilt.

A neuroanatomical and physiological explanation can be given for this clinical manifestation known as "paradoxical vestibular syndrome". As mentioned above, the normal position of the head is maintained by information which is "fired off" by both vestibuli. When an inner ear "fires" at a lower threshold than normal due to a pathological change, then the head tilt is aimed at the vestibule on this side. As a consequence, a direct lesion of the vestibular structures provokes head tilt in this direction. There is a close relationship between the cerebellum (especially the archicerebellum) and the vestibular system. The cerebellum has an inhibitory effect on the vestibular nuclei. In a lesion that affects the archicerebellum (flocculonodular lobe) or the fibres that run between the

15

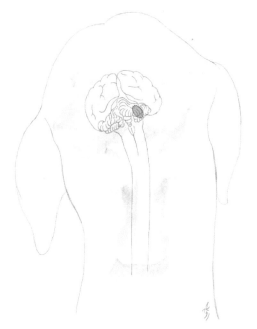

Fig. 15.1
Schematic representation of a lesion in the flocculonodular region, which can induce a paradoxical vestibular syndrome. Typical clinical deficits include head tilt to the contralateral side of the lesion (red area) and other neurological disturbances ipsilateral to the lesion (e. g. deficits in posture and placement reactions, dysfunction of the cranial nerves and gait abnormalities).

cerebellum and the vestibular nuclei (caudal cerebellar peduncle), there is a loss of this inhibitory effect. The vestibular system on the affected side begins to fire with a higher threshold (particularly a higher threshold than the contralateral side). Subsequently, if it is assumed that the head tilt is always to the side with the weakest firing vestibulum, then the head tilt in this case is to the side contralateral to the lesion (see Table 1.2).

15.2.2 Clinical symptoms with bilateral disease

Excessive "throwing" or swinging of the head from side to side characterises a bilateral vestibular syndrome. The animal either crawls or moves in a squatting position so that it does not lose its balance. Physiological nystagmus is normally absent.

15.3 Neurological examination of a vestibular syndrome

One of the most important aids in the neurological examination is to answer the question: "Where is the neuroanatomical localisation of the lesion?" The clinical signs of a vestibular syndrome are very typical and therefore easy to recognise, so that the examiner can usually quickly localise the lesion to the vestibular system. The subsequent question is whether the lesion is peripheral or central. As mentioned before, proprioception plays a decisive role in the differentiation between the two syndromes. Consideration of the other clinical signs such as type of nystagmus, paresis, etc., makes the determination of the location easier. The correct answer to the neuroanatomical question allows the clinician to set up a usable list of differential diagnoses and to choose those adjunct diagnostic aids which are necessary for a definitive diagnosis.

It can be, however, very difficult or even impossible to localise a vestibular disease because:

a) a sudden occurrence of vestibular disease causes such a severe ataxia that the affected animal is unable to stand and is hyperexcited. Under such conditions, a trustworthy and rapid neurological examination is very difficult and the proprioception tests are not interpretable. A second test, a couple of hours or a day later, can help to characterise the neuroanatomical lesion.

b) some slowly progressive intracranial or even extracranial lesions, such as meningioma of the cerebellopontine angle, can induce the slow development of a mild vestibular syndrome with no nystagmus and normal proprioception. In such cases, a false diagnosis of a peripheral vestibular syndrome can be made, and only after a long period of further progression is the clinical manifestation of a central lesion seen.

c) a peripheral lesion can develop into a central lesion (e.g. otitis interna that leads to the development of meningitis via the internal auditory meatus).

15

Table 15.1: Differential diagnoses for peripheral vestibular diseases

I	<ul><li>Otitis media-interna</li><li>Polyps (nasopharyngeal)</li><li>Tinnitus (complication?)</li></ul>

T	<ul><li>Traumatic rupture of the ear drum</li><li>Fracture of the petrous temporal bone</li><li>Intoxication with:
	  – Antibiotics
	  – Antiseptics (local treatment)
	  – Heavy metals</li></ul>

A	<ul><li>Congenital vestibular syndrome</li></ul>
M	<ul><li>Hypothyroidism</li></ul>
I	<ul><li>(Geriatric) idiopathic vestibular syndrome</li></ul>
N	<ul><li>Adenocarcinoma</li><li>Ceruminous gland adenoma</li><li>Cholesteatoma</li><li>Chondrosarcoma</li><li>Fibrosarcoma</li><li>Melanoma</li><li>Neurofibroma</li><li>Osteosarcoma</li><li>Squamous cell carcinoma</li></ul>

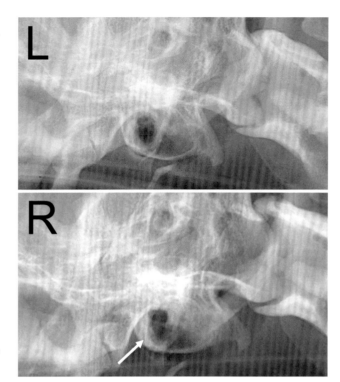

Fig. 15.2a
Radiograph of chronic otitis with bulla osteitis. Six weeks after the start of the clinical symptoms, increased radiodensity in the right bulla could be seen. The bulla wall is thickened and has slightly irregular contours (arrow).

15.4 Diseases of the peripheral vestibular apparatus

Differential diagnosis: Usually the examiner determines the neuroanatomical localisation during the work-up of a neurological case and then formulates a list of differential diagnoses according to the VITAMIN D scheme. Differential diagnoses for peripheral vestibular diseases are shown in Table 15.1.

Diagnosis: The recording of the anamnesis is essential in finding out whether ototoxic substances have been administered or not. Haematology and blood biochemistry are the second diagnostic step. If there are no specific signs of metabolic disease (hypercholesterolaemia, etc.), then this is a reason for undertaking specialised blood investigations (thyroid values: TSH, fT4, etc.)

A careful **otoscopic examination** is done in the sedated / anaesthetised patient. It should not be done in the conscious animal as the results are inexact. An otoscope with the aid of an endoscope is the best method of investigating the ear drum and its pathological changes. When an inflammatory lesion is suspected, a myringotomy can be done with a 22-gauge spinal needle. The tympanic bulla should be washed out with sterile saline; the washing solution can be then used for bacteriological investigations.

The bony structures of the middle ear including the tympanic bulla can be visualised **radiographically** (Fig. 15.2a). For a complete radiographic study, it is necessary to take views in four different planes: VD, through the open mouth as well as obliquely from the left and right. The radiographs can reveal fluid accumulation in the bulla, sclerosis or lysis of the bone, as well as fractures of the petrous bone. Despite this, radiographs which appear normal can be taken even when the bulla is filled with fluid due to an acute infection as the inflammatory fluid is not very radiodense. In such cases, CT (Fig. 15.2b, c) or MRI studies may be necessary to visualise the lesion (2).

15

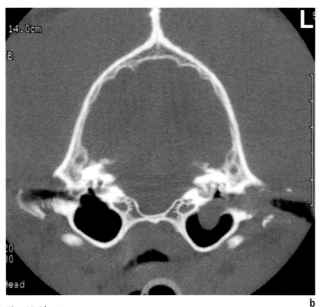
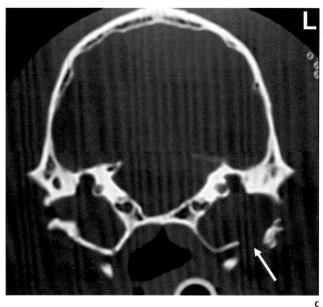

b

c

Fig. 15.2b, c
Otitis media and otitis media / interna with bulla osteitis on CT. (b) Fluid in the area of the ear drum and in the left bulla (animal in sternal recumbency). Well-depicted internal acoustic meatus. (c) Cocker Spaniel: both bullae filled with fluid. Fine foci of osteolysis in the wall of the right bulla. Left: extensive destruction of the bulla wall and the semi-circular canals (arrow). (Pictures: Johann Lang, Berne.)

15

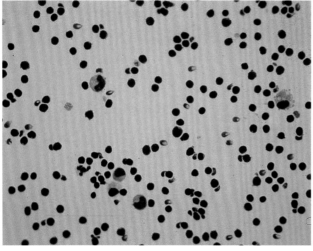

Fig. 15.3
Smear (HE stain) of exudate from the middle ear of a seven-year-old Cocker Spaniel with acute vestibular disturbance showing a mixed population of cells (e.g. macrophages, lymphocytes and neutrophilic granulocytes). The dog had a head tilt to the right, vestibular strabismus on the right, paralysis of the right facial nerve, Horner's syndrome on the right (miosis, ptosis and enophthalamus), severe gait abnormalities with drifting to the right, and from time to time falling down on the left side.

15.4.1 Otitis media / interna

Occurrence: Common. In two retrospective studies on the peripheral vestibular syndrome, otitis media was diagnosed in 49% and 41% of the cases (2, 3).

Aetiology: In the majority of cases, infection penetrates a damaged tympanic membrane from the external auditory canal (4). However, it is not uncommon for middle ear infections to occur without any involvement of the outer ear and the ear drum is intact (Fig. 15.3). Indeed, infection can diffuse up through the eustachian tube from the pharynx or be haematogenous in origin. Frequently, the path of infection remains unclear. Factors such as foreign bodies (grass awns), ear mite allergy, fungal infections (*Malassezia* spp.) or stenosis of the ear canal play a decisive role in chronic otitis externa. They can cause a perforation of the ear drum with extension of the inflammatory processes into the middle ear. Bacteria are the most common causative agents and mainly *Staphylococcus* spp., *Escherichia coli*, *Pseudomonas* spp, *Proteus* spp. and *Enterococci* have been isolated.

Clinical: Vestibular symptoms occur as soon as inflammatory-induced fluid accumulates in the tympanic bulla and the inflammation extends to the labyrinth or the petrous bone. Asymmetrical ataxia, head tilt and positional nystagmus are observed. Hearing damage may be found on occasion. The infection is mainly unilateral but bilateral infections can occur, whereby there can be a complete loss of vestibular sys-

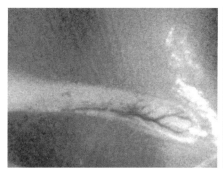

Fig. 15.4a
Otoscopic investigation of the right ear of a two-year-old Boxer. Normal view of the malleus (first auditory ossicle) with its blood vessel.

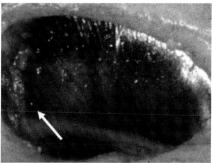

Fig. 15.4b
Otoscopic investigation of a 12-year-old female Cocker Spaniel. The results show an erythematous ear drum and part of the outer auditory canal. Malleus is still visible (arrow). Acute otitis externa/media/interna.

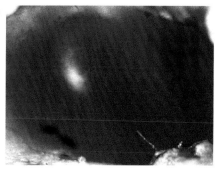

Fig. 15.4c
Otoscopic results showing a markedly erythematous ear drum. The malleus is blurred. Chronic otitis media/interna.

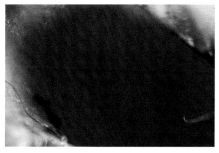

Fig. 15.4d
Otoscopic results showing a markedly erythematous ear drum and outer auditory canal. The malleus can no longer be seen. Chronic otitis media/interna.

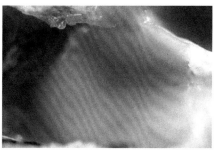

Fig. 15.4e
Otoscopic results of the left ear of a six-year-old Labrador Retriever. Normal view of the milk-white coloured ear drum.

tem function (5). The sympathetic innervation of the eye which runs through the tympanic bulla is often involved, too. As a consequence, a partial or complete Horner's syndrome develops.

The disease process can also invade the petrous bone through the canal of the facial nerve and induce a facial nerve paralysis. This mainly occurs in association with otitis externa. In some cases of severe infection, it is possible to elicit a pain reaction by pressing on the region of the tympanic bulla.

Diagnosis: When there are signs of a middle ear infection associated with otitis externa, the otoscopic examination has both a diagnostic and therapeutic use. As with severe chronic infections the external auditory canal is often displaced by a mixture of fluid and cell debris as well as oedema of the mucosa, a careful washing and aspiration with warm saline is undertaken until the ear drum region is visible (if possible). In the worse case, the ear drum is perforated; this must be assumed even if the tympanic membrane cannot be clearly seen. If the ear drum is perforated, there is no need for myringot-

omy. The cleaning fluid aspirated from the auditory canal is used for cytological and bacteriological investigations.

If there are no indications of otitis externa, the tympanic membrane is carefully investigated (Figs. 15.4a–e). If there is middle ear inflammation, the membrane can appear hyperaemic or opaque, and it may partially protrude into the canal (Fig. 15.5). In such situations, it is sensible to do a myringotomy to confirm the presence of otitis media. A 22-gauge spinal needle is pushed through the membrane, whereby care should be taken not to injury the manubrium of the malleus. With careful aspiration, material is collected for cytological and bacteriological investigations and the bulla is then gently washed out with 0.5–1.0 ml sterile saline.

It is especially wise to take routine radiographic studies of the middle/inner ear which can reveal chronic inflammatory conditions that are associated with dense empyema or sclerosis of the bone. Sadly, false negative results are not uncommon if the disease situation is acute (see Fig. 6.38). CT or MRI offer the best imaging nowadays; even acute processes

15

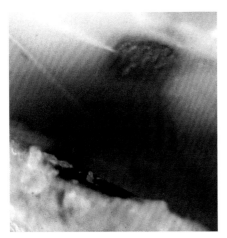

Fig. 15.5
Otoscopic investigation of the right ear of a four-year-old Boxer. The ear drum is coloured milk-white and has a small area of brown discolouration in the upper right quadrant (scarring after iatrogenic perforation: myringotomy).

and their extent can be recognised. MRI is useful in the recognition of brain stem structures and the possible dissemination of disease through the internal auditory canal in the direction of the meninges (see Fig. 6.39).

A hearing test is additionally helpful in the recognition of the lesions in the auditory system and to determine whether the inflammatory process has extended to the brain stem or not (see Chap. 7.1.3).

Therapy: Otitis media/interna can be treated either with medication or by surgery. Systemic antibiotics must be given over a long period of time (2 months) and should be chosen according to the results of the bacterial culture. In the first days of therapy when no bacterial culture results are available, chloramphenicol (30 mg/kg TID), first-generation cephalosporins (20–30 mg/kg TID) or enrofloxacin (10 mg/kg SID; cats ≤ 5 mg/kg SID) are good choices. When otitis externa is present, the external auditory canal should be repeatedly washed out with saline, and debridement should be undertaken. If there is a possible tear in the ear drum, then the local application of antibiotics is recommended.

In cases of severe infection, steroids can be given for 5 to 6 days (prednisolone 0.5 mg/kg SID).

If there appears to be no response to the medication or associated lesions are present (tumour, ear canal stenosis), then surgery should be taken into consideration. Two different methods have been established for bullectomy: (1) ventral bullectomy is indicated when no otitis externa is present; (2) lateral bullectomy is the method of choice when severe

lesions are present in the external auditory canal (stenosis, neoplasia, polyps). In such severe cases, a total external auditory canal ablation with a bullectomy (TECABU) should be considered (6). After surgery, a drain must be left in place for 1 week and antibiotics should be given for 1 month (see Chap. 10.6).

Prognosis: The prognosis of otitis media/interna is guarded. Many animals recover if an aggressive therapy is undertaken and antibiotics are given consequently for the suggested periods of time; however, the more chronic the disease, the more guarded the prognosis. In some patients, the only remaining clinical sign is a slight head tilt. An associated facial nerve paralysis can certainly be remedied if the treatment is started in the early stages of the disease.

A rare complication of middle ear inflammation is tinnitus. An "objective" tinnitus is not only heard by the animal but also by the owner. These are noises which are made by the body itself, e.g. sounds due to turbulence in blood vessels, noises made by movements of the temporomandibular joint, contractions of the middle ear muscles, etc. The cause of such sounds can mostly not be determined. Spontaneous healing is possible.

15.4.2 Congenital vestibular diseases

Occurrence: A congenital peripheral syndrome has been described in various dog and cat breeds (see Table 15.2).

Aetiology: The disease becomes apparent between birth and the fourth month of life. The clinical signs are head tilt and vestibular ataxia (falling over, rolling around the body's longitudinal axis). Nystagmus is not seen. A congenital vestibular disturbance combined with deafness has been described in the Doberman (7). The deafness could be diagnosed by a hearing test at the age of 3 weeks. Pathological investigations revealed a degeneration of the cochlear neuroepithelium and a lack or abnormality of the otoliths in the macula. It is presumed that this disease is inherited as an autosomal recessive. In another study, congenital vestibular disturbances were described in puppies of related breeding lines, which were affected by a lymphocytic labyrinthitis.

Clinical: The first clinical signs begin at an age of 3 to 4 weeks or directly after birth with the neonates making rolling movements. In addition, there is head tilt and a mild ataxia, and sometimes deafness. An abnormal vestibular nystagmus cannot be determined nor can a physiological nystagmus be elicited by passively moving the head (5).

Diagnosis: When there are no other neurological deficits (apart from the symptoms mentioned above), radiography and other investigations (e.g. CSF) are unremarkable, and other vestibular diseases can be excluded (8). With respect to the

15

Table 15.2: Dog and cat breeds affected by congenital peripheral vestibular syndrome

Dog	Cat
■ Akita Inu	■ Burmese
■ Beagle	■ Siamese
■ Cocker Spaniel	
■ Doberman Pinscher	
■ German Shepherd	
■ Tibetan Terrier	

previously described association between vestibular disturbances and deafness (even unilateral), a hearing test should always be undertaken when young animals show signs of vestibular problems.

Prognosis: The prognosis in congenital vestibular disturbances is variable. These diseases are usually not progressive and an improvement is mainly seen at an age of 2 to 3 months as the animals learn to compensate through visual and proprioceptive influences (5). Other cases remain stationary or show periods of improvement; any associated deafness naturally remains.

The affected animals should not be used for breeding.

15.4.3 Metabolic causes

Hypothyroidism
Occurrence: Hypothyroidism is a well-known cause of neurological disturbances in the dog, which particularly affect the peripheral nervous system (9, 10).

Aetiology: Peripheral vestibular disease can be a manifestation of primary hypothyroidism. Older dogs of any breed can be affected; a sex predisposition is not present. From a pathogenetic point of view, the vestibular syndrome appears to be caused by an accumulation of mucinous material around the respective nerves in the internal auditory meatus leading to a direct compression of the nerves.

Clinical: The clinical signs begin acutely and are characterised by head tilt, positional strabismus and vestibular ataxia. In a few cases, the disease is chronic progressive. The vestibular disturbances are rarely associated with generalised LMNS symptoms such as weakness, reduced spinal reflexes and proprioceptive deficits.

Diagnosis: The otoscopic and radiographic investigations of the bulla do not reveal any abnormalities. Clinicopathological investigations such as the determination of fT4 and TSH in the serum are necessary to confirm hypothyroidism.

Interestingly, EMG can show abnormal results such as PSWs or fibrillations in the proximal extensors, even in those patients that only have vestibular disturbances. Finally, these results make it clearly apparent that the vestibular disturbance is only the clinical expression of a more generalised disease involving the whole of the PNS. In such cases, a nerve and muscle biopsy can be helpful (see Chap. 7.3). A biopsy usually reveals the presence of inflammatory changes in the nerves and/or necrotising muscle abnormalities. These histological deficits indicate the presence of an active inflammatory destructive process, but they are not pathognomomic for hypothyroidism.

Therapy: The therapy is based on a supplementation with levothyroxin at a dosage of 20 µg/kg, PO, BID for the dog and 10–20 µg/kg, PO, SID in the cat.

Prognosis: The clinical signs usually disappear within 2 to 4 months; however, the hormone supplementation must be continued for the rest of the animal's life.

Ototoxicity
Occurrence: Iatrogenic damage of the auditory and vestibular functions can occur due to the application of various substances (11) (see Table 15.3).

Aetiology: Ototoxic substances cause a loss of the hair cells and the peripheral receptors of both the auditory and vestibular systems. Little is known about the biochemical mechanism of this toxicity. The damage to the auditory system is normally irreversible, though the patient often recovers from the vestibular disturbances.

Substances: The aminoglycosides are the most notorious ototoxic agents. Streptomycin is the most toxic, while netilmycin, one of the newer ones, is the least toxic. The biochemical mechanism of the aminoglycoside toxicity appears to be an inhibition of the glucose mechanism or the "turnover" of the polyphosphoinositide mechanism.

15

Table 15.3: Overview of ototoxic medications in the dog and cat

Antibiotics

Aminoglycosides
■ Gentamycin
■ Kanamycin
■ Neomycin
■ Streptomycin

Fluorinated quinolonese (topical)
■ Ciprofloxacin
■ Enrofloxacin

Antiseptics
■ Chlorhexidine
□ Quaternary ammonia (e.g. benzalkonium chloride)

Even the topical use of fluorinated quinolones (e.g. enrofloxacine) can have ototoxic effects.

Some disinfectants such as chlorhexidine and quaternary ammonium products (e.g. benzalkonium chloride) also have a high degree of ototoxicity and can induce a complete destruction of the auditory and vestibular apparatus. The rule is that none of these substances should be used topically in the ear canal if there is any suspicion of damage to the ear drum.

Substances such as furosemide can cause a reversible ototoxicity. This increases the toxic effects of aminoglycosides and so the use of both types of substances together should be avoided.

15.4.4 Idiopathic causes (geriatric or idiopathic vestibular syndrome)

Occurrence: An idiopathic vestibular disease can be observed in cats of every age and in older dogs. In an overview of 75 cats, a high incidence in the months of July and August was found. This type of disease is also called "geriatric vestibular syndrome" in the dog.

Clinical: The peracute start of the disease is characterised by head tilt, horizontal or rotatory nystagmus, and severe vestibular ataxia. A few episodes of vomiting may occur just before the vestibular symptoms begin. The ataxia is normally dramatic in the first hours; sometimes it is so severe that a correct neurological examination cannot be done. Facial nerve paresis, Horner's syndrome or other associated lesions are never found with this disease. Usually, a spontaneous and rapid recovery occurs within the first 48 to 72 hours. The head tilt is the last sign which disappears, or it may remain in a mild form for the rest of the animal's life.

Diagnosis: The diagnosis is based on the exclusion of other diseases (otitis media, neoplasia, etc.), and on the dramatic appearance of the clinical signs with their quick recovery.

Therapy: As spontaneous healing occurs, no treatment is necessary. Often the patients become extremely excited or show massive neurological deficits with sudden collapse may be, so it necessary to give diazepam 1–2 mg, TID. A good alternative for treating the disturbance in consciousness is stugerone at a dosage of 4 mg/kg, PO, BID.

Prognosis: The prognosis is good, though relapses are possible.

15.4.5 Neoplastic disease

Neoplasia is rarely the cause of vestibular disturbances in the dog and cat.

15.4.5.1 Neurofibroma

Occurrence: The neurofibroma affecting CN VIII often found in human medicine (acoustic neuroma) is rare in veterinary medicine. The trigeminal nerve (CN V) is the most commonly affected nerve in the dog.

Clinical: A peripheral vestibular syndrome is observed with neoplasia of the vestibular nerve. With progression of the disease, the clinical signs may become typical for those of a central lesion because the cerebellopontine angle and the brain stem become affected.

15.4.5.2 Osteosarcoma/fibrosarcoma

Occurrence and aetiology: Osteosarcomas / fibrosarcomas represent aggressive forms of neoplasia. They originate in the petrous bone. Carcinomas arise from the epithelium of the external auditory canal or the tympanic bulla (squamous cell carcinoma, ceruminous gland adenocarcinoma). A secondary infiltration of the neighbouring soft tissues is also possible and a secondary otitis media can also occur.

Clinical: Symptoms of a vestibular disease, sometimes pain in the area of the ear.

Diagnosis: The signs of osteolysis / osteogenesis are recognisable on a radiograph. CT or MRI studies are necessary to gain more complete information about the morphology and extent of the tumour.

Therapy: Surgery can be promising. If the tumour is limited to the external auditory canal, then a total canal ablation can be a therapeutical option.

Prognosis: The prognosis for extensive tumours is poor.

15.4.5.3 Tumour in the cerebellopontine angle

Tumours in the cerebellopontine angle, especially the slow-growing meningiomas, provoke symptoms of a central vestibular disturbance or compression of the brain stem. However, the peripheral symptoms may be present for a long time before the brain stem compression becomes obvious (see Chap. 15.5.2.1).

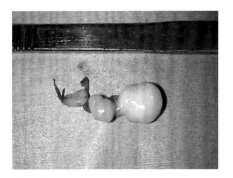

Fig. 15.6
Ear polyp from a cat with chronic disequilibrium. The cat had a conspicuous head tilt to the left, positional nystagmus (horizontal), ventral strabismus and generalised ataxia (www.vetsurgerycentral.com).

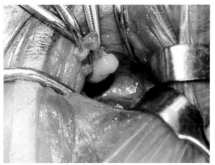

Fig. 15.7
Surgical removal of a nasopharyngeal polyp after opening of the bulla (www.vetsurgerycentral.com).

15.4.5.4 Cholesteatoma

Occurrence and aetiology: The cholesteatoma is a form of epidermoid cyst that consists of keratin layers mixed with inflammatory granulation tissue. It can be the cause of peripheral vestibular disease (12). In the dog, it has been described as a collection of sacks formed from the tympanic membrane and inflammatory products which arise in the middle ear. Indeed, the cholesteatoma can be a complication of otitis media. In a retrospective study of 62 dogs with middle ear infection, this type of tumour was diagnosed in 11%.

Clinical: Affected animals can show pain when the mouth is opened, and vestibular symptoms.

Diagnosis: Resorption and proliferation of bony material in the tympanic bulla and the temporomandibular joint can be seen radiographically.

Therapy: Surgery is the therapy of choice. A total excision promises a low relapse rate and a good prognosis. A total auditory canal ablation with bulla osteotomy (see Chap. 10.6) is the most useful surgical method. The removal of a cholesteatoma through a caudal approach to the bulla to protect the auditory ossicles has been described. It this case the animal's hearing was retained.

15.4.5.5 Ear polyps

Occurrence and aetiology: Inflammatory polyps can be found in young cats (mainly less than 2 years old) in the nasopharynx, middle ear and in the outer auditory canal. In the majority of cases, they are formed in the ear canal to which they are joined by a fine stalk (Fig. 15.6).

Clinical: The signs are those of an otitis externa / media that progresses to an inflammation of the petrous bone, and the development of vestibular disturbances.

Diagnosis: Otoscopy.

Therapy: Depending on the localisation, the polyps can be surgically removed from the nasopharyrnx or the external auditory canal. When the polyps extend into the bulla (Fig. 15.7), a lateral or ventral bullectomy is necessary (13). The thick and fine tissue connections to the tuba or the ear canal tear easily with careful traction.

Prognosis: The prognosis is good.

15.5 Diseases of the central vestibular apparatus

Causes of central vestibular disease are shown in Table 15.4 organised according to the VITAMIN D scheme. In the majority of cases, these diseases affect more than one part of the brain and are dealt with in different ways in other chapters in this book (see Chaps. 17.2 and 18). In this section, only the few central diseases that are definitely responsible for a central vestibular syndrome are described.

15.5.1 Metabolic causes

Thiamine deficiency

Occurrence: A deficiency of thiamine can cause encephalopathy in many mammals including ruminants, human beings (Wernicke-Korsakof syndrome), dogs and cats.

15

Table 15.4: Differential diagnoses for central vestibular diseases

V	▪ Infarct ▪ Haemorrhage
I	▪ Distemper ▪ Granulomatous meningoencephalitis ▪ Necrotizing meningoencephalitis ▪ Bacterial meningoencephalitis ▪ Rickettsia ▪ Protozoa ▪ FIP ▪ Fungal disease
T	▪ Cranial brain stem trauma
M	▪ Thiamine deficiency ▪ Metronidazole intoxication
N	▪ Meningioma ▪ Choroid plexus papilloma/carcinoma ▪ Medulloblastoma ▪ Glioma ▪ Lymphoma ▪ Metastases
D	▪ Storage diseases

Aetiology: Thiamine is essential for the oxidative pyruvic acid decarboxylation in the Krebs cycle – an essential reaction in glucose metabolism. Thiamine deficiency leads to a degeneration of those tissues that almost exclusively get their energy from glucose; e.g. the brain. In the cat, starvation or a thiaminase-rich diet (fresh fish) are the main causes of deficiency.

Clinical: Specific areas in the brain – such as the caudal colliculus, lateral geniculate body, vestibular nucleus and oculomotor nucleus – are often affected. The lesions are characterised by oedema, haemorrhages and necrosis. Sometimes other areas of the brain stem are affected such as the basal nuclei, the cerebral cortex and the cerebellar vermis.

The clinical symptoms consist of vestibular disturbances such as ventroflexion of the head (see Fig. 14.13), non-responsive pupils, and seizures.

Diagnosis: The diagnosis may be based on the anamnesis and the clinical symptoms, even though they can be – theoretically – confirmed by determining the transketolase activity, a thiamine-dependent coenzyme.

Therapy: The administration of 50 mg thiamine/kg for dogs and 20 mg/kg for cats is indicated even when there is just a suspicion of thiamine deficiency. The therapy must be given for 3 to 5 days and coupled with an intravenous administration of glucose.

15.5.2 Neoplastic diseases

15.5.2.1 Neoplasms in the cerebellopontine angle

Occurrence: These are very common in the dog and cat; they are mainly meningiomas

Clinical: These tumours tend to be slow-growing and cause a progressive central vestibular syndrome. In the advanced stages of the disease, dramatic consequences of brain stem compression such as tetraparesis or multiple cranial nerve deficits become obvious.

Diagnosis: MRI is very suitable for diagnosing causal lesions of the fossa, including tumours. It is more sensitive for this than CT.

Therapy: The surgical removal of a tumour in the cerebellopontine angle is not easy. The classical occipital approach can be a satisfactory option for meningiomas in the cat. In this species, the meningioma is fibrous and can be easily separated from the surrounding tissues due to its well-demarcated capsule. In the dog, meningiomas infiltrate the surrounding tissues more and a combined occipital/rostrotentorial approach with removal of the nuchal ligament may be necessary to provide a satisfactory surgical solution.

Prognosis: The prognosis is always reserved. It is perhaps slightly better in the cat.

15.5.2.2 Choroid plexus papilloma

Occurrence: Common.

Aetiology: The choroid plexus papilloma originates from the fourth ventricle.

Clinical: Mainly central vestibular symptoms. Combined cerebellar/vestibular signs can be also seen with this type of tumour due to its mass effect dorsally and ventrolaterally.

Therapy: Surgery via a median occipital approach.

Prognosis: The prognosis is guarded.

Other tumours
Tumours such as the medulloblastoma, lymphoma, etc., can occur in the caudal fossa and also induce vestibular symptoms. Basically, the prognosis for a tumour in the caudal fossa is worse than a tumour in the prosencephalon (see Chap. 18.7).

15

Literature

1 THOMAS, W.B. (2000): Vestibular dysfunction. Vet Clin North Am. Small Anim Pract. **30**: 227–246.

2 GAROSI, L.S, DENNIS, R. (2001): Results of magnetic resonance imaging in dogs with vestibular disorders: 85 cases (1996–1999). J Am Vet Med Assoc. **218**: 385–391.

3 SCHUNK K.L, AVERILL D.R. (1983): Peripheral vestibular syndrome in the dog: a review of 83 cases. J Am Vet Med Assoc. **182**: 1354–1357.

4 BRUYETTE, D.S, LORENZ, M.D. (1993): Otitis externa and otitis media: Diagnostic and Medical Aspect. Semin Vet Med Surg. (Small Anim) **8**: 3–9.

5 De LAHUNTA, A. (1977): Veterinary Neuroanatomy and Clinical Neurology, 2ed. Philadephia, Chap 11.

6 SMEAK, D.D., KERPSACK, S.J. (1993): Total ear ablation and lateral bulla osteotomy for management of end stage otitis. Semin Vet Med Surg. (Small Anim) **8**: 30–41.

7 WILKES, M.K., PALMER, A.C. (1992): Congenital deafness and vestibular deficit in the Dobermann. J Small Anim Pract. **33**: 218–224.

8 VANDEVELDE, M., JAGGY, A., LANG, J. (2001): Veterinär-medizinische Neurologie, 2. Auflage. Parey, Berlin.

9 JAGGY, A., OLIVER, J.E. (1994): Neurological manifestations of hypothyroidism: A retrospective study of 29 dogs. J Vet Int Med. **8**: 328–336.

10 JAGGY, A., OLIVER, J.E. (1994): Neurological manifestations of thyroid disease. Vet Clin North Am Small Anim Pract. **24**: 487–493.

11 PICKRELL, J.A., OEHME, F.W., CASH, W.C. (1993): Ototoxicity in dogs and cats. Semin Vet Med Surg Small Anim. **8**: 42–49.

12 LITTLE, C.J, LANE, J.G. (1991): Inflammatory middle ear disease of the dog: the clinical and pathological features of cholesteatoma, a complication of otitis media. Vet Rec. **128**: 319–322.

13 TREVOR, P.B, MARTIN, R.A. (1993): Tympanic bulla osteotomy for treatment of middle-ear disease in cats: 19 cases (1984–1991). J Am Vet Med Assoc. **202**: 123–128.

15

16 Cerebellum

Sigitas Cizinauskas
André Jaggy

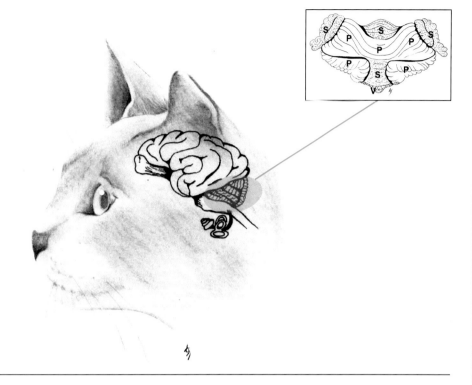

16.1 Anatomy and physiology

The cerebellum forms the dorsal part of the metencephalon. It lies in the caudal cranial fossa and is separated from the cerebrum by the tentorium cerebelli (Fig. 16.1). It is joined to the brain stem via the rostral, middle and caudal peduncles. The cerebellum can be divided into three parts (1). The smallest part, the flocculonodular lobe, is separated from the rest of the cerebellum (corpus cerebelli) by the uvulonodular fissure. The corpus cerebelli is further divided by the primary fissure into the rostral and caudal lobes. On its surface, the vermis can be seen lying in the median plane between the two small cerebellar hemispheres. The cerebellum itself consists of the superficial cortex and the central white matter, which contains the three bilaterally symmetrical cerebellar nuclei (dentate, fastigial and interpositus) (Fig. 16.2) (2).

The cerebellum is responsible for the coordination of all somatic motor functions (see Fig. 1.4a). Movements are planned and initiated in the upper motor centres (pyramidal and extrapyramidal systems). They are controlled and correctly "prescribed" by the cerebellum before they are carried out. Coordination of the motor activities by the cerebellum is performed by comparison of the planned movement in the upper motor centres with the movements that actually take place. This occurs as follows:

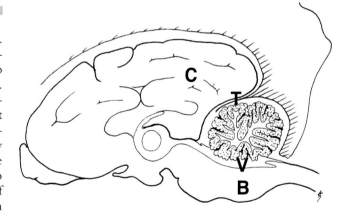

Fig. 16.1
Anatomy of the cerebellum. The cerebellum is a roundish structure that lies in the caudal cranial fossa. It is separated from the cerebrum (C) by the tentorium cerebelli (T) and lies on top of the caudal brain stem (B). Together with the rostral and caudal medullary velum, it forms the roof of the fourth ventricle (V).

16

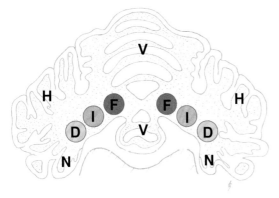

Fig. 16.2
Histology of the cerebellum. The intensely folded cerebellar cortex is divided into numerous folia oriented perpendicular to the longitudinal axis of the brain. The cortex surrounds the coral-reef-like central medulla which contains the bilaterally symmetrical cerebellar nuclei (dentate [D], fastigial [F], interpositus [I]). Its phylogenetically oldest part, which lies closest to the brain stem, is the flocculonodular lobe (N). This is smaller than the large dorsal part of the cerebellum formed by the vermis (V) and the two lateral hemispheres (H).

Somatic motor function is determined by the sensory and motor information tracts in the cerebellum. The ascending (afferent) tracts inform the cerebellum of the spatial position of individual parts of the body (via the spinocerebellar tracts). In addition, the vestibular and the visual systems inform the cerebellum of the body's posture and orientation in three-dimensional space. At the same time, the cerebellum receives signals from the upper (cerebral) motor centres, which inform it of motor impulse initiation (Fig. 16.3). By combining incoming sensory and motor information, the cerebellum has a regulatory role. It is the main coordinator of all movements, but it cannot initiate any movement itself. The cerebellum also plays an important role in balance and the regulation of muscle tone at rest and during movement (1, 2).

The ontogenetic development of the cerebellum is not complete at the time of birth although it correlates strongly with the motor abilities of the species at birth (3). For example, prey animals such as foals or calves stand up immediately after birth and can run. They have a more strongly developed cerebellum than a puppy or kitten (nidicolous animals). In the dog and cat (and also human beings), the brain, including the cerebellum, has to finish its development during the postnatal period. The perinatal phase is very important as many infectious, toxic and other factors can hamper the normal development of the cerebellum or even completely stop it (4).

16.2 Symptomatology and localisation of cerebellar lesions

Theoretically three cerebellar syndromes can be differentiated due to the specific localisation of lesions within the cerebellum: these are the vestibulocerebellar, spinocerebellar and pontocerebellar syndromes (1). They are observed when the lesion occurs in the respective region of the cerebellum. The names of these three syndromes describe the origin of the afferent projections into the cerebellum (vestibulocerebellum = vestibular nuclei; spinocerebellum = spinal cord: pontocerebellum = higher motor centres; Fig. 16.4). This information has been mainly gleaned from animal experimental models (5). Destructive lesions of the flocculonodular lobe induce problems with balance (e.g. head tilt, wide-legged stance, ataxia); lesions in the spinocerebellum are associated with increased muscle tone (hypertonus) and disturbances in proprioception; while lesions in the pontocerebellum are manifested as asynergia (the components of movement are not harmonious, but isolated and disproportionate), dysmetria (abnormal length and height of the strides) and intention tremor (tremor during precise movements of the head or limbs) (5, 6).

These syndromes are rarely seen in isolation in either human or veterinary medicine. Animals are rarely presented early enough so that isolated small lesions can be localised to a single cerebellar region. Usually the disease is extensive by the time of presentation and the clinical picture indicates involvement of two or even three regions of the cerebellum. Additionally, diffuse diseases of the cerebellum are more often seen in small animals than focal lesions (4, 5, 6).

The following clinical signs are frequently observed with cerebellar lesions:
- Abnormal posture (wide-legged stance, and rarely opisthotonus of head and neck).
- Abnormal gait (generalised ataxia, dysmetria, hypermetria, intention tremor) (Fig. 16.5).
- Abnormal postural and placement reactions.

Cranial nerve functions can also be abnormal in association with diseases of the cerebellum. A reduced menace response is the most common finding. Nystagmus is less commonly seen, but can be observed. Behaviour, consciousness and autonomic functions are not influenced by diseases of the cerebellum (5, 6).

The dynamics with which a lesion develops is also of importance (5) (Table 16.1). Increased muscle tone is typical of acute cerebellar lesions, as in cranial trauma, and is increased over the whole body. If the lesion affects the whole of the cerebellum, opisthotonus and hyperextension in all four limbs can be seen (decerebellate rigidity). The animal cannot stand to walk (although initiation of motor function is not affected by pure cerebellar lesions), and spinal reflexes may appear to be increased due to the increased muscle tone.

Fig. 16.3
Communication pathways of the cerebellum. The cerebellum receives impulses from both the sensory and motor systems: (1) from the upper motor centres (the cerebral cortex projects via the nuclei of the pons [pyramidal system] and the extrapyramidal system [especially the red nucleus]) over the caudal olives); (2) from the visual and auditory systems; (3) from the vestibular nuclei; and (4) over the spinocerebellar tracts in the spinal cord, which run mainly on the sides of the lateral tracts. The unconscious appreciation of the body's position takes place via the proprioceptive fibres from the dorsal tracts of the spinal cord, which are relayed in the dorsal tract nuclei and enter the cerebellum at the same time.

The cerebellum projects mainly via the central cerebellar nuclei to: (1) The red nucleus (most important efferent of the cerebellum; extrapyramidal system) and the cerebral cortex (pyramidal system) via the thalamus; (2) The motor centres in the reticular formation; (3) The vestibular system; from the cortex of the flocculonodular lobe to the vestibular nuclei.

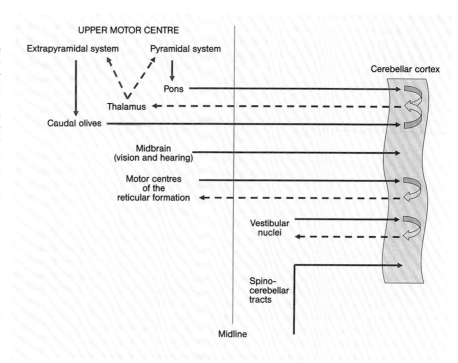

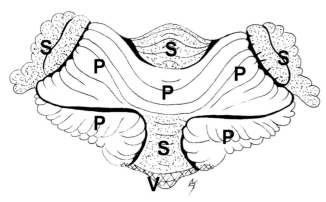

Fig. 16.4
Functions of the cerebellum. The cerebellum can be differentiated into three separate parts according to their function: vestibulocerebellum (V; flocculonodular lobe), spinocerebellum (S; rostral and caudal parts of the vermis and the paraflocculus) and the pontocerebellum (P; middle part of the vermis and the rest of the two hemispheres). The names "vestibulo", "spino" and "ponto" describe the origin of the afferent projections to the cerebellar cortex.

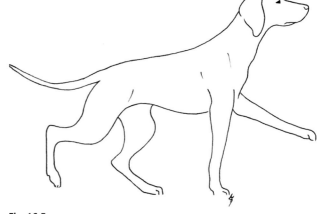

Fig. 16.5
Cerebellar ataxia: hypermetria. A severe ataxia is noticeable when the animal walks, though it is not accompanied by either motor weakness or a basic disturbance of targeted movements. Whilst walking, the animal lifts its limbs up excessively high and then "throws" them too far forwards.

16

Intention tremor is not present with acute cerebellar lesions. Compensation for the abnormal cerebellar functions can take days or weeks after the injury. The brain learns to suppress the abnormal (increased) muscle tone and such animals can develop normal muscle tone, and can stand to walk. Despite this improvement, the posture and gait remain neurologically abnormal (5).

In early small animal neurology literature, it was often stated that cerebellar rigidity can be clinically differentiated from cerebral rigidity (decerebrate rigidity) by examining the hindlimbs. Increased flexor muscle tone was described in cerebellar rigidity and hypertonus of the extensor muscles in cerebral lesions. Since then, clinical observations and experimental studies have shown that both phenomena can be accompanied by hyperextension in all four limbs if the lesion is large and complete (5).

Table 16.1: Description of the clinical symptoms of acute and chronic cerebellar disease

| | Bilateral/diffuse lesions of the cerebellum | |
	Acute	Chronic
■ Consciousness	Normal	Normal
■ Posture	Cannot stand	Able to stand, wide-legged stance
Head	Opisthotonus	Normal
Neck	Opisthotonus	Normal
Forelimbs	Hypertonus of the extensors	Normotonus
Hindlimbs	Hypertonus of the extensors	Normotonus
■ Gait	Not able to walk	Able to walk
Coordination	Generalised ataxia	Generalised ataxia
Dysmetria	Hypermetria	Hypermetria
■ Tremor	–	Intention tremor
■ Postural and positioning reflexes	Generally reduced	Generally reduced
■ Menace response	Reduced bilaterally	Reduced bilaterally
■ Pathological nystagmus	Absent/pendulous	Absent/pendulous
■ Spinal reflexes	Normal/reduced (very rare)	Normal

The rostroventral parts of the cerebellum (lingual and central lobes) responsible for the regulation of muscle tone in the hindlimbs are often spared when trauma of the cerebellum occurs. In such cases, the tone in the hindlimbs may remain normal. This is, therefore, more indicative of a partial cerebellar lesion than differences between the two phenomena. In addition, decerebrate rigidity is normally accompanied by coma and multiple deficits in the cranial nerves: the prognosis is unfavourable (3, 6).

Focal lesions are less common than diffuse ones in small animals, but they do occur (Table 16.2). Specifically, the vestibulocerebellum can be affected by focal processes such as tumours. It is important to bear in mind that the function of the cerebellum is basically ipsilateral. This means that the right side of the cerebellum controls the movements on the right side of the body and vice versa. This is explained more clearly in Fig. 16.3. The ipsilateral function of the cerebellum is due to (i) the decussation of the afferent (input) *and* efferent (output) cerebellar projections to the higher motor centres, and (ii) the ipsilateral input from the vestibular system and spinal cord. A lesion in the flocculonodular lobe or caudal cerebellar peduncle is neurophysiologically interesting as this can induce a so-called paradoxical vestibular syndrome. In this syndrome, the components of the vestibular syndrome (head tilt, leaning, positional strabismus) are contralateral to the lesion. The rapid component of the nystagmus in this syndrome is *toward* the side of the lesion. Despite all this, the postural and placement reactions are abnormal (with respect to rate, range and force) *ipsilaterally*, as is the menace response. Therefore, postural reactions help in the determination of the lateralisation of the lesion. Focal pathological processes in the vermis and/or cerebellar hemispheres are associated with neurological deficits ipsilateral to the lesion. The clinical symptomology of focal cerebellar lesions are summarised in Table 16.2.

It is important to note that clinical signs such as hypermetria, tremor and ataxia are not just present with diseases of the cerebellum. Diseases of the spinal cord, brain stem and cerebrum can also be manifested as generalised tremor and/or dysmetria. Degenerative diseases of the CNS, such as hypomyelinogenesis or storage diseases, can look similar to cerebellar disease. The cerebellum can also be affected by such degenerative diseases, but the pathological changes are part of a diffuse CNS disorder (4). In addition, diseases of the PNS (i.e. sensory polyneuropathies) are often accompanied by dysmetria, hypermetria, tremor and ataxia. Only a complete neurological examination and correct interpretation of the results make it possible to differentiate between the aforementioned groups of diseases. Polyneuropathies can almost always be recognised by the presence of reduced spinal reflexes. Hypomyelinogenesis and storage diseases often cause multiple cranial nerve deficits or can be diagnosed tentatively because of the diffuse/multifocal localisation of a disease in the CNS (4, 6).

Table 16.2: Description of the clinical symptoms of unilateral cerebellar disease

| | Unilateral lesions of the cerebellum | |
	Vermis and hemisphere	Flocculonodular lobe
■ Consciousness	Normal	Normal
■ Posture	Able to stand	Able to stand
Head	Normal	Tilted (contralateral)
Body	Ipsilateral scoliosis	Contralateral scoliosis
Limbs	Unilateral hypotonus or normotonus of the extensors	Wide-legged stance
■ Gait	Able to walk	Able to walk
Coordination	Generalised ataxia	Generalised ataxia
Drifting	To the side of the lesion	Contralateral to lesion
■ Tremor	–	–
■ Postural and positioning reflexes	Generally reduced/intact	Generally reduced/intact
■ Menace response	Reduced ipsilateral	Reduced ipsilateral
■ Nystagmus	Missing	Rapid component to the side of the lesion
■ Spinal reflexes	Normal	Normal

16

16.3 Differential diagnoses (VITAMIN D) and investigation methods

Information about signalment (breed, age, gender) and anamnesis (time when the disease started and its progression), together with the neuroanatomical localisation (focal or diffuse), is important for the development of a complete list of differential diagnoses. With the help of the VITAMIN D scheme, no important group of diseases will be overlooked (Table 16.3). Vascular, traumatic and neoplastic diseases are, from a pathophysiological point of view, focal processes and are often to seen as unilateral focal processes in the cerebellum. In contrast, metabolic-toxic, idiopathic and degenerative diseases have a tendency to affect the cerebellum dif-

Table 16.3: VITAMIN D and a list of cerebellar diseases (the more common diseases are printed in bold)

	Bilateral diffuse lesions	Focal lesions
V	■ –	■ Infarct (dog, cat) ■ Haemorrhage (dog, cat)
I	■ **Feline panleucopaenia** (cat) ■ **Granulomatous meningoencephalitis** (dog) ■ Distemper (dog) ■ Herpes virus (dog) ■ Feline infectious peritonitis (cat) ■ *Cryptococcus neoformans* (dog, cat) ■ *Toxoplasma gondii* (dog, cat) ■ *Neospora caninum* (dog)	■ **Granulomatous meningoencephalitis, Necrotizing meningoencephalitis** (dog)
T	■ –	■ **Contusion / laceration / herniation** (dog, cat)
A	■ **Agenesis** (dog, cat) ■ **Hypoplasia** (dog, cat) ■ **Dysplasia** (dog) Australian Kelpie, Beagle, Bull Mastiff, Chow Chow, English Pointer, Fox Terrier, Irish Setter, Labrador Retriever, Samoyed, Toy Poodle	■ Dandy Walker Syndrome (dog, cat) ■ Chiari-like Syndrome (dog)
M	■ **Metronidazole intoxication** (dog) ■ Lead (dog, cat) ■ Organophosphates (dog, cat) ■ Hexachlorophene (dog, cat)	■ –
I	■ **Idiopathic cerebellitis or White shaker syndrome** (dog)	■ –
N	■ –	■ Primary tumours (dog, cat) – **medulloblastoma** – other CNS tumours ■ Secondary tumours (dog, cat) – metastatic tumours – cranial nerve tumours – bone tumours
D	■ **Abiotrophy** (dog, cat) Airedale, Bernese Cattle Dog, Border Collie, Brittany Spaniel, Chow Chow, Finnish Harrier, Fox Terrier, Gordon Setter, Great Dane, Kerry Blue Terrier, Labrador and Golden Retrievers, Rhodesian Ridgeback, Rough-haired Collie, Samoyed ■ Storage diseases (dog, cat) – GM1 gangliosidosis Beagle Crosses, English Springer Spaniel, Portuguese Water Dog; Siamese, European Shorthair – GM2 gangliosidosis German Short-haired Pointer, Japanese Spaniel; European domestic cat – Globoid cell leukodystrophy Basset, Cairn Terrier, Pomeranian, Poodle, West Highland White Terrier; European domestic cat – Sphingomyelinosis Balinese, European domestic cat, Siamese – Mannosidosis Persian, European domestic cat	■ –

16

fusely. Inflammatory diseases can focally or diffusely affect the cerebellum. Anomalies of cerebellar structure can be either focal or bilaterally symmetrical.

A list of probable cerebellar diseases is very important for the planning of further investigations. Blood and urine analyses can provide important information about metabolic, inflammatory, infectious, toxic and degenerative (sometimes) processes.

Radiography can be diagnostically valuable if the cerebellar lesion is associated with radiographically depictable changes in the surrounding bony structures (malformation, trauma) (3). Sadly, at present there are no electrophysiological methods available in small animal practise that can be used for diagnosing cerebellar function. Investigation of CSF can be very useful and may help to differentiate infectious (viral, fungal, protozoal, rickettsial and bacterial) from immune-mediated processes (e.g., GME). In some cases, serological or immunocytochemical investigations of the CSF or serum are reasonable options (e.g., feline panleucopaenia, distemper). The cerebellar tissue itself can only be visualised using imaging techniques such as CT or MRI. MRI is currently the best method of investigation for studying the integrity and anatomy of the cerebellum. However, the cerebellum may still appear normal under MRI despite the presence of a degenerative disease. Even a normal result is important in the determination of a diagnosis. In rare cases, an ante-mortem diagnosis is impossible without taking a cerebellar biopsy. This is rarely undertaken even in specialised neurology practises as the results of the biopsy (e.g. with degenerative disease) will rarely make any difference to the therapeutic plan or the long-term prognosis for the patient.

16.4 Diseases

As it has been already mentioned, the development of the cerebellum in small animals is not complete at the time of birth, making it very susceptible to disease in the perinatal phase. Many cerebellar diseases in small animals are, however, manifested in the neonatal or early postnatal phase. It is, therefore, possible and clinically important to divide cerebellar disease into congenital and acquired forms (3, 4, 6). Both groups will be discussed in short in the following sections.

16.4.1 Congenital cerebellar disease

Congenital diseases can be inherited or acquired. Inherited cerebellar diseases are usually manifested shortly after birth and become particularly apparent when the animal starts to move around more. Inherited diseases of the cerebellum can also become first apparent after weeks or months; therefore,

inherited processes can never be excluded, even in adult animals.

16.4.1.1 Cerebellar hypoplasia associated with viral diseases

Occurrence: Relatively frequent in the cat; very rare in the dog.

Aetiology: Perinatal infection with a virus (feline panleucopaenia virus [7, 8, 9] and canine parvovirus [10]) can lead to the destruction of the outer germinal layer of the cerebellum in an animal during its development. The virus has a predilection for the actively dividing cells in this layer. The cerebellar cortex remains underdeveloped and the size of the cerebellum is much reduced. The exact time of the infection is not known, but it is considered most likely to be a transplacental infection rather than a postnatal one. Canine herpes virus can also infect the cerebellum (11).

Clinical: One or more animals in a litter can be affected. The clinical signs are first notable when the kittens / puppies start to walk. Cerebellar hypoplasia is normally bilaterally symmetrical and so causes bilaterally symmetrical cerebellar symptoms. These are not progressive and a certain degree of compensation is possible with time. Mildly affected animals can survive for years (3).

Diagnosis: Cerebellar hypoplasia can be presumed in kittens / puppies with cerebellar disturbances that do not appear to be progressive. Suggestion of the diagnosis is possible with CT or MRI, which show the presence of a small cerebellum (Fig. 16.6). CSF may be necessary to rule out inflammatory disorders.

Therapy: Vaccination against feline and canine parvoviruses is the only prevention against these relatively common diseases. A therapy for cerebellar hypoplasia is not known.

Prognosis: Fair in most cases if they are able to sustain themselves after three months of age, as it is a non-progressive disease.

16.4.1.2 Malformation of the cerebellum

Occurrence: Malformation of the cerebellum has been more often described in the dog than in the cat.

Aetiology: These diseases are inherited (mode of inheritance known), presumably inherited (mode of inheritance unknown) or of unknown aetiology. Cerebellar malformations can be divided anatomically and histologically into hypoplasia, dysplasia and aplasia (12). These diseases have been described in numerous dog breeds and in the majority of cases the whole of the cerebellum is affected (Table 16.3). In such

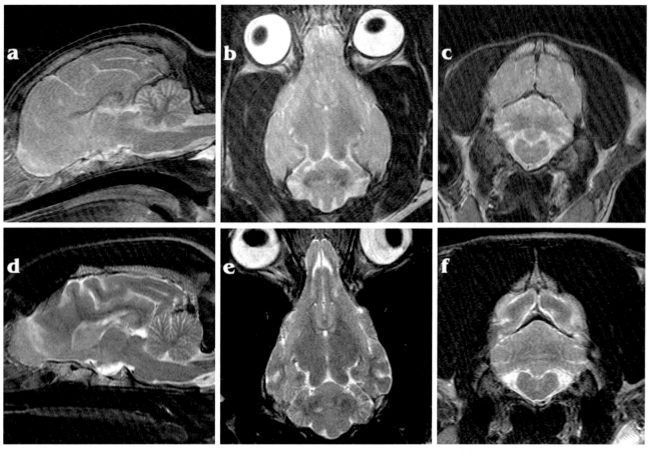

Fig. 16.6a–f
Cerebellar hypoplasia. (a, b, c) MRI of a 2-year-old male mixed-breed dog with symptoms of diffuse disturbance of the cerebellum. (a) T1w sagittal and (b) T2w dorsal sequences. Very definite folia formation in the cerebellum with conspicuously large CSF spaces, hypointense on the T1w and hyperintense on the T2w sequences (Fig. Johann Lang, Bern.) (c) Cerebellar abiotrophy. The T2w sequences show a slight reduction in the size of the cerebellum, especially of the cerebellar cortex. A reduction in the folia of the cortex and widening of the fissures are visible; (d, e, f) the same sequences in a healthy dog. A histopathological investigation confirmed the abiotrophic changes in the cerebellum. These results show that atrophy of the cerebellum can be observed using MRI.

patients, the cerebellum can be completely missing (aplasia), is under-developed (hypoplasia) or is incorrectly organised (dysplasia). Normally only the cerebellum is affected; however, in the Irish Setter and the Wire-haired Fox Terrier cerebellar hypoplasia is combined with lissencephaly of the prosencephalon.

In the dog, two other very rare and complex cerebellar malformations have been described: the Dandy Walker Syndrome and the Chiari-like Malformation. The names of these diseases are taken from the scientists who first described them in children. Dandy Walker Syndrome, which includes a complete lack of the vermis, is very rare but is known to occur in the dog and cat (13, 14, 15). The agenesis of the vermis is often combined with hydrocephalus, stenosis of the aqueduct and lack of the corpus callosum. The Chiari-like malformation is a complex malformation of the caudal cerebellum and the brain stem (16). In these cases, the foramen magnum is widened, the suboccipital bone is hypoplastic and the

flat caudal cerebellum is herniated into the spinal canal, and the medulla oblongata makes a Z-shaped curve over the rostral segments of the spinal cord.

Clinical: The clinical symptoms associated with malformations of just the cerebellum are characteristic for a bilateral or diffuse lesion of the organ. Generally, the clinical signs of cerebellar malformation are observed in puppy- or kittenhood, are not progressive and can affect one or more animals in a litter. Often such animals are euthanised early, though others can compensate for the ataxia and tremor to a certain degree. Even dogs with Dandy Walker Syndrome predominantly demonstrate a cerebellar symptomology. However, affected animals (and also human beings) can also suffer from increased ICP (hydrocephalus), while in others the cerebellar symptoms may occur after months or years, if at all. The Chiari-like malformation can theoretically cause a mixture of cerebellar, brain stem and spinal cord symptoms. Interestingly, this syndrome causes hyperaesthesia-like symp-

16

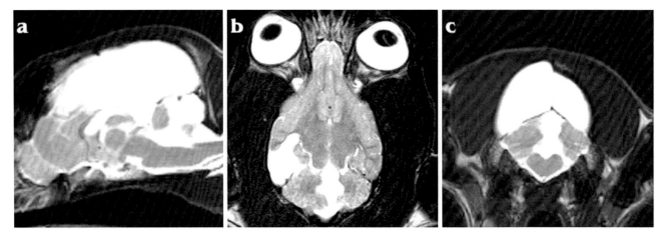

Fig. 16.7a–c
Anomaly of the cerebellum. MRI of a one-year-old male mixed-breed dog with symptoms of diffuse disturbance of the cerebellum and partial blindness. T2w sequences: the sagittal (a), dorsal (b) and transverse (c) sections show that the vermis is completely lacking. The occipital and also part of the temporal and frontal regions of the cerebrum have been replaced by CSF. Despite the complex and significant changes in its brain, this animal could live a normal life as a family dog.

16

toms around the nape of the neck in the dog, which can be misdiagnosed as pruritis or pain. Cerebellar disturbances, similar to those seen with the Chiari-like malformation have rarely been observed in the domestic cat, though they have been seen in a number of Lion cubs (*Panthera leo*) (17).

Diagnosis: A definitive diagnosis is difficult to achieve without the use of CT or MRI (Fig. 16.7). In the absence of these modalities, cisternography in combination with normal radiography or linear tomography can help to visualise cerebellar defects. In this method, 0.2 ml/kg water-soluble iodine contrast agent is injected into the cistern magna with the patient under anaesthesia. After the injection, the radiography table is tilted by 30° for 5 minutes (with the head of the patient pointing downwards), and then VD and lateral views are taken of the head. This technique enables not only the structures of the caudal fossa (brain stem, cerebellum) to be visualised, but also the pituitary and the optic chiasm (13). This procedure has risks related to the injection of contrast around the CNS and so should be performed with extreme care and only if it can be readily justified.

Therapy: There is no specific therapy for cerebellar malformations such as hypoplasia, agenesis or dysplasia. In animals with Dandy Walker Syndrome and increased ICP, medical (glucocorticoid, diuretic) or surgical (ventriculoperitoneal shunts) treatment can be attempted. Decompressive surgery is possible in patients affected by the compression of neural structures associated with Chiari-like malformations.

Prognosis: Guarded. Some animals are euthanised due to their neurological problems, while others can lead virtually a normal life.

16.4.1.3 Cerebellar atrophy

Occurrence: This disease is known to occur in a number of dog breeds. In the cat, it is an inherited syndrome (mode of inheritance is known or presumed). Cerebellar atrophy can also be seen in older animals as a sporadic disease.

Aetiology: Cerebellar atrophies are also known as cerebellar cortical abiotrophies. The term abiotrophy means growth affected by the lack of an important factor (18). In these diseases, normal development of the cerebellum occurs at first and is followed by early and progressive degeneration of the nerve cells, especially the purkinje cells (19). A metabolic defect is presumed to be involved in cerebellar atrophy, though the exact mechanism is not known.

Clinical: Animals with cerebellar atrophy have normal clinical signs at birth and have a normal cerebellum. The cerebellar symptoms are typically seen later (after months or even years) when the majority of the purkinje cells have degenerated (Gordon Setter: usually from 18 months onwards; Rough Collie: 1 to 2 months; Kerry Blue Terrier: 3 to 4 months; Brittney Spaniel: 7 to 13 years) (20, 21, 22). The progressive course of the disease is characteristic, but in some cases the disease can stabilise.

Diagnosis: The cerebellum becomes macroscopically smaller after months to years; therefore, a diagnosis of cerebellar atrophy can only be made pre-mortem with CT or MRI in the later stages of the disease (23, 24, 25) (Fig. 16.6c). In such cases, atrophy of the cerebellum, reduction in the size of the cortical folia and widening of the fissures is visible. Microscopically, cerebellar atrophy is recognisable in the early stages and could theoretically be diagnosed with a cerebellar biopsy. A cerebellum which weighs less than 10% of the total brain mass is most probably atrophic.

Therapy: There is no therapy described.

Prognosis: Guarded. Some animals are euthanised due to neurological problems, while others can live an almost normal life.

16.4.1.4 Storage diseases

Occurrence: Rare (see Chap. 18.8).

Aetiology: The majority of the lysosomal storage diseases are inheritable diseases in which the gene carrying the genetic information of a particular enzyme is defective. With time, the end-products or intermediary products of the faulty metabolism are stored in the affected cells until finally the function of these cells changes (4). Principally, this can affect all the cells in the organism, but the nerves cells are affected in a special manner as the proliferation of these cells and so the re-instatement of the function of the organ is impossible. The whole of the CNS is usually affected by storage diseases; however, the clinical symptoms that arise are extremely variable. In this section only those storage diseases that have predominantly cerebellar symptoms are discussed (4).

Clinical: Gangliosidosis is a storage disease in which there is a defect in the enzyme for the degradation of gangliosides (oligosaccharide). Two groups of gangliosides are known: GM1 (defect in β-galactosidase) and GM2 (defect in β-hexosamidase). GM1 and GM2 gangliosidoses have been described in various dog breeds and the cat (Table 16.3). Diffuse cerebellar symptoms are to be observed early in the disease and occur at an age of 3 to 6 months. Cerebral (depression, behavioural changes, whole body tremor) and brain stem / spinal cord symptoms (stupor, tetraparesis, tetraplegia) are seen later and normally determine the time point for the euthanasia of animals affected by this progressive problem.

Globoid cell leukodystrophy is a storage disease due to deficiency of galactosylceramidase 1 and has an autosomal-recessive inheritance in the West Highland White and Cairn Terriers. The mode of inheritance is not known in the other dog breeds and the European domestic cat (Table 16.3). The clinical signs of this disease occur at an age of 3 to 5 months and include paraparesis, generalised ataxia, intention tremor, and / or spastic hypermetria in the forelimbs. Later, the multifocal character of the disease becomes clear with paraplegia, reduced spinal reflexes and blindness.

Sphingomyelinosis has mainly been described in the cat and can cause cerebellar disturbances (Table 16.3). The enzyme sphingomyelinase is deficient in affected cats or may even be completely missing.

A deficiency of α- or β-mannosidase causes mannosidosis in the cat (Table 16.3). Cerebellar disturbances occur as a rule in Persian kittens at an age of 1 to 3 months. Skeletal abnormalities and hepatomegaly may also be found.

Diagnosis: A diagnosis can be presumed when cytoplasmic inclusion bodies are found in the leukocytes or liver cells. The determination of the enzyme activity in a leukocyte homogenate or cultivated skin fibroblasts provides a definitive diagnosis.

Therapy: None.

Prognosis: Poor.

16.4.1.5 Degenerative diseases of the CNS associated with cerebellar symptoms

Occurrence: Rare.

Aetiology: Degenerative diseases such as leukodystrophies, neuroaxonal dystrophies and the different forms of hypomyelinogenesis are sometimes difficult to differentiate from primary diseases of the cerebellum. These diseases have an unknown aetiology and normally affect the CNS as a whole (4).

Clinical: Leukodystrophy, hypomyelinogenesis and neuroaxonal dystrophy normally cause generalised ataxia and body tremor. Neurological examination reveals their multifocal or diffuse characteristics and aids in the formation of a list of differential diagnoses. As a rule, these diseases occur in puppyhood / kittenhood or while the animal is still young. Degenerative diseases of the spinal cord, which due to their localisation and diagnosis appear to be of cerebellar origin include (a) ataxia and myelopathy of Terriers and (b) axonopathy of the Labrador Retriever. In both these diseases, there is initially a notable ataxia of the hindlimbs. Later, hypermetria and spasticity of the forelimbs develop, followed by body tremor. These diseases occur in young dogs and are normally progressive.

Diagnosis: A definitive diagnosis of the aforementioned disease is sadly only possible *post mortem*.

Therapy: These diseases are progressive and cannot be influenced by therapy.

Prognosis: Poor.

16

16.4.2 Acquired diseases of the cerebellum

Acquired diseases of the cerebellum can be observed in young animals, but are more often found in adult or old patients. Vascular diseases of the cerebellum, trauma and tumours are more common than focal cerebellar processes. In contrast, inflammatory, metabolic-toxic and idiopathic diseases have the tendency to affect the cerebellum diffusely. Naturally, there are exceptions.

16.4.2.1 Vascular diseases of the cerebellum

Occurrence: Rare.

Aetiology: To aid understanding, it is sensible to first discuss the blood supply to the cerebellum in both the dog and cat (1). The arterial blood supply of the cerebellum is via two bilateral arteries; the cranial and caudal cerebellar arteries. These respectively supply the cranial and caudal parts of the organ. The cranial cerebellar artery originates in the caudal communicating part of the basal artery. The anatomical relationships for this are identical in both species. Differences between the dog and cat occur in the blood supply to the circular cerebral artery and the basal artery and accordingly, to the cerebellar arteries (called just arteries in the following). In the dog, these arteries are supplied with blood exclusively by the basal artery. This runs on the floor of the spinal canal and forms a continuation of the vertebral arteries. In contrast, in the cat, the maxillary artery supplies the whole of the brain with blood (including the cerebellum). The maxillary artery arises from the external carotid artery. Interestingly, the internal carotid artery is completely obliterated shortly after birth in the cat.

The blood supply outline explained in the previous paragraph is necessary for understanding, for example, how obstruction of the basal artery or its terminal arteries, after trauma in the neck region or a thromboemboli (septic or fibrocartilaginous) in the dog, can theoretically lead to cerebellar ischemia. In the cat, by comparison, diseases of the external carotid artery (maxillary artery) have similar consequences (1).

Luckily, in comparison to human beings, infarcts of the cerebrum or cerebellum are very rare in animals. The infrequency of predisposing factors such as arteriosclerosis, atherosclerosis and hypercholestrolaemia in the dog and cat may be an explanation for this. Dogs with secondary hyperlipidaemia (hypercholesterolaemia) as a consequence of hypothyroidism or primary (hereditary) hyperlipidaemia may be at risk of such infarcts, as are patients with hyperadrenocorticism, renal disease and neoplasia. Spontaneous haemorrhages are rare in small animals unless there is an underlying primary or secondary coagulopathy (4).

Clinical: The clinical symptoms associated with vascular diseases of the cerebellum are typically peracute, non-progressive and in the majority of cases asymmetrical.

Diagnosis: MRI is necessary for determining the definitive diagnosis.

Therapy: Supportive therapy (fluid therapy, turning, feeding, rest, emptying the bladder) and physiotherapy.

Prognosis: Animals can either recover completely after such an injury or the neurological deficits persist.

16.4.2.2 Cerebellar inflammation and infections

Occurrence: Apart from a perinatal infection with feline infectious peritonitis (FIP) virus, which has a predilection for the cerebellum, other infectious or immune-mediated diseases rarely selectively attack the cerebellum.

Aetiology: It is well known that the cerebellum is one of a number of predilection sites for the distemper virus (others are the optic nerve and the spinal medulla). Despite this, the distemper virus, as with other infections of the CNS, often causes a systemic disease and is multifocal or diffuse in its dissemination. Various infectious agents can infect the cerebellum: viruses (distemper, FIP), bacteria (gram-positive, gram-negative and anaerobes), fungi (common in the US but rare in Europe with the exception of *Cryptococcus neoformans*) and protozoa (*Neospora caninum, Toxoplasma gondii*; see Chaps. 20.2 and 20.3, respectively). Granulomatous meningoencephalitis (GME), a presumed immune-mediated inflammation of the CNS, can in rare cases cause primarily cerebellar symptoms, though it is more often seen as a brain stem or cerebral disease.

Clinical: Clinically, infectious CNS diseases may cause focal lesions in which case, clinical signs may be predominantly cerebellar.

Diagnosis: The diagnosis of CNS infections is often not easy. Systemic signs (e.g. hyperthermia) may be absent and haematological changes such as leukocytosis are infrequent. Fortunately, CSF investigations are usually diagnostic for the presence of inflammation based on pleocytosis and cell differentiation abnormalities. For example, neutrophilic pleocytosis is often found with bacterial and FIP infections, mononuclear pleocytosis is possible with distemper and GME, while a mixed pleocytosis may be common with GME and FIP. Information from serological, PCR, immunohistochemical and bacteriological investigations of the CSF and/or blood help in the determination of a definitive or tentative diagnosis of infectious disease. MRI investigations can help support the diagnosis and the extent of the disease (Fig. 16.8).

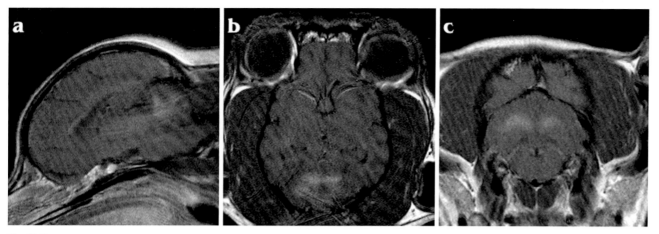

Fig. 16.8a–c
Granulomatous meningoencephalitis. MRI of a male ten-year-old Bishon Havanese with symptoms of diffuse disturbance of the cerebellum. T1w sequences after IV injection of gadodiamide (0.1 mmol/kg). The slightly paramedian sagittal (a), dorsal (b) and transverse (c) sections all show a hyperintense and irregular lesion in the white matter of the cerebellum due to an uptake of contrast. The investigation of the CSF revealed a mononuclear pleocytosis (36 cells/μl; 97% lymphocytes, 3% monocytes). The dog was euthanised due to deterioration of its symptoms. The histopathological investigation confirmed a diagnosis of granulomatous meningoencephalitis.

Therapy: Prevention of viral diseases by vaccination is very important as there is no direct therapy for these types of infections. Infections due to bacteria, fungi or parasites can often be treated effectively with antibiotics if a definitive diagnosis can be confidently made.

Prognosis: Therapy success or failure and long-term prognosis are dependent on the severity of the neurological deficits, the diagnosis, and the early recognition and therapy of the disease.

16.4.2.3 Cerebellar Trauma

Occurrence: Injury just affecting the cerebellum is rare following cranial trauma in the dog and cat. More frequently, the cerebrum and/or the brain stem are concurrently affected.

Aetiology: Contusion, laceration and haemorrhage can occur. In combination with the secondary consequences of brain trauma (ischaemia, oedema), these primary injuries can lead to an increase in ICP, especially in the caudal cranial fossa. In such cases, caudal displacement (herniation) of the cerebellum into the foramen magnum is possible. This can then cause injury to the cerebellar tissue and subsequent compression of the brain stem, both of which play a major role in such cases. Compression at the foramen magnum can affect the important centres in the reticular formation (especially the respiratory centre) and so lead to respiratory arrest (3, 6).

Clinical: Patients with cranial trauma are emergencies and as such should be treated as quickly as possible. Cerebellar dysfunction is possible during the recovery of such patients. In addition, an increase in ICP can lead to herniation of the cerebrum under the tentorium, which in turn causes caudal displacement of the cerebellum. In such cases, the cerebellum is secondarily injured and the before-mentioned brain stem compression may also occur.

The diagnostic methods, therapy and prognosis of patients with cranial trauma are extensively described in Chap. 10.2.

16.4.2.4 Metronidazole intoxication

Occurrence: Relatively frequent in patients subjected to metronidazole therapy.

Aetiology: A whole list of substances has been described in veterinary literature that can cause cerebellar dysfunction, though practically, metronidazole poisoning is the only such intoxication seen in the dog. Metronidazole is often used for the treatment of gastrointestinal disease, although it is also used to treat anaerobic infections affecting other organ systems. Experiments have shown that a high dose of metronidazole (250 mg/kg/d) can cause nystagmus, opisthotonus, ataxia, hypertonus of the extensors, tetraparesis and even death. These clinical signs occur after 4 to 6 days (26). However, clinically, total daily doses of as little as 30 mg/kg can result in signs of central vestibular dysfunction.

16

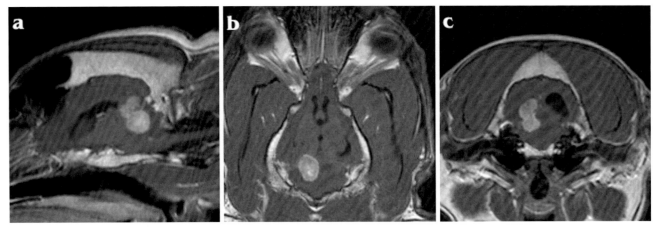

Fig. 16.9a–c
Meningioma. MRI of a seven-year-old male Bernese Cattle Dog with symptoms of a diffuse disturbance of the cerebellum and epileptic seizures. T1w sequences after the injection of gadodiamide (0.1 mmol/kg). Due to the uptake of the contrast agent, the right slightly paramedian sagittal (a), dorsal (b) and transverse (c) sections all show a hyperintense lesion starting at the tentorium cerebelli on the right. The lesion runs in two directions: to the right cerebral cortex and to the right cerebellar hemisphere. The right lateral ventricle is effaced and the left one is slightly dilated.

16

Clinical: The clinical signs may arise after a relatively short period of time on metronidazole (3 days) or could take weeks to months.

The affected dog is usually acutely ill and exhibits generalised ataxia, hypermetria and tremor of the head and body. Some animals can no longer stand, exhibit opisthotonus, epileptic seizures and vertical nystagmus. Often the animals walk or stand with their noses pointed into the air and their eyes are also directed upwards (dorsal strabismus).

Diagnosis: Diagnosis is simply based on anamnesis. Other investigations such as blood and urine analyses, CSF analysis and MRI normally show no changes.

Therapy: Cessation of the medication and supportative therapy (infusion, turning, feeding, rest, emptying the bladder) is usually sufficient in the majority of cases. Low-dose oral diazepam therapy has also been described as adjunctive treatment.

Prognosis: Good. Usually partial recovery occurs after 2 to 3 days and full recovery after 2 to 3 weeks.

16.4.2.5 Idiopathic tremor (cerebellitis) or White Shaker Syndrome

Occurrence: Relatively frequent in the dog; rare in the cat.

Aetiology: Idiopathic cerebellitis is an inflammatory disease of unknown aetiology.

Clinical: This disease occurs most commonly in West Highland White and Maltese Terriers. It causes a whole body tremor, dysmetria and generalised ataxia. Exaggerated cranial nerve test responses can occur. This disease has also been found in other breeds (dogs that are not white-haired) (27). The authors have also seen this syndrome in white cats. Its course is normally acute and progressive. Some dogs cannot walk at all. Characteristic for this disease is that picking up the dog increases the magnitude of the body tremor.

Diagnosis: The diagnosis is not easy and is mainly achieved by a process of elimination of other diseases. Blood and urine analyses usually do not show any changes, nor does MRI. A mild pleocytosis may be seen in the CSF, but this result is not specific. In euthanised animals, individual mononuclear perivascular infiltrates can occasionally be found. However, it is questionable whether these changes are responsible for the clinical symptoms.

Therapy: Treatment consists of a combination of prednisolone 1–2 mg/kg PO, daily) and diazepam (0.25–0.5 mg/kg PO, q 8 h). Diazepam can normally be stopped after a week. The prednisolone should be given for a longer time (approx. 2 months) and then slowly tapered. This therapy protocol is empirical and different regimens have been published.

Prognosis: Affected animals are often much better after 2 to 3 days of the start of therapy and can recover completely after approx. 2 weeks. Relapses are possible.

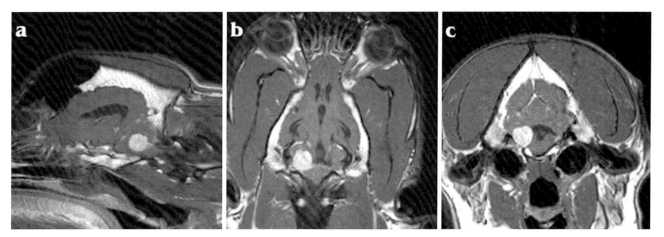

Fig. 16.10a–c
Nerve root tumour. MRI of a six-year-old male Rottweiler with symptoms of a paradoxical vestibular syndrome. T1w sequences after IV injection of gadodiamide (0.1 mmol/kg). The right slightly paramedian sagittal (a), dorsal (b) and transverse (c) sections all show a hyperintense lesion between the cerebellum and the brain stem following uptake of the contrast agent. The fourth ventricle is dilated.

16.4.2.6 Cerebellar tumours

Occurrence: Relatively common in both species.

Aetiology: The medulloblastoma is the only tumour that occurs in the cerebellum alone. It has been described in both the dog and cat. The tumour has its origin in the germinal layer of the cerebellum, grows quickly and is therefore more commonly found in young animals. It causes massive disturbances of cerebellar function. A similar situation is found in human medicine. Medulloblastomas are malignant tumours, have invasive and rapid growth, can be disseminated throughout the CNS and have a very poor prognosis in animals.

Other primary CNS tumours such as meningioma, astrocytoma and oligodendroglioma are only sporadically found in the cerebellum, particularly in older dogs and cats (see Chap. 18.7). These types of tumours are more frequently supratentoral than infratentoral. Meningiomas can arise from the tentorium cerebelli (Fig. 16.9). Tumours such as the choroid plexus papilloma and ependymoma, which originate in the fourth ventricle, can also primarily cause cerebellar symptoms if they grow into the cerebellum.

Metastatic tumours (lymphoma, sarcoma, carcinoma, etc.) can be found sporadically in the cerebellum. Cranial nerve tumours (e.g. schwannoma / neurofibroma of the trigeminal nerve) can also cause cerebellomedullary symptoms if they grow in a dorsal direction (Fig. 16.10).

Clinical: Tumours can induce either uni- or bilateral cerebellar symptomatology. Although these tumours tend to have a slow rate of growth, an acute and a chronic course of disease is possible.

Diagnosis: The diagnosis of cerebellar tumours is similar to that of tumours in other areas of the brain. Radiographic investigation can only help in those rare cases where there is tumour mineralisation or osteosclerosis of the bones. The results of CSF investigations are rarely specific with cerebellar tumours as tumour cells are extremely rare in cytology preparations. Protein increases and a mild mixed-cell pleocytosis (neutrophilic pleocytosis with meningiomas) are the most common results, but they are not specific and can only support a tentative diagnosis. CT and MRI are the best diagnostic methods. MRI has more indications for diseases of the caudal cranial fossa than CT as it is associated with less artefact production and better three-dimensional imaging. Despite this, MRI can only help provide a tentative diagnosis of the type of tumour. A biopsy of the tumour is necessary if one wants to achieve a definitive diagnosis.

Therapy: The surgical excision of operable tumours (superficial position, non-invasive) is the treatment of choice. Surgical removal can be combined with radiation therapy. Radiation therapy in combination with chemotherapy is the only method of treatment for inoperable tumours.

Prognosis: The long-term prognosis is poor.

16

Literature

1 KING, A.S. (1994): Physiological and clinical anatomy of the domestic mammals. Oxford science publications, Oxford.

2 DE LAHUNTA, A. (1983): Veterinary neuroanatomy and clinical neurology, 2nd ed. W.B. Saunders, Philadelphia.

3 VANDEVELDE M., JAGGY A., LANG J. (2001): Veterinärmedizinische Neurologie. 2. Aufl. Parey, Berlin.

4 SUMMERS, B.A., CUMMINGS, J.F., DE LAHUNTA, A. (1994): Veterinary Neuropathology, 1st ed. Mosby, St. Louis.

5 HOLLIDAY, T.A. (1979): Clinical signs of acute and chronic experimental lesions of the cerebellum. Vet Sci Communic. **11**: 259–278.

6 OLIVER, J.E., LORENZ, M.D., KORNEGAY, J.N. (1997): Handbook of Veterinary Neurology. 3rd ed. W.B. Saunders, Philadelphia.

7 HERRINGHAM, W.P., ANDREWS, F.N. (1888): Two cases of cerebellar disease in cats with staggering. St Bartolomews Hosp Rep. **24**: 241–248.

8 KILHAM, L., MARGOLIS, G. (1996): Viral etiology of spontaneous ataxia of cats. Am J Path. **48**: 991–1011.

9 JOHNSON, R.H., MARGOLIS, G., KILHAM, L. (1967): Identity of feline ataxia virus with feline panleukopenia virus. Nature **241**: 175–177.

10 SCHATZBERG, S.J., HALEY, N.J., BARR, S.C., PARRISH, C., STEINGOLD, S., SUMMERS, B.A., DE LAHUNTA, A., KORNEGAY, J.N., SHARP, N.J.H. (2003): Polymerase chain reaction (PCR) amplification of parvoviral DNA from the brains of dogs and cats with cerebellar hypoplasia. J Vet Intern Med. **17**: 538–544.

11 PERCY, D.H., CARMICHAEL, L.E., ALBERT, D.M. (1971): Lesions in puppies surviving infection with canine herpesvirus. Vet Path. **8**: 37–53.

12 SUMERS, B.A., CUMMINGS, J.F., DE LAHUNTA, A. (1994): Veterinary Neuropathology, 1st ed. Mosby, St. Louis.

13 SCHMID, V., LANG, J., WOLF, M. (1992): Dandy-Walker-like Syndrome in four dogs: cisternography as a diagnostic aid. J Am Anim Hosp Assoc. **15**: 355–360.

14 DOW, R. (1940): Partial agenesis of the cerebellum in dogs. J Comp Neur. **2**: 569–586.

15 KORNEGAY, J.N. (1986) Cerebellar vermian hypoplasia in dogs, Vet Path. **23**: 374–379.

16 RUSBRIDGE, C., MACSWEENY, J.E., DAVIES, J.V., CHANDLER, K., FITZMAURICE, S.N., DENNIS, R., CAPPELLO, R., WHEELER, S.J. (2000): Syringomyelia in Cavalier King Charles Spaniels. J Am Anim Hosp Assoc. **36**: 34–41.

17 SHAMIR, M.H., HOROWITZ, I.H., YAKOBSON, B., OFRI, R. (1998): Arnold-Chiari malformation in a captive African lion cub. J Wildl Dis. **36**: 661–666.

18 DE LAHUNTA, A. (1990): Abiotrophy in domestic animals. A review. Can J Vet Res. **54**: 65–76.

19 DE LAHUNTA, A. (1980): Comparative cerebellar disease in domestic animals. Compend Contin Educ. **2**: 8–19.

20 DE LAHUNTA, A., AVERILL, D.R. (1976): Hereditary cerebellar cortical and extrapyramidal nuclear atrophy in Kerry blue terriers. J Am Vet Med Assoc. **168**: 1119–1124.

21 STEINBERG, H.S., TRONCOSO, J.C., CORK, L.C., PRICE, D.L. (1981): Clinical features of inherited cerebellar degeneration in Gordon Setters. J Am Vet Med Assoc. **179**: 886–890.

22 TATALICK, L.M., MARKS, S.L., BASZLER, T.V. (1993): Cerebellar abiotrophy characterized by granular cell loss in a Brittany. Vet Pathol. **30**: 385–388.

23 VAN DER MERWE, L.L., LANE, E. (2001): Diagnosis of cerebellar cortical degeneration in a Scottish terrier using magnetic resonance imaging. J Small Anim Pract. **42**: 409–412.

24 SANDY, J.R., SLOCOMBE, R.F., MITTEN, R.W., JEDWAB, D. (2002): Cerebellar abiotrophy in a family of Border Collie dogs. Vet Pathol. **39**: 736–738.

25 STEINBERG, H.S., VAN WINKLE, T., BELL, J.S., DE LAHUNTA, A. (2000): Cerebellar degeneration in Old English Sheepdogs. J Am Vet Med Assoc. **217**: 1162–1165.

26 DOW, S.W., LECOUTEUR, R.A., POSS, M.L., BEADLESTON, D. (1989): Central nervous system toxicosis associated with metronidazole tretment of dogs: five cases (1984–1987). J Am Anim Vet Med Assoc. **195**: 365–368.

26a EVANS, J., LEVESQUE, D., KNOWLES, K., LONGSHORE, R., PLUMMER, S. (2003): Diazepam as a treatment for metronidazole toxicosis in dogs: a retrospective study of 21 cases. J Vet Intern Med. **17** (3): 304–310.

27 WAGNER, S.O., PODELL, M., FENNER, W.R. (1997): Generalized tremors in dogs: 24 cases (1984–1995). J Am Anim Vet Med Assoc. **211**: 731–735.

16

17 Brain Stem

Frank Steffen
Thomas Gödde
Anne Muhle
Bernhard Spiess

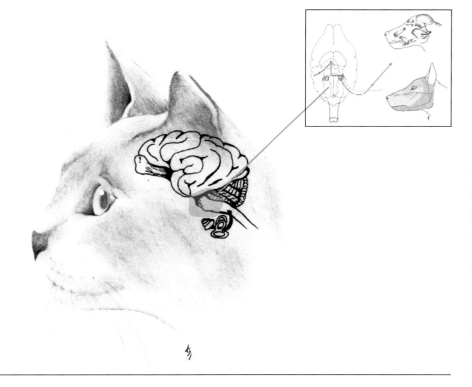

17.1 Anatomy

Anatomically, the brain stem consists of the mesencephalon (midbrain), the pons and medulla oblongata.

Functionally, the vital centres are found in the brain stem, and include the respiratory and cardiac centres. The central control of urination and defaecation, swallowing and vomiting are also found in the brain stem.

Body posture and movement are controlled to a significant degree via the brain stem. Ascending and descending tracts, for example, the tracts responsible for proprioception, run and crossover within the brain stem. Between these tracts lie the locomotor centres, cellular areas, which play a role in the initiation and steering of movement. The reticular formation is located diffusely throughout the brain stem; this is a net-like system of nerve cells that plays a central role in consciousness and sleep-wake behaviour.

The nuclei of cranial nerves III to XII lie amongst the tracts of the brain stem, especially in the medulla oblongata (see Fig. 1.14). Diseases affecting the intra- and extracranial locations of the cranial nerves and nerve roots often induce similar deficits seen with focal lesions of the cranial nerve nuclei (Fig. 17.1, Table 17.1; see also Chap. 15). For this reason we also discuss peripheral diseases of the cranial nerves in this chapter (Chap. 17.2.6).

17.2 Diseases

17.2.1 Infarct of the brain stem

Occurrence: Infrequent.

Aetiology: Blockage of the basal artery by a thrombus or embolus; usually of unknown aetiology. Association with chronic inflammatory lesions (e.g. prostate infection), neoplasia, endocrine disease, hypertension or renal disease is possible (1).

Clinical: Acute with severe brain stem symptoms (see Chap. 1.4.8.2). Disturbances of consciousness, generalised UMN weakness (more severe ipsilateral to the lesion), asymmetrical deficits of cranial nerves such as head tilt or facial nerve paralysis, and reduced postural and placement reactions (ipsilateral) can all be seen.

Diagnosis: Imaging techniques (MRI, CT) can be confirmatory. CSF analysis can help exclude CNS inflammatory causes. A search for associated diseases should take place with CBC, blood biochemistry, radiographs, ultrasonography including that of the heart, and ECG, blood pressure evaluations and endocrine testing.

17

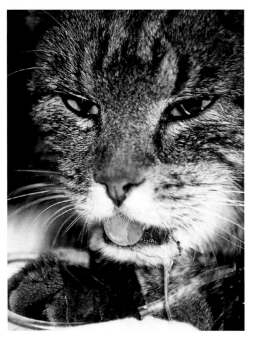

Fig. 17.1
Cat with brain stem lesion. The conspicuous symptoms in this case were severe apathy, dysphagia, jaw and tongue paralysis.

Table 17.1: Overview of the diseases of the brain stem

V	■ Infarct of the basal artery (dog/cat)
	■ Post-traumatic haemorrhage (dog/cat)
I	■ Feline infectious peritonitis (cat)
	■ Rabies (dog/cat)
	■ Post-vaccination rabies (dog)
	■ Granulomatous meningoencephalitis
	■ Necrotising meningoencephalitis (Yorkshire Terrier, Chihuahua)
	■ Distemper (dog)
	■ Protozoal encephalitis (dog/cat)
	■ Feline polioencephalomyelitis (cat)
	■ Mycosis (dog/cat)
	■ *Herpes canis* encephalitis (dog)
	■ Parvovirus encephalitis (dog)
	■ Bacterial encephalitis (dog/cat)
	■ Pseudorabies (Aujeszky's disease) (dog)
	■ Feline spongiform encephalopathy (cat)
	■ Feline immunodeficiency (FIV) (cat)
	■ Post-vaccination distemper encephalitis (dog)
	■ Unclassified viral meningoencephalomyelitis (dog)
	■ Steroid-responsive meningoencephalomyelitis (dog)
T	■ Compression of brain stem due to herniation (dog/cat)
	■ Contusion (dog/cat)
	■ Haemorrhage (dog/cat)
A	■ Meningeal cysts (dog/cat)
	■ Dandy Walker Syndrome (dog)
	■ Thiamine deficiency (dog/cat)
M	■ Encephalopathy (dog/cat)
	■ Metronidazole intoxication (dog/cat)
N	■ Astrocytoma (dog/cat)
	■ Ependymoma (dog/cat)
	■ Glioblastoma (dog/cat)
	■ Medulloblastoma (dog/cat)
	■ Meningioma (dog/cat)
	■ Oligodendroglioma (dog/cat)
	■ Primary lymphoma (dog/cat)
	■ Choroid plexus tumour (dog/cat)
	■ Epidermoid cyst (dog/cat)
D	■ Storage disease (dog/cat)

Therapy: There is no specific treatment for CNS infarction. Supportive care and physiotherapy is essential. Improvement may initially take 2 to 3 weeks to be noted.

Prognosis: Guarded; unfavourable if secondary to inflammatory or neoplastic diseases.

17.2.2 Inflammatory diseases of the brain stem

17.2.2.1 Distemper

Occurrence: Frequent, worldwide. Occurs endemically in dogs, mustelidae and exotic cats (e.g. Lions). Related viruses occur in sea lions and dolphins.

Aetiology: Morbillivirus, Paramyxoviridae. The dissemination of the virus occurs via aerosol, urine and faeces.

According to recent studies, puppies and dogs under 10 months of age are more commonly affected. In these animals, a noninflammatory form of distemper with demyelination affecting the cerebellum, brain stem and optic tract maybe found. The disease course is usually acute progressive and lethal. In surviving animals or immunocompetent older animals, the main form of distemper is inflammatory with lesions affecting the spinal cord, cerebrum or brain stem. The latter is often associated with central vestibular deficits.

Clinical: A febrile generalised systemic disease with conjunctivitis, tonsillitis, bronchopneumonia and gastroenteritis is only seen in two-thirds of affected dogs and is not necessarily seen before the neurological symptoms. Vaccination break-downs have also been described in a third of patients.

These are presumably due to poor vaccination status as well as an antigenic variation between the vaccination virus and the wild type.

The PNS is less frequently affected than the CNS. Exceptions include the demyelinating neuropathies, or neuritis, of the optic tract or nerves, and ganglioneuritis of the nerve roots causing paravertebral muscle spasms and intermittent lameness.

Myoclonus (i.e. a rhythmical repetitive twitching of individual muscle groups) can also be recognised. It is, however, important to note that this phenomenon can also be seen in other neurological diseases and is not pathognomonic for distemper.

Extraneural signs in dogs infected with distemper include defects in the dental enamel and hyperkeratosis of the foot pads and tip of the nose. In acute cases, multifocal oedematous lesions of the retina maybe seen. With a protracted disease course, chronic chorioretinitis may be seen.

Diagnosis: The combination of anamnesis and neurological symptoms in addition to the presence of extraneural signs increases the clinical suspicion of distemper. **NB:** A normal vaccination history does not exclude distemper!

The CBC may initially reveal leukopaenia with lymphopaenia, particularly when distemper affects young dogs. In the chronic form, lymphopaenia with leukocytosis and a left shift may be seen in combination. Anaemia and thrombocytopaenia are rare.

Demonstration of the virus in the noninflammatory form of young dog distemper is possible with immunofluorescence or RT-PCR on the buffy coat or conjunctival, preputial or vaginal swabs, urine and skin biopsies. The demonstration of the antigen in the inflammatory form of distemper is possible with CSF cytospin using either immunofluorescence or RT-PCR.

False-negative results have been described with immunofluorescence investigations of the inflammatory form due to antibody "coating" of the virus. A false-negative result can also arise in the noninflammatory form due to inadequate antigen concentration in the test preparations.

False-positive results are virtually impossible with RT-PCR, while false-negative results mainly depend on choosing the incorrect time point for taking the samples, i.e. during the presence of the virus.

Therapy: Symptomatic with fluid therapy, phenobarbital and diazepam (if seizures) and antibiotics (for secondary bacterial infections, especially of the lungs). The use of high doses of dexamethasone may in some cases provide temporary relief, but continual immunosuppressive therapy is not helpful.

Prognosis: Guarded with focal lesions and a non-progressive course; otherwise poor (2, 3, 4, 5, 6).

17.2.2.2 FIP encephalomyelitis

Occurrence: Frequent. Cats.

Aetiology: Feline corona virus. Genetic predispositions may exist. A corona virus variant associated with immunosuppression and selective infection of the macrophages play an important part in the development of this disease. Young and young adult cats of all breeds can become ill, with cats from multi-cat households particularly at risk. Histopathologically, the neurological form of FIP is a dry granulomatous inflammation, which mainly affects the brain stem and cerebellum including the choroid plexus and the ventricles.

Clinical: Two thirds of all patients exhibit nonspecific abnormalities including disturbances in consciousness and behaviour, loss of weight and generalised weakness; rarely is there an increase in body temperature. In a third of the patients, only neurological deficits are found, usually consisting of central vestibular and cerebellar symptoms. In addition, there is a purely spinal form described with lesions of the pelvic limb LMNS. Ocular lesions such as keratitis, iritis and chorioretinitis are found in a third of the patients. The disease is usually chronic progressive in nature. Short-term improvement may be possible with the administration of steroids.

Diagnosis: A tentative diagnosis can be attained based on extraneural laboratory tests revealing hyperproteinaemia and hypergammaglobulinaemia. An IFT corona virus titre is not significant on its own; in some histologically proven cases of FIP, it can even be negative. The causes of this are most probably immunosuppression or attachment of antibodies to immune complexes. CSF analysis forms the basis of the diagnosis usually revealing a moderately to severely increased cell count and increased total protein in association with a predominantly neutrophilic pleocytosis. In cases in which there are only slight changes, repeat CSF investigation is necessary or advanced imaging techniques are indicated. Secondary hydrocephalus is frequently diagnosed in association with this disease by CT or MRI. PCR and immunoperoxidase tests for FIP are being developed, but are not 100% suitable for a definitive diagnosis of the neurological form of FIP.

Therapy: Symptomatic.

Prognosis: Poor (7, 8).

17

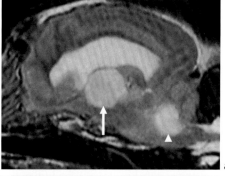

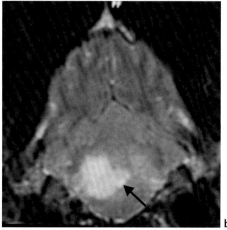

Fig. 17.2a, b
(a) Sagittal and (b) transverse T2w sequences of a five-year-old Boxer with multifocal GME. (a) Visible in the sagittal section are two large hyperintense foci lying in the thalamus (thalamic adhesion, arrow) and the brain stem (arrowhead). The focus in the brain stem extends into the cerebellum and lies dorsal and to the right of the fourth ventricle (arrow). There is only mild mass effect. (b) Moderately dilated lateral ventricle (arrow) possibly due to a congenital hydrocephalus or it may be the result of an obstruction of CSF drainage. (Fig. Johann Lang, Bern.)

17.2.2.3 Granulomatous meningoencephalitis (GME)

Occurrence: Dogs: sporadic, world-wide.

Aetiology: Unknown. There is a characteristic histological picture of a perivascular granulomatous inflammation with a high proportion of histiocytes in addition to a variable proportion of lymphocytes, neutrophils and eosinophilic granulocytes. A massive lesion can result from the fusion of these inflammatory foci. The disease is often localised to the brain stem, and less commonly the cerebrum, optic nerve (see Chap. 17.3.1) or the spinal cord. If the inflammatory components are absent, the histological picture is that of a reticulocytosis, about which there is still no consensus as to whether this is a histological variation of GME or neoplasia (9, 10).

Clinical: All dog breeds can be affected. However, middle-aged to older small dogs are preferentially affected in Europe, while a study in the USA found that young dogs between 1 to 3 years and especially Poodles and Terriers were over-represented. In addition to other neurological deficits, some of the patients had a high cervical hyperaesthesia. Increased body temperatures are rarely found (3). Cases in which only the optic nerves are affected (especially in the region of the optic chiasm) can occur. This ocular form manifests itself as a unilateral or bilateral blindness in combination with a reduced or absent pupillary light reflex. The ophthalmological investigation is typically unremarkable.

In addition to the acute progressive form, a chronic progressive form has also been observed; the former can sometimes be characterised by an increase in mast cells on histopathological investigation. As a rule, the prognosis for the chronic form is often better.

Diagnosis: The diagnosis can only be reached by histopathology or biopsy. A clinical suspicion of the disease arises from the CSF results – usually there is a moderate to severe change in the Pandy reaction; the cell count is over 500 cells per µl. **NB**: Pre-treatment with cortisone causes the pleocytosis to be variable: a third of the patients have a lymphocytic pleocytosis, while a mixed cell pleocytosis with eosinophilic granulocytes can be seen in others.

Imaging techniques such as MRI and CT show focal to multifocal contrast enhancement. A mass lesion is present in some in the later stages of the disease, which can make it difficult to differentiate from a tumour (Fig. 17.2).

A biopsy of focal forms may be required but is technically difficult and risky to achieve. The prerequisites for this technique in cerebral disease are high-resolution imaging methods, stereotactic apparatus and personnel experience. A biopsy can be taken in the region of the spinal cord via a routine hemilaminectomy but is often associated with more morbidity than a brain biopsy.

Therapy: Glucocorticoids at immunosuppressive dosages after exclusion of other granulomatous inflammations of the CNS, especially those of parasitic, fungal or protozoal meningoencephalitis (3).

Irradiation can be tried with the focal form. The treatment protocol is the same as that for a brain tumour (11).

Chemotherapy can be attempted, especially the cytosine-arabinoside protocol with selective lesions of the optic nerve (13). Cyclosporine, mycophenolate, and procarbazine have all been recommended as adjunctive treatments to corticosteroids.

Prognosis: Guarded to poor depending on initial response to medications.

17

17.2.2.4 Tick-borne encephalitis (TBE)

Occurrence: Dogs. Rare, in endemic areas; transmitted by infected ticks.

Aetiology: Flavivirus, Arboviridae.

Clinical: The causative agent causes a febrile generalised illness with brain-stem symptoms, cervical hyperaesthesia and generalized tonic-clonic seizures. The disease course is acute progressive and lethal. Another form with predominantly LMNS deficits in the forelimbs has been described and in this form reconvalescence is possible, though prolonged (14).

Diagnosis: Distemper, rabies, Aujeszky's disease, rickettsial meningoencephalitides and bacterial meningoencephalitis should be considered as differential diagnoses.

There are nonspecific changes in the CBC; leukopaenia with lymphopaenia may be seen on rare occasions.

There is a moderate to severe Pandy reaction in the CSF and a predominantly mononuclear cell reaction can be seen.

Direct demonstration of the virus is currently not possible. Serological determination is performed via repeat tests noting an increase or rise in antibody titres. Residual titres that do not change are not indicative of an infection, just exposure.

Therapy: Analgesia with butorphanol, anti-inflammatory treatment with methylprednisolone or NSAIDs, fluid therapy, parenteral nutrition (when necessary by stomach tube).

Prognosis: Unfavourable. Be aware that this can be a disease causing a LMNS-type syndrome limited mainly to the forelimbs (15).

17.2.2.5 Protozoal meningoencephalitis

Neospora caninum

Occurrence: Dogs. Subclinical infection: frequent; clinical infection: rare.

Aetiology: *N. caninum* is a parasite found throughout the world. The final host according to recent studies is the dog. *N. caninum* causes abortion in cattle, while in the dog young animals are mainly affected by a polyneuritis / polymyositis with spastic muscle contractions, especially of the hindlimbs. In addition, *N. caninum* can be found in inflammatory foci in the liver, lungs, pancreas and skin as a generalised systemic disease (see Chap. 20.2).

Clinical: The clinical symptoms are typical of an inflammatory brain stem disease and they cannot be clinically differentiated from the other causes of brain stem encephalitis (19).

Diagnosis: CSF with mixed cell pleocytosis and variable proportions of eosinophilic granulocytes. If the animal has been pre-treated with steroids, the CSF may be normal.

Titre determination in the serum using indirect fluorescence or ELISA is possible (see Chap. 20.2). PCR enables the antigen to be determined in the CSF, blood or faeces.

Electrophysiology and nerve-muscle biopsies are indicated if there is a concomitant LMNS disease.

Microscopic determination using fine needle aspiration of the diseased organs or more rarely scraping of affected skin regions (ulcerative dermatitis), or from CSF samples can be possible. The differentiation of this organism from *Toxoplasma gondii* is only feasible histopathologically using electron microscopy

Therapy: Clindamycin, 15–22 mg/kg, PO, BID, especially if there is neuromuscular disease; good effectivity in combination with pyrimethamine 1 mg/kg, SID PO; otherwise azithromycin 5–10 mg/kg, PO, BID in combination with pyrimethamine; or even trimethoprim / sulphonamide 15 mg/kg, BID PO in combination with pyrimethamine can be used.

Prognosis: Guarded to to poor, depending on how early treatment can be initiated; relapses are possible.

Toxoplasma gondii

Occurrence: Dog / cat. Rare.

Aetiology: Protozoa closely related to *N. caninum*. It has a broad intermediate host spectrum, but the final host is the cat. Transmission can be transplacental, smear infection or via contaminated meat.

Clinical: The neurological symptoms are part of a systemic disease (see Chap. 20.3). The eyes are frequently affected in the cat, though rarely in the dog. A combination with immunosuppressive diseases, such as FIV in cats or distemper in dogs, is possible.

Diagnosis: See Chap. 20.3. If there is suspicion of this disease, then it is recommended to do serological testing for both *Toxoplasma* spp. and *Neospora* spp. as a cross reaction between these two infectious agents does not exist.

Therapy: Clindamycin, azithromycin, sulfadiazine, pyrimethamine (dosage as above for *Neospora canis*), brewer's yeast to prevent folic acid deficiency (100 mg/kg/d) or folic acid.

All the puppies in a litter should be treated prophylactically when an animal develops this disease.

Prognosis: Guarded to poor (20, 21).

17

17.2.2.6 Rabies

Occurrence: Dog, cat. Frequent throughout the world; especially the Indian subcontinent, North and South Africa; rare in Central Europe. In addition to Great Britain, Sweden, Norway, Portugal and Switzerland are classed as free of rabies (situation: March 2004). Imported disease due to travelling is possible.

Aetiology: Lyssa virus of the family Rhabdoviridae. Transmission usually occurs via bite inoculation due to infected saliva. With bats, the transmission can also occur via aerosol (bat colonies, enclosed caves).

The skunk, coyote, racoon and possum are the main wildlife vectors in North America. The fox is the main infection reservoir in the northern half of the world, especially in Central Europe. The sylvan form of rabies is present in this region. This term, however, requires amending as the fox can be found in urban areas, too. The direct danger for human beings is small. At greater risk are pets, horses and cattle, which reside outdoors; human beings can become infected through these. Very good success has been achieved in immunising fox populations in Europe to prevent epidemic spread of this disease using vaccination with an attenuated live virus (23).

The dog is the main disease reservoir of the Indian subcontinent, Indonesia and North and South Africa. The disease is particularly strongly disseminated in the slums of urban settlements where there is great danger of infection for the human population. Accordingly, there is a large number of deaths, with estimations of between 40000 and 70000 per year (the number of unreported cases is, however, also thought to be high) (25). The importation of infected and then vaccinated animals by tourists from these areas presents a high degree of risk. **NB:** Beware all imported animal with neurological deficits!

Clinical: The incubation time depends mainly on the location of the bite wound. After local replication of the virus in the muscle cells, it then goes into the PNS via the neuromuscular endplates and muscle spindles. Afterwards, the virus spreads via centripetal axonal transport to the motor neurons in the spinal cord. From there, the virus ascends via the bilateral axons to the brain stem and so on to the cerebrum. The virus replicates here and finally spreads centrally via the sensory and autonomic nerves. Infection of the salivary glands is particularly common. As infection of the CNS and the brain stem occurs before that of the salivary glands, it is possible that peracute death can occur without any release of virus and infectivity. This is known as silent rabies.

The incubation period is variable and can be from 3 weeks to 6 months, though in the majority of cases it ranges from 3 to 8 weeks. Usually, the incubation period in the cat is shorter than that of the dog (22).

The prodromal stage is associated with altered behaviour, particularly restlessness, irritability and erratic social behaviour. Some animals lick the bite wound so intensively that self-mutilation occurs.

During the course of the disease, the behavioural changes can increase to include generalised hyperaesthesia and increased irritability. Restless running around, aggression towards animate and inanimate objects, and a depraved appetite are often observed. Due to pharyngeal paresis or injuries in the buccal cavity, some animals show profuse salivation. These clinical signs are defined as being the excitatory or "furious" phase of rabies. In addition, wide-opened eyes and a continuous vocalising in an abnormal tone can be observed in cats. As the disease progresses, seizures occur, usually followed by death. A paralytic form of rabies when a LMNS-type paresis follows the prodromal stage has been described. This can initially affect the cranial nerves or may ascend from the limbs to the brain stem. The animals may then die during the course of the disease without showing any furious phase (3, 22).

Diagnosis: NB: Notifiable disease. This means that the rules for dealing with animals suspected of having rabies should be taken from the veterinary laws in force in the respective country.

Basically, animals with behavioural changes and multifocal neurological deficits, especially in the head region, should be suspected of having rabies. If a human has been bitten as well, then the local veterinary officer should be immediately notified. If he / she decides on euthanasia of the animal, then the corpse should be transferred as quickly as possible (ideally cooled) to the official pathology laboratory. Demonstration of the virus is performed using either direct immunofluorescence on an impression preparation of the brain stem, Ammon's horn and cerebrum, or by demonstration in a cell culture.

Due to the usually rapidly lethal course of the disease, animals with good vaccination protection can be kept in quarantine to see what happens.

In the few cases investigated, the CSF shows a positive Pandy reaction and a lymphocytic pleocytosis with a moderate increase in cell count (24). Virus isolation is not possible due to its neurotropism (22).

Therapy: None.

Prognosis: Hopeless.

Rabies as zoonosis: Basically, post-exposure therapy should be started in humans as soon as possible if there is a proven case of rabies. This includes wound treatment, injecting rabies antiserum around the site of the wound, and a series of vaccinations with an inactive vaccine. It is important to build up a neutralising antibody titre before the virus enters the PNS in order to prevent development of a CNS infection. Once the infectious disease has developed, its course is, as a rule, lethal.

17.2.2.7 Aujeszky's (Pseudo-rabies) disease

Occurrence: Dog, cat. Rare.

Aetiology: Herpes virus. Infection occurs due to the ingestion of contaminated raw meat. The virus reservoir is the pig.

Clinical: Peracute course with disturbances in the general well-being of the animal, a significant rise in body temperature, vomiting, **intensive pruritis** in the head and neck region with secondary self-mutilation due to scratching. There is a tendency for one-sided cranial nerve deficits, especially affecting the eye muscles and pharyngeal nuclei, resulting in hypersalivation; tetraparesis.

Diagnosis: Clinical tentative diagnosis. Disease can only be determined using histopathology. There is a nonpurulent encephalomyelitis (especially in the caudal brain stem) and a ganglionitis.

NB: Rabies is a differential diagnosis.

Therapy: None.

Prognosis: Unfavourable, usually rapidly lethal. **NB: Notifiable disease.** There are indications that inapparent infections occur in pig herds.

17.2.2.8 Necrotising encephalitis of Yorkshire Terriers

Occurrence: Dog. Rare.

Aetiology: Immune-mediated with a presumed viral origin in combination with genetic predisposition. The disease is similar to the encephalitis found in Pugs, Chihuahuas and Maltese Terriers, but in the Yorkshire Terrier the disease localisation is more often in the brain stem than the cerebrum. Adult animals of both sexes are particularly affected. The course is acute to chronic progressive. Histologically, this disease consists of disseminated, mononuclear inflammatory foci with central necrosis.

Clinical: The clinical signs are usually specific for brain stem disease. Asymmetrical deficits such as head torticollis and hemiparesis are possible, depending on the lesion.

Diagnosis: Signalment, course, CSF with significantly positive Pandy Test and lymphocytic pleocytosis. Differentiate from distemper, GME and some other infectious encephalitides. Imaging techniques (CT and MRI) reveal a multifocal distribution with contrast enhancement.

Therapy: Prednisolone in immunosuppressive doses; adjunctive therapy with cytosine, mycophenolate or cyclosporine may be warranted.

Prognosis: Guarded to poor (26).

17.2.2.9 Focal bacterial meningoencephalitis

Occurrence: Very rare. Cat and dog.

Aetiology: Extension of inflammation mainly arising from otitis media / interna and subsequent osteomyelitis of the petrosal bone.

Clinical: Febrile disease. Usually a lateralised lesion with deficits of multiple cranial nerve functions, hyperaesthesia in the head region, sometimes in combination with peripheral vestibular deficits and later severe central brain stem symptoms.

Diagnosis: CSF, bacteriological investigation, radiography of the bulla, CT or MRI.

Therapy: Initial intravenous antibiotics. Suitable ones are those with a good penetration of bone tissue such as cephalosporins or penicillinase-resistant penicillins. The antibiotic therapy should be continued for 6 to 8 weeks. Surgical treatment (with concurrent tissue culture for bacterial determination and sensitivity) in the form of a ventral bulla osteotomy ± the insertion of a drain is indicated in cases of purulent otitis media / interna. An initial administration of steroids (dexamethasone or prednisolone 1–2 mg/kg SID for 3 days) can have a positive effect on the disease course in some cases.

Prognosis: Guarded to poor.

17.2.2.10 Post-vaccination encephalitis

Occurrence: Rare. Dog.

Aetiology: Due to vaccination with an attenuated live virus during gestation, during an immunosuppressed state or during chemotherapy; also possible when dogs are vaccinated younger than 8 weeks of age. Usually, according to the history, vaccination was given between 1 to 3 weeks prior to the onset of clinical signs.

Clinical: Post-vaccination distemper usually has an acute progressive course, which is characterised by brain stem symptomology and poorly controlled tonic-clonic spasms. Although the prognosis is poor, remissions have been reported.

Diagnosis: Pathologically, most of the changes can be found in the transitional region between the mesencephalon and the metencephalon.

Therapy: See distemper (Chap. 17.2.2.1).

Prognosis: Poor.

17.2.2.11 Post-vaccination rabies

In dogs, an ascending LMNS-type paresis starting from the site of vaccination is usually observed over a variable time-period like rabies itself. Recovery is possible but takes time. In cats, by comparison, there is spastic hyperextension initially of the hindlegs and then usually of the forelimbs. Spinal reflexes and superficial pain appreciation are reduced. With further progression of the disease, the brain stem may be involved, which tends to make the prognosis more unfavourable.

Therapy: None (3).

Prognosis: Poor.

17.2.2.12 Feline immunodeficiency virus (FIV) encephalopathy

Occurrence: Cats. Rare as primarily neurological patient.

Aetiology: Lentivirus of the family Retroviridae. Transmission is via bite or transplacental, although other routes are possible. The disease is widely disseminated in southern Europe and the feral cat population living there. Mainly adult uncastrated male animals are affected.

Clinical: The neurological deficits occur mainly in the late phase of the disease and are usually restricted to changes in urination / defaecation and behaviour. More rarely, seizures and gait disturbances develop. At this time, the clinical picture is complicated by obturation, chronic wasting, opportunistic infections and FIV-associated neoplasia, so that the neurological symptoms are rarely notable. A correlation between FIV and an increased occurrence of opportunistic CNS infections such as toxoplasmosis or cryptococcus has been presumed to occur in the cat.

Diagnosis: Definitive diagnosis using serology or CSF.

Therapy: Symptomatic / supportive.

Prognosis: Poor (3).

17.2.2.13 Feline spongiform encephalopathy (FSE)

Occurrence: Cats. Rare; at the moment restricted to Great Britain (although no cases have been reported for several years); one case each has been proven in Norway, Luxemburg and Switzerland. As there is no *in vitro* test on the market, diagnosis is only possible post-mortem, so the true number of cases is unknown.

Aetiology: The first cases of FSE occurred within the time period of the BSE epidemic, so the presumption is that the infection is due to the ingestion of contaminated food. This disease has also been demonstrated in wild large felids in zoos. In contrast, the species barrier to the dog does not appear to have been crossed. The uptake of the virus is most probably oral. The infection of the brain is presumably neurogenic. Under the influence of the prion protein, there is an accumulation of amyloid fibrils resulting in a spongiform appearance of the cells in the histopathological sections. The majority of affected cats were older than 5 years due to the disease's long incubation period.

Clinical: The course of the disease is chronic progressive and deadly. The main symptoms are behavioural including gait disturbances (generalised ataxia and tetraparesis). Changes in personality in the form of shyness or aggression are also typical. Due to the changes in the laws governing food and feedstuffs and the diagnostic advances in the elimination of subclinically infected cattle, a definite reduction in the cases of BSE and FSE are expected. The success of these measures, however, must be awaited.

Diagnosis: Diagnosis by process of elimination, clinical signs, and necropsy.

Therapy: None.

Prognosis: Unfavourable (29).

17.2.2.14 Herpes virus encephalitis

Occurrence: Dog. Rare.

Aetiology: Canine herpes virus.

Clinical: The infection usually occurs shortly after birth. It is rarely transplacental or gestational.

Puppies of 1 to 3 weeks of age become systemically ill with an acute progressive, mainly lethal disease. Due to multiple organ failure and hypothermia, there is high morbidity, weakness and mortality. Specific neurological deficits are rarely seen. A nonpurulent necrotising vasculitis in the brain stem and cerebellar regions has been seen on histopathology. Surviving animals can exhibit a retinal or cerebellar dysplasia.

17

Diagnosis: Clinical signs and post-mortem histopathology.

Therapy: If the disease occurs in a litter, then passive intraperitoneal immunisation of the puppies with the antiserum of a female dog that has been infected with herpes virus is recommended. This measure is purely prophylactic and does not change the clinical progression of the disease.

Prognosis: Guarded to poor.

17.2.2.15 Unclassified viral meningoencephalomyelitis

Occurrence: Dog. Rare.

Aetiology: In a study of 220 dogs with inflammatory diseases of the CNS, 27 cases had histopathological lesions which were consistent with a viral meningoencephalomyelitis of unknown aetiology.

Clinical: In the aforementioned study, the clinical symptoms consisted of seizures, disturbances of consciousness, cranial nerve deficits, gait disturbances and hyperaesthesia.

Diagnosis: The haematological investigations in the affected dogs of the aforementioned study were unremarkable. Lymphocytes and other mononuclear cells were found in the CSF and the protein content varied between normal to high.

Therapy: Palliative; initially steroids in immunosuppressive doses.

Prognosis: Guarded.

17.2.2.16 Steroid-responsive meningoencephalomyelitis (SRME)

Occurrence: Dog. Sporadic.

Aetiology: SRME is a collective term sometimes used for those cases that do not clinically fit into the other categories of meningoencephalomyelitis, such as GME or unclassified viral meningoencephalomyelitis; some refer to this group of diseases as meningitides of unknown aetiology (MUA). This is not the same as the breed-related steroid-responsive meningitis seen in Beagles and Boxers, which is a specific condition. SRME patients can vary in their clinical presentation, in their CSF cytology or in their response to a particular therapy. These cases reflect our momentary inability to determine the cause of the inflammation and represent most probably a variety of as yet unclassified CNS inflammations that respond well to immunosuppressive steroid administration and can recover without any relapses.

Clinical: The clinical symptoms often develop acutely and can appear to be located in the cerebrum, brain stem or spinal cord and affect dogs of every age and breed. The disease is not always associated with head or back pain. The body temperature is usually normal but can be slightly increased.

Diagnosis: Infectious diseases need to be excluded from the disagnosis. The CBC is usually unremarkable or there may be a stress leukogram with a slight increase in the segmented neutrophils and lymphopaenia. The cell count in the CSF is increased and ranges from 20–1000 cells/µl. Lymphocytes, macrophages or mixed cell populations are usually found with a few neutrophils on CSF cytological examinations. The protein content is increased. CT and MRI are usually normal.

Therapy: Severely affected dogs can be treated initially with methylprednisolone sodium succinate (10–15 mg/kg, IV, TID during the first 24 hours) followed by prednisolone (1–2 mg/kg, IV, SID–BID). This latter dosage is maintained for 3 to 4 weeks and then reduced stepwise by 25% every 3 to 4 weeks. If a relapse occurs, the initial introductory dosage can be given for a few days and then the animal is given the last effective dosage. Protection of the gastrointestinal tract and initial prophylaxis with antibiotics is recommended until an infectious disease can be ruled out

Prognosis: The majority of these patients recover within 3 to 6 months and then may remain normal.

17.2.3 Tumours of the brain stem

Occurrence: Rare; more common in the dog than cat; mainly in animals older than 5 years.

Aetiology: The most common primary tumours of the brain stem are basal meningiomas, choroid plexus tumours of the fourth ventricle and trigeminal nerve sheath tumours (Fig. 17.3) (33, 36). Rare tumours include gliomas, ependymomas, lymphomas (especially in the cat) and nerve root tumours of the other cranial nerves. Secondary tumours reach the brain stem through haematogenous metastasis or local invasion (osteosarcoma, fibrosarcoma). In addition to the tumour localisation, secondary effects such as peritumoural oedema, haemorrhage, necrosis and even obstructive hydrocephalus are usually responsible for the clinical symptoms (45).

Diagnosis: Radiography of the thorax, CSF analysis, CT, MRI and brain stem evoked potentials (34, 40, 41, 42, 43, 44, 45).

Therapy: Palliative glucocorticoids for reduction of the peritumoural oedema; radiation therapy (brain tumour protocol).

Surgical resection via a basioccipital craniectomy or caudotentorial craniectomy is difficult (39).

Prognosis: Unfavourable; with increasing improvements made in radiation therapy: guarded (38).

17

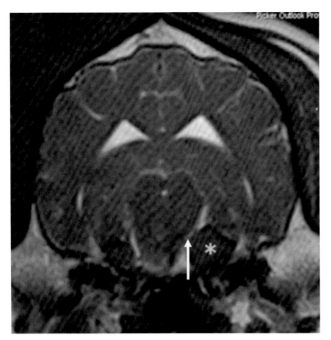

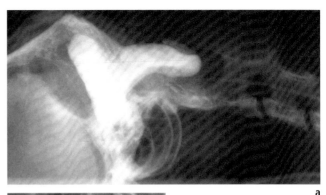

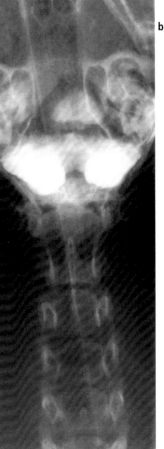

Fig. 17.3
Trigeminal schwannoma in a dog. Transverse CBASS sequence at the level of the cerebellopontine angle. The tumour is a hypointense space-occupying lesion in the typical location for trigeminal tumours (*) and is compressing the mesencephalon (arrow). Note the muscle atrophy of the ipsilateral temporal muscles. (Fig. Johann Lang, Bern.)

17.2.4 Malformations of the brain stem and the caudal cranial fossa

Occurrence: Rare.

Aetiology: Sporadic malformations occur spontaneously in this region. Hereditary causes are possible. Sub-(intra)arachnoid cysts and meningoceles (Fig. 17.4) in the caudal cranial fossa are found as rarities and can lead to various degrees of brain stem symptoms.

An increased incidence of cerebellomedullary malformation which has similarities to the Chiari Syndrome in human beings has been associated with syringo(hydro)myelia in the Cavalier King Charles Spaniel and several other small dog breeds. A hereditary cause has been presumed in this disease (46). The caudal cranial fossa of affected animals shows an abnormally small volume relative to the cranial fossa volume and the cerebellum is partially herniated through the foramen magnum (Fig. 17.5). The medulla oblongata is also longer than normal and extends into the first cervical segments. The brain stem is compressed at the craniocervical transition and the CSF outflow is hindered.

Clinical: The affected animals develop different degrees of neurological deficits, ranging from pain in the occipital region, pruritis around the neck (especially when the animal is

Fig. 17.4a, b
(a) Lateral and (b) ventrodorsal radiographs of the craniocervical junction of a cat after an injection of contrast into the cisterna magna. A complex contrast-filled cavity fills practically the whole of the caudal cranial fossa and extends through the foramen magnum to underneath the vertebral arch of C1. The cyst obviously communicates with the central canal, which is also filled with contrast. Histologically, the structure could be diagnosed as a subarachnoid cyst. The changes are similar to Dandy Walker Malformation. (Fig. Johann Lang, Bern.)

17

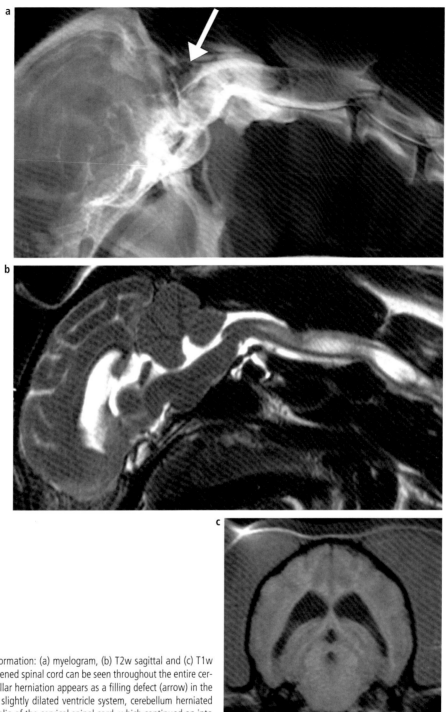

Fig. 17.5a–c
Cavalier King Charles Spaniel with Chiari-like Malformation: (a) myelogram, (b) T2w sagittal and (c) T1w transverse sequences. (a) In the myelogram, the widened spinal cord can be seen throughout the entire cervical spine, especially at the level of C2. The cerebellar herniation appears as a filling defect (arrow) in the cisterna magna. (b) In the sagittal T2w sequence: slightly dilated ventricle system, cerebellum herniated through the foramen magnum and syringohydromyelia of the cervical spinal cord, which continued on into the lumbar spinal cord (not shown). (c) The transverse T1w image of the brain shows a moderate hydrocephalus of the supratentorial ventricular system and a fluid-filled left tympanic bulla. (Fig. Johann Lang, Bern.)

17

"pulled" by its collar) to severe generalised ataxia, scoliosis and personality changes. Due to the lesions in the medulla oblongata, cranial nerve deficits (VIII to XII) and disturbances in consciousness have been observed but these are infrequent and other causes should be investigated.

Another malformation which is sometimes associated with anomalies of the medulla oblongata is the Dandy Walker Syndrome (see Chap. 16.4.1.2).

In human beings, malformations of the nervous tissue are frequently associated with anomalies in the bony parts of the caudal cranium. In animals, respective investigations are lacking.

Clinically, occipital malformations are mainly associated with cervical cord symptoms, though they can also involve brain stem symptoms in the form of disturbances of consciousness (47).

Occipital dysplasia is a congenital malformation of the caudal cranium resulting in an abnormally large foramen magnum. An obvious broadening of the foramen magnum in toy dogs such as the Yorkshire Terrier, Toy Spitz and Chihuahua has been associated with a neurological syndrome consisting of generalised ataxia, reduced consciousness and various cranial nerve deficits (48). Morphometrical studies of the foramen magnum in clinically normal dogs have, however, revealed that the varying shapes and sizes of the foramen magnum can just be individual variations and are not clinically relevant (49). Dogs with deficits that indicate caudal brain stem, cerebellum or the high cervical region localisations should therefore undergo a thorough work up (CSF analysis, CT, MRI) before occipital dysplasia is documented as responsible for the clinical problem.

Diagnosis: Radiography, CT, MRI.

Therapy: There is no specific therapy for the majority of these malformations. Syringo(hydro)myelia: restrict movement, palliative steroids, diuretics, gabapentin. Surgical intervention in the form of a decompression of the caudal cranial fossa via a suboccipital approach, C1 dorsal laminectomy and the positioning of a ventriculoperitoneal shunt has been described with reasonable success in the dog (50).

Prognosis: Guarded.

17.2.5 Metabolic-toxic diseases of the brain stem

17.2.5.1 Metronidazole intoxication

Occurrence: Dog and cat.

Aetiology: Metronidazole (Flagyl®) is a nitroimidazole chemotherapeutic, which is used against anaerobic infections,

protozoa (Giardia, trichomonads), gastrointestinal inflammation and hepatoencephalopathy. Disturbances of the CNS can arise with chronic therapy or the application of high dosages > 60 mg/kg/d (e.g. treatment of gastrointestinal parasites). The mechanism is unknown. Metronidazole crosses the blood-brain barrier and accumulates in the CNS. It is metabolised in the liver and excreted via the urine and faeces (54).

Clinical: The clinical symptoms are acute severe ataxia, hypermetria, tremor, weakness, disturbances in balance, disorientation, reduced positioning and placement reflexes, reduced menace reaction, nystagmus, apathy, and seizures (51, 52, 53). Histopathological lesions (swelling of axons, leukomalacia) have been observed in the central vestibular system and the brain stem.

Diagnosis: Anamnesis, improvement of the clinical symptoms within 48 hours after stopping metronidazole.

Therapy: Immediate stoppage of metronidazole, supportative therapy.

Prognosis: Favourable; slow recovery within 1 to 2 weeks, neurological deficits may persist (52).

17.2.5.2 Thiamine or Vitamin B₁ deficiency encephalopathy

Occurrence: Especially in cats with diets of raw fish. Rare in the dog. Can also occur secondary to liver, pancreatic or gastrointestinal disease.

Aetiology: Thiamine is a water-soluble vitamin. It is found in the food as thiamine pyrophosphate particularly in yeast, cereals, liver, kidneys and meat. The body must have a continuous supply of this vitamin. It is resorbed in the duodenum. Dietary thiamine deficiency occurs due to (1) reduced food intake (inappetence, anorexia), (2) thiamine deficiency in the food due to excessive conservation of tinned food or the conservation of fresh food with sulphur-containing substances (SO_2) (56, 57, 60), and (3) uptake of thiaminases associated with the feeding of raw fish. If fur-bearing animals are fed only fish offal (mackerel, carp), then Chastek paralysis can develop (55, 56).

Thiamine has an important function as a coenzyme of a series of enzymes involved in energy metabolism, especially those of carbohydrate metabolism. Both mitochondrial pyruvate dehydrogenase, which channels the final products of aerobic glycolysis in the citrate cycle, and transketolase in the pentose phosphate cycle are thiamine-dependent enzymes. A disturbed energy supply resulting from dysfunctions of these enzymes results in CNS symptoms.

Thiamine deficiency causes bilateral symmetrical vascular disease of the brain stem; specifically, there are petechial haemorrhages in the brain stem nuclei, individually shrivelled and degenerated neurons, and swollen axons. The areas affected include the paraventricular and periaqueductal nuclei: vestibular nucleus, oculomotor nucleus, red nucleus, caudal quadrigeminal plate, lateral geniculate body, basal nuclei and the cerebellar vermis (55, 59).

Clinical: As clinical symptoms, cats initially show anorexia and occasional vomiting, followed by vestibular ataxia, dilated poorly responsive pupils, seizures, ventroflexion of the head / neck, coma and death. In the dog, thiamine deficiency manifests itself as spastic paresis, ataxia, torticollis, circling and seizures (56, 58, 59).

Diagnosis: Anamnesis, clinical symptoms, increased concentration of pyruvate and lactate in the blood and CSF, reduced activity of transketolase in the erythrocytes, and disappearance of the signs following thiamine administration.

Therapy: Thiamine 10–100 µg/kg/d.

Prognosis: Good with immediate treatment, although dependent on the severity of the clinical signs.

17.2.6 Diseases of the cranial nerves

Table 17.2: Diseases of the cranial nerves and musculature

V	■ Intraneural haemorrhage (dog / cat) ■ Trigeminal neuritis (dog)
I	■ Polyneuritis ■ Cranial neuropathy (cat) ■ Focal myasthenia gravis (dog / cat) ■ Mastication muscle myopathy ■ Myositis (dog) ■ Polymyositis (dog / cat)
T	■ Nerve trauma (dog / cat)
M	■ Hypothyroidism (dog) ■ Botulinum toxin (dog) ■ Tetanus toxin (dog / cat)
I	■ Idiopathic facial nerve paralysis (dog, rare cat) ■ Megaoesophagus (dog / cat) ■ Laryngeal paralysis (dog) ■ Idiopathic cricopharyngeal dysphagia (dog)
N	■ Schwannoma (dog / cat) ■ Neurofibroma (dog / cat) ■ Neuroepithelioma (dog / cat)
D	■ Congenital laryngeal paralysis (dog / cat) ■ Acquired laryngeal paralysis (dog / cat)

17.2.6.1. Trigeminal neuritis (Idiopathic trigeminal neuropathy)

Occurrence: Sporadic. There is possibly an increased risk in the Golden Retriever. This disease is extremely rare in the cat.

Aetiology: Idiopathic. Inflammation of all parts of the trigeminal nerve can be found in some cases, while in others neuropraxia has been found.

Clinical: The most common clinical signs include an inability to close the lower jaw, difficulty ingesting water and food, and hypersalivation. Less common signs include sensory deficits in the area supplied by the trigeminal nerve, Horner's syndrome, muscle atrophy and facial nerve deficits. Depression, vomiting, dehydration, dyspnoea and injected scleral vessels can be seen as extraneurological symptoms. Corneal lesions as a consequence of a neuroparalytic keratitis are sporadic complications of the disease.

Diagnosis: Clinical symptoms. CSF changes in the form of a mild increase in protein and a slight mononuclear pleocytosis may arise. EMG changes in the form of denervation potentials can be expected a week after the occurrence of the clinical symptoms. The differential diagnoses include bilateral luxation of the mandibular joints, oral foreign bodies, mandibular fractures or disease of the masticatory muscles.

Therapy: Spontaneous resolution can be expected in 4 to 9 weeks. Steroids do not speed up the remission. Affected animals must be supported by being fed with moistened pieces of food placed directly in the mouth and water supplied by syringe in the mouth. Tear replacement therapy is necessary with neuroparalytic keratitis.

Prognosis: Favourable. Animals with sensory deficits may require somewhat longer periods of recovery. Relapses are extremely exceptional (61).

17.2.6.2 Idiopathic facial nerve paralysis

Occurrence: Frequent in the dog; rare in the cat.

Aetiology: Unknown. Swelling of the nerve within its bony canal (facial nerve canal in the petrous bone) has been purported as a possible cause (analogous to Bell's facial nerve paralysis in human beings). Histological investigations of the nerve in two diseased dogs revealed degeneration of the nerve fibres and demyelination of large diameter fibres (62, 63).

Clinical: Generally, there seems to be an increased risk of this disease in dogs with large, hanging ears and in the Cocker Spaniel in particular.

Facial nerve paralysis usually occurs acutely and on one side. The contralateral side may become affected during the course

17

Table 17.3: Diseases causing megaoesophagus

Neuromuscular
- Congenital (dog: Shar Pei, Newfoundland; cat: Siamese)
- Idiopathic (dog/cat)
- Hereditary (dog: Fox Terrier, Miniature Schnauzer)
- Myasthenia gravis (dog/cat)
- Dysautonomia (dog/cat)
- Systemic lupus erythematosus (dog)
- Polymyositis (dog/cat)
- Glycogen storage diseases (dog/cat)
- Polyradiculoneuritis (dog)
- Spinal muscle atrophy (cat/dog)
- Bilateral vagus lesions (dog/cat)
- Brain stem diseases (dog/cat)

Poisoning
- Lead (dog/cat)
- Thallium (dog/cat)
- Anticholinesterase (dog/cat)

Others
- Hypoadrenocorticism (dog)
- Hypothyroidism (dog)
- Mediastinitis – inflammatory (dog/cat)
- Pylorus stenosis (dog/cat)
- Persistent Botallo's duct (dog/cat)
- Hiatal hernia (dog/cat)
- Oesophageal foreign bodies (dog/cat)
- Stricture due to scarring – post inflammatory (dog/cat)
- Oesophageal tumours (dog/cat)

of the disease in some cases. Typical for this disease is the lack of other deficits such as vestibular disease or Horner's syndrome.

Diagnosis: Diagnosis by process of elimination using otoscopy, radiography (bullae series) or as more sensitive methods, CT or MRI. Thyroid tests to exclude hypothyroidism should be considered (64).

EMG of other cranial muscles and the skeletal musculature helps in differentiating this disease from a more generalised polyneuropathy.

Therapy: A specific treatment for idiopathic facial paralysis is not known. Steroids do not have any influence on the disease course.

Prognosis: Spontaneous remission can be expected within 6 weeks. In some cases, the deficits can persist throughout life. Fibrotic contracture of the face muscles can occur with chronic disease. Monitoring tear production (Schirmer tear test) is recommended, so that tear replacement therapy can be initiated to prevent the development of keratoconjunctivitis sicca.

17.2.6.3 Megaoesophagus

Occurrence: Frequent in the dog; rare in the cat.

Aetiology: Idiopathic or as a symptom of various diseases (Table 17.3).

Clinical: Regurgitation is the cardinal symptom of megaoesophagus. Affected animals often exhibit drooling of saliva from their mouths. Secondary aspiration pneumonia is common (65, 66, 67, 68, 69).

Diagnosis: Clinical symptoms (see above). Radiography of the thorax. Other investigations in individual cases include: (1) CBC, blood biochemistry, urinalysis; (2) endoscopy, possibly fluoroscopic swallowing tests; (3) thyroid function tests, antiacetylcholine receptor antibody titre, ACTH stimulation test, antinuclear antibody titre, electromyography of the head and skeletal musculature, nerve-muscle biopsy; (4) CSF investigation, MRI, CT when brain stem lesions are suspected.

Therapy: Treatment of the causal disease. Symptomatic: feeding with head and neck elevated, e.g. on stairs or with the food bowl on a chair. Feeding via percutaneous stomach tube. Systemic antibiosis for aspiration pneumonia. Pro-motility drugs such as cisapride are often recommended.

Prognosis: Unfavourable. Megaoesophagus is reversible in some cases of myasthenia gravis, hypothyroidism, hypoadrenocorticism and some intoxications if the causal disease can be treated successfully (70).

17.2.6.4 Idiopathic cricopharyngeal dysphagia (achalasia)

Occurrence: Rare; in various dog breeds in puppyhood.

Aetiology: Due to an unknown mechanism, there is inadequate relaxation of the cricopharyngeal muscle (sphincter of the proximal oesophagus) during swallowing. Some dogs have an additional complication involving motility disturbances in the cranial oesophagus. These symptoms indicate that there is a disturbance in the afferent signal transmission from the pharynx or there is a lesion in the swallowing centre in the brain stem (nucleus ambiguus).

Clinical: Affected puppies demonstrate repeated swallowing movements when sucking, followed by choking, coughing and nasal regurgitation.

Diagnosis: The clinical symptoms, fluoroscopic swallowing studies with contrast-containing food, EMG of the pharyngeal muscles, muscle biopsy of the pharyngeal muscles. Determination of anti-acetylcholine receptor antibodies to rule out possible focal myasthenia gravis (71, 72, 73, 76).

Therapy: Symptomatic surgical resection of the dorsal part of the cricopharyngeal muscle (74, 75). This operation is, however, contraindicated in animals with oral or pharyngeal swallowing disturbances (risk of making the symptoms worse).

Prognosis: Unfavourable without treatment (aspiration pneumonia).

17.2.6.5 Idiopathic laryngeal paralysis

Occurrence: Frequent. A greater incidence is seen in aged dog from large breeds (e.g. Afghan, Irish Setter Labrador Retriever, St. Bernard). Castrated male animals have an increased tendency for this disease.

Aetiology: Idiopathic neuropathy of the recurrent laryngeal nerve with atrophy of the laryngeal muscles. It is possibly part of a subclinical polyneuropathy (77). The differential diagnoses include all other diseases that cause laryngeal paralysis (Table 17.4).

Clinical: Exertion intolerance, inspiratory stridor, dyspnoea, hoarseness, dysphagia, choking and coughing.

Diagnosis: By process of elimination; signalment, anamnesis, laryngoscopy.

Therapy: Different surgical methods have been described. Lateral fixation of the arytenoid cartilage and of the vocal cords usually leads to a satisfactory result (79).

Prognosis: Favourable after surgical therapy.

17.2.6.6 Hereditary laryngeal paralysis

Occurrence: Rare. Dog: affected breeds include Alaskan Malamute, Bouvier des Flandres, Dalmatian, Rottweiler and Siberian Husky (68).

Aetiology: Inherited disease. Histopathological findings include degenerative neuropathy of the recurrent laryngeal nerve and degenerative lesions in the neurons of the brain stem. The disease is autosomal recessive in the Bouvier des Flandres and leads to a uni- or bilateral laryngeal paralysis. Stress can lead to laryngeal spasm and life-threatening hyperthermia.

Table 17.4: Differential diagnoses of idiopathic laryngeal paralysis

- Laryngitis (bacterial or viral)
- Laryngeal trauma
- Congenital malformation (brachycephalic breeds)
- Myasthenia gravis (focal form)
- Neoplasia in region of the larynx

Clinical: See idiopathic laryngeal paralysis (Chap. 17.2.6.5).

Diagnosis: Signalment, anamnesis, laryngoscopy, EMG.

Therapy and Prognosis: Analogous to idiopathic or acquired laryngeal paralysis. Selective breeding.

17.2.7 Deafness

Occurrence: Deafness is particularly well described in the Australian Sheepdog, Bull Terrier, Dalmatian, English Bulldog, English Setter, Great Dane, Norwegian Dunker Hound, Old English Sheepdog and Sealyham Terrier. White cats.

Aetiology: In addition to inflammatory, traumatic, toxic, neoplastic and age-associated causes of deafness at the level of the PNS, animals can be affected by congenital deafness in association with degenerative changes or malformations of the peripheral auditory apparatus. This is especially frequent in cats with white fur and blue irises. In the dog, there is a positive correlation with certain pigmentation genes (merle and piebald genes).

Diagnosis: Hearing is a difficult sensory function to test in animals. It can only be objectively investigated in clinical animal neurology by electrophysiological means such as auditory evoked potentials (Chap. 7.1.3). Only total deafness or extremely reduced hearing can be determined clinically.

Therapy and Prognosis: Selective breeding measures are considered the only prophylaxis. The prognosis of hearing defects in congenital deafness is poor as there is no treatment.

Literature

1 AXLUND, T.W., ISAACS, A.M., HOLLAND, M., O'BRIEN, D.P. (2004): Fibrocathilaginous embolic encephalomyelopathy of the brainstem and midcervical spinal cord in a dog. J. Vet. Intern Med 18: 765–7

2 GREENE, C.E. (1998): Infectious Diseases of the Dogs and Cat. WB Saunders, Philadelphia, pp. 114–126.

3 TIPOLD, A. (1997): Entzündliche Erkrankungen des Nervensystems. Enke Verlag, Stuttgart.

4 STEFFEN, F.: Mündliche Mitteilung aus eigenem Patientengut.

5 STETTLER, M., ZURBRIGGEN A. (1995): Nucleotide and deduced amino acid sequences of the nucleocapsid protein of the virulent. A75/17-CDV strain of canine distemper virus, Vet Microbiol. **44:** 11–217.

6 MORITZ, A. (1998): Beurteilung diagnostischer Möglichkeiten bei der Staupevirusinfektion des Hundes. Kleintierprax. **43:** 153–172.

17

7 BARONI, M., HEINOLD Y. (1995): A review of the clinical diagnosis of Feline Infectious Peritonitis viral meningoencephalomyelitis. Vet Neurol. **6, 3:** 88–94.

8 FOLEY, J.E., LAPOINTE J.M, KOBLIK P., POLAND A., PEDERSEN N.C. (1998): Diagnostic features of neurologic feline infectious peritonitis. J Vet Intern Med. **12:** 415–423.

9 SUMMER, B.A., CUMMINGS, J.F., DE LAHUNTA, A. (1994): Veterinary Neuropathology pp. 110–111.

10 BRAUND, K.G. (1998): Granulomatous meningoencephalitis. J Am Vet Med Assoc. **186:** 138–141.

11 KASER-HOTZ, B.: Institut für Radiologie und Radioonkologie, Vetsuisse Fakultät Universität Zürich; personal communication.

12 BAILEY, C.S., HIGGINS, R.J. (1986): Characteristics of cerebrospinal fluid associated with canine granulomatous meningoencephalitis. J Am Vet Med Assoc. **188:** 418–421.

13 NUSHBAUM, M.T., POWELL, C.C., GIONFRIDDO, J.R., CUDDON, P.A. (2001): Treatment of granulomatous meningoencephalitis in a dog. Vet Ophthalmol. in press.

14 TIPOLD, A. (1993): Zentraleuropäische Zeckenenzephalitis beim Hund, Kleintierprax. 38, 619–628.

15 FISCHER, A. (1998): Proc ECVN, Vienna.

16 LINDSAY D.S., RITTER D.M., BRAKE D. (2001): Oocyst excretion in dogs fed mouse brains containing tissue cysts of cloned line of *Neospora caninum*. J Parasitol. **87:** 1171–1173.

17 BASSO, W., VENTURINI, L., MORRE, P., RAMBEAU, M., UNZAGA, C., CAMPERO, C., BACIGALUPE, D., DUBEY, J.R. (2001): Prevalance of *Neospora caninum* infection in dogs from beef-cattle farms, dairy farms, and from urban areas of Argentina J Parasitol. **87:** 906–907.

18 DUBEY, J.P., METZGER, F.L., HATTEL, A.L.(1995): Canine cutaneous neoprosis clinical improvement with clindamycin. Vet Derm. **6:** 37–43.

19 GREIG, B., ROSSOW, K.D., COLLINS, J.E. (1995): *Neospora caninum* pneumonia in an adult dog. J Am Vet Med Assoc. **206:** 1000–1001.

20 DUBEY, J.P., LAPPIN M.R. (1998): Neosporosis. In: GREENE, C.E. (ed.): Infectious Diseases of the Dog and Cat. W.B. Saunders, Philadelphia, pp. 503–509.

21 WOLF, M., CACHIN, M., VANDEVELDE, M. (1991): Zur klinischen Diagnostik des protozoären Myositissyndroms (*Neospora caninum*) des Welpen. Tierärztl Prax. **19:** 302–306.

22 GREENE, C.E., DREESEN, D.W. (1998): Rabies. In: GREENE, C.E. (ed): Infectious Diseases of the Dog and Cat, W.B. Saunders, Philadelphia, pp. 114–126.

23 KELLER, D.: Landesuntersuchungsamt Südbayern in Unterschleißheim; personal communication.

24 GÖDDE, T. (2004): Personal communication.

25 WHO Bericht (1998): Rabies.

26 VANVELDE, M. (1998): Pseudorabies. In: GREENE C.E. (ed.) Infectious diseases of the dog and cats, WB Saunders, Philadelphia, pp. 126–128.

27 TIPOLD, A., FATZER, R, JAGGY, A. (1993): Necrotizing encephalitis in Yorkshire terriers. J Small Anim Pract. **34:** 623–28.

28 CORNWELL, H.J., THOMPSON, H., MCCANDLISH, I.A., MACARTNEY, L., NASH A.S. (1998): Encephalitis in dogs associated with a batch of canine distemper vaccine. Vet Rec. **122:** 54–59.

29 DEMIERRE, S., BOTTERON, C., CIZINAUSKAS, S., DOHERR, M.G., FATZER, R., JAGGY, A. (2002): Feline Spongyform Encephalopahty: first clinical case in Switzerland. Schweiz Arch Tierheilkd. **144:** 550–557.

30 APPEL, M. (1987): Canine herpesvirus. In: Appel M (ed.) Virus infections of carnivores. Amsterdam, Elsevier.

31 TIPOLD, A. (1995): Diagnosis of inflammatory and infectious diseases of the central nervous system in dogs: a retrospective study. J Vet Intern Med. **9:** 304–314.

32 CHRISMAN, C.L (2001): When titers are negative – meningoencephalomyelitis retrospectively. Proceedings 19th ACVIM, Denver, 390–392.

33 BAGLEY, R. S., WHEELER, S. J., KLOPP, L. (1998): Clinical features of trigeminal nerve-sheath tumor in 10 dogs. J Am Anim Hosp Assoc. **34:** 19–25.

34 BAILEY, C.S., HIGGINS, R.J. (1986): Characteristics of cisternal cerebrospinal fluid associated with primary brain tumors in the dog: A retrospective study. J Am Vet Assoc. **188:** 414–417.

35 CIZINAUSKAS, S., LANG, J., MAIER, R. (2001): Paradoxical vestibular disease with trigeminal nerve-sheath tumor in a dog. Schweiz Arch Tierheilkd. **143:** 419–425.

36 DEWEY, C.W., BAHR, A., DUCOTÉ, J.M. (2000): Primary brain tumors in dogs and cats. Compend Contin Educ Pract Vet. **22:** 756–762.

37 FISCHER, A., OBERMAIER, G. (1994): Brainstem auditory-evoked potentials and neuropatholgic correlates in 263 dogs with brain tumors. J Vet Int Med. **8:** 363–369.

38 HEIDNER, G.L., KORNEGAY, J.R., PAGE, R. L. (1991): Analysis of survival in a retrospective study of 86 dogs with brain tumors. J Vet Int Med. **5:** 219–226.

39 KLOPP, L.S., SIMPSON, S.T., SORJONEN, D.C. (2000): Ventral surgical approach to the caudal brain stem in dogs. Vet Surg. **29:** 533–542.

40 KORNEGAY, J.N. (1990): Imaging brain neoplasms: Computed tomography and magnetic resonance imaging. Vet Med Rep. **2:** 372–390.

41 KRAFT, S.L., GAVIN, P.R., DE HAAN, C., et al. (1997): Retrospective review of 50 canine intracranial tumors evaluated by magnetic resonance imaging. J Vet Intern Med. **11:** 218–225.

42 LECOUTEUR, R.A. (1999): Current conceps in the diagnosis and treatment of brain tumors in dogs and cats. J. Small Anim Pract. **40:** 411–416.

43 MOORE, M.P., BAGLEY, R.S., HARRINGTON, M.L., et al (1996): Intracranial tumors. Vet Clin North Am Small Anim Pract. **26:** 759–777.

44 STEISS, J.E., COX, N.C., HATHCOCK, J.T. (1994): Brain stem auditory-evoked response abnormalities in 14 dogs with confirmed central nervous system lesions. J Vet Int Med. **8:** 293–298.

17

45 THOMAS, W.B., WHEELER, S.J., KRAMER, R. (1996): Magnetic resonance imaging features of primary brain tumors in dogs. Vet Radiol Ultrasound **37**: 20–27.

46 RUSBRIDGE, C., M.C., SWEENY, J.M., DAVIS, J.V., CHANDLER, K., FITZMAURICE, S.N., DENNIS, R., CAPELLO, R., WHEELER, S.J. (2000): Syringohydromyelia in Cavalier King Charles Spaniels: J Am Anim Hosp Assoc. **36**: 34–41.

47 JAGGY, A., HUTTO, C., OLIVER, J.R. (1991): Occipito-atlanto-axial malformation in a cat. J Small Anim Pract. **32**: 366–372.

48 PARKER, A.J., PARK, R.D. (1974): Occipital dysplasia in the dog. J Am Anim Hosp Assoc. **10**: 520–526.

49 SIMONES, P., POELS, P., LAUWERS, H. (1994): Morphometric analysis of the foramen magnum in pekingese dogs. Am J Vet Res. **55 (1):** 43–49.

50 VERMEERSCH, K., VAAN HAM, L.; CAEMAERT, J., TSHAMALA, M., TAEYMANS, O., BHATTIS, S., POLIS, I., (2004): Suboccipital craniectomy, dorsal laminectomy of C1, durotomy and dural gratt placement as a treatment for syringomyenia with cerebella tonsil nermiation in CKC-Spaniels. Vet Surg (33)4: 355–60.

51 CAYLOR, K.B., CASSIMATIS, M.K.v (2001): Metronidazol neurotoxicosis in two cats. J Am Anim Hosp Assoc. **37**: 258–262.

52 DOW, S.W., LECOUTEUR, R.A., POSS, M.L., BEADLESTON, D. (1989): Central nervous system toxicosis associated with metronidazole treatment of dogs: Five cases (1984–1987). J Am Vet Med Assoc. **195**: 365–368.

53 FITCH, R., MOORE, M., ROEN, D. (1991): A warning to clinicians: Metronidazole neurotoxicity in a dog. Prog Vet Neurol. **4:** 307–309.

54 KAPOOR, K., CHANDRA, M., NAG, D., PALIWAL, J.K., GUPTA, R.C., SAXENA, R.C.(1999): Evaluation of metronidazole toxicity: a prospective study. Int J Pharmacol Res. **19(3):** 83–88.

55 JUBB, K.V., SAUNDERS, L.Z., COATES, H.V. (1956): Thiamine deficiency encephalopathy in cats. J Comp Pathol Bacteriol. **66:** 217.

56 LOEW, F.M., MARTIN, C.L., DUNLOP, R.H., MAPLEHOF, R.J., SMITH, S.I. (1970): Naturally-occuring and experimental thiamin deficiency in cats recieving commercial cat food. Can Vet J. **11:** 109.

57 READ, D.H., HARRINGTON, D.D. (1981): Experimentally induced thiamine deficiency in Beagle dogs: Clinical observations. Am J Vet Res. **42:** 989.

58 READ, D.H., HARRINGTON, D.D. (1981): Experimentally induced thiamine deficiency in Beagle dogs: Clinicopathologic findings. Am J Vet Res. **43:** 1258–1267.

59 READ, D.H., JOLLY, R.D., ALLEY, M.R. (1977): Poliencephalomalacia in dogs with thiamine deficiency. Vet Pathol. **14:** 103.

60 STUDDERT, V.P., LABUC, R.H. (1991): Thiamin deficiency in cats and dogs associated with feeding meat preserved with sulfur dioxide. Aust Vet J. **68:** 54–57.

61 MAYHEW, P.D., BUSH, W.W., GLASS, E.N. (2002): Trigeminal neuropathy in dogs: a retrospective study of 29 cases. J Am Anim Hosp Assoc. **38:** 262–270.

62 KERN, T.J., ERB, H.N. (1987): Facial neuropathy in dogs and cats: 95 cases, 1975–1985. J Am Vet Med Assoc. **191:** 1604–1609.

63 BRAUND, K.G., LUTTGEN, P.J., SORJONEN, D.C. (1979): Idiopathic facial paralysis in the dog. Vet Rec **105:** 927–929.

64 JAGGY, A., OLIVER, J.E., FERGUSON, D.C. (1994): Neurological manifestations of hypothyroidism: A retrospective study of 29 dogs. J Vet Intern Med **8:** 328–336.

65 COX, V.S., WALLACE, L.J., ANDERSON, V.E. (1980): Hereditary eosophageal dysfunction in the miniature schnauzer dog. Am J Vet Res **41:** 326–330.

66 GUILFORD, W.G. (1990): Megaoesophagus in the dog and cat. Semin Vet Med Surg. **5:** 37–45.

67 SCHWARTZ, A., RAVIN, C.E., GREENSPAN, R.H. (1976): Congenital neuromuscular eosophageal disease in a litter of Newfoundland puppies. J Vet Radiol **17:** 101–105.

68 KNOWLES, J.E., O'BRIEN, D.P., AMANN, J.F. (1990): Congenital idiopathic megaoesophagus in a litter of Chinese Shar Peis: Clinical, electrodiagnostic an pathological findings. J Am Anim Hosp Assoc. **26:** 313–318.

69 BOUDRIEAU, R.J., ROGERS, W.A. (1985): Megaoesophagus in the dog: A review of 50 cases. J Am Anim Hosp Assoc. **26:** 182–183.

70 WASHABAU, R.J. (1986): Pathogenesis and therapy of canine megaoesophagus. Proc. Amer.Coll. Vet. Intern. Med. **10:** 671–674.

71 SUTER, P.F., WATROUS, B.J. (1980): Oropharyngeal dysphagias in the dog: a cinefluorographic analysis of experimentally induced an spontaneously occuring swallowing disorders. Vet Radiol **21:** 24–39.

72 WATROUS, B.J., SUTER, P.F. (1983): Oropharyngeal dysphagias in the dog: a cinefluorographic analysis of experimentally induced and spontaneously occuring swallowing disorders, II: cricopharyngeal stage and mixed oropharyngeal dysphagias. Vet Radiol. **24:** 11–24.

73 VENKER-VAN HAAGEN, A.J. (2000): Neural regulation of swallowing: Relevance to swallowing disorders. Proc 18th Ann Vet Med Forum, pp. 71–573.

74 WEAVER, A.D. (1983): Cricopharyngeal achalasia in Cocker Spaniels. J Small Anim Pract. **24:** 209–214.

75 NILES, J.D., WILLIAMS, J.M., SULLIVAN, M., CROWSLEY, F.E. (2001): Resolution of dysphagia following cricopharyngeal myectomy in six young dogs. J Small Anim Pract **42:** 32–35.

76 SHELTON, G.D., WILLARD, M.D., CARDINET G.H., LINDSTROM J. (1990): Acquired myasthenia gravis: selective involvement of esophageal, pharyngeal, and facial muscles. J Vet Intern Med. **4:** 218–284.

77 BRAUND, K.G., STEINBERG, H.S., SHORES, A. (1989): Larnygeal paralysis in immature and mature dogs as one sign of a diffuse polyneuropathy. J Am Vet Med Asooc. **194:** 1735–1740.

17

78 VENKER-VAN HAGEN, A. (1992). Diseases of the larynx. Vet Clin North Am Small Anim Pract. **22:** 1155.

79 WHITE, R.A.S. (1989): Unilateral arytenoid lateralisation: An assessment of technique and long-term results in 62 dogs with laryngeal paralysis. J Small Anim Pract. **30:** 543.

17.3 Neuro-ophthalmology

Bernhard Spiess

Neuro-ophthalmological patients are presented not only because of disturbances of vision but also due to abnormal positioning and/or mobility of the globes. In addition to the assessment of vision, therefore, the testing of the pupillary light reflex is of central importance. It is simple to do and quickly provides indications of the most important and frequent neuro-ophthalmological problems in small animals.

17.3.1 Abnormal pupillary light reflexes (PLR)

The direct and indirect PLR can be tested in both eyes using the swinging light test. In addition, the size of the pupils must be compared to determine the presence of unequal sizes (anisocoria).

17.3.1.1 Lesions of the retina or the optic nerve

Prechiasmal lesions can be localised with the swinging light test as long as they are unilateral. A positive swinging light test is always an indication of an ipsilateral prechiasmal lesion, i.e. the lesion is on the side of the absent or reduced PLR (Fig. 17.6).

Bilateral lesions are characterised by absent or delayed PLR and associated visual disturbances. They can be easily diagnosed using ophthalmoscopic and electroretinographic investigations.

Retinal degeneration

Occurrence: Dogs and cats. In addition to the inflammatory changes found in the choroid and retina, retinal heredodegeneration is playing a greater and greater role in retinal degeneration. As this is a bilateral change, the swinging light test is not meaningful. However, the retinal changes are often diagnostic.

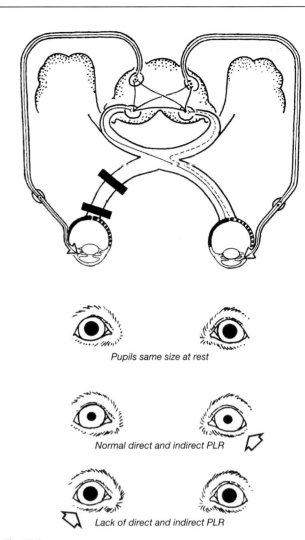

Pupils same size at rest

Normal direct and indirect PLR

Lack of direct and indirect PLR

Fig. 17.6
Prechiasmic lesions of the optic nerve cause a positive swinging flashlight test.

Aetiology: In some breeds the cause of this heredodegeneration is known. In the Collie, for example, it is associated with a deficiency of cAMP phosphodiesterase in the area of the outer segment of the photoreceptors (1). In recent years, the research in this field has been concentrated on the affected gene loci (1, 2, 3, 4, 5, 6).

Clinical: The disease begins, depending on the breed, at 1 to 4 years of age. It is initially expressed as night blindness. Later, the visual acuity is reduced during the day, too. Parallel to this, mydriasis and increased reflectivity of the tapetum lucidum occurs (7). The degeneration follows the loss of the rods and cones as well as their associated neurons. This is seen ophthalmoscopically as a hyperreflectivity of the retina, atrophy of the retinal venules and arterioles, and finally by demyelination and atrophy of the optic papilla (Fig. 17.7).

17

Diagnosis: The diagnosis is usually based on the typical clinical picture, the time of development and the breed of the affected patient. In equivocal cases, the diagnosis can be ascertained using ERG (8).

Therapy: As there is no treatment for this heredodegeneration, selective breeding is of great importance. Nowadays, molecular genetic investigations are being undertaken in addition to the standard ophthalmoscopic investigations (5, 9, 10, 11, 12, 13, 14, 15).

Prognosis: Hopeless.

Naturally, numerous other inflammatory and infectious changes in the retina and choroid can also lead to uni- or bilateral blindness (16).

Retrobulbar (optic) neuritis

Occurrence: In the dog, independent of age, breed and sex.

Aetiology: The causes of retrobulbar (optic) neuritis can be traumatic, infectious, neoplastic, toxic, metabolic and immunological (17). Traumatic neuropathy is mainly observed as a consequence of proptosis in brachycephalic dogs (18). The abrupt displacement of the bulbus leads to massive traction on the optic nerve with its subsequent degeneration. The lesion is usually one-sided. Granulomatous meningoencephalitis has also been described as a cause of retrobulbar neuritis (19). However, in the dog, the aetiology is unknown (20, 21).

Clinical: Retrobulbar (optic) neuritis manifests as an acute bilateral blindness with dilated pupils. In some cases, oedema of the papilla and the surrounding retina can be seen in addition to haemorrhages in this area.

Diagnosis: The diagnosis is based on the clinical picture, anamnesis and the ERG results.

Therapy: If diagnosed in time, retrobulbar (optic) neuritis can be successfully treated with prednisolone (2 mg/kg, PO, SID; tapering off over 4 to 5 weeks) (21).

Prognosis: Favourable if diagnosed and treated aggressively in time. In the majority of cases, vision returns within a few hours. Relapses should be considered; therefore long-term therapy with sequentially reduced prednisolone dosages is recommended.

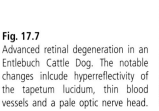
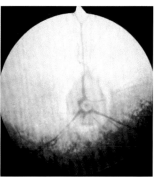

Fig. 17.7
Advanced retinal degeneration in an Entlebuch Cattle Dog. The notable changes inlcude hyperreflectivity of the tapetum lucidum, thin blood vessels and a pale optic nerve head.

Acute retinal necrosis (Sudden acquired retinal degeneration – SARD)

Occurrence: Dog. Mainly adult, obese, castrated female dogs from small breeds are affected. The diagnosis is most common in the Dachshund. Historically, the affected animals often have polyphagia and polydipsia. Recently, a similar syndrome has also been observed in the cat (22, 23, 24, 25).

Aetiology: The cause of SARD is still not known (22, 23, 24, 25).

Clinical: Rapidly developing blindness over a period of a few days. The animals are disorientated, have fixed, dilated pupils and their eyes are notably wide open. The animals have no abnormalities on ophthalmoscopic examination. Signs of diffuse retinal degeneration occur within a few weeks (26).

Diagnosis: The diagnosis is confirmed with ERG. Whereas the ERG remains normal with retrobulbar (optic) neuritis, it is completely absent in SARD (8).

Therapy: There is none (27).

Prognosis: Hopeless for return of vision.

17

Aplasia / Hypoplasia of the optic nerve

Occurrence: Aplasia or hypoplasia of the optic nerve has been described as an inherited problem in a number of dog breeds. It is more commonly found in Toy and Miniature Poodles (28, 29, 30).

Aetiology: Inherited malformation. It has also been described in cattle as a consequence of hypovitaminosis A (31).

Clinical: The animals are blind at birth and have fixed dilated pupils. The optic papilla is conspicuously small and round (Fig. 17.8).

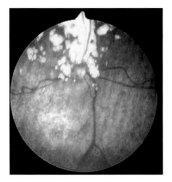

Fig. 17.8
Hypoplasia of the optic nerve in a Poodle puppy. There is a conspicuously small, round optic nerve head with normal-sized retinal blood vessels.

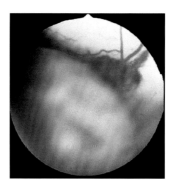

Fig. 17.9
Myxosarcoma of the optic nerve in a dog. The tumour extends far into the vitreous body. An increase in the width of the optic nerve could be seen using ultrasound.

Diagnosis: The clinical picture is usually typical. The mesodermal part of the optic nerve (i.e. the meninges and the glia) is physiologically normal but the axons of the ganglia are missing. The ganglion cell layer of the retina is completely missing. The outer layers of the retina are normal and so the ERG is unchanged (30). The ganglion cells are not involved in the biogenesis of the normal flash ERG. As a rule the changes are bilateral, however, unilateral hypoplasia of the optic nerve has been described (32).

Therapy: None.

Prognosis: Hopeless. Breeding programs may be of prophylactic assistance.

Neoplasia of the optic nerve

Occurrence: In dogs, rarer in cats. Meningioma, ganglioglioma, medulloepthelioma and astrocytoma can all affect the optic nerve (17, 21, 33).

Clinical: If only the intraorbital or intraocular part of the optic nerve is affected, then blindness is unilateral (34). Due to the normal afferent supply in the contralateral eye, the pupil is normal in size or only slightly dilated. The direct and consensual PLR are missing. With extensive neoplasms, the chiasm is also affected and in such cases, the blindness is often bilateral. As a rule, orbital tumours of the optic nerve are associated with an obvious exophthalmos (33, 34). In some cases, intraocular tumour growth can be observed (Fig. 17.9).

Diagnosis: The clinical symptoms usually indicate the presence of a retrobulbar space-occupying lesion. The lesion can be visualised and localised with imaging techniques, which also facilitates the taking of a biopsy (35, 36, 37, 38).

Therapy and Prognosis: In individual cases, an attempt can be made to remove the tumour surgically (34). However, usually the diagnosis has been made too late, so that an operation is no longer possible and only euthanasia can be considered. Recently, radiotherapy of such tumours has become possible in small animals (39, 40, 41).

17.3.1.2 Lesions of the optic chiasm
Lesions of the optic chiasm are rare in small animals as pituitary tumours tend to grow in the direction of the hypothalamus and the chiasm is infrequently affected (Fig. 17.10) (21, 33).

17.3.1.3 Lesions of the optic tract

Occurrence: Rare. Dog.

Aetiology: Bilateral, inflammatory lesions of the optic tract caused by the distemper virus have been described (42).

Clinical: Unilateral lesions of the optic tract cause similar symptoms as prechiasmal lesions, whereby the dilated pupil is on the contralateral side (Fig. 17.11).

Diagnosis: The swinging light test is negative. Clinically, a unilateral lesion of the optic tract causes a uniocular hemianopia of the contralateral eye, which is very difficult to determine with the standard visual tests.

17.3.1.4 Lesions of the oculomotor nerve (CN III)
Lesions of CN III lead to a dilated pupil on the side of the lesion. The direct PLR is lacking, while the indirect PLR is normal. At the same time, the eye may be rotated laterally, which means that there is an exotropia because the lateral rectus muscle (CN VI) has no active opponent (medial rectus muscle [CN III]) (Fig. 17.12) (21, 42).

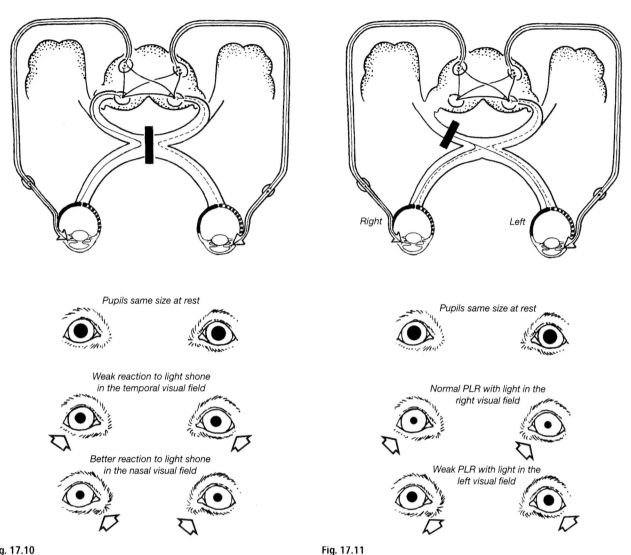

Fig. 17.10
The crossed axons that arise from the medial half of the retina are affected with central lesions of the optic chiasm. The PLR of the medial (i.e. tested by shining a focal light source onto the lateral part of the retina) causes a brisker and more complete PLR.

Fig. 17.11
With one-sided lesions of the optic tract, the swinging flashlight test is negative. Using a focal light source, a more notable PLR can be elicited from the ipsilateral visual field than from the contralateral one.

17.3.1.5 Lesions of the oculomotor (Edinger-Westphal) nucleus

If only the parasympathetic segments of the oculomotor nerve are affected, then a dilated pupil is found on the side of the lesion, though the position of the globe remains unchanged (Fig. 17.13). This is internal ophthalmoplegia (42).

17.3.2 Central blindness

Central blindness is a uni- or bilateral blindness in the presence of a normal pupillary reflex. Unilateral lesions of the optic radiation or the visual cortex cause a hemianopia, i.e. a loss of the contralateral visual field. The cause can be trau-

matic, inflammatory, vascular or neoplastic (42). The different storage diseases can also manifest themselves as a central blindness (27). Complete blindness with retained PLR is typical for a bilateral lesion of the visual cortex, such as can occur after herniation or cranial trauma. One of the most common causes of central blindness in the dog is, however, anaesthetic accident. Anoxia which lasts for more than 3 minutes can lead to damage in the visual cortex (27).

17.3.3 Internal ophthalmoplegia

Internal ophthalmoplegia is also called tonic pupil syndrome or Adie's syndrome (42, 44).

17

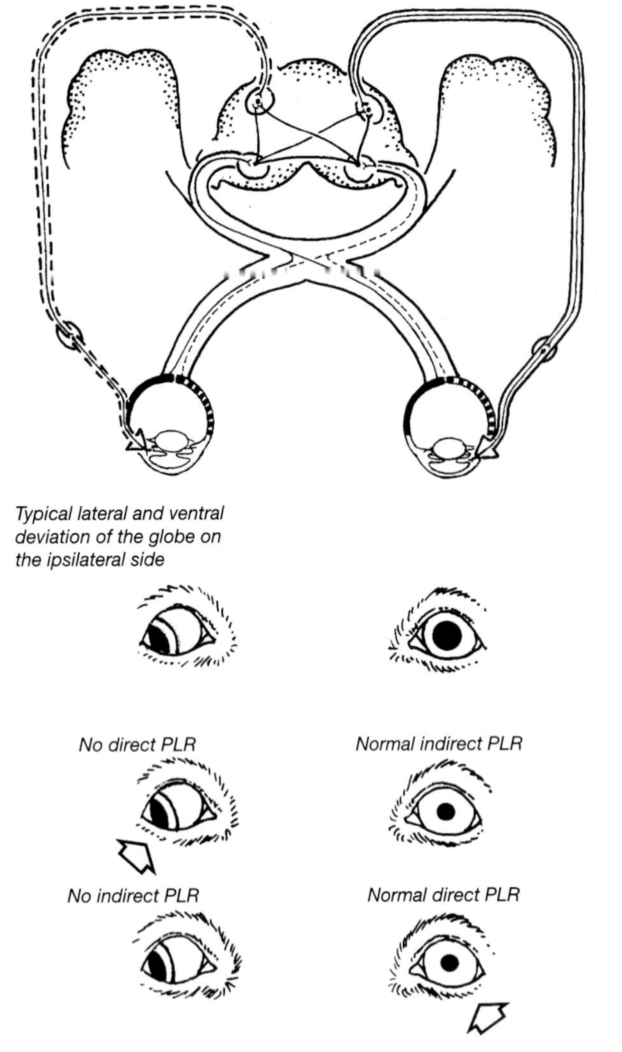

Typical lateral and ventral deviation of the globe on the ipsilateral side

No direct PLR

Normal indirect PLR

No indirect PLR

Normal direct PLR

Fig. 17.12
Lesions of the oculomotor nerve cause a dilated, non-responsive pupil on the same side. At the same time, there can be a lateral and ventral deviation of the ipsilateral globe.

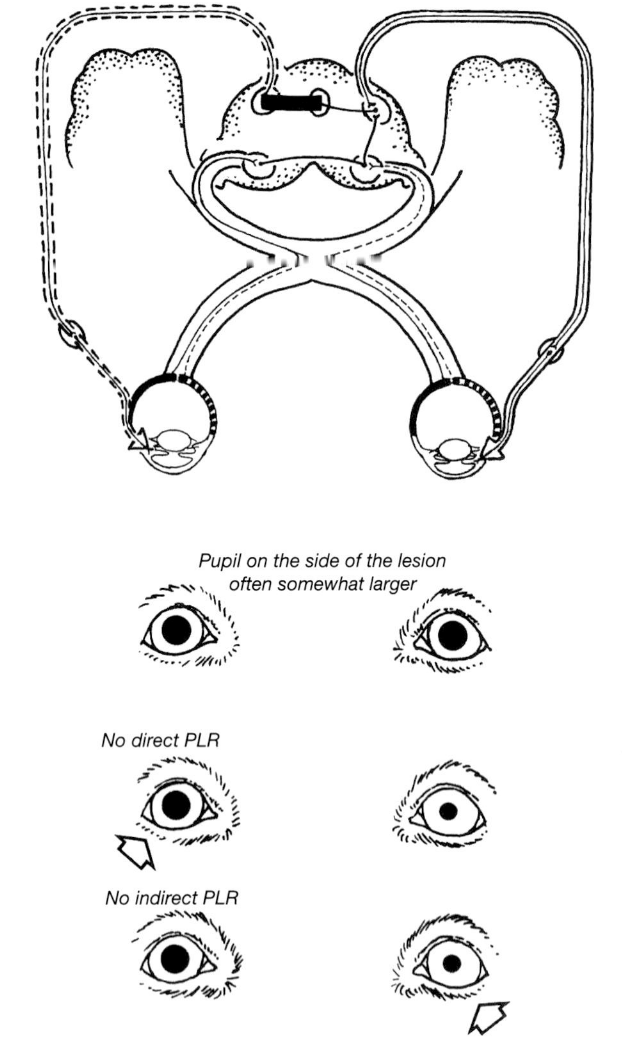

Pupil on the side of the lesion often somewhat larger

No direct PLR

No indirect PLR

Fig. 17.13
With internal ophthalmoplegia, the ipsilateral pupil does not respond directly or indirectly. The anisocoria is stronger in bright light and disappears in the dark.

Occurrence: Rare in the dog.

Aetiology: The aetiology is unknown though inflammatory lesions in the ciliary ganglia have been assumed.

Clinical: The animal is presented with a dilated pupil on one side. Vision is not disturbed. The animal has no direct PLR, but a good indirect PLR, which indicates an efferent problem. The anisocoria is more obvious in bright light. Both pupils are the same width in the dark, indicating a parasympathetic efferent problem.

Diagnosis: The differential diagnosis includes atropinisation of one pupil, atrophy of the pupillary sphincter muscle or the rare Pourfour du Petit syndrome (45). Atropinisation can

usually be historically excluded. Atrophy of the pupillary sphincter muscle can be determined with a biomicroscope. As a rule, the affected animals have a hypersensitivity to parasympathomimetics at low concentrations. Pilocarpine 0.1% induces a strong miosis on the affected side within 20 minutes, while the normal side develops no miosis. This miosis is lacking with both atropinisation of a pupil or atrophy of the pupillary sphincter muscle (Table 17.5).

The differentiation between preganglionic or central lesions from postganglionic lesions can be achieved using physostigmine. A positive test result with pilocarpine confirms the neurological origin of internal ophthalmoplegia. All these tests are negative with either structural changes of the iris or with pharmacological dilatation of the pupil.

17

Therapy: None.

Prognosis: The mydriasis associated with internal ophthalmoplegia decreases with time, although the direct PLR continues to be absent.

17.3.4 External ophthalmoplegia

External ophthalmoplegia is the complete lack of globe movements due to paralysis of the extraocular muscles (21). A bilateral external ophthalmoplegia can also be seen with extraocular polymyositis (Fig. 17.14) (46).

An internal and partial external ophthalmoplegia occurs with lesions of the oculomotor nerve (see Chap. 17.3.1.4). In addition, an internal and external ophthalmoplegia has been described in conjunction with blindness and Horner's syndrome in a cat that had an extensive squamous cell carcinoma (47).

17.3.5 Horner's syndrome

Occurrence: More common in the dog than in the cat.

Aetiology: Horner's syndrome is the result of damage to the sympathetic pupillomotor tract. Differentiation is made between central, preganglionic and postganglionic lesions (27, 48).

The causes of Horner's syndrome are manifold: hypothyroidism, intracranial and intrathoracic tumours, otitis media and interna, and avulsion of the brachial plexus have been reported in both the dog and cat (49). Injuries of the head, neck and thorax in addition to aggressive irrigation of the external auditory canal have also been documented to result in Horner's (50). No cause could be found in approx. 50% of dogs and 42% of cats affected with Horner's syndrome. An idiopathic preganglionic Horner's syndrome has been described in the Golden Retriever (51, 52). The clinical signs disappear spontaneously within 6 months at the most. Rare causes of Horner's syndrome include a leukaemic myelomonocytic leukaemia, surgical operations on the cervical spine and in the orbit, intrathoracic tube drainage and infections with *Neospora canis* (53, 54, 55, 56, 57).

Clinical: Horner's syndrome is characterised by ipsilateral miosis, ptosis and prolapse of the nictitating membrane (Fig. 17.15) (21).

Usually there is also a slight enophthalmos present, whereby the palpebral fissure is also narrowed. The direct PLR is lacking on the side of the lesion or is barely visible. The indirect PLR (on the "normal" side) is present. Anisocoria in this case is more obvious in the dark. In bright light both pupils are the same size. This indicates the presence of an efferent sympathetic lesion. The miosis is due to a denervation of the dilator pupillae muscle. It is reversible when the cranial cervical ganglia have not been destroyed. The ptosis is the result of a lack of action of the Müller muscles in the upper lid. The reduced sympathetic tone of the orbital smooth musculature that is part of the periorbita leads to a slight enophthalmos, which additionally narrows the palpebral fissure. As a result, the nictitating membrane prolapses; this latter symptom is more severe in the cat (Fig. 17.16).

Diagnosis: The diagnosis is made possible by the clinical picture. The localisation of the lesion can be determined using pharmacological tests (Table 17.6) (27). However, the pharmacological tests are not always practically meaningful (49).

Therapy: Treatment of the cause. Specific therapy for Horner's is not possible. The ocular symptoms disappear after the local application of phenylephrine.

Prognosis: Dependent on the causal disease. Idiopathic Horner's syndrome in the Golden Retriever has a favourable prognosis. A spontaneous resolution occurs over several months.

17.3.6 Feline and canine dysautonomia

An autonomic syndrome of unknown aetiology was first described in the UK in 1982 (58).

Occurrence: In the cat, independent of age, breed or sex. The syndrome has been observed mainly in the UK, though occasionally it has also been seen in continental Europe. Since its first description, this syndrome appears to have become rare. A similar syndrome has been described in the dog, particularly in rural USA (59).

Aetiology: A disturbance of the autonomic nervous system.

Clinical: The ocular symptoms include hyposecretion of the tear glands, fixed and dilated pupils, prolapse of the nictitating membrane, photophobia and blepharospasm (27, 42).

Diagnosis: The diagnosis is based on the clinical symptoms and can be ascertained by histology of the autonomic ganglia.

Therapy: Specific treatment is not possible. Supportive care is essential.

Prognosis: Guarded to poor.

17

Table 17.5: Pharmacological localisation of efferent parasympathetic lesions

Active substance	Normal	Central/preganglionic	Postganglionic	Atrophy of the pupillary sphincter muscle or atropinisation
■ Physostigmine	Miosis	Miosis	No miosis	No miosis
■ Pilocarpine	Miosis	Miosis	Miosis	No miosis

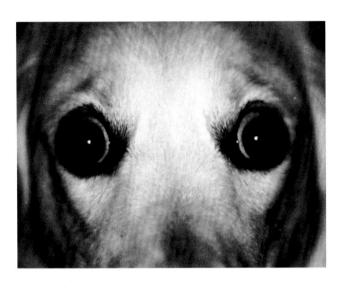

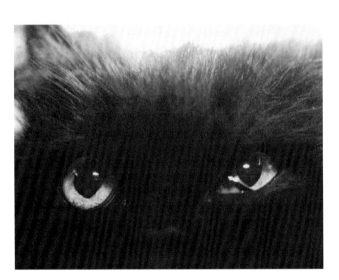

Fig. 17.14
External ophthalmoplegia and exophthalmus in a young Hovawart with extraocular polymyositis.

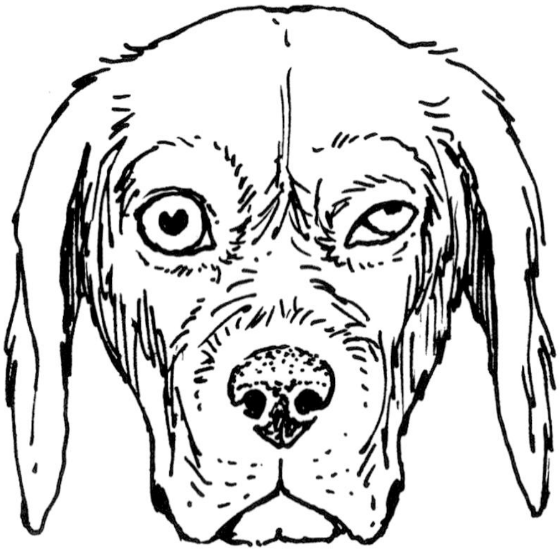

Fig. 17.15
The three most important symptoms of Horner's syndrome: miosis, ptosis and prolapse of the nictitating membrane.

Fig. 17.16
Horner's syndrome on the left in a cat.

Table 17.6: Pharmacological localisation of efferent sympathetic lesions

Active substance	Central	Preganglionic	Postganglionic
■ Cocaine 6%	Slight mydriasis	No dilatation	No dilatation
■ Phenylephrine 10%	No dilatation	No dilatation	Normal mydriasis
■ Hydroxyamphetamine 1%	Normal mydriasis	Normal mydriasis	No or incomplete mydriasis

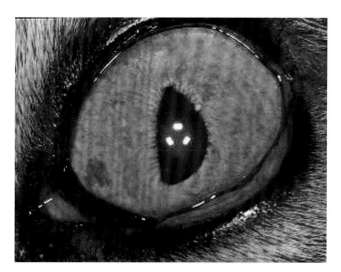

Fig. 17.17
Hemidilation of the pupil in a cat (D pupil). (Fig. Barbara Nell, Vienna.)

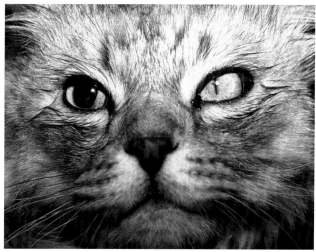

Fig. 17.18
Pourfour du Petit syndrome in a cat. The right pupil is dilated; the lid fissure is slightly enlarged. There is a slight exophthalmos. The anisocoria is especially conspicuous in bright light and is reduced in the dark.

17.3.7 Feline spastic pupils

Spastic pupils have been described in FeLV-positive cats (60). Affected cats have normal vision and show no symptoms of any structural changes in the pupillary sphincter muscles or the pupillary dilator muscles. The pupils are immobile and do not dilate in the dark.

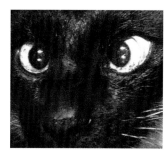

Fig. 17.19
Esotropia in a Siamese Cat.

17.3.8 Hemidilatation of the pupils in the cat

In contrast to the dog, the cat has two distinct short ciliary nerves that emerge from the ciliary ganglia: the ciliaris latralis s. malaris nerve and the ciliaris medialis s. nasalis nerve. The former innervates the lateral half of the pupillary sphincter muscle, while the latter innervates the nasal half. With lesions that affect only one of these nerves, there is only a partial dilatation of the pupil so that a D-shaped or reverse-D-shaped pupil occurs (Fig. 17.17) (61). Affected cats are often positive for FeLV. The D-shaped pupil must be differentiated from dyscoria which can occur due to caudal synechia.

17.3.9 Facial nerve paralysis

Occurrence: Facial nerve neuropathy is seen both in the cat and dog.

Aetiology: Along with trauma, neoplasia and otitis media / interna are the most common causes of facial nerve paralysis. In a retrospective study, 75% of dogs and 25% of cats with this neuropathy were classed as idiopathic (62). In the dog, keratoconjunctivitis sicca has also been observed in many cases. The neurological deficit most commonly noted in association with facial nerve paresis of peripheral or central origin, is vestibular dysfunction.

Clinical: The clinical signs include a widened palpebral fissure (lack of tone of the orbicularis oculi muscle), ipsilateral drooping facial muscles, salivation and possibly a slight drooping of the ear. In many cases, there is a concomitant reduction in tear secretion (42).

Diagnosis: Clinical symptoms.

Therapy: Until the facial nerve has regenerated, drying out of the surface of the eye must be prevented: artificial tear products are used.

17

Usually a temporary tarsorrhaphy is necessary. If the facial nerve does not regenerate, then either a permanent tarsorrhaphy or even enucleation must be considered if supportive care with artificial tears is not effective and secondary ulceration occurs (27).

Prognosis: Good to fair.

17.3.10 Pourfour du Petit syndrome

Hyperactivity of the sympathetic nerve has been observed in the cat after flushing out the middle ear (45). This syndrome, which was first described by Pourfour du Petit, is manifested as a dilatation of the pupils, wide palpebral fissure and a slight exophthalmos (Fig. 17.18). The symptoms can disappear spontaneously or progress into Horner's syndrome.

17.3.11 Strabismus

Strabismus is not uncommon in the Siamese. Usually it is an esotropia, i.e. a squint toward the midline (Fig. 17.19). The majority of these cats have little pigment in their eyes and fur. Their visual acuity is undisturbed (63, 64). Isotropy has also been described in other cats, in which there was also malformation of the optic tracts (65). Many cats with esotropia also have a horizontal nystagmus.

A progressive esotropia has been described in the Shar Pei, which can lead to blindness (42). The problem occurs bilaterally and is characterised by an increasingly inwards rotation of the eyes.

Literature

1 WANG, W., ZHANGA, Q., ACLANDA, G.M., MELLERSHB, C., OSTRANDERB, E.A., RAYA, K., GUSTAVO, D. (1999): Molecular characterization and mapping of canine cGMP-phosphodiesterase delta subunit (PDE6D). Gene, **236** (2): 325–332.

2 RAY, K., BALDWIN, V.J., ZEISS, C., ACLAND, G.M., AGUIRRE G.D. (1997): Canine rod transducin alpha-1: cloning of the cDNA and evaluation of the gene as a candidate for progressive retinal atrophy. Current Eye Research **16** (1): 71–77.

3 ACLAND, G.M., FLETCHER, R.T., GENTLEMAN, S., CHADER, G., AGUIRRE, G. (1989): Non-allelism of three genes (rcd1, rcd2 and erd) for early-onset hereditary retinal degeneration. Experimental Eye Res. **49**(6): 983–998.

4 DEKOMIEN, G., RUNTE, M., GODDE, R., EPPLEN, J.T. (2000): Generalized progressive retinal atrophy of Sloughi dogs is due to an 8-bp insertion in exon 21 of the PDE6B gene. Cytogen Cell Gen. **90**(3–4): 261–267.

5 AGUIRRE, G.D., BALDWIN, V.J., WEEKS, K.M., ACLAND, G., RAY, K. (1999): Frequency of the codon 807 mutation in the cGMP phosphodiesterase beta-subunit gene in Irish setters and other dog breeds with hereditary retinal degeneration. J Heredity **90**(1): 143–147.

6 RUNTE, M., DEKOMIEN, G., EPPLEN, J.T. (2000): Evaluation of RDS/Peripherin and ROM1 as candidate genes in generalised progressive retinal atrophy and exclusion of digenic inheritance. Anim Gen. **31**(3): 223–227.

7 SPIESS, B.M. (1994): Vererbte Augenkrankheiten beim Entlebucher Sennenhund. Schweiz Arch Tierheilk. **136**(3): 105–110.

8 SPIESS, B.M. (1994): Elektrophysiologische Untersuchungen des Auges bei Hund und Katze. Stuttgart: Enke Copythek, p. 351.

9 PETERSEN-JONES, S.M., F.X. ZHU (2000): Development and use of a polymerase chain reaction-based diagnostic test for the causal mutation of progressive retinal atrophy in Cardigan Welsh Corgis. Am J Vet Res. **61**(7): 844–846.

10 DU, F., ACLAND, G.M, RAY, J. (2000): Cloning and expression of type II collagen mRNA: evaluation as a candidate for canine oculoskeletal dysplasia. Gene **255**(2): 307–316.

11 RAY, K., WHANG, W., CZARNECKI, J., ZHANG, Q., ACLAND, G., AGUIRRE, G. (1999): Strategies for identification of mutations causing hereditary retinal diseases in dogs: evaluation of opsin as a candidate gene. J Heredity, **90**(1): 133–137.

12 RAY, K., BALDWIN, V.J., ACLAND, G., BLANTON, S.H., AGUIRRE, G. (1994): Cosegregation of codon 807 mutation of the canine rod cGMP phosphodiesterase beta gene and rcd1. Invest Ophthalmol Vis Sci. **35**(13): 4291–4299.

13 ZEISS, C.J., ACLAND, G.M., AGUIRRE, G.D. (1999): Retinal pathology of canine X-linked progressive retinal atrophy, the locus homologue of RP3. Invest Ophthalmol Visual Sci. **40**(13): 3292–3304.

14 ZHANG, Q., ACLAND, G., ZANGERL, B., JOHNSON, J.L., MAO, Z., ZEISS, C.J., OSTRANDER, E.A., AGUIRRE, G. (2001): Fine mapping of canine XLPRA establishes homology of the human and canine RP3 intervals. Invest Ophthalmol Visual Sci. **42**(11): 2466–2471.

15 ZHANG, Q., BALDWIN, V.J., ACLAND, G., PARSHALL, C.J., HASKEL, J., AGUIRRE, G., RAY, K. (1999): Photoreceptor dysplasia (pd) in Miniature Schnauzer dogs: evaluation of candidate genes by molecular genetic analysis. J Heredity **90**(1): 57–61.

17

16 NARFSTRÖM, K., EKESTEN, B. (1999): Diseases of the canine ocular fundus, In: Gelatt, K. (ed.): Veterinary Ophthalmology, Lippincott, Williams & Wilkins: Philadelphia, pp. 869–933.

17 BROOKS, D.E. (1999): The canine optic nerve, In: Gelatt, K. (ed.): Veterinary Ophthalmology, 1999, Lippincott, Williams & Wilkins: Philadelphia.

18 FRITSCHE, J., SPIESS, B.M., RÜHLI, M.B., BOLLIGER, J. (1996): Prolapsus bulbi in small animals: A retrospective study of 36 cases. Tierärztl Prax. **24**(1): 55–61.

19 CUDDON, P., SMITH-MAXIE, L. (1984): Reticulosis of the central nervous system in dogs. Comp Cont Educ. **6**: 23–32.

20 BISTNER, S. (1994): Allergic- and immunologic-mediated diseases of the eye and adnexae. Vet Clin North Am Small Anim Pract. **24**(4): 711–734.

21 SLATTER, D. (1990): Fundamentals of Veterinary Ophthalmology, 2nd ed. Vol. 1. W.B. Saunders Co, Philadelphia.

22 GRÄNITZ, U. (1994): Visusschwäche und Blindheit beim Hund – eine retrospektive Studie. Berl Münch Tierärztl Wochenschr. **107** (9): 295–299.

23 VENTER, I.J., PETRICK, S.W. (1995): Acute blindness in a dog caused by sudden acquired retinal degeneration. J S Afr Vet Assoc. **66**(1): 32–34.

24 ACLAND, G., IRBY, N.L., AGUIRRE, G.D. (1984): Sudden acquired retinal degeneration in the dog: clinical and morphologic characterization of the "silent retina" syndrome. Trans Am Coll Vet Ophthalmol. **15**: 86–104.

25 ACLAND, G., AGUIRRE, G.D. (1986): Sudden acquired retinal degeneration: clinical signs and diagnosis. Trans Am Coll Vet Ophthalmol. **17**: 58–63.

26 MARTIN, C.L. (1999): Ocular manifestations of systemic disease. Part 1: The dog. In: Gelatt, K. (ed.): Veterinary Ophthalmology, Lippincott, Williams & Wilkins: Philadelphia.

27 GELATT, K. (2000): Essentials of Veterinary Ophthalmology. Lippincott, Williams & Wilkins, Philadelphia.

28 ERNEST, J.T. (1976): Bilateral optic nerve hypoplasia in a pup. J Am Vet Med Assoc. **168**(2): 125–128.

29 KERN, T.J., RIIS, R.C. (1981): Optic nerve hypoplasia in three Miniature Poodles. J Am Vet Med Assoc, **178**(1): 49–54.

29a TIPOLD, A. (1995): Diagnosis of inflammatory and infectious diseases of the central nervous system in dogs: a retrospective study. J Vet Intern Med. **9** (5): 304–314.

30 SPIESS, B., LITSCHI, B., LEBER-ZÜRCHER, A.C., STELZER, S. (1991): Bilaterale Hypoplasie der Nervi optici bei einem Pudelwelpen. Kleintierprax. **36**: 173–178.

31 MARTIN, C.L. (1999): Ocular manifestations of systemic disease. Part 4: Food animals, In: GELATT, K. (ed.): Veterinary Ophthalmology, Lippincott, Williams & Wilkins: Philadelphia, 1404–1504.

32 TURNQUIST, S.E., PACE, L.W., SARDINAS, J. (1991): Unilateral optic nerve hypoplasia and hydrocephalus in a Pekingese. Cornell Veterinarian, **81**(3): 305–311.

33 SPIESS, B.M., WILCOCK, B.P. (1987): Glioma of the optic nerve with intraocular and intracranial involvement in a dog. J Comp Pathol. **97**(1): 79–84.

34 SPIESS, B.M., RUHLI, M.B., BAUER, G.A. (1995): Zur Therapie von retrobulbären Neoplasien beim Kleintier. Tierärztl Prax. **23**(5): 509–514.

35 BOYDELL, P. (1991): Fine needle aspiration biopsy in the diagnosis of exophthalmos. J Small Anim Pract. **32**: 542–546.

36 RUEHLI, M., SPIESS, B.M. (1995): Retrobulbar space-occupying lesions in dogs and cats: Clinical signs and diagnostic work-up. Tierärztl Prax. **23**: 306–312.

37 CARLTON, W. (1983): Orbital Neoplasms, In: Peiffer, R. (ed.): Comparative Ophthalmic Pathology, C.C. Thomas Publisher: Springfield. pp. 47–63.

38 MARTÍN, E., PÉREZ, J., MOZOS, E., LÓPEZ, R., MOLLEDA, J.M. (2000): Retrobulbar anaplastic astrocytoma in a dog: clinicopathological and ultrasonographic features. J Small Anim Pract. **41**(8): 354–357.

39 KASER-HOTZ, B., FODOR, G., CORDT-RIEHLE, I., BLATTMANN, H., MUNKKEL, G., EGGER, E., LA RUE, S.M., SUTER, P.F. (1994): Radiotherapie in der Kleintiermedizin: Grundlagen, Indikationen und Bedeutung. Schweiz Arch Tierheilk. **136** (10): 319–328.

40 KASER-HOTZ, B., REINER, B., HAUSER, B., ARNOLD, P., LIEB, A., CORDT, L., LANG, J., BLATTMANN, H. (2000): Strahlentherapie bei zwei Katzen mit Hypophysentumoren. Schweiz Arch Tierheilk. **142**(11): 631–637.

41 KASER-HOTZ, B., ROHRER, C.R., FIDEL, J.L., NELT, C.S., HÖRAUF, A., HAUSER, B. (2001): Radiotherapy in three suspect cases of feline thymoma. J Am Anim Hosp Assoc. **37**(5): 483–488.

42 SCAGLIOTTI, R. (1998): Comparative Neuro-ophthalmology, In: Gelatt, K. (ed.): Veterinary Ophthalmology, Lippincott Williams & Wilkins: Philadelphia, 1307–1400.

43 SPIESS, B. (1988):, What is your diagnosis? Idiopathic internal ophthalmoplegia (Adie's Syndrom) in a dog. Can Vet J. **29**: 73–74.

44 GERDING, P.A., BRIGHTMAN, A.H., BROGDON, J.D. (1986): Pupillotonia in a dog. J Am Vet Med Assoc. **189**(11): 1477.

45 BOYDELL, P. (2000): Iatrogenic pupillary dilation resembling Pourfour du Petit syndrome in three cats. J Small Anim Pract. **41**(5): 202–203.

46 SPIESS, B., WALLIN-HÅKANSON, N. (1999): Disease of the canine orbit. In: Gelatt, K. (ed.): Veterinary Ophthalmology, Lippincott, Williams & Wilkins: Philadelphia. pp. 511–533.

47 MURPHY, C.J., KOBLIK, P., BELLHORN, R.W., PINO, M., HACKER, D., BURLING, T. (1989): Squamous cell carcinoma causing blindness and ophthalmoplegia in a cat. J Am Vet Med Assoc. **195**(7): 965–968.

17

48 JONES, B.R., STUDDERT, V.P. (1975): Horner's syndrome in the dog and cat as an aid to diagnosis. Austr Vet J. **51**(7): 329–332.

49 KERN, T.J., AROMANDO, M.C., ERB, H.N. (1989): Horner's syndrome in dogs and cats: 100 cases (1975–1985). J Am Vet Med Assoc. **195**(3): 369–373.

50 MORGAN, R.V., ZANOTTI, S.W. (1989): Horner's syndrome in dogs and cats: 49 cases (1980–1986). J Am Vet Med Assoc. **194**(8): 1096–1099.

51 BOYDELL, P. (2000): Idiopathic Horner's syndrome in the Golden Retriever. J Neuro Ophth. 20(4): 288-290

52 BOYDELL, P. (1995): Idiopathic Horner's syndrome in the Golden Retriever. J Small Anim Pract. **36**(9): 382–384.

53 CARPENTER, J.L., KING, N.W., Jr., ABRAMS, K.L. (1987): Bilateral trigeminal nerve paralysis and Horner's syndrome associated with myelomonocytic neoplasia in a dog. J Am Vet Med Assoc. **191**(12): 594–596.

54 BOYDELL, P. (1995): Horner's syndrome following cervical spinal surgery in the dog. J Small Anim Pract. **36**(11): 510–512.

55 BOYDELL, P. (2001): Horner's syndrome following vertical ramus osteotomy in a dog. Vet Rec. **148**(4): 113–114.

56 BOYDELL, P., PIKE, R., CROSSLEY, D., TORRINGTON, A. (1997): Horner's syndrome following intrathoracic tube placement. J Small Anim Pract. **38**(10): 466–467.

57 BOYDELL, P., BROGAN, N. (2000): Horner's syndrome associated with Neospora infection. J Small Anim Pract. **41**(12): 571–572.

58 KEY, T.J., GASKELL, C.J. (1982): Puzzling syndrome in cats associated with pupillary dilatation. Vet Rec. **110**(7): 160.

59 SCHULZE, C., SCHANEN, H., POHLENZ, J. (1997): Canine dysautonomia resembling the Key-Gaskell syndrome in Germany. Vet Rec. **141**: 496–497.

60 SCAGLIOTTI, R.H. (1980): Current concepts in veterinary neuro-ophthalmology. Vet Clin North Am, Small Anim Pract. **10**(2): 417–436.

61 DE LAHUNTA, A. (1973): Small animal neuro-ophthalmology. Vet Clin North Am Small Anim Pract. **3**(3): 491–501.

62 KERN, T.J., ERB, H.N. (1987): Facial neuropathy in dogs and cats: 95 cases (1975–1985). J Am Vet Med Assoc. **191**(12): 1604–1609.

63 RENGSTORFF, R.H. (1976): Strabismus measurements in the Siamese cat. Am J Optometry Physiol Optics **53**(10): 643–646.

64 BLAKE, R., COOL, S.F., CRAWFORD, M.L. (1974): Visual resolution in the cat. Vision Res. **14**: 1211–1271.

65 VON GRUNAU, M.W., RAUSCHECKER, J.P. (1983): Natural strabismus in non-Siamese cats: lack of binocularity in the striate cortex. ExpT Brain Res. **52**(2): 307–310.

17

18 Cerebrum

Gualtiero Gandini
André Jaggy
Iris Challande-Kathmann
Thomas Bilzer
Christophe Lombard

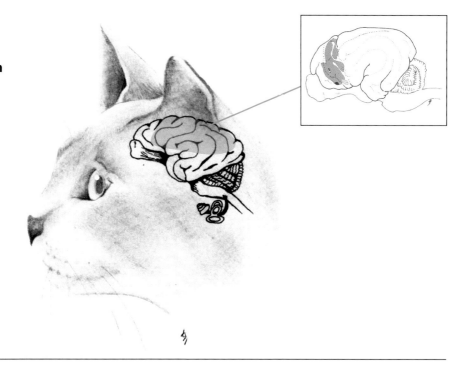

Diseases of the cerebrum are very complex and extensive, and may affect the whole of the **central nervous system (CNS)** (Fig. 18.1). Due to the differences in brain function between human beings and animals, the symptoms of brain disease in the latter tend to be different to those found in human patients. In veterinary medicine, the clinical symptoms of cerebral dysfunction are relatively mild despite often being associated with a severe lesion. The most common clinical signs of cerebral disease include disturbances in consciousness, behavioural changes, loss of vision with retention of intact pupillary reflexes, seizures, deficits in placement and positioning reflexes, and gait abnormalities.

From a clinical point of view, diseases that affect the cerebrum (telencephalon) are difficult to differentiate from lesions in the diencephalon, because both structures are closely related functionally. Diseases of the cerebrum are therefore often termed forebrain diseases, whereby the forebrain (**prosencephalon**) is the region containing the **telencephalon** and **diencephalon**.

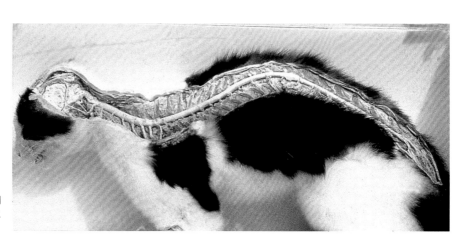

Fig. 18.1
Macroscopic *in situ* preparation of the central nervous system of an eight-year-old domestic cat. (Fig. Marc Vandevelde, Bern.)

18

The following chapter describes the diseases of the cerebrum. For didactic reasons, the section in the first part is subdivided into a short discussion of the most important anatomical structures of the cerebrum and the diagnostics available that can lead the clinician to a definite diagnosis. The second part is a description of the most important cerebral diseases organised according to the VITAMIN D scheme.

18.1 Anatomy and physiology

Anatomically, the brains of domestic animals are subdivided into five parts. Moving rostrocaudally, they are the **telencephalon** (cerebrum), **diencephalon**, **mesencephalon** (midbrain), **metencephalon** (pons and cerebellum) and the **myelencephalon** (medulla oblongata).

The **cerebrum** is formed by two hemispheres separated by a deep longitudinal furrow in which lies the cerebral falx. A bridge of white matter, the corpus callosum, connects both hemispheres. The cerebral cortex forms the outer part of the cerebrum and consists of neurons that collectively form the **grey matter**. The inner part of the cerebrum contains both grey and white matter. In the subcortical areas, the grey matter is formed by the **basal nuclei**, while the white matter consists of nerve fibres that, depending on their function, are called **projection**, **association** or **commissural** fibres.

Both hemispheres are subdivided into four anatomically poorly defined lobes: frontal, parietal, temporal and occipital. The **temporal lobes** receive and process acoustic and sensory signals, the **occipital lobes** contain the visual cortex, and the **frontal lobes** are of importance for motor and learning functions.

Functionally, the cerebral cortex is subdivided into the **projection areas**, **association areas** and the **rhinencephalon** (limbic and olfactory systems). The association areas are only partially developed in human beings and primates. They receive information and decide on its significance through the influx of previously made experiences. They then select a suitable response and can predict consequences (1).

The **rhinencephalon** is the phylogenetically oldest part of the forebrain. It lies on the ventral surface of the cerebral hemispheres and is divided in two parts: the **olfactory** (olfactory bulb, peduncle, tract and tubercle; and the piriform lobe) and the **limbic** (hippocampus, amygdala, the septum and habenular nuclei). The limbic system is responsible for the visceral processes, especially those that are involved in the control and expression of emotion, behaviour, personality and memory (1).

In the literature, there is still no consensus about which structures actually belong to the limbic system; the more studies that are done on this region, the more apparent it becomes

that various structures in the telencephalon and diencephalon are also involved in its functions.

The cerebral cortex is less important in the dog and cat than in human beings. It appears that a dog or cat can retain normal motor functions without its cerebrum, though it loses the ability to recognise its owner or to learn anything new.

18.2 Neuroanatomical localisation

A great variety of clinical symptoms can be seen with diseases of the forebrain, depending on the duration and severity of the particular aetiology. As mentioned before, diseases that result in slowly progressive forebrain lesions are only accompanied by mild clinical symptoms. Seizures may be the only sign in a dog with a supratentorial tumour. The most commonly found abnormalities in the neurological examination of patients with diseases of the forebrain are reduced consciousness, seizures, slight gait abnormalities, deficits in placement and positioning responses, and/or reduced to no menace response with an intact pupillary light reflex. The clinical signs can be bilateral or unilateral according to whether the lesion is diffuse or focal.

Consciousness is rarely reduced with lesions of the forebrain. Usually such damage causes obtundation and apathy. Stupor and even coma are the consequences of severe, diffuse bilateral cerebral damage (Fig. 18.2). The animal's **behaviour** is often changed. Depending on the localisation of the lesion, dogs and cats can exhibit circling (ipsilateral to lesion) (Fig. 18.3), compulsive pacing (Fig. 18.4), hyperexcitability, aggression and attacks of anxiety.

Forgetting what has been learnt can lead to the animal being unable to recognise its owner or to follow simple commands. **Seizures** are the consequence of cortical dysfunction and are typical of forebrain lesions. They can be primary or secondary sequelae of cerebral disease. **Blindness** can result from lesions that affect the lateral geniculate body, the optic radiations or the occipital visual cortex.

The animal's **posture** sometimes reveals ipsilateral pleurothotonus.

During the examination, the animal's **gait** evaluation *may* reveal a slight to moderate tetra- or hemiparesis (the latter contralateral to the lesion); however, motor deficits are not common and are usually associated with brainstem and/or spinal cord disease Compulsive pacing is usually exhibited by patients with forebrain disease. The gait abnormalities also include the aforementioned circling and changes in behaviour.

Deficits in proprioception (abnormal positioning and placement reactions; Fig. 18.5) can be obvious during the neurological examination – despite the presence of (almost) nor-

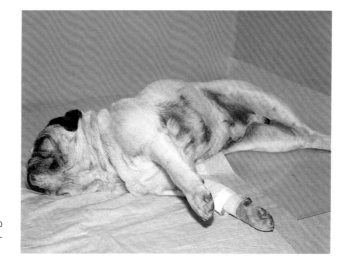

Fig. 18.2
Pug, 12-year-old, castrated male, in lateral recumbency and coma (no reaction to external stimuli) after a car accident. The histopathology revealed a massive bilateral cerebral haemorrhage.

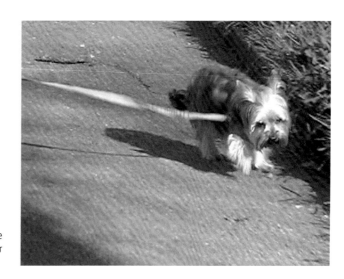

Fig. 18.3
Yorkshire Terrier, 12-year-old male. Acute cerebral symptoms with circling to the right and behavioural disturbances. The dog was suffering from "Yorkshire Terrier encephalitis".

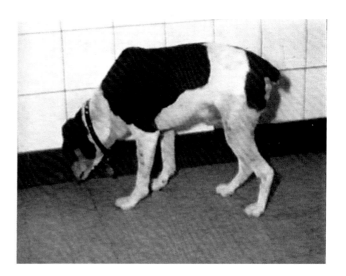

18

Fig. 18.4
Hound dog with compulsive pacing. The patient suffered from symptoms of epilepsy for two years, after that the dog did not recognise its owner and central blindness with compulsive pacing became apparent. The dog could remain for hours stuck by a wall or furniture, but began to walk without stopping following slight manipulation.

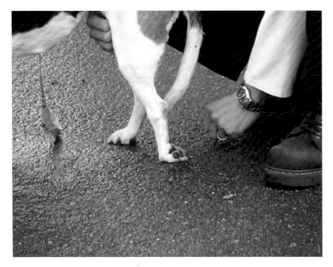

Fig. 18.5
Ten-year-old hound with marked abnormalities of the positioning and placement reactions. Proprioception was no longer present in any of its limbs (here shown as knuckling). The dog also showed pacing and bilateral deficits of the menace response.

mal gait. Obviously, the spinal reflexes are not influenced by forebrain disease. The examination of the cranial nerves can reveal a uni- or bilateral reduction / lack of the menace response, although the pupillary light reflex is normal. In addition, there may be a hypalgesia of the face. Usually, the other cranial nerves function normally due to their origin in the brain stem (with the exception of the olfactory nerve). Intracranial diseases can sometimes cause cervical or head pain, so careful palpation of these structures is indicated.

18.3   Adjunct investigations

Haematological investigation should include a CBC and the determination of the biochemical profile (most important biochemical parameters).

Various encephalopathies with a metabolic aetiology are accompanied by changes in haematology (see Chap. 4). Under certain circumstances, specific blood analyses are necessary: the determination of bile acids and blood ammonium concentrations can be helpful in the diagnosis of hepatic encephalopathy; while serology may be necessary for diagnosing infectious disease (e.g. FeLV, FIV, distemper, toxoplasmosis, etc.).

The **analysis of CSF** is the most important method in the diagnosis of inflammatory disease of the CNS (see Chap. 2.3). **Electroencephalography** (**EEG**) reveals the electrical activity of the brain. EEG can be performed under general anaes-

thesia using a standard protocol (see Chap. 7.2.1). **CT** and **MRI** are considered to be the best diagnostic aids for visualising brain structures (see Chap. 6).

A **brain tissue biopsy** is undertaken in some specialised clinics to obtain an aetiological diagnosis and information about which treatment methods may be used, particularly with respect to brain tumours. This necessarily invasive method must be weighed up against the advantages of the information gained (2).

18.4   Diseases of the cerebrum

18.4.1   Vascular disease

Cerebrovascular disease is a very frequent reason for neurological dysfunction in human beings and it is the third most common cause of death in industrialised countries (3). In veterinary medicine, by contrast, cerebrovascular disease has been infrequently described, and the true incidence is simply not known (4). Until recently, the diagnosis of cerebrovascular disease could only be made *post mortem*. The modern development of imaging techniques has greatly improved the ability of demonstrating such a disease in the living animal.

18.4.1.1   Ischemia and infarct

Aetiology: Vascular disturbances of the nervous system can arise due to a loss of adequate blood supply (ischemia / infarct) or haemorrhage into the nervous tissue (5). The initial process is focal in the majority of cases. However, it is possible with a disturbance in systemic perfusion that there is a multifocal, or diffuse vascular process in the brain.

Vascular damage to the nervous system can be due to various different causes such as neoplasia, CNS infections, aneurysms, arthrosclerosis, arteriovenous malformations, carcinogenic emboli, vasospasm, atrial fibrillation, mitral stenosis, haematological disturbances, vasculitis, hyperviscosity syndrome, hypertension, coagulopathy, immune deficiency, disseminated intravascular coagulation (DIC) or sepsis (5).

Ischemia means the reduction of blood flow to a level which is not compatible with normal function (6). A large and continual reduction in the blood flow results in tissue necrosis called an **infarct** (7). Hypoxia / ischemia initially affects the most sensitive elements of the tissue and then subsequently disturbs all the surrounding tissue components. Neurons are the most sensitive to these influences especially those of laminae II, III and IV of the cerebral cortex, the amygdala in the hippocampus, some of the basal and thalamic nuclei, and the Purkinje cells of the cerebellar cortex (6). The main mechanism of cell damage found in an infarct is reduced energy metabolism caused by the lack of synthesis of adenosine triphosphate (ATP), which is needed for maintaining homeostasis by

18

ion exchange through the cell membrane. During hypoxia, anaerobic glycolysis occurs and the concentrations of H^+ ions and lactic acid increase. The subsequent dysfunction of the membrane pumps allows an uncontrolled increase in Ca^{2+} that in turn activates proteases and phospholipases. Finally, there is formation of free radicals that damage the cell membrane leading to its rupture. Progressive necrosis is the ultimate consequence (8).

Spontaneous intracranial **haemorrhage** is caused by a bleed within the brain or in its immediate surroundings without accompanying trauma. A brain haemorrhage can be epidural, subarachnoid, intraparenchymal or intraventricular. Epi- or subdural haemorrhages are always associated with cranial trauma. Although it has not been well documented, hypertension appears to play a role in the development of primary intraparenchymal haemorrhage in the dog and cat. Secondary intraparenchymal haemorrhages are associated with reperfusion disturbances after infarcts, congenital arteriovenous malformations, intracranial tumours and coagulopathies. Damage to the brain is the result of compression or destruction of the surrounding brain tissue. In addition, reduced blood flow to the brain, increased intracranial pressure (ICP) and obstructive hydrocephalus can be consequences of intracranial haemorrhage.

Clinical: Generally, cerebrovascular diseases start suddenly and have a nonprogressive course. The brain dysfunction due to an infarct is usually focal. The neurological deficits depend on the size of the lesion and are usually asymmetrical. The forebrain symptoms include seizures, possibly in clusters, with contralateral visual and proprioceptive deficits. Behavioural changes are common and involve compulsive pacing, disorientation and sudden attacks of anxiety or aggression. Ipsilateral circling or head turn are usually seen. Specific clinical signs can be seen in association with an increase in ICP (see Chap. 5.1.1). Systemic haemorrhaging can lead to multifocal and at times progressive neurological deficits.

Diagnosis: CBC, biochemistry profile, coagulation tests and a urinalysis are helpful in excluding renal disease, sepsis, hyperviscosity syndrome or coagulopathy. ECG and an ultrasonography investigation of the heart may be necessary to diagnose heart disease.

The most useful diagnostic methods are imaging techniques such as CT or MRI. (see Table 6.8) Abnormalities in patients with brain infarcts can be visualised with CT within a few hours. These changes depend on the age of the lesion and are normally present as a slightly hypodense region with a mass effect. An increase in contrast can occur after a few days at the periphery of the lesion which reflects local capillary proliferation. CT investigation is also a sensitive method of imaging acute haemorrhage. These appear as hyperdense regions which become better demarcated over the next 72 hours and attain a homogenous pattern after approx. 4 weeks (9).

On MRI, an infarct is hypointense on T1w sequences and hyperintense on T2w sequences. These changes can be seen an hour after the onset of an infarct, meaning that MRI is more sensitive for the visualisation of an infarct than CT (10). In comparison, the depiction of a haemorrhage with MRI is more complicated and depends on the age of the lesion. CT used to be preferred in the acute stages to differentiate between infarction and haemorrhage but with the addition of gradient echo sequences to the MR imaging repertoire; this is no longer the case (4) (Fig. 18.6).

Therapy: The aim of treatment is to ensure an adequate oxygen supply to the tissue, to treat specific neurological problems (such as seizure activity) and to treat the causative disease where this can be identified (4).

Oxygen supplementation is often sufficient in many cases. Hypovolaemia should be treated with fluids, though the administration of large volumes of crystalloids should be avoided as they may cause worsening of cerebral oedema and can increase the ICP; however, the danger associated with over-hydration is far less than the risks to the brain associated with hypoperfusion Hypertension, if present, should be *carefully* corrected to avoid the risk of a reduction of cerebral perfusion if performed aggressively.

The control of ICP is achieved by a combination of oxygenation and mannitol administration, once euvolaemia has been achieved (see Chap. 5.1.1). Mannitol is given at a dosage of 0.5 to 2 g/kg, IV (if necessary, every 4 hours) over 15 to 20 minutes. Although the use of mannitol for the treatment of intracranial haemorrhage has been contraindicated in veterinary literature, there is evidence that this substance can reduce intracranial haemorrhaging and not actually worsen it. Osmotic diuresis is routinely used for the control of ICP in suitable patients in human medicine (4, 11).

Diazepam (0.5–2.0 mg/kg, IV × 2–3 doses) and barbiturates (phenobarbital 2–5 mg/kg, IV, IM or PO, q 4–12h) can be used to control seizure activity and reduce the brain's metabolism, protecting it from a low oxygen and glucose supply.

Even though there are different opinions as to the use of glucocorticoids in cerebrovascular disease, there is no evidence that they are beneficial.

18.4.2 Inflammatory/infectious diseases

Inflammatory/infectious diseases of the CNS usually have an acute onset and progressive course. The lesions can be multifocal or diffuse. The clinical signs reflect the localisation of the lesion; accordingly, inflammatory diseases are characte-

18

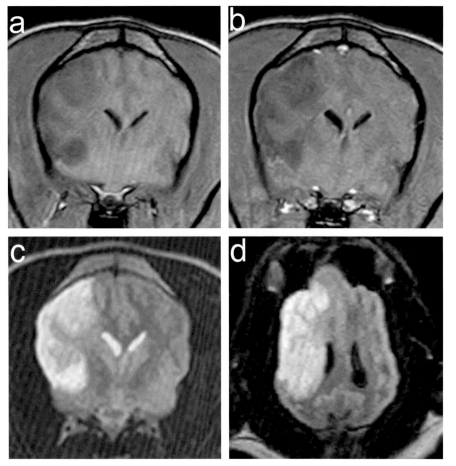

Fig. 18.6a–d
Brain infarct in the region of the vascular supply of the medial cerebral artery. The MRI was performed 24 hours after clinical signs occurred. T1w sequence (a) pre-contrast, (b) after IV contrast agent and (c) transverse T2w sequence. The right cerebral hemisphere is hypointense with a moderate mass effect (a). After the administration of intravenous contrast, the meninges over the lesion and the normal brain tissue showed a higher degree of contrast enhancement than the lesion, which increased the contrast between the infarcted and normal brain tissue. The infarct is hyperintense on the T2w sequence. (d) The dorsal FLAIR sequence shows the rostrocaudal extension of the infarct, which corresponds to the vascular supply of the medial cerebral artery. The CSF signal in the ventricles is suppressed with the use of this sequence. (Fig. Johann Lang, Bern.)

rised by neurological deficits that reflect their multifocal or diffuse pattern.

In the following, only the most important inflammatory diseases of the cerebrum are considered. Particular attention is paid to the clinical signs and diagnostic tools. Due to the basically similar manner in which inflammatory / infectious processes lead to CNS lesions, their diagnostic determination is discussed generally, underlining the most important measures. As the majority of inflammatory CNS diseases have a multifocal clinical picture, some of them are also discussed in other chapters (e.g. Chap. 17 Brain stem).

Inflammation of the CNS can be infectious or noninfectious. In small animals infectious aetiologies tend to be rare, most probably due to the blood-brain barrier. Infection (and infestation) of the CNS can be caused by viral, bacterial, protozoal, rickettsial or fungal agents. The most important ones affecting the dog and cat are given in Table 18.1. However, many well known inflammatory diseases of the dog and cat do not have an infectious background (Table 18.2).

Inflammation within the CNS has the same characteristics as inflammation in other organs and is therefore characterised by increased blood flow, leucocyte migration in the direction of the lesion, endothelial changes, exudation and dysfunction in the affected area.

CNS inflammation can be **disseminated** or **local**. An **abscess** is the most common form of focal disease and is characterised by local necrosis and pus formation – usually as a consequence of bacterial infection. Clinical symptoms develop quickly and can be similar to the progressive course of other focal lesions, for example, primary aggressive CNS tumours. The majority of brain abscesses occur in combination with a neighbouring infection, e.g. otitis externa (5).

Granulomas are collections of inflammatory cells mixed with fibrotic reactionary tissue. They are the consequence of the body's attempt to defend itself against fungi, protozoa, parasites or foreign bodies, etc. (5). Depending on the aetiology, these can be solitary (foreign bodies) or multifocal (fungal infection). Granulomas are normally slowly progressive. Their clinical symptoms depend on their anatomical location.

Table 18.1: Causes of infectious encephalitis in the dog and cat

Viruses
- Distemper encephalomyelitis (dog)
- Rabies (dog/cat)
- Aujeszky's disease (dog/cat)
- Feline infectious peritonitis [FIP] (cat)
- Feline immunodeficiency virus [FIV] (cat)
- Feline leukaemia virus [FeLV] (cat)
- Tick-borne encephalitis (dog)
- Canine herpes virus (dog)
- Parvovirus (dog/cat)
- Canine parainfluenza virus (dog)

Bacteria
- Aerobes (dog/cat)
- Anaerobes (dog/cat)

Rickettsia
- Ehrlichiosis (dog)
- Anaplasmosis (dog)
- Rocky Mountain Spotted Fever (dog)

Protozoa
- Toxoplasmosis (dog/cat)
- Neosporosis (dog)
- Encephalitozoonosis (dog)
- Babesiosis (dog)

Fungi
- Cryptococcosis (dog/cat)
- Blastomycosis (dog)
- Histoplasmosis (dog)
- Coccidiomycosis (dog)
- Aspergillus (dog/cat)
- Phaeohyphomycosis (dog/cat)

Parasites
- Dirofilariosis (dog)
- *Toxocara canis* (dog)
- *Ancylostoma caninum* (dog)
- Cuterebra (dog)

Table 18.2: Non-infectious encephalitis in the dog and cat

- Granulomatous meningoencephalomyelitis [GME] (dog)
- Necrotising encephalitis (dog)
  - Pug encephalitis
  - Maltese encephalitis
  - Chihuahua encephalitis
  - Yorkshire Terrier encephalitis
- Steroid-responsive meningitis-arteritis [SMRA] (dog)
- Pyogranulomatous meningoencephalitis of the Pointer (dog)
- Feline polioencephalomyelitis (cat)

Disseminated inflammation can have an infectious aetiology (often haematogenous dissemination), though it can also arise due to disturbances in the immune system or be of an unknown cause (5). It is important to diagnose the cell type which is infiltrating the CNS in the inflammation. The most common pathways of an infection are haematogenous, direct invasion, extension through neighbouring tissues and along a nerve root (5). The blood-brain barrier is an anatomical and physiological barrier between the systemic circulation and the brain tissue. An infection can, however, cross this barrier through an anatomical defect or as with virus infections such as distemper, via infected lymphocytes.

18.4.2.1 Borna disease

Aetiology: In the last few years, individual reports on the incidence of Borna disease (BD) in the dog and cat have become more frequent. These reports appear to be plausible as the neurotrophic Borna disease virus (BDV; single strand RNA virus; own genus) can be experimentally transmitted to many different species – from birds to primates – and its occurrence in psychiatric patients has been repeatedly documented. Classical BD is a florid subacute to chronic T-cell-transmitted polio-encephalomyelitis (Fig. 18.7), with loss of nerve cells leading to severe neurological symptoms. Typically, the so-called Joest degenerate intranuclear inclusion bodies are formed in the affected neurons. Atypical courses have been described in the cat associated with muscle fasciculation and proprioceptive deficits. This is significant as atypical and partially inapparent courses have been observed in sheep, a species that has always been counted as one of the natural hosts of BDV. The epidemiology of BD is completely unknown.

18.4.2.2 Contagious canine hepatitis

Aetiology: CNS complications can arise with contagious canine hepatitis caused by adenoviruses (CAC 1). On the one hand, liver insufficiency induced by the virus can lead to hepatic encephalopathy and on the other hand, the virus has a strong affinity for vessel endothelium and can directly destroy brain capillaries, so that intracerebral haemorrhages and inflammatory reactions may occur.

18.4.2.3 Tick-borne encephalitis

Aetiology: The so-called tick-borne encephalitis (TBE) is caused by arboviruses (Family: Flaviviridae) in mainland Europe. It occurs mainly in the early summer (spring-summer encephalitis) and causes a meningitis and partially necrotising encephalitis, which is usually progressive leading to death within a few days. The viruses are transmitted by *Ixodes ricinus* (see Chap. 17.2.2.4).

18

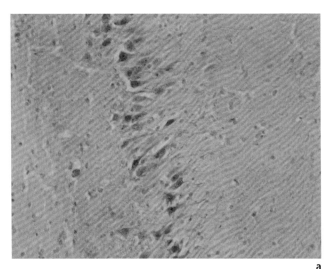 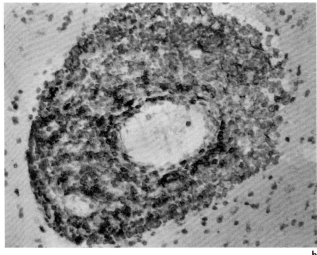

a
b

Fig. 18.7a, b
Virus infection of the brain. (a) Band of cells belonging to Ammon's horn showing neurons infected with Borna virus (immunohistochemistry; brown substrate: virus protein). (b) Marked perivascular lymphocytic infiltration in the region of the virus-infected Ammon's horn (immunohistochemistry; brown substrate: CD8+ T-cells).

18.4.2.4 Feline polioencephalomyelitis

Aetiology: This disease, which is known both as feline polioencephalomyelitis and as staggering disease, is a subacute to chronic process in cats without any age or sex predisposition. A nonpurulent inflammation of the meninges, brain and spinal cord occurs, with a predilection for the grey matter.

Nerve cell necrosis, glial accumulations and diffuse astrogliosis can be found in the thoracic and cervical spinal cord and in the medulla oblongata. The other parts of the brain are less conspicuously affected. The aetiology is unclear, though a neurotrophic virus has been presumed, such as the feline panleucopaenia virus (which can cause leukodystrophy and inflammatory changes), BDV (see Chap. 18.4.2.1), FIV and FeLV.

18.4.2.5 Feline spongiform encephalopathy (FSE)

Aetiology: The first case of naturally occurring scrapie-like spongiform encephalopathy was described in 1990. Since then, this disease has been reported in almost 100 cats in Great Britain. FSE has sporadically occurred in other European countries such as Ireland, Liechtenstein, Norway and Switzerland.

It is assumed that FSE is transmitted by BSE-contaminated food. BSE is caused by the ingestion of food contaminated by the scrapie prion. The disease begins gradually and has a slowly progressive course lasting for weeks or even months. The clinical symptoms are **changes in behaviour** such as aggression or (in contrast) shyness, followed by **progressive locomotory dysfunction**, **hyperaesthesia**, overreaction to auditory stimuli, hypersalivation and fine tremor. A definitive diagnosis can only be achieved *post mortem*. The neuropath-

ological changes include vacuolation of the neurons in the basal nuclei, thalamus and other regions of the brain stem. The incidence of this disease appears to have fallen since BSE has become less frequent (see Chap. 17.2.2.13).

18.4.2.6 General overview of inflammatory cerebral disease

Clinical: In the majority of cases, cats and dogs with CNS disease show signs of a generalised illness. Usually hyperthermia occurs – in the form of fever – and is the result of endogenous and exogenous pyrogens. Respiratory and gastrointestinal symptoms can be seen in many cases, e.g. in distemper and FIP. Ophthalmological changes such as conjunctivitis, choroiditis, uveitis or retinitis are also common. Heart problems, either due to brain stem damage or direct damage to the myocardium, can be associated with increased ICP.

Usually it is apparent that the **meninges** are involved in the processes associated with inflammatory CNS disease. The resulting meningitis causes severe cervical and paraspinal pain, stiff neck and a stiff gait with short strides (5) (Fig. 18.8).

Abnormal CNS signs reflect the localisation of a process and as inflammatory processes are usually progressive and cause multifocal or diffuse lesions, it is relatively common to see clinical signs which indicate that more than one region is affected. On the other hand, it is well known that multifocal inflammatory diseases may be recognised as focal disturbances on neurological examination (12). Forebrain signs include **seizures** (generalised or partial), **changes in behaviour** (aggression, anxiety, soiling, disorientation, circling, compulsive pacing), **abnormal positioning and placement reac-**

tions, **abnormal menace response** and **reduced facial sensation**.

Diagnosis: CBC, blood biochemistry profile and urinalysis are important for the work-up of presumed CNS inflammation. The number of white blood cells can be either increased as a consequence of a systemic bacterial infection or reduced due to a viral disease (distemper, FIV). The lymphocyte count can be very low with viraemias due to the presence of immunosuppressive agents. Together with a leucocytopaenia, lymphopaenia is a significant characteristic of a clinical FIV in the cat. Hyperproteinaemia and hyperglobulinaemia (specific) represent the body's battle against chronic infection (see Chap. 4.3).

Serology is an important diagnostic aid. Positive serum antibody titres help in the diagnosis of diseases such as **distemper**, **toxoplasmosis**, **neosporosis**, **ehrlichiosis** and **FIV**. The presence of **FeLV** is proven by the demonstration of the antigen (protein p27) in the blood of the host. Serology can also be performed on CSF, revealing the presence of intrathecal antibody production (e.g. in chronic distemper encephalomyelitis). Blood, urine and CSF can be used to culture and isolate infectious bacteria and fungi.

The most important diagnostic method in inflammatory CNS disease is the CSF analysis. Coarse macroscopic changes can be present, as can changes in the protein content and in the cell count (see Chap. 2.3).

Therapy: If possible, therapy should be directed against the causal agent. With bacterial meningoencephalitis, an aggressive intravenous antibiotic therapy must be instigated as quickly as possible (see Chap. 9).

Suitable nursing and symptomatic treatment must be undertaken in addition to therapy aimed at the causal agent. Control of ICP must be ensured using a combination of steroids (anti-inflammatory doses) and mannitol (0.5–2.0 g/kg IV). Any tendency toward seizures must be controlled using diazepam (0.5–2.0 mg/kg, IV, to effect) and barbiturates (phenobarbital 2–5 mg/kg, IV, IM, PO q 4–12 hrs).

18.4.3 Trauma

Trauma is an injury with kinetic energy affecting the head causing damage to its soft tissues as well as causing brain contusion, concussion, laceration, oedema, intracranial and/or extracranial haemorrhages, and skull fractures. Skull fractures are often linear or compression fractures. Intracranial haemorrhages can theoretically be in the epidural, subdural, subarachnoid space or in the brain parenchyma. Due to the anatomical characteristics of the meninges, subarachnoid or intraparenchymal haemorrhages usually occur in veterinary medicine.

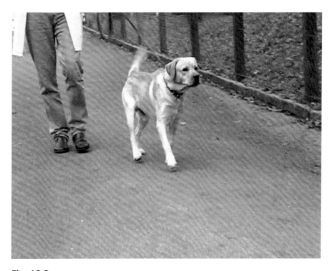

Fig. 18.8
Dog with acute meningitis. The symptoms include stiff trotting gait (notable in the picture) with mild generalised deficits in the positioning and placement reflexes.

Pathophysiology: The biological, chemical and physiological processes involved in association with cranial trauma are very complex and have still not been completely elucidated. The following section provides an overview of these pathological mechanisms, so that the treatment possibilities and constraints can be made understandable to the veterinary surgeon.

The lesions caused by trauma can be divided into **primary** and **secondary injuries** (13). Primary injury consists of haemorrhage and acute cell death due to the direct effects of force. These lesions attain their maximum severity at the time of the accident and can, therefore, not be reduced by treatment. The situation is different with secondary injury as this occurs in the first hours to days *after* the accident and can be curtailed by specific treatments.

Under normal conditions, the brain lies in a unique physiological environment. Protected, but at the same time enclosed, within the cranial cavity, there is a balance between the brain parenchyma, CSF and blood. The pressure difference between the bony calvarium and this internal balance is responsible for the ICP. Intracranial disease changes the volume of at least one of the three components: parenchyma, CSF or blood. Due to the rigidity of the calvarium, there is no room available to cope with a change in volume, therefore the body tries initially to compensate for the increase in the volume of one component (e.g. brain parenchyma in brain oedema) by a reduction in the volume of one or both of the other components (CSF and blood) in order to keep the intracranial balance and so the ICP constant.

18

This involves complex biochemical reactions such as activation of the complement cascade, the kinin-angiotensin system and the arachidonic acid cascade. As a consequence, free oxygen radicals are formed and the intracellular calcium concentration rises. The latter appears to promote the inflammatory reaction, which in turn potentiates the ischemia and oedema formation in the brain. If the compensatory mechanisms for maintaining pressure are exhausted, an increase in ICP occurs that does not allow for any physiological feedback and a vicious cycle starts. The increasing ischemia and hypoxia induce neuronal dysfunction, autolysis and cell death. Nowadays, it is assumed that part of the induced damage is due to reversible axon lesions, but these are only reversible if they occur in an advantageous biochemical milieu. Inflammatory reactions that are instigated by trauma have a negative influence on previously damaged axons and change reversible into irreversible damage. It is the role of treatment to maintain as advantageous an intracranial biochemical constellation as possible to prevent secondary injury, which then causes autolysis of the brain.

An increase in ICP primarily reduces the perfusion of the brain. The reduced blood perfusion allows CO_2 to accumulate at the receptors of the vasomotor centres in the brain stem. This accumulation sets an "alarm signal" off, which causes a rise in systemic blood pressure and so increases brain perfusion via stimulation of the sympathetic nervous system. This physiological reaction is described as the cerebral ischemic response. The increase in systemic blood pressure stimulates the baroreceptors of the circulatory system. These send their information about hypertension to the vagal centres in the brain stem resulting in bradycardia (Cushing's reflex). A further increase in ICP leads to a release of catecholamines, which possibly can lead to myocardial damage and ventricular arrhythmias.

Clinical: A traumatised animal should be handled with extreme care as there may be spinal instabilities present. Manipulation of the cervical spine and especially compression of the jugulars should be avoided to prevent further increase in ICP. The general / systemic condition of the animal should be stabilised first. This is done according to the standard rules of emergency medicine: treatment of shock with concurrent stabilisation of respiration and circulation.

The use of heavy and long-acting sedatives and narcotics should be avoided as far as possible, as they may increase ICP and reduce **brain perfusion** via a series of complex mechanisms; short-acting and partial agonists are preferred. Death may arise as a consequence of over-sedation. If an animal cannot be examined, a sedative (e.g. diazepam) can be given at a **low dose**. Morphine derivatives must be used with extreme care due to their depressant action on the respiration. We caution most strongly against the use of **phenothiazines** and **alpha-adrenergics** because of their hypotensive and arrythmogenic effects.

The most common cause of death after cranial trauma is **hypoxia**. Ensuring that the respiratory tract is functioning and that respiration is adequate is a basic necessity. Adequate oxygenation is indicated in the majority of cranial trauma patients. Hyperventilation is also desired, but this is only possible and safe in unconscious animals, whereby the resulting PCO_2 can be closely monitored. **Hyperventilation** can reduce cerebral blood volume by 36%; in contrast, hypoventilation can increase the normal cerebral blood volume by 170%. The possibilities and usage of oxygen is described below. Basically, the method of administering oxygen is chosen according to the animal's conscious state and its level of cooperation. Principally, after cranial trauma all comatose animals should be intubated, either endotracheally, or transtracheally if the upper airway has been displaced, and given artificial respiration. A great advantage of intubation is the reduction of the **PaCO$_2$** that is subsequently possible, so that a substantial reduction in ICP can be created. The standard values for arterial $PaCO_2$ and end-expiratory CO_2 lie between 25–35 mmHg. As a rule, artificial respiration requires 10 to 20 breaths per minute.

The type of respiration exhibited by animals with cranial trauma can provide an indication about the localisation of the lesion and its prognosis. The frequency, depth and type of respiration should be assessed. First of all, life-threatening trauma of the airways or pulmonary parenchyma must be excluded. If the respiratory pattern is obviously abnormal despite the presence of only a mild pathological insult to the airways, then it must be assumed that this is the result of a central, intracranial lesion. **Cheyne-Stokes respiration** is found with lesions of the cerebrum and diencephalon. Characteristic for this type of respiration are episodes of hyperventilation that slowly reduce in frequency until the animal is apnoeic. The **apnoea** can last for different periods of time before another episode of hyperventilation occurs.

With lesions in the midbrain, animals hyperventilate with more then 25 breaths per minute. In contrast to a pure airway problem, this type of breathing does not alter in an oxygen-enriched environment. Extremely irregular respiratory patterns with frequent apnoeic phases have been observed with lesions of the brain stem. In such cases, the prognosis is poor. This is a cyclic form of respiration with periods of prolonged inspiration followed by expiration and finally apnoea.

A very incoordinated, gasping form of respiration is seen when extensive damage has occurred to the **respiratory centres** in the medulla oblongata.

Diagnosis: Notice should certainly be taken of bleeding from the nose, nasopharynx and orbits as these are often associated with fractures of the base of the skull. The places where blood exits are also places where bacteria can gain entrance. **Skullbase fractures** are relatively common as this is the weakest point of the calvarium. The cauterization of rup-

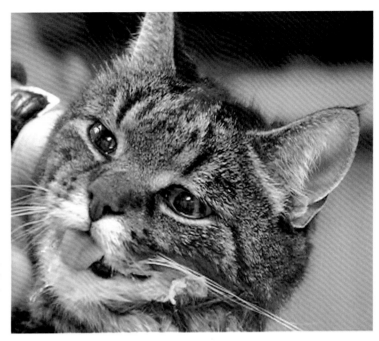

Fig. 18.9
Cat with severe disturbances in consciousness, anisocoria and hypersalivation after a car accident. The cat was presented as an emergency and immediately treated; however, it died within a short time. Histopathology revealed a massive cerebral haemorrhage with herniation of parts of the cerebrum and secondary compression of the brain stem.

tured superficial blood vessels that bleed profusely should be performed as quickly as possible.

Regular examination of **consciousness**, **pupils** (size, symmetry and responsiveness) and **proprioception** is important for the assessment and prognosis of the patient (Fig. 18.9). The deterioration of one or more of these parameters is an indicator of increasing oedema, hypoxia or continual intracranial haemorrhage, and is life threatening. Such patients require aggressive therapy.

As heavy sedation and narcosis should be avoided where possible, only poor-quality pictures can be taken with the imaging techniques available. As a result, **radiographs** taken immediately after the trauma are only used for assessing whether or not there is cervical instability / fracture or fractures of the calvarium. If the general condition of the patient allows it, radiography of the skull in cranial trauma patients is indicated (Chap. 6.5.3). Explanations about changes in the bony cervical spine can be found in Chap. 6.3. Fractures of the base of the skull have a direct influence on the prognosis and treatment: massively indented compression fractures in which bone fragments have been displaced inside the skull and open cranial fractures require surgery. This is done after the initial stabilisation phase. Before such animals are given anaesthesia, thorax radiographs and a peritoneal lavage are indicated to help recognise any occult injuries.

Therapy: Sedatives should only be given to animals that are in a hysterical-hyperreactive state and cannot be examined or treated. These animals can be treated with **diazepam** 0.5–40 mg total dose (given to effect), IV or per-rectally. If no effect is seen or the animal exhibits epileptiform seizures, then phenobarbital 2–10 mg/kg can be given IV or IM. The maximal effect of this medication, however, occurs after about 35 minutes. The advantage of giving barbiturates is the drop in ICP due to the reduction of the brain's need for oxygen and glucose, and especially due to the **decline in blood pressure** and increased resistance of the cerebral blood vessels. This mechanism can be used in patients with massive brain oedema to prevent the viscous cycle of secondary damage in the brain parenchyma (so-called **artificial coma**). If the condition of the patient does not allow time for the phenobarbital to work, then anaesthesia can be induced with pentobarbital (3–5 mg/kg, slow IV, to effect) or propofol (0.1–0.6 mg/kg/min titrated to effect or up to 6 mg/kg/h), though this approach requires intubation and artificial respiration of the patient.

The priorities in treatment of cranial trauma patients are the maintenance of adequate ventilation and the treatment of shock. The patient must be placed in lateral recumbency with its head stretched out and its neck slightly elevated (up to 30°). This position can improve cerebral blood "backflow" and reduce the ICP. **Hyperventilation** of the intubated animal is a rapid and effective method of reducing ICP. **Hypocapnia** should be avoided as it leads to strong vasoconstriction in the brain and subsequently to ischemia. **Fluid**

18

therapy should be used for patients with shock, but excessive hydration should be avoided due to the danger of brain oedema. At the moment, the use of corticosteroids is controversial, though despite this many different authors advise the early administration of **methylprednisolone sodium succinate** to stabilise the cell membranes and reduce oedema. In human medicine, corticosteroids are now contraindicated for patients with head trauma. **Benzodiazepines** and **barbiturates** are of use when the patient has seizures or for inducing a reduction in brain metabolism and to prevent excitotoxicity.

Mannitol is still the drug of choice for reducing ICP. It should be given intravenously (0.5–2.0 g/kg) over a period of 5 to 30 minutes. Mannitol draws water from the cells, reduces the blood viscosity and cerebral vasoconstriction. With respect to intracranial haemorrhag, there are different opinions on the concurrent use of mannitol. If there is an increased ICP, then mannitol should be given despite the possible presence of a bleed (13). **Furosemide** is then administered, usually after the mannitol, with the aim of maintaining the osmotic gradient for a longer period of time. Craniotomy is the last recourse for reducing ICP (see Chap. 10.2.2). This should be done after CT or MRI with the aim of removing bone fragments from inside the skull and to reduce an increased ICP.

The management of comatose patients after the initial treatment must ensure adequate hydration, nutrition, normal body temperature, adequate ventilation, avoidance of decubitus (by frequent turning), and control of micturition and defaecation (5).

Prognosis: The prognosis for a craniocerebral trauma depends on the severity and localisation of the injury. A prognostically unfavourable sign is a significant **loss in consciousness** within minutes after the accident; usually a massive brain stem lesion is present in such patients. The presence of open skull factures is also unfavourable, as the complications are severe. Cerebral symptoms are prognostically better than brain stem symptoms, which may be accompanied by an impairment of vital functions. If the cerebral symptoms become progressively worse, then it may be assumed that oedema has occurred, which must and can be treated immediately. Prognostically poor signs include the presence of decerebrate rigidity and apnoeic respiration in comatose patients.

The correct treatment given within the first 30 minutes after an accident is decisive in limiting secondary damage. A long convalescent period must be considered; the patient may require intensive nursing for weeks. Impatience often leads to premature euthanasia. During the convalescent period, complications such as infection, sepsis, DIC, fistula formation to the CSF space, encephalitis or epileptiform seizures can occur. If despite aggressive conservative therapy the symptoms worsen, then surgical decompression should be performed without delay as this is most probably the only life-saving measure available that can improve the prognosis of a medically refractory case.

18.4.4 Anomalies

In addition to genetic abnormalities, viruses play the biggest role in defects of the neural tube (e.g. parvoviruses – panleucopaenia in the cat). Defects of different severities occur dependent on the stage of development which is damaged: **anencephaly** (complete lack of brain) and **amyelia** (complete lack of a spinal cord) can occur independently of each other, but occur in association with skull defects and/or spinal defects (cranioarchischisis). **Porencephaly** is a defect in the substance of the brain that produces a connection between the ventricle system and the brain surface, sometimes in association with cavity formation in the brain.

Hydroencephaly is an extreme case of this. Different forms of protrusions of brain or spinal cord tissue through bony defects belong to this complex. They consist of leptomeningeal protrusions – covered by epidermis and filled with fluid – that extend over the open cranium or spinal canal. If nervous tissue elements are included in the protrusion then they are called **encephalo- or myelomeningoceles**; when these are absent, then they are known as **meningoceles**. The most important brain anomalies in the dog and cat are hydrocephalus and less commonly lissencephaly, encephalocele, agenesis of the corpus callosum, and hydranencephaly.

Lissencephaly is a rare disease seen in the Lhasa Apso, Wirehaired Fox Terrier and Irish Setter. The cerebrum has a smooth surface and the formation of the gyri and sulci is abnormal. The lesion only affects the neopallium and the cortex is thicker than normal (pachygyria), with an abnormal pattern of laminar neuronal organisation (14).

The protrusion of brain parenchyma through a defect in the calvarium, though it is covered by skin, is known as **encephalocele**. It is inherited in the Burman. In addition, it is thought that the administration of griseofulvin during pregnancy can cause such a teratogenic change (14).

Agenesis of the corpus callosum has been described sporadically in the Labrador Retriever. **Hydranencephaly** means an almost complete destruction and loss of the neocortex. It has been described rarely in young cats as a consequence of a panleukaemia virus infection during gestation (14).

18.4.4.1 Hydrocephalus
The term hydrocephalus is usually used to describe an abnormal enlargement of the ventricular system within the cranium (15).

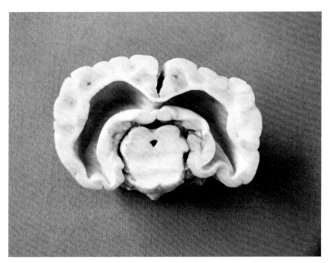

Fig. 18.10a
Dalmatian, six-month-old female, with delayed growth and a mild generalised ataxia from 3 months of age onwards. These symptoms then developed into a severe gait abnormality with falling over and falling down the stairs. The brain section showed moderate congenital internal hydrocephalus.

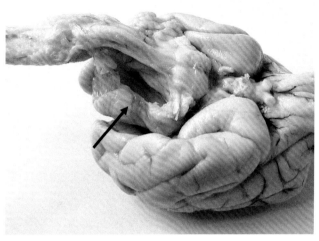

Fig. 18.10b
Labrador, eight-month-old male, with an abnormal swaying and hopping gait since puppyhood. From 6 months of age onwards, the dog developed frequent regurgitation and then aspiration pneumonia. A complex malformation of the cerebellum (hypoplasia [arrow] and partial aplasia) was found on brain section.

Aetiology: Congenital internal hydrocephalus is the most common malformation of the brain (Figs. 18.10a, b) and is caused by a disturbance to the CSF circulation. The CSF is produced in the choroid plexi and flows through the intraventricular (Monro) foramen into the third ventricle and then through the mesencephalic aqueduct to the fourth ventricle, which also has its own choroid plexus. From the fourth ventricle, the CSF enters the subarachnoid space via Luschka's and Magendi's foraminae. There the CSF is resorbed by the arachnoid villi and granulations (Pacchionian bodies), as well as in the nerve root sacs. Displacement of the CSF outflow leads to a blockage and a widening of the CSF channels above / rostral to the blockage. Internal hydrocephalus can be manifested in the fetal stage or postnatal (though often months or years after birth). Neonatal internal hydrocephalus is usually associated with a poor life expectancy and neural function deficits, as brain regions close to the ventricles such as the septum pellucidum, hippocampus, thalamus and hypothalamus are affected by pressure atrophy. With a late manifestation of the disease, the animals initially develop normally and then suddenly have ataxia, changes in behaviour or epileptic seizures. In addition to fetal noxious agents such as viral infections, inherited causes also play a role. The latter include brain malformations (Bullmastiff) and breed-associated head shapes in the brachycephalic breeds (e.g. Boxer or Toy Poodle), where due to a narrowing of the space within the cranium, craniostenosis develops leading to CSF drainage problems.

Hydrocephalus can be **congenital** or **acquired**. **Obstructive hydrocephalus** occurs as a consequence of a displacement of the CSF outflow or a disturbance in the CSF resorption. Aqueductal stenosis is the most common congenital malformation (14). An acquired stenosis can be induced by inflammation, tumours, granulomas or haemorrhage. Often the neighbouring regions / parenchyma around the ventricular system are affected; e.g. the mesencephalic aqueduct and the interventricular foramen (15). Congenital hydrocephalus is usually symmetrical; in contrast, the acquired form is often asymmetrical.

Congenital hydrocephalus occurs most commonly in toy breeds (Chihuahua, Toy Poodle, Toy Spitz, Yorkshire Terrier) and brachycephalic breeds (Boston Terrier, English Bulldog, Lhasa Apso, Pekingese, Pug). The causes of congenital hydrocephalus (not including the speculative ones) have not been fully elucidated. Some dog breeds are known to develop an asymptomatic ventricular dilatation.

Clinical: The severity of the clinical symptoms of hydrocephalus is not necessarily related to the degree of ventricular dilatation; however, they reflect the abrupt onset of the process, the associated increase in ICP and the possible underlying disease. Hydrocephalus can be presumed in puppies when they have a dome-shaped cranial cavity (Fig. 18.11). These animals usually exhibit learning difficulties, behavioural changes such as compulsory circling and sterotypies, dementia and visual deficits. Later on, seizures can occur. Ventral and/or lateral strabismus has been observed in human beings and animals with hydrocephalus and is termed "sunset gaze" or downcast eye gaze; it is due to the abnormal skull conformation accom-

18

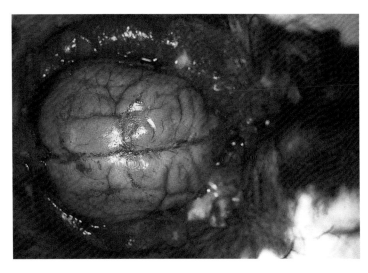

Fig. 18.11
Cocker Spaniel, one-year-old male, with congenital hydrocephalus. The dome-shaped curvature of the brain is notable.

panying hydrocephalus (15). In congenital hydrocephalus, the course is usually slowly progressive and some patients even remain stable for some time. However, acute, dramatically deteriorating symptoms have been described in a small percentage of cases due to intraventricular haemorrhage (5). Secondary hydrocephalus is accompanied by acute progressive symptoms. In such patients, it is difficult to differentiate between the symptoms of the primary disease and those of the hydrocephalus (5).

Diagnosis: In the past years, the development of new imaging technologies for brain diagnostics (CT and MRI) has significantly improved the determination of hydrocephalus. In contrast, the older well-established diagnostic imaging methods are rarely used nowadays. These are radiography of the skull, ventriculography and EEG. Radiography can reveal the thin calvarium, the loss of gyri and persistent fontanelles associated with congenital hydrocephalus (16). Ventriculography is rarely used as CT and MRI are less invasive and deliver better images of the ventricular system.

Electroencephalography is practically not used anymore. One reason for this is that the equipment is expensive. In addition, the typical pictures associated with hydrocephalus (increased amplitudes and slow frequent waves) can also be found with other encephalopathies and so are not diagnostic.

In young animals with open fontanelles, ultrasonography can be used focussing the beam through this "acoustic window" to characterise the size of the ventricles and to diagnose hydrocephalus (Fig. 18.12) (17).

CT and MRI scans are, therefore, the methods of choice for confirming hydrocephalus. Both methods can optimally visualise the ventricles and brain parenchyma, and in secondary hydrocephalus provide indications about the underlying causal disease. Dilated ventricles are hypodense in comparison to the parenchyma on CT. It must be emphasized once again that the severity of the clinical symptoms is not correlated to the size of the ventricles and the clinical significance cannot be predicted by the degree of ventricular dilatation (15).

Therapy: Acetazolamide reduces the CSF pressure by reducing CSF production. This diuretic is especially important in the initial treatment of patients with raised ICP associated with hydrocephalus. The use of steroids can also reduce CSF production (5). Prednisolone is initially given at a dose of 0.25–0.5 mg/kg, PO, BID. This dosage is reduced stepwise weekly until 0.1 mg/kg, PO, is given every second day. Some patients can be effectively treated with chronic low-dose steroid therapy. Despite this, such treatment cannot be effective in the long term if the specific cause of the hydrocephalus is not known and not specifically treated (15).

Surgery must be used in animals if the condition does not improve within 2 weeks of starting steroid treatment. The aim is to control the CSF flow. **Shunt systems** developed for human medicine also work in animal patients and allow drainage from the lateral ventricles to the peritoneal cavity or less commonly to the right atrium (see Chap. 10.2.3).

The most common complication with using shunts in human beings is **infection** (18). A so-called undershunting must be assumed when the condition of the patient after surgery does not improve. This can arise as a consequence of catheter blockage due to obstruction by proteinaceous plugs, blood or cellular deposits (15). Animals with severe thinning of the cerebral cortex are not candidates for a shunt as they have a high risk of brain collapse and extra-axial haemorrhage at the time of shunt insertion.

18

18.4.5 Metabolic/toxic diseases

Numerous metabolic, toxic and nutritional disturbances that result in neurological symptoms are summarised under the term "metabolic" diseases.

Changes in **homeostasis**, e.g. in **oxygen transport** or **glucose** and **electrolyte metabolism**, can have severe effects on the nervous system; for example, **hepatic or uraemic encephalopathy**.

Nutritional deficits are relatively rare nowadays in pets. The most important type seen in the dog and cat is **vitamin B complex deficiency**, which leads to neurological dysfunction.

In addition, the toxin-associated diseases are important causes of metabolic dysfunction leading to neurological deficits. The different groups that have the ability to affect the forebrain in domestic animals include **pesticides**, **rodenticides**, **heavy metals**, **drugs** and less commonly **poisonous plants**.

Metabolic disturbances cause nerve cell dysfunction, which in the worst cases can lead to neuronal death. Theoretically, the neurological deficits are **reversible with successful treatment of the causal disease** (19). Metabolic diseases can be manifold and induce either acute or chronic clinical symptoms. However, **forebrain symptoms** are the most commonly described manifestations of metabolic encephalopathies.

18.4.5.1 Oxygen deficiency

Aetiology: The brain has an enormously high metabolic rate as it requires 20% of the total oxygen (O_2) requirements of the whole body (20). The grey matter needs 94% of this O_2, particularly the cerebrocortical pyramidal cells and cerebellar purkinje cells (19).

Oxygen deficiency in the brain can be caused by reduced blood flow with reduced cerebral perfusion (ischemia) or low arterial O_2 concentration (hypoxia). **Hypoxia** is defined as **hypoxic hypoxia** when the O_2 concentration is reduced or **anaemic hypoxia** when there is a reduced haemoglobin concentration in the blood (19). An acute drop in arterial PaO_2 to less than 40–50 mm Hg means that there is reduced cerebral function; below 20–30 mm Hg there is loss of consciousness (21).

Cerebral ischemia is accompanied by glucose deficiency in the brain and increased CO_2 concentration. Accordingly, there is a greater probability of irreversible neuronal damage than with a simple hypoxia. With absolute ischemia, there is an exhaustion of O_2 within 10 seconds, while the ATP stores are exhausted within 2 to 4 minutes (22). Afterwards, energy is provided by anaerobic glycolysis producing lactic acid, which is totally incapable of covering the energy requirements of the brain. After complete ischemic/hypoxic damage, loss of consciousness occurs within 10 seconds, though

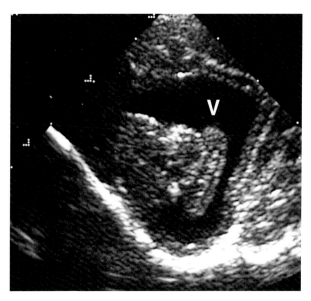

Fig. 18.12
Ultrasonography of hydrocephalus. Sagittal section through the open fontanelles of the right lateral ventricle in a Yorkshire Terrier. The individual sections of the lateral ventricle (V) are clearly visualised. (Fig. Johann Lang, Bern.)

irreversible neuronal damage does not occur before 15 minutes after the start of ischemia (23).

In small animals, the **causes** of severe hypoxia include **acute vascular damage, anaesthetic accidents, cardiopulmonary damage, shock, sepsis, severe anaemia** and more rarely, **carbon monoxide poisoning** and **asphyxiation**.

Therapy: Acute hypoxic/ischemic damage necessitates immediate and aggressive therapy. The systemic causes should be treated. The first therapeutic steps are O_2 administration and reduction of the ICP. Accordingly, adequate hydration and appropriate ventilation must be ensured. If there are no contraindications, the patient should be placed in lateral recumbency with its head extended and slightly raised: this prevents a further increase in ICP. Highly potent glucocorticoids (methylprednisolone sodium succinate: 30 mg/kg, IV as bolus; followed by an infusion with 5 mg/kg/h over 24 to 48 hours) should be administered to reduce the ICP and to stabilise the cell membranes; the patient must be euvolaemic prior to mannitol use. The diuretic effect of mannitol can be prolonged by giving furosemide (0.75–1 mg/kg, IV, q 6 h).

18.4.5.2 Disturbances in glucose metabolism

18.4.5.2.1 Hypoglycaemia

Aetiology: Hypoglycaemia can occur in both young and old animals (Table 18.3). Puppies are affected secondary to **parasite infestations, malnutrition, stress, gastrointestinal**

18

diseases, sepsis and more rarely **glycogen storage diseases**.

The affects of hypoglycaemia on the brain cells are very similar to those seen with hypoxia.

In adult animals, hypoglycaemia is often caused by a functional tumour of the pancreatic β-cells (insulinoma) (Fig. 18.13) (2). The excessive insulin production by these tumours leads to systemic hypoglycaemia and neurological symptoms. A similar situation occurs with the **paraneoplastic syndrome** described with various tumours; for example, **hepatic carcinoma, haemangiosarcoma, lymphosarcoma, mammary gland carcinoma, melanoma** and **adenocarcinoma** of the lungs (24). It is thought that these tumours produce an insulin-like substance that causes hypoglycaemia.

Clinical: The clinical symptoms can progress with the development of a peripheral polyneuropathy, and are characterised by weakness, exercise intolerance, reduced spinal reflexes and muscle atrophy. The severity of the clinical symptoms depends on the degree of glucose concentration reduction (2). **Seizures** and **coma** are the result of a sudden drop in the glucose concentration, while weakness, LMNS symptoms and depression are the most common consequences of a gradually developing hypoglycaemia.

Therapy: Specific therapy consists of removal of the causative tumour. Symptomatic therapy includes a protein- and fat-rich diet and low doses of prednisolone (0.25–0.5 mg/kg, PO, BID). Diazoxide (3–20 mg/kg, TID, in the food) can also be given as this is an inhibitor of insulin secretion and promoter of hepatic gluconeogenesis.

18.4.5.2.2 Hyperglycaemia
Diabetes mellitus can be associated with many different clinical symptoms that arise due to persistent hyperglycaemia. A **peripheral neuropathy** as a consequence of demyelination and axon degeneration has been observed in patients with prolonged noncompensated diabetes mellitus (2). **Intracranial disturbances** (depression to coma) are known to occur with two syndromes associated with the later stages of diabetes mellitus: **diabetic ketoacidosis** and **hyperosmolar non-ketotic diabetes mellitus**. It is assumed that the neurological symptoms are a consequence of the blood's hyperosmolarity, dehydration, renal insufficiency and acidosis.

18.4.5.3 Hepatic encephalopathy (HE)
Aetiology: The normal function of the liver is essential for maintenance of normal brain metabolism as it indirectly provides glucose and removes substances that are toxic to the CNS. Liver insufficiency can lead to problems in the detoxification of dangerous substances and to an inadequate supply of energy to the brain. HE is the neurological syndrome of a

Table 18.3: Causes of hypoglycaemia in small animals
(modified after CUDDON, 1996 [19])

Glucose deficiency
- Iatrogenic: insulin overdose
- Iatrogenic: inadequate glucose supply
- Insulinoma
- Extra-pancreatic tumours that produce insulin-like substances

Glucose underproduction
- Neonatal hypoglycaemia
- Transient juvenile hypoglycaemia
- Starvation
- Malabsorption
- Addison's disease
- Liver disease
  - Portosystemic shunt
  - Cirrhosis
  - End-stage hepatitis
- Glucose storage diseases
  - Glucose-6-phophatase deficiency
  - Amylo-1,6-glucosidase deficiency
  - α-glucosidase deficiency

Glucose underproduction and increased requirement
- Sepsis

complex metabolic disturbance developing from abnormal liver function (2).

HE can be congenital or acquired. **Portosystemic shunts,** due to different types of congenital vascular defects, are the most common causes of such pathology. The most commonly affected dog breeds are Australian Cattle Dog, Irish Wolfhound, Maltese Terrier, Miniature Schnauzer and the Yorkshire Terrier (25, 26). **Extrahepatic shunts** occur frequently in small dog breeds, while **intrahepatic shunts** have been described in medium-sized and large breeds (25). Congenital portosystemic shunts tend to be rare in the cat and usually consist of a single extrahepatic portocaval shunt. The abnormal blood vessels can be demonstrated using either ultrasonography or jejunum contrast portography (Fig. 18.14).

Acquired shunts are associated with severe liver cirrhosis and are usually a consequence of chronic hepatitis in the dog or hepatic lipidosis in the cat (19). The portal hypertension that causes the changes in the liver tissue leads to the formation of new venous vessels on the liver surface that then lead to portosystemic shunting of the mesenteric blood.

The present theory about the pathogenesis of HE is based on four factors: (1) **ammonia,** with or without a synergistic toxin, is thought to be the actual neurotoxin; (2) an **abnormal metabolism of aromatic amino acids** leads secondarily to a disturbance of the cerebral monoamine neurotransmitters; (3) the monoamine neurotransmitter concentrations (**γ-aminobutyric acid** (GABA) and/or **glutamate)** are sig-

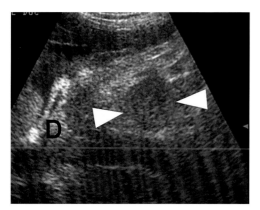

Fig. 18.13
Ultrasonography of an insulinoma in the right lobe of the pancreas. The duodenum (D) is in cross-section. Insulinomas are typically seen as hypoechogenic round foci. The sensitivity of the investigation depends on the size of the tumour, its localisation and the experience of the investigator. If there are metastases in the regional lymph nodes, these are often more easily recognised than the tumour in the pancreas. (Fig. Johann Lang, Bern.)

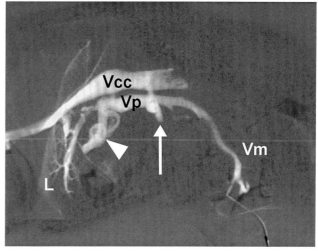

Fig. 18.14
Intraoperative portogramme (subtraction) via the mesenteric vein (Vm). Two extra-hepatic shunt vessels (arrow and arrowhead), initially lead ventrally from the portal vein (Vp) and then finally, after forming a curve, they enter the caudal vena cava (Vcc). They fill this and at the same time parts of the liver tissue with contrast. The liver (L) is perfused by the left branch of the portal vein especially in its ventral areas. (Fig. Johann Lang, Bern.)

nificantly altered in the brain; and (4) the cerebral concentration of endogenous **benzodiazepine-like substances** is increased (19, 26). Ammonia is produced in the intestines by urease-producing bacteria and a healthy liver transforms it into uric acid. In liver insufficiency, ammonia reaches the systemic blood circulation in excess and can easily pass through the blood-brain barrier, where it disturbs the cerebral metabolism. This appears to play an important role in the regulation of the relationship between GABA and glutamate metabolism. Potential synergistic toxins include the mercaptans, short-chain fatty acids, phenols and the bile acids (26). The increase in aromatic amino acids in HE patients can potentially lead to an increase in serotonin and a reduction in dopamine and noradrenaline. The central role of the benzodiazepine-like substances has been supported by the observation that patients in human medicine show a clinical improvement when they are treated with flumazenil in the acute stages, a benzodiazepine antagonist (26). There does not seem to be the same success with its use in chronic cases.

Clinical: Animals with a portosystemic shunt and HE are usually smaller than their littermates and appear to be undernourished. The most commonly described neurological abnormalities include chronic, intermittent periods of reduced consciousness (depression to stupor or even coma), behavioural changes (disorientation, compulsive pacing, anxiety, aggression) and proprioception deficits. Seizures tend to be rather rare but can occur. Hypersalivation occurs in cats more commonly than dogs. The symptoms of hepatic dysfunction can include vomiting, loss of weight, polyuria / polydipsia and diarrhoea.

Therapy: Treatment is either with medication and / or surgery. Ligation of the abnormal vessel is the method of choice for a simple portosystemic shunt.

Special care must be taken during the anaesthesia and the first phase after the operation. Postoperative status epilepticus is a well described fatal complication although its aetiology and its prevalence is not known. Nonsurgical treatment consists of dietary management, whereby easily digestible food with a small amount of high-quality protein should be used. The oral administration of lactulose makes the milieu in the colon more acidic which reduces the number of ammonia-producing bacteria and converts ammonia to the poorly absorbable ammonium ion.

Oral antibiotics (neomycin, doxycycline, metronidazole) are used to inhibit bacterial multiplication in the colon (see Chap. 9). If antibiosis is necessary for life, then the antibiotics should be alternated every 2 to 3 months.

18.4.5.4 Uraemic encephalopathy (UE)
Aetiology: Acute or chronic renal insufficiency can lead to neurological consequences similar in intensity and temporal development to the metabolic disturbances. Numerous factors play a role in the development of UE. These include arterial hypertension, uraemic toxaemia (methylguanidine,

18

guanidine succinate, phenolic acid), an increased concentration of parathormone, increased calcium concentration in the brain, reduced cerebral blood flow and a neurotransmitter imbalance (19). In addition, uraemic vasculitis occurs which increases the permeability of the blood-brain barrier so that uraemic substances can pass through it and damage the neurons.

Clinical: The symptoms can be episodic and include seizures, disturbances in consciousness, disorientation and delirium. The respiration can also be affected – Kussmaul's breathing may be seen as a consequence of acidosis. Irregular breathing is a sign of a hyposensitivity of the brain stem chemoreceptors (19).

Diagnosis: The diagnosis is based on the systemic clinical signs and haematological changes.

Therapy: The therapy of renal failure depends on the type of disturbance and can be read about in the relevant literature. When renal disease is chronic and irreversible, the prognosis is poor – unless dialysis or a renal transplant is considered. Potentially, the neurological symptoms can disappear if the causal disease is treated.

18.4.5.5 Toxic encephalopathies

Many substances can induce neurological symptoms. The following chapter provides an overview of the consequences of the most common intoxications that can lead to cerebral dysfunction. Many toxins cause biochemical changes that are potentially reversible, while others cause structural defects. The most common toxins that are dangerous for the brain are listed in Table 18.4. The observation by the owner that his or her animal has been poisoned is significant for the diagnosis. However, any animal that is presented with seizures, stupor / coma, tremor and ataxia may have potentially been poisoned. The differential diagnoses can naturally include inflammatory or metabolic diseases.

The most common CNS symptoms in poisoned animals include seizures. These can occur in clusters or as status epilepticus. The most common seizure-inducing toxins are listed in Table 18.5; particular attention is paid to some pesticides (organochlorines, organophosphates, carbamates, pyrethrins), metaldehyde, strychnine and lead.

18.4.5.5.1 Pesticides

The most common pesticide poisonings in small animals occur due to the ingestion of organophosphates or carbamates. These compounds cause dysfunction of the autonomic system (salivation, miosis, gastrointestinal motility disturbances, diarrhoea, bronchospasm and continual dyspnoea) and neuromuscular symptoms (tremor, fasciculations). Excitement and seizures may also be seen. They can be treated by administering atropine (0.2–0.4 mg/kg IV over 5 minutes) to counter the muscarinic effects and symptomatic therapy can

Table 18.4: The most common CNS-damaging toxins in domestic animals (modified after OLIVER et al., 1997 [2])

Pesticides
- Chlorinated hydrocarbons
- Organophosphates
- Carbamates
- Pyrethrins
- Metaldehyde

Rodenticides
- Strychnine
- Warfarin
- ANTU (α naphthylthiourea)
- Sodium fluoroacetate
- Zinc phosphide
- Bromethalin

Herbicides and fungicides
- Many

Heavy metals
- Lead

Drugs
- Narcotics
- Amphetamine
- Barbiturates
- Tranquilisers
- Ivermectin
- Aspirin
- Marijuana

Poisonous plants
- Many

Animal origin
- Snake bite
- Toads (*Bufo* spp.)
- Tick paralysis

Anti-freeze agents
- Ethylene glycol

Detergents and disinfectants
- Hexachlorophene
- Phenols

be accomplished with diazepam, phenobarbital and / or pentobarbital. With organophosphate poisoning, cholinesterase-reactivating oximes such as pralidoxime chloride (2-PAM) may need to be administered to control the neuromuscular abnormalities. The dose of 2-PAM (given as a 10% solution) is 10–20 mg/kg for cats and 40 mg/kg for dogs, given IV slowly with fluids over a 30-minute period.

18.4.5.5.2 Metaldehyde

Metaldehyde is a commonly used pesticide for controlling snails. It can cause continual seizures or status epilepticus. Treatment consists of emptying and washing out the stomach and colon, binding of the residual toxin in the stomach with activated charcoal (0.5–4.0 g/kg) and symptomatic therapy (e.g. treatment of hyperthermia).

Table 18.5: List of toxins that most commonly cause seizures in domestic animals (modified after OLIVER et al., 1997 [2])

Pesticides
- Organic chlorines
- Organophosphates
- Carbamates
- Pyrethrins
- Metaldehyde

Rodenticides
- Strychnine
- Sodium fluoroacetate
- Zinc phosphide
- Bromethalin

Heavy metals
- Lead

Drugs
- Amphetamine
- Methylxanthine

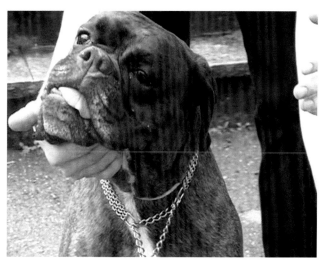

Fig. 18.15
Boxer, twelve-year-old male, with proven ivermectin intoxication. The notable symptoms were head tilt, ventral strabismus on the right, stupor and deficits in positioning and placement reactions in all four limbs.

18.4.5.5.3 Strychnine

Strychnine at one time was commonly used as a rodenticide but it is now forbidden in many countries. However, intentional poisoning of dogs with contaminated meat has sometimes been reported. Strychnine blocks the inhibitory interneurons. Hyperexcitement, fasciculations, tonic-clonic spasms and an increased reaction to acoustic and tactile stimuli occur. Strychnine tends to cause tetany rather than seizures. The poisoned animal is fully conscious. Prognosis is guarded, depending on the amount of poison ingested and/or promptness of treatment. The main objectives of treatment are to keep the muscles relaxed and to prevent asphyxia. The drug of choice in dogs has been pentobarbital, at 30 mg/kg, IV (or via intraperitoneal or intrathoracic routes if the animal is difficult to manage or is having seizures). The muscle relaxants recommended include methocarbamol (Robaxin®) at a dose of 150 mg/kg IV, repeated as needed. Supportive treatment includes prompt gastric or enterogastric lavage using 1 to 2% tannic acid or 1:2000 potassium permanganate and enemas, followed by administration of activated charcoal. Forced diuresis with 5% mannitol in isotonic saline and acidification of urine with 150 mg/kg body weight of ammonium chloride PO, will enhance the urinary elimination of strychnine.

If the animal survives 24 hours, the prognosis for complete recovery is very good.

18.4.5.5.4 Lead

Lead poisoning following ingestion can occur particularly in young dogs. The diagnosis is often difficult as the neurological symptoms usually develop following chronic poisoning. A high lead concentration in the blood is diagnostic. Although stupor and coma can occur in the end stage of lead poisoning, earlier on in the disease severe depression may be noticed and with small amounts of lead, behavioural changes may be more prominent. Treatment with the chelating agent, calcium disodium ethylene diamine tetra acetate (EDTA), using a dose of 25 mg/kg IV, QID for 2 to 5 days, often results in rapid recovery within 36 to 48 hours. Oral administration using the same dosage is also effective. Alternatively, oral penicillamine may be given (100 mg/kg, daily, for 1 to 2 weeks). Treatment is repeated over another 5-day period if signs persist. The prognosis is favorable in the majority of lead poisoning cases treated with chelating agents. Recent studies in dogs with naturally acquired lead poisoning indicated that succimer (meso-2,3-dimercaptosuccinic acid), administered orally for 10 days (10 mg/kg of body weight, PO, q 8 h), also effectively reduced blood lead concentrations and eliminated clinical signs of lead poisoning. Succimer is also effective in cats. Succimer may also be given rectally as a solution in patients that are vomiting.

18.4.5.5.5 Medications

In pets, it is fairly common that ingestion of the owner's medication leads to poisoning; e.g. narcotics, barbiturates, sedatives and marijuana. The treatment consists of eliminating the poison, combined with antagonistic and symptomatic therapy. Emergency and intensive medicine is necessary when respiratory function is adversely affected.

Ivermectin can pass through the blood-brain barrier in the Collie, Old English Sheepdog, and related breeds. In these dogs, administration of ivermectin can lead to coma or even death (Fig. 18.15). Treatment is supportive, including activated charcoal and a saline cathartic, fluids, and shock doses of corticosteroids (in severely affected dogs).

18

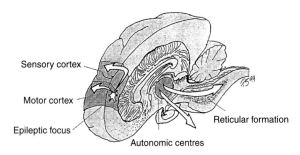

Fig. 18.16
Schematic representation of an epileptic focus. Longitudinal section through the right cerebral hemisphere of a dog. The epileptic focus lies in the motor cortex. From here it spreads to the sensory cortex, and then it extends via the connections between the two hemispheres to the left half of the brain and also to the autonomic centres and the reticular formation (From: JAGGY and STEFFEN, 1995 [32]).

18.5 Epilepsy

18.5.1 Idiopathic or primary epilepsy

A differentiation is made between primary or idiopathic epilepsy in which no obvious structural or metabolic changes can be determined in the brain, and secondary (or symptomatic) epilepsy in which the seizures are a consequence of organic changes in the cerebrum (vascular insult, infection, trauma, malformation, neoplasia, degenerative disease) or extracerebral metabolic disturbances (including intoxication). Epilepsy can also occur as a late consequence of any insult to the brain even though the original brain lesion has long since healed clinically and has been anatomically replaced by scar tissue (most commonly known as so-called post-traumatic epilepsy).

Pathophysiology: Epilepsy was first described in domestic animals in the first half of the nineteenth century (27). Its historical roots in human beings can be traced back to 2080 BC, when it was mentioned in Hammurabi's Babylonian Laws. It took until the first half of the nineteenth century to scientifically prove the 2000-year-old statement that the brain is the starting point of every epileptic seizure (28).

In veterinary medicine, idiopathic epilepsy is of great importance in small animal medicine. The reason for epilepsy's importance is its relatively frequent occurrence in the total dog population in general (1–2%; 5–6% experience at least one fit during their lives) and in certain breeds in particular (prevalence < 17%). Additionally, the social aspects of the disease make this an important neurological issue as an epileptic fit is extremely frightening for the affected animal's owner (29, 30). As epilepsy is also common in human beings (1%) and the pathogenesis and cause is still unknown for various forms of epilepsy, the dog can serve as a research model for the pathogenesis of this disease (31).

According to definition, epileptic seizures, spasms and epileptiform fits are initiated by uncontrolled, synchronised electrical discharges of single groups of neurons in the brain. The term epilepsy should technically only be used for idiopathic epilepsy in which chronic relapsing epileptic seizures occur without an identifiable underlying cause (32).

Epileptic seizures develop as a consequence of a sudden excessive discharge of neurons in the grey matter of the brain. An increased irritability of the neurons is an essential quality for the abnormality, which is either inherited or acquired. The disturbance in electrical discharge is due to either an intracellular or synaptic mechanism. This leads primarily to an abnormal distribution of electrolytes at the cell membrane; in particular, a massive influx of calcium ions occurs. There is also a relative deficiency of the inhibitory neurotransmitter GABA and an increased release of the excitatory neurotransmitters, glutamate and aspartate. Beginning with a series of discharges from these individual neurons – also known as the focus – synchronisation of different groups of nerve cells occurs, leading to an extension of the discharge into individual regions of the brain (Fig. 18.16) (33).

The seizure manifests itself clinically according to which section of the brain is stimulated in this manner. Motor, sensory and even autonomic disturbances can be seen either in combination or isolation, with or without changes in consciousness. The "kindling phenomenon" plays an important role in the therapeutic basis for epilepsy: every epileptic seizure potentiates the occurrence of the next one as it causes facilitation or acclimatisation of the neurons to chronic relapsing stimulation (34). The end of a seizure is usually not due to neuronal exhaustion or oxygen deficiency, but is the result of active inhibition (35).

Morphological changes secondary to seizures have been found in the brain both in human beings and dogs; this includes neuronal degeneration in the cerebrum, hippocampus and the amygdala (36).

Classification: In human medicine, many attempts have been made to classify epileptic seizures. In 1989, a classification was defined by the International League against Epilepsy, which has been accepted by neurologists world wide. Three categories have been differentiated according to the clinical picture, aetiology, and ictal and interictal EEG results: localisation-related (focal or partial), generalised and unclassifiable epileptic seizures. The difference in the dog is that EEG results are often lacking, especially those of the ictal period. A definite differentiation on the grounds of clinical symptoms alone is very difficult as it is virtually impossible to determine whether or not the animal is affected by disturbances in consciousness during the seizures. Without EEG results, it is not possible to differentiate between seizures that are generalised and those that begin focally and later generalise (30).

18

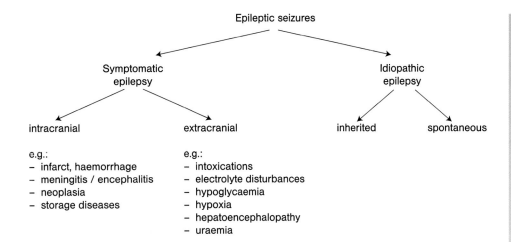

Fig. 18.17
Differentiation of seizures according to their aetiology

At the moment in veterinary medicine, there is no internationally recognised classification for epilepsy. Accordingly, in the following, a classification is introduced that follows that of the International League against Epilepsy but has been adapted for animals.

Two groups are differentiated according to the aetiology of the epileptic seizures (Fig. 18.17).
1. Symptomatic epilepsy with an intracranial or extracranial instigating factor.
2. Idiopathic epilepsy without any recognisable cause. Idiopathic epilepsy is usually inherited, though it can occur spontaneously in individual animals.

Basically, two groups of seizure types are differentiated according to their clinical manifestation: partial and generalised (Fig. 18.18). Partial seizures are subdivided further into complex (also known as psychomotor seizures) and simple partial seizures. Generalised seizures may begin as partial seizures.

In general, simple partial seizures do not influence consciousness; in reality this is a very difficult determination to make confidently. These seizures are usually motor disturbances manifested as twitching of the facial muscles, individual limbs or a turning of the neck or head. More rarely, purely autonomic or sensory partial / focal disturbances can occur in the dog and cat. It should be noted that sensory seizures in an animal are difficult to appreciate by owners. Complex partial seizures involve changes in consciousness and can manifest themselves as "absences", fits of temper, unprovoked barking or screaming, anxiety or wild circling (= running fit). A frequently observed form of this seizure type is the so-called "fly catching" seizure in which the animal snaps at an imaginary fly and even swallows it in some cases. This form is more frequent in the Cavalier King Charles Spaniel, though it is also seen in other breeds such as the Bernese Cattle Dog, Dachshund, Miniature Schnauzer and Old English Sheepdog (37). These types of events are difficult to differentiate from the so-

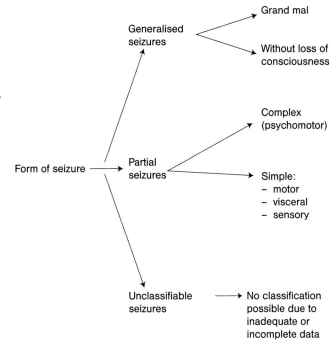

Fig. 18.18
Differentiation of seizures according to their clinical picture

called behavioural or neuropsychiatric disorders without an EEG evaluation. A partial form of seizures is seen as the manifestation of idiopathic epilepsy in the Viszla. The affected dogs exhibit a combination of limb tremor, staring, mydriasis or hypersalivation without any disturbance in consciousness (38). Partial seizures that are very difficult to recognise can frequently be seen in cats (39, 40).

18

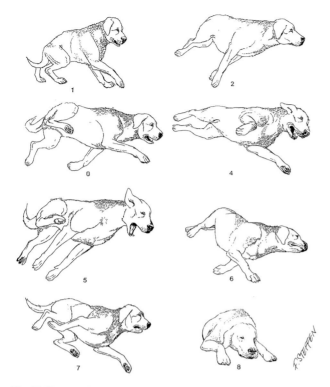

Fig. 18.19
Schematic drawing showing an epileptic seizure in a Labrador Retriever. (1) Aura as partial seizure: (2) extensor spasm of the forelimbs; (3) coordinated paddling movements of all limbs, so-called automatisms; (4) automatisms of the forelimbs; (5) extensor spasm of the forelimbs and the head musculature (jaw clamping); (6) automatisms of the forelimbs: (7) tonic-clonic seizures; (8) recovery phase (from: JAGGY and HEYNOLD, 1996 [44]).

18

Generalised seizures are the most common form of seizure activity recognised in dogs (80%; though they include many that start focally and then generalise).
If the animal loses consciousness during a generalised seizure, the event is sometimes called a grand mal. Generalised seizures are often mixed seizures, though usually motor deficits are prominent either as tonic, clonic or tonic-clonic symptoms. Very often, the abnormal motor activity is accompanied by autonomic deficits such as salivation, micturition and defecation (30, 41).

Often an impending epileptic seizure is indicated by a prodromal phase. This can last for hours to days and is manifested by behavioural changes such as restlessness, nervousness, staring into space, excited snuffling or barking. An aura is occasionally observed in animals. This is a very short episode of psychic or motor abnormalities seen immediately before the actual seizure ("the seizure before the seizure"). Nowadays, the aura is considered to be a partial seizure. In one study, fifteen Labrador Retrievers with idiopathic epilepsy were recorded using a video camera and an aura was observed in each of

them (Fig. 18.19) (42). The seizure itself, the ictus, starts suddenly and lasts for between a few seconds and a number of minutes. The time required for the dog to recover is called the postictal phase; it can last for up to 24 hours. The animals are disorientated and show compulsive pacing and aggression; central blindness may also be exhibited.

The frequency of seizures can vary greatly from animal to animal. Some have them in a regular cyclical fashion, whilst others have them at very irregular intervals. The intensity (duration and severity) varies greatly, too. In some animals, the seizures occur in groups (clusters). In large dog breeds, the course is usually severe and the incidence of the seizures tends to become more frequent with time. The course of a seizure can be variable, though each patient usually exhibits the same pattern of seizures, which indeed may be breed-specific (37, 43, 44).

A dog's first seizure occurs, in the majority of cases, between the ages of 1 to 3 years. Idiopathic epilepsy, however, can be found in both younger and older animals. In the Golden and Labrador Retrievers, 40% of the dogs are older than 3 years when they have their first seizure (45, 46), whereas in the Bernese Cattle Dog, 20% are younger than 1 year and 18% are older than 3 years (47).

Mode of inheritance: Idiopathic epilepsy occurs in all breeds and in mixed-breed dogs, too. Roughly half of all dogs suffering from epileptic seizures are affected by idiopathic epilepsy (41). However, there are some breeds that are more commonly affected than others (and in these certain families are especially affected): Border Collie, Cocker Spaniel, Rough Collie, Dachshund, Greater Swiss Mountain Dog, Horak's Laboratory Hound, Irish Setter, Miniature Schnauzer, Poodle, St. Bernard, and Wire-haired Fox Terrier, (2, 48). A genetic basis has been be determined in the Beagle (49), Belgian Sheepdog (52), Bernese Cattle Dog (47), Boxer (53), German Shepherd (50), Golden Retriever (45), Keeshond (51), Labrador Retriever (46), Shetland Sheepdog (54) and Viszla (38).

With exception of the Keeshond (in which idiopathic epilepsy is inherited as autosomal recessive), the mode of inheritance is complex. It appears that more than one gene is responsible for the inheritance of epilepsy in most breeds and that environmental factors may also play a role. A so-called multi-factoral inheritance is responsible. Gender appears to play a role in some breeds. A significant predisposition for male dogs has been found in the Beagle, Golden Retriever and Bernese Cattle Dog (45, 47, 49). In the Bernese Cattle Dog, it has been found that animals with affected parents become affected with idiopathic epilepsy earlier than animals with healthy parents (47). In an epidemiological study on Labrador Retrievers looking into the effect of environmental factors on epilepsy, it was discovered that the dogs tended to develop seizures in certain specific situations, especially after stress (42). Castration to remove an additional source of

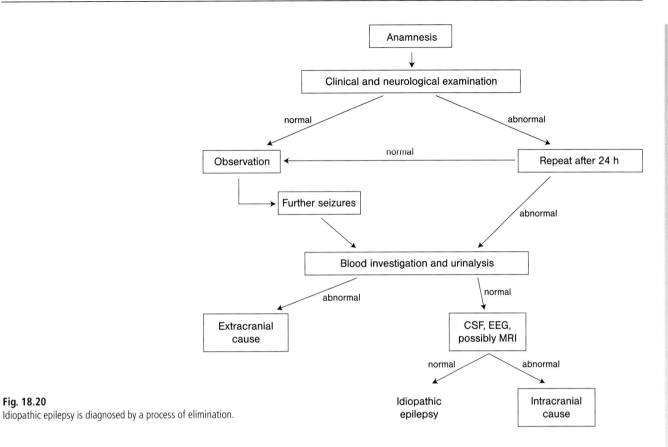

Fig. 18.20
Idiopathic epilepsy is diagnosed by a process of elimination.

"stress" had no influence on the seizures in the Golden Retriever (55).

Idiopathic epilepsy can also occur in cats, though rarely. Approx. 5–10% of all cats with epileptic seizures have been reported to be affected by idiopathic epilepsy (40).

The fact that the inheritance of idiopathic epilepsy in the majority of breeds involves a number of genes, makes elimination of the disease by breeding difficult. Many animals are carriers of one of the genes but do not become affected and so remain unknown. It is, therefore, recommended that at least affected animals should not be used for breeding, and matings that have lead to the production of an affected animal should not be repeated again. In addition, it is recommended to completely avoid breeding from siblings of epileptics. An attempt should be made to determine the mode of inheritance and heritability of this disease for every breed, and then to develop unaffected breeding lines.

Diagnosis: According to its definition, idiopathic epilepsy implies the occurrence of recurrent epileptic seizures that have no recognisable cause. Diagnosis is made possible by a process of elimination and it is recommended that a practical method as shown in Fig. 18.20 should be used. Even if only a single seizure is observed, a thorough clinical and neurological examination is indicated. If the results are normal, further investigations may not be immediately necessary. Historically,

poisoning should be excluded and the owner should report back once another epileptic seizure occurs. If the results of clinical and neurological examinations are abnormal 24 hours after the seizure, then further investigations must be undertaken (37). In the first 24 hours following seizure activity, the neurological examination can be falsely abnormal.

If a number of seizures have already been observed, then clinical investigation is required to exclude other diseases which can manifest themselves outside of the CNS, such as cardiac insufficiency. If deficits are found during the neurological examination, then this often indicates the presence of an intracranial process such as neoplasia (frequently lateralised deficits) or diffuse involvement of the cerebrum as in HE (associated with symmetrical deficits). Clinical investigations should include CBC, biochemical profile and urinalysis. The blood biochemical profile should at least include the determination of glucose, calcium, urea, creatinine, the electrolytes, liver specific enzymes (ALT, AST, GLDH, GGT) and liver function tests such as pre- and postprandial ammonia and bile acid concentrations (see Chap. 4) (37, 56).

If the results of these investigations are all normal and the animal is between 1 to 3 years of age, then the diagnosis is likely to be idiopathic epilepsy and antiepilepsy therapy can be started. In animals older than this, cats and therapy-resistant patients, further diagnostic investigations must be undertaken.

18

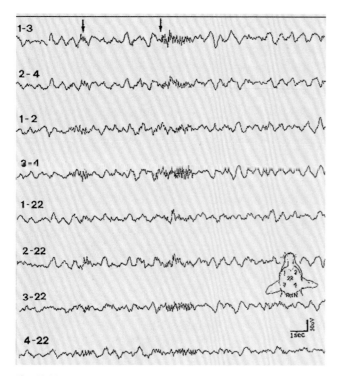

Fig. 18.21
Schematic representation of an EEG. Interictal EEG recording with spindle activity (arrows) under standardised conditions of anaesthesia in a three-year-old Golden Retriever. Recordings: 1–3 = LF-LO; 2–4 = RF-RO; 1–2 = LF-RF; 3–4 = LO-RO; 1–22 = LF-V; 2–22 = RF-V; 3–22 = LO-V; 4–22 = RO-V (L: left; F: frontal; O: occipital; R: right; V = vertex) (from JAGGY and HEYNOLD, 1996 [44]).

The results of CSF analysis often provide an indication that neoplastic, degenerative or inflammatory / infectious diseases are present as well as providing information about the "health" of the blood-brain barrier. The Pandy reaction is used to test the protein content of the CSF. Cloudiness after the addition of carbolic acid to the CSF sample is associated with abnormal protein content due to organic disturbances of the CNS. An increased cell count (normal < 10^3 cells/mm³, mononuclear) is often seen with inflammatory, neoplastic and destructive processes. Important additional information with irritating (inflammation, neoplasia) and degenerative processes in the cerebrum can be obtained using EEG, which records the sum of the cortical and subcortical resting potentials as well as the excitatory and inhibitory potentials in these areas (43). In a family of Golden Retrievers with idiopathic epilepsy, a typical interictal EEG pattern was recorded under standard anaesthesia. The EEG pattern consisted of spindle activity of 12 Hz with different amplitudes and duration (Fig. 18.21; 57). In another study, 125 dogs from different breeds with idiopathic epilepsy were investigated and it was found that approx. 90% of the animals had interictal paroxysmal activity (41). The complete exclusion of space-occupying processes is only possible with either CT or MRI; MRI can more exactly depict the characteristics of lesions within the CNS than CT.

Therapy: The treatment of idiopathic epilepsy consists of symptomatic treatment using anticonvulsants and is a continual life-long therapy. The therapy only leads to success if the owner is well informed, understanding and willing. A comprehensive consultation concerning the therapeutic effects and the expected side-effects is essential, and helps to prevent disappointment. The serum concentration of the anticonvulsant being used and its effects on the patient's liver enzymes (when using phenobarbital) should be investigated at regular intervals. In addition the owner should keep a "seizure diary" so that the therapy can be optimised (dosage adjustment, change of drug, combination therapy). HEYNOLD et al. (1997) (42) demonstrated that therapy in Labrador Retrievers with phenobarbital had the best prospects of success when started early in the course of disease.

There are basically three groups of anticonvulsants, divided according to their mechanism of reducing seizure activity:
1. Reduction of the transmission of neuronal excitement.
2. Increasing the inhibitory processes by potentiating the effect of GABA.
3. Modulation of the ion exchange on the cell membrane (39).

There are many anticonvulsants available on the market, however, only a limited number can be used in the dog and cat. Two substances have found wide use in veterinary medicine and are relatively well tolerated. These are phenobarbital, which is cheap and usually very effective, and potassium bromide which is now being used more frequently than in the past. The latter has no negative influence on the liver and is effective as a sole anticonvulsant. Initially, these drugs should be used on their own, but eventually can be used in combination. If success is not achieved, then treatment with other anticonvulsants should be attempted (primidone, felbamate, gabapentin, levetiracetam, zonisamide, pregabalin, carbamazepine or clorazepate) though they must all be administered carefully and with knowledge of their dosing regimens and possible side-effects (37, 39, 58). The same treatment principles should be applied to the cat, however it should be noted that phenytoin (half-life in cats 24 to 108 hours vs. 3 to 4 hours in the dog!) and primidone are toxic for this species. Additionally, diazepam can be used in cats as the half-life in these animals is significantly longer than in dogs and there is no development of tolerance as is seen in dogs. Diazepam can particularly be used at the start of therapy with another compound until the other medication (such as phenobarbital) has reached an effective serum concentration. The characteristics, recommended dosages and possible side-effects of phenobarbital, potassium bromide and diazepam are listed in Table 18.6 (37).

There is no strict treatment schedule as each patient responds differently to different medications. This seems understandable in consideration of the huge variation in types of seizure, frequency and intensity as well as the affected breeds. Every animal with idiopathic epilepsy should therefore be treated

18

Table 18.6: Characteristics, dosages and side-effects of phenobarbital, potassium bromide and diazepam

Phenobarbital
- Excretion via hepatic biotransformation; maintenance dosage must be adapted to the serum concentration due to individual variation
- Sudden withdrawal can lead to status epilepticus
- Dosage: 2–5 mg/kg, PO, BID
- Half-life: 70 +/– 16 hours
- Time required before steady state is reached: 10 to 18 days
- Desired serum concentration: 15–45 µg/ml
- Formulation: tablets and injectable solutions

Advantages	Disadvantages
■ Effective	■ Side effects especially in the first three weeks of use:
■ Short time before effective	
■ Short half-life	■ Sedation
■ Different application forms	■ Polyuria
■ Cheap	■ Polydipsia
■ Few side effects	■ Polyphagia
■ Can be used in both cats and dogs	■ Possible liver damage; do not use if already present

Potassium bromide
- Excretion via kidneys
- Dosage: 20–50 mg/kg, BID, PO; in combination with phenobarbital, 15–30 mg/kg, PO, BID
- Half-life: 25 days in the dog
- Time required before steady state is reached: 3 months
- Desired serum concentration: 1–3 mg/ml
- Formulation: tablets, capsules or liquid

Advantages	Disadvantages
■ Wide therapeutic range	■ Expensive
■ Not metabolised by liver	■ Long time before effective
■ Can be used in both cats and dogs	■ Sedation possible
■ Few side effects	

Diazepam
- Excretion via hepatic biotransformation
- Dosage: 0.5–1 mg/kg, PO, BID
- Half-life: 1.5 to 3 hours in the dog and 5 to 12 hours in the cat
- Desired serum concentration: 200–500 ng/ml
- Application: tablets, suppositories and injectable solutions

Advantages	Disadvantages
■ Immediately effective	■ Tolerance can develop in the dog
■ Different formulations	■ Very short half-life
	■ Side-effects

individually and therapy should be adapted to each respective situation. It is important to have both a well-diagnosed patient and a good knowledge of the different antiepileptics with their effects, side-effects and combination possibilities.

Prognosis: Seizures can usually be well controlled with anticonvulsant medications, though complete cessation is only rarely achieved. The aim of therapy is a reduction in the number of seizures down to a few mild ones in association with minimal side-effects. If the treatment is a success, then the quality of life for both the animal and its owner will be ensured, while the life expectancy of the patient will not be reduced (43). However, seizures in some animals can be extremely therapy-resistant and even increase in frequency in the face of medication. This is more common in large dog breeds. In addition, large breeds are often used as working dogs and the possible sedative side-effects of the anticonvulsants can affect their working abilities. Furnishings in a home may be damaged during a grand mal seizure, which is more of a problem in large dogs than small ones. The aggression that can occur in the postictal phase is also more of a danger for the animal's surroundings when the patient is a large dog (37).

Individual seizures with prolonged intervals between them have a better prognosis than groups of seizures within a certain period (such as a number of seizures per day = cluster). The potential danger of clusters is that the animal may progress to status epilepticus (see chap. 18.5.2). Neither castration nor the intensity of the seizures appear to have any effect on the outcome of therapy (37, 42). In the Labrador Retriever, freedom from seizures was achieved in a third of the dogs, a third showed significantly fewer seizures and a third did not respond to the treatment. However, it should be noted that this was with monotherapy with phenobarbital (47).

18.5.2 Secondary or symptomatic epilepsy

Aetiology: Many pathological processes in the cerebrum can lead to seizures. They are listed in Table 18.7 and discussed in this chapter. The seizures can be focal or generalised. The severity, duration and frequency are often not correlated with the size of the lesion. Extraneural metabolic disease may cause other neurological symptoms in addition to seizures (see Chap. 18.4.5): these diseases include hypoglycaemia, hypocalcaemia, hypoxia, liver and renal disease. As reported in the section on metabolic encephalopathies, liver disease is the most common cause of cerebral symptoms which can include seizures (see Chap. 18.4.5.3). The possibility of a portosystemic shunt should be considered in young dogs, while chronic destructive liver damage, especially cirrhosis, is more frequent in older animals.

18

Table 18.7: Differential diagnoses in patients with symptomatic epilepsy divided according to their most common causes

V	■ Arrhythmia, hypoxia, infarct ■ Haemorrhage
I	■ Viral, bacterial, rickettsial, protozoal, fungal ■ Immune-mediated
T	■ Acute ■ Chronic (scar tissue)
A	■ Hydrocephalus ■ Lissencephaly ■ Cysts
M	■ Uraemic, hepatic encephalopathies ■ Hypo- or hyperglycaemia, hypocalcaemia, hypothyroidism, disturbances in osmolarity or acid-base metabolism ■ Electrolyte abnormalities ■ Heat stroke, thiamine deficiency, intoxication
I	■ Idiopathic epilepsy ■ (Hyperaesthesia syndrome)
N	■ Primary, metastatic tumours
D	■ Storage diseases

Hypoglycaemia can occur in puppies in association with malnutrition, cold, and severe parasite infestations (see Chap. 18.4.5.2.1). In toy-breed puppies, congenital, metabolic-related hypoglycaemia has been described (e.g. glucose-6-phophatase deficiency). Exhaustion-related hypoglycaemia can occur in working dogs after extreme exercise (e.g. prolonged hunting). Hypoglycaemia has also been seen in conjunction with pregnancy and parturition. Pancreatic islet cell tumours (insulinomas) occur in older dogs (5 years and older), which cause a reduction in blood glucose concentration due to their hormonal activity. These are more common in the Boxer, Poodle and Terrier breeds. Seizures often occur before feeding when the blood glucose concentration is normally at its lowest.

Hypocalcaemia is sometimes seen in lactating bitches, especially shortly after parturition, and more rarely after extreme exertion. The main cause of hypocalcaemia in the dog is hypoparathyroidism.

Other metabolic problems that lead to seizures, though rarely, include severe uraemia in association with renal failure, hypoxia with heart-lung disease, hyperkalaemia with adrenal cortical insufficiency (Addison's disease or chronic cortisone treatment), hyperlipoproteinemia (e.g. familial lipid metabolism disturbance in Miniature Schnauzers). In cats, thiamine deficiency can also sometimes lead to seizures (see Chap. 15.5.1). Finally, there is an immense number of poisonous substances that can cause seizures, though these tend to be unique occurrences.

Diagnosis: As stated above, seizures can have many causes and the diagnostic expense would be too great to determine all possibilities; therefore it is recommended that a practical method of determining the diagnosis is adopted.

If only a single seizure has been seen, then a general and neurological examination is indicated. If there are no abnormal results found, then further investigations are not necessary; the course of the disease should be monitored. Historical information is always of importance in order to exclude any possibility of poisoning. If pathological results are attained, then the investigation must be continued in the direction indicated.

If repeated seizures are observed, then a general and neurological examination is again initially undertaken. If objective abnormalities are noted, then the investigation is continued in the indicated direction. If not, then liver enzymes, blood ammonia, bile acids, glucose, blood urea and electrolytes should be determined. If there are no abnormalities to be found and the dog is up to 3 years of age, then a tentative diagnosis of primary epilepsy can be made and administration of anticonvulsant therapy should be considered. If the seizures are therapy-resistant or they initially occur in a dog older than 5 years, additional tests such as blood insulin-glucose ratios, liver function tests, CSF analysis and EEG are indicated.

Special consideration should be given to those animals that are affected by seizures that occur rapidly one after another or are in **status epilepticus**. The vital treatment aim is to obviously stop the seizures immediately. Only when the animals are free of seizures for at least 24 hours can additional meaningful investigations be undertaken.

Therapy: Treatment of secondary epilepsy is aimed at controlling the primary cause. Status epilepticus (SE) can be treated as follows:

Intravenous injection of 10 mg diazepam or an IV or IM injection of midazolam (0.2 mg/kg) is initially administered to stop the seizures. If there is no success within 5 minutes, repeat this approach up to two times. The use of parenteral phenobarbital (2–4 mg/kg IV or IM) should be considered if there is no or just a temporary response. This can take 20 to 30 minutes to be effective and can be repeated every 30 minutes up to a maximum of 24 mg/kg/24 hours. If the initial dose is effective, parenteral dosing should be repeated every 4 to 6 hours for 24 hours, after which oral maintenance dosing should be initiated. When parenteral phenobarbital does not work, then the patient should be anaesthetised with pentobarbital or propofol. This will allow time for either the parenteral phenobarbital to become effective or an underlying toxicity to be treated or metabolised. Afterwards, a blood sample is taken to determine the blood calcium and glucose concentrations. If hypoglycaemia or hypocalcaemia is present, then suitable replacement and fluid therapy should be administered. If there is a suspicion of poisoning (e.g. metaldehyde:

proof from stomach contents), the stomach should be emptied and the antidote given where possible. Gastric lavage may be of some risk to the patient though, if multiple doses of an anticonvulsant have been administered, compromising respiration and consciousness. Finally, palliative therapy consisting of fluid therapy, oxygen and possibly mannitol should be administered where appropriate. As soon as the animal has recovered, further investigations and oral anticonvulsant therapy should be undertaken.

The diagnostics and treatment of epilepsy in the cat follows principally the same philosophies that are applied to the dog.

18.5.3 Hyperaesthesia syndrome in the cat ("Running fits")

Aetiology: Unknown (presumed to be a form of idiopathic epilepsy; so-called running fits). Found in cats manifesting **just hyperaesthesia** of the spinal muscles and paravertebral skin (triggered by palpation; an inclusion body myopathy has been found in some cats).

Clinical: The predominant signs of this disease are behavioural disturbances and "hallucinations". The majority of these cats start with an uncontrolled licking of a limb. This can last for a few seconds or minutes. Afterwards a fine or jerky movement of the thoracolumbar muscles occurs. These spasms become more pronounced with contractions that affect the whole of the thoracic epaxial muscles and can last for several seconds. The cats appear not to be responsive to external stimuli (a possible change in consciousness is inferred) and then begin to run around uncontrollably. The whole episode can last for a few seconds or minutes.

Diagnosis: Diagnosis is by process of elimination. The work-up is as with idiopathic epilepsy (see Chap. 18.5.1).

Therapy: Occasionally, these cats respond positively to phenobarbital therapy. Other anticonvulsants should be considered if phenobarbital is not effective.

Prognosis: In the long term, this is guarded to poor.

18.6 Differential diagnoses for primary and secondary epilepsy

Hypersomnia (narcolepsy / cataplexy), movement disorders and syncope are the most important differential diagnoses for epilepsy.

18.6.1 Cataplexy / narcolepsy

Aetiology: Narcolepsy is a very rare disease in the dog and is principally a disturbance in the sleep regulation mechanism. It has been described in various breeds of dogs. In the Doberman and Labrador Retriever it is an inherited syndrome. The first symptoms occur usually before 6 months of age and are characterised by sudden generalised muscle weakness (cataplexy), whereby the animal collapses but does not lose consciousness (the eyes remain open). It occurs often in association with excitement, such as feeding or play. The events can last for a few seconds up to 2 minutes, and can be very frequent ($<$ 100 events per day!). Even rarer is partial cataplexy whereby only the hindlimbs are affected. With longer lasting cataplectic attacks, sleep behaviour may accompany the muscle involvement (= narcolepsy). The animal's eyes close and twitching of the distal muscles occur; the EEG shows a normal REM sleep pattern.

Diagnosis: Clinical picture. The events can be provoked by offering food (put pieces of food at certain distances from each other on the floor) or by the intravenous injection of physostigmine salicylate (Antilirium®) 0.025–0.1 mg/kg, IV. The cataplectic events occur 5 to 10 minutes after the injection.

Therapy: The frequency of the events can be reduced using dextroamphetamine 5–10 mg/kg, TID PO, and methylphenidate (Ritalin) 5–10 mg, BID PO. Pure cataplectic events can be relatively well controlled with imipramine 0.5–10 mg/kg, TID PO. Pure narcoleptic events respond well to protriptylin 10 mg/d PO or imipramine 0.5–1.0 mg/kg TID, PO.

Prognosis: The disease reaches a plateau after the first events and is not progressive. However, the frequency of the events can be debilitating and affect the animal's quality of life. Lifelong therapy may be required and side-effects of the required treatments may be of concern in the long term.

18.6.2 Syncope

Christophe Lombard

Syncope is generally accepted medically as a transient, self-limiting loss of consciousness with collapse due to the loss of muscle tone necessary to maintain the animal upright. Classic syncopal "attacks" occur suddenly, last only for a short time and recovery is complete (59). According to the definition used in human medicine, attacks of syncope occur due to a sudden reduction or short-term cessation of the blood supply to the CNS (60), while in veterinary medicine reduced oxygen or nutritional supply to the brain are also accepted causes (61). Syncope should be differentiated from collapse

18

Table 18.8: Nonsyncopal loss of consciousness (59)

Diseases with loss of consciousness
- Migraine (human beings, animals [?])
- Metabolic problems including hypoxia, hypoventilation
- Hypoglycaemia
- Epilepsy
- Transient ischemic attack (TIA, humans, animals [?])

Diseases with apparent loss of consciousness
- Cataplexy/narcolepsy
- "Somatisation" problems

(simple collapse or neuromuscular weakness), epileptiform seizures or narcolepsy / cataplexy; which is not always easy from the description or anamnesis provided by the owner (Table 18.8). The symptoms of a classical epileptiform seizure (spastic movements of the limbs and jaw) are described in Chap. 18.5. Syncope and collapse/loss of consciousness can appear to be very similar to the owner. The exact classification of an "attack" event is only possible after a complete work-up of the patient.

Anamnesis: Understandably, the first attack of syncope in a pet is shocking for its owner and consequently the duration of unconsciousness or fainting is generally overestimated. In reality, such attacks only last for a few seconds. Rarely is the owner able to describe the signs prior to the syncope. These signs can include a stiff posture and a short period of mental "absence". Sometimes an abnormal, "vacant" facial expression is described. Sometimes these may be the only signs and complete syncope with loss of muscle tone and collapse does not occur. Usually, these prodromal signs are followed by hindlimb weakness, followed by collapsing of the hind limbs then the forelimbs, with the head hitting the floor toward the end. The animal falls in lateral recumbency, with its head on the floor, though sometimes the dog remains in sternal recumbency. If the dog is already lying down or resting, the dog may be seen to roll on to its side. The animal lies flaccid for a few seconds without any movement of its limbs and then unconsciousness occurs, as per definition of syncope. If this final stage is absent, then the "attack" or event is "only" described as weakness and/or collapse. As the definition of these two conditions is very difficult for the layperson, it may be impossible to differentiate between them on the basis of the anamnesis alone. Micturition and defaecation only occur during prolonged attacks of syncope. Respiration is usually normal, i.e. slow with deep breaths. Virtually nothing dependable can be learnt about the pulse or heart beat, nor about the colour of the mucosal membranes as they are virtually never noticed by the owner. If noted properly, however, the pulse is slow and the mucosal membranes are normal to pale.

Typically, the animal stands up slowly after a few seconds. It is at first uncertain on its legs and then appears fully normal within seconds. Certain owners do not wait this long, but raise their animal's head, talk to it or even try to resuscitate by blowing air through its nose. Although nothing definite can be said about these actions, the owner can be completely convinced that this has saved the animal's life. The degree of truth or the correlation between the resuscitation attempts of the owner and the animal returning to normal consciousness is totally unimportant and does not need to be discussed here.

The causes of syncope involve physical exertion or psychological excitement such as greeting a known member of the family, or the anticipation of a walk. However, it is not uncommon for the owner to report that the animal woke up out of its sleep or stood up from resting and then collapsed.

The degree of activity and the behaviour of the patient between the attacks of syncope are also important for determining the underlying aetiology. With cardiac causes of paroxysmal bradycardia, tachycardia or abnormal vagal reflexes, the patient generally exhibits normal activity and exercise tolerance between the attacks. Coughing can be a common factor inducing syncope due to vaso-vagal causes. Additionally, straining during defaecation or micturition can sometimes lead to vaso-vagal-related syncope. The so-called micturition syncope is a common disease in human beings (60). Severe pain is also known to be the cause of syncope in human beings; however, this has not been documented in animals.

By contrast, the causative abnormalities associated with metabolic or neuromuscular causes of syncope are constant rather than intermittent. For this reason, these patients often show a continual lack of interest in moving or a constant weakness; the owner may complain about the animal being permanently "tired".

Breed: The epidemiological knowledge about the frequency of some heart diseases in specific breeds has diagnostic advantages. It is known that Boxers and German Shepherds have a tendency for myocardial disease associated with tachyarrhythmias, while Miniature Schnauzers have preponderance for sick sinus syndrome (SSS). AV blocks and increased vaso-vagal reflexes with bradyarrhythmias occur particularly in brachycephalic breeds. Cardiomyopathies of large breeds are more common in the Great Dane, Newfoundland, Irish Wolfhound and Doberman.

Ingested medications: A complete log of all possible ingested medications is essential. The following classes of medications can cause syncope due to their bradycardic or hypotensive effects: vasodilators (i.e. ACE inhibitors), beta blockers, digitalis glycosides, diuretics and sedatives.

Aetiopathogenesis: As has already been mentioned, a sudden, severe reduction in CNS blood flow leads to syncope.

18

Accordingly, syncope can be caused by all arrhythmias that cause a reduction in the cardiac output, heart diseases with reduced cardiac output (pulmonary stenosis, aortic stenosis, cor pulmonale), and sudden vasodilation or redistribution of the circulating blood volume.

With respect to arrhythmias, it is the bradyarrhythmias (2nd and 3rd degree AV block, sinus arrest in association with SSS) that have been found in association with syncope in the dog (Fig. 18.22). Other forms of bradycardia can be induced by hyperkalaemia or medications (digitalis intoxication, beta blockers, calcium antagonists). Suddenly occurring tachyarrhythmias (especially paroxysmal ventricular tachycardia > 260 beats/min) can induce syncope due to the severely reduced diastolic filling time and a severe reduction in cardiac output. With hypertrophic cardiomyopathy, severe pulmonary stenosis, pulmonary hypertension (Eisenmenger's syndrome, heart worm disease, thromboemboli), aortic stenosis and large pericardial effusions, it is impossible for the cardiac output to be increased when required, which can then lead to syncope. The latter two heart diseases are relatively common causes of syncope.

Vaso-vagal syncope often occurs in human beings, whereby a reflex-induced high vagal and reduced sympathetic tone lead to both hypertension and a reduction in heart rate at the same time, resulting in reduced CNS perfusion. It is much less common in the dog, but a few cases of coughing-associated syncope have been reported.

Clinical: In addition to a general examination, syncope patients should be subjected to a special cardiovascular examination and a neurological examination. Often during the first series of examinations, no physical abnormalities can be found in syncope patients. Highly significant abnormal features include altered resting heart rates: either bradycardia (< 50–60 beats/min) or tachycardia (> 160 beats/min). These indicate the presence of a possible heart rhythm disturbance. Increased capillary filling time together with pale or cyanotic mucosal membranes, tachypnoea and/or dyspnoea and increased heart rate (> 120 beats/min), weak pulse and "rattling" pulmonary sounds are classical signs of congestive cardiac insufficiency. They indicate that a general cardiovascular disease may be the cause of the syncope. Other indicators of primary heart disease are abnormal heart sounds (consequence of valve insufficiency or malformations), gallop rhythms (indication of ventricular filling anomalies in cardiomyopathies), irregularities of the heart rhythm (with or without pulse deficits) and the volume of the heart sounds as indicators of an arrhythmia (e.g. atrial fibrillation or extra systoles). These latter two types of arrhythmia are relatively dependable signs of myocardial disease (cardiomyopathy or myocarditis). Dampened heart sounds coupled with venous congestion ± ascites is very suspicious for pericardial effusion. Finally, the recognition of a severely accentuated or even split heart tone is a relatively dependable indicator of pulmonary hypertension and so a cor pulmonale.

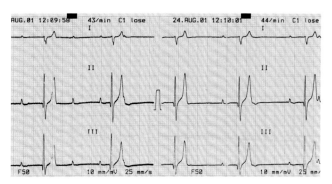

Fig. 18.22
Example of a third-degree AV block with a ventricular escape rhythm on the right and a frequency of approx. 43 beats/minute. Many more P-waves with a frequency of approx. 100 beats/minute are apparent.

Weakness or reduced muscle tone indicate a neurological or neuromuscular cause of the collapse. In Table 18.9, the factors that serve to differentiate syncope from seizure, weakness and narcolepsy are described.

Diagnosis: A CBC and complete biochemical profile are indispensable as anaemia, hyperkalaemia and hypoglycaemia need to be excluded. In a patient with syncope and a normal heart rate and rhythm, an ECG should still be performed and the blood pressure measured. Abnormal ECG results can indicate the causal primary heart disease. Many machines are suitable for measuring the blood pressure noninvasively and the normal values for dogs and cats have been published; the reader is referred to an authoritative cardiology text for further details. Whole-body tilting manoeuvres, utilised in human beings to cause a sudden drop in blood pressure via receptor discharging, are used to indicate the lability of the vagus-controlled blood pressure receptors and the regulation of the blood pressure. These manoeuvres are unfortunately not possible in the dog, and especially not in the cat. Long-term ECG recording can be done using portable recorders (event recorders) if there is suspicion of intermittent arrhythmias (62). These machines record the ECG continually, though they continuously record over themselves. If there is an event (attack of weakness or obvious syncope), the observer or accompanying person presses a button and the ECG is then recorded on an external machine for several minutes (63).

Modern recorders have enough capacity to record 20 to 30 events. These are then interpreted later. In this manner, event recording can be performed on patients with rarely occurring events over a number of weeks.

BRIGHT and CALI (2000) reported on the impact of such event recorders in a series of 60 patients with syncope (62). A definitive diagnosis could be made in 51 animals. In 18 of these (35%), a definite arrhythmia with known haemody-

18

Table 18.9: Factors to aid differentiation of syncope from a seizure, weakness or narcolepsy
(From DAVIDOW, PROULX and WOODFIELD, 2001 [61])

Factor	Syncope	Seizure	Episodic weakness	Narcolepsy
Loss of consciousness	Yes	Yes	No	Yes (REM sleep)
Immediate preceding signs	Sometimes tripping over, ataxia or nothing	Very variable, depends on patient	Can trip over before collapsing	None
Trigger factors	Exertion, excitement, coughing	Usually none ±excitement	Often exertion	None
Clonic movements	No	Almost always yes	No	No
Tonic movements	Possible (towards the end of the period of unconsciousness)	Yes	No	No
Urinary and faecal incontinence	Rarely	Often, depends on severity	No	No
Postictal phase with abnormal behaviour	No	Yes	No	No
Duration	Usually seconds	Seconds to minutes	Minutes (variable)	Seconds to minutes

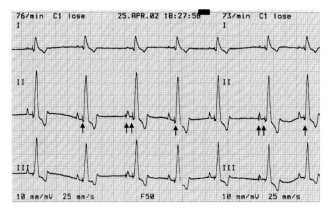

Fig. 18.23
Pacemaker rhythm in a dog with a two-chamber pacemaker implant. Small electrical impulse waves (arrows) are visible before the P waves and the QRS complexes. In the present demand mode, the atrial stimulation is shut off in some of the spontaneous sinus beats (no stimulation waves before the P wave), when the frequency goes above the set basal frequency of 70 beats/minute.

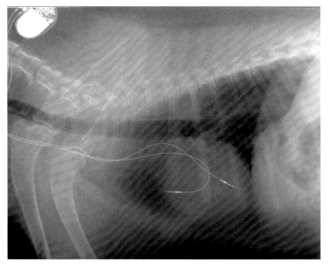

Fig. 18.24
Implanted pacemaker in a nine-year-old Labrador with a third-degree AV block. The pulse generator is implanted laterally on the neck just in front of the shoulder blade in a subcutaneous pocket. The two transvenous electrodes were inserted through the jugular vein. The cranial electrode has an angle of 180° and lies with its tip in the right atrial auricle and the caudal electrode is anchored endocardially on the tip of the right ventricle.

18

namic effects severe enough to induce syncope could be found. In the other 65%, no arrhythmias could be seen at the time of the event(s) and so arrhythmia as a cause of the syncope could be excluded with certainty. Ambulatory blood pressure recorders that register blood pressure automatically at regular intervals are currently only available for use in human beings.

Therapy: With disturbances of electrolytes, blood glucose and other metabolic causes of syncope, therapy and prognosis depends on the primary disease. It is guarded to poor with insulinoma, while it is fair to good with hyperkalaemia secondary to hypoadrenocorticism (Addison's disease).

As little is known about the incidence of vaso-vagal-induced syncope in the dog and cat, no comments can be made as to its therapy or prognosis.

Individual treatment with vasoconstrictors can increase the blood pressure; the circulating blood volume can be cautiously increased by enriching the animal's food with salt. Stabilisation of the blood pressure may be achieved using this method.

Prognosis: The prognosis is naturally determined by the primary cause of the syncope and is usually guarded. With structural and difficult to treat heart diseases such as cardiomyopathy, tumours and stenoses of the semilunar valves, palliative treatment can be used, although a reduction in the incidence of the syncope is all that can be achieved. The underlying heart disease often has a poor prognosis and is usually progressive. High-grade AV blocks can, however, have a favourable prognosis once structural changes are excluded and a pacemaker has been successfully implanted (Fig. 18.23). Dogs with such implants can live for many years without problems and without experiencing any further attacks of syncope (Fig. 18.24).

18.7   Neoplasia

The diagnosis of intracranial tumours in the dog and cat has been significantly improved by the development of special imaging techniques such as CT and MRI. Brain tumours are quite frequent in dogs, and tend to be infrequent in cats. Objective data about the incidence of brain tumours may be inaccurate, especially regarding the presence of secondary metastatic tumours, which may have been underestimated in the past (5).

In the following section, tumours of the cerebrum will be discussed. Brain tumours usually occur in dogs from the age of 5 years onwards, with the average age being 9 years (64). Brachycephalic breeds appear to have a predisposition for glial and pituitary tumours, while meningiomas are more commonly found in dolicocephalic breeds (65). Boxer, Doberman, Golden Retriever, Old English Sheepdog and the Scottish Terrier are renowned for tending to develop intracranial tumours more than other breeds (65). Intracranial tumours may be sporadically seen in young animals; these include teratoma, medulloblastoma and epidermoid cysts (66).

Aetiopathogenesis: In dogs, the incidence of brain tumours is similar to that of human beings; however, as stated before the frequency and type of tumour can be breed-specific. Gliomas occur more commonly in breeds with short skulls, and meningiomas in breeds with longer skulls. Cats are generally less frequently affected, with preponderance for benign meningiomas and lymphomas. As there are breed predispositions, it may be assumed that a genetic basis is present; though proving this is very difficult. Definitive sex predisposition has not been observed so far. Clinical onset is usually during the second half of an animal's life, with increasing frequency noted with age. In the dog and cat, brain tumours occur more commonly than tumours of the spinal cord or PNS.

Classification: Comprehensive overviews of CNS tumours can be found in the WHO classification from 1999 and 2007. The classification in animals follows that used for human beings, with a few exceptions, The determining criteria for tumour classification are the predominant cell type and the growth behaviour. The cell type determines the type of tumour (e.g. astrocytoma, schwannoma, ependymoma, etc.), while the growth determines the grade (benign or malignant; Grades I to IV). Brain tumours can arise from neurocctodermal or mesenchymal cells.

Neuroepithelial tumours
- Astrocytoma (Grades I–III)
- Glioblastoma (Grade IV)
- Oligodendroglioma (Grades I–II)
- Mixed glioma (Oligoastrocytoma) (Grade II)
- Gliosarcoma (Grade IV)
- Gliomatosis cerebri
- Spongioblastoma
- Ependymoma (Grades I–III)
- Plexus tumours (papillomas and carcinomas of the choroid plexus) (Grades I–III)
- Gangliocytomas, ganglioglioma, olfactory neuroblastoma
- Primitive neuroectodermal tumour (PNET) (Grade IV)
- Medulloblastoma (Grade IV)
- Neuroblastoma
- Ependymoblastoma
- Thoracolumbar spinal tumour of young dogs (nephroblastoma)
- Pineocytoma (Grade I) and pineoblastoma (Grade (IV)

Meningiomas (Grades I–III)

Tumours of the sellar region
- Pituitary adenoma and carcinoma
- Craniopharyngioma (Grade I)
- Germal cell tumours

Secondary tumours
- Metastases
- Tumours from surrounding tissues

Clinical: As has already been mentioned, intracranial tumours generally have a slow rate of growth resulting in chronic progressive symptoms. However, with respect to tumours of the forebrain, it is not uncommon to have a sudden onset of clinical symptoms. Dogs with tumours of the forebrain exhibit an increased susceptibility to seizures, either tonic-clonic or complex partial in nature. Seizures are one of the most common clinical symptoms that have been described in association with cerebral neoplasia (5).

Seizure activity leads to suspicion of a tumour in middle-aged or older dogs, especially when the seizure incidence is high and the type of seizure indicates the presence of a focal process. In patients with forebrain tumours, there are often no other problems such as behavioural abnormalities (the second

18

most common symptom). Dogs and cats affected by behavioural abnormalities exhibit compulsive pacing (circling to the side of the lesion), head pressing, forgetting learned behaviour, disorientation and depression. The involvement of the limbic system can lead to anxiety, hyperexcitability and increased aggression. In the cat, piloerection and spitting can seen when tumours affect this area.

Apart from these behavioural changes, the neurological examination may reveal only subtle abnormalities: reduced/lack of menace response (uni- or bilateral) and proprioceptive deficits (contralateral to the lesion) despite a normal gait. It is not unusual to find patients with cerebral tumours that only have a reduction in the menace response or even no neurological deficits at all. In the final stages, cerebral tumours can cause a contralateral paresis. Severe symptoms are usually the consequence of secondary complications, e.g. increased ICP, acute haemorrhage or obstructive hydrocephalus.

Diagnosis: Neoplasia should be placed at the top of the list of differential diagnoses when there is a sudden onset of seizures in animals over 7 years of age without any other symptoms. The definitive diagnosis is based on laboratory tests (5). CBC and a biochemical profile including bile acids and/or blood ammonia are necessary to exclude metabolic disease (HE, UE). Due to the increasing incidence of metastatic neoplasia, patients suspected of having a brain tumour should be subjected to a complete investigation for the primary tumour (Table 18.10). Careful palpation, ultrasonography of the abdomen, and three-view radiography of the thorax and abdomen should be part of the diagnostic protocol.

The most conspicuous change seen on CSF analysis is an increase in protein concentration. Many intracranial tumours are associated with normal CSF cell count and cytology. Some tumours can induce an inflammatory response (particularly meningiomas, lymphomas, choroid plexus tumours), which leads to an obvious increase in CSF leucocytes. Despite everything, CSF analysis is rarely diagnostic for cerebral tumours. Suspicion of raised ICP is a contraindication for a cisternal tap, due to the risk of herniation. If a brain tumour is presumed, then CT or MRI should be performed initially. If the presence of a tumour is not confirmed by these imaging modalities, then CSF should be collected and analysed (66).

Special imaging techniques, in combination with contrast agent administration, have proven to be the diagnostic method of choice for CNS tumours (5). **CT** and **MRI** enable determination of the localisation of the tumour, the involvement of the blood-brain barrier and any secondary damage such as oedema, hydrocephalus and herniation (see Chap. 6).

Other diagnostic aids include **ophthalmological investigations** and **EEG**. Some patients with a cerebral tumour can have uni- or bilateral oedema of the optic nerve (papillary oedema), which can be seen by looking at the fundus (5). On

Table 18.10: Classification of primary brain tumours according to their origin

Meninges
- Meningioma/meningiosarcoma

Neuroepithelium
- Astrocytoma
- Choroid plexus papilloma/carcinoma
- Ependymoma
- Medulloblastoma
- Gllublastoma multiforme
- Oligodendroglioma
- Pinealoma

Lymphoid tissue
- Lymphoma/lymphosarcoma

Vascular
- Haemangiosarcoma

Germ cells
- Teratoma

Malformation
- Craniopharyngioma

Nerve sheath
- Neurofibroma/neurofibrosarcoma

EEG, the majority of domestic animals with brain tumours exhibit a low frequency wave activity. Asymmetrical amplitudes or frequencies occur, though these changes do not allow any conclusions with respect to the presence of tumours or their precise localisation. The size of the skull cavity with its overlying muscle tissue, the necessity for a general anaesthesia, the lack of specificity and the cost and availability of the equipment all decrease the utility of EEG as an aid in the diagnosis of brain tumours (66).

Therapy: The treatment of brain tumours has two different aims. The first is palliative to reduce and control the secondary clinical symptoms caused by the tumour. The second is definitive, to destroy or remove the tumour tissue.

Palliative therapy consists of **glucocorticoids** and when necessary **anticonvulsants**. Glucocorticoids appear to reduce the blood flow through the tumour and so its size. In addition, they reduce CSF production while increasing its resorption (5). These effects result in a reduction in the ICP and so an improvement of the clinical symptoms.

If secondary epilepsy occurs, this must be treated with anticonvulsants. These types of epileptic patients are treated routinely, though as can be expected they tend to respond more poorly to the therapy.

Definitive therapy for brain tumours consists of **surgical** removal, **radiation** therapy or **chemotherapy**; or a combination of these (5). Meningiomas are the types of tumours

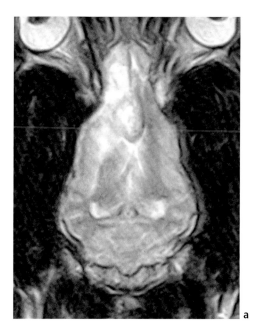

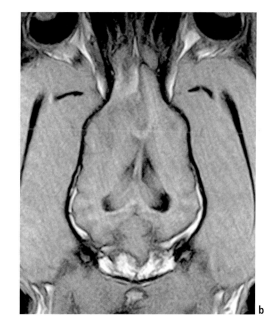

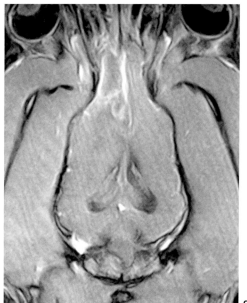

Fig. 18.25a–c
Astrocytoma in the region of the rhinencephalon. (a) Dorsal T2w sequence and dorsal T1w sequence: (b) pre-contrast and (c) after gadolinium. (a) In the T2w sequence, there is a hyperintense lesion extending from the rhinencephalon into the frontal lobe, which has a moderate mass effect (displacement of the midline). (b) There is a small hyperintense focus in the rhinencephalon in the T1w sequence, otherwise the lesion is hypotense and poorly demarcated. (c) After gadolinium, there is a strong inhomogeneous ring-shaped uptake of contrast around the lesion. Diagnosis: astrocytoma with extensive peritumoural oedema. (Fig. Johann Lang, Bern.)

18

which can be removed most successfully from both cats and dogs. In many cats, a symptom-free survival period of 18 to 24 months without any additional treatment has been seen. Surgery can indeed be combined with radiation or chemotherapy to delay relapse of the tumour. Radiation appears to be very effective in the improvement of the patient's quality of life and survival rate (67). Cytosine arabinoside has been used to treat CNS lymphosarcoma in the dog but definitive protocols and long terms outcomes are lacking in the veterinary literature.

18.7.1 Neuroepithelial tumours

Astrocytoma (Fig. 18.25) is probably the most common type of brain tumour in the dog. It occurs in a number of different subtypes (pilocytic, fibrillary, protoplasmic [Fig. 18.26a], gemistocytic) and locations (mainly cerebrum).

Most patients are middle-aged to older, though sometimes young animals can be affected. The majority of these tumours have a moderate malignancy, meaning that they grow slowly

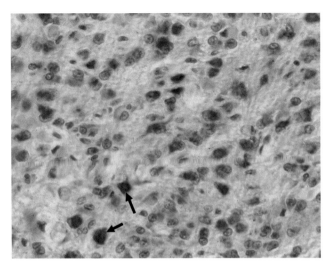

Fig. 18.26a
Progressive disorientation occurred in a twelve-year-old Boxer, which finally developed into reduction of the visual field with the dog running into objects and circling to the left. The dog was euthanised when it developed somnolence. Histopathology of the brain revealed a large astrocytoma in the area of the piriform lobe of the left hemisphere with extension into the frontal lobes and the basal ganglia. Immunohistochemistry revealed the presence of glial fibrillary acid protein (GFAP) in the tumour astrocytes (arrows).

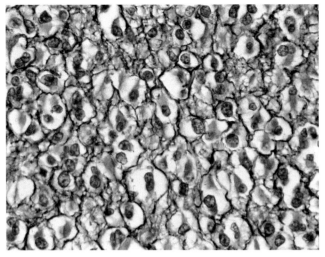

Fig. 18.26b
A seven-year-old Boxer exhibited changes in personality (extremely frightened, hiding). Finally, the animal developed severe anxiety with uncontrolled compulsive movements and then apathy. The dog was euthanised. During the brain inspection, a cherry-sized tumour was found in the left parietal lobe. Its histological structure showed the honeycombing typical of an oligodendroglioma: immunohistochemical representation of growth factor receptors in the cell membranes of the tumour cells.

but are diffusely infiltrative. Severely malignant (anaplastic) courses rarely occur. Astrocytomas are very rare in the cat. A special form of malignant glial tumour is the glioblastoma (WHO Grade IV), which is less common in the dog than in humans.

Oligodendrogliomas are frequent in the Boxer and other brachycephalic breeds; they are found mainly in the cerebrum (Fig. 18.26b) and often adjacent to the ventricles. Oligodendrogliomas, similar to astrocytomas, grow slowly but infiltratively.

The **olfactory neuroblastoma** is the most frequent of all the neuronal tumours. It grows from the olfactory mucosa in the nasal cavities and can infiltrate the brain, as do **medulloblastomas**.

Ependymomas of the brain ventricles or spinal cord are rare. **Papillomas and carcinomas of the choroid plexus** (Fig. 18.27) are more common.

All the other forms of neuroepithelial tumours are extremely rare.

18.7.2 Meningiomas

Tumours of the enveloping tissues of the brain are the most common tumours in the cat and most probably in the dog, too. They predominantly occur in the second half of life, are more frequent in dog breeds with long skulls, grow mainly in the parietal lobe over the convex surface of the brain or basal in the area of the sphenoid bone. They are more rarely found in the area of the cerebellum or pons. Meningiomas are not uncommonly found adjacent to the tentorium cerebelli. They can be single or multiple (cat). Their size can range from a few millimetres to a number of centimetres. They grow almost exclusively expansile and are well demarcated, which tends to make them more operable (especially in comparison to the gliomas). There are many different cell variants, though the majority belong to WHO Grade I; malignant forms are very rare.

18.7.3 Tumours from surrounding tissues and metastases

Tumours of the **pituitary** are not uncommon in the dog. They may be endocrinologically active (Cushing's disease!) or inactive adenomas. They may also be rarely found as infiltrating pituitary carcinomas.

18

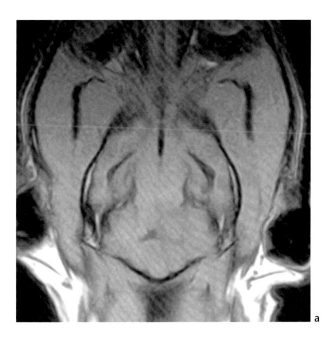

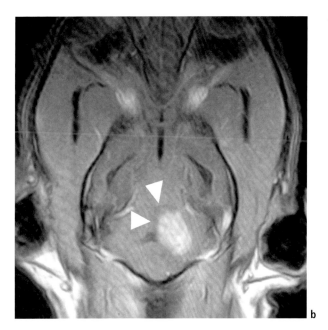

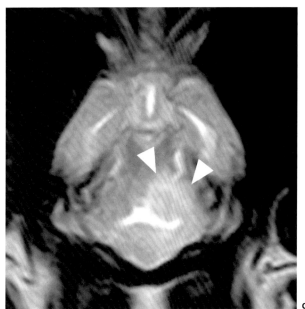

Fig. 18.27a–c
Choroid plexus papilloma in a three-year-old mixed-breed dog. Dorsal T1w sequence (a) before and (b) after gadolinium; (c) T2w sequence. Choroid plexus papilloma in its typical location in the fourth ventricle with slight mass effects. The tumour is hypointense on the pre-contrast T1w sequence (a) and hyperintense on the T2w sequence. The tumour shows strong, well-demarcated contrast enhancement (b). There is moderate peri-tumoural oedema, which is particularly obvious on the T2w sequence (b, c: arrowheads). (Fig.: Johann Lang, Bern.)

18

Haemangiomas and **haemangioendotheliomas** belong to the mesenchymal tumours. They can be localised primarily in the CNS or be metastases.

Lymphatic tumours can be also be primary, but are more commonly metastatic. This also applies to the melanoma. In addition, lymphatic tumours can occur in the CNS as a part of malignant histiocytosis. Basically, all peripheral carcinomas and sarcomas can metastasise to the CNS; however, experience has shown that they tend to do this after having first metastasised to the lungs.

18.8   Degenerative diseases

Those degenerative diseases of the brain that are presumed or known to be genetic will be discussed in the following section (68). Other causes which have been associated with degenerative brain disease include age, nutrition, toxins and metabolic disturbances (see Chap. 18.4.5). Particular attention has been paid in the last few years to cognitive dysfunction in older dogs as a consequence of neuronal degeneration in the brain. Degenerative brain disease consists of a process in which the brain tissue **initially develops normally** and then due to a disturbance in metabolism **degenerates prema-**

turely (69). This type of disease can be inherited, i.e. **lysosomal storage disease** (LSD) and **neuronal abiotrophy**.

The definitive diagnosis of an inherited degenerative disease of the brain requires histopathological investigation. Swollen cells are seen in association with LSD pathology, whereas degeneration / loss of individual cell types is characteristic of abiotrophic diseases.

18.8.1 General criteria

Aetiopathogenesis: Storage diseases (lysosomal enzymopathies) are rare degenerative processes caused by enzymatic defects that lead to intracellular deposits in postmitotic cells such as the neurons. Usually, storage diseases occur within the first few months of life and have a poor prognosis. The symptoms of all of these diseases are similar to each other: personality change, problems with balance, ataxia and tremor. Later, paresis and visual disturbances can develop.

The following storage diseases have been described in the dog and cat:
- Leukodystrophies
- Lipidosis / gangliosidosis
- Galactocerebrosidosis (Gaucher's disease)
- Sphingomyelinosis (Niemann-Pick disease)
- Fucosidosis
- Mannosidosis
- Galactosidase
- Mucopolysaccharidosis (Types I, II, IIIA and B, VI, VII)
- Glycogenosis (Types I, II, III, IV, VII)
- Ceroid lipofuscinosis
- Lafora disease (myoclonic epilepsy)

Clinical: The clinical symptoms that are seen with the majority of these neurodegenerations are normally inconspicuous at birth; progressive neurological symptoms occur later in life (69). All these diseases are inherited as an autosomal recessive and as a consequence are mostly seen in pure breeds. The symptoms first occur after weaning and are progressive. Not uncommonly, the disease is first seen in adulthood. The progression of the symptoms is irreversible and ultimately leads to death within 4 to 6 months after the start of disease (5). Cerebellar symptoms are often more prominent especially with the abiotrophies. In addition, there are diffuse cerebrocortical symptoms manifested as personality change, blindness, seizures, dementia, circling and proprioception deficits (69). As LSD affects more than one group of neurons, it is possible to find neurological disturbances indicative of brain stem and/or spinal cord lesions.

Apart from affecting the CNS, LSD can affect other systems, which can be found on clinical investigation.

Diagnosis: The definitive diagnosis is usually confirmed with histopathology. As this group of diseases can also affect other organs, a diagnosis can be made in the living animal in some cases using biopsy and histology of tissues outside of the CNS (e.g. liver), haematological analysis or urinalysis.

Therapy: There is no effective clinical therapy for these diseases; bone marrow transplantation is being investigated in research colonies. Due to their autosomal recessive inheritance, population control and breeding advice are important for disease prevention.

18.8.2 Specific diseases

18.8.2.1 Leukodystrophies
In globoid cell leukodystrophy, there is a galactosylceramidase (β-galactosidase) deficiency which leads to the accumulation of psychosine (galactosylsphingosine), a lipid which is highly toxic for oligodendrocytes and Schwann cells. Degeneration and dissolution of the myelin sheath occurs with a bilaterally symmetrical, demyelinating encephalopathy. The term globoid cell leukodystrophy is taken from the morphological appearance of the macrophages / microglia that are filled with storage material. The clinical symptoms include weakness, cerebellar ataxia, ascending hindlimb paralysis, para- and tetraplegia, reflex disturbances, nystagmus, disturbances in sensation, reduced muscle tone, muscle atrophy and personality changes. The disease has been reported in the Basset, Beagle, Cairn Terrier, Irish Setter, Pomeranian, Poodle and West Highland White Terrier as well as European Short- and Longhaired cats. Usually the disease occurs a few weeks or months after birth.

18.8.2.2 Lipidoses and gangliosidoses
In the lipidoses / gangliosidoses, there are defects in the catabolism of ganglioside (glycosphingolipids). GM1 gangliosidosis (deficiency of β-galactosidase) has been described in dogs (Alaskan Husky, Beagle, English Springer Spaniel, Portuguese Water dog, Shiba Inu, mixed-breed dogs) and cats (Korat, Siamese, European Shorthair). GM2 gangliosidosis (deficiency of hexosaminidase) occurs in the German Shorthaired and Japanese Pointers, as well as the Korat and other cats, as different variants similar to the human subtypes B (Tay-Sachs disease), O (Sandhoff disease), AB and B^{-1}; but they also form their own subtypes. There is marked accumulation of various substrates in the abdominal organs and particularly in the brain. These diseases manifest themselves clinically at a few months of age with cerebellar ataxia and dysmetria, head tremor, vestibular disturbances, nystagmus, para- and tetraplegia, visual weakness and seizures. They usually quickly result in death.

18

18.8.2.3 Glucocerebrosidoses

A glucocerebrosidosis equivalent to Gaucher's disease has been reported in the Australian Silky Terrier. Deficiency of glucocerebrosidase leads to the deposition of small storage granules in the neurons and to cell degeneration, especially in the thalamus and hippocampus. Cell degeneration is cleaned up by foamy cells (macrophages, Gaucher cells).

18.8.2.4 Sphingomyelinosis (Niemann-Pick disease)

This is a group of lysosomal enzymopathies in which a prominent enlargement of systemic organs occurs. Types A, B, C, D and E are differentiated in human beings, whereby A, C and D have neurodegenerative components. Sphingomyelinoses have been seen in the Toy Poodle, as well as Siamese, Balinese and domestic cats. There is a genetic deficiency of sphingomyelinase – similar to Niemann-Pick disease Type A. Membranous storage material accumulates in the neurons, glial cells, endothelial cells and periocytes. This leads to neuronal swelling and vacuolisation in the CNS and PNS (axonal spheroids). Foamy cells (Niemann-Pick cells) are conspicuous in this disease. The clinical symptoms include ataxia, dysmetria and tremor, with later development of visual weakness and paresis.

18.8.2.5 Glycoproteinoses

Glycoproteinoses are very rare, though again cerebellar disturbances such as ataxia, dysmetria and tremor are the predominant symptoms. Morphologically, variously sized accumulations of storage material can be found in neurons and glial cells with different patterns of intracellular vacuolation, axonal spheroids, cell death and attempts at regeneration.

18.8.2.6 Fucosidosis

Fucosidosis with an autosomal recessive inheritance has been seen world wide in the English Springer Spaniel. Deficiency of α-L-fucosidase leads to an accumulation of fucoglycoproteins, oligosaccharides and glycosaminoglycans in the CNS, and PNS.

18.8.2.7 Galactosidoses

Galactosidoses initially occur with adulthood. Up to now they have been rarely seen in dogs and cats.

18.8.2.8 Mannosidoses

Mannosidoses have been reported in domestic (Shorthair and Longhair) and Persian cats. Due to a deficiency of α-D-mannosidase, there is intralysosomal accumulation of oligosaccharides particularly in the brain, liver and kidneys.

18.8.2.9 Mucopolysaccharidoses

Mucopolysaccharidosis (MPS) occurs in various types (Type I, II, III A and B, VI, VII), whereby the catabolic metabolism of glycosaminoglycans and acidic mucopolysaccharides (such as dermatan, heparin, chondroitin) is inherently deficient. There is an accumulation of storage material in the connective tissues and the brain. Usually a large amount of storage material is excreted via the urine. Affected human patients are mentally retarded and also suffer from disturbances in the growth of the skeleton, joints and the cornea, with the development of hepatomegaly and splenomegaly. The neurological symptoms in the dog and cat are not as extreme as in human beings. MPS I has been reported in Shorthaired cats and the Plott Hound,; MPS II in Labrador Retrievers; MPS III A in the Wire-haired Dachshund and New Zealand Huntaway Hunting Dog; and MPS III B has been found in the Schipperke. MPS VI occurs in Siamese, and MPS VII in Shorthaired cats. The latter form has also been described in a mixed-breed dog.

18.8.2.10 Glycogenoses

Glycogenoses tend to be rare in the dog and cat. In these diseases, there is a defect in the glycogen metabolism which leads to accumulation of glycogen in different tissues, particularly in the liver, muscle and nervous tissues (neurons and glial cells). Usually there is a fine PAS-positive, diatase-resistant material distributed throughout the cytoplasm, bearing no relationship to the lysosomes. Cell death occurs in the CNS and PNS, as well as the skeleton and heart muscle. Glycogenosis Type Ia (Gierke disease, glucose-6-phosphatase deficiency) has been reported in toy breeds, especially in the Maltese Terrier. Glycogenosis Type II (Pompe's disease; acidic α-glucosidase deficiency) occurs in Lapland dogs, Type III (Cori's disease; deficiency of amylo-1,6-glucosidase) in the German Shepherd and Akita, Type IV (Anderson's disease; deficiency of amylopekinose, α−1,4-glycan-6-glycosysl-transferase) in the Norwegian Forest Cat and Type VII (deficiency of phosphofructokinase) in the English Springer Spaniel.

18.8.2.11 Ceroid lipofuscinosis

Ceroid lipofuscinosis results from an accumulation of membranous storage material (lipofuscin in combination with the pigment ceroid) in the neurons and glial cells (and other cell types) in the CNS and PNS leading to degenerative changes (Fig. 18.28). The pathogenesis is unclear. Most probably this is a mitochondrial disturbance rather than a lysosomal one. The symptoms vary greatly, although ataxia, personality changes, aggression, hyperactivity and visual loss are predominant. The majority of animals become affected under the age of two. An autosomal recessive inheritance has been described for the English Setter, Tibetan Terrier and Border Collie. However, the disease occurs in many other dog breeds (Blue Heeler, Chihuahua, Cocker Spaniel, Corgi, Dachshund, Dalmatian, Gordon Setter, Japanese Retriever, Miniature Schnauzer, Owtcharka, Poodle, Saluki, Yugoslavian Sheepdog) and in cats.

18

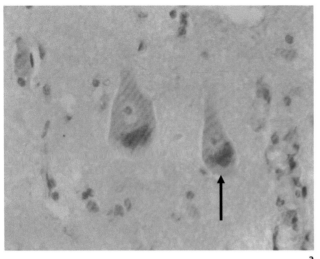

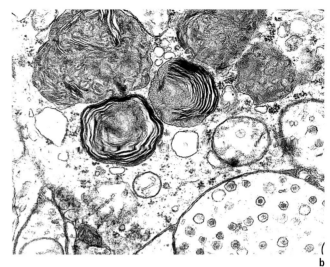

Fig. 18.28a, b
Initially disorientation occurred in a three-year-old Doberman (eating next to its food bowl); then the dog developed increasing attacks of aggression with the biting of objects. The dog had to be euthanised. The brain was macroscopically normal, though neurohistological investigation revealed intracytoplasmic deposits of ceroid lipofuscin (arrow) in almost all areas of the brain. The pictures show the basal nuclei with ceroid-lipofuscin-containing intracytoplasmic inclusion bodies: (a) luxol fast blue stain and (b) electron microscopy.

18.8.2.12 Lafora disease

Lafora disease is an autosomal recessive myoclonic epilepsy. The disease involves the formation of intraneuronal, round glycoprotein-mucopolysaccharide inclusion bodies (Lafora bodies) in the CNS and PNS, less commonly in the heart, liver and striated muscle. The disease leads to somnolence/dementia and to changes in the retina (blindness). It occurs in the dog (especially Beagle, Miniature Wire-Haired Dachshund and Basset) and cats. With the exception of the Miniature Wire-haired Dachshund, in which the prognosis is fair, the prognosis is guarded to poor.

18.8.2.13 Ammon's horn necrosis (polioencephalomalacia)

Aetiology: This syndrome can occur in every breed and age group. It is an acute degeneration of the nerve cells, especially in the cerebral cortex, and leads to "softening" of the cortex.

The cortex is often diffusely and bilaterally affected, though in individual cases there is selective necrosis of the Ammon's horns in the dog and cat, while the rest of the cortex (neocortex) remains normal. The cause and pathogenesis of this disease is basically not known. In some cases of Ammon's horn necrosis there has been an association with the ingestion of iodoxychinoline derivatives (clioquinol: intestinal antiseptic; this has now been removed from the market) or distemper infections. Ischemic necrosis of the cerebral cortex can also

occur after a prolonged respiratory or cardiac arrest (e.g. anaesthetic accident or prolonged syncope). Finally, it is thought that cerebrocortical necrosis, and especially Ammon's horn necrosis, can be a consequence of status epilepticus. Contrary to this is the fact that many dogs that have had a severe attack of seizures do not develop any changes in their Ammon's horn.

Clinical: The symptoms of polioencephalomalacia are acute, with severe epileptic seizures being predominant (prolonged seizures developing into status epilepticus, or short repetitive generalised spasms, sometimes only jaw spasms). Between and after the seizures, there are other severe cerebral symptoms such as personality changes, listlessness to dementia, compulsive pacing, etc. Increased aggression is conspicuous in cats with Ammon's horn necrosis (N.B. rabies!).

Diagnosis: Acute, severe, often generalised seizures; CSF: increased protein, slight to severe pleocytosis with mainly neutrophils.

Therapy: None apart from palliative and anticonvulsant therapy.

Prognosis: Even when the seizures can be stopped, there is irreversible, diffuse damage to the cortex with the respective neurological deficits (e.g. central blindness, dementia).

18

Literature

1 KING, A.S. (1987): Physiological and clinical anatomy of the domestic mammals – Volume 1: central nervous system. Oxford University Press, Oxford.

2 OLIVER, J.E., LORENZ, M.D., KORNEGAY, J.N. (1997): Systemic or multifocal signs. In: Handbook of veterinary neurology. 3rd ed, W.B. Saunders, Philadelphia, pp. 341–402.

3 TOOLE, J.F., BURROW, D.D. (1990): Pathophysiology and clinical evaluation of ischemic vascular disease. In: YOUMANS, J.R. (ed.): Neurological Surgery, 3rd ed. W.B. Saunders, Philadelphia, pp. 1463–1515.

4 THOMAS, W.B. (1996): Cerebrovascular disease. Vet Clin North Am Small Anim Pract. **26**(4): 925–943.

5 FENNER, W.R. (2000): Diseases of the brain. In: ETTINGER, S.J. (ed.): Textbook of Veterinary Internal Medicine, 5th ed. Vol 1, W.B. Saunders, Philadelphia, pp. 552–602.

6 SUMMERS, B.A., CUMMINGS, J.F., DE LAHUNTA, A. (1995): Degenerative diseases of the central nervous system: central nervous system hypoxia, ischemia and related disorders. In: Veterinary Neuropathology. Mosby, St Louis, pp. 237–249.

7 HETCH, S.T., EELKEMA, E.A., LATCHAW, R.E. (1991): Cerebral ischemia and infarction. In: LATCHAW, R.E. (ed.): MR and CT imaging of the head and neck. Mosby Year Book, St. Louis, pp. 145–169.

8 SIESJO, B.K. (1992): Pathophysiology and treatment of focal cerebral ischemia, Part 1: Pathophsiology. J Neurosurg. **77**: 169–184.

9 GROSSMAN, R.I. (1991): Intracranial Hemorrage. In LATCHAW, R.E. (ed.): MR and CT imaging of the head and neck. Mosby Year Book, St. Louis, pp. 171–202.

10 BRANT-ZAWADZKI, M., PEREIRA, B., WEINSTEIN, P., MOORE, S., KUCHARCZYK, W., BERRY, I., MCNAMARA, M., DERUGIN, N. (1986): MR imaging of acute experimental ischemia in cats. Am J Neuroradiol. **7**: 7–11.

11 DIRINGER, M.N. (1993): Intracerebral hemorrage: Pathophysiology and management. Crit Care Med. **21**: 1591–1603.

12 TIPOLD, A. (1995): Diagnosis of inflammatory and infectious diseases of the central nervous system in dogs: a retrospective study. J Vet Intern Med. **9**: 304–314.

13 HOPKINS, A.L. (1996): Head trauma. Vet Clin North Am Small Anim Pract. Intracranial disease **26**(4): 875–891.

14 SUMMERS, B.A., CUMMINGS, J.F., DE LAHUNTA, A. (1995): Malformations of the central nervous system. In: Veterinary Neuropathology. Mosby, St Louis, pp. 68–94.

15 HARRINGTON, M.L., BAGLEY, R.S., MOORE, M.P. (1996): Hydrocephalus. Vet Clin North Am Small Anim Pract. Intracranial disease **26**(4): 843–856.

16 FEW, A.B. (1966): The diagnosis and surgical treatment of canine hydrocephalus. J Am Vet Med Assoc. **149**: 286–293.

17 RIVERS, W.J., WALTERS, P.A. (1992): Hydrocephalus in the dog: utility of ultrasonography as an alternative diagnostic imaging technique. J Am Anim Hosp Assoc. **28**: 333–343.

18 GREENBERG, M.S. (1991): Treatment of hydrocephalus. In: Handbook of neurosurgery. Lakeland, FL, Greenberg Graphics.

19 CUDDON, P.A. (1996): Metabolic encephalopathies. Vet Clin North Am Small Anim Pract. **26**(4): 893–924.

19a RAMSEY, D.T., CASTEEL, S.W., FAGGELLA, A.M., et al. (1996): Use of orally administered succimer (meso-2,3-dimercaptosuccinic acid) for treatment of lead poisoning in dogs. J Am Vet Med Assoc. **208**: 371–375.

19b KNIGHT, T.E., KENT, M., JUNK, J.E. (2001): Succimer for treatment of lead toxicosis in two cats. J Am Vet Med Assoc. **218**: 1946–1948.

20 SIESJO, B.K. (1988): Mechanisms of ischemic brain damage. Crit Care Med. **16**: 954–963.

21 O'BRIEN, D.P., KROLL, R.A. (1992): Metabolic encephalopathies. In: KIRK, R.W., BONAGURA, J.D. (eds.): Current veterinary therapy XI: small animal practice. W.B. Saunders, Philadelphia, pp.998–1003.

22 MUIR, W.W. (1989): Brain hypoperfusion post-resuscitation. Vet Clin North Am Small Anim Pract. **19**: 1151–1166.

23 RAICHLE, M.E. (1983): The pathophysiology of brain ischemia. Ann Neurol. **13**: 2–10.

24 LEIFER, C.E., PETERSON, M.E., MATUS, R.E., PATNAIK, A.K. (1985): Hypoglycemia associated with non-islet cell tumors in 13 dogs. J Am Vet Med Assoc. **186**: 53–55.

25 MADDISON, J.E. (1988): Canine congenital portosystemic encephalopathy. Austr Vet J. **65**: 245–249.

26 MADDISON, J.E. (1992): Hepatic encephalopathy: current concepts of the pathogenesis. J Vet Intern Med. **6**: 341–353.

27 FORSTER, F.M. (1962): Synopsis of neurology. C.V. Mosby Co, St Louis, MO.

28 MATTHES, A., SCHNEBLE, H. (1992): Geschichte der Epilepsie. In: Epilepsien. Georg Thieme Verlag Stuttgart. pp. 3–5.

29 CUNNINGHAM, J.C., FARNBACH, G C. (1988): Inheritance and idiopathic canine epilepsy. J Am Anim Hosp Assoc. **24**: 421–424.

30 JAGGY, A., BERNARDINI, M. (1998): Idiopathic epilepsy in 125 Dogs: A long-term study. Clinical and electrophysiologic findings. J Small Anim Pract. **39**: 23–29.

31 STRAUB, H., SPECKMANN, E.J. (1992): Genetically determed epileptic seizures in animals. In: Benign localized and generalized epilepsies of early childhood (Epilepsy Res. Suppl. 6). Elsevier Science Publishers **6**: 26–39.

32 JAGGY, A., STEFFEN, F. (1995): Epileptische Krampfanfälle beim Hund, Teil 1: Klassifikation, Symptomatik und Diagnose. Der Prakt Tierarzt **2**: 95–102.

33 MELDRUM, B.S. (1990): Anatomy, physiology and pathology of epilepsy. Lancet, pp. 11–14.

34 ENGEL, J., CAHAN, L. (1993): Potential relevance of kindling to human partial epilepsy. In: Kindling. Raven, New York, pp. 37–57.

35 HEINEMANN, U., JONES, R.S.G. (1990): Neurophysiology. In: Comprehensive Epileptology. Raven, New York, pp. 17–42.

36 MELDRUM, B.S. (1991): Exitotoxicity and epileptic brain damage. Epilepsy Res. **10**: 55–61.

18

37 KATHMANN, I., JAGGY, A. (2003): Idiopathische oder symptomatische Epilepsie? Der Prakt Tierarzt **84**: 588–592.

38 PATTERSON, E.E., MICKELSON, J.R., DA, Y., ROBERTS, M.C., MC VEY, A.S., O'BRIAN, D.P., JOHNSON, G.S., ARMSTRONG, P.J. (2003): Clinical Characteristics and Inheritance of Idiopathic Epilepsy in Vizslas. J Intern Med. **17**: 319–325.

39 PODELL, M. (1998): Antiepileptic drug therapy. Clinical Tech Small Anim Pract. **13**: 185–192.

40 CIZINAUSKAS, S., JAGGY, A. (2004): Idiopathic epilepsy in cats: a retrospective study. J Fel Med.Surg. *In press.*

41 JAGGY, A., BERNARDINI, M. (2004): Idiopathic epilepsy in 125 dogs: a long term study. Clinical and electroencephalographic findings. J Small Anim Pract. **39**: 23–29.

42 HEYNOLD, Y., FAISSLER, D., STEFFEN, F., JAGGY, A. (1997): Clinical, epidemiological and treatment results of idiopathic epilepsy in 54 Labrador retrievers: a long-term study. J Small Anim Pract **38**: 7–14.

43 STEFFEN, F., JAGGY, A. (1995): Epileptische Krampfanfälle beim Hund, Teil 3: Intrazerebrale Ursachen, Idiopathische Epilepsie und Behandlung. Der Prakt Tierarzt **4**: 304–314.

44 JAGGY, A., HEYNOLD, Y. (1996): Die idiopathische Epilepsie des Hundes. Schweiz Arch Tierheilk. **138**: 523–531.

45 SRENK, P., JAGGY, A., GAILLARD, C., BUSATO, A., HORIN, P. (1994): Genetische Grundlagen der idiopathischen Epilepsie beim Golden Retriever. Tierärztl Prax. **22**: 574–578.

46 JAGGY, A., FAISSLER, D., GAILLARD, C., SRENK, P., GRABER, H., HEYNOLD, Y. (1998): Genetic aspects of idiopathic epilepsy in the Labrador retriever. J Small Anim Pract. **39**: 275–280.

47 KATHMANN, I., JAGGY, A., BUSATO, A., BÄRTSCHI, M., GAILLARD, C. (1999): Clinical and genetic investigations of idiopathic epilepsy in the Bernese mountain dog. J Small Anim Pract. **40**: 319–325.

48 DE LAHUNTA, A. (1983): Seizures-convulsions. In: Veterinary neuroanatomy and clinical neurology, 2nd ed. W.B. Saunders, Philadelphia, pp. 326–343.

49 BIELFELT, S.W., REDMAN, H.C., MCCLELLAN, R.O. (1971): Sire- and sex-related differences in rates of epileptiform seizures in a purebred beagle dog colony. Am J Vet Res. **32**: 2039–2048.

50 FALCO, M.J., BARKER, J., WALLACE, M.E. (1974): The genetics of epilepsy in the British Alsatian. J Small Anim Pract. **15**: 685–692.

51 HALL, S.J.G., WALLACE, M.E. (1996): Canine epilepsy: a genetic counselling programme for keeshonds. Vet Rec. **138**: 358–360.

52 FAMULA, T.R., OBERBAUER, A.M., BROWN, K.N. (1997): Heritability of epileptic seizures in the Belgian tervueren. J Small Anim Pract. **38**: 349–352.

53 NIELEN, A.L.J., JANSS, L.L.G., KNOL, B.W. (2001): Heritability estimations for disease, coat color, body weight and height in a birth cohort of Boxers. Am J Vet Res. **62**: 1198–12006.

54 MORITA, T., SCHIMADA, A., TAKEUCHI, T., HIKAS, Y., SAWADA, M., OHIWA, S., TAKAHASHI, M., KUBO, N., SHIBAHARA, T., MIYATA, H., OHAMA, E. (2003): Clinicoeuropathological findings of familial frontal lobe epilepsy in Shetland sheepdogs. Can J Vet Res. **66**: 35–41.

55 LENGWEILER, C., JAGGY, A. (1999): Klinische, epidemiologische und therapeutische Aspekte der idiopathischen Epilepsie bei 25 Golden Retrievern: Resultate einer Langzeitstudie. Schweiz Arch Tierheilk. **141**: 231–238.

56 STEFFEN, F., JAGGY, A. (1995): Epileptische Krampfanfälle beim Hund, Teil 2: Extrazerebrale Ursachen der Epilepsie beim Hund. Der Prakt Tierarzt **3**: 191–204.

57 SRENK, P., JAGGY, A. (1996): Interictal electroencephalographic findings in a family of golden retrievers with idiopathic epilepsy. J Small Anim Pract. **37**: 317–321.

58 FORRESTER, S.D. (1989): Current concepts in the management of canine epilepsy. Comp Contin Educ. **11**: 811–820.

59 BLANC, J.J., L'HER, C., TOUIA, A., GARO, B., L'HER, E., MANSOURATI, J. (2002): Prospective evaluation and outcome of patients admitted for syncope over a 1 year period. Eur Heart J. **23**: 815–820.

60 KAPOOR, W.N. (2000): Syncope. N Engl J Med. **343**: 1856–1862.

61 DAVIDOW, E.B., PROULX, J., WOODFIELD, J.A. (2001): Syncope: Pathophysiology and differential diagnosis. Comp Cont Educ. **23**: 608–620.

62 BRIGHT, J.M., CALI, J.V. (2000): Clinical usefulness of cardiac event recording in dogs and cats examined because of syncope, episodic weakness, or intermittent weakness: 60 cases (1997–1999). J Am Vet Med Assoc. **216**: 1110–1114.

63 COTE, E., CHARUVASTRA, E., RICHTER, K. (1999): Event-based cardiac monitoring in small animal practice. Comp Cont Educ. **21**: 1025–1033.

64 HEIDNER, G.L., KORNEGAY, J.N., PAGE, R.L., DODGE, R.K., THRALL, D.E. (1991): Analysis of survival in a retrospective study of 86 dogs with brain tumors. J Vet Intern Med. **5**: 219–226.

65 PRATA, R.G., CARRILLO, J.M. (1985): Oncology – nervous system. In: SLATTER, D.H. (ed.): Textbook of Small Animal Surgery. W.B. Saunders, Philadelphia, p. 2449.

66 MOORE, M.P., BAGLEY, R.S., HARRINGTON, M.L., GAVIN, P.R. (1996): Intracranial Tumors. Vet Clin North Am Small Anim Pract. **26**(4): 759–777.

66a LOUIS, D.N., OHGAKI, H., WIESTLER, O.D., CAVENEE, W.K., BURGER, P.C., JOUVET, A., SCHEITHAUER, B.W., KLEIHUES, P. (2007): The 2007 WHO classification of tumours of the central nervous system. Acta Neuropathol. **114** (2): 97–109.

67 GALLAGHER, J.G., BERG, J., KNOWLES, K.E., WILLIAMS, L.L., BRONSON, R.T. (1993): Prognosis after surgical excision of cerebral meningiomas in cats: 17 cases (1986–1992). J Am Vet Med Assoc. **203**: 1437–1440.

68 SUMMERS, B.A., CUMMINGS, J.F., DE LAHUNTA, A. (1995): Degenerative diseases of the central nervous system: Lysosomal storage diseases. In: Veterinary Neuropathology., Mosby, St Louis, pp. 214–236.

69 MARCH, P.A.: (1996): Degenerative brain disease. Vet Clin North Am Small Anim Pract.: Intracranial disease **26**(4): 945–971.

18

19 Behavioural Problems and Abnormal Behaviour

Petra Mertens

19.1 Aggression in the dog

The assessment of aggressive behaviour in the dog is predominantly based on the context in which the behaviour occurs. This especially includes interactions with people or other animals at the time of the attack. Aggressive behaviour is, as a rule, explicable in connection with certain environmental influences and can be completely normal according to the ethology of the dog; however, this behaviour is absolutely unacceptable and certainly not usually wanted. Only when such associations are absent (e.g., manipulating the dog, the appearance of unknown people, etc.) can there be a well-founded suspicion that aggression is a medical problem. However, it is important in every case of aggression in the dog to systematically exclude all possible differential diagnoses, as medical, neurological and even orthopaedic problems can influence aggressive behaviour or induce it. Examples of such problems include encephalitis (distemper, rabies, etc.), neoplasia, congenital defects (fucidosis, lipofuscinosis, etc.), senile degeneration, hypoxic encephalopathy, hydrocephalus, hepatoencephalopathy / hepatic shunt, endocrine disease (hypothyroidism, Cushing's syndrome, etc.), breeding status (puberty, oestrus, pseudopregnancy) and painful conditions of different aetiologies (polyarthritis, neoplasia, meningitis, otitis, arthrosis, etc.). Table 19.1 provides an overview of the different forms of aggression in the dog.

19.1.1 Dangerous dogs and prognosis

Owners of aggressive dogs ask for veterinary advice for a number of reasons. Some owners are trying to get a confirmation of their own feelings that the dog should be euthanized, especially when feelings of guilt or pressure from third parties are making the decision difficult. Some owners are well aware that a problem can only be partially resolved and that the dog will always be a danger. Other owners are trying to get a quick solution and are not ready or in a position to assess the situation realistically or to control it. Descriptions of the situation are often varied when different members of a household give their opinions.

If pressure is being applied for a therapy programme to be immediately successful or for the dog to be euthanized, then it is important to devise some boundaries and guidelines. Problems do not usually arise spontaneously – changes require time, patience and work. In some cases, the owner must work with their dog over a period of years and change the management or husbandry of their animal.

19

Table 19.1 Different forms of aggressive behaviour in the dog

Form of aggression	Expression	External conditions	Type of biting	Behaviour after biting	Victim	Place	Other behavioural characteristics	Frequency	Development
Status-associated aggression	Offensive head position (stiff, staring look, upright) tail held upright, etc.	Interactions that the dog considers offensive or challenging	Often severe injuries; single or multiple bites	Depending on its earlier experiences, the dog appears "normal" or shows submissive behaviour (after punishment)	People known to the dog (often family members) or people who challenge the dog	Independent of place	Active, challenging, controlling but also anxiety or fear	Often episodic; after particular interactions which provoke aggression	Begins often between 6 and 12 months of age (puberty) or up to 36 months (social maturity)
Anxiety-associated aggression	Tends to be defensive (ears laid back, tail lowered, crouching)	Interactions that the dog considers threatening	Single snaps followed by behaviour resulting in increasing distance	Submissive behaviour; goes away from victim	Unknown people or people who appear to be threatening	Independent of place	Scared, often other behavioural patterns instigated by fear	Every time when the situation occurs	Often starts early in life and then increasing degree of aggression; cause is often lack of socialisation or negative experiences
Territorial aggression	Tends to be defensive; with increasing experience also offensive	Possible or actual penetration of the dog's territory	Single snaps followed by behaviour resulting in increasing distance	Often vocalisation	Everyone who comes close to the dog's territory	Areas considered by the dog as its territory (sleeping place, room, house, garden, car, etc.)	Often in association with anxiety-associated aggression or other forms of aggressive behaviour	Dependent on the number of interactions	Increasing frequency and intensity with experience
Play aggression	Neither defensive nor offensive	Part of play behaviour	Increasing jaw pressure	Independent of problem	Aimed at play partner	Independent of place	Can occur with status-associated aggression	Dependent on frequency of playing	Incitement to rough biting games and lack of bite inhibition
Hunting aggression	Neither defensive nor offensive	Sequence: lying in wait, hunting, catching, shaking	Single or multiple bites	No reaction (apart from consequence of earlier punishment)	Individuals who incite this behaviour (runners, cyclists, etc.)	Independent of place	Anxiety-associated aggression and territorial behaviour	Every time when the stimulus occurs	Experience increases the behaviour
Pain-induced aggression	Mix of defensive and offensive	In association with pain-inducing interactions	Usually single, quick snap	Pain vocalisation	Individuals who induce pain	Dependent on situation or independent	Anxiety-associated aggression	Every pain-inducing interaction	Expectation of pain can incite reaction

19

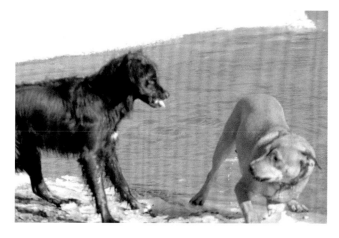
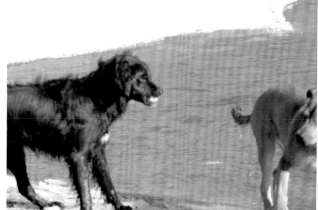
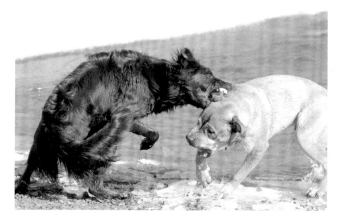
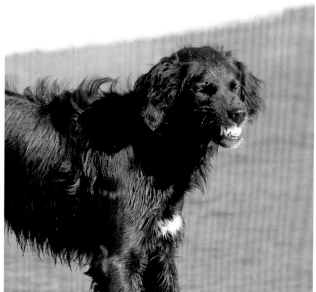

Fig. 19.1
Intraspecific competitive aggression over a piece of ice which is being "defended" by the black dog. Black dog: threat mimic and ritualized aggression, which often makes the owner nervous but as a rule is usually without any serious consequences. Brown dog: submissive behavior, which serves to reduce the aggressive behavior.

19

Some owners want a 100% guarantee that their dog will never bite again. No one is in a position to give such a guarantee, especially if the dog has bitten someone in the past.

The prognosis varies enormously and depends on the following factors:

- Diagnosis (the motivation underlying the dog's aggression).
- Duration of the problem.
- Intensity and frequency of the biting behaviour.

- The dog's irritability threshold and impulsiveness, and the predictability of the dog's aggressive behaviour.
- Size and weight of the dog.
- Characteristics of the victim (child, adult, family member, stranger, etc.)
- Other behavioural problems.
- Family structure and dog husbandry (especially if children are living in the household).
- Ability and willingness of the owner to work with the dog and to undertake the therapeutic measures.

Once the diagnosis has been made, the veterinarian can only make suggestions for therapy and management, provide information about alternatives, and present the owner with a realistic prognosis when they are willing to work under the prescribed conditions. As the diagnosis and treatment of aggressive dogs is not easy and is associated with many ethical and legal risks, it is advisable to exclude any medical / neurological problems and refer such cases to a specialist when the veterinarian responsible for the case is not absolutely certain how to deal with it. Specialists can decide which therapy is suitable and set up the necessary measures (behaviour modification, medication, referral to a trainer).

Successful behavioural therapy is based on a good follow-up of the cases over an average of 6 to 12 months. The time and work needed are often not compatible with the limitations of a small animal practise.

19.1.2 Status-related aggression

The term dominance aggression was often used in the past to describe behaviour that arises within the framework of conflicts over resources. This term is misleading and so will not be used here.

Social dominance should not be confused with aggression or be equated with it as dogs try to avoid aggressive disputes wherever possible (Fig. 19.1). Ritualised gestures can signalise threat and submission so that a fight, which is associated with a high degree of risk, is avoided. Biting represents the tip of the iceberg in behavioural medicine. The origin of aggression should be investigated with respect to the cause of the problem, the development of the behaviour and the number of previous social interactions. When the outcome of a conflict can be foreseen, the normal behavioural repertoire of submission and threat in dogs is perfectly adequate to prevent an attack. In such situations, two factors should be taken into consideration: the value of the resource being fought over (e.g. food), and the motivation of the dog to get the resource (e.g. hunger). A dog which has a greater motivation to eat is more interested in obtaining a piece of meat which has been dropped on the floor by the owner. Aggression is less probable when the dog has just eaten than when a dog that has had nothing to eat for two days. Dogs whose position in the past with respect to the owner has been unclear are more likely to react aggressively in such situations than a dog which is generally known to be submissive. When the dog has reacted aggressively in the past and was placed in the position, for example, to force the owner to let it have the food that has fallen on the floor, it is more likely that the dog will repeat its aggressive behaviour.

There are also other types of motivation that play a role in a dog reacting aggressively. Fear, territorial behaviour or irritability due to medical problems can increase the probability of biting, depending on the situation. Finally, it is possible that neurotransmitter imbalances can increase aggression or irritability. In the past, reduced serotonin concentrations in the CNS have been associated with so-called disturbed impulse control. This problem affects a very small number of dogs with status-related aggression so that use of drugs which influence the concentration of serotonin usually do not have any effect on this condition. Anxiolytic drugs can cause a dysinhibition (as well as other effects) that can increase the risk of aggressive behaviour (see Chap. 19.7).

The description of the situations during which aggression occurs is usually typical. Answers to the following questions must be determined:
- Body position before and after the attack.
- Position of people and other animals in the environment.
- Detailed description of the interactions of all the participants.
- Interventions before, during and after the biting behaviour
- Environmental conditions (place, visitor, noise, etc.).
- Endogenous influences (reproductive status, disease, medication, etc.)
- Other behavioural problems.

It is not uncommon that anxiety-associated and status-related aggression overlap or occur in the same dog, but in different situations. The ambivalent behaviour of such dogs can make diagnosis difficult and complicate the treatment. Dogs which show status-related aggression often react "spontaneously", "without visible warning" and have a "vacant look about them". Specific questioning can show that the owner of the dog was doing something that the dog interpreted as being competitive at the time of the aggressive behaviour.

Miscommunication, which is usually due to a lack of knowledge about dog behaviour, consists for example, of the following situations:
- Standing over the dog.
- Staring at the dog / direct eye contact.
- Continual stroking of the dog's head or back.
- Hugging the dog or kissing it.
- Touching and manipulation of parts of the dog's body (combing, drying, putting on the lead, etc.).
- Verbal or physical punishment.
- Taking something away from the dog (or trying to).
- Pushing or pulling the dog away from something.
- Being close to the dog's food or toys, or threatening to take them away from the dog.

19

Therapy: The treatment of the problem is based on a combination of principles that must be adapted to each specific case:

■ Prevention of every physical confrontation (verbal punishment, turning the dog on its back, shaking the dog by its nape, etc.).
■ Control all resources which the dog considers important.
  – The access to all these resources is controlled by the owner and their family members only (N.B.: children should only be involved or allowed to interact with the dog under strict control and with consideration of all safety measures).
  – Typical resources are food, attention, toys, access to preferred resting places, walks, etc.
  – These resources are only available to the dog when the person who is working with the dog initiates and finishes the interaction (this means that demands for attention must be strictly ignored). The dog must follow a command given once and receives access to the particular resource (small amount, short duration). This allows the owner and other people to clarify their status with respect to the dog without confrontation which would increase the risk of biting.

Example:
■ The dog goes to the owner and obviously wants to be stroked.
■ The dog is ignored.
■ Later – independent of this situation – the owner calls the name of the dog and gives it the command to come.
■ The dog obeys. The owner praises the dog verbally and strokes the dog or gives it small amount of its daily food ration, which is not given as a meal but in portions throughout the training as reinforcement.
■ Before the dog stops the interaction, the owner gives the command which finishes the interaction. After that the dog is again ignored until the owner decides to interact with the dog as described above.
■ When the dog does not obey the command, it is not repeated. Instead the dog is ignored for a significant period of time before it is again given the opportunity to receive the things that it likes or considers necessary by displaying obedience.
■ This principle should be strictly and consequently implemented when attention is given to the dog and by every person involved. The response to disobedience and aggressive behaviour is a deprivation of attention (immediately turning around and going away, leaving the dog isolated).

Counter-conditioning and systemic desensitization. This is based on the principle that an undesired behaviour is replaced by another behaviour that is not compatible with the original behaviour (counter-conditioning). In addition, the aggression-inducing stimulus is weakened to the extent that the reaction no longer occurs. Then it is incrementally increased so that the dog is able to tolerate the stimulus without reacting aggressively (desensitization).

A dog which, for example, reacts aggressively when an attempt is made to clean its ears can become used to having its ears cleaned and is rewarded for nonaggressive behaviour (steps that can be used in this example are short-term stroking over the head, prolong the stroking, stroke closer to the ear, lift up the ear for a short time, the length of time when the ear is lifted up is increased stepwise, lift up ear and gently manipulate the pinna, increase the manipulation of the ear, then repeat all of these steps with the bottle of cleaning fluid, and so on). It is important that the steps are small and are frequently repeated, and are below the dog's threshold which elicits aggression.

Castration of a male dog. The early castration of male dogs (before puberty; under 6 months of age) reduces the risk that, when reaching adulthood, they demonstrate status-related aggression either toward other dogs or humans. Castration of a dog which already exhibits this behaviour will not solve the problem. The earlier the surgery is done, the better the chance that the castration reduces the aggression-enhancing effects of testosterone with respect to normal social development (social maturity). Castration has no effect on other forms of aggression.

Neutering a female dog. Neutering female dogs does not have the same aggression-reducing effect as does castration of a male, except in those cases when aggression occurs in association with oestrus or pseudopregnancy. Bitches that show status-related aggression tend to react more aggressively after neutering and the associated reduction in the sex hormones. This potential risk must be weighed up against the advantages of neutering (prevention of disease and avoidance of unwanted pregnancies).

19.1.3 Status-related aggression between dogs in the same household

Aggression between dogs that live together can appear to begin suddenly and lead to apparently unprovoked attacks.

Fights are more frequent when:
■ A dog has reached sexual or social maturity.
■ Disease- or age-related changes make it impossible for a dog to maintain its status.
■ Dogs want to maintain control over things that reflect their status (attention from the owner, toys, resting places, food, etc.).
■ Situations occur that increase the general level of excitement (feeding time, arrival of guests, excitement before a walk, dogs find themselves in a narrow passageway).
■ The owner unintentionally or intentionally supports the subdominant dog and punishes the dominant dog (which is often the attacker).

19

Fights occur sporadically at first and increase both in frequency and intensity, when the dogs are not able to sort out the dominance relationship on their own. The confrontations can cause a great deal of injury, especially when two bitches are involved. Intervention by the owner is dangerous as the dogs often then change the target of their aggression.

The majority of cases involve two bitches, followed in frequency by households with two male dogs and then mixed-sex pairs. The probability of confrontation is increased during oestrus. Factors such as age, seniority in the household, size and body weight often do not play a role in the establishment of dominance. More important is the ability of the dog to ensure its access to important resources. Dogs have often been observed cutting off the pathway of other (sub-dominant) dogs with whom they live or are visiting; or they put themselves in a T-position in front of the other dogs. These observations are an important basis on which an attempt is made to determine the dominance relationships. The owner is advised not to interfere with the situation and to support the dominant dog. Attempts at changing the dominance order not infrequently result in increasing the aggression.

19.1.4 Aggression between dogs that meet by chance

Confrontations between dogs that do not live together and possibly do not know each other can be seen frequently. These fights often occur between male dogs (uncastrated or castrated late in life). As long as the dogs have normal social behaviour, such fights rarely result in serious injury.

The following causes can lead to aggression (they can occur in combination, too):
- Fear and social deprivation due to inadequate socialisation during the first 3 to 4 months of life and in the juvenile phase of life (< 1 year) (see Chap. 19.1.5).
- Experience from earlier fights.
- Hierarchical arguments (see Chap. 19.1.2).
- Frustration due to lack of being able to have a normal confrontation (in a car, on a lead, behind a fence).
- Territorial behaviour (see Chap. 19.1.7).
- Mood transfer from owner, whose fear subconsciously increases and can lead to a worsening of the dog's behaviour.

The diagnosis can usually be made using direct observation or video recordings of the specific social behaviour, the description of the dog's early socialisation and development during the juvenile period, the development of the problem, and the interventional actions of the owner.

Good socialisation of dogs and castration of male dogs before sexual maturity are important elements which reduce the

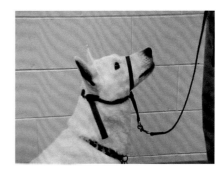

Fig. 19.2
Gentle leader head collar.

probability of aggressive behaviour toward other dogs during walks.

Therapy: The basis of successful treatment of aggressive behaviour toward other dogs is the dog's obedience and the ability of the owner to control the dog physically. The use of a head collar is preferable to a standard neck collar as they allow a better control of the dog (Fig. 19.2). The effect is comparable with the use of a head collar in the horse.

In dogs which are repeatedly and extremely aggressive to other dogs the unwanted reaction (aggression) should be replaced by another behaviour (e.g. "sit" and food reward) not compatible with the previous behaviour (counter-conditioning; see Chap. 19.1.2). At the beginning, the training is performed far away from other dogs, so that the dog cannot react aggressively. The distance between the aggressive dog and other dogs is then reduced stepwise until the dog is able to tolerate other dogs walking past it (systematic desensitization). After systematic training, instead of attacking the other dog, the patient will have learnt to associate the command "sit" with the presence of another dog and await a reward.

19.1.5 Fear-related aggression

Aggressive behaviour can be associated with fear of people, other animals or particular situations. The characteristics of a frightened dog (lowered head, diverted gaze, ears flat to the head, crouching, tail under the stomach, lip commissures drawn backwards) can be overlaid by aggressive elements if the dog attacks, after which it usually quickly withdraws to a safe distance. Misinterpretation of the normal behaviour of a dog can commonly lead to biting behaviour which is not foreseen by the victim and so they assume it is pathological behaviour.

Examples of misinterpretation which can lead to fear-related aggression:

- *"Dogs which are lying on their backs want to be stroked."* This gesture is an appeasement or submissive gesture that serves to inhibit the aggressive behaviour of the social partner. When a person leans over a dog that is frightened and has turned itself on its back to reduce aggression, stroking can be interpreted by the dog as an attack and lead to defensive biting.
- *"Dogs love to be hugged."* Stroking on the back and hugging are principally dominant gestures which can provoke or frighten a dog.
- *"A good form of punishment is shaking the dog's nape and to try and lay the dog down on its back."* Dogs that are punished physically often react aggressively (defensively) especially when the attempt of the aggressor (person) to appease the dog is unsuccessful.

Even when a dog is well socialised with, for example, men, little or no experience with women and children, infers inadequate socialisation; fear in the presence of these types of people may lead to aggressive behaviour. When the dog has learnt that aggression forces a person to retreat, then this behaviour is reinforced and usually escalates. This process can be broken using behavioural (therapeutic) measures based on the principles of counter-conditioning and systematic desensitisation (see Chap. 19.1.2).

19.1.6 Pain-related aggression

Pain or the danger of experiencing pain or injury often leads to aggressive behaviour, which may be preceded by submission or threatening behaviour. Aggression as a consequence of unexpected or extreme pain occurs without any specific warning and can appear abnormal when it is not known that the dog is ill. This behaviour is aimed at anyone who actually causes pain or in the eyes of the dog is the cause. This form of defensive behaviour can also occur in connection with physical punishment (see Chap. 19.1.5).

Professional handling, the treatment of medical or orthopaedic problems, pain therapy and attempts to prevent fear in the dog are the elementary principles of treatment for these dogs. When the dog reacts aggressively (e.g. during the cleaning of its ears) despite the fact the disease (otitis) is being successfully treated, a systematic training programme can help the dog to associate the touching of its ears with pleasure (praise, food, etc.; see Chap. 19.1.2) rather than pain.

19.1.7 Territorial aggression

Territorial aggression is usually motivated by fear that is more apparent close to the dog's resting place, garden or car. In other cases, territorial behaviour can occur as part of status-related aggression when the dog defends an area because it considers it to be an important resource. Fences, leads and other barriers increase the aggressive behaviour, often due to increasing frustration and apparent safety.

The fact that postmen, pedestrians, cars or other dogs continue walking away and disappear increases the behaviour, as in the eyes of the dog it has successfully driven its foe away. In unusual surroundings, it may take some time for this behaviour to recur; however, some dogs react territorially, even when the owner has sat down on a park bench. The treatment of this problem is based on treating the motivation underlying the dog's aggressive behaviour (see Chaps. 19.1.2 and 19.1.5).

19.1.8 Maternal aggression, abnormal or lack of maternal behaviour, and infanticide

Maternal aggression is the result of hormonal changes during the preparation for birth, the *post-partum* period or during pseudopregnancy.

The behaviour serves to protect the puppies and can be directed towards people who the bitch knows well and whom she would not attack under normal circumstances. The aggression is directed towards anyone who approaches the nesting box, the puppies, or objects which a pseudopregnant female is mothering. This is connected to nesting behaviour, general disquiet and swelling of the mammary glands.

The aggression usually disappears on its own within 2 weeks or at the time when the puppies begin to be more active and to leave the nesting box on their own.

Maternal aggression is normally not directed towards the puppies. Commotion and continual disturbances can, however, lead to the aggression being directed towards them.

Inadequate nursing and aggression towards the puppies occurs more commonly in primiparous bitches (infantophobia) and fearful animals.

Excessive nursing can lead to injury of the puppies (e.g. continual licking or careless severing of the umbilical cord). Eating of one's own offspring is as a rule considered abnormal. In individual cases, this behaviour is the result of the puppies being ill. More frequently, however, it is the consequence of continual disturbances that do not allow the (inexperienced) bitch to feel secure. Even medically necessary inter-

19

ventions can disturb the birth and prevent the dog's maternal behaviour from occurring with normal intensity (oxytocin release, appreciation of pheromones, mother-child relationship).

When careful monitoring of the birth and good preparation do not prevent aggressive behaviour and there is danger for the puppies, then the puppies should be removed from the bitch and either raised by hand, or be only brought to the mother under observation or after the female has been fitted with a muzzle.

19.1.9 Aggression as a part of hunting behaviour

Hunting aggression is normally part of a typical behaviour sequence (lying in wait, creeping towards prey, chasing prey, springing on prey, biting, shaking, killing and eating). This behaviour occurs more strongly in some dogs than others due to their breed (hunting dogs). Other dog breeds typically exhibit only part of hunting behaviour due to their breeding or training, (e.g. Border Collie: creeping towards prey and partially chasing; Retriever: no creeping towards prey and lying in wait but chasing and catching, then taking prey back to owner).

This behaviour is often a problem in conjunction with other forms of aggressive behaviour (see Chaps. 19.1.5 and 19.1.7); for example, when a dog chases after people who cause it fear. The treatment of aggression that is part of hunting behaviour is based on excellent obedience, continual supervision of the dog, and the treatment of problems that lie at the core of the aggression. The utilisation of so-called taste aversion conditioning (application of emetics such as LiCl after the ingestion of mutton in dogs that attack sheep) has only limited clinical use. The use of electrical punishment stimuli that are applied by a collar is not allowed in many countries and should only be used in individual cases when all other possibilities have been exhausted. In addition, this method should only be used by people who are well-trained.

19.1.10 Aggression as part of play behaviour

Play aggression appears to be a contradiction in terms. It refers to injuries that occur during play. Lack of biting inhibition is a common problem in puppies that persists when the dog is continually invited to play with people's hands or feet. Instead of punishing the dog, it is more sensible to react with a high-pitched yell and as punishment to simply ignore the dog (turn away and leave the room without a word). Attempts at punishing the dog directly (verbally or physically) can – dependent on the type of dog – lead to an escalation or

the development of fear in the puppy. The dog should be given adequate opportunity to fulfil its daily requirement for physical movement and to play with other dogs, so that it can practise well-adjusted social behaviour.

19.2　Aggression in the cat

Aggressive behaviour in the cat can occur unexpectedly for the owner and may be the result of a medical or neurological problem.

Aggressive behaviour is, with the exception of hunting aggression, either offensive or defensive. It is aimed at other cats, animals or humans. A detailed anamnesis can help to determine whether the behaviour is really spontaneous or the consequence of an interaction that has caused the cat to attack (Table 19.2).

The information that should be included in the anamnesis is:
- People and animals present during the aggression.
- The place where the attack occurred.
- Interaction and external factors or influences.
- A neutral description of the cat's body posture and expression.
- When possible, a video recording of the behaviour.

19.2.1　Territorial aggression

Cats that live in groups (multiple cat households) behave similarly to cats which live in colonies. Although aggressive behaviour is reduced by the members of a group, it can occur when the members of the group determine their status using individual conflict. If an attempt is made to introduce new cats to the group, then severe fights and attacks on the interloper may occur.

Castrated tom cats are usually treated by other cats as females. However, male cats do not always dominate female cats. The social position of a queen within a group in not always determined by her size, strength or matriarchal connections. The mechanism of the status-related disputes in cats is usually unknown. Fights are usually avoided due to the risk of injury and it appears that disputes are settled by using control of important resources and the expression of social behaviour.

In cohabitation with humans, status-related aggression is seen when the owner of the cat continually strokes it. Attacks appear to be sudden and unprovoked. A cat which has just approached its owner and sat itself on his or her knee suddenly turns around and bites hard. This behaviour appears to be due to overstimulation (in addition to other causes). Stroking imitates the typical sexual behaviour of cats and is limited to regions that induce tolerance behaviour for a period of time

Table 19.2: Different forms of aggressive behaviour in the cat and diagnostic criteria

Form of aggression	Diagnostic criteria
Anxiety-associated aggression	■ The cat is frightened, thinks that it is being attacked and cannot see any possibility of getting away. ■ As a reaction to being attacked by another cat. ■ As a reaction to other fear-inducing stimuli (being held by the owner, loud sounds, etc.).
Aggression as a consequence of disease	■ Medical and neurological problems can induce aggression (rare). Basic investigation: general examination, neurological examination, where necessary serum biochemistry, CBC, urinalysis, thyroid tests and other tests depending on the results of the preceding ones.
Irritable aggression	■ Some cats only liked to be stroked for a short time (differential diagnosis: social status/fear/pain). ■ Stroking is equivalent to social cleaning or sexual behaviour under cats and can lead to overstimulation. ■ Owners are often not capable of ascertaining their cat's mood (upright vibrissae, flicking of the tail, ear position, widening of the pupils, etc.).
Hunting aggression	■ Typical sequence of behaviour (lying in wait, creeping, tensing up, springing and biting). ■ The control of hunting behaviour and feeling of hunger are independent (even a well-nourished cat needs to hunt).
Maternal aggression	■ Queens with newborn kittens are very protective. ■ Aggressive behaviour occurs more commonly during the first two weeks after birth. ■ Maternal aggression can be observed lasting up to two weeks.
Pain-induced aggression	■ Painful disease can induce irritability; painful manipulations can also instigate aggressive behaviour.
Play aggression	■ Rough (hunting) games with attacking of other cats, pets or the owner. ■ Often young animals which have not learnt to use suitable objects for their games or whose behaviour has unknowingly been reinforced by the owner.
Territorial aggression	■ Consequence of the intrusion of an unknown cat (stray cats, new cat in the house, a cat living in the house that has reached sexual maturity). ■ The cat lies in wait and/or attacks. ■ Victim of attack tries to stop contact and goes away. ■ Same in male and female cats.
Re-directed aggression	■ Aggression is transferred to another animal, object or person who/which is not the cause of the aggressive behaviour. ■ The tension and excitement lasts for a prolonged period of time and so makes it difficult to ascertain the cause.

(back, hips and nape). Signs that indicate an increasing degree of excitement (whipping the tail around, tense body posture, raising the vibrissae) and which occur before an attack are often overlooked by the owner or misinterpreted.

The size of the so-called "home range" of a cat is regionally variable as it is dependent on food availability and the population density. A cat's "home range" can vary between 0.1 hectare to 170 hectares (queens) or 1000 hectares (toms) (1 hectare = 2.47 acres). The territory of an uncastrated male cat is usually 3.5 times larger than that of a castrated male or a queen. The male:female sex ratio within a tom cat's range varies between 1:1 and 1:10. A spatial or temporal division of the range is possible with cats that have freedom of movement, especially since subdominant cats can wander out.

A number of problems will occur in the case of a house cat that possibly has to share its restricted range – the home of the owner – with other cats, as the loser of aggressive disputes cannot avoid the aggressor and so permanently invades its range. The consequence of this is persistent attacks with increasing intensity.

19.2.2 Fear-related aggression

Cats that grow up isolated or due to their husbandry have little or no contact with other cats, animals or humans, frequently show aggressive behaviour to other cats, dogs and humans during their lives. Even when the cat has been kept with its littermates until the end of its socialisation period and has regular contact with the breeder, the learned behaviour usually disappears if the cat does not have an opportunity to refresh this experience with the help of other contacts. As a rule, the frequency and intensity of fear-related aggressive behaviour increases with time as the cat learns that aggressive behaviour allows it to get away from the instigating stimulus.

19

19.2.3 Play and hunting aggression

Cats that are not allowed to go outside and move freely about only have a limited possibility of satisfying their natural needs for movement and play. Play generally serves to allow the practising of behavioural patterns and to improve their precision. Play behaviour can be observed in the cat in all age groups and especially during the first year of life. The natural tendency of a cat to play is mainly limited to hunting games. When there are no interactive toys and the cat has no recourse to prey, the cat's play or hunting behaviour may target other cats or humans. Cats which do not tolerate this behaviour will react aggressively towards the attacker and serious fights may occur. In such cases, the attacks have a typical behavioural pattern: (1) creeping towards the target, (2) lying in wait, (3) ducking down, (4) jumping on the target, and (5) biting the target.

Human reactions (invitation to play with a hand, but also crying out after the bite or punishment) strengthen the behaviour of the cat or induce fear. Cat owners should therefore be instructed to avoid games that include the hands or other parts of the body to prevent future aggressive behaviour of their cats.

19.2.4 Maternal aggression

The aggressive behaviour of queens raising a litter is particularly strong towards tom cats; this is because male cats kill the litters of other toms to ensure that the female cats within their territory come into oestrus again and so allow them to mate. In this period of time, the queen will spontaneously leave the nesting box and take the litter to a safer place if she feels threatened. Maternal aggressive behaviour is adaptive and disappears when the queen has weaned her litter.

The killing of a litter by its own mother may arise due to the queen thinking that there is a disturbance or disease in the kittens. Primiparous queens, queens that are anxious and nervous, or those that have poor mothering qualities have a greater tendency toward infanticide. Cats that show these behaviour patterns without any apparent reason (e.g. repeated disturbance by people or other animals) should be separated from their kittens (which should be raised by hand) and not used for breeding in the future.

19.2.5 Re-directed aggression

Re-directed aggression is a behavioural problem in which the aggressive behaviour is aimed towards an individual who is not the original cause of the behaviour. (Example: two cats are sitting on a window-sill and see a cat outside. Cat 1 is extremely excited and turns its aggression towards Cat 2, who just happens to be sitting next to it.) Due to the process of classical conditioning, the individual who is attacked (cat or person) is then associated with the feeling of excitement and aggression, so that the attacks occur repeatedly when the victim of aggression comes into sight without the original trigger for the aggression having induced the behaviour.

19.2.6 Therapy

Enrichment of the animal's environment
- Allow the cat to use the home in all three dimensions (sitting places by the window, cat trees, permission to go into cupboards, etc.).
- Avoid playing with the hand (instead use toys on strings, etc.)
- Re-direct aggression towards suitable toys.
- Social isolation as the only suitable method of punishment (aggression is punished by turning around and going away without a word).
- Provision of suitable play facilities.

Games that allow the cat to attack, scratch or bite the hands or other parts of the human body must be avoided. Instead toys can be attached to strings or flexible rods to allow for interactive play. The following are examples to give the owner ideas for enriching the environment of house cats:
- Weekly rotation of toys (offer only a few toys at the same time).
- Provision of different types of toys (something to roll, a toy for biting, a toy on a string for hunting, etc.).
- "Hiding" of toys in different places.

Suitable toys
- Large domestic objects made of plastic.
- Plastic balls that have some form of filling that makes a sound (e.g. bell). The balls can be put in some form of vessel (e.g. bath or clothes basket) to make them more attractive.
- Paper bags (after removal of the handles; no plastic bags) which are laid on their side or cardboard boxes with an opening for the cat (pull toy on a string through the box).
- Self-made scratching posts with toys (e.g. feather on a rod).
- Cardboard rolls (e.g. kitchen paper or toilet rolls), closed at one end and holes punched in the sides, with food placed in them that falls out during play (whilst "hunting").
- Dried cat mint (active ingredient: neptolactone) makes toys more attractive (genetic variation means that some cats cannot smell this substance; other cats react aggressively and exhibit mating behaviour).
- Stuffed toys and tennis balls are large enough so that a cat can bite them and make the typical scratching movements with the hindlegs (hunting behaviour).

19

Systematic desensitization and counter-conditioning

The owner should never try to leave the cats to fight without intervention as the tension between the animals increases instead of leading to a cessation of the conflict. If an attempt is made to separate fighting cats, methods should be chosen which ensure that the owner is not injured (distracting noises, throwing a blanket over the fighters so they cannot see, etc.). Once the cats have stopped fighting, it is not uncommon for them to still be excited and aggressive. If during this time an attempt is made to examine them for injuries or to just quieten them down, there is a danger that the cats will redirect their aggression and react aggressively towards the owner.

The fearful behaviour of the subdominant cat strengthens the aggression of the attacker. In cases in which tensions are more chronic, cats tend to mark and secure their territory with urine. A prerequisite for the successful treatment of marking behaviour or spraying is that the true cause – intraspecific aggression – is treated.

The owner of fighting cats should separate them immediately. The more often the fights take place, the more difficult it is to modify the behaviour successfully. The following therapy programme can be used for the treatment of ongoing problems and in an abbreviated form, can be used for prophylaxis. As fights often occur following the introduction of a new cat into a household or after the return of a cat back into the house (e.g. after a prolonged stay at a veterinary clinic), the owner should be advised to introduce the cat slowly.

The following principles should be considered:
- Step 1: The cats should be housed in separate rooms without direct or visual contact.
- Step 2: The animals should be taken from one room to the other daily or more than once daily (exchange of territories) so that no territorial disputes arise and the cats remain in olfactory contact. The cat litter tray as well as the food and water bowls should be cleaned as usual, though left in the room.
- Step 3: Exchange of pheromones (Felifriend® CEVA; or the transmission of the smell of the facial pheromones using a cloth and the establishment of a group scent within the household).
- The cats should be kept apart for at least 2 weeks before they are (re-)introduced to each other (e.g., after a stay at a veterinary clinic: a few days). With cats that have fought over a long period of time, the time of separation before Step 4 is started should be related to the duration of the dispute (e.g. 3 months fighting = 3 weeks separation; 5 months fighting = 5 weeks separation).
- Step 4: After the separation period, the cats should be brought into contact with each other at least once a day under control conditions, so they can be (re-)introduced to each other. During this phase, the cats should still be kept apart outside of the training period (see Steps 1 and 2).

- During this time the principles of systematic desensitization and classical counter-conditioning should be used:
  - Training is done during feeding (association of the other cat with food).
  - The cats are kept so far apart that they do not show any aggressive behaviour.
  - The owner must ensure that the cats cannot attack each other either by using chest harnesses (to which the cats have become accustomed during the period of separation) or a screen.
  - The cats are only allowed to see each other during feeding time. Once they have eaten, they are separated again.
  - Over a period of weeks, the distance between the cats during feeding is reduced slowly until they are finally able to eat side-by-side without showing any aggression. The speed with which the programme can be completed depends primarily on the reactions of the cats. As soon as fear or aggression is seen, the owner must place the cats further apart (so far that no reactions are visible). A renewed attempt at bringing the cats together should be done more slowly.
  - Now the time in which the cats are together should be carefully prolonged.
  - The owner allows the cats to be together in different places until they can have an unlimited access to the whole house (again).

19.3 Problems associated with excretory behaviour of cats

19.3.1 Excretory behaviour outside of the litter tray

The use of a litter tray is partially inherited. It is formed from the behaviour of the cat's mother and litter mates as well as through play. Young animals that show a significant variation from normal excretory behaviour may be affected by inherited or acquired neurological diseases. It is possible that other diseases which affect the cat's mobility or its appreciation of its environment can lead to urine or faeces being deposited outside of the litter tray (Table 19.3).

Preferences or aversions for a certain type of litter tray (size, roof), the position of the tray and the type of substrate are often causes of irritating excretory behaviour. Preferences or aversions can also occur as secondary phenomena; for example, as a consequence of a disease that induces pain on micturition. Due to the pain, the cat avoids the litter tray and urinates, for example, on the carpet. Even after the successful treatment of the medical cause of the disturbing behaviour, the unwanted behaviour (cat-litter tray aversion or a learned substrate or position preference) may remain.

19

19.3.1.1 Rudiments of treatment

Punishment
- Avoid punishment totally, as by increasing its fear the probability that the cat will avoid the litter tray increases.
- The danger is that the cat will search for another place and will only urinate or defecate when the owner is not there.

Cleaning
- Look for soiled places and cover them with plastic.
- Do not use a steam cleaner as the heat causes permanent protein binding of the fibres with chemical substances within the urine.
- Chemical cleaners such as ammonia-containing substances or vinegar have a similar smell to urine and cause the cat to soil in the same place or to mark it.
- Wash materials that can be cleaned in the washing machine according to the manufacturer's instructions and dry them in fresh air.
- The surfaces of wood or walls must be removed, treated and sealed.
- Wipe up urine on the carpet or furniture with hand towels and then dilute with water before wiping up again with hand towels; repeat this procedure until the largest possible amount of urine is removed from the material or furnishings.
- Enzymatic cleaners that have been specifically made for treating urine stains are only effective when there are no chemicals in the treated material. These cleaners are ideal for the treatment of soiled surfaces and should be used according to the instructions.

19.3.1.2 The optimal cat litter tray/box location

- Put a cat litter tray on every floor in the house or flat.
- Choose places that are easily accessible but do not lie in the main pathways through the house or where they can be affected by other disturbances (e.g. next to a washing machine that suddenly turns on).
- Take into account the special requirements of kittens and older cats.
- Place the cat litter tray in places that the cat has already used for urinating or defaecating.
- Place the cat litter tray as far away as possible from food and water bowls.
- Prevent access to cat litter tray by other pets and children (disturbances).

Substrate
- Owners whose cats do not cause a problem should avoid changing the make of substrate.
- Choose fine, dust-free substrate.
- Cats mainly prefer substrates that clump.
- Do not use scents or scent inhibitors.
- If the cat has a preference for an atypical and non-commercially produced substrate (e.g. sand, carpet), this substrate can be used at first, then slowly but surely the new substrate is added until just the commercial substrate is accepted.

Number of cat litter trays
- The ideal number of litter trays depends on the number of cats in the household; there should me one more litter tray than there are cats.
- The cat toilets or litter trays should not be placed next to each other but be distributed throughout the home.

Type of cat litter tray
- The cat toilet or litter tray must be suitable for the size of cat (at least as long as the body length of the cat).
- The edge must be high enough to contain enough substrate but low enough to allow the cat easy access.
- Roofs are often not to the liking of the cat as the smell is more concentrated and the cat cannot see its surroundings adequately.
- Electrical, self-cleaning toilets can frighten the cat.

Cleaning
- Remove faeces and urine at least twice daily.
- Clumping substrate: the contents should be renewed at least once a week.
- Non-clumping substrate: the contents of the cat toilet should be renewed every 3 days.
- Renew the plastic box at least every 6 months.
- Clean the plastic box thoroughly with (scent-free) soap and rinse well.

19.3.1.3 Medical treatment

- This only makes sense when medical causes of spraying are the reasons for the soiling problem, or it is due to aggression between rival cats (see Chaps. 19.2.1 and 19.3.2).
- Localisation, substrate or position preferences or aversions cannot be successfully treated using medication.

19.3.2 Marking with urine (spraying)

The cat usually sprays urine at vertical surfaces so that the owner finds relatively small amounts of urine on walls and furniture in strategically important places in the home (windows, doors, passageways, etc.). The urine is either at the height of the hips of the cat on the vertical surface or directly underneath it on the floor. Cats often smell the surface first, rub their heads or cheeks on the surroundings, turn around, raise the tail vertically in the air, dance with their hind feet, whip the distal part of their tails backwards and forwards, and spray short spurts of urine. Spraying on horizontal surfaces is rarely seen and difficult to differentiate from disturbed micturition behaviour (Table 19.4).

19

Table 19.3: Different causes which can lead to irritating excretory behaviour and spraying in the cat

Cause	Examples of diagnostic criteria
Medical problems	■ General examination, laboratory investigations, difficulty in defaecation or urination, urinary incontinence, haematuria, increased frequency of urination, neurological disease, age-related changes and cognitive dysfunction.
Location preference	■ Cat urinates/defaecates independent of the surface. ■ Possibly in a place where the litter tray used to be. ■ Uses litter tray when placed in this position. ■ Uses litter tray when cat is kept in one room. ■ Cat chooses a particular place to urinate/defaecate (part of the house, room, furniture, or part of a room).
Substrate preference	■ Training during kittenhood or later. ■ Uses another place when the substrate has been changed. ■ Does not use cat toilet when the litter tray is put in a dirty place. ■ Uses litter tray when cat is kept in one room.
Conflict between cats	■ The aggressor does not allow the subdominant cat to leave a particular place where it has removed itself or to enter a particular room. ■ Due to its social position, the cat cannot use a litter tray which is used by the aggressor.
Cat litter tray aversion	■ Behaviour of cat in the litter tray. ■ Urination or defaecation near to the litter tray but outside it. ■ Anamnesis: aversive experience with respect to litter tray. ■ Cleanliness of the litter tray, type of litter tray, type of cat litter, depth of cat litter. ■ Pain on urination or defaecation. ■ The cat is disturbed whilst using the litter tray. ■ The cat associates the litter tray with punishment (e. g. the owner punishes the cat for urination/defaecation outside the litter tray and then puts it into the litter tray).
Fear	■ General nervousness. ■ Fear-induced stimuli in the region of the litter tray. ■ Confrontation between cats in the household. ■ Punishment by the owner.
Spraying	■ Context (often in combination with aggression/conflict between cats within the household or in the neighbourhood). ■ Body position (usually standing, tail upright, dancing on the hindlegs). ■ Contact with other cats; conditions within the household. ■ Olfactory stimuli. ■ Amount of urine/place.

Table 19.4 Diagnostic criteria for spraying and irritating urination

	Spraying	Irritating urination
Body position	Standing, tail upright, dancing with the hindlimbs, urine sprayed backwards	Usually in crouching position
Amount of urine	Small	Complete emptying of bladder contents
Place of urination	Usually vertical surfaces	Usually horizontal surfaces
Motivation	Territorial behaviour, aggression between cats in household, sexual behaviour	Urination

19

Marking with faeces is comparatively rare. The faeces are released in places or on objects that are associated with a particular person (e.g. clothes, places where the person sits or sleeps).

Detection of the urine marks

As urine fluoresces under UV light, a Wood's lamp can be used to find soiled places.

Causes

Even after many years of cats living in harmony in a household, territorial conflict can arise suddenly (see Chap. 19.2.1). However, other stimuli can be possible causes of marking behaviour such as the presence of stray cats in the garden, cats that come into the home through the cat flap, disturbances due to workmen in the home, changes in the family structure, absence of the owner, changes in the daily routine, new furniture and smells which the cat can detect on clothes or objects that are brought into the home.

Therapy

The successful treatment of unwanted spraying requires that the original motivation of the cat to start marking is recognised. When it is not possible to remove this conflict, then the prognosis for successful treatment of spraying should be guarded.

Castration

Cats that are not castrated spray more often than castrated animals (intact tom > intact queen > castrated tom > neutered queen). In these cases, the first step in reducing the disturbing behaviour is castration or neutering, which in 80–90% of cases successfully inhibits further spraying. To prevent spraying completely, castration must be done before puberty at an age of up to 6 months (1). Long-term studies that investigated the consequences of early castration at an age of 3 to 4 months have shown that neutering cats of this age from a behavioural point of view should be encouraged and is both medically and surgically routine.

Cleaning

Once the places have been thoroughly cleaned (see Chap. 19.3.1.1), attempts must be made to prevent the cat from using the place again for defaecation or micturition. This can be achieved by placing a litter tray at the site or a piece of furniture or plastic sheeting as a protective device.

Pheromone analogues

A synthetic pheromone analogue, Feliway® (CEVA), has been shown in clinical studies to be successful in 74–98% of cases of spraying after specialist diagnosis and correct use. The affected cats reduced their marking behaviour significantly. Only in a few cases could the preparation alone effectively result in the cats not spraying any more. Accordingly, in individual cases it is sensible to use psychotropic drugs in addition to the above-mentioned therapies.

Medical therapy

Table 19.5: Medications that can be used for the successful treatment of urine marking

	Dosage	Effect
Buspirone Selective serotonin antagonist (5-HT1$_A$)	0.5 mg/kg BID PO	Reduces or prevents marking in 55–74% of cases
Clomipramine Tricyclic antidepressant	0.5 mg/kg SID PO	In the third month of treatment, an 85% reduction in the marking behavior can be observed if a dosage of 0.5–1 mg/kg is given
Fluoxetine Selective serotonin reuptake inhibitor	1 mg/kg SID PO	Reduces the marking behavior by 90% within 8 weeks (6/9 cats)

19.4 Fears and phobias in the dog and cat

Anxiety describes the feeling that an individual has when potential danger threatens. Anxiety is manifested in animals in the form of somatic symptoms such as increased excitability, tension and activity.

Fear is an adaptive response to a specific environmental stimulus. The intensity of the fear which is felt is individually variable but it is usually proportional to the distance from the fear-inducing stimulus.

A phobia is a profound, non-adaptive reaction that is based on an excessive fear of a specific situation or thing. Both dogs and cats try to flee the causative stimulus. In some cases, affected animals react catatonically (freezing).

In addition to a bad experience which an animal has in a certain situation, the most common cause of fears and phobias is a lack of experience. Dogs and cats live through a relatively short period in which they are particularly receptive to learning specific things. The so-called socialisation period (dog: 3rd–12th week of life; cat: 2nd to 7th week of life) allows the animals to collect experiences under the protection of the mother, which then later form their basis of differentiating potentially dangerous environmental stimuli from those which are harmless. Things that are not seen or experienced in this period will induce fear later on. Repeated experience of the fear-inducing stimulus after the end of the socialisation period allows the animal to learn that there is no danger involved. The duration of this training, however, is prolonged and generally proportional to the degree of deprivation during the socialisation period. For example, dogs that are only cared for by adult people during the development phase later react fearfully when confronted with children. If a dog grows up with a cat, there is a low probability that it will demonstrate hunting behaviour towards this species, as long as it is not trained to do so by play. Dogs which come from solitary dog kennels and are then later given up as juvenile or adult dogs, often suffer from generalised fear as common things have never occurred in their environment and the dog has not been allowed to develop the confidence to investigate new things through this type of husbandry.

19.4.1 Fear of animate and inanimate stimuli

Lack of experience and bad experience can lead to dogs and cats reacting with fear in the presence of people, other animals or environmental stimuli (places, noises, smells, etc.). This type of fear includes fear of thunder, fireworks, and even visits to the veterinary surgeon. Dogs quickly learn to associate these things with other stimuli; for example, the sound of thunder is associated with wind and lightening. Some dogs even learn that the changes in atmospheric pressure that occur before a storm are actually associated with a storm. This phenomenon is known as generalisation and it becomes a problem as the fear is no longer just induced by the original stimulus but from a variety of stimuli. Therapy of this situation requires that all possible fear-inducing stimuli are treated. This can be a problem when the fear of thunder is being treated, for example. The use of systematic desensitisation and counter-conditioning can help to overcome fear of thunder. In this situation, the fear-inducing stimulus (thunder) is minimised (playing the sound of thunder from CD at a level that does not induce fear, even though at full power it would cause fear) so that the dog remains calm. Thereafter during the course of the training sessions, an attempt is made to incrementally increase the level of sound. Care should be taken that the dog is not caused to react with panic – such a reaction indicates that the process has been performed too quickly. The aim is to get the dog to cope with the stimulus at its normal intensity (desensitisation). Classical counter-conditioning is aimed at bringing a previously fear-inducing stimulus (thunder) into association with another stimulus (e.g. food) assuming that fear and food intake are incompatible. It is, however, impossible to imitate the drop in pressure during such a training programme. Even if the dog no longer reacts to thunder, it will still react with fear to a drop in air pressure (if it already reacts with fear when a storm is brewing). In such cases, it is imperative to use medication. Fears and phobias that only occur sporadically (thunder) can be treated with the help of benzodiazepines as long-term therapy is not needed. As these substances inhibit short-term memory and the ability, in the sense of conditioning, to couple associations, they should not be used when counter-conditioning is being used. In such cases, it is sensible to use a substance that works on the serotonergic system. Such drugs

include tricyclic antidepressants or selective inhibitors of serotonin reuptake (SSRIs; see Chap. 19.7.4). The spectrum of effects and the selectivity for certain neurotransmitters should be taken into account when selecting a medication. It can be sensible in individual cases to select a drug that is less selective for serotonin when antihistamine effects (doxepin) or anticholinergic effects (amitriptyline) are preferred to serotonin effects (clomipramine or SSRIs).

Transdermal application of antidepressants must be undertaken with great care as the "first-pass effect" is avoided which can increase blood levels of the drug. As yet there is no information about the plasma concentrations following transdermal administration of these drugs.

19.4.2 Situation-related fears and phobias

Separation anxiety in the dog has been given the most attention of all the situation-related fears and phobias. Separation anxiety also occurs in cats if they are very close to their owners. Affected animals behave destructively, are excessively excited or are active and vocal when their reference person is absent. Risk factors that are commonly found in dogs suffering from separation anxiety are change of owners, a stay in an animal home or kennel (because of being put there or the result of being separated from the owner), inadequate acclimatisation to separation as a puppy or kitten, isolation from the owner without step-wise acclimatisation (e.g. 8-hour working day without the dog, following a prolonged period of unemployment), generalised fear of other fear-associated behavioural problems or episodes of separation anxiety that were successfully treated in the past.

Dogs which suffer separation anxiety often show non-specific symptoms such as salivation, tremor, increased locomotion and aggression. For the owner, this is often not a problem unless the dog starts to bark when the owner is away, or does damage to doors or windows, or urinates / defecates in the home.

The degree of separation anxiety differs from case to case:
- The dog will only remain with someone at home.
- The dog will only remain with someone who it knows at home.
- The dog will only remain at home with a specific person.
- No symptoms are seen when the dog can move freely throughout its home.
- The dog can remain alone as long as it can stay in a particular place.
- Clinical signs occur at home but not in the car.
- The dog reacts nervously when it is isolated even though the owner is at home.

19

Before a diagnosis can be made, it is important to eliminate all other differential diagnoses (Table 19.6). It is not uncommon that dogs are presented which, for example, destroy objects whilst the owner is away. Video tapes of the dog in the absence of the owner can either show that suspicion of separation anxiety is correct or that the dog's behaviour is due to another cause (play, lack of training, etc.).

Treatment of separation anxiety is based primarily on behavioural modification. In individual cases it may be sensible to use drugs to support this therapy. Sometimes it is necessary to find short-term solutions when, for example, barking or destructive behaviour forces the owner to find a quick solution (day-care by the neighbour or a friend, doggy day care, etc.). The use of punishment (anti-barking collars, nagging when destroyed objects are found on returning home) is useless and tends to potentiate the fear.

Instead the owner must try not to potentiate the animal's fear by his or her own behaviour. Accordingly, before leaving the dog and on returning home, the dog should be strictly ignored. The majority of owners of dogs with separation anxiety feel uneasy themselves or have a bad conscience due to the daily separation – this feeling can be transferred to the dog and start a viscious circle.

The basis of successful treatment is therefore the establishment of a healthy emotional distance. The interaction between the dog and its owner must be limited. The dog may not continually follow the owner; it must learn to wait behind a closed door and should not be continually rewarded with attention.

The owner must be encouraged to continually leave the house for a short period of time and to return. These "separations" should be variable in their duration and will help the dog to get used to the owner's comings and goings without feeling any fear. This type of training is equivalent to what is normally done when the dog is taken shopping (leave the car for a few minutes, return, drive off, leave the car for a few minutes, etc.).

The dog must be acclimatised to the stimuli which signal separation whilst the owner is at home (keys in hand, putting on of shoes or coat, opening garage door, etc.). As these stimuli reliably occur before a separation, the dog is sub-consciously conditioned (key = separation). The owner must make a list of all the associated stimuli and then present them to the dog in different combinations without leaving the house, until such time as the dog no longer reacts. The aim is that the dog will no longer be able to predict whether the owner is going to leave the house or just going to the post box. Repetition of these exercises leads to acclimatisation so that reactions that are based on fear do not occur.

The use of tricyclic antidepressants (see Chap. 19.7.3) can be anxiolytic and should be used to support the therapy. However, drugs cannot replace training. If the behaviour of the dog makes rapid resolution necessary, they can be treated with a combination of an antidepressant (amitriptyline or clomipramine) or with a benzodiazepine (alprazolam). The anxiolytic effect of antidepressants is usually expected 4 to 6 weeks after the therapy has been started. In contrast, side-effects that are more frequently seen with older medications such as amitriptyline (sedation, dry mouth, etc.) occur immediately. Such side-effects may actually be desirable in individual cases.

The benzodiazepines are reduced stepwise when the effect of the antidepressants start, as dogs can develop tolerance to these compounds. The antidepressants are also reduced stepwise after successful treatment (25% dosage reduction / week for 4 weeks), even though there is no potential for dependency to develop with these drugs.

19.5 Compulsive disturbances

Repetitive behavioural patterns that occur outside of their natural context and serve no specific reason are often described as compulsive disturbances or disturbed impulse control due to their similarity to obsessive-compulsive behaviour in humans (trichotillomania, hand washing, compulsive counting, etc.). According to DSM IV (*Diagnostic and Statistical Manual of Mental Disorders*, American Psychiatric Association, 1994 / 2000), obsessive-compulsive behaviour is an

Table 19.6: Typical symptoms of separation anxiety and examples of differential diagnoses

Symptom	Other causes
Destructive behaviour	Play behaviour, lack of training, environmental stimuli which induce anxiety or territorial behaviour.
Urination	Diseases of the urinary tract, PU/PD (e. g. Cushing's syndrome, corticosteroids), soiling, marking behaviour, submissive urination, cognitive dysfunction.
Defaecation	Changes in diet, parasite infestation, diarrhoea, marking behaviour, soiling, not enough possibilities for animal to relieve itself outside.
Vocalisation	Appreciation of other stimuli, territorial aggression, lack of training.
Excessive grooming	Dermatological disease, acral lick dermatitis.
Hypersalivation	Diseases of the teeth or oral cavity, nausea.
Anorexia	General disease.
Locomotion or lethargy	Age-related behaviour, fear of other stimuli, general disease.

19

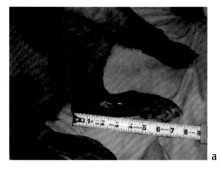 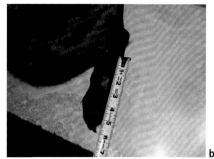 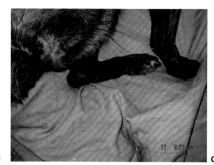

Fig. 19.3a–c
Acral lick dermatitis in a five-year-old Golden Retriever.

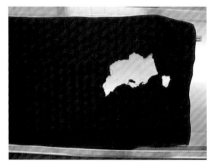 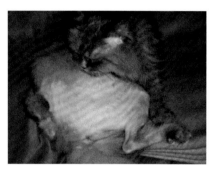

Fig. 19.4
Towel with a hole in it due to compulsive wool chewing in a Siamese.

Fig. 19.5
Cat with psychogenic alopecia. The localised hair loss is a consequence of the cat's continual licking of its abdomen.

anxiety-related behavioural disturbance. As with people, affected animals are significantly more commonly affected by other fear-related behavioural problems. Suboptimal husbandry and stress may be connected with the start of the disturbances or accelerate their progression. They are, however, not the only causes of these types of behavioural problems.

At the moment, due to the similarity of compulsive disturbances in animals with those found in humans and the successful therapy of these conditions with antidepressants that increase the serotonin concentration, it is thought that serotonin plays an important role in the development of compulsive disturbances.

The dopaminergic system is certainly also involved in the development of these problems because experimental application of dopamine agonists can induce sterotypies, while dopamine antagonists suppress this behaviour.

19.5.1 Manifestations of compulsive disturbances in the dog and cat

Acral lick dermatitis was one of the first behavioural problems in the dog that was compared to compulsive hand washing in humans and successfully treated with clomipramine (Fig. 19.3). Other typical compulsive disturbances in the dog include circling, fly catching, licking, sucking at the flanks and aerophagia. Cats exhibit pica (wool chewing) (Fig. 19.4), psychogenic alopecia (Fig. 19.5) and feline hyperaesthesia. Even though changes sometimes occur during the life of any dog or cat, breed-specific predispositions are evident (Doberman: flank sucking and acral lick dermatitis); Bull Terrier and German Shepherd: circling; Siamese: wool chewing), with individual lines or families often affected.

Diagnosis
The diagnosis is attained on the basis of the clinical signs (quality and quantity) and after the elimination of differential

19

diagnoses (neurological or medical, e.g. infection, neoplasia, cauda equina syndrome, pain-related problems, infections of the anal glands, skin diseases, etc.). The repetitive behaviour must be ritualised and the ability of the animal to show normal behavioural patterns with species-specific frequency must be limited.

As dogs respond easily to intermittent rewards it is not uncommon that an owner unknowingly has trained their pet to show a specific behavioural pattern. The effect of the owner can be positive (praise, quietening, etc.) or tend to be more negative (reprimands). Every form of attention can lead to a situation where the behaviour will occur more frequently in the future. So-called attention-seeking behaviour is often considered to be compulsive behaviour. Usually this type of behaviour occurs more often or more intensively in the presence of the owner. A video tape of the dog without the owner being present at home or in the clinic can be diagnostically helpful.

Compulsive running can be connected to a breed-specific need for movement; only in rare cases are dogs clinically hyperactive. Hyperactive dogs react paradoxically. The application of methylphenidate (0.5 mg/kg PO) is used as a diagnostic test (normal reaction: raised cardiac and respiratory rate, increased body temperature and activity). Dogs which show a reduction of these parameters (approx. 15% or more) are classed as hyperactive and treated throughout their life with this substance.

Therapy
The treatment of compulsive disturbances includes a combination of medication and behavioural modification.
- Avoid unconscious reinforcement of unwanted behavioural patterns (extinction) by reacting to the behaviour (praise, quietening, or even rebukes can be interpreted as attention and reinforce the unwanted behaviour).
- Reinforce wanted behaviour (counter-conditioning) helps to replace unwanted behaviour by other behavioural patterns.
- Punishment for unwanted (repetitive or compulsive) behaviour is to be strictly avoided.
- An enrichment of the animal's environment (training, being able to go outside, etc.) and also stress reduction are important components of the therapy when suboptimal husbandry has been determined to have played a role in the development of the problem.
- Medical behavioural therapy is an important component of a successful programme. Substances such as clomipramine, fluoxetine and fluvoxamine have proven to be effective. If no significant improvement has been attained after 6 to 8 weeks, then another substance should be used. When serotonergic substances do not provide the desired result, an attempt to reduce the repetitive behavioural pattern using selegiline should be made (see Chaps. 19.6 and 19.7.6).
- When an effective treatment has been found, the therapy should be continued until success is maintained for a number of weeks. An attempt can then be made to reduce the dosage of the medication in step-wise fashion (10–20% dosage reduction/week). It is often not possible to completely stop the medication, so long-term or lifelong treatment is necessary.

19.6 Cognitive dysfunction in the dog and cat

The term cognitive dysfunction (CD) describes changes in behaviour that occur in the dog and cat late in life, but which cannot be explained by other medical diseases.

Clinical signs that have been found in affected animals include:
- Reduced interest in food.
- Non-recognition of known people, places or other animals.
- Reduced activity or apathy.
- Confusion and disorientation.
- Disturbances in the sleep-wake cycle (night active, disquiet, vocalisation).
- Repetitive or stereotypical behaviour.
- Sudden house soiling or loss of other learned abilities that the animal once had.

The age at which these changes occur varies. Cats are affected at an older age than dogs. About 60% of all 11-year-old dogs show clinical signs of CD. It may already be conspicuous in large breed dogs at an age of 7 years; smaller breeds, in contrast, are first affected at an age of 10 years.

The causes of these changes include reduced organ function and reduced ability of the animal to respond to changes. Cats and dogs that show the aforementioned symptoms have diffuse amyloid plaques which are similar to those found in patients with Alzheimer's disease but are not accompanied by neurofibrillary tangles typical of this disease in humans.

Other problems of older animals associated with behavioural changes are:
- Arteriosclerosis (arterial fibrosis, endothelial proliferation, mineralisation, amyloid deposits).
- Cerebral ischemia.
- Chronic hypoxia as a result of reduced cardiac function.
- Anaemia.
- Hypertension (resulting from other diseases such as diabetes mellitus, hyperthyroidism, renal disease, heart disease).
- Reduction in the number of neurons and increase in number of glial cells.
- Reduction in serotonin concentration in the CNS in comparison to normal adult animals.

19

- Increase in monoamine oxidase B (MAOB) concentration (reduction in dopamine concentration).
- Increase in free radicals.

In addition to the exclusion or treatment of medical and orthopaedic problems, and adaptation of the animal's husbandry to accommodate the requirements of an older animal (increased excretion frequency, problems with climbing stairs, reduced vision and hearing ability, etc.), the treatment of choice is medication to slow down the process and to bring about changes that enable the owner to keep their animal having a good quality of life.

The MAOB inhibitor **selegiline** or **L-deprenyl** is registered for use in several countries for the treatment of fear-related behavioural disturbances in the dog. In some countries (e.g. the USA and Canada), this drug is registered for use in the treatment of CD and Cushing's syndrome (see Chap. 19.7.6). This substance leads to an inhibition of the enzyme MAO, which is localised in various places throughout the body (brain, kidneys, adrenals, liver or thrombocytes) and catalyses the decomposition of dopamine there. The inhibition of MAO leads to an increase in the concentration of cerebral neurotransmitters. MAO is present in two forms, type A and type B. The de-amination of noradrenaline (norepinephrine), adrenaline (epinephrine) and serotonin are predominantly catalysed by MAOA. In comparison, MAOB preferentially catalyses the decomposition of dopamine and phenylethylamine. In the dog, selegiline selectively inhibits MAOB (at least with the administration of daily doses no higher than 1 mg/kg). In some species (e.g. dog and rat), MAOA is responsible for the decomposition of all catecholamines (noradrenaline, adrenaline and dopamine) as well as serotonin, so that selegiline administration induces an increase in the concentration of phenylethylamine but not of dopamine.

Selegiline is mainly metabolised in the liver by the microsomal P450 system to the metabolites N-desmethylselegiline and L-metamphetamine, which are then metabolised to L-amphetamine. The elimination half-life ($t_{1/2}$) is approx. 1.5 hours, but this is increased fourfold when selegiline is given repeatedly (as is the elimination of its metabolite N-desmethylselegiline).

The effects of selegiline (L-deprenyl) include:
- Irreversible (at low doses) selective inhibition of MAOB with a subsequent increase in the concentration of dopamine (human) and phenylethylamine (human, dog and rat).
- It usually takes more than 2 weeks before recovery of the enzyme activity due to renewed synthesis of MAO.
- Strengthening of the catecholaminergic activity due to increase in phenylethylamine caused by inhibition of MAOB.
- Increased turn-over of dopamine.
- Reduced production of free radicals.

- A neuroprotective effect and reduced apoptosis (programmed cell death).
- Increased release of dopamine due to the selegiline metabolite L-metamphetamine.

Side-effects and contraindications associated with selegiline treatment:
- Gastrointestinal disturbances (vomiting and diarrhoea).
- Stereotypical behaviour.
- Hypersalivation (bitter taste).
- Should not be given in combination with substances that also increase the availability of serotonin (SSRIs, tricyclic antidepressants, tryptophan as a serotonin precursor, serotonin antagonists or St. John's Wort extract).
- Serotonin syndrome (characterised by confusion, tremor, fever, ataxia, myoclonia, etc.) when a MAO inhibitor is combined with a serotoninergic substance.
- Should not be given in combination with ephedrine, other MAO inhibitors, other substances with an effect on MAO (e.g. amitraz), pethidine or other opioids.
- When changing from selegiline to the use of a SSRI, there must be a treatment-free period of 2 weeks.
- There must be a treatment-free period when changing from fluoxetine (5 weeks), or any SSRI or tricyclic antidepressant (1 week) to selegiline.

Selegiline should be given for at least 4 to 6 weeks before the efficacy of the treatment can be assessed. If the treatment leads to an obvious improvement in the symptoms, then it should be given for the rest of the animal's life.

The treatment can be supported by changing the animal's diet to a prescription feed (e.g. Hill's b/d) as these feeds are adapted to the requirements of older animals and are thought to biochemically slow down the aging process.

19.7 Medical behavioural therapy

Drugs can be effectively used to support behavioural therapy, when they are utilised in a specific manner (see Table 19.9).

Before using drugs, the following points should be considered:
- A complete list of differential diagnoses must be made on the basis of the symptoms which are causing the problem(s).
- The problem(s) underlying the core of the behaviour are based on a neurotransmitter imbalance. The veterinarian must have a good understanding of the mechanisms of the drugs used as well as knowing their side-effects and interactions. This understanding of the mechanisms is the basis for the choice of suitable substances.
- In order not to create false hopes, the veterinarian must explain the effects of the drugs to the owner as well as their possible side-effects, the duration of the therapy and the prognosis.

19

- Great care is recommended in animals that also have other medical problems, which are old or are being treated with other medications.
- All animals must be carefully examined before the treatment is started (general examination, blood and additional investigations when indicated).

Medical behavioural therapy must be considered as part of a complex integrated treatment programme so that the desired effect is attained. Drugs are not a replacement for behavioural modification under the care of an experienced behavioural therapist. Owners who are expecting a quick solution will not see their hopes fulfilled with the use of drugs alone.

19.7.1 Important neurotransmitter systems

Serotonin (5-hydroxytryptamine or 5-HT) binds to fourteen different receptors. A prominent role is played by the 5-HT1 receptors in the region of the dorsal and medial raphe nuclei, the hippocampus and various regions in the cortex that predominantly influence emotion and behaviour.

The second messenger effects (cAMP, Ca^{++}, cGMP, IP3) are a consequence of a temporary inhibition of serotonin synthesis and serotonin release from the neuron as well as reduced activation of the postsynaptic receptors.

Noradrenaline influences a series of behavioural patterns such as depression (reduced concentration) and manic behaviour (increased concentration). Noradrenaline also plays a role in connection with internal feedback systems that reward behaviour patterns endogenously. The centres for these mechanisms lie in the area of the locus coeruleus, the pons and the lateral tegmental nucleus.

Dopamine plays an important role in the coordination of movements (substantia nigra and striatum, corpus striatum, extrapyramidal system, nucleus accumbens and other areas of the limbic system). Of all the dopamine receptors (D1–D4), the D1 receptors play a special role in connection with stereotypical movements as well as anxiety and depression.

Dopamine is metabolised using MAO (DOPAC and HVA). This enzyme is an important target in the use of selegiline, a MAO inhibitor (see Chap. 19.6).

GABA is a neurotransmitter that has an effect (inhibition) on two receptors (GABA-A and GABA-B) in over 30% of all neurons. Benzodiazepines and barbiturates potentiate the effects of GABA-A.

19.7.2 Benzodiazepines

All benzodiazepines potentiate the effects of GABA by increasing the affinity of the receptors for the neurotransmitter at the GABA-A receptors. The most commonly used substances are diazepam, alprazolam and oxazepam. The effects of diazepam are greatest in the cortex, followed by the limbic system and the brain stem.

The effects of benzodiazepines are mainly dose-dependent:
- Low dose: low degree of sedation.
- Moderate dose: anxiolytic effect and dysinhibition.
- High dose: hypnotic effect (ataxia, muscle relaxation, sedation, etc.).

These substances are often used to treat fears and phobias that tend to occur more rarely (e.g. noise phobia with fireworks). Their use for other fears or phobias should be especially avoided during continual behavioural therapy as it is based on learning and benzodiazepines reduce learning ability.

Therapeutic dosages should provide a calming effect without the occurrence of ataxia or other motor deficits except during the adaptation phase which should only last a few days. Animals can have problems with proprioception during this initial phase and can injure themselves when they try, for example, to jump.

As benzodiazepines are associated with tolerance with continual use and withdrawal symptoms when they are abruptly stopped, the dosage should be reduced stepwise (10–25%/week) once therapy has been completed.

Side-effects
- Increased appetite.
- Temporary ataxia.
- Paradoxically increased excitement (cat).
- Tolerance.
- Impairment of short-term memory.
- Dysinhibition (dangerous when used in already aggressive animals).
- Reduced ability to learn conditioned behavioural patterns (basis for many therapy programmes).
- Idiopathic hepatic necrosis (rare: cat).

Table 19.7: Duration of the effects of diazepam and its active intermediate metabolite, N-desmethyldiazepam, after oral administration to emphasize the danger of accumulation (especially in obese cats)

	Diazepam	N-desmethyldiazepam
Dog	3.2 hours	3–6 hours
Cat	5.5 hours	21 hours

19

The effects of diazepam and especially its active intermediate metabolite, N-desmethyldiazepam, last much longer in cats than in dogs (Table 19.7). There is, therefore, a greater danger of accumulation in cats than in dogs and care must be taken when using diazepam in this species. Oxazepam (cat: 0.2–1.0 mg/kg, BID, PO) has no active intermediary metabolites and is not oxidised so that it should be preferentially used in cats and in animals with liver disease.

19.7.3 Tricyclic antidepressants

Tricyclic antidepressants (TCAs) are closely related to phenothiazine and block the reuptake of monoamines (serotonin, dopamine, norepinephrine and histamine) at the presynaptic level. All antidepressants induce modification of receptors and therefore have a delayed onset of action (4 to 6 weeks) even when the pharmacological effect on the receptor is immediate. Dogs that are treated with clomipramine demonstrate a steady-state plasma concentration within 3 to 5 days. The peak concentration is reached 1 to 3 hours after administration. The half-life of clomipramine in the dog is 1 to 16 hours. The $t_{1/2}$ of the active metabolites is 1 to 2 hours.

Cats cannot metabolise TCAs as well due to their lack of the glucuronidation process. The consequence is a slower drug metabolism, so caution must be taken when using these compounds.

Side-effects
The side-effects of TCAs vary depending on their selectivity for individual neurotransmitter systems (serotonin, noradrenaline, histamine, etc.). Clomipramine acts more selectively on the serotoninergic system than the other drugs within this group (Table 19.8). Accordingly, the side-effects mentioned below are expected to be less with clomipramine than, for example, amitriptyline.

The following side-effects have been described:
- Sedation (antihistamine effect).
- Dry mouth (antimuscarinic effect).
- Constipation (antimuscarinic effect).
- Urine retention (careful in cats: reduced muscle tone and weakness, so urine excretion is reduced).
- Tachycardia and arrhythmia (mainly amitriptyline).
- Ataxia (high dosages).
- Reduced tear production.
- Mydriasis.
- Increased liver enzymes and hepatotoxicity (high dosages).

These side effects are mainly seen in the first weeks of treatment and often disappear during the rest of the therapy.

Contraindications
- Dysrhythmias.
- Urine retention.
- Use with hypertensive drugs.
- Narrow-angle glaucoma.
- Seizures.
- Utilisation within the first 2 weeks after the use of MAO inhibitors.
- Animals that receive thyroid hormone supplements.

19.7.4 Selective serotonin reuptake inhibitors

Selective serotonin reuptake inhibitors (SSRIs) have similar effects as TCAs but they are selective for the serotonin system so that unwanted side-effects (muscarinergic or histaminergic effects) are less problematic, and are especially useful when their slight sedative and antipruritic effects, etc. are not required.

Fluvoxamine reduces the clearance of diazepam and its active metabolites (nordiazepam and alprozolam) so the combined use of these compounds is to be undertaken with care.

Side-effects
- Nausea and vomiting.
- Lethargy.
- Inappetence and loss of weight.
- Tremor and increased excitability (especially fluoxetine).
- Raised liver enzymes.
- Constipation (cat).

Contraindications
- Not in combination with MAO inhibitors (stop at least 2 weeks before the therapy is started; for fluoxetine wait 5 weeks before MAO inhibitors are used).
- Epilepsy.

Table 19.8: Selectivity of the three most commonly used tricyclic antidepressants, and the selective serotonin reuptake inhibitor, fluoxetine, with respect to the neurotransmitters noradrenaline, serotonin and histamine

	Noradrenaline	Serotonin	Histamine
Amitriptyline	++	+	+
Clomipramine	+	+++	++
Doxepin	+	+	+++
Fluoxetine	–	++++	–

19

19.7.5 Buspirone

Buspirone is an azapirone and selective serotonin agonist. It works selectively on the serotonergic 5-HT1$_A$ receptors. The compound has an anxiolytic effect that is comparable to that of the benzodiazepines. Its advantages in comparison with the benzodiazepines include the lack of tolerance development, lack of potential abuse by the owner, and less potential side-effects. A disadvantage of this compound is the delayed onset of action (4 to 6 weeks), so buspirone is more recommended for long-term treatment in combination with behavioural therapy.

Side effects
- Bradycardia / tachycardia.
- Increased excitability.
- Vomiting.
- Diarrhoea.

Contraindications
As with all anxiolytic substances, a reduction in anxiety can lead to an increase in aggressive behaviour when dysinhibition occurs.

19.7.6 Monoamine oxidase B inhibitors

Selegiline is the only monoamine oxidase B (MAOB) inhibitor used at the moment for the treatment of fear-related behavioural problems, compulsive disorders and cognitive dysfunction (see Chap. 19.6). At a therapeutic dosage (< 1mg/kg), the compound is selective for the enzyme MAOB, inhibiting it irreversibly. The MAOB inhibition therefore leads to an increase in dopamine concentration in the CNS. Selegiline also has neuroprotective effects.

Side-effects (see also Chap. 19.6.)
- Hypersalivation (bitter taste).
- Vomiting.
- Diarrhoea.
- Stereotypies (high dosage).

Contraindications (see also Chap. 19.6.)
- Do not give substances that influence the serotonergic system for at least 2 weeks after the cessation of selegiline.

Table 19.9: Overview of the standard recommended dosages of drugs that are routinely used in behavioural therapy

Type	Drug	Recommended oral dosage – dog	Recommended oral dosage – cat
Azapirone / 5-HT1$_A$ agonist	Buspirone	1 mg/kg, SID	0.5 mg/kg, BID
Tricyclic antidepressants	Amitriptyline	2–4 mg/kg, BID	0.5 mg/kg, BID
	Clomipramine	2–4 mg/kg, BID	0.5 mg/kg, SID
	Doxepin	3–5 mg/kg, SID	0.5–1 mg/kg, BID
Selective serotonin reuptake inhibitors	Fluoxetine	1 mg/kg, SID	0.5–1 mg/kg, SID
	Fluvoxamine	1 mg/kg, SID	0.25–1 mg/kg, SID
	Paroxetine	1 mg/kg, SID	0.5–1 mg/kg, SID
Monoamine oxidase B inhibitor	Selegiline	0.5–1 mg/kg, SID	1 mg/kg, SID
Benzodiazepines	Diazepam	0.5–2.2 mg/kg, SID; ideally 1 hour before anxiety-inducing stimulus (e. g. fireworks)	0.5–2.2 mg/kg, SID or BID*
	Alprazolam	0.01–0.1 mg/kg as needed for phobias (no more than 4 mg/dog/day)	0.01–1.0 mg/kg, SID or BID
	Oxazepam	0.2–1.0 mg/kg, SID or BID	0.2–1.0 mg/kg, SID or BID

* Should be given with caution

19

Further reading

BERNAUER-MÜNZ, H., QUANDT, CH. (1995): Problemverhalten beim Hund. Gustav Fischer Verlag, Jena.

LANDSBERG, G., HUNTHAUSEN, W., ACKERMAN, L. (2003): Handbook of Behaviour Problems of the Dog and Cat. W.B. Saunders, Philadelphia.

BOWEN, J., HEATH, S. (2005): Behaviour Problems in Small Animals. Practical Advice for the Veterinary Team. Elsevier Saunders, New York.

HORWITZ, D., MILLS, D., HEATH, S. (2002): BSAVA Manual of Canine and Feline Behavioural Medicine. The British Veterinary Association, Gloucester.

SERPELL, J., JAGOE, J.A. (1995): Domestic Dog: Its evolution, behaviour and interactions with people. Cambridge University Press, Cambridge.

THORNE, C. (1992): The Waltham book of dog and cat behaviour. Waltham centre for pet nutrition, Melton Mowbray.

19

20 Parasitic Neurological Diseases of the Dog and Cat

Peter Deplazes

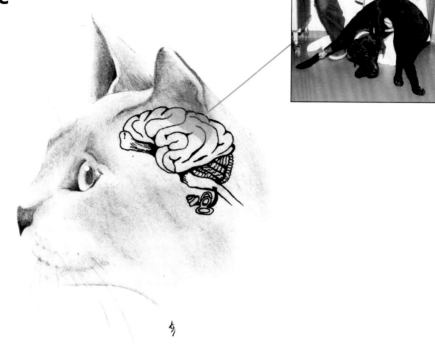

Various helminth and protozoal species are capable of infesting nervous tissue either transiently or permanently. The following overview includes information about a selection of clinically relevant parasites that affect the nervous tissues directly or indirectly via pathophysiological or immunopathological mechanisms.

20.1 Trypanosomiasis in the dog

General information and epidemiology: Trypanosomiasis of the dog is a rare imported disease. Trypanosomes in tropical Africa (*Trypanosoma brucei* and *T. congolense*) are transmitted by the tsetse fly; while in the subtropical areas of Africa, Asia and South America, *T. evansi* is transmitted by tabanid flies and *Stomoxys* spp. Dogs can also become infected by *T. evansi* by ingesting meat from infected herbivores. Another trypanosome species present in South and Central America is *T. cruzi*, which is transmitted by ticks, and is found in up to 30% of dogs and 20% of cats (Chaga's disease). However, as stated at the start, imported trypanosome infections are very rare.

Clinical: Trypanosomiasis can be acute or chronic in the dog. In the acute form, the main symptoms are a febrile, rapidly deteriorating systemic disease causing a loss of condition, anaemia, leukopaenia, thrombocytopaenia, circulatory and respiratory symptoms, multiple generalised haemorrhages and oedema, conjunctivitis and corneal clouding (1, 2). Except for *T. congolense*, CNS symptoms can occur due to a meningoencephalomyelitis associated with the presence of extravascular trypanosomes (3). In such cases, death takes only a few days. Neurological signs may also occur as part of a chronic clinical picture and are determined by the location of the parasitic migration.

Diagnosis: The extracellular trypanosomes in the blood can be diagnosed by staining them in blood smears with Giemsa.

Therapy: Treatment can be tried with quinapyramine sulphate (5 mg/kg, SC) or isomethamidium (0.25–1 mg/kg, IM). Both medications, however, are associated with severe side-effects (4).

20.2 Neosporosis in the dog

General information: The taxonomic position of *Toxoplasma gondii* and *Hammondia heydorni* are very close, while that of *Neospora caninum*, a species described in 1984, remains controversial (4, 5). Infection with *N. caninum* is increasingly associated with paralysis and death in the dog, as well as abortion and neonatal deaths in cattle and small ruminants.

20

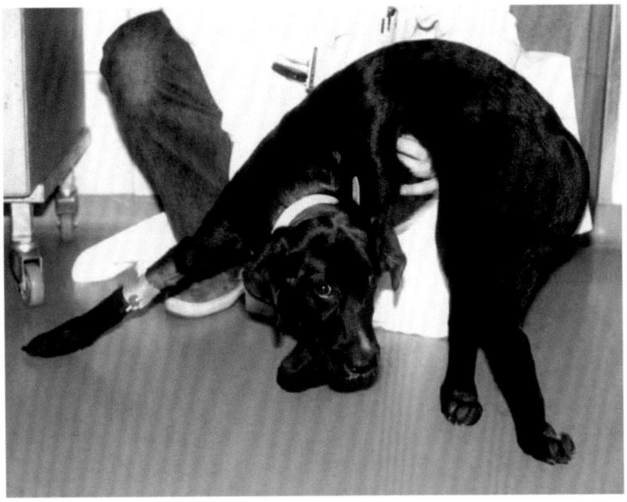

Fig. 20.1
Young dog with acute neosporosis showing severe generalised weakness (had to be supported), spontaneous knuckling and increased proximal extensor tone of the hindlimbs. (Fig.: Institute for Parasitology, Zurich.)

The latest data convincingly demonstrate that *N. caninum* is one of the most important causes of abortion in cattle in Europe and is widely geographically distributed (6). Infections with *Neospora* have not as yet been reported in humans.

Epidemiology: Using experimental infections, it has been shown that the dog can be a final host of *N. caninum*. In addition, naturally infected dogs have been shown to excrete *Neospora* oocytes (8). In comparison, the fox does not appear to be a suitable final host (9). The epidemiological importance of the dog as final host is still unclear; however, seroepidemiological studies in the dog and cattle have consolidated the fact that the dog must be considered as being an infection risk for cattle (10). Extensive studies of the prevalence of oocyte excretors are not available; however, the number of excretors is thought to be very small (4, 7). Serological investigations in different European countries revealed a large difference in prevalence (< 1% to approx. 50%) depending on the dog population and the origin of the animal (4, 6, 7, 11). The interpretation of serological results in the dog is additionally made difficult by the fact that an intestinal infestation does not always lead to seroconversion (12).

20

Two different modes of transmission have been recorded in the dog: the oral uptake of cysts with ingestion of tissue from an intermediate host (mainly cattle and small ruminants), and intrauterine infection of the foetus. The epidemiological significance of an infection due to the intake of sporulated oocysts from the environment is uncertain. Infection through the ingestion of intermediate host tissues with cysts has been experimentally proven. After the feeding of infected placenta to dogs, all animals excreted *N. caninum* oocytes for three days

after the first infection. After a repeated infection 5 weeks later, there was no oocyte excretion, which indicates the development of a protective intestinal immunity (12). Sources of infection especially include muscle tissue, nervous tissue, placenta and aborted foetuses from cattle, though other herbivores should also be considered as potential sources.

Transplacental transmission has been presumed in the majority of previously described clinical cases in young dogs (13). It is especially remarkable that repeated transplacental transmission can occur in the same bitch (14). An epidemiological study in England, however, came to the conclusion that transplacental transmission of *Neospora* is not sufficient to maintain the parasite within a dog population. More than 80% of puppies born to bitches chronically infected with *Neospora* were not infected (15).

Clinical: Clinical cases of neosporosis in the dog have been described throughout the world in various breeds (see for example 13, 14, 16, 17, 18). The disease is particularly severe in puppies and young dogs (< 1 year old) and results in high mortality rates. Several siblings in a litter can be seropositive; however, they are often affected with differing degrees of disease severity and progression. The most common neurological symptom, especially in young dogs, is an ascending paralysis of the hindlimbs caused by polymyositis and polyradiculoneuritis (Fig. 20.1). In 21 dogs proven to have neosporosis and that were starting to show ascending hindlimb weakness, BARBER and TREES (17) observed the following clinical symptoms: muscle atrophy (78%); spastic hyperextension (53%); paralysis (52%); pain in the lumbar and pelvic or quadriceps muscles (35%); head tilt, dysphagia and incontinence (24% each). In the generalised form, changes in various organs can occur and are manifested as myositis, myocarditis, ulcerative dermatitis, pneumonia and meningoencephalomyelitis, etc. In chronic cases, aggression, depression and other changes in behaviour has also been observed in older dogs.

Asymptomatic infections can persist for years. Outbreak of the disease, or even clinical deterioration, has been described in various cases as being associated with partial immunodeficiency due to some other aetiology; for example, in association with leishmaniasis in conjunction with steroid therapy or high doses of immunosuppressive medication. The clinical manifestation of neosporosis has been associated with vaccination in a number of cases (19); although as vaccination is in the anamnesis of many young dogs, this should be interpreted with care.

Diagnosis: Routine CBC and blood biochemistry are of little significance in the diagnosis of neosporosis.

In the neuromuscular form of neosporosis, the diagnostic methods of choice in the dog are serology (IFAT, ELISA) and the use of PCR. The demonstration of specific antibodies or antigen, is highly sensitive and specific. However, in assessing the results of serology, it is important to take into consideration that specific antibodies against *N. caninum* can be found in clinically sound dogs.

Direct demonstration of the parasite in the live dog is less sensitive than serology. In acute infections (in untreated animals), the parasite can be cultivated *in vitro* from the CSF or muscle biopsies (endozoites = tachyzoites) or can be demonstrated using specific antibodies. Endozoites (5–7 × 1–5 μm) replicate in macrophages, granulocytes, myocytes, neurocytes and other cells. These *N. caninum* stages differ from *T. gondii* with respect to their molecular and antigenic make-up, and in their fine structure. The cytozoite-containing cysts that are present in the chronic disease are up to 100 μm long and have a relatively thick cyst wall (in contrast to *T. gondii*). These less pathogenic stages can be demonstrated using immunohistochemistry. They can be found in nerve and muscle tissues and in the retina; however, they are difficult to demonstrate in the living animal (20). The most sensitive and specific demonstration of *N. caninum* in tissue samples can be achieved with the previously mentioned tissues using PCR, though the developmental stages cannot be differentiated using this method (21).

In intestinal infestations, the presence of oocytes (10–11 μm) can be proven with a sedimentation-flotation method. The differentiation of the morphologically identical oocytes from *Hammondia* and *Toxoplasma* (only excreted in the cat) can currently only be done by animal testing in rodents or by specific PCR (8, 12).

Therapy: DUBEY and LINDSAY (14) achieved clinical recovery in dogs infected with *N. caninum* with a 4-week treatment of sulfadiazine / trimethoprim (Tribrissen®, Pittman-Moore) 15 mg/kg, BID, PO combined with pyrimethamine (Daraprim®, Wellcome) 1 mg/kg PO, daily. A similar success was achieved with sulfadiazine / trimethoprim combined with clindamycin (Antirobe®, Upjohn) at a dosage of 13.5 mg/kg, BID, PO for 10 days. Ten of sixteen animals with neuromuscular symptoms responded well to treatment using the sulfadiazine / trimethoprim and clindamycin combination, though over a period of 13 to 60 days (independent of the clinical course and the medication given) (17). Toltrazuril and panazuril in the drinking water (20 mg/kg) prevented cyst production in treated mice by approx. 90% (22); however, the chemotherapeutic and curative use of these substances have not be tested in the dog.

Prognosis: The prognosis for the success of the medical treatment of neosporosis is dependent on the time and clinical course of the disease. The probability of recovery with an early diagnosis can be more favourable. Puppies with the acute form of disease leading to paresis within a few days respond less well to treatment than animals with a more chronic form. Dogs suffering from relapses respond well clinically to repeating the chemotherapy. Currently, it is not clear whether complete elimination of the parasite is possible.

Prophylaxis: Dogs should not be fed with raw meat and brain tissue. They should also not be allowed access to material from abortions or placentas. Different authors have recommended that infected females should not be used for breeding.

20.3 Toxoplasmosis in the cat and dog

General information: *Toxoplasma gondii* is found throughout the world and causes chronic persistent infections in a broad range of mammals and birds. Usually this protozoal parasite has a very low pathogenicity in immune-competent hosts (including humans) and induces a protective immunity of long duration in its host. In Europe up to 57% of pregnant women are seropositive (23). *T. gondii* is, however, one of the most important zoonotic organisms that causes prenatal infections, abortion and foetopathies. It can also cause generalised and cerebral forms of toxoplasmosis in AIDS patients. Both dogs and humans rarely become infected with an active *Toxoplasma* infection. The cat is the only final host and excretor of oocysts; however, this species can also become affected by an extra-intestinal infection with this organism.

Epidemiology: The cat is the only relevant final host of *T. gondii* and so it is at the hub of the organism's epidemiology. Excretion occurs 3 to 9 days after the ingestion of tissue oocytes. The prepatent period after the ingestion of oocysts is 20 to 35 days. Oocyst excretion lasts for 1 to 20 days after a first infection and up to 600 million oocysts can be released. In Central Europe, 0.1–6.0% of cats excrete *T. gondii* oocysts in their faeces. BEELITZ et al. (24) showed the presence of *Toxoplasma / Hammondia* oocytes in 12 / 70 litters of kittens (17.1%) born on farms. Specific antibodies could be found in the serum of up to 71% of cats and 85% of dogs in Europe (23).

Extreme differences in the prevalence of the organism are to be expected in both species due to the different age structures and origins of the investigated populations (urban and rural populations, pets, feral, etc.).

Infection of the cat and dog occurs due to the ingestion of either *T. gondii* cysts in raw meat from the intermediate hosts (sheep, goat, pig, rabbit or wild animals such as rodents and birds) or sporulated oocysts. Another form of transmission found both in the cat and dog is intrauterine infection of the foetus (4).

20

Clinical: In young cats, a massive first time infection can lead to diarrhoea during the **intestinal phase** due to parasite replication. Such animals excrete millions of oocysts over just a few days. Older cats rarely show any signs of disease after a first infection, and clinical disease hardly ever occurs in such animals, even after re-infection.

The **parenteral phase** of the infection (cat as intermediate host) is rarely associated with clinical signs. In the evaluation of 100 lethal cases in cats in the USA (aged 2 weeks to 16 years), 36 cases of generalised toxoplasmosis, 26 pulmonary, 16 abdominal, 7 neurological and 6 other forms could be differentiated (25). In another 9 cases, the toxoplasmosis was neonatal. Intra-ocular inflammation was diagnosed in 22 of 27 cats investigated.

After inducing experimental first time infections during pregnancy, DUBEY *et al.* (26) observed no clinical signs in five queens, though 16 to 31 days after infection, 22 living and 3 dead kittens were born to these cats. Within the following 2 to 16 days, 21 kittens died (or had to be euthanised). Disseminated toxoplasmosis could be diagnosed in all these animals. The pathology results in the 21 kittens included: interstitial pneumonia (21 / 21), necrotising hepatitis (20 / 21), myocarditis (21 / 21), myositis of the skeletal musculature (21 / 21), generalised nonpurulent encephalitis (18 / 18), uveitis (19 / 19) and interstitial nephritis (16 / 21). It is probable that the significance of neonatal toxoplasmosis in weak neonates is underestimated both in the cat and dog, and is often not clarified aetiologically. After reinfection, usually no clinical signs occur in immune-competent animals, and oocyte excretion in the cat is very much reduced or ceases totally.

Simultaneous infections with feline leukaemia virus (FeLV) or the feline immunodeficiency syndrome virus (FIV) appear to unfavourably influence the course of a toxoplasmosis infection in a few exceptional cases (25). In reactive forms, a renewed oocyst excretion can occur in the cat.

As *Toxoplasma* and *Neospora* infections in the dog were not differentiated before 1986, some clinical information regarding toxoplasmosis in this species still requires confirmation. According to ROMMEL (4), three forms of toxoplasmosis can occur in the dog: (1) a generalised form that occurs in 7- to 12-month-old dogs with clinical signs of intermittent fever, tonsillitis, dyspnoea, diarrhoea and vomiting; (2) a CNS form that occurs in dogs over 4 months of age; and (3) a radiculoneuritis in puppies under 3 months of age that is characterised by progressive paralysis or paresis. A massively disseminated toxoplasmosis infection has been reported in dogs with neuromuscular symptoms in association with distemper (27).

Diagnosis: Cats can be investigated with respect to the excretion of *Toxoplasma / Hammondia* oocytes in their faeces, serologically, or with PCR. As *Toxoplasma* and *Hammondia* oocytes cannot be differentiated morphologically, they are referred to as *Toxoplasma*-like oocytes under practical conditions due to their potential zoonotic danger. A parenteral infection in the cat can be diagnosed serologically. An attempt at diagnosing a new infection can be done by the determination of IgM or with an avidity test (4). The demonstration of tachyzoites is rarely successful in active infections, e.g. respiratory or CNS forms (microscopic investigation or PCR on nasal or bronchial secretions, or the CSF).

In the **dog**, neosporosis must be considered in the differential diagnosis of clinical toxoplasmosis in the living animal. As a large proportion of healthy adult dogs have specific antibodies against *T. gondii*, serological results must be considered with care and only in association with the clinical picture.

Therapy: Intestinal toxoplasmosis in the **cat** is usually self-limiting; 80–95% of the oocytes are excreted within the first 3 days of the patent period! Chemotherapy is usually not required; however, it can be attempted with sulphonamides, spiramycin or clindamycin.

Chemotherapy of extra-intestinal toxoplasmosis makes sense when there are clinical signs. An asymptomatic infestation with tissue cysts cannot be influenced with the currently available medications and so is not necessary. According to ROMMEL (4), the following treatments are available: clindamycin hydrochloride (10–12 mg/kg, BID, PO for 4 weeks), clindamycin phosphate (12.5–25 mg/kg, BID, IM for 4 weeks) or sulphadiazine plus trimethoprim (12.5 plus 2.5 mg/kg, BID, PO for 4 weeks).

Treatment in the **dog**: as for neosporosis (see Chap. 20.2).

Prophylaxis: Prophylaxis used mainly for the prevention of oocyte excretion in the cat (chemoprophylaxis and immunoprophylaxis) has been shown to be promising under experimental conditions (4). It is to be expected that in the near future suitable products will appear on the market.

20.4 Babesiosis in the dog

General information: *Babesia canis* is a large species of Babesia (approx. 4–5 µm). It is a strict intracellular parasite of canine erythrocytes. Two subspecies occur in Europe, *B. canis canis* transmitted by the tick *Dermacentor reticulates* (rarely by *D. marginatus*) and *B. canis vogeli* transmitted by *Rhipicephalus sanguineus*. These subspecies cannot be differentiated from each other morphologically. Babesia infections are often imported to Central Europe in dogs or ticks. *Babesia canis* (*B. canis canis*, *B. canis vogeli*, *B canis rossi*) and *B. gibsoni* are reported in the USA and are often spread by *Ixodes* ticks, the brown dog tick (*Rhipicephalus sanguineus*) and *Dermacentor variabilis*.

Epidemiology: The endemic areas of canine babesiosis are dependent on the distribution of the carrier tick. Southern Europe, parts of Western and Eastern Europe and south eastern, central and western states in the USA are considered as being endemically affected. Indigenous endemic foci are known to occur north of the Alps, e.g. in France, the Netherlands and in Germany (28). The indigenous occurrence of *B. canis* in Switzerland has also been ascertained. It is known from general practice that the number of babesiosis cases in the Swiss cantons of Genf and Jura, including the surrounding midlands, have increased greatly.

Pathogenesis: *B. canis vogeli* is less pathogenic than *B. canis canis* (29). The most important disease characteristic of babesiosis is intravascular haemolysis with the subsequent development of anaemia. The increased adhesion of erythrocytes to the capillary endothelium leads to "clumping" of blood in the capillaries, with subsequent circulatory stasis and vasodilatory shock (30). The cerebral disturbances seen in this disease are also due to the adhesion of the erythrocytes in the cerebral capillaries and the resulting capillary occlusion.

Clinical: The incubation period for *B. canis* is 7 to 21 days. Dogs of all breeds and ages are susceptible, although at least in the USA, Greyhounds seem to be predisposed. Puppies tend to be more severely affected, as are dogs which are taken into endemic areas (anamnesis including travelling and/or tick exposure).

Acute and peracute forms: High fever with exhaustion and inappetence, loss of weight, progressive anaemia and thrombocytopaenia, as well as reduced haemoglobin and haematocrit values dominate the clinical picture. Usually icterus and splenomegaly are notable. Massive haemoglobinuria is due to the destruction of the erythrocytes. Less common complications include gastrointestinal and respiratory disturbances, oedema, ascites, muscle inflammation and mucosal haemorrhages. Acute renal failure has also been described as a consequence of acute babesiosis.

The cerebral form of babesiosis, caused by capillary occlusion and subsequent ischemia, is characterised by incoordination, paresis, muscle tremor, nystagmus, epileptiform seizures, disturbances in consciousness and coma. In the peracute form the symptoms occur within 24 hours. Without therapy, both the peracute and acute forms can be lethal.

The clinical signs of **chronic babesiosis** are variable. Affected dogs are usually very weak and obtunded. The predominant sign is anaemia; increases in body temperature or icterus are usually less significant signs.

Therapy: A single dose of 3–6 mg/kg, SC of imidocarb diproprionate (Imizol® or Carbesia®, Schering-Plough) is adequate for successful therapy in many cases. If the clinical signs remain, the treatment can be repeated after 14 days. Phenamidine (Oxipirvedine®, Rhône Mérieux) 15 mg/kg, SC, single dose (repeat after 48 hours) has a comparable effect. Both preparations have relatively strong side-effects and must be dosed exactly (4). In the majority of cases, the dogs respond well to the medication within 24 hours. In advanced stages of the disease, the patient should be also treated symptomatically (e.g. for shock).

Prophylaxis: Different prophylactic strategies can be chosen for dogs living in endemic areas or for animals going to such areas. Tick prophylaxis can be recommended in all cases. An inactivated vaccine, Piradog® (Merial), is sold in many countries. The time factor for basic immunisation of a dog with this vaccine must be taken into consideration, as its effect starts 1 to 2 weeks after the booster. The vaccine protects against severe clinical disease though not against infection. In addition, the vaccine is not equally effective against all *B. canis* strains (30).

Dogs can be protected against babesiosis with chemotherapy especially for short trips. A single dose of imidocarb at a dose of 2.4–6 mg/kg protects dogs for 2 to 6 weeks, depending on the *B. canis* strain and the sensitivity of the dog (30). No clinical symptoms occurred in experimentally infected dogs given a daily dose of doxycycline (20 mg/kg, PO), though parasite invasion was not totally suppressed (31). The daily oral application of doxycycline protects against ehrlichiosis at the same time, which is also transmitted by ticks (see Table 20.1).

20.5 Acanthamoeba infections

Free-living amoeba of the genus Acanthamoeba and other genera can sometimes be found as pathogens in animals and humans. Acanthamoeba was isolated and cultivated from a lung biopsy taken from a puppy with a lethal pneumonia and granulomatous encephalitis (32).

The diagnosis of this disease is achieved by culture isolation and PCR in a specialised laboratory (human medicine). The infrequent occurrence of such rare, lethal cases must also be considered.

20.6 Encephalitozoonosis

General information: Microsporidia are spore-producing eukaryotes with an obligatory intracellular development. They have only just been designated taxonomically as being related to fungi. The most important species in veterinary medicine, *Encephalitozoon cuniculi*, infects a broad spectrum of mammals including humans (it is important as an opportunistic pathogen in immune-deficient patients) (33). *E. cuniculi* is particularly important in rabbits, rodents, monkeys and carnivores. *E. cuniculi* has been divided into three strains according to epidemiological data and by using immunological and molecular methods. In Europe, the rabbit strain occurs in AIDS patients and is often found in domestic and pigmy rabbits. Encephalitozoonosis is the most common cause of neu-

20

rological symptoms in rabbits, and is mainly manifested as head tilt. In the USA, there is a highly pathogenic dog strain that affects dogs, but which has also been found in AIDS patients and in South American monkeys. In the latter, it induced high mortality in young animals in Zurich Zoo. The mouse strain occurs in mice and rats, and it has been responsible for large losses in the breeding colonies of farm foxes in Scandinavia. However, the mouse strain has not been found in any other domestic animals or in humans.

Epidemiology: A common characteristic of all microsporidia is the formation of resistant, 2-μm long exospores that are excreted in the urine of affected animals. After oral infection, there is dissemination of *E. cuniculi* throughout the body, most probably by passive transfer in the blood or in migrating host cells. Another method of transmission is the intrauterine infection of the foetus. This mode of transmission is especially important in foxes, monkeys and dogs. As with neosporosis, the dam can infect her young of subsequent pregnancies. Experimentally orally infected dogs remain chronically infected without becoming ill.

Clinical: The majority of cases of encephalitozoonosis that have been described in carnivores affected young dogs and puppies in the USA and South Africa, more rarely cats and caged fur animals (blue and silver foxes, mink). The clinical signs in affected puppies result from meningitis, encephalitis and nephritis, and must be differentiated from distemper. The main symptoms include anorexia, loss of weight, weakness, depression, ataxia, tremor, blindness, convulsions and sometimes aggression (34). The mortality in affected litters can be up to 100%. These parasites are often found disseminated throughout the whole brain and can be demonstrated in the kidneys, spleen, liver, eyes, spinal cord and urine (35).

At present, only individual cases of microsporidiosis have been reported in the cat; for example, in a Siamese with neurological disturbances. A nonpurulent meningoencephalitis and interstitial nephritis were diagnosed on histological investigation. Encephalitozoon-like spores were observed in the animal's brain, kidneys, spleen and lymph nodes (33).

Diagnosis: The diagnostic methods of choice in carnivores include the very specific and sensitive serological tests (IFAT, ELISA). Demonstration of exospores in the urine sediment is infrequent but possible. Using various special stains with specific antibodies or PCR, an attempt at demonstrating *E. cuniculi* in the live animal can be made using urine or biopsy material.

Therapy and Prophylaxis: At the moment, no experience with respect to treatment and prophylaxis of encephalitozoonosis in canids is available. It is known from human medicine that albendazole has a good efficacy. In rabbits, the prophylactic application of fenbendazole in the food prevented clinical signs after experimental infection with *E. cuniculi* exospores (36). Fenbendazole treatment (20 mg/kg, daily, PO) for 4 weeks, in combination with corticosteroids in some cases, induced clinical improvement in some rabbits affected by head tilt.

20.7 Neurological diseases caused by helminths

Helminths can damage nervous tissue either by inducing space-occupying effects (e.g. cestode larvae) or by larval migration (e.g. cestodes or nematodes).

20.7.1 Infection with space-occupying cysticerci

In dogs, rare infections of the brain with tape worm cysticerci (e.g. from *Taenia solium, T. pisiformis, T. multiceps* or *Echinococcus granulosus*) have been described (37). The clinical symptoms are variable and depend on the location of the infection. A tentative diagnosis can be achieved using imaging techniques. A definite parasitological diagnosis can be achieved using histopathological samples (morphology, specific antigen test or PCR). Measuring the antibody titre against various larval antigens can be attempted serologically. The diagnosis of these very rare parasites can only be done in specialised laboratories.

These very rare infections of the brain have also been diagnosed in the cat; for example, an infection with a cenurus from *Taenia serialis* (38).

20.7.2 Infection with migrating larvae

During their complicated migration through the body, nematode larvae can sometimes cross the blood-brain barrier and enter the CNS. The consequences of larval migration (which may last for months) include haemorrhage, tissue destruction and inflammatory reactions with the formation of granulomatous foci. The neurological clinical picture described in humans due to visceral larval migrans of the dog and cat roundworms (*Toxocara canis* and *T. mystax*) is not known in the dog and cat, although these larvae have been found in the CNS of both species (37).

20.7.3 Angiostrongylosis of the dog

General information: *Angiostrongylus vasorum* is a nematode of the vascular system and the lungs. It occurs in the fox and also in the dog. Various endemic areas for the disease in the fox are known to occur in Europe; for example, in Italy

(Toscana), west and south France, Ireland, Great Britain and Denmark (region around Copenhagen) (37). This worm has also been reported in naturally infected animals in the Canadian provinces on the Atlantic coast but not in the USA. Imported cases have been described from various European countries, though in the past few years increasingly more indigenous cases in Switzerland have been observed (39). Due to the large increase in the fox population, there is a danger that angiostrongylosis will also become more disseminated in the dog population in Europe.

Epidemiology: The adult worms live in the pulmonary artery and in the right chamber of the heart. The larvae reach the alveoli of the lungs via the circulation. They penetrate here and then travel to the gastrointestinal tract via the trachea. Finally, they are excreted in the faeces. The sources of infection for the final host are the slugs, snails (e.g. *Arion* spp.) or frogs that act as intermediate hosts.

Clinical: The main symptoms are cardiopulmonary with a chronically progressive course after a month-long incubation period. Infected dogs show progressive weight loss, coughing, vomiting, dyspnoea and tire quickly. The infection is often lethal due to the increasingly severe circulatory disturbances and pneumonia (37).

The neurological manifestation of angiostrongylosis can be due to either cerebral hypoxia or hemorrhagic diathesis with subdural haemorrhages (37, 39, 40). In dogs with *A. vasorum*, however, the larvae have been found disseminated throughout the CNS or spinal cord, and were seen to be the cause of haemorrhage and inflammatory changes (40, 41). The neurological symptoms are manifold and can occur independently of the typical cardiopulmonary symptoms. A very progressive course has been reported in various cases, leading to complete paresis, loss of consciousness and coma.

Diagnosis: The larvae of *A. vasorum* can be demonstrated in the faeces or from bronchial secretion using the Baermann Test.

Therapy: Fenbendazole has been used successfully at a dosage of 20–50 mg/kg PO once or twice daily for 1 to 3 weeks (37). Milbemycin (0.5 mg/kg, PO) once a week for 4 weeks was also effective in 15 of 16 naturally infected male dogs (30, 37, 39).

20.8 Neurological diseases caused by arthropods

Tick paralysis is a toxicosis that has been described clinically as a localised or generalised disease of the peripheral nervous system in mammals and birds. It is transmitted by roughly 40 species of ticks found in the US, Australasia, the Tropics and Subtropics. Tick paralysis has not been described in cats and dogs in Europe. A similar neurological disease can occur

after a massive infection with *Neotrombicula autumnalis* (Harvest mite). In two Yorkshire Terriers infested with at least 2,000 *N. autumnalis*, paresis of the hindlimbs with concomitant reddy orange deposits all over the skin was seen a few hours after the infestation with the mites began. The clinical picture worsened within 24 hours, ending in a total collapse of both animals. The condition of the dogs improved (within a few days) only after bathing with acaricides (42). A similar case of *Neotrombicula* toxicosis was reported from a private practice: a massively infested cat developed epileptiform seizures and progressive paresis.

Ticks can also transmit viral, bacterial and eukaryote disease agents to dogs and cats. A selection of such diseases found in the dog and cat in Europe are shown in Table 20.1.

20.9 Borreliosis

General information: The spirochete *Borrelia burgdorferi* is the causative agent of Lyme's disease (43). This tick-transmitted bacterial zoonosis has a wide distribution in Central Europe and the USA in both humans and animals (44). Within the *B. burgdorferi* group, 142 isolates from Europe could be subdivided into the following species: *B. garinii* (44%), *B. afzelii* (27%), *B. burgdorferi* sensu stricto (15%) and *B. valaisiana* (10.5%) (45). In comparison, *B. burgdorferi* is the most common species in the USA.

Epidemiology: According to investigations in Central Europe up to 34% of ticks (*I. ricinus*) are infected with *Borrelia* (46, 47). *Borrelia* have also been found in the hedgehog tick (*I. hexagonus*). Serological studies in dogs in Central Europe reveal a prevalence of up to 35%; however, in such studies the chosen dog population and the tests used should be considered critically.

Clinical: It is known from experimental infections and serological studies that asymptomatic carriers often occur in the dog. The incubation period is 2 to 5 months (48). The subdivision of Lyme's disease into three main stages as is done in humans is not suitable for the dog. The clinical picture in the dog has only been determined for *B. burgdorferi*. It mainly involves a disturbed general well-being with anorexia, fever and a relapsing lameness due to arthritis which responds to antibiotic therapy (48). The chronic erythema migrans frequently found in humans is only rarely seen in the dog (49).

An occurrence of neurological symptoms in combination with canine borreliosis is presumed to occur by some (50); however, this is doubted by many authors. In 20 dogs experimentally infected with *B. burgdorferi* given dexamethasone, 12 dogs became ill with fever and intermittent lameness. The histopathological investigation showed that three of these dogs had meningitis, one dog developed a mild focal encephalitis, and 18 dogs had perineuritis (51).

20

Table 20.1: Infectious diseases of the dog transmitted by ticks[1]

Disease: Infectious disease (tick responsible for transmission)	Main clinical picture and neurological symptoms
■ **Anaplasmosis** (ehrlichiosis): *Anaplasma* (*Ehrlichia*) *phagocytophilum*, causative agent of granulocytic ehrlichiosis (*Ixodes ricinus* in Europe; *Ixodes scapularis* and *Ixodes pacificus* in USA)	Febrile, transient thrombocytopaenia, mild anaemia, disturbed well-being, unwillingness to move and lameness (55). Meningitis and meningoencephalitis reported in dogs.
■ **Babesiosis:** *Babesia canis vogeli*, (*Rhipicephalus sanguineus*), *B. canis canis* (*Dermacentor reticularis*) in Europe; *Babesia canis* (*B. canis canis; B. canis vogeli; B canis rossi*) and *B. gibsoni* are reported in the USA and are often spread by *Ixodes* ticks, the brown dog tick (*Rhipicephalus sanguineus*) and *Dermacentor variabilis*.	Acute febrile generalised disease with increasing anaemia and thrombocytopaenia, haemoglobinuria, acute renal failure. The cerebral form, caused by capillary occlusion and subsequent ischemia, although rare, is characterised by paresis, nystagmus, epileptiform seizures, disturbances in consciousness and coma (4).
■ **Borreliosis:** *Borrelia burgdorferi* sensu lato (*Ixodes ricinus, I. hexagonus, Dermacentor* spp.)	For *B. burgdorferi* sensu stricto: disturbed general well-being, fever and recurrent arthritis; central and peripheral neurological symptoms are presumed to occur, however, this is contentious (50, 51).
■ **Ehrlichiosis** (tropical pancytopaenia and canine monocytic ehrlichiosis): *Ehrlichia canis* (*Rhipicephalus sanguineus*); *Ehrlichia chaffeensis* and *Ehrlichia ewingii* (*Amblyoma americanum*)	Febrile, generalised disease with obtundation, and lymphadenopathy. The chronic course is characterised by fever, pancytopaenia, anaemia and the tendency for spontaneous haemorrhaging (nose, eyes). It is particularly severe in the German Shepherd. The neurological symptoms are associated with meningitis: hyperaesthesia, ataxia, vestibular deficits (54, 55) Meningoencephalitis causing seizures, paraparesis or tetraparesis, vestibular dysfunction, generalized or localized hyperesthesia, cranial nerve deficits, intention tremors of the head, and coma. Fundic lesions, including retinal hemorrhage, chorioretinal exudate, or retinal detachment.
■ **Filariasis:** *Ceropithifilaria grassi, Dipetalonema dracunculoides* (*Rhipicephalus sanguineus*)	Subclinical infestation (37).
■ **Hepatozoonosis:** *Hepatozoon canis* (*Rhipicephalus sanguineus*)	Febrile generalised disease with unwillingness to move, muscle weakness, muscle pain, paresis and paralysis with extensive myositis (4, 56, 57).
■ **Rocky Mountain Spotted Fever:** *Rickettsia rickettsii* (*Dermacentor andersoni* and *Dermacentor variabilis*)	Febrile, obtundation, and lymphadenopathy. Meningoencephalitis causing seizures, paraparesis or tetraparesis, vestibular dysfunction, generalized or localized hyperesthesia, cranial nerve deficits, intention tremors of the head, and coma. Fundic lesions, including retinal hemorrhage, chorioretinal exudate, or retinal detachment.
■ **Spring-summer meningoencephalitis:** SSME virus (*Ixodes ricinus, Dermacentor* spp.)	Febrile generalised disease which within a few days can lead to massive CNS deficits: nausea, nervousness, seizures, ataxia, tetraparesis, tetraplegia (53).

[1] Selection of parasites only; not included are *Anaplasma* (*Ehrlichia*) *platys, Rickettsia conorii*, etc.

Diagnosis: Anamnesic information such as tick infestation in known *Borrelia* endemic areas, clinical symptoms, serology and response to antibiotic therapy all enable a tentative diagnosis of borreliosis to be made. The **direct demonstration** of *Borrelia* can be made from synovial fluid under a dark-field microscope or in culture. *Borrelia* can be isolated from the urine, blood and internal organs in febrile dogs. The most sensitive test is PCR and, nowadays this is recommended as being the method of choice.

Indirect demonstration of *Borrelia* can be performed with serological methods (IFAT, ELISA, haemagglutination or Western blot). High genus specificity is attained with Western blot. Infections with different *Borrelia* spp. and genotypes, however, cannot be distinguished serologically. After experimental infection of dogs with infected ticks, the infection can last for 12 months and the antibody titre for up to 18 months afterwards. The clinical relevance of serological results is difficult to interpret as up to 50% of healthy dogs in an endemic region can be seropositive. Indeed, the higher the seroprevalence in a region, the less significant a positive serological result is.

Therapy and Prognosis: Ampicillin, tetracycline and doxycycline appear to be the most effective antibiotics. Ampicillin (25mg/kg, PO, TID, for 10 days), for example, has been used with success in dogs with acute polyarthritis and fever. Clinical improvement occurred as early as 24 hours; after 3 days the dogs were free of fever and after 7 days clinically resolved.

Prophylaxis: Tick prophylaxis and the removal of ticks within 24 hours can prevent the transmission of *Borrelia*. The experimental transmission of *B. burgdorferi* in dogs using infected ticks has been prevented by using amitraz-impregnated collars (52). The vaccine against borreliosis in the dog available in many countries (Merilym®) is aimed at *B. burgdorferi* (46). However, further investigations into the degree of protection provided by this vaccine in endemic areas, the possible induction of autoimmune mechanisms, and its efficacy against other *Borrelia* spp. and genotypes are still needed.

20

Literature

1 HELLEBREKERS, L.J., SLAPPENDEL, R.J. (1982): Trypanoso-miasis in a dog imported in the Netherlands. Vet Quart. **4**: 182–186.

2 NWOSU, C.O., IKEME, M.M. (1992): Parasitaemia and clinical manifestations in *Trypanosoma brucei* infected dogs. Rev Elev Med Vet Pays Trop. **45**: 273–277.

3 IKEDE, B.O., LOSOS, G.J. (1972): Trypanosomal meningo-en-cephalomyelitis with localization *of T. brucei* in the brain of a dog. Trans Royal Soc Trop Med Hyg. **66**: 357.

4 TENTER, A.M:, DEPLAZES, P. (2006): Protozoeninfektionen von Hund und Katze. In: Schnieder T. (ed.), Veterinärmedizinische Parasitologie, 6. Auflage. Paul Parey, Berlin S. 409–443.

5 DUBEY, J.P., HILL, D.E., LINDSAY, D.S., JENKINS, M.C., UGLA, A., SPEER, C.A. (2002): *Neospora caninum* and *Hammondia heydorni* are separate species. Trends Parasitol. **18**: 66–69.

6 HEMPHILL, A., GOTTSTEIN, B. (2000): A European perspec-tive on *Neospora caninum*. Int J Parasitol. **30**: 877–924.

7 SAGER, H., MORET, C.S., MULLER, N., STAUBLI, D., ES-POSITO, M., SCHARES, G., HASSIG, M., STARK, K., GOTT-STEIN, B. (2006): Incidence of *Neospora caninum* and other intesti-nal protozoan parasites in populations of Swiss dogs. Vet Parasitol. **139**: 84–92.

8 BASSO, W., VENTURINI, L., VENTURINI, M.C., HILL, D.E., KWOK, O.C.H., SHEN, S.K., DUBEY, J.P. (2001): First isolation of *Neospora caninum* from the feces of a naturally infected dog. J Parasitol. **87**: 612–618.

9 SCHARES, G., HEYDORN, A.O., CÜPPERS, A., MEHL-HORN, H., GEUE, L., PETERS, M., CONRATHS, F.J. (2002): In contrast to dogs, red foxes (*Vulpes vulpes*) did not shed *Neospora caninum* upon feeding of intermediate host tissues. Parasitol Res. **88**: 44–52.

10 DIJKSTRA, T., BARKEMA, H.W., EYSKER, M., WOUDA, W. (2001). Evidence of post-natal transmission of *Neospora caninum* in Dutch dairy herds. Int J Parasitol. **31**: 209–215.

11 KLEIN, B.U., MÜLLER, E. (2001): Seroprävalenz von Antikör-pern gegen *Neospora caninum* bei Hunden mit und ohne klinischen Neosporoseverdacht in Deutschland. Prakt Tierarzt **82**: 473–440.

12 DIJKSTRA, T., EYSKER, M., SCHARES, G., CONRATHS, F. J., WOUDA, W., BARKEMA, H.W. (2001): Dogs shed *Neospora caninum* oocysts after ingestion of naturally infected bovine placenta but not after ingestion of colostrum spiked with *Neospora caninum* tachyzoites. Int J Parasitol. **31**: 747–752.

13 DUBEY, J.P. (1999): Recent advances in Neospora and neosporosis. Vet Parasitol. **84**: 349–367.

14 DUBEY, J.P., LINDSAY, D.S. (1993): Neosporosis. Parasitol Today **9**: 452–458.

15 BARBER, J.S., TREES, A.J. (1998): Naturally occurring vertical transmission of *Neospora caninum* in dogs. Int J Parasitol. **28**: 57–64.

16 WOLF, M., CACHIN, M., VANDEVELDE, M., TIPOLD, A., DUBEY, J.P. (1991): Zur klinischen Diagnostik des protozoären Myositissyndroms (*Neospora caninum*) des Welpens. Tierärztl Prax. **19**: 302–306.

17 BARBER, J.S., TREES, A.J. (1996): Clinical aspects of 27 cases of neosporosis in dogs. Vet Rec. **139**: 439–443.

18 PETERS, M., WAGNER, F., SCHARES, G. (2000): Canine neos-porosis: clinical and pathological findings and first isolation of *Neos-pora caninum* in Germany. Parasitol Res. **86**: 1–7.

19 LÖSCHENBERGER, K., RÖSSEL, C., EDELHOFER, R., SUCHY, A., PROSEL, H. (2000): Diagnose von *Neospora caninum* beim Hund anhand eines Fallbeispiels. Tierärztl Prax. **28**: 390–394.

19a SPENCER, J.A., WITHEROW, A.K., BLAGBURN, B.L. (2000): A random amplified polymorphic DNA polymerase chain reaction technique that differentiates between Neospora species. J Parasitol. **86**: 1366–1368.

19b STILES, J., PRADE, R., GREENE, C. (1996): Detection of To-xoplasma gondii in feline and canine biological samples by use of the polymerase chain reaction. Am J Vet Res. **57**: 264–267.

20 PETERS, M., LUTKEFELS, E., HECKEROTH, A.R., SCHARES, G. (2001): Immunohistochemical and ultrastructural evidence for *Neospora caninum* tissue cysts in skeletal muscles of nat-urally infected dogs and cattle. Int J Parasitol. **31**: 1144–1148.

21 MÜLLER, N., ZIMMERMANN, V., HENTRICH, B., GOTT-STEIN, B. (1996): Diagnosis of *Neospora* sp. and *Toxoplasma gondii* by PCR and DNA-hybridization Immuno-Assay (DIA). J Clin Microbiol. **34**: 2850–2852.

22 GOTTSTEIN, B., EPERON, S., DAI, W.J., CANNAS, A., HEM-PHILL, A., GREIF, G. (2001): Efficacy of toltrazuril and ponazuril against experimental *Neospora caninum* infection in mice. Parasitol Res. **87**: 43–48.

23 TENTER, A.M., HECKEROTH, A.R., WEISS, L.M. (2000): *To-xoplasma gondii*: from animals to humans. Int J Parasitol. **30**: 1217–1258, erratum **31**: 217–220.

24 BEELITZ, P., GÖBEL, E., GOTHE, R. (1992): Fauna und Befalls-häufigkeit von Endoparasiten bei Katzenwelpen und ihren Müttern unterschiedlicher Haltung in Süddeutschland. Tierärztl Prax. **20**: 297–300.

25 DUBEY, J.P., CARPENTER, J.L. (1993): Histologically con-firmed clinical toxoplasmosis in cats: 100 cases (1952–1990): J Am Vet Med Assoc. **203**: 1556–1566.

26 DUBEY, J.P., MATTIX, M.E., LIPSCOMB, T.P. (1996): Lesions of neonatally induced toxoplasmosis in cats. Vet Pathol. **33**: 290–295.

27 DUBEY, J.P., CHAPMAN, J.L., ROSENTHAL, B.M., MENSE, M., SCHUELER, R.L. (2006): Clinical *Sarcocystis neurona*, *Sarcocys-tis canis*, *Toxoplasma gondii*, and *Neospora caninum* infections in dogs. Vet Parasitol. **137**: 49–49.

28 ZAHLER, M., GOTHE, R. (2001): Ein neuer Naturherd der Buntzeckenart *Dermacentor reticulatus* in Bayern – Risiko einer wei-teren endemischen Ausbreitung der Hundebabesiose. Tierärztl Prax. **29**: 121–123.

29 HAUSSCHILD, S., SCHEIN, E. (1996): Zur Artspezifität von *Babesia canis*. Berl Tierärztl Wschr. **109**: 216–219.

20

30 DEPLAZES, P., STAEBLER, S., GOTTSTEIN, B. (2006): Reisemedizin parasitärer Erkrankungen des Hundes. Schweiz Arch Tierheilk. **148**: 447–461.

31 VERCAMMEN, F., DE DEKEN, R., MAES, L. (1996): Prophylactic activity of Imidocarb against experimental infection with *Babesia canis*. Vet Parasitol. **63**: 195–198.

32 BAUER, R.W., HARRISON, L.R., WATSON, C.W., STYER, E.L., CHAPMAN Jr., W.L. (1993): Isolation of *Acanthamoeba* sp. from a greyhound with pneumonia and granulomatous amebic encephalitis. J Vet Diag Invest. **5**: 386–391.

33 MATHIS, A., WEBER, R., DEPLAZES, P. (2005): Zoonotic potential of the Microsporidia. Clin Microbiol Rev. **18**: 423–445.

34 BOTHA, W.S., VAN DELLEN, A.F., STEWART, C.G. (1979): Canine encephalitozoonosis in South Africa. J South Afr Vet Assoc. **50**: 135–144.

35 SZABO, J.R., SHADDUCK, J.A. (1987): Experimental encephalitozoonosis in neonatal dogs. Vet Pathol. **24**: 99–108.

36 SUTER, C., MÜLLER-DOBLIES, U.U., HATT, J.-M., DEPLAZES, P. (2001): Prevention and treatment of *Encephalitozoon cuniculi* infection in rabbits with fenbendazole. Vet Rec. **148**: 478–480.

37 DEPLAZES, P. (2006): Helminthosen von Hund und Katze. In: Schnieder T. (ed.), Veterinärmedizinische Parasitologie. 6. Aufl. Paul Parey, Berlin S. 444–520.

38 SMITH, M.C., BAILEY, C.S., BAKER, N., KOCK, N. (1988): Cerebral coenurosis in a cat. J Am Vet Med Assoc. **192**: 82–84.

39 STAEBLER, S., OCHS, H., STEFFEN, F., NAEGELI, F., BOREL, N., SIEBER-RUCKSTUHL, N., DEPLAZES, P. (2005): Autochthone Infektionen mit *Angiostrongylus vasorum* bei Hunden in der Schweiz und Deutschland. Schweiz Arch Tierheilk. **147**: 121–127.

40 BOLT, G., MONRAD, J., KOCH, J., JENSEN, A.L. (1994): Canine angiostrongylosis: a review. Vet Rec. **135**: 447–452.

41 REIFINGER, M., GRESZL, J. (1994): Pulmonale Angiostrongylose mit systemischer Ausbreitung und zentralnervaler Manifestation bei einem Hund. J Vet Med. **41**: 391–398.

42 PROSL, H., RABITSCH, A., BRABENETZ, J. (1985): Zur Bedeutung der Herbstgrasmilbe – *Neotrombicula autumnalis* (Shaw 1790) – in der Veterinärmedizin: Nervale Symptome bei Hunden nach massiver Infestation. Tierärztl Prax. **13**: 57–64.

43 HORST, H. (1993): Einheimische Zeckenborreliose (Lyme-Krankheit) bei Mensch und Tier. Primed-Spitta, Nürnberg.

44 GERN, L., HUMAIR, P.F. (1998): Natural history of *Borrelia burgdorferi* sensu lato. Wien Klin Wochenschr. **110**: 856–858.

45 SAINT GIRONS, I., GERN, L., GRAY, J.S., GUY, E.C., KORENBERG, E., NUTTALL, P.A., RIJPKEMA, S.G., SCHONBERG, A., STANEK, G., POSTIC, D. (1998): Identification of *Borrelia burgdorferi* sensu lato species in Europe. Int J Med Microbiol. **287**: 190–195.

46 WIEDEMANN, C., MILWARD, F. (1999): Wirksamkeit- und Verträglichkeitsprüfung mit einem neuen Impfstoff gegen Lyme-Borreliose beim Hund (Merilym®). Tierärztl Umschau. **54**: 242–249.

47 LIEBISCH, A. (1993): Biologie und Oekologie der Zecken. In: Einheimische Zeckenborreliose (Lyme-Krankheit) bei Mensch und Tier. HORST, H. (ed.), Primed-Spitta, Nürnberg. pp. 31–47.

48 APPEL, M.J., ALLAN, S., JACOBSON, R.H., LAUDERDALE, T.L., CHANG, Y.F., SHIN, S.J., THOMFORD, J.W., TODHUNTER, R.J., SUMMERS, B.A. (1993): Experimental Lyme disease in dogs produces arthritis and persistent infection. J Infect Dis. **167**: 651–664.

49 PFISTER, K., BIGLER, B., NESWADBA, J., GERN, L., AESCHLIMANN, A. (1989): *Borrelia burgdorferi* infections of dogs in Switzerland. Zbl Bakt Suppl. **18**: 26–31.

50 HEIM, U., WEBER, A. (1991): Nachweis von Antikörpern gegen *Borrelia burgdorferi* bei Hunden mit neurologischen Krankheitserscheinungen: Fallberichte zur Lyme-Borreliose. Kleintierprax. **36**: 561–564.

51 CHANG, Y.F., NOVOSEL, V., CHANG, C.F., SUMMERS, B.A., MA, D.P., CHIANG, Y.W., ACREE, W.M., CHU, H.J., SHIN, S., LEIN, D.H. (2001): Experimental induction of chronic borreliosis in adult dogs exposed to *Borrelia burgdorferi*-infected ticks and treated with dexamethasone. Am J Vet Res. **62**: 1104–1012.

52 ELFASSY, O.J., GOODMAN, F.W., LEVY, S.L., CARTER, L.L. (2001): Efficacy of an amitraz-impregnated collar in preventing transmission of *Borrelia burgdorferi* by adult *Ixodes scapularis* to dogs. Am Vet Med Assoc. **219**: 185–189.

53 TIPOLD, A., FATZER, R., HOLZMANN, H. (1993): Zentraleuropäische Zeckenenzephalitis beim Hund. Kleintierprax. **38**: 619.

54 GLAUS, T., JAGGY, A. (1992): Ehrlichiose beim Hund: Literaturübersicht und Fallbeschreibung. Schweiz. Arch. Tierheilk. **134**: 319–323.

55 PUSTERLA, N., BRAUN, U., LEUTENEGGER, C.M., REUSCH, C., LUTZ, H. (2000): Ehrlichiosis in Switzerland – significance for veterinary medicine. Schweiz. Arch. Tierheilk. **142**: 367–373.

56 FISCHER, S., HARTMANN, K., GOTHE, R. (1994): *Hepatozoon canis*: Eine importierte parasitäre Infektion bei Hunden. Tierärztl Prax. **22**: 172–180.

57 ARNOLD, P., DEPLAZES, P., MÜLLER, A., KUPPER, J., LUTZ, H., GLAUS, T. (1998): Importierte Hepatozoonose beim Hund: 3 Fälle. Schweiz Arch Tierheilk. **140**: 287–293.

20

Appendices

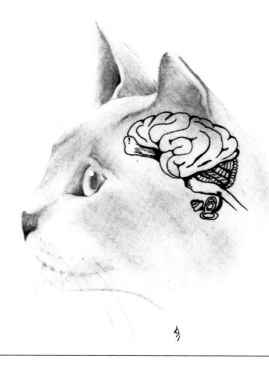

Appendix 1: Comparative sectional anatomy of the canine and feline brain

Appendix 2: Breed-specific diseases of the dog

Appendix 3: List of inheritable neurological diseases of the dog

Appendix 4: List of inheritable neurological diseases of the cat

Appendix 5: Drugs

Appendix 6: Epidemiological overview of the neurological diseases seen in dogs between 1989 and 2000 at the Small Animal Clinic in Bern, Switzerland

Appendix 1:
Comparative sectional anatomy of the canine and feline brain

Nicole Gassner
Federica Rossi
Martin Konar
Johann Lang
Marc Vandevelde

A1

The aim of the following pages is to reproduce those structures in the skull and brain which are most important for neurological diagnosis, thereby contributing to the understanding of sectional anatomy. Accordingly, magnetic resonance, computer tomographic, and macroscopic sections of the canine and feline brains are compared. Transverse, sagittal, and dorsal projections have been chosen to describe the anatomical structures. An overview of the most popular sequences in neurological MRI diagnostics is given and their use explained in case studies. Last but not least, by doing this the reading and understanding of the pathological conditions presented in this atlas and textbook should be made easier. The main anatomical structure for understanding brain anatomy is the ventricle system as it provides the radiologist and pathologist with the most important points for orientation.

The MRI pictures were taken with a low-field machine (0.3 Tesla), the CT images with a spiral CT (single slice) system.

Dog transverse axis

A1

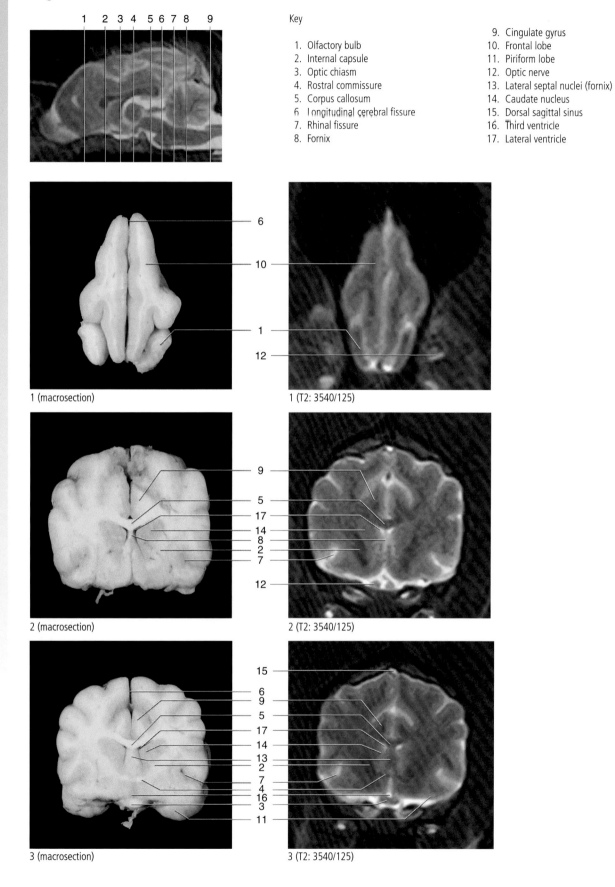

Key

1. Olfactory bulb
2. Internal capsule
3. Optic chiasm
4. Rostral commissure
5. Corpus callosum
6. Longitudinal cerebral fissure
7. Rhinal fissure
8. Fornix

9. Cingulate gyrus
10. Frontal lobe
11. Piriform lobe
12. Optic nerve
13. Lateral septal nuclei (fornix)
14. Caudate nucleus
15. Dorsal sagittal sinus
16. Third ventricle
17. Lateral ventricle

1 (macrosection)

1 (T2: 3540/125)

2 (macrosection)

2 (T2: 3540/125)

3 (macrosection)

3 (T2: 3540/125)

a. Basisphenoid
b. Optic canal
c. Body of the basisphenoid
d. Body of the presphenoid
e. External sagittal crest

f. Endoturbinate IV
g. Orbital fissure
h. Rostral alar foramen
i. Ethmoid bone
j. Frontal bone

k. Palatine bone
l. Septum of the frontal sinus
m. Frontal sinus
n. Vomer

A1

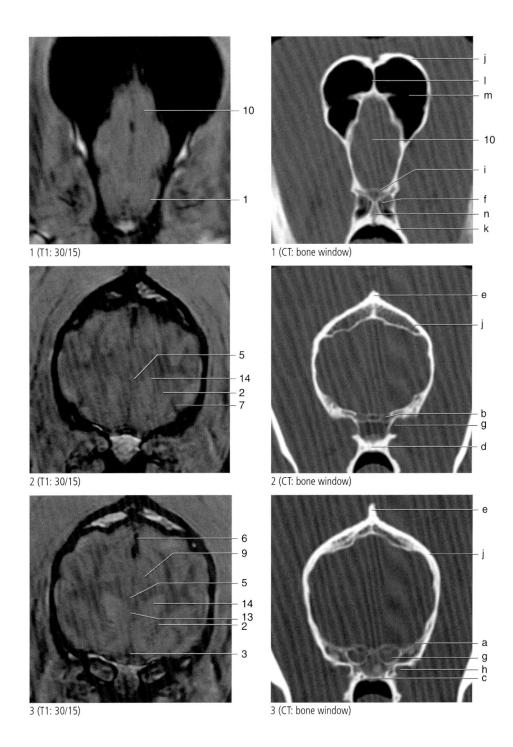

1 (T1: 30/15)

1 (CT: bone window)

2 (T1: 30/15)

2 (CT: bone window)

3 (T1: 30/15)

3 (CT: bone window)

Dog transverse axis

A1

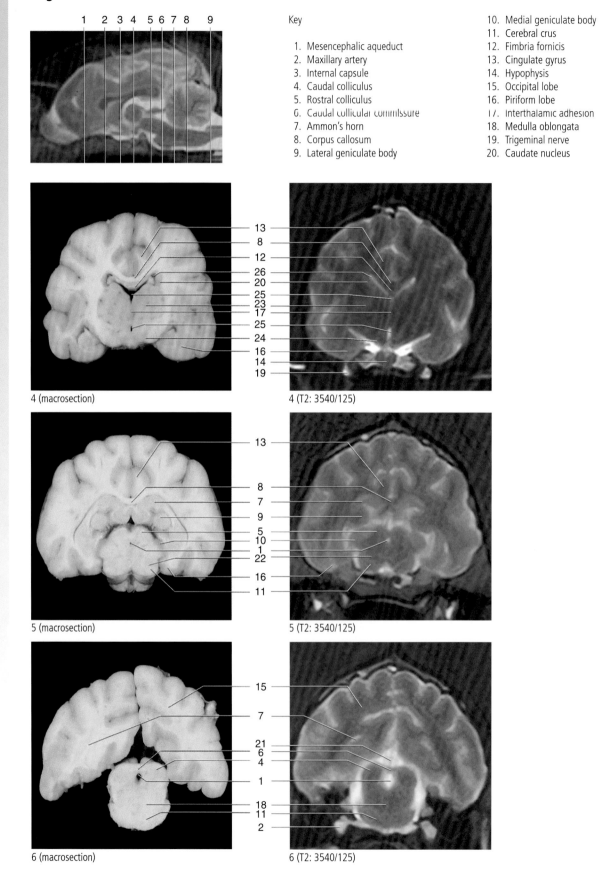

Key

1. Mesencephalic aqueduct
2. Maxillary artery
3. Internal capsule
4. Caudal colliculus
5. Rostral colliculus
6. Caudal collicular commissure
7. Ammon's horn
8. Corpus callosum
9. Lateral geniculate body
10. Medial geniculate body
11. Cerebral crus
12. Fimbria fornicis
13. Cingulate gyrus
14. Hypophysis
15. Occipital lobe
16. Piriform lobe
17. Interthalamic adhesion
18. Medulla oblongata
19. Trigeminal nerve
20. Caudate nucleus

4 (macrosection)

4 (T2: 3540/125)

5 (macrosection)

5 (T2: 3540/125)

6 (macrosection)

6 (T2: 3540/125)

21. Suprapineal recess
22. Substantia nigra
23. Thalamus
24. Optic tract
25. Third ventricle
26. Lateral ventricle

a. Temporomandibular joint
b. Rostral alar canal
c. Musculotubal canal
d. Body of the basisphenoid bone
e. External sagittal crest
f. Dorsum sellae

g. Foramen lacerum with carotid canal
h. Foramen ovale
i. Frontal bone
j. Parietal bone
k. Temporal bone
l. Retroarticular process

A1

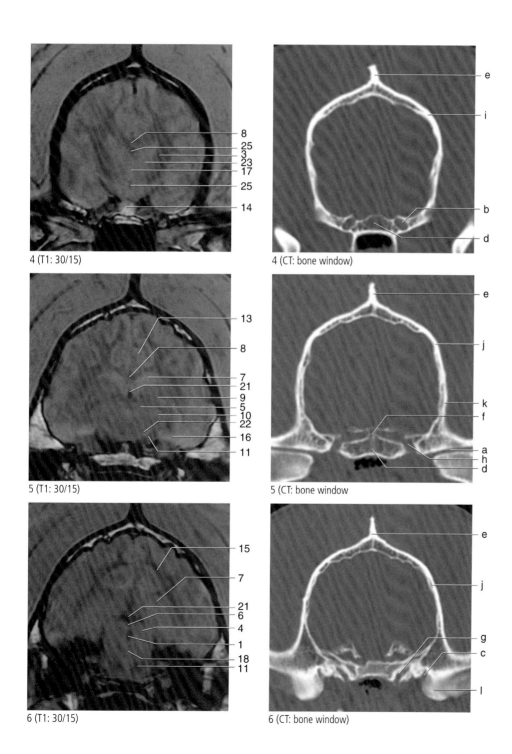

4 (T1: 30/15)

4 (CT: bone window)

5 (T1: 30/15)

5 (CT: bone window

6 (T1: 30/15)

6 (CT: bone window)

A1

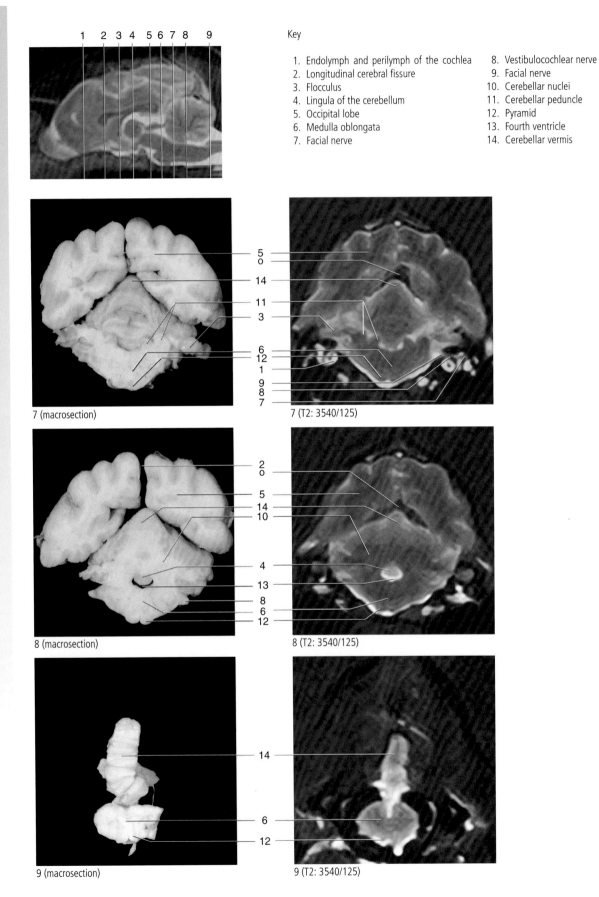

Key

1. Endolymph and perilymph of the cochlea
2. Longitudinal cerebral fissure
3. Flocculus
4. Lingula of the cerebellum
5. Occipital lobe
6. Medulla oblongata
7. Facial nerve

8. Vestibulocochlear nerve
9. Facial nerve
10. Cerebellar nuclei
11. Cerebellar peduncle
12. Pyramid
13. Fourth ventricle
14. Cerebellar vermis

7 (macrosection)

7 (T2: 3540/125)

8 (macrosection)

8 (T2: 3540/125)

9 (macrosection)

9 (T2: 3540/125)

a. Carotid canal
b. Condyloid canal
c. Hypoglossal canal
d. Tympanic cavity
e. Occipital condyle
f. External sagittal crest

g. Vestibular window
h. Cerebellar fossa
i. External auditory meatus
j. Internal auditory meatus
k. Parietal bone
l. Temporal bone

m. Paracondyle process
n. External occipital protuberance
o. Tentorium ossium
p. Muscular tubercle

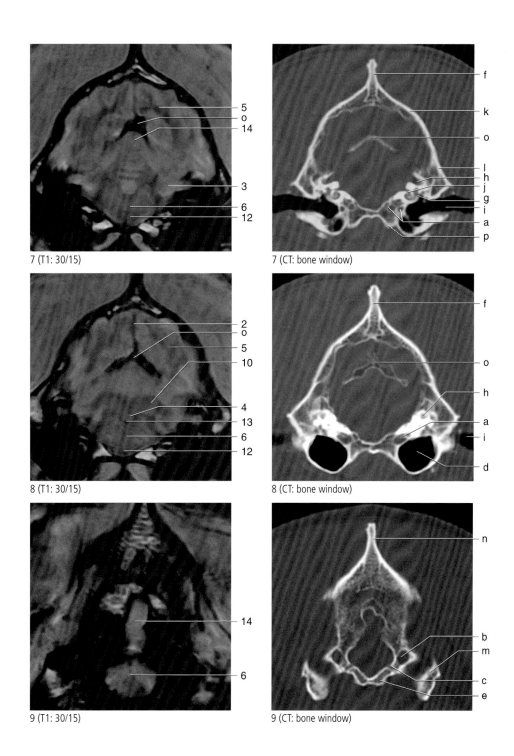

7 (T1: 30/15)

7 (CT: bone window)

8 (T1: 30/15)

8 (CT: bone window)

9 (T1: 30/15)

9 (CT: bone window)

Dog sagittal axis

A1

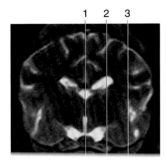

Key

1. Mesencephalic aqueduct
2. Arbor vitae
3. Olfactory bulb
4. Optic chiasm
5. Caudal colliculus
6. Rostral colliculus
7. Rostral commissure
8. Ammon's horn
9. Mammillary body
10. Cerebellar cortex
11. Fimbria fornix
12. Fissura prima
13. Fornix
14. Basal ganglia
15. Genu of the corpus callosum
16. Cingulate gyrus
17. Hypophysis
18. Interthalamic adhesion
19. Medulla oblongata
20. Obex
21. Choroid plexus of fourth ventricle
22. Pons
23. Pyramid
24. Suprapineal recess
25. Splenium of the corpus callosum
26. Cruciate sulcus
27. Thalamus
28. Trunk of the corpus callosum
29. Third ventricle
30. Fourth ventricle
31. Lateral ventricle

a. Inner ear
b. Optic canal
c. Transverse sinus canal
d. Body of the basisphenoid bone (medulla)
e. Dorsum sellae
f. Second ectoturbinate
g. First to fourth ectoturbinates
h. Orbital fissure
i. Internal carotid foramen
j. Cerebellar fossa
k. Cribriform plate
l. Internal lamina of the frontal bone
m. Basisphenoid bone
n. Frontal bone
o. Interparietal bone
p. Occipital bone
q. Parietal bone
r. Presphenoid bone
s. Temporal bone
t. Nasal septum
u. Frontal sinus
v. Tentorium ossium
w. Musclular tubercle

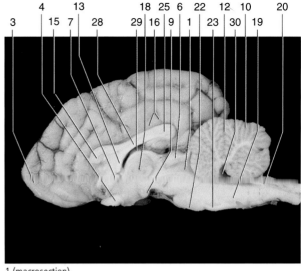

1 (macrosection)

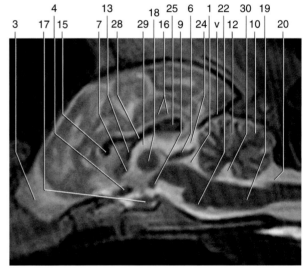

1 (T2: 4000/120)

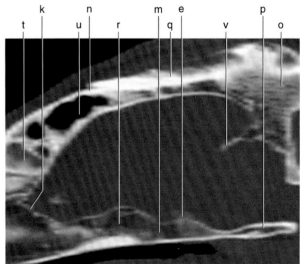

1 (CT: bone window)

A1

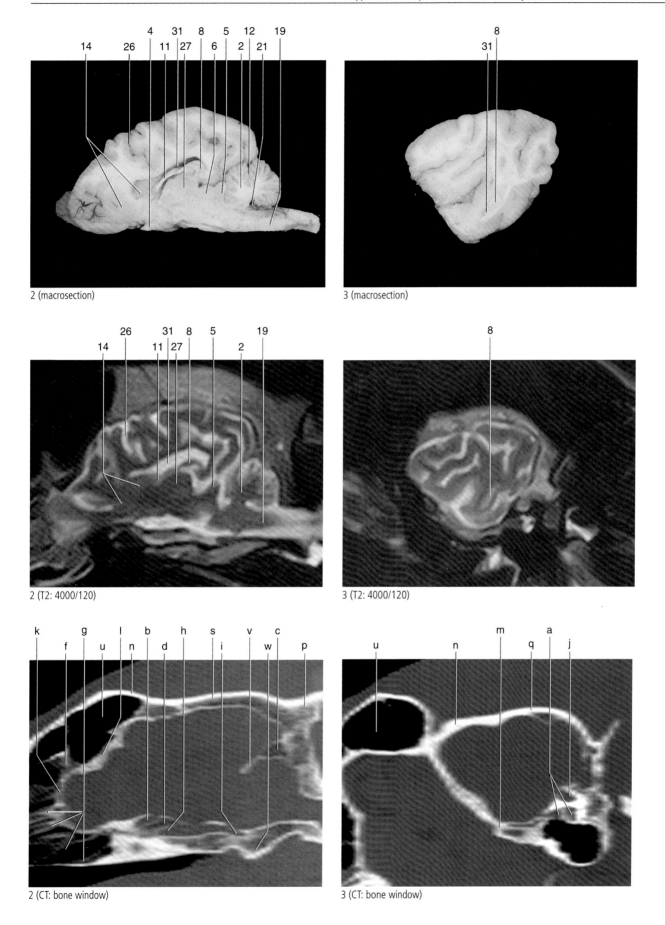

2 (macrosection)

3 (macrosection)

2 (T2: 4000/120)

3 (T2: 4000/120)

2 (CT: bone window)

3 (CT: bone window)

Dog dorsal axis

A1

Key

1. Mesencephalic aqueduct
2. Olfactory bulb
3. Optic chiasm
4. Caudal colliculus
5. Rostral colliculus
6. Ammon's horn
7. Temporal horn of the lateral ventricle
8. Lateral geniculate body

9. Cerebral crus
10. Longitudinal cerebral fissure
11. Lateral cerebral hemisphere
12. Hypothalamus
13. Transition between hypothalamus and hypophysis
14. Cerebellar lingula
15. Temporal lobe

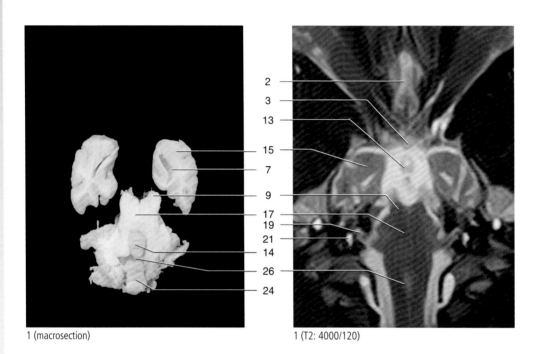

1 (macrosection)

1 (T2: 4000/120)

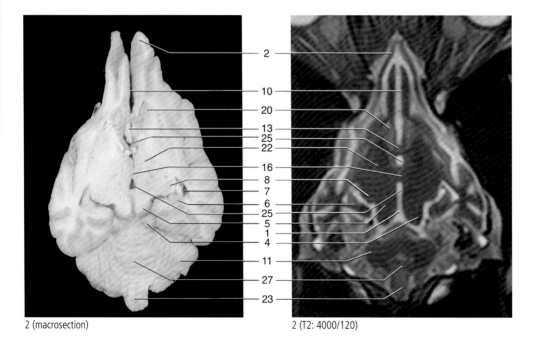

2 (macrosection)

2 (T2: 4000/120)

16. Interthalamic adhesion
17. Medulla oblongata
18. Facial nerve
19. Vestibulocochlear and facial nerve
20. Caudate nucleus
21. Perilymph and endolymph of the cochlea
22. Thalamus
23. Tuber vermis

24. Cerebellar uvula
25. Third ventricle
26. Fourth ventricle
27. Cerebellar vermis

a. Inner ear
b. Condylar canal
c. Optic canal

d. Second endoturbinate
e. Cribriform plate
f. Frontal bone
g. Sphenoid bone
h. Temporal bone
i. Rostral clinoidal process
j. Nasal septum

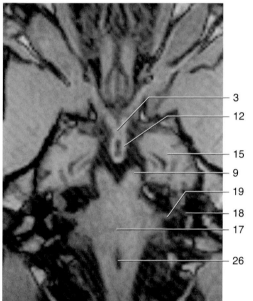

1 (T1w: 30/12)

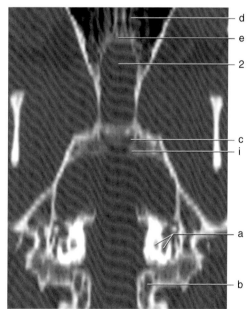

1 (CT: bone window)

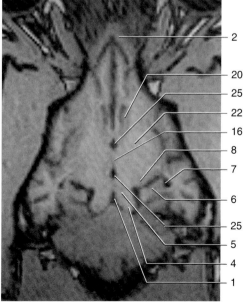

2 (T1: 30/12)

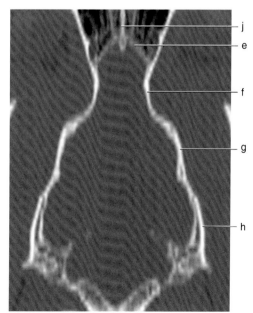

2 (CT: bone window)

A1

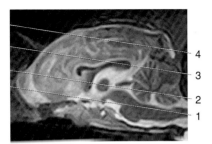

Key

1. Cerebellum with primary fissure
2. Ammon's horn
3. Corpus callosum
4. Longitudinal cerebral fissure
5. Marginal fissure
6. Superior frontal gyrus

7. Frontal lobe
8. Caudate nucleus
9. Splenium of the corpus callosum
10. Cruciate sulcus
11. Lateral ventricle

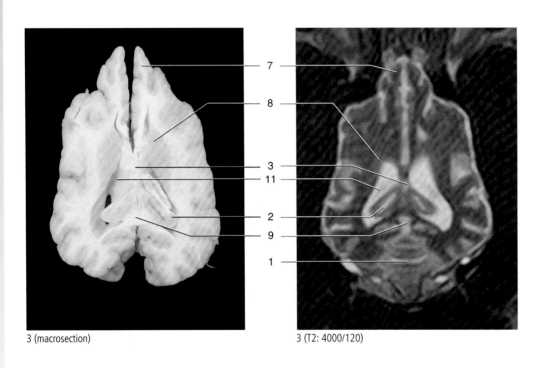

3 (macrosection)

3 (T2: 4000/120)

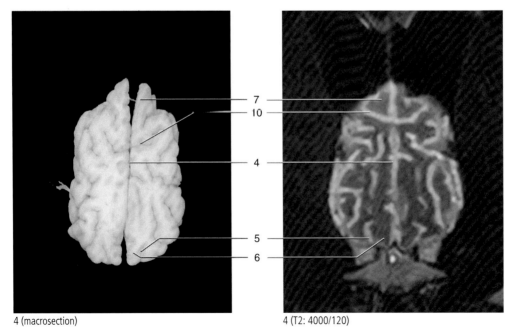

4 (macrosection)

4 (T2: 4000/120)

a. Transverse cranial sinus
b. Internal occipital crest
c. Vermiform impression
d. Cribriform plate

e. Internal lamina of the frontal bone
f. Frontal bone
g. Parietal bone
h. Temporal bone

i. Septum of the frontal sinus
j. Frontal sinus
k. Tentorium ossium

A1

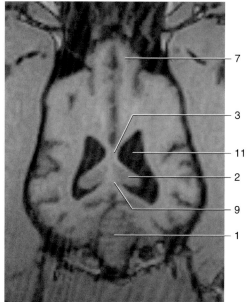

3 (T1w: 30/12)

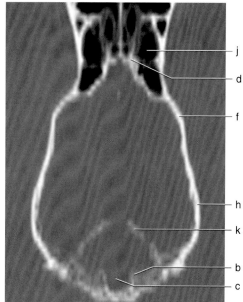

3 (CT: bone window)

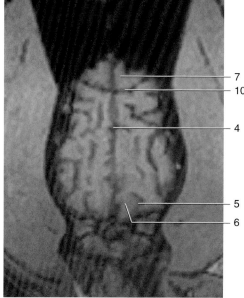

4 (T1: 30/12)

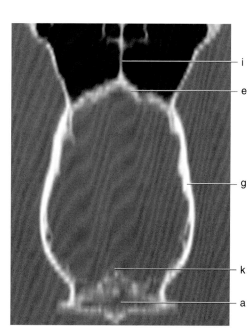

4 (CT: bone window)

Dog cervical vertebrae

A1

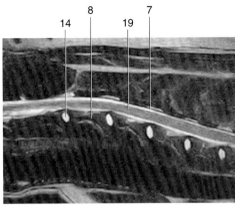

T2 sag (2500/120): L2–S1

Key

1. Wing of ilium
2. Aorta
3. C6 vertebral arch
4. L5 vertebral arch
5. Intervertebral articulation
6. Epidural space
7. Subarachnoid space
8. C3 vertebral body
9. C7 vertebral body
10. L2 vertebral body
11. L4 vertebral body
12. L7 vertebral body
13. S1 vertebral body

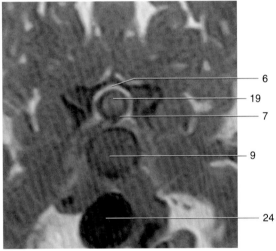

T1 tra (5000/18.3): C6/7

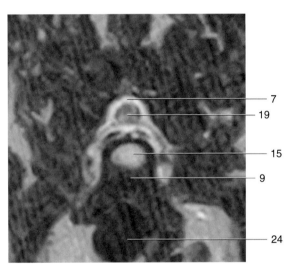

T2 tra (3540/100): C6/7

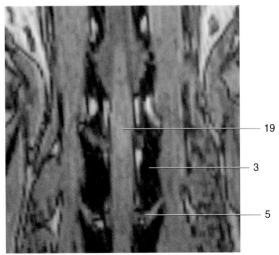

MPR dor (30/12): C5–C7

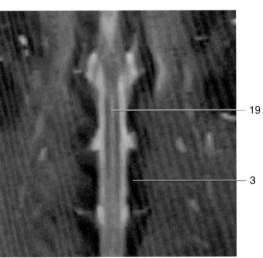

STIR dor (4000/25): C5–C7

Dog lumber vertebrae

14. C2/3 intervertebral disc
15. C6/7 intervertebral disc
16. L3/4 intervertebral disc
17. L5/6 intervertebral disc
18. L7/S1 intervertebral disc
19. Spinal medulla
20. Root of spinal nerve L7
21. Root of spinal nerve S1
22. L4 vertebral process
23. L7 vertebral process
24. Trachea
25. Lumbar trunk

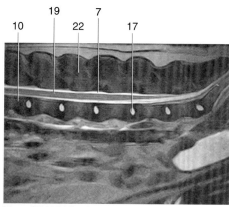

T2 sag (2500/120): L2–S1

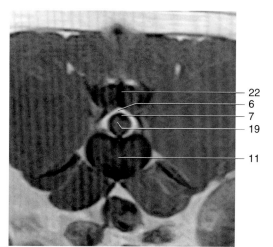

T1 tra (500/18.3): L3/L4

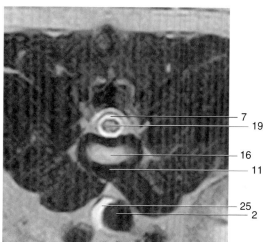

T2 tra (3540/100): L3/4

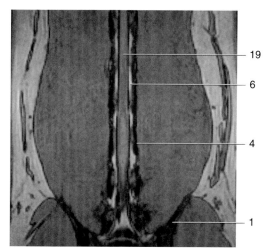

MPR dor (30/12): L2–L7

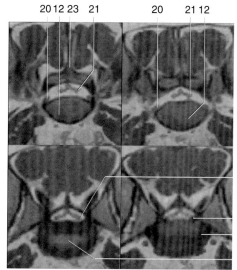

BASG tra (13.6/16.8): lumbosacral junction

Cat transverse axis

A1

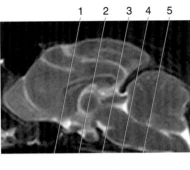

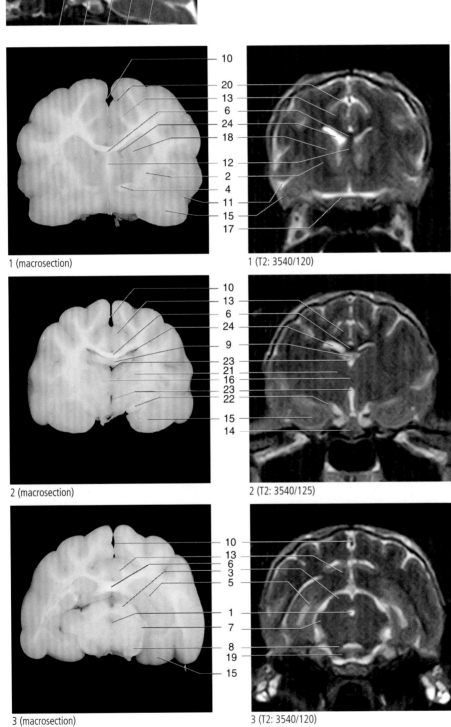

1 (macrosection)

1 (T2: 3540/120)

2 (macrosection)

2 (T2: 3540/125)

3 (macrosection)

3 (T2: 3540/120)

16. Interthalamic adhesion
17. Optic nerve
18. Caudate nucleus
19. Pons
20. Cruciate sulcus
21. Thalamus
22. Optic tract

23. Third ventricle
24. Lateral ventricle

a. Tympanic cavity
b. Body of the basisphenoid bone
c. Foramen ovale
d. Foramen rotundum

e. Cerebellar fossa
f. Hypophyseal fossa
g. Ethmoid bone
h. Frontal bone
i. Palatine bone
j. Parietal bone
k. Temporal bone
l. Zygomatic process

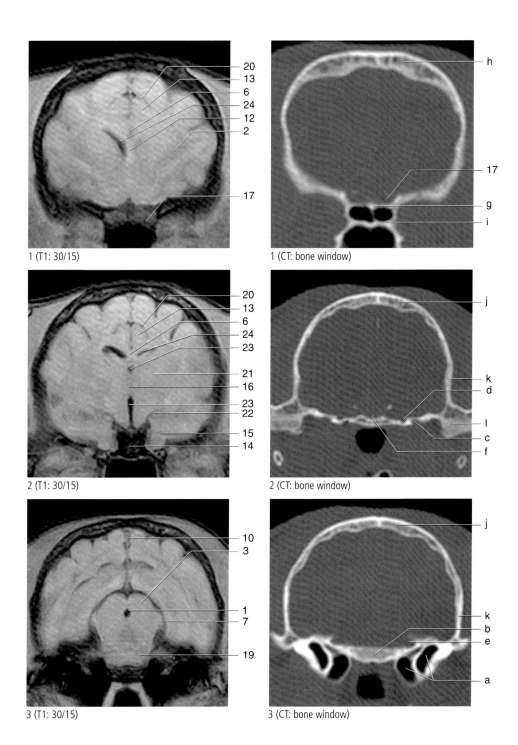

1 (T1: 30/15)

1 (CT: bone window)

2 (T1: 30/15)

2 (CT: bone window)

3 (T1: 30/15)

3 (CT: bone window)

A1

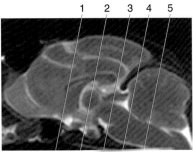

1 2 3 4 5

Key

1. Endolymph and perilymph of the cochlea
2. Flocculus
3. Lingula of the cerebellum
4. Occipital lobe
5. Rostral cerebellar lobe
6. Medulla oblongata
7. Hypoglossal nerve
8. Vestibulocochlear and facial nerve
9. Cerebellar peduncle
10. Pyramid
11. Fourth ventricle
12. Cerebellar vermis

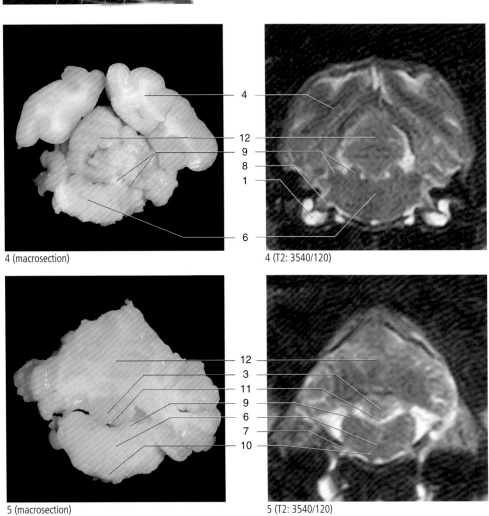

4 (macrosection)

4 (T2: 3540/120)

5 (macrosection)

5 (T2: 3540/120)

a. Carotid canal
b. Tympanic cavity
c. External sagittal crest
d. Vestibular window
e. Hyploglossal foramen
f. Internal auditory meatus
g. Parietal bone
h. Temporal bone
i. Tentorium ossium

A1

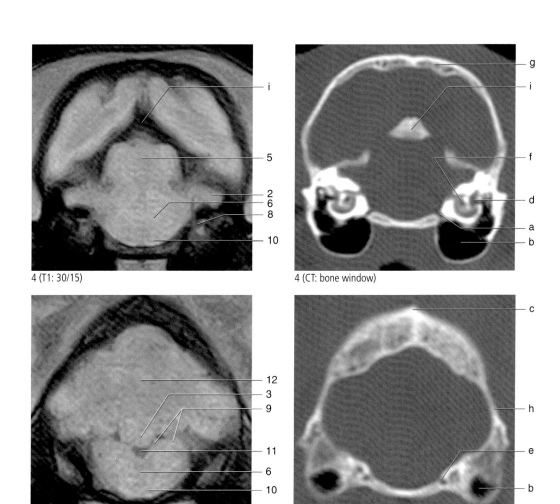

4 (T1: 30/15)

4 (CT: bone window)

5 (T1: 30/15)

5 (CT: bone window)

Cat sagittal axis

A1

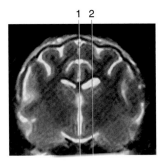

1 2

Key

1. Mesencephalic aqueduct
2. Arbor vitae
3. Olfactory bulb
4. Cerebellum
5. Optic chiasm
6. Caudal colliculus
7. Rostral colliculus
8. Rostral commissure
9. Ammon's horn
10. Mammillary body
11. Cerebellar cortex
12. Fimbria fornix
13. Fornix
14. Genu of the corpus callosum
15. Cingulate gyrus
16. Hypophysis
17. Interthalamic adhesion
18. Optic nerve
19. Caudate nucleus
20. Pons
21. Pyramid
22. Splenium of the corpus callosum
23. Cruciate sulcus
24. Mesencephalic tectum
25. Thalamus
26. Third ventricle
27. Fourth ventricle
28. Lateral ventricle

a. Atlanto-occipital joint
b. Carotid canal (with internal carotid foramen)
c. Tympanic cavity
d. Dorsum sellae
e. Second to fourth endoturbinates
f. Hypoglossal canal
g. Hypophyseal fossa
h. Cribriform plate
i. Basisphenoid bone
j. Frontal bone
k. Occipital bone
l. Parietal bone
m. Presphenoid bone
n. Septum of the frontal sinus
o. Frontal sinus
p. Tentorium ossium

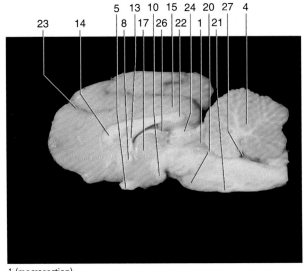

1 (macrosection)

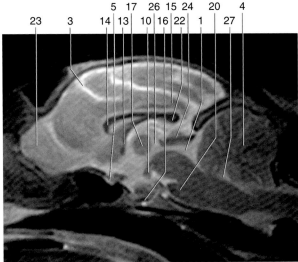

1 (T2: 3540/125)

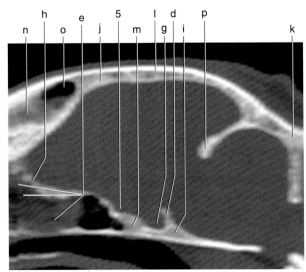

1 (CT: bone window)

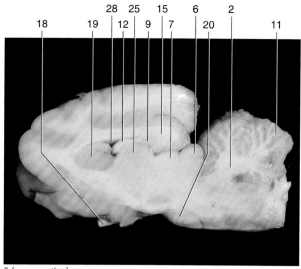

2 (macrosection)

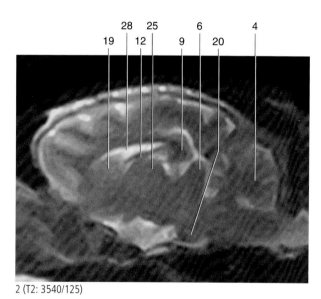

2 (T2: 3540/125)

2 (CT: bone window)

Cat dorsal axis

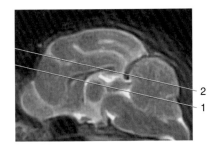

Key

1. Mesencephalic aqueduct
2. Olfactory bulb
3. Cerebellum
4. Caudal colliculus
5. Rostral colliculus

6. Caudal collicular commissure
7. Ammon's horn
8. Corpus callosum
9. Longitudinal cerebral fissure
10. Interthalamic adhesion

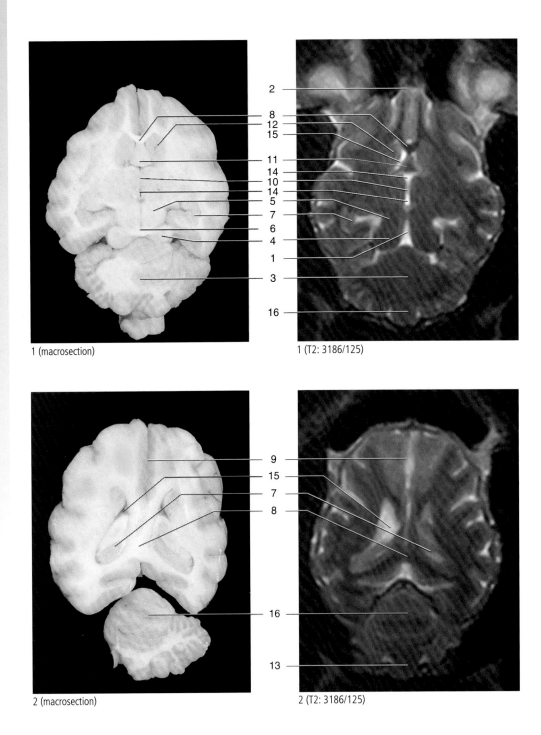

1 (macrosection)

1 (T2: 3186/125)

2 (macrosection)

2 (T2: 3186/125)

11. Lateral septal nuclei (fornix)
12. Caudate nucleus
13. Tuber vermis
14. Third ventricle

15. Lateral ventricle
16. Cerebellar vermis

a. Third ectoturbinate
b. Frontal bone

c. Occipital bone
d. Temporal bone
e. Tentorium ossium

A1

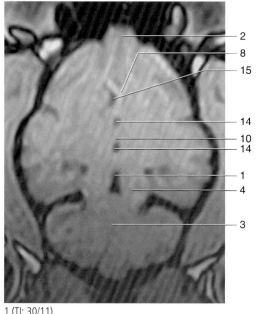

— 2
— 8
— 15

— 14
— 10
— 14

— 1
— 4

— 3

1 (TI: 30/11)

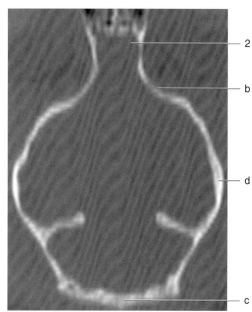

— 2

— b

— d

— c

1 (CT: bone window)

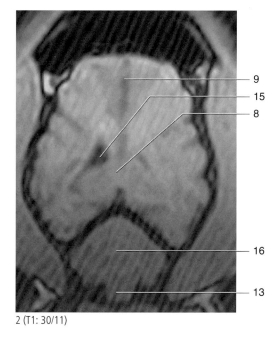

— 9
— 15
— 8

— 16

— 13

2 (T1: 30/11)

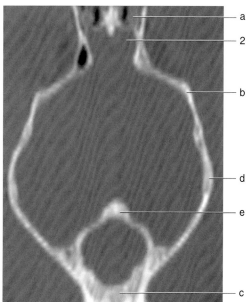

— a
— 2

— b

— d

— e

— c

2 (CT: bone window)

A1

Standard sequences in MRI diagnostics

T1-weighted sequences

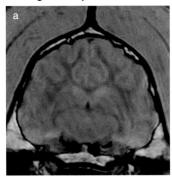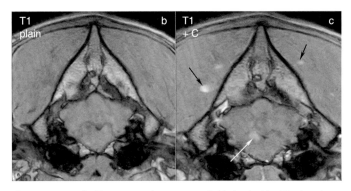

(a) T1w sequences demonstrate a good contrast between grey and white matter and so are very suitable for the identification of anatomical structures in the brain. On T1w sequences grey matter has a lower signal intensity than white matter. Fat has a high signal intensity, while CSF has, like other liquids, a low signal intensity. As a consequence, T1w sequences are not really suitable for finding pathological changes such as oedema. Paramagnetic contrast agents result in a shortening of the T1 relaxation time. If the blood-tissue barrier is more permeable than normal due to disease, the contrast agent can enter the surrounding tissue and increases the signal intensity of that tissue. Hemangiosarcoma metastases are shown in the example given above. (b) In the right cerebellar peduncle, in the transitional area with the medulla oblongata, there is a poorly demarcated lesion, which is slightly hypointense in the plain T1w sequence. (c) The lesion demonstrates a strong contrast accumulation in the center (white arrow). Miliary lesions are present in the musculature, which also show contrast accumulation (black arrows).

Gradient-Echo 3-Dimensional T1w MultiPlanar Reconstruction

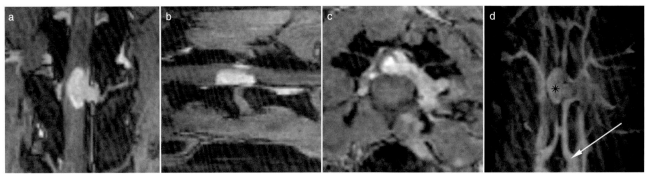

In these sequences, a three-dimensional T1w gradient echo sequence with high definition (possible in low-field MRI of 1 mm³). This allows a **m**ulti**p**lanar **r**econstruction (MPR). In the sequences of the third and fourth cervical vertebrae of a dog following the administration of contrast, a nerve root tumour is visible which demonstrates strong contrast enhancement (see also Fig. 6.30). Figure (a) shows the original dorsal plane section, while Figs. (b) and (c) are the reconstructed sagittal and transverse sections, respectively. Figure (d) shows a maximum intensity projection (MIP) of the subtraction images. For this, the plain sequences are subtracted from the enriched ones and the pixels with the highest signal intensity (SI) after the contrast-enriched images are used for a three-dimensional reconstruction. This allows a good angiographic effect to be achieved, which reveals both the tumour (black star) and the vertebral plexus (white arrow).

T2-weighted sequences

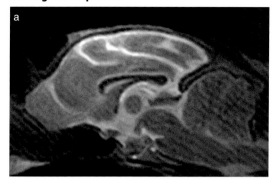 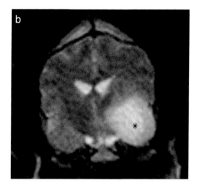

T2w sequences depict fluids, such as CSF, with a high SI. White matter has a low SI in comparison to the grey matter. Basal nuclei and nuclei in the brain stem and cerebellum have a high SI. Pathological tissues also often have a high SI due to prolongation of the T2 relaxation time.
(a) Medial sagittal section of a normal cat brain. (b) Glioma in the left piriform lobe (star).

STIR and T1-weighted FS sequences

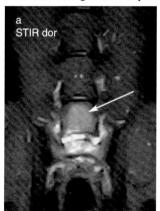 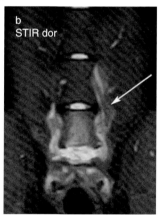 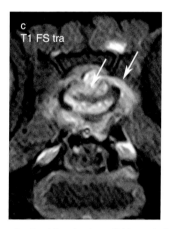

The **s**hort **t**au **i**nversion **r**ecovery (STIR) sequence is a sequence that selectively suppresses the signal from fat tissue. Fluids are depicted as being hyperintense. This type of sequence is especially sensitive for pathological changes as the majority cause an increase in the fluid signal.
The T1w **f**at-water **s**eparation (FS) sequence suppresses the signal from fat tissue by a mathematical process. Normally, this type of sequence is undertaken after the administration of a contrast agent, so that tissues with a higher SI can be differentiated from hypointense fat tissue.
This four-year-old female German Shepherd has discospondylitis in the area of L7 / S1. Figures (a) and (b) show the STIR sequence. The normal fat-containing bone marrow is dark. Due to the inflammation, both the vertebral body of L7 (a: white arrow) and the surrounding soft tissues (b: white arrow) have a high SI.
(c) In the T1w FS sequence after the injection of contrast, the intervertebral cleft and the surrounding soft tissues exhibit a high SI (white arrows).

A1

Gradient echo sequence BASG

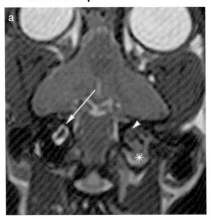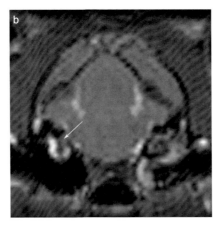

The BASG sequence (balanced spoiled steady state acquistion rewinded gradient echo) is a gradient echo sequence whose contrast results from the relationship of the T1 relaxation time to the T2 relaxation time. It has a high definition and depicts fluids as being particularly hyperintense. As a result, BASG is especially suitable for depicting nerve exits (Fig. a: * = vestibulocochlear nerve) and the inner ear. Depending on the manufacturer of the machine, this sequence type has different names (e.g. true FISP or CBASS).

(a) In this section, the left tympanic cavity is filled with an inhomogenous hyperintense material (white star). The SI of the endolymph of the cochlea of the healthy right inner ear (arrow) is also considerably higher than that of the left (arrowhead).

(b) This image is a transverse reconstruction from the original sequence at the height of the inner ear. The hyperintense filling of the tympanic cavity can also be seen here. The left inner ear has a lower SI than the healthy right ear (arrow). These changes are typical of inflammation in the middle and inner ear.

FLAIR

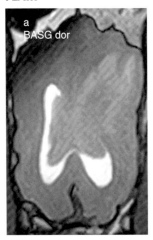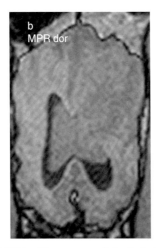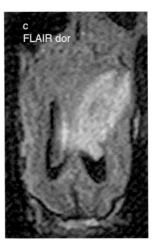

Fluid attenuation inversion recovery (FLAIR) is a T2w sequence which selectively suppresses the CSF signal so that lesions close to the subarachnoid space can be recognised and differentiated from the CSF.

(a) In the dorsal BASG, the CSF in the intraventricular area is hyperintense. More cranially, an irregular hyperintense, poorly demarcated area can be seen. (b) The dorsal GE T1w MPR (multiplanar reconstruction) sequence shows these changes as an area that is hypointense in comparison to the surrounding parenchyma. The CSF is dark. It is only in Fig. c that the true extent of the frontoparietal intraparenchymal lesion can be visualized. With the suppression of the CSF signal, the lesion appears strongly hyperintense and shows finger-like extensions pointing rostrally. On the caudal left side, the lesion is well demarcated from the suppressed hypointense CSF in the lateral ventricle.

Appendix 2:
Breed-specific diseases of the dog

Breed	Disease	Breed	Disease	Comments
A		Belgian Tervueren	Epilepsy Muscular dystrophy	
Afghan Hound	Degenerative spinal cord disease Hereditary myelopathy	Bernese Mountain Dog	Hepato-cerebellar degeneration Dysmyelination[27] Steroid responsive meningitis-arteritis Head and limb tremors[29]	
Airedale Terrier	Cerebellar cortical atrophy			
Akita Inu	Deafness Glycogenosis (Type III) Progressive retinal atrophy[43]	Bichon Frisé	Epilepsy	
Alaskan Husky	Necrotizing encephalopathy	Border Collie	Central progressive retinal atrophy[61]	
Alaskan Malamute	Chondrodysplasia[4] Hereditary polyneuropathy Idiopathic polyneuropathy		Cerebellar cortical degeneration Ceroid lipofuscinosis[63] Epilepsy Nemaline rod myopathy Peripheral sensory neuropathy	
American Cocker Spaniel	Glycogen storage disease			
American Foxhound	Deafness	Border Terrier	Hemivertebrae Oligodendroglioma[36] Progressive retinal atrophy	
American Staffordshire Bull Terrier	Deafness	Borzoi	Hereditary cervical spondylomyelopathy	[1] Starts at an age of 9–16 weeks; stiffness of the hindlimbs, mild head tremor, progresses to paralysis.
Australian Cattle Dog	Ceroid lipofuscinosis Deafness Polioencephalomyelopathy	Boston Terrier	Craniomandibular osteopathy[30] Deafness Hemivertebrae[21] Hydrocephalus[22] Oesophageal achalasia Oligodendroglioma[36] Pituitary tumour "Swimmers"[57] Vascular compression of the oesophagus	[2] Deformed vertebral bodies cause pressure necrosis of the overlying spinal cord. Age: birth to 6 months. [3] Congenital. [4] Together with anaemia, deformed forelimbs, lateral deviation of the paws, and enlarged carpus. [5] Signs: marked creatinuria and reduced muscle mass. Onset at 6 weeks to 7 months. Presents with 'bunny-hopping gait', cervical ventroflexion, depressed spinal refelexes; condition stabilises by 8–12 months.
Australian Shepherd Dog	Inherited deafness[60] Progressive retinal atrophy[46] Retinal detachment Retinal dysplasia Spina bifida[51]			
Australian Silky Terrier	Gaucher's disease I	Bouvier des Flandres	Idiopathic laryngeal paralysis	[6] Strongly convoluted retinal blood vessels, chorioretinal dysplasia, excavation of the optic disc, retinal detachment, intraocular haemorrhage.
B		Boxer	Centroperipheral neuropathy Deafness Intervertebral disc degeneration Niemann-Pick type C Oligodendroglioma[36] Polymyositis (immune mediated) Progressive axonopathy Spondylosis deformans Steroid responsive meningitis-arteritis	[7] Hereditary canine spinal muscular atrophy. [8] Diagnosis at a young age with EEG possible. [9] Starts at adulthood. [10] Occurs after strenuous exercise: stiff gait followed by collapse; consciousness maintained. [11] Possible predisposition caused by breeding and other factors
Basenji	Coloboma of the optic disc			
Bassett Hound	Cervical vertebral malformation (cervical spondylomyelopathy) [2] Lafora's disease			
Beagle	Bundle block Cerebellar cortical atrophy Deafness Epilepsy[8] GM1 gangliosidosis Lafora's disease Necrotising panostitis[34] Progressive retinal atrophy[43]			[12] Begins at an age of 8–18 months; characterised by frequent and persistent snapping at non-existent flies. [13] Progressive signs begin at an age of 3–6 months: stiffness of pelvis or cerebellar symptoms, increased total protein in CSF, enzyme deficiency in globoid cells in CNS.
		Briard	Progressive retinal atrophy[46] Progressive retinal degeneration type II[44]	
Bearded Collie	Epilepsy Progressive retinal atrophy[43]	Brittany Spaniel	Epilepsy Hereditary spinal muscular atrophy[7] Retinal dysplasia	[14] β-galactosidase deficiency. [15] Inherited, persistent aortic arches.
Bedlington Terrier	Retinal dysplasia[46]			
Belgian Malinois	Epilepsy			
Belgian Shepherd Dog	Epilepsy			

A2

Breed	Disease	Breed	Disease	Comments
Brussels Griffon	Hydrocephalus Spinocerebellar degeneration Syringomyelia		Polygenetic behavioural abnormalities Progressive retinal atrophy Progressive retinal degeneration Retinal dysplasia	
Bulldog	Cranial spina bifida Deafness Hydrocephalus[23] Oligodendroglioma[36] Spina bifida[52] "Swimmers"[57]	Collie	Cerebral degeneration[40] Choroidal hypoplasia Deafness Dermatomyositis Epilepsy[8] Neuraxonal dystrophy Optic nerve hypoplasia Progressive retinal atrophy Progressive retinal degeneration type I/II[44] Recessive ectasia (Collie eye anomaly)[47] Retinal dysplasia	
Bull Mastiff	Cerebellar degeneration Deformation of the cervical vertebrae Degeneration of spinal cord grey matter Glaucoma[17] Progressive retinal atrophy			
Bull Terrier	Deafness[58] Tail chasing syndrome[54]			
C		**D**		
Cairn Terrier	Cerebellar hypoplasia[28] Galacterocerebrosidosis Globoid cell leukodystrophy[18] Multisystem neuronal degeneration Progressive retinal atrophy	Dachshund	Congenital myasthenia gravis Deafness Hypoplasia (or aplasia) of the optic nerve Idiopathic epilepsy Intervertebral disc disease[11] Lafora's disease Mucopolysaccharidosis IIIa Narcolepsy / cataplexy Progressive retinal atrophy Sensory neuropathy[50] Scleral ectasia[6]	[16] Reduced number of retinal blood vessels; increased reflectivity of tapetum lucidum in young dogs; characteristic night blindness, which progresses to complete blindness. [17] Increased intraocular pressure with subsequent retinal atrophy; blindness possible. [18] Progressive signs beginning at an age of 3–6 months: stiffness of the pelvis or cerebellar symptoms, increased total protein in CSF, enzyme deficiency in globoid cells in CNS.
Canaan Hound	Epilepsy Progressive retinal atrophy			
Cardigan Welsh Corgi	Generalised progressive retinal atrophy[16] Degenerative myelopathy Luxated thoracic and lumbar discs	Dalmatian	Deafness[59] Galactocerebrosidosis / Globoid cell leukodystrophy[18] Hypertonic myopathy-polyneuropathy Laryngeal paralysis-polyneuropathy complex Cerebral and spinal leukodystrophies Muscular dystrophies[32]	[19] Protruding tongue. [20] Anterior uveitis, dermatitis, CNS involvement. [21] Asymmetrical, abnormal development of a vertebra; can cause neonatal death or spinal cord compression in older puppies; individual vertebra are wedge-shaped due to developmental retardation of one half of the vertebra; leads to scoliosis or an abnormal tail form; displacement of ribs in the thoracic region. [22] Dilatation of brain ventricles with increased CSF pressure.
Cavalier King Charles Spaniel	Chiari-like malformation Episodic weakness and collapse syndrome[10] Fly-catching syndrome[12] Syringomyelia			
Chihuahua	Ceroid lipofuscinosis Hydrocephalus[22] Hypoglycaemia[24] Hypoplasia of the dens axis[25]	Dandie Dinmont Terrier	Bilateral sensorineural deafness Intervertebral disc syndrome Narcolepsy	[23] Recessive gene with grave consequences: dilatation of brain ventricle with increased CSF pressure. [24] Stress-associated hypoglycaemia in young dogs: subnormal blood glucose concentration. [25] Dens hypoplasia or non-union of the dens with C2 causes atlantoaxial subluxation; onset not age-dependent; causes anything from pain originating from the neck to quadriplegia.
Chow Chow	Cerebellar cortical abiotrophy Cerebellar hypoplasia[28] Dysmyelinogenesis Myotonia congenita Retinal folds	Doberman Pinscher	Congenital vestibular disease Dancing Doberman disease Deafness Narcolepsy Wobbler syndrome[55]	
Clumber Spaniel	Mitochondrial myopathy (pyruvate dehydrogenase deficiency)	Dunker	Deafness	[26] Dilatation of brain ventricles with increased CSF pressure. [27] Ataxia and hypermetria at an age of 12 weeks.
Cocker Spaniel	Cerebellar degeneration Congenital vestibular disease[45] Deafness[39] Hypoplasia (or aplasia) of the optic nerve Idiopathic facial nerve paralysis Internal hydrocephalus[26] Intervertebral disc disease[11] Neuronal degeneration Oesophageal achalasia	**E** English Bulldog	Cerebellar cortical abiotrophy Hemivertebrae Spina bifida[53]	[28] Defect or incomplete development.
		English Cocker Spaniel	Congenital vestibular disease Deafness Generalised progressive retinal atrophy[16] "Swimmers"[57]	[29] First seen at an age of 8–12 weeks; can remain throughout whole life, but gets weaker.

Breed	Disease	Breed	Disease	Comments
English Foxhound	Deafness Osteochondrosis of the spinous process[37]		Cerebellar hypoplasia Epilepsy Hypomyelinating neuropathy Myasthenia gravis Retinal dysplasia X-linked muscular dystrophy	
English Setter	Ceroid lipofuscinosis Craniomandibular osteoarthropathy Deafness Progressive retinal atrophy	Gordon Setter	Cerebellar cortical abiotrophy Generalised progressive retinal atrophy	
English Springer Spaniel	Epilepsy[48] Episodic collapse Fucosidosis (alpha) Gangliosidosis GM1[14] Glycogen storage disease type VII[19] Myasthenia gravis Primary retinal dystrophy Progressive central retinal atrophy[61] Progressive retinal degeneration type II Central retinal atrophy Retinal dysplasia	Great Dane	Central core-like myopathy Cervical calcinosis circumscripta Cerebellar hypoplasia Deafness Distal symmetrical polyneuropathy Megaoesophagus Myasthenia gravis Myotonic myopathy Necrotising myelopathy Chronic progressive ataxia Retinal dysplasia Spondylolisthesis / Wobbler Stockard paralysis[65] syndrome	
F				
Finnish Spitz	Epilepsy[9] Ectasia	Great Pyrenees Dog	Deafness	
Flat-coated Retriever	Epilepsy Megaoesophagus	Greyhound	Deafness Megaoesophagus Oesophageal achalasia Retinal dystrophy Short spinal processes Steroid responsive meningitis-arteritis	[30] Irregular bony proliferation of the mandibles and the tympanic bullae; difficulties in eating possibly leading to malnutrition; intermittent fever up to 40°C; starts at an age of 4–7 months; can regress or stop.
French Bulldog	Hemivertebra[21]			
G		Groenendaler	X-linked muscular dystrophy	[31] Congenital lack of cerebrocortical gyri: signs in first year of life; changes in behaviour and ability to see; seizures.
German Shepherd Dog	Congenital vestibular disease Deafness Degenerative myelopathy Epilepsy[8] Giant axonal neuropathy Glycogenosis Type III Hereditary fibrotic myopathy Immune-mediated polymyositis Megaoesophagus Myasthenia gravis Mucopolysaccharidosis VII Oesophageal achalasia Pituitary dwarfism Progressive posterior paralysis[42] Spinal muscular atrophy Vascular anomalies with oesophageal compression	**I** Ibizan Hound Irish Setter	Deafness Seizures Cerebellar dysplasia Epilepsy Generalised myopathy General progressive retinal atrophy Globoid cell leukodystrophy Lissencephaly Megaoesophagus Persistent aortic arches[41]	[32] X-linked myopathy. [33] Generalised muscle atrophy; reduced spinal reflexes; bunny-hopping gait. [34] Genetic predisposition. [35] Signs at an age of 3–9 months: characteristic biting of the toes, self-mutilation; poor sensation in distal limbs; vascular degeneration; demyelination of the spinal cord. [36] CNS tumour. [37] Craniocaudal herniation of the intervertebral endplate into the vertebral body; stiff gait prevents normal gallop; starts from an age of 7–10 months.
		Irish Terrier	Muscular dystrophy[32]	[38] Clinically similar to "swimmer" pups. Uniformly dense bones and abnormal zones of bony resorption can be seen on a radiograph.
		Irish Wolfhound	Progressive retinal atrophy	[39] Arises due to the ears lying flat on the head; irritation.
German Short-haired Pointer	Acral mutilation CNS storage disease[64] Gangliosidosis GM2 Steroid responsive meningitis-arteritis X-linked muscular dystrophy	Italian Greyhound **J** Jack Russell Terrier	Epilepsy Persistent right aortic arch[44] Congenital myasthenia gravis Deafness Hereditary ataxia (spinocerebellar degeneration) Neuroaxonal dystrophy	[40] Low grade: characterised by partial agnathy, hydrocephalus and partial defects of the fontanelles. High grade: characterised by agenesis of all structures rostral to the medulla. [41] Development of the right aortic arch instead of a left one, which crosses the oesophagus and forms a ring with the pulmonary artery and the arterial ligament resulting in oesophageal stenosis.
Golden Retriever	Central progressive retinal atrophy Central retinal degeneration	Japanese Spaniel	Gangliosidosis GM2 (type AB)	

A2

Breed	Disease	Breed	Disease	Comments
K		**O**		
Kerry Blue Terrier	Cerebellar cortical abiotrophy and extra pyramidal nuclei degeneration[1] Cerebral degeneration Spiculosis	Old English Sheepdog	Cytochrome c oxidase deficiency Muscular dystrophy	
Kelpie	Cerebellar cortical abiotrophy	**P** Papillon	Deafness Neuroaxonal dystrophies (only one litter reported)	
King Charles Spaniel	Episodic collapse syndrome	Pekingese	Diseases of the intervertebral discs[11] Progressive retinal atrophy "Swimmers"[57]	
Kuvasz	Deafness	Pembroke Welsh Corgi	Degenerative myelopathy	
L Labrador Retriever	Abnormal nystagmus Axonopathy Central progressive retinal atrophy[62] Cerebellar cortical abiotrophies Cortex degeneration Deficit of type II muscle fibres / familial myopathy[5] Degenerative myelopathy Epilepsy Familial reflex myoclonus Fibrinoid leukodystrophy Hereditary myelopathy Type II Megaoesophagus Mucopolysaccharidosis II Muscular dystrophy[33] Narcolepsy-cataplexy Retinal detachment Retinal dysplasia[20] Spongy degeneration of the white matter	Plott Hound Pointer Pomeranian	Mucopolysaccharidosis I Deafness Epilepsy Neurogenic muscle atrophy Neurotrophic osteopathy[35] Progressive retinal atrophy Progressive retinal degeneration Sensory neuropathy Progressive retinal atrophy Hydrocephalus	
		Poodle (miniature: no bigger than 38.10 cm; toy: no bigger than 25.40 cm)	Behavioural abnormalities Cerebrospinal demyelination Congenital deafness Epilepsy[8] Globoid cell leukodystrophy Hypoplasia or aplasia of the optic nerve Intervertebral disc degeneration Narcolepsy-cataplexy Neonatal encephalopathy Progressive degeneration of the rods and cones Progressive retinal atrophy Retinal detachment	[42] Affects dogs in middle and old age, possible predisposition in males, gradual asymmetrical start in hindlimbs. [43] Dilated pupils react slowly to stimuli, night blindness progressive to complete blindness, atrophy of retinal vessels, increased reflectivity of the tapetum lucidum. [44] Central retinal atrophy. [45] (= mental retardation) progressive – starts as "swimmer" at an age of 3 days, later inability to stand and amblyobia; can be accompanied by tremor and nystagmus; vascular anomaly with compression of the oesophagus. [46] Recessive; disordered and abnormally formed layers of the retina with retinal detachment; causes blindness. [47] Strongly convoluted retinal blood vessels, chorioretinal dysplasia, excavation of the optic disc, retinal detachment, intraocular haemorrhage. [48] Depression and reduced ability to see at an age of 12–15 months; at 18 months old, muscle spasms develop that may result in seizures. [49] Recessive; hyperkinetic functional disturbance characterised by an apparently painless rigidity of the limbs, back and tail musculature; can affect both sexes; the head may be lowered between the forelegs; the dog recovers in 15–30 seconds. Oral administration of diazepam 0.5 mg/kg TID is very effective in controlling episodes. [50] Long-haired breed. [51] Spinal canal remains open.
Lhasa Apso	Lissencephaly[31] Progressive retinal atrophy			
M Maltese	Blindness[3] Deafness Glycogen storage disease Type IA Hydrocephalus Malonic aciduria Necrotizing encephalitis Shaker dog / idiopathic tremors	Poodle (standard)	Behavioural abnormalities Epilepsy Niemann-Pick disease type A/B Progressive retinal atrophy	
		Pug	Hemivertebrae Necrotizing Meningo-encephalitis	
Manchester Terrier	Epilepsy	**R**		
Miniature Pinscher	Progressive retinal atrophy Mucopolysaccharidosis VI	Rhodesian Ridgeback	Aggression Cerebellar cortical abiotrophies Congenital deafness Deformation of cervical vertebrae / Wobbler's syndrome Hypothyroidism Lumbosacral transitional vertebrae	
Miniature Schnauzer	Ceroid lipofuscinosis Megaoesophagus Oesophageal achalasia Progressive retinal atrophy X-linked muscular dystrophy X-linked myopathies			
N Newfoundland	Megaoesophagus[15] Myasthenia gravis Polymyositis (immune mediated)	Rottweiler	Congenital deafness Distal myopathy Laryngeal	

Breed	Disease	Breed	Disease	Comments
	Leucoencephalomalacia Muscular dystrophy Neuraxonal dystrophy paralysis-polyneuropathy complex Progressive Polyneuropathy Retinal dysplasia Spinal (neurogenic) muscular atrophy Spinal subarachnoid cyst	Smooth Coated Fox Terrier	Ataxia Congenital myasthenia gravis Congenital vestibular disease Deafness Oesophageal achalasia Persistent aortic arches[41]	
		Springer Spaniel	Congenital myasthenia gravis Dysmyelination	
S		Staffordshire Bull Terrier	L-2-hydroxyglutaric aciduria	
Saluki	Progressive retinal atrophy Retinal detachment Spongy degeneration of the grey matter	Sussex Spaniel	Pyruvate dehydrogenase deficiency (metabolic myopathy)	[52] Neural arches do not bear any relationship to each other. Possible consequences: herniation of the meninges and / or the spinal cord (spina bifida manifesta) or no herniation (spina bifida occulta). Hemivertebrae: asymmetrical abnormal development of a vertebra leading to neonatal death or spinal cord compression in older puppies. Individual wedge-shaped vertebrae due to developmental retardation in one half of the vertebra leading to scoliosis or an abnormal tail form; displacement of ribs in the thoracic region.
Samoyed	Cerebellar cortical degeneration Deafness Hypomyelination Lissencephaly X-linked muscular dystrophy Progressive retinal degeneration Retinal detachment Spongy degeneration of the grey matter	**T** Tibetan Mastiff Tibetan Spaniel Tibetan Terrier	Hypertrophic neuropathy Progressive retinal atrophy Ceroid lipofuscinosis	
Scottish Terrier	Alexander's disease Cerebellar cortical abiotrophy Deafness Fibrinoid leukodystrophy Hypotonic myopathies Intervertebral disc disease Progressive tetraparesis Scotty cramp[49]	**V** Vizsla	Epilepsy Facial nerve paralysis Focal polymyositis	[53] Starts at an age of 4–6 weeks, not progressive; abduction of one limb, hopping gait, abnormal proprioception in the hindlimbs. [54] Form of epilepsy. [55] The cranial ventral canal is narrower than the caudal part; dorsoventral between C3 and C7. [56] Preganglionic sympathetic degeneration.
Sealyham Terrier	Blindness Deafness Retinal detachment Retinal dysplasia[46]	**W** Weimaraner	Dysmyelination Myasthenia gravis Spinal dysraphism[53] Steroid responsive meningitis-arteritis	[57] Characteristic inability to stand at an age of 4–6 weeks; flat chest. [58] Often associated with white coat, but not so in the Bull Terrier. [59] Cochlear degeneration.
Schipperke	Mucopolysaccharidosis IIIB	Welsh Corgi	Central retinal atrophy Dermatomyositis Progressive retinal degeneration[38]	[60] Associated with the genes for Merle colouration and dappling.
Shar Pei	Primary megaoesophagus			
Siberian Husky	Congenital pharyngeal paralysis Epilepsy Gangliosidosis GM1 Eosinophilic granuloma Progressive retinal atrophy	West Highland White Terrier	Deafness Globoid cell leukodystrophy / Galactocerebrosidosis (Krabbe's disease)[13] Myotonia Shaker dog / idiopathic tremors	[61] Affects dogs between 3–5 years. Presumably dominant with incomplete penetrance; patchy and increased reflection in the central area leads to loss of sight; difficulty in seeing non-moving objects; can see best in poor lighting conditions.
Silky Terrier	Glucocerebrosidosis (Gaucher disease) Hydrocephalus Occipital dysplasia White matter spongy degeneration	Wire-haired Dachshund Wire-haired Fox Terrier	Lafora's disease Mucopolysaccharidosis III Cerebellar hypoplasia Epilepsy Lissencephaly Megaoesophagus	[62] Possibly dominant with incomplete penetrance. [63] Changes in behaviour; hyperactivity followed by aggression starting between 16–23 months of age; motor abnormalities; blindness.
Sky Terrier	Enlarged foramen magnum / occipital dysplasia Megaoesophagus	**Y** Yorkshire Terrier	Hydrocephalus Retinal dysplasia Necrotizing encephalitis Necrotizing encephalopathy (Leigh's disease)	[64] Characteristic nervousness and reduced possibility of training at an age of 6 months; between 9–12 months of age: ataxia and reduced ability to stand.

Appendix 3:
List of inheritable neurological diseases of the dog[1]

Hereditary defect or disease	Breeds	Mode of inheritance	References
Acral mutilation	English and German Pointers	autosomal recessive	CUMMINGS et al. (1983)
Alexander's disease	Bernese Cattle Dog; also seen in Miniature Poodle, Scottish Terrier and Labrador Retreivers (single case reports)		WEISSENBOCK et al. (1996)
Ataxia and myelopathy	Jack Russell Terrier, Smooth-haired Fox Terrier	autosomal recessive	HARTLEY and PALMER (1973)
Bilateral sensorineural deafness	Doberman Pinscher	autosomal recessive	GARASHI et al. (1972), WILKES and PALMER (1987)
Black hair follicle	Great Munsterland	autosomal recessive	SCHMUTZ et al. (1998)
Central core-like myopathy	Great Dane		NEWSHOLME and GASKELL (1987), TARGETT et al. (1994)
Cerebellar cortical abiotrophies	Airedale Terrier, Beagle, Chow Chow, Harrier, Kelpie, Labrador Retriever, Rhodesian Ridgeback		SUMMERS et al. (1995)
Cerebral hypoplasia	Airedale Terrier	familial	CORDY et al. (1952)
Cerebral degeneration	Bernese Cattle Dog, Gordon Setter, Kerry Blue Terrier, Rough Collie	autosomal recessive	DE LAHUNTA and AVERILL (1976), HARTLEY et al. (1978), STEINBERG et al. (1981), CARMICHAEL et al. (1996)
Ceroid lipofuscinosis	Australian Cattle Dog, Border Collie, English Setter, Miniature Schnauzer, Tibetan Terrier, and others	autosomal recessive	KOPPANG et al. (1965), ARMSTRONG et al. (1982), LINGAAS et al. (1998)
Congenital myasthenia gravis	Danish Chicken Dog	autosomal recessive	FLAGSTAD (1989)
Congenital myasthenia gravis	Jack Russell Terrier, Smooth-Haired Miniature Dachsunds		WALLACE and PALMER (1984), DICKINSON et al. (2005)
Congenital myasthenia gravis	Smooth-haired Fox Terrier	autosomal recessive	JENKINS et al. (1976)
Deafness	Beagle, Bulldog, Bull Terrier, Dalmatian, English Setter, Greyhound, Great Pyrenee Dog, Samoyed	oligogene	STRAIN (1996), MUHLE et al. (2001)
Deafness	American Foxhound, Collie, Dachshund, Dunker, Great Dane, Old English Sheepdog, Shetland Sheepdog	autosomal, incomplete dominance and incomplete penetrance	REETZ et al. (1977), STRAIN (1996)
Degenerative myelopathy	Afghan, Boxer, Chesapeake Bay Retriever, German Shepherd, Labrador Retriever, Welsh Corgi	autosomal recessive	BARCLAY and HAINES (1994), DE LAHUNTA et al. (1994), SUMMERS et al. (1995)
Dermatomyositis	Collie, Shetland Sheepdog, Welsh Corgi	autosomal dominant	HARGIS and MUNDELL (1992), WHITE et al. (1992), FERGUSON et al. (2000)
Distal polyneuropathy	Rottweiler		BRAUND et al. (1994a)
Dysmyelination	Bernese Cattle Dog, Chow Chow, Weimaraner	autosomal recessive	VANDERVELDE et al. (1978), KORNEGAY et al. (1987), PALMER et al. (1987)

Hereditary defect or disease	Breeds	Mode of inheritance	References
Epilepsy	Many breeds	autosomal recessive / polygenic	CROFT and STOCKMANN (1964), MARTINEK (1980), HALL and WALLACE (1996), FAMULA et al. (1997), JAGGY et al. (1998), KATHMANN et al. (1999)
Fibrinoid leukodystrophy	Labrador Retriever, Scottish Terrier		McGRATH (1979), SORJONENE et al. (1987)
Fucosidosis (alpha)	English Springer Spaniel		HARTLEY et al. (1982), KELLY et al. (1983), OCCHIODORO et al. (1996), SKELLY et al. (1996), HOLMES et al. (1998)
Galactocerebrosidosis	Beagle, Blue Tick Hound, Cairn Terrier, Dalmatian, Miniature Poodle, West Highland White Terrier	autosomal recessive / familial	FANKHAUSER et al. (1963), HIRTH et al. (1967), BOYSEN et al. (1974), JOHNSON et al. (1975), BJERKAS et al. (1977)
Galactosidosis	Schipperkee		KNOWLES et al. (1993)
Gangliosidosis GM1 (β-galactosidase deficiency)	English Springer Spaniel, Portuguese Water Dog, Shiba, Siberian Husky	autosomal recessive	READ et al. (1976), SAUNDERS et al. (1988), MULLER et al. (1998), YAMATO et al. (2000)
Gangliosidosis GM2	German Short-haired Pointer		KARBE and SCHIEFER (1967), SINGER and CORK (1989)
Gangliosidosis GM2 (Type AB)	Japanese Spaniel		CUMMINGS et al. (1983), ISHIKAWA et al. (1987)
Gaucher's disease I	Australian Silky Terrier		HARTLEY and BLAKEMORE (1973), FARROW et al. (1982)
Giant axonal neuropathy	German Shepherd	autosomal recessive	DUNCAN et al. (1981)
Glycogen storage disease type Ia (Gierke disease)	Maltese	autosomal recessive	BRIX et al. (1995), KISHNANI et al. (1997)
Glycogen storage disease type II (Pompe's disease)	Lapland Dog	autosomal recessive	MOSTAFA (1970), WALVOORT et al. (1984)
Glycogen storage disease type VII	American Cocker Spaniel, English Springer Spaniel	autosomal recessive	GIGER and HARVEY (1987), GIGER et al. (1992), SMITH et al. (1996)
Grey matter spongy degeneration	Bull Mastiff, Saluki	autosomal recessive	SUMMERS et al. (1995)
Hereditary canine spinal muscular atrophy	Brittany Spaniel	autosomal dominant	BLAZEJ et al. (1998)
Hereditary myopathy	Afghan, German Shepherd	autosomal recessive	BRAUND and VANDEVELDE (1978), CUMMINGS and DE LAHUNTA (1978)
Hereditary myopathy	Labrador Retriever	autosomal recessive	McKERRELL and BRAUND (1987), AMMAN et al. (1988)
Hereditary necrotising myelopathy	Kooikerhund	autosomal recessive	MANDIGERS et al. (1993)
Hereditary polyneuropathy	Alaskan Malamute	autosomal recessive	MOE (1992)
Hypomyelinating neuropathy	Golden Retriever	autosomal recessive	MATZ et al. (1990
Hypertonic collapse	Cavalier King Charles Spaniel, Dalmatian, Scottish Terrier		PETERS and MEYERS (1977), WOODS (1977), WRIGHT et al. (1987)
Hypertrophic neuropathy	Tibetan Mastiff	autosomal recessive	CUMMINGS et al. (1981), SPONENBERG and DE LAHUNTA (1981)
Idiopathic polyneuropathy	Alaskan Malamute		BRAUND et al. (1997)
Laryngeal paralysis – neuropathy	Dalmatian, Rottweiler	autosomal recessive	BRAUND et al. (1994b), MAHONEY et al. (1998)
Laryngeal paralysis	Bouvier de Flandres	autosomal dominant	VENKER-VAN HAAGEN (1981)
Leukodystrophies	Dalmatian	autosomal recessive	BJERKAS (1977, 1979)
Leucoencephalomyelopathy	Rottweiler		WOUDA and VAN NESS (1986)
Lissencephaly	Lhasa Apso		GREENE et al. (1976)
Mitochondrial myopathy	Clumber Spaniel, Sussex Spaniel		SHELTON (2000)
Mitochondrial myopathy	Old English Sheepdog		BREITSCHWERDT et al. (1992), VIJAYASARTHY et al. (1994)

A3

A3

Hereditary defect or disease	Breeds	Mode of inheritance	References
Mucopolysaccharidosis I	Plott Hound		SHULL et al. (1982), SPELLACY et al. (1983), MENON et al. (1992)
Mucopolysaccharidosis II	Labrador Retriever	autosomal recessive	WILKERSON et al. (1998)
Mucopolysaccharidosis IIIa	Wire-haired Dachshund		FISCHER et al. (1998)
Mucopolysaccharidosis VI	Miniature Pinscher		NEER et al. (1995)
Mucopolysaccharidosis VII	German Shepherd		HASKINS et al. (1984), SCHUCHMAN et al. (1989), RAY et al. (1998)
Myopathy and generalized Neuropathy	Doberman Pinscher		BRAUND (1995)
Myotonia	Chow Chow	autosomal recessive	JONES et al. (1977), FARROW and MALIK (1981)
Narcolepsy	Doberman, Labrador Retriever	autosomal recessive	LIN et al. (1999)
Niemann-Pick disease type A/B	Poodle		BUNDZA et al. (1979)
Niemann-Pick disease type C	Boxer		KUWAMURA et al. (1993)
Nemaline rod myopathy	Border Collie, Schipperkee		DELAUCHE et al. (1998)
Neuroaxonal dystrophy	Jack Russell Terrier, Papillon, Rottweiler	autosomal recessive	CHRISTMAN et al. (1984), SACRE et al. (1993), FRANKLIN et al. (1995)
Neurogenic muscular atrophy	Pointer, Rottweiler	autosomal recessive	IZUMO et al. (1983), SHELL et al. (1987)
Neurodegeneration	Cairn Terrier		ZAAL et al. (1997)
Neurodegeneration	Cocker Spaniel		JAGGY and VANDEVELDE (1988)
Neuronal abiotrophy	Swedish Lappenhund	autosomal recessive	SANDEFELDT et al. (1976)
Neuronal vacuolation	Rottweiler		PUMAROLA et al. (1999)
Polioencephalomyelopathy	Australian Cattle Dog		BRENNER et al. (1997)
Primary sensory neuropathy	Long-haired Dachshund		DUNCAN and GRIFFITHS (1982)
Progressive axonopathy	Boxer	autosomal recessive	GRIFFITHS et al. (1987)
Sensorineural deafness	Pointer	autosomal recessive	STEINBERG et al. (1994)
Shaking pup	Springer Spaniel	sex-linked recessive	NADON et al. (1990)
Spinal Ataxia	Many breeds	familial	BJORCK et al. (1957), JAGGY et al. (1988), DENIS et al. (1994)
Spinal cerebellar degeneration	Brittany Spaniel		HIGGINS et al. (1998)
Spinal muscular atrophy	Brittany Spaniel, German Shepherd	autosomal dominant	CORK et al. (1979), CUMMINGS et al. (1989), BLAZEJ et al. (1998)
White matter spongy degeneration	Labrador Retriever, Samoyed, Silky Terrier		ZACHARY and O'BRIEN (1985), SUMMERS et al. (1995)
X-linked myopathy	German Shorthair, Golden Retriever, Groenendaler, Irish Terrier, Pigmy Schnauzer, Rottweiler, Samoyed	X-linked	WENTINK et al. (1972), HAM et al. (1993), PAOLA et al. (1993), PRESTHUS and NORDSTOGA (1993), SCHATZBERG et al. (1998, 1999)

---

[1] A large part of this data comes from BROOKS M., SARGAN D. (2001): Genetic aspects of the disease in dogs. In: Ruvinsky A., Sampson J. (eds.), The Genetics of the Dog. CABI Publishing, Oxon, U.K., pp. 191–266.

Appendix 4:
List of inheritable neurological diseases of the cat[1]

Hereditary defect or disease	Breeds	Mode of inheritance[2]	References[3]
Axonopathy	Burmese		MOREAU et al. (1991)
Cerebellar abiotrophy	Siamese		SHAMIR et al. (1999)
Cerebellar ataxia			KOCH et al. (1955), DE LAHUNTA (1971)
Cerebellar cortical atrophy			TANIYAMA et al. (1994), AYE et al. (1998)
Cerebral degeneration		autosomal recessive	INADA et al. (1996)
Cerebral hypoplasia			BLOOD (1946), SCHEIDY (1953)
Ceroid lipofuscinosis	Siamese		GREEN and LITTLE (1974), WEISSENBOCK and ROSSEL (1997)
Dandy-Walker Syndrome			REGNIER et al. (1993)
Dysautonomia			SYMONDS et al. (1995), McNULTY et al. (1999)
Encephalomyelopathy	Burmese		JONES et al. (1992)
Deafness	White cats	associated with dominant hair colouration	BAMBER (1933), BERGSMA et al. (1971), HEID et al. (1998)
Epilepsy			QUESNEL et al. (1997), FATZER et al. (2000)
Exencephaly	Manx		FIELD and WANNER (1975)
Fucosidosis (alpha)			GILBERT et al. (1988)
Gangliosidosis GM1	Siamese		BAKER et al. (1971), GILBERT et al. (1988), DEMARIA et al. (1998)
Gangliosidosis GM2	Siamese		CORK et al. (1977), GILBERT et al. (1988), MULDOON et al. (1994)
Glycogen storage disease type II			SANDSROM et al. (1969), GILBERT et al. (1988), REUSER (1993)
Glycogen storage disease type IV	Norwegian Forest Cat		FYFE et al. (1992), COATES et al. (1996)
Hindlimb paralysis			LANSDOWN and PATE (1992)
Hydrocephalus			SILSON and ROBINSON (1969), SHELL (1996)
Hypomyelination of the central nervous system			STOFFREGEN et al. (1993)
Krabbe's disease (globoid cell leukodystrophy)			JOHNSON (1970)
Lysosomal storage disease	Abyssinian, Persian		HEGREBERG and NORBY (1973), KRAMMER et al. (1975), BLAND VAN DEN BERG et al. (1977)
Mannosidosis, alpha			BURDITT et al. (1980), BERG et al. (1997)
Megacolon			DIETZMANN (1968), EGGERT et al. (1998), WASHABAU and HOLT (1999)
Megaoesophagus			MADDISON and ALLAN (1990), MEARS and JENKINS (1997)
Mucolipidosis II		autosomal recessive	BOSSHARD et al. (1996), HUBLER et al. (1996)
Mucopolysaccharidosis I		autosomal recessive	HASKINS et al. (1979), HE et al. (1999)
Mucopolysaccharidosis VI			COWELL et al. (1976), HASKINS et al. (1992), BYERS et al. (2000)

A4

Hereditary defect or disease	Breeds	Mode of inheritance[2]	References[3]
Mucopolysaccharidosis VII			HASKINS et al. (1992), FYFE et al. (1999)
Muscular dystrophies: Duchenne and Becker types		X-linked	CARPENTER et al. (1989), GASCHEN et al. (1992, 1999)
Myasthenia gravis			DAWSON (1970), MASON (1976)
Myelocele			KITCHEN et al. (1972)
Myopathy			MALIK et al. (1993), LANTINGA et al. (1998)
Myotonia			HICKFORD et al. (1998), TOLL et al. (1998)
Neuroaxonal dystrophy	Siamese		WOODARD et al. (1974), RODRIGUEZ et al. (1996)
Niemann-Pick disease type C	Siamese		CRISP et al. (1970), WENGER et al. (1980), MARCH et al. (1997)
Olivopontocerebellar hypoplasia			BROUWER (1934)
Sacral dysgenesis	Manx		KITCHEN et al. (1972)
Sacrococcygeal agenesis			FRYE (1967)
Spastic syndrome	Devon Rex		ROBINSON (1992)
Spina bifida	Manx		KERRUISH (1964), LEUPOLD et al. (1974), CLARKE and CARLISLE (1975)
Spina bifida occulta			FRYE (1967)
Spina bifida with raduschisis			FRYE and McFARLAND (1965)
Spinal dysplasia			LANSDOWN and PATE (1992)
Strabismus	Siamese		KALIL et al. (1971), DISTLER and HOFFMANN (1996), YIN et al. (1996)
Syringomyelia			CLARK and CARLISLE (1975), BAGLEY et al. (2000)
Short tail	Manx	dominant	TODD (1961), ADALTEINSSON (1980), ROBINSON (1993)
Tremor			NORBY and THULINE (1970)
Vertebral anomalies			PARSONS and STEIN (1955–1956)
Visual acuity, abnormal	Siamese		GUILLERY et al. (1974)
Visual pathway, abnormal	Siamese		JOHNSON (1991)
Wardenburg syndrome			FAITH and WOODARD (1973)

---

[1] A large part of this data comes from the databank "Online Mendelian Inheritance in Animals (OMIA)"; http://www.angis.su.oz.au/Databases/BIRX/omia/.

[2] The mode of inheritance in the cat has not been elucidated in many of the diseases in this list, but as in the majority of them analogue genetic diseases have been described in humans, they have been included in this summary.

[3] As a rule, the oldest and the newest publications are included.

Literature about inheritable neurological diseases in the dog and cat

ADALSTEINSSON S. (1980): Establishment of equilibrium for the dominant lethal gene for Manx taillessness in cats. Theoretical and Applied Genetics 58: 49.

AMMAN J.F., LAUGHLIN M.H., KORTHUIS R.J. (1988): Muscle hemodynamics in hereditary myopathy of Labrador Retrievers. American Journal of Veterinary Research 49: 1127–1130.

ARMSTRONG D., KOPPANG N., NILSSON S.E. (1982): Canine hereditary ceroid lipofuscinosis. European Neurology 21: 147–156.

AYE M.M., IZUMO S., INADA S., ISASHIKI Y., YAMANAKA H., MATSUMURO K., KAWASAKI Y., SAWASHIMA Y., FUJI-YAMA J., ARIMURA K., OSAME M. (1998): Histopathological and ultrastructural features of feline hereditary cerebellar cortical atrophy – a novel animal model of human spinocerebellar degeneration. Acta Neuropathologica 96: 379–387.

BAGLEY R.S., GAVIN P.R., SILVER G.M., MOORE M.P., KIPPENES H., CONNORS R. (2000): Syringomyelia and hydromyelia in dogs and cats. Compendium on Continuing Education for the Practicing Veterinarian 22: 471–479.

BAKER J.J., LINDSEY J.R., MCKHANN G.M., FARRELL D.F. (1971): Neuronal GM1 gangliosidosis in a Siamese cat with beta-galactosidase deficiency. Science 174: 838–839.

BAMBER R.C. (1933): Correlation between white coat colour, blue eyes, and deafness in cats. Journal of Genetics 27: 407–413.

BARCLAY K.B., HAINES D.M. (1994): Immunohistochemical evidence for immunoglobulin and complement deposition in spinal cord lesions in degenerative myelopathy in German shepherd dogs. Canadian Journal of Veterinary Research 58: 20–24.

BERG T., TOLLERSRUD O.K., WALKLEY S.U., SIEGEL D., NILSSEN O. (1997): Purification of feline lysosomal alpha-mannosidase, determination of its cdna sequence and identification of a mutation causing alpha-mannosidosis in Persian cats. Biochemical Journal 328: 863–870.

BERGSMA D.R., BROWN K.S. (1971): White fur, blue eyes and deafness in the domestic cat. Journal of Heredity 62: 171–185.

BJERKAS I. (1977): Hereditary 'cavitating' leucodystrophy in Dalmatian dogs: light and electron microscopic studies. Acta Neuropathologia 40: 163–169.

BJERKAS I. (1979): Hereditary leukodystrophy in Dalmatian dogs in Norway. Norsk Veterinaertidsskrift 91: 167–170.

BJORCK G., DRYENDAHL S., OLSSON S.E. (1957): Hereditary ataxia in smooth haired Fox Terriers. Veterinary Record 69: 871–876.

BLAND VAN DEN BERG P., BAKER M.K., LANGE A.L. (1977): A suspected lysosomal storage in Abyssinian cats, Part I: genetic, clinical and clinical pathological aspects. Journal of the South African Veterinary Association 48: 195–199.

BLAZEJ R.G., MELLERSH D.S., CORK L.C., OSTRANDER E.A. (1998): Hereditary canine spinal muscular atrophy is phenotypically similar but molecularly distinct from human spinal muscular atrophy. Journal of Heredity 6: 531–537.

BLOOD D.C. (1946): Cerebellar hypoplasia and degeneration in the kitten. Australian Veterinary Journal 22: 120–121.

BOSSHARD N.U., HUBLER M., ARNOLD S., BRINER J., SPYCHER M.A., SOMMERLADE H.J., VONFIGURA K., GITZELMANN R. (1996): Spontaneous mucolipidosis in a cat – an animal model of human i-cell disease. Veterinary Pathology 33: 1–13.

BOYSEN B.G., TRYPHONAS L., HARRIES N.W. (1974): Globoid cell leucodystrophy in the Bluetick Hound dog. I. Clinical manifestations. Canadian Veterinary Journal 15: 303–308.

BRAUND K.G., VANDEVELDE M. (1978): German Shepherd dog myelopathy – a morphologic and morphometric study. American Journal of Veterinary Research 39: 1309–1315.

BRAUND K.G., TOIVIO-KINNUCAN M., VALLAT J.M., MEHTA J.R., LEVESQUE D.C. (1994a): Distal sensorimotor polyneuropathy in mature Rottweiler dogs. Veterinary Pathology 31: 316–326.

BRAUND K.G., SHORES A, COCHRANE S., FORRESTER D., KWIECIEN J.M., STEISS J.E. (1994b): Laryngeal paralysis-polyneuropathy complex in young Dalmatians. American Journal of Veterinary Research 55: 534–542.

BRAUND K.G. (1995): Disorders of peripheral nerves. In: Ettinger S.J. and Feldman E.C. (eds.): A Textbook of Veterinary Internal Medicine, 4th edn. S.B. Saunders, Philadelphia, pp. 701–728.

BRAUND K.G., SHORES A, LOWRIE C.T., STEINBERG H.S., MOORE M.P., BAGLEY R.S., STEISS J.E. (1997): Idiopathic polyneuropathy in Alaskan malamutes. Journal of Veterinary Internal Medicine 11: 243–249.

BREITSCHWERDT E.B., KORNEGAY J.N., WHEELER S.J., STEVENS J.B., BATY C.J. (1992): Episodic weakness associated with exertional lactic acidosis and myopathy in Old English Sheepdog littermates. Journal of the American Veterinary Medical Association 201: 731–736.

BRENNER O., DELAHUNTA A., SUMMERS B.A., CUMMINGS J.F., COOPER B.J., VALENTINE B.A., BELL J.S. (1997): Hereditary polioencephalomyelopathy of the Australian Cattle dog. Acta Neuropathologica 94: 54–66.

BRIX A.E., HOWERTH E.W., MCCONKIEROSELL A., PETERSON D., EGNOR D., WELLS M.R., CHEN Y.T. (1995): Glycogen storage disease type Ia in two littermate maltese puppies. Veterinary Pathology 32: 460–465.

BROUWER B.A. (1934): Familial olivo-ponto-cerebellar hypoplasia in cats. Psychiatry and Neurology B1 38: 352–367.

BUNDZA A., LOWDEN J.A., CHARLTON K.M. (1979): Niemann-Pick disease in a Poodle dog. Veterinary Pathology 16: 530–538.

BURDITT L.J., CHOTAI K., HIRANI S., NUGENT P.G., WINCHESTER B.G., BLACKMORE W.F. (1980): Biochemical studies on a case of feline mannosidosis. Biochemical Journal 189: 467–473.

BYERS S., CRAWLEY A.C., BRUMFIELD L.K., NUTTALL J.D., HOPWOOD J.J. (2000): Enzyme replacement therapy in a feline model of MPS VI: Modification of enzyme structure and dose frequency. Pediatric Research 47: 743–749.

CARMICHAEL K.P., MILLER M., RAWLINGS C.A., FISCHER A., OLIVER J.E., MILLER B.E. (1996): Clinical, hematologic, and biochemical features of a syndrome in Bernese mountain dogs characterized by hepatocerebellar degeneration. Journal of the American Veterinary Medical Association 208: 1277–1280.

CARPENTER J.L., HOFFMAN E.P., ROMANUL F.C.A., KUNKEL L.M., ROSALES R.K., MA N.S.F., DASBACH J.J., RAE J.F., MOORE F.M., MCAFEE M.B., PEARCE L.K. (1989): Feline muscular dystrophy with dystrophin deficiency. American Journal of Pathology 135: 909–919.

CHRISMAN C.L., COK L.C., GAMBLE D.A. (1984): Neuroaxonal dystrophy in Rottweiler. Journal of the American Veterinary Medical Association 184: 464–467.

CLARK L., CARLISLE C.H. (1975): Spina bifida with syringomyelia and meningocele in a short-tailed cat. Australian Veterinary Journal 51: 392–394.

COATES J.R., PAXTON R., COX N.R., BRAUND K.G., STEISS J.E., BAKER H.J., SIMPSON S.T. (1996): A case presentation and discussion of type IV glycogen storage disease in a Norwegian forest cat. Progress in Veterinary Neurology 7: 5–11.

CORDY D.R., SNELBAKER H.A. (1952): Cerebellar hypoplasia and degeneration in a family of Airedale dogs. Journal of Neuropathology and Experimental Neurology 11: 324–328.

COWELL K.R., JEZYK P.F., HASKINS M.E., PATTERSON D.F. (1976): Mucopolysaccharidosis in a cat. Journal of the American Veterinary Medical Association 169: 334–339.

CORK L.C., MUNNELL J.F., LORENZ M.D., MURPHY J.V., BAKER H.J., RATTAZZI M.C. (1977): GM-2-ganglioside lysosomal storage disease in cats with beta-hexosaminidase deficiency. Science 196: 1014–1017.

CORK L.C., GRIFFIN J.W., MUNNELL J.F., LORENZ M.D., ADAMS R.J., PRICE D.L. (1979): Hereditary canine spinal muscular atrophy. Journal of Neuropathology and Experimental Neurology 38: 209–221.

CRISP C.E., RINGLER D.H., ABRAMS G.D., RADIN N.S., BRENKERT A. (1970): Lipid storage disease in a Siamese cat. Journal of the American Veterinary Medical Association 156: 616–622.

CROFT P.G., STOCKMAN M.J.R. (1964): Inherited defects in dogs. Veterinary Record 76: 260–261.

CUMMINGS J.F., DE LAHUNTA A. (1978): Hereditary myelopathy of Afghan Hounds, a myelinolytic disease. Acta Neuropathologia 42: 173–181.

CUMMINGS J.F., COOPER B.J., DELAHUNTA A., WINKLE T.J. VAN (1981): Canine inherited hypertrophic neuropathy. Acta Neuropathologia 53: 137–143.

CUMMINGS J.F., DELAHUNTA A., MITCHELL W.J. Jr. (1983): Ganglioradiculitis in the dog. A clinical light and electromicroscopic study. Acta Neuropathologica 60: 29–39.

CUMMINGS J.F., GEORGE D., DELAHUNTA A., VALENTINE B.A., BOOKBINDER P.F. (1989): Focal spinal muscular atrophy in two German shepherd pups. Acta Neuropathologica 79: 113–116.

CUMMINGS B.J., SU J.H., COTMAN C.W., WHITE R., RUSSELL M.J. (1993): b-amyloid accumulation in aged canine brain – A model of early plaque formation in Alzheimers disease. Neurobiology of Aging 14: 547–560.

DAWSON J.R.B. (1970): Myasthenia gravis in a cat. Veterinary Record 86: 562–563.

DELAUCHE A.J., CUDDON P.A., PODELL M., DEVOE K., POWELL H.C., SHELTON G.D. (1998): Nemaline rods in canine myopathies: 4 case reports and literature review. Journal of Veterinary Internal Medicine 12: 434–440.

DELAHUNTA A. (1971): Comments on cerebellar ataxia and its congenital transmission in cats by feline panleukopenia virus. Journal of the American Veterinary Medical Association 158: 901–906.

DELAHUNTA A., AVERILL D.A. (1976): Hereditary cerebellar cortical and extrapyramidal nuclear abiotrophy in Kerry Blue Terriers. Journal of the American Veterinary Medical Association 179: 886–890.

DELAHUNTA A., INGRAM J.T., CUMMINGS J.F., BELL J.S. (1994): Labrador retriever central axonopathy. Progress in Veterinary Neurology 5: 117–122.

DEMARIA R., DIVARI S., BO S., SONNINO S., LOTTI D., CAPUCCHIO M.T., CASTAGNARO M. (1998): Beta-glactosidase deficiency in a Korat cat – a new form of feline G(M1)-gangliodosis. Acta Neuropathologica 96: 307–314.

DENIS B., MARESCAUX L. (1994): Heredity of a medullary cervical ataxia syndrome (Wobbler Syndrome) in the Mastiff. Recueil de Médecine Vétérinaire 170: 245–247.

DIBARTOLA S.P., TARR M.J., WEBB D.M., GIGER U. (1990): Familial renal amyloidosis in Chinese Shar-Pei dogs. Journal of the American Veterinary Medical Association 197: 483–487.

DIETZMANN V.U. (1968): Über das Vorkommen des kongenitalen Megakolons (Hirschsprungsches Megakolon) bei der Katze. Monatshefte für Veterinarmedizin 23: 349–352.

DISTLER C., HOFFMANN K.P. (1996): Retinal slip neurons in the nucleus of the optic tract and dorsal terminal nucleus in cats with congenital strabismus [Review]. Journal of Neurophysiology 75: 1483–1494.

DUNCAN I.D., GRIFFITHS I.R., CARMICHAEL S., HENDERSON S. (1981): Inherited canine giant axonal neuropathy. Muscle Nerve 4: 223–227.

DUNCAN K.D., GRIFFITHS I.R. (1982): A sensory neuropathy affecting long-haired dachshund dogs. Journal of Small Animal Practice 23: 381–390.

FAITH R.E., WOODARD J.C. (1973): Waardenburg's syndrome (deafness and pigment abnormalities in cat): Comparative Pathology Bulletin 2: 3–4.

EGGERT A., HAIDE E., NIEWERTH B., PREM J. (1998): Idiopathic megacolon in a cat [German]. Praktische Tierarzt 79: 816.

FAMULA T.R., OBERBAUER A.M., BROWN K.N. (1997): Heritability of epileptic seizures in Belgian Trevueren. Journal of Small Animal Practice 38: 349–352.

FANKHAUSER R., LUGINBUHL H., HARTLEY W.J. (1963): Leukodystrophie von Typus Krabbe beim Hund. Schweizer Archiv für Tierheilkunde 105: 198–207.

FARROW B.R.H., MALIK R. (1981): Hereditary myotonia in the Chow Chow. Journal of Small Animal Practice 22: 451–465.

FARROW B.R.H., HARTLEY W.J., POLLARD A.C., FABBRO D., GRABOWSKI G.A., DESNICK R.J. (1982): Gaucher disease in the dog. In Gaucher Disease: A Century of Delineation and Research. Alan R. Liss Inc., New York. pp. 645–653.

FATZER R., GANDINI G., JAGGY A., DOHERR M., VANDEVELDE M. (2000): Necrosis of hippocampus and piriform lobe in 38 domestic cats with seizures: A retrospective study on clinical and pathologic findings. Journal of Veterinary Internal Medicine 14: 100–104.

FERGUSON E.A., CERUNDOLO R., LLOYD D.H., REST J., CAPPELLO R. (2000): Dermatomyositis in five Shetland sheepdogs in the United Kingdom. Veterinary Record 146: 214–217.

FIELD B., WANNER R.A. (1975): Cerebral malformation in a Manx cat. Veterinary Record 96: 42–43.

FISCHER A., CARMICHAEL K.P., MUNNELL J.F., JHABVALA P., THOMPSON J.N., MATALON R., JEZYK P.F., WANG P., GIGER U. (1998): Sulfamidase deficiency in a family of Dachshunds – a canine model of mucopolysaccharidosis IIIAa (Sanfilippo A). Pediatric Research 44: 74–82.

FLAGSTAD A. (1989): Congenital mysthenic syndrome in the dog breed Gammel Dansk Honsehund. An animal model for research in neuromuscular disorders. Scandinavian Journal of Laboratory Animal Science 16: 89–95.

FRANKLIN R.J.M., JEFFERY N.D., RAMSEY I.K. (1995): Neuroaxonal dystrophy in a litter of papillon pups. Journal of Small Animal Practice 36: 441–444.

FRYE F.L., MCFARLAND L.L. (1965): Spina bifida with raduschisis in a kitten. Journal of the American Veterinary Medical Association 146: 481–482.

FRYE, F.L. (1967): Spina bifida occulta with sacro-coccygeal agenesis in a cat. Animal Hospital 3: 238–242.

FYFE J.C., GIGER U., VANWINKLE T.J., HASKINS M.E., STEINBERG S.A., WANG P., PATTERSON D.F. (1992): Glycogen storage disease type-IV – inherited deficiency of branching enzyme activity in cats. Pediatric Research 32: 719–725.

FYFE J.C., KURZHALS R.L., LASSALINE M.E., HENTHORN P.S., ALUR P.R.K., WANG P., WOLFE J.H., GIGER U., HASKINS M.E., PATTERSON D.F., SUN H.C., JAIN S., YUHKI N. (1999): Molecular basis of feline beta-glucuronidase deficiency: An animal model of mucopolysaccharidosis VII. Genomics 58: 121–128.

GASCHEN F.P., HOFFMAN E.P., GOROSPE J.R.M., UHL E.W., SENIOR D.F., CARDINET G.H., PEARCE L.K. (1992): Dystrophin deficiency causes lethal muscle hypertrophy in cats. Journal of the Neurological Sciences 110: 149–159.

GASCHEN L., LANG J., LIN S., ADE-DAMILANO M., BUSATO A., LOMBARD C.W., GASCHEN F.P. (1999): Cardiomyopathy in dystrophin-deficient hypertrophic feline muscular dystrophy. Journal of Veterinary Internal Medicine 13: 346–356.

GERRITSEN R.J., VANNES J.J., VANNIEL M.H.F., VANDENINGH T.S.G.A.M., WIJNBERG I.D. (1996): Acute idiopathic polyneuropathy in nine cats. Veterinary Quarterly 18: 63–65.

GIGER U., HARVEY J.W. (1987): Hemolysis caused by phosphofructokinase deficiency in English Springer Spaniels: seven cases. Journal of the American Veterinary Medical Association 191: 453–459.

GIGER U., SMITH B.F., WOODS C.B., PATTERSON D.F., STEDMAN H. (1992): Inherited Phosphofructokinase Deficiency in an American Cocker Spaniel. Journal of the American Veterinary Medical Association 201: 1569–1571.

GILBERT D.A., O'BRIEN J.S., O'BRIEN S.J. (1988): Chromosomal mapping of lysosomal enzyme structural genes in the domestic cat. Genomics 2: 329–336.

GREEN P.D., LITTLE P.B. (1974): Neuronal ceroid lipofuscin storage in Siamese cats. Canadian Journal of Comparative Medicine and Veterinary Science 38: 207–212.

GREENE C.E., VANDEVELDE M., BRAUND K. (1976): Lissencephaly in two Lhasa Apso dogs. Journal of the American Veterinary Medical Association 169: 405–410.

GRIFFITHS I.R., MCCULLOCH M.C., ABRAHAMS S. (1987): Progressive axonopathy: an inherited neuropathy of boxer dogs: 4. Myelin sheath and Schwann cell changes in the nerve roots. Journal of Neurocytology 16: 145–153.

GUILLERY R.M., CASAGRANDE V.A., OBERDORFER M.D. (1974): Congenitally abnormal vision in Siamese cats. Nature 252: 195–199.

HALL S.J.G., WALLACE M.E. (1996): Canine epilepsy – a genetic counselling programme for Keeshonds. Veterinary Record 138: 358–360.

HAM L.M.L., DESMIDT M., TSHAMALA M., HOORENS J.K., MATTHEEUWS D.R.G. (1993): Canine X-linked muscular dystrophy in Belgian Groenendaeler shepherds. Journal of the American Animal Hospital Association 29: 570–574.

HARGIS A.M., MUNDELL A.C. (1992): Familial canine dermatomyositis. Compendium on Continuing Education for the Practicing Veterinarian 14: 855–865.

HARTLEY W.J., PALMER A.C. (1973): Ataxia in Jack Russell terriers. Acta Neuropathologica 26: 71–74.

HARTLEY W.J., BLAKEMORE W.F. (1973): Neurovisural glucocerebroside storage (Gaucher's disease) in a dog. Veterinary Pathology 10: 191–201.

HARTLEY W.J., BARKER J.S.F., WANNER R.A., FARROW B.R.H. (1978): Inherited cerebellar degeneration in the Rough Coated Collie. Australian Veterinary Practitioner 8: 79–85.

HARTLEY W.J., CANFIELD P.J., DONNELLY T.M. (1982): A suspected new canine storage disease. Acta Neuropathologia 56: 225–232.

HASKINS M.E., JEZYK P.F., DESNICK R.J., MCDONOUGH S.K., PATTERSON D.F. (1979): Alpha-L-iduronidase deficiency in a cat: a model of mucopolysaccharidosis I. Pediatric Research 13: 1294–1297.

A4

HASKINS M.E., DESNICK R.J., DIFERRANTE N., JEZYK P.F., PATTERSON D.F. (1984): Beta-glucuronidase deficiency in a dog: a model of human mucoploysaccharidosis VII. Pediatric Research 18: 980–984.

HASKINS M.E., OTIS E.J., HAYDEN J.E., JEZYK P.F., STRAMM L. (1992): Hepatic storage of glycosaminoglycans in feline and canine models of mucopolysaccharidose-I, mucopolysaccharidose-VI, and mucopolysaccharidose-VII. Veterinary Pathology 29: 112–119.

HE X.X., LI C.M., SIMONARO C.M., WAN Q., HASKINS M.E., DESNICK R.J., SCHUCHMAN E.H. (1999): Identification and characterization of the molecular lesion causing mucopolysaccharidosis type I in cats. Molecular Genetics & Metabolism 67: 106–112.

HEGREBERG G.A., NORBY D.E. (1973): An inherited storage disease of cats. Federation Proceedings 32: 821.

HEID S., HARTMANN R., KLINKE R. (1998): A model for prelingual deafness, the congenitally deaf white cat – population statistics and degenerative changes. Hearing Research 115: 101–112.

HICKFORD F.H., JONES B.R., GETHING M.A., PACK R., ALLEY M.R. (1998): Congenital myotonia in related kittens. Journal of Small Animal Practice 39: 281–285.

HIGGINS R.J., LECOUTEUR R.A., KORNEGAY J.N., COATES J.R. (1998): Late onset progressive spinocerebellar degeneration in Brittany spaniels. Acta Neuropathologica 96: 97–101.

HIRTH R.S., NIELSEN S.W. (1967): A familial canine globoid cell leukodystrophy (Krabbe type): Journal of Small Animal Practice 8: 569–575.

HOLLAND C.T. (1996): Horners syndrome and ipsilateral laryngeal hemiplegia in three cats. Journal of Small Animal Practice 37: 442–446.

HOLMES N.G., ACHESON T., RYDER E.J., BINNS M.M. (1998): A PCR-based diagnostic test for fucosidosis in English Springer Spaniels. Veterinary Journal 155: 113–114.

HUBLER M., HASKINS M.E., ARNOLD S., KASERHOTZ B., BOSSHARD N.U., BRINER J., SPYCHER M.A., GITZELMANN R., SOMMERLADE H.J., VONFIGURA K. (1996): Mucolipidosis type II in a domestic shorthair cat. Journal of Small Animal Practice 37: 435–441.

IGARASHI M., ALFORD B.R., COHN A.M., SAITO R., WATANABE T. (1972): Inner ear anomalies in dogs. Annals of Otology, Rhinology and Laryngology 81: 249–255.

INADA S., MOCHIZUKI M., IZUMO S., KURIYAMA M., SAKAMOTO H., KAWASAKI Y., OSAME M. (1996): Study of hereditary cerebellar degeneration in cats. American Journal of Veterinary Research 57: 296–301.

ISHIKAWA Y., LI S.C., WOOD P.A., LI Y.T. (1987): Biochemical basis of type AB GM2 gangliosidosis in a Japanese spaniel. Neurochemistry 48: 860–864.

IZUMO S., IKUTA F., IGATA A., OSAME M., YAMAUCHI C., INADA S. (1983): Morphological study on the hereditary neurogenic amyotrophic dogs: accumulation of lipid compound-like structures in the lower motor neuron. Acta Neuropathologica 61: 270–276.

JAGGY A., GAILLARD C., LANG J., VANDEVELDE M. (1988): Hereditary cervical spondylopathy (wobbler syndrome) in the Borzoi dog. Journal of the American Animal Hospital Association 24: 453–460.

JAGGY A., VANDEVELDE M. (1988): Multisystem neuronal degeneration in Cocker spaniels. Journal of Veterinary Internal Medicine 2: 117–120.

JAGGY A., FAISSLER D., GAILLARD C., SRENK P., GRABER H. (1998): Genetic aspects of idiopathic epilepsy in labrador retrievers. Journal of Small Animal Practice 39: 275–280.

JENKINS W.L., DYK E. VAN, MCDONALD C.B. (1976): Myasthenia gravis in a Fox Terrier litter. Journal of the South African Veterinary Association 47: 59–62.

JOHNSON K.H. (1970): Globoid leukodystrophy in the cat. Journal of the American Veterinary Medical Association 157: 2057–2064.

JOHNSON G.R., OLIVER J.E., SELCER R. (1975): Globoid cell leukodystrophy in a Beagle. Journal of the American Veterinary Medical Association 167: 380–384.

JOHNSON B.W. (1991): Congenitally abnormal visual pathways of Siamese cats. Compendium on Continuing Education for the Practicing Veterinarian 13: 374–378.

JONES B.R., ANDERSON L.J., BARNES G.R.G., JOHNSTONE A.C., JUBY W.D. (1977): Myotonia in related Chow Chow dogs. New Zealand Veterinary Journal 25: 217–220.

JONES B.R., ALLEY M.R., SHIMADA A., LYON M. (1992): An encephalomyelopathy in related Birman kittens. New Zealand Veterinary Journal 40: 160–163.

KALIL R.E., JHAVERI S.R., RICHARDS W. (1971): Anomalous retinal pathways in the Siamese cat: an inadequate substrate for normal binocular vision. Science 174: 302–305.

KARBE E., SCHIEFER B. (1967): Familial amaurotic idiocy in male German Shorthair Pointers. Pathologia Veterinaria 4: 223–232.

KATHMANN I., JAGGY A., BUSATO A., BARTSCHI M., GAILLARD C. (1999): Clinical and genetic investigations of idiopathic epilepsy in the Bernese mountain dog. Journal of Small Animal Practice 40: 319–325.

KELLY W.R., CLAGUE A.E., BARNS R.J., BATE M.J., MACKAY B.M. (1983): Canine alpha-L-fucosidosis: a storage disease of Springer Spaniels. Acta Neuropathologica 60: 9–13.

KERRUISH D.W. (1964): The Manx cat and spina bifida. Journal of Cat Genetics 1: 16–20.

KISHNANI P.S., BAO Y., WU J.Y., BRIX A.E., LIN J.L., CHEN Y.T. (1997): Isolation and nucleotide sequence of canine glucose-6-phosphatase mRNA – identification of mutation in puppies with glycogen storage disease type Ia. Biochemical & Molecular Medicine 61: 168–177.

KITCHEN H., MURRAY R.E., COCKRELL B.Y. (1972): Spina bifida, sacral dysgenesis and myelocele in Manx cats. American Journal of Pathology 68: 203–206.

KNOWLES K., ALROY J., CASTAGNARO M., RAGHAVAN S.S., JAKOWSKI R.M., FREDEN G.O. (1993): Adult-onset lysosomal storage disease in a Schipperke dog – clinical, morphological and biochemical studies. Acta Neuropathologica 86: 306–312.

KOPPANG N. (1965): Familial glycosphingolipidosis or juvenile amaurotic idiocy in the dog. Ergebnisse der allgemeinen Pathologie und pathologischen Anatomie 47: 1–45.

KOCH P., FISCHER H., STUBBE A.E. (1955): Heredity congenital cerebellar ataxia in cats. Berliner und Münchener Tierärztliche Wochenschrift 68: 246–249.

KORNEGAY J.N., GOODWIN M.A., SPYRIDAKIS L.K. (1987): Hypomyelination in Weimaraner dogs. Acta Neuropathologica 72: 394–401.

KRAMMER J.W., DAVIS W.C., PRIEUR D.J., BAXTER J., NORSWORTHY G.D. (1975): An inherited disorder of Persian cats with intracytoplasmic inclusion in neutrophils. Journal of the American Veterinary Medical Association 166: 1103–1104.

KUWAMURA M., AWAKURA T., SHIMADA A., UMEMURA T., KAGOTA K., KAWAMURA N., NAIKI M. (1993): Type C Niemann-Pick disease in a boxer dog. Acta Neuropathologica 85: 345–348.

LANSDOWN A.B.G., PATE P. (1992): Spinal dysplasia with stump tail and hind limb paralysis in a laboratory bred cat. Laboratory Animals 26: 299–300.

LANTINGA E., KOOISTRA H.S., VANNES J.J. (1998): Periodic muscle weakness and cervical ventroflexion caused by hypokalemia in a Burmese cat [Dutch]. Tijdschrift voor Diergeneeskunde 123: 435–437.

LEIPOLD H.W., HUSTON K., BLAUCH B., GUFFY M.M. (1974): Congenital defects of the caudal vertebral column and spinal cord in Manx cats. Journal of the American Veterinary Medical Association 164: 520–523.

LIM G.P., RUSSELL M.J., CULLEN M.J., TOKES Z.A. (1997): Matrix metalloproteinases in dog brains exhibiting Alzheimer-like characteristics. Journal of Neurochemistry 68: 1606–1611.

LIN L., FARACO J., LI R., KADOTANI H., ROGERS W., LIN X.Y., QIU X.H., DE JONG P.J., NISHINO S., MIGNOT E. (1999): The sleep disorder canine narcolepsy is caused by a mutation in the hypocretin (orexin) receptor 2 gene. Cell 98: 365–376.

LINGAAS F., AARSKAUG T., SLETTEN M., BJERKAS I., GRIMHOLT U., MOE L., JUNEJA R.K., WILTON A.N., GALIBERT F., HOLMES N.G., DOLF G. (1998): Genetic markers linked to neuronal ceroid lipofuscinosis in English Setter dogs. Animal Genetics 29: 371–376.

MADDISON J.E., ALLAN G.S. (1990): Megaesophagus attributable to lead toxicosis in a cat. Journal of the American Veterinary Medical Association 197: 1357–1358.

MAHONY O.M., KNOWLES D.E., BRAUND K.G., AVERILL D.R., FRIMBERGER A.E. (1998): Laryngeal paralysis-polyneuropathy complex in young Rottweilers. Journal of Veterinary Internal Medicine 12: 330–337.

MALIK R., MEPSTEAD K., YANG F., HARPER C. (1993): Hereditary myopathy of Devon Rex cats. Journal of Small Animal Practice 34: 539–546.

MANDIGERS P.J.J., VANNES J.J., KNOL B.W., UBBINK G.J., GRUYS E. (1993): Hereditary necrotising myelopathy in Kooiker dogs. Research in Veterinary Science 54: 118–123.

MARCH P.A., THRALL M.A., BROWN D.E., MITCHELL T.W., LOWENTHAL A.C., WALKLEY S.U. (1997): Gabaergic neuroaxonal dystrophy and other cytopathological alterations in feline niemann-pick disease type c. Acta Neuropathologica 94: 164–172.

MARTINEK Z. (1980): Epilepsy in dogs due to genetic causes. Kleintierpraxis 25: 44–46.

MASON K.V. (1976): A case of myasthenia gravis in a cat. Journal of Small Animal Practice 17: 467–472.

MATZ M.E., SHELL L., BRAUND K. (1990): Peripheral hypomyelinization in two golden retriever littermates. Journal of the American Veterinary Medical Association 197: 228–230.

MCGRATH J.T. (1979): Fibrinoid leukodystrophy (Alexander Disease): In: Andrews E.M., Ward B.C., Altman N.H. (eds): Spontaneous Animal Models of Human Disease. Academic Press, New York.

MCKERRELL R.E., BRAUND K.G. (1987): Hereditary myopathy in Labrador Retrievers: clinical variations. Journal of Small Animal Practice 28: 479–489.

MCNULTY E.E., SCHMIDT M.L., GILES A.M. (1999): Successful treatment of feline dysautonomia. Feline Practice 27: 8–11.

MEARS E.A., JENKINS C.C. (1997): Canine and feline megaesophagus. Compendium on Continuing Education for the Practicing Veterinarian 19: 313 ff.

MENON K.P., TIEU P.T., NEUFELD E.F. (1992): Architecture of the canine IDUA gene and mutation underlying canine mucopolysaccharidosis-I. Genomics 14: 763–768.

MOE L. (1992): Hereditary polyneuropathy of Alaskan malamutes. In: Kirk R.W. and Bonagura, J.D. (eds): Current Veterinary Therapy XI, Small Animal Practice. W.B. Saunders, Philadelphia, pp. 1038–1039.

MOREAU P.M., VALLAT J.M., HUGON J., LEBOUTET M.J., VANDEVELDE M. (1991): Peripheral and central distal axonopathy of suspected inherited origin in Birman cats. Acta Neuropathologica 82: 143–146.

MOSTAFA I.E. (1970): A case of glycogenic cardiomegaly in a dog. Acta Veterinaria Scandinavica 11: 197–208.

MUHLE A.C., JAGGY A., STRICKER C., STEFFEN F., DOLF G., BUSATO A., KRONBERG M., MARISCOLI M., SRENK P., GAILLARD C. (2001): Further contributions to the genetic aspect of congenital sensorineural deafness in dalmatians. The Veterinary Journal 163: 311–318.

MULDOON L.L., NEUWELT E.A., PAGE M.A., WEISS D.L. (1994): Characterization of the molecular defect in a feline model for type II G(M2)-gangliosidosis (Sandhoff disease): American Journal of Pathology 144: 1109–1118.

MÜLLER G., BAUMGARTNER W., MORITZ A., SEWELL A., KUSTERMANNKUHN B. (1998): Biochemical findings in a breeding colony of Alaskan huskies suffering from GM(1)-gangliosidosis. Journal of Inherited Metabolic Disease 21: 430–431.

NADON N.L., DUNCAN I.D., HUDSON L.D. (1990): A point mutation in the proteolipid protein gene of the 'shaking pup' interrupts oligodendrocyte development. Development 110: 529–537.

NEER T.M., DIAL S.M., PECHMAN R., WANG P., OLIVER J.L., GIGER U. (1995): Clinical vignette. Mucopolysaccharidosis VI in a miniature pinscher. Journal of Veterinary Internal Medicine 9: 429–433.

NEWSHOLME S.J., GASKELL C.J. (1987): Myopathy with core-like structure in a dog. Journal of Comparative Pathology 97: 597–600.

NORBY D.E., THULINE H.C. (1970): Inherited tremor in the domestic cat (Felis catus L): Nature 227: 1262–1263.

OCCHIODORO T., ANSON D.S. (1996): Isolation of the canine alpha-l-fucosidase cDNA and definition of the fucosidosis mutation in English Springer Spaniels. Mammalian Genome 7: 271–274.

PALMER A.C., BLAKEMORE W.F., WALLACE M.E., WILKES M.K., HERRTAGE M.E., MATIC S.E. (1987): Recognition of trembler, a hypomyelinating condition in the Bernese mountain dog. Veterinary Record 120: 609–612.

PAOLA J.P., PODELL M., SHELTON G.D. (1993): Muscular dystrophy in a Miniature Schnauzer. Progress in Veterinary Neurology 4: 14–18.

PARSONS T.S., STEIN J.M. (1955–1956): A cat with an anomalous third hind leg and abnormal vertebrae. Harvard College Museum of Comparative Zoology Bulletin 114: 293–317.

PETERS R.I., MEYERS K.M. (1977): Regulation of serotonergic neuronal systems affecting locomotion in Scottish terrier dogs. Federation Proceedings 36: 1023.

PRESTHUS J., NORDSTOGA K. (1993): Congenital myopathy in a litter of Samoyed dogs. Progress in Veterinary Neurology 4: 37–40.

PUMAROLA M., FONDEVILA D., BORRAS D., MAJO N., FERRER I. (1999): Neuronal vacuolation in young Rottweiler dogs. Acta Neuropathologica 97: 192–195.

QUESNEL A.D., PARENT J.M., MCDONELL W. (1997): Clinical management and outcome of cats with seizure disorders – 30 cases (1991–1993): Journal of the American Veterinary Medical Association 210: 72ff.

RAY J., BOUVET A., DESANTO C., FYFE J.C., XU D.B., WOLFE J.H., AGUIRRE G.D., PATTERSON D.F., HASKINS M.E., HENTHORN P.S. (1998): Cloning of the canine beta-glucuronidase cDNA, mutation identification in canine MPS VII, and retroviral vector-mediated correction of MPS VII cells. Genomics 48: 248–253.

READ D.H., HARRINGTON D.D., KEENAN T.W., HINSMAN E.J. (1976): Neuronal visceral GM-1 glangliosidosis in a dog with beta galactosidase deficiency. Science 194: 442–445.

REETZ I., STECKER M., WEGNER W. (1977): Audiometrische Befunde in einer Merlezucht. Deutsche tierärztliche Wochenschrift 84: 273–277.

REGNIER A.M., DELAHITTE M.J.D., DELISLE M.B., DUBOIS G.G. (1993): Dandy-Walker syndrome in a kitten. Journal of the American Animal Hospital Association 29: 514–518.

REUSER A.J.J. (1993): Molecular biology, therapeutic trials and animal models of lysosomal storage siseases – type-II glycogenosis as an example. Annales de Biologie Clinique 51: 218–219.

RIVAS A.L., TINTLE L., MEYERS-WALLEN V.N., SCARLETT J.M., VANTASSELL C.P., QUIMBY F.W. (1993): Inheritance of renal amyloidosis in Chinese Shar-Pei dogs. Journal of Heredity 84: 438–442.

ROBINSON R. (1992): Spasticity in the Devon Rex cat. Veterinary Record 130: 302.

ROBINSON R. (1993): Expressivity of the Manx gene in cats. Journal of Heredity 84: 170–172.

RODRIGUEZ F., DELOSMONTEROS A.E., MORALES M., HERRAEZ P., JABER J.R., FERNANDEZ A. (1996): Neuroaxonal dystrophy in two siamese kitten littermates. Veterinary Record 138: 548–549.

ROTHUIZEN J., INGH TH.S.G.A.M. VAN DEN, VOORHAUT G., LUER R.J.T. VAN DER, WOUDA W. (1982): Congenital porto systemic shunts in sixteen dogs and three cats. Journal of Small Animal Practice 23: 67–81.

SACRE B.J., CUMMINGS J.F., DELAHUNTA A. (1993): Neuroaxonal dystrophy in a Jack Russell terrier pup resembling human infantile neuroaxonal dystrophy. Cornell Veterinarian 83: 133–142.

SANDEFELDT E., CUMMINGS J.F., DELAHUNTA A., BJORCK G., KROOK L.P. (1976): Animal model of human disease. Infantile spinal muscular atrophy, Werdnig-Hoffman disease. Animal model: Hereditary neuronal abiotrophy in Swedish Lapland dogs. American Journal of Pathology 82: 649–652.

SANDSTROM B, WESTMAN J., OCKERMAN P.A. (1969): Glycogenesis of the central nervous system in the cat. Acta Neuropathologia 14: 194–200.

SAUNDERS G.K., WOOD P.A., MYERS R.K., SHELL L.G., CARITHERS R. (1988): GM1 gangliosidosis in Portuguese water dogs: pathologic and biochemical findings. Veterinary Pathology 25: 265–269.

SCHATZBERG S.J., ANDERSON L.V., WILTON S.D., KORNEGAY J.N., MANN C.J., SOLOMON G.G., SHARP N.J. (1998): Alternative dystrophin gene transcripts in golden retriever muscular dystrophy. Muscle Nerve 8: 991–998.

SCHATZBERG S.J., OLBY N.J., BREEN M., ANDERSON L.V., LANGFORD C.F., DICKENS H.F., WILTON S.D., ZEISS C.J., BINNS M.M., KORNEGAY J.N., MORRIS G.E., SHARP N.J. (1999): Molecular analysis of a spontaneous dystrophin 'knockout' dog. Neuromuscular Disorders 5: 289–295.

SCHEIDY S.F. (1953): Familial cerebellar hypoplasia in cats. North American Veterinarian 34: 118–119.

SCHMUTZ S.M., MOKER J.S., CLARK E.G., SHEWFELT R. (1998): Black hair follicular dysplasia, an autosomal recessive condition in dogs. Canadian Veterinary Journal – Revue Veterinaire Canadienne 39: 644–646.

A4

SCHUCHMAN E.H., TOROYAN T.K., HASKINS M.E., DESNICK R.J. (1989): Characterization of the defective beta-glucuronidase activity in canine mucopolysaccharidosis type-VII. Enzyme 42: 174–180.

SCHUNK C.M. (1997): Feline portosystemic shunts. Seminars in Veterinary Medicine & Surgery (Small Animal) 12: 45–50.

SHAMIR M., PERL S., SHARON L. (1999): Late onset of cerebellar abiotrophy in a Siamese cat. Journal of Small Animal Practice 40: 343–345.

SHELL L.G., JORTNER B.S., LEIB M.S. (1987): Familial motor neuron disease in Rottweiler dogs: neuropathologic studies. Veterinary Pathology 24: 135–139.

SHELL L.G. (1995): Diabetic polyneuropathy. Feline Practice 23: 27.

SHELL L.G. (1995): Horners syndrome. Feline Practice 23: 28–29.

SHELL L.G. (1996): Congenital hydrocephalus. Feline Practice 24: 10–11.

SHELTON G.D. (2000): Disorders of muscle and neuromuscular junction. In: Birchard, S.G. and Sherding, R.G. (eds): Saunders Manual of Small Animal Practice. W.B. Saunders, Philadelphia, pp. 1302–1310.

SHULL R.B., MUNGER R.J., SPELLACY E., HALL C.W., CONSTANTOPOULOS G., NEUFELD E.F. (1982): Mucopolysaccharidosis I. American Journal of Pathology 109: 244–248.

SILSON M., ROBINSON R. (1969): Hereditary hydrocephalus in the cat. Veterinary Record 84: 477.

SINGER H.S., CORK L.C. (1989): Canine GM2 Gangliosidosis – Morphological and biochemical analysis. Veterinary Pathology 26: 114–120.

SKELLY B.J., SARGAN D.R., HERRTAGE M.E., WINCHESTER B.G. (1996): The molecular defect underlying canine fucosidosis. Journal of Medical Genetics 33: 284–288.

SORJONEN C.C., COX N.R., KWAPIEN R.P. (1987): Myeloencephalopathy with eosinophilic refractile bodies (Rosenthal fibers) in a Scottish Terrier. Journal of the American Veterinary Medical Association 190: 1004–1006.

SPELLACY E., SHULL R.M., CONSTANTOPOULOS F., NEUFELD E.F. (1983): A canine model of human alpha-L-iduronidase deficiency. Proceedings of the National Academy of Sciences USA 80: 6091–6095.

SPONENBERG D.P., DELAHUNTA A. (1981): Hereditary hypertrophic neuropathy in Tibetan Mastiff dogs. Journal of Heredity 72: 287.

STEINBERG H.S., TRONCOSO J.C., CORK L.C., PRICE D.L. (1981): Clinical features of inherited cerebellar degeneration in Gordon Setters. Journal of the American Veterinary Medical Association 179: 886–890.

STEINBERG S.A., KLEIN E., KILLENS R.L., UHDE T.W. (1994): Inherited deafness among nervous pointer dogs. Journal of Heredity 85: 56–59.

STOFFREGEN D.A., HUXTABLE C.R., CUMMINGS J.F., DELAHUNTA A. (1993): Hypomyelination of the central nervous system of 2 Siamese kitten littermates. Veterinary Pathology 30: 388–391.

STRAIN G.M. (1996): Aetiology, prevalence and diagnosis of deafness in dogs and cats [Review]. British Veterinary Journal 152: 17–36.

SUMMERS B.A., CUMMINGS J.F., DELAHUNTA A. (1995): Veterinary Neuropathology. Mosby, St. Louis, Missouri, 527–612.

SYMONDS H.W., MCWILLIAMS P., THOMPSON H., NASH A., SANCHEZ S., ROZENGURT N. (1995): A cluster of cases of feline dysautonomia (Key-Gaskell syndrome) in a closed colony of cats. Veterinary Record 136: 353–355.

TANIYAMA H., TAKAYANAGI S., IZUMISAWA Y., KOTANI T., KAJI Y., OKADA H., MATSUKAWA K. (1994): Cerebellar cortical atrophy in a kitten. Veterinary Pathology 31: 710–713.

TARGETT M.P., FRANKLIN R.J.M., OLBY N.J., DYCE J., ANDERSON J.R., HOULTON J.E.F. (1994): Central core myopathy in a Great Dane. Journal of Small Animal Practice 35: 100–103.

TODD N.B. (1961): The inheritance of taillessness in Manx cats. Journal of Heredity 52: 228–232.

TOLL J., COOPER B., ALTSCHUL M. (1998): Congenital myotonia in 2 domestic cats. Journal of Veterinary Internal Medicine 12: 116–119.

VANDEVELDE M., BRAUND K.G., WALDER T.L., KORNEGAY J. (1978): Dysmyelination of the central nervous system in the Chow-Chow dog. Acta Neuropathologica 42: 211–215.

VENKER-VAN HAAGEN A.J., BOUW J., HARTMANN W. (1981): Hereditary transmission of laryngeal paralysis in Bouviers. Journal of the American Animal Hospital Association 17: 75–76.

VIJAYASARATHY C., GIGER U., PROCIUK U., PATTERSON D.F., BREITSCHWERDT E.B., AVADHANI N.G. (1994): Canine mitochondrial myopathy associated with reduced mitochondrial mRNA and altered cytochrome c oxidase activities in fibroblasts and skeletal muscle. Comparative Biochemistry and Physiology A – Physiology 109: 887–894.

WALLACE M.E., PALMER A.C. (1984): Recessive mode of inheritance in myasthenia gravis in the Jack Russell terrier. Veterinary Record 114: 350.

WALVOORT H.C., SLEE R.G., SLUIS K.J., KOSTER J.F., REUSER A.J. (1984): Biochemical genetics of the Lapland dog model of glycogen storage disease type II (acid-alpha-glucosidase deficiency). American Journal of Medical Genetics 19: 589–598.

WASHABAU R.J., HOLT D. (1999): Pathogenesis, diagnosis, and therapy of feline idiopathic megacolon. Veterinary Clinics of North America – Small Animal Practice 29: 589–603.

WEISSENBOCK H., OBERMAIER G., DAEHME E. (1996): Alexanders disease in a Bernese mountain dog. Acta Neuropathologica 91: 200–204.

WEISSENBOCK H., ROSSEL C. (1997): Neuronal ceroid-lipofuscinosis in a domestic cat – clinical, morphological and immunohistochemical findings. Journal of Comparative Pathology 117: 17–24.

WENGER D.A., SATTLER M., KUDOH T., SYNDER S.P., KINGSTON R.S. (1980): Niemann-Pick disease: a genetic model in Siamese cats. Science 208: 1471–1473.

WENTINK G.H., LINDE-SIPMAN J.S. VAN DER, MEIZER A.E.F.H., KAMPHUISEN H.A.C., VORSTENBOSCH C.J.A.H.V. VAN, HARTMAN W., HENDRIKS H.J. (1972): Myopathy with a possible recessive X-linked inheritance in a litter of Irish Terriers. Veterinary Pathology 9: 328–349.

WHITE S.D., SHELTON G.D., SISSON A., MCPHERRON M., ROSYCHUK R.A.W., OLSON P.J. (1992): Dermatomyositis in an adult Pembroke Welsh Corgi. Journal of the American Animal Hospital Association 28: 398–401.

WILKES M.K., PALMER A.C. (1987): Deafness in Dobermanns. Veterinary Record 120(26): 624.

WILKERSON M.J., LEWIS D.C., MARKS S.L., PRIEUR D.J. (1998): Clinical and morphologic features of mucopolysaccharidosis type II in a dog: Naturally occurring model of Hunter syndrome. Veterinary Pathology 35: 230–233.

WOLSCHRIJN C.F., MAHAPOKAI W., ROTHUIZEN J., MEYER H.P., VAN SLUIJS F.J. (2000): Gauged attenuation of congenital portosystemic shunts: Results in 160 dogs and 15 cats. Veterinary Quarterly 22: 94–98.

WOODARD J.C., COLLINS G.H., HESSLER J.R. (1974): Feline hereditary neuroaxonal dystrophy. American Journal of Pathology 74: 551–560.

WOODS C.B. (1977): Hyperkinetic episodes in two Dalmatian dogs. Journal of the American Animal Hospital Association 13: 255–257.

WOUDA W., VAN NESS J.J. (1986): Progressive ataxia due to central demyelination in Rottweiler dogs. Veterinary Quarterly 8: 89–97.

WRIGHT J.A., SMYTH J.B., BROWNLIE S.E., ROBINS M. (1987): A myopathy associated with muscle hypertonicity in Cavalier King Charles Spaniels. Journal of Comparative Pathology 97: 559–565.

YAMATO O., OCHIAI K., MASUOKA Y., HAYASHIDA E., TAJIMA M., OMAE S., IIJIMA M., UMEMURA T., MAEDE Y. (2000): GM1 gangliosidosis in Shiba dogs. Veterinary Record 146: 493–496.

YIN Z.Q., CREWTHER S.G., YANG M., CREWTHER D.P. (1996): Distribution and localization of nmda receptor subunit 1 in the visual cortex of strabismic and anisometropic amblyopic cats. Neuroreport 7: 2997–3003.

ZAAL M.D., VAN DEN INGH T.S. GOEDEGEBUURE S.A., VAN NES J.J. (1997): Progressive neuronopathy in two Cairn terrier litter mates. Veterinary Quarterly 19: 34–36.

ZACHARY J.F., O'BRIEN D.P. (1985): Spongy degeneration of the central nervous system in two canine littermates. Veterinary Pathology 6: 561–571.

Appendix 5:
Drugs

Active substance	Activity	Indication	Dosage	Contraindication/ interactions	Side effects
Acepromazine phenothiazine	Blockage of postsynaptic dopamine receptors	Sedation, premedication	Dog/cat: 0.005–0.03 mg/kg, IV, IM, SC	Myelography, epilepsy	Reduced threshold for epileptic seizures, although this is contentious
Acetazolamide carbonic anhydrase inhibitor	Reversible inhibitor of carbonic anhydrase	Glaucoma, diuretic, metabolic alkalosis	Dog: 5–10 mg/kg PO, IV, TID Dog/cat: 50 mg/kg IV once, then 7 mg/kg, PO, TID	Liver, renal and adrenal insufficiency; hyponatraemia; hypokalaemia; hyperchloraemic acidosis; chronic non-congestive closed-angle glaucoma. Amphotericin B, corticosteroids, insulin, phenobarbital, phenytoin, primidone	CNS depression or hyperexcitation, crystalluria, polyuria, dysuria, bone marrow suppression, hypokalaemia, hyponatraemia, hyperglycaemia
Acetylsalicylic acid NSAID	Cyclic oxygenase inhibitor (analgesic, antipyretic, antiinflammatory, inhibition of thrombocyte aggregation)	Ischemic myelopathy, conservative management of disc disease	Dog: 0.5 mg/kg, PO, BID Cat: 10–25 mg/kg, PO, q 48–72 h	Hypersensitivity, Von Willebrand's disease, liver and renal insufficiency, GI disease (haemorrhage, ulceration)	Gastrointestinal problems; vomiting, diarrhoea, intestinal haemorrhage
Activated charcoal GI absorbent		GI intoxication, diarrhoea	Small dog/cat: 100–150 mg, PO, TID Large dog: 200–500 mg, PO, TID–QID Poisoning: mix 1 g with 5 ml water, give 1–2 g (= 5–10 ml)/kg over stomach tube	In cases of poisoning, only use when consciousness and swallowing reflexes are retained, and there are no seizures. Do not give with other tablets PO	
Alfuzosin α_1-sympatholytic	Blockage of the α_1-receptors in smooth muscle of the lower urinary tract	Hypertonus of the urethral sphincter	Dog/cat: 0.01–0.1 mg/kg, BID–TID	Hypotension	Headache, dizziness (only known from human medicine)
Alphadolone/ Alphaxolone steroid anaesthetic		Induction and maintenance of anaesthesia	Cat: 3–9 mg/kg IV, IM	Contraindicated in dogs	Hyperaemia and oedema of ears and paws, laryngospasm, oedema of larynx and lungs, choking, vomiting, sneezing
Alprazolam Benzodiazepine	GABA antagonist, serotonin antagonist, reduced release of acetylcholine in CNS	Phobias	Dog: 0.01–0.1 mg/kg, PO before the angst-inducing stimulus or BID–TID; no more than 4 mg/dog/day Cat: 0.01–0.1 mg/kg, PO, SID–BID	Careful with liver insufficiency. Analgesics; potentiates other sedatives	Sedation, ataxia

A5

Active substance	Activity	Indication	Dosage	Contraindication / interactions	Side effects
Aminocaproic acid	Inhibition of fibrinolysis by inhibiting plasminogen activator substance and antiplasminogen activity; antiprotease activity	Degenerative myelopathies (not proven as efficacious)	Dog: 500 mg, PO, TID	Active intravascular coagulation; careful with liver and renal insufficiency	Gastrointestinal irritation
Aminophylline / theophylline xanthine derivatives	Increase epinephrine release due to inhibition of cyclic AMP metabolism	Bronchospasm, asthma, congestive cardiac insufficiency, cerebral hypoxia	Dog: 5–10 mg/kg, PO, SC, IM, IV, TID Cat: 5 mg/kg, PO, SC, IM, IV, BID–TID	Stomach ulcer, hyperthyroidism, liver and renal insufficiency, severe hypoxia and hypertension. Reduced efficacy with barbiturates, beta blockers; increased efficacy with cimetidine, erythromycin, clindamycin; additive effects with isopreternol and ephedrine	Vomiting, anorexia, excitement, excitability, tachyarrhythmia
Amitriptyline tricyclic antidepressant	Blockage of the amino acid pumps leading to increase in serotonin concentration; central and peripheral anticholinergic activity	Separation anxiety	Dog: 2–4 mg/kg, PO, BID Cat: 0.5 mg/kg, PO, SID	Monoamine oxidase inhibitors	Sedation, hyperexcitation, bone marrow depression, vomiting, diarrhoea
Amoxicillin + clavulanic acid antibiotic	Bactericidal, β-lactamase resistant penicillin, broad spectrum	Bacterial meningoencephalitis, otitis media / interna	Dog / cat: 20 mg/kg, IV, PO, BID		
Amphotericin B antimycotic	Fungiostatic; affinity to the sterols (ergosterol > cholesterol) in cell membranes; destroys membrane permeability	Only in systemic fungal infections: *Aspergillus, Blastomyces, Coccidiodes, Cryptococcus, Cygomyces, Histoplasma, Mucor, Sporothrix*	Dog / cat: 0.25 mg/kg in 30 ml 5% glucose solution IV over 5 min; then repeat 0.25–0.5 mg/kg in same dilution 3 × a week until a total dose of 9–12 mg/kg is attained	Renal failure. Gentamycin B, polymycin B, colistin, cisplatin, methoxyflurane, vancomycin, cardiac glycosides, corticosteroids, thiazide	Nephrotoxic
Ampicillin antibiotic	Bactericidal; non-β-lactamase resistant penicillin used against gram-negative (*E. coli, Haemophilus, Klebsiella*) and anaerobic bacteria (*Clostridia*)	Hepatoencephalopathy (targets the proliferation of ammonia-producing bacteria in the GI tract)	Dog / cat: 20 mg/kg, PO, TID	Poor absorption from GI tract	
Apomorphine emetic	Central stimulation of the dopamine receptors in the chemoreceptor centre of the medulla oblongata	Emptying of the stomach to treat intoxication	Dog: 0.04 mg/kg, IM, IV, once	Hypoxia, shock, dyspnoea, coma, premature vomiting. Anti-emetics, opioids	Depression; overdosage leads to respiratory depression, seizures, protracted vomiting
Asparaginase chemotherapeutic	Inhibition of the DNA and proteosynthesis in post mitotic G_1 phase	Chemotherapy protocol	Dog: 20 000 IU/m², IM, IV, intraperoniteal, once/week Cat: 10 000 IU/m², IM, SC, IV, intraperoniteal, once/week	Pancreatitis, liver and renal insufficiency, severe bone marrow suppression. Can effect methotrexate reduction	Nausea, vomiting, diarrhoea, pruritis, nervousness, hypotension, collapse, hepatotoxicity, pancreatitis

Active substance	Activity	Indication	Dosage	Contraindication/ interactions	Side effects
Atipamezole α_2-adrenergic antagonist	Competitive inhibition of the α_2-adrenergic agonists	Antagonisation of the α_2-adrenergic agonists	Half to same dosage of medetomidine used	Pregnancy	Tachycardia, overexcitement
Atracurium muscle relaxant	Competitive binding to choline receptors of the neuromuscular endplate	Muscle relaxation during anaesthesia	Dog/cat: 0.22 mg/kg, IV; 1/10 as first dose then the rest after 5 min	Careful with severe cardiovascular diseases, asthma (can cause histamine release). Effects of atracurium are potentiated by procainamide, quinidine, verapamil, amidoglycosides, clindamycin, polymyxin B, thiazide diuretics and isoflurane	Hypotension, vasodilation, bradycardia, tachycardia, dyspnoea, bronchospasm, urticaria
Atropine sulphate Parasympatholytic	Inhibition of acetylcholine at the postganglionic muscarinic receptors	Antidote for pyridostigmine and in organophosphate and carbamate intoxication. Diagnostic uses: oral test for taste, mydriatic	Dog/cat: 0.02–0.05 mg/kg, SC, IM, IV, QID 1 drop on tongue or in the eye	Glaucoma, tachycardia, tachyarrhythmia, hyperthyroidism, paralytic ileus. Parasympathomimetics	Initial bradycardia then tachycardia; reduced salivation and bronchial secretion; intestinal atony
Azathioprine cytostatic	Antagonist of purine metabolism resulting in inhibition of RNA and DNA synthesis	Immunosuppression; for reducing the dosage of concomitantly used glucocorticoids	Dog: 2–2.5 mg/kg, PO, SID Cat: 1.1 mg/kg, PO q 48 h	Liver insufficiency. Allopurinol	Myelosuppression with neutropaenia and thrombocytopaenia; anaemia, acute pancreatitis and liver damage
Benzyl penicillin sodium antibiotic	Bactericidal, non-β-lactamase resistant penicillin	Tetanus	Dog/cat: initial dosage 40000–100000 IU/kg, IV, then 20000 IU/kg, IV slowly, QID		Vomiting after rapid application
Betamethasone corticosteroid	Inhibition of phospholipase A$_2$; effect < 48 h	Anti-inflammatory, otitis externa, intensive pruritis	Dog/cat: 0.15–0.3 mg/kg, IM; maximal 4 × local as ear drops	Gastrointestinal ulceration, liver and renal insufficiency	PU/PD, polyphagia, fluid retention, vomiting/diarrhoea, gastrointestinal ulceration
Bethanecol parasympathomimetic	Stimulation of the muscarinic receptors	Increased contractility of the bladder detrusor muscle	Dog/cat: 0.5–1 mg/kg, PO, BID–TID	Urethral obstruction, mechanical damage to bladder wall, gastrointestinal ulceration and inflammation. Do not give with carbechol, neostigmine, atropine, sympathomimetics.	Vomiting, diarrhoea, salivation; overdosage leads to arrhythmia, hypotension
Buprenorphine opioid	Partial agonist	Analgesia, sedation	Dog/cat: 0.005–0.01 mg/kg, IV, IM, SC, TID	Potentiation of other sedatives; antagonises morphine and morphine derivatives	Respiratory depression after high doses
Buspirone benzodiazepine	Effect not totally understood; affinity to serotonin receptors	Behaviour problems (anxiety)	Dog: 1 mg/kg, PO, SID cat: 0.5 mg/kg, PO, BID	Liver and renal insufficiency	Nausea, anorexia, restlessness, headache
Butorphanol opioid	Agonist/antagonist	Analgesia, sedation	Dog/cat: 0.1–0.05 mg/kg, IV, IM, SC, q 2–4 h	Potentiated effects of other sedatives, analgesics and anaesthetics	Respiratory depression
Calcium EDTA	Binds heavy metal ions	Intoxication	Dog/cat: 25 mg/kg, SC	Renal insufficiency and failure	Nephrotoxic, vomiting, diarrhoea

A5

A5

Active substance	Activity	Indication	Dosage	Contraindication / interactions	Side effects
Calcium gluconate	Calcium is an essential ion for muscle contraction, nerve excitability and enzymatic reactions	Hypocalcaemia	Dog / cat: 50–150 mg/kg, IV	Hypercalcaemia, ventricular fibrillation; careful with renal insufficiency. Careful with digitalis glycosides	Hypercalcaemia
Carpofen NSAID	Cyclic oxygenase inhibitor	Analgesia, anti-inflammatory, antipyretic	Dog / cat: initial dosage 4 mg/kg, IV, PO, then 2 mg/kg, BID	Von Willebrand's disease, liver and renal insufficiency, intestinal disease	Gastrointestinal problems with vomiting, diarrhoea, haemorrhage
Cephalexin antibiotic	Bactericidal, first generation cephalosporin, broad spectrum	Bacterial meningoencephalitis, otitis interna / media, preoperatively	Dog / cat: 20–30 mg/kg, IV, PO, BID–TID		Vomiting
Cefatoxime antibiotic	Bactericidal, third generation cephalosporin, broad spectrum	Bacterial meningoencephalitis, otitis interna / media,	Dog / cat: 20–40 mg/kg, IV, PO, BID–TID		Vomiting
Chlorazepate benzodiazepine	GABA agonist, serotonin antagonist, reduced release of acetylcholine in CNS	Antiepileptic Separation anxiety	Dog: 1–2 mg/kg, PO, BID Dog: 11.25–22.5 mg/dog, PO, SID–BID	Closed-angle glaucoma. Potentiates effects of other analgesics, sedatives and analgesics; cimetidine and erythromycin reduce metabolism of benzodiazepines	Sedation, ataxia
Chloramphenicol antibiotic	Bacteriostatic, broad spectrum	Otitis media, bacterial meningoencephalitis	Dog / cat: 30 mg/kg, PO, TID	Contraindicated in puppies / kittens and pregnancy. Disturbs liver metabolism of various drugs, particularly barbiturates, phenytoin and primidone. Do not give with myelosuppressive drugs especially in cats	Can inhibit bone marrow
Chlorpromazine phenothiazine	Blocks postsynaptic dopamine receptors	Sedation, premedication, tetanus	Dog / cat: 2 mg/kg, IV, IM, SC, BID	Myelography, epilepsy	Reduced threshold for epileptic seizures
Cinarizine calcium antagonist	Inhibition of increased calcium influxes in hypoxic cells, causing antivasoconstrictive effects without influencing blood pressure; depressive effects on labyrinth	Disturbances of inner ear or cerebral perfusion	Dog: 4 mg/kg, PO, BID	Not with antihypertensives or cardioglycosides	Tiredness
Cisapride prokinetic drug	Increases release of acetylcholine in mesenteric plexus and blocks dopaminergic receptors	Oesophagitis, increases stomach emptying, colonic obstipation	Dog / cat: 0.5 mg/kg, PO, BID–TID	Mechanical GI obstruction, perforation, haemorrhage. Increased rapidity of GI passage can influence the absorption of other drugs; anticholinergics; increases effects of cimetidine, ranitidine and benzodiazepines; increased cisapride concentration with ketoconazole, itraconazole and miconazole	Diarrhoea and abdominal pain observed in human medicine

Active substance	Activity	Indication	Dosage	Contraindication/ interactions	Side effects
Clindamycin antibiotic	Bacteristatic against gram-positive bacteria and *Toxoplasma gondii*	Discospondylitis and osteomyelitis, otitis media/interna, toxoplasmosis	Dog/cat: 10 mg/kg, PO, BID Toxoplasmosis: 20 mg/kg, PO, BID		Vomiting, diarrhoea
Clomipramine tricyclic antidepressant	Blockage of norepinephrine and serotonin uptake at the neuronal membrane	Separation anxiety, dominant behavioural traits, soiling problems	Dog: 2–4 mg/kg, PO, BID Cat: 0.5 mg/kg, PO, SID	Epilepsy, careful with reduced gastrointestinal motility and cardiac arrhythmia. Not with monoamine oxidase inhibitors	Sedation, tachycardia, dry oral mucosa
Clonazepam benzodiazepine	GABA agonist, serotonin antagonist, reduced release of acetylcholine in CNS	Antiepileptic, muscle relaxant	Dog/cat: 0.5 mg/kg, PO, BID–TID	Closed-angle glaucoma. Potentiates effects of other analgesics, sedatives and analgesics; cimetidine and erythromycin reduce metabolism of benzodiazepines	Sedation, ataxia
Colchicine cytostatic	Inhibition of cell division during metaphase	Hepatic cirrhosis, fibrosis, myopathy	Dog: 0.03 mg/kg, PO, SID	Renal insufficiency, cardiac insufficiency, pregnancy	Nausea, vomiting, diarrhoea
Cyclophosphamide chemotherapeutic, immunosuppression	Interference with DNA replication and RNA transcription and replication	Chemotherapy protocol	Dog: 50 mg/m², PO, IV, for 4 days a week Cat: 100 mg/m², PO, on 3rd, 4th and 6th day after doxorubicin	Careful with liver and renal insufficiency. Phenobarbital increases cyclophosphamide metabolism; allopurinol and thiazides increase the bone marrow suppression caused by cyclophosphamide; doxorubicin potentiates its cardiotoxicity	Nausea, vomiting, diarrhoea, bone marrow suppression, alopecia
Cyproheptadine antihistamine	Competative inhibition of H_1 receptors, serotonin antagonist	Antihistamine, ischemic myopathy	Dog: 1.1 mg/kg, PO, BID–TID Cat: 2–4 mg/cat, PO, SID–BID	Prostatic hypertrophy, urinary bladder obstruction, cardiac insufficiency, closed-angle glaucoma. Potentiates barbiturates and tranquilisers; with monoamine oxidase potentiation of anticholinergic effects	Depression of CNS; anticholinergic effects: dry mouth, vomiting, diarrhoea, anorexia, urine retention
Dantrolene muscle relaxant	Inhibition of calcium release from sarcoplasmic reticulum	Malignant hyperthermia	dog/cat: 2–5 mg/kg IV	Liver and cardiac insufficiency	Sedation, headache, nausea, vomiting, diarrhoea, hypotension, hepatotoxicity
Dexamethasone corticosteroid	Inhibition of phospholipase A_2, effects > 48 h	Anti-inflammatory Swelling of brain and spinal cord Immunosuppression	Dog/cat: 0.25–0.5 mg/kg, IV Dog/cat: 1–2 mg/kg, IV Dog/cat: 2 mg/kg, IV	Infections, gastrointestinal ulceration, liver and renal insufficiency	PU/PD, polyphagia, fluid retention, vomiting/diarrhoea, gastrointestinal ulceration
Diazepam benzodiazepine	GABA agonist, serotonin antagonist, reduced release of acetylcholine in CNS	Antiepileptic Muscle relaxation, sedation, reduction of the external urethral sphincter tone Appetite stumulant, behavioural problems (anxiety)	Dog/cat: 1–2 mg/kg, IV Dog/cat: 0.2–0.5 mg/kg, PO, IV, TID Dog/cat: 0.5–2 mg/kg, PO, BID or once before anxiety-causing stimulus	Potentiates effects of other analgesics, sedatives and analgesics; cimetidine and erythromycin, ketoconazole and valproic acid reduce metabolism of benzodiazepines	Paradoxical reaction (excitement)

A5

Active substance	Activity	Indication	Dosage	Contraindication/ interactions	Side effects
Diazoxide thiazide diuretic	Vasodilation of the peripheral arterioles, inhibits secretion of pancreatic insulin	Insulinoma	Dog/cat: 5 mg/kg, PO, BID	Careful in patients with congestive hear failure and renal insufficiency (diazoxide can cause sodium and water retention). Phenothiazine, phenytoin, phenylbanzamine, hydralizine, prazosin	Anorexia, vomiting, diarrhoea
Dihydrotachysterol vitamin D	Increases absorption of calcium from GI tract, resorption from renal tubuli	Hypocalcaemia due to secondary hyperparathyroidism or renal failure	Dog: 0.02–0.05 mg/kg, PO, SID for 2 to 3 days, then 0.01–0.03 mg/kg SID	Hypercalcaemia, hyperphosphataemia, malabsorption	Anorexia, polydipsia, polyuria, hypercalcaemia, hyperphosphataemia, nephrocalcinosis
Diphenhydramine antihistamine	Competitive inhibition of histamine on H_1 receptors, additional anticholinergic effect	Organophosphate or carbamate intoxication, antiemetic, angioedema, urticaria, antipruritic	Dog/cat: 1–4 mg/kg, PO, BID–TID	Closed-angle glaucoma, pyloric or duodenal obstruction, bladder obstruction, careful with hyperthyroidism and cardiovascular diseases. Increases effects of sedatives, epinephrine; interaction with heparin	CNS depression; anticholinergic effects: dry mouth, vomiting, diarrhoea, anorexia, urine retention
Dopamine sympathomimetic	Precursor of norepinephrine, α- and β_1-agonist, dopamine receptor agonist	Improvement of renal blood perfusion, Increased cardiac output per minute	Dog/cat: < 5 µg/kg/min, IV Dog/cat: < 10 µg/kg/min as continuous intravenous infusion in 5% glucose	Pheochromocytoma, tachyarrhythmia. Inactivated in alkali solutions	Tachycardia
Doxepin tricyclic antidepressant	Antihistamine, anticholinergic and anti-α_1-adrenergic activity; blocks norepinephrine and serotonin uptake at the presynaptic membrane	Psychogenic dermatosis Antihistamine	Dog: 2–5 mg/kg, PO, q 12–24 h Cat: 0.55–1 mg/kg, PO, BID Dog/cat: 0.5–1 mg/kg, PO, BID	Glaucoma, urine retention. Do not give with monoamine oxidase inhibitors or other anticholinergic medications; cimetidine may inhibit doxepin metabolism	Ventricular arrhythmias, hyperexcitation
Doxorubicin chemotherapeutic	Inhibition of DNA and RNA synthesis and proteosynthesis	Chemotherapy protocol	Dog: 30 mg/m², IV, every 21 days or 10 mg/m², IV, every 7 days Cat: 30 mg/m², IV, every 3 to 4 weeks	Cardiac insufficiency, liver insufficiency. Cyclophosphamide potentiates the effects of doxorubicin	Bone marrow suppression, cardiotoxic, nausea, vomiting, diarrhoea, alopecia, perivascular necrosis; skin irritation (work with gloves)
Doxycycline antibiotic	Bacteristatic, broad spectrum	Ehrlichiosis, borreliosis, toxoplasmosis	Dog/cat: 10 mg/kg, PO, SID; possibly 5 mg/kg, PO, BID	Not during growth until tooth eruption finished	Nausea, vomiting (especially in cats), discolouration of teeth in puppies and kittens
Edrophonium chloride parasympathomimetic	Short-acting acetylcholinase inhibitor	Myasthenia gravis	Dog: 0.1–0.2 mg/kg, IV Cat: 0.25–052 mg/kg, IV	Atropine antagonist	Ptyalism, diarrhoea, vomiting, miosis, tachycardia, hypotension, respiratory disturbances, muscle spasms, weakness

A5

Active substance	Activity	Indication	Dosage	Contraindication / interactions	Side effects
Enrofloxacin antibiotic	Bactericidal, broad spectrum, mainly gram-negative bacteria	Otitis media / interna	Dog / cat: 5–10 mg/kg, PO, IM, SID	Do not use in puppies / kittens. Antacids and sucralfate may prevent resorption of enrofloxacin	Cartilage damage in growing dogs; blindness in cats
Ephedrine sympathomimetic	α- and $\beta_{1,2}$-agonist	Urinary incontinence: increases urethral sphincter tone	Dog / cat: 2 mg/kg, PO, SID; after 10 days, 1–2 mg/kg, PO, SID	Hypertonia, tachycardia, cardiac arrhythmias, glaucoma, hyperthyroidism, diabetes mellitus	Increased irritability, nervousness, sleeplessness, hypertonia
Esmolol sympatholytic	β_1-adrenergic inhibitor	Supraventricular tachycardia	Dog / cat: 0.25–0.5 mg/kg, IV; 0.02–0.05 mg/kg/min, IV	Bradycardia	Hypertension, bradycardia
Ethanol 20% alcohol	Competitive inhibition of alcohol dehydrogenase	Ethylene glycol and methanol intoxication	Dog / cat: 5.5 ml/kg, IV every 4 h five times; then every 6 h four times	Barbiturates, benzodiazepines, cephalosporins, furazolidone, phenothiazine	Ataxia, depression, polyuria, dehydration
Etodolac NSAID	Cyclic oxygenase 2 inhibitor	Analgesia, anti-inflammatory	Dog / cat: < 10–15 mg/kg, PO, SID	Cardiovascular disease, liver and renal insufficiency, GI disease	Vomiting, diarrhoea, depression, hypoproteinaemia, urticaria, behavioural disturbances
Etomidate intravenous anaesthetic	Imidazole, intravenous hypnotic, effects have not been elucidated	Induction of anaesthesia	Dog / cat: 1–3 mg/kg, IV	Avoid in epileptic seizures	During induction of anaesthesia: spontaneous movements, muscle tremors and hypertonus
Famotidine H$_2$-antagonist	Blocks H$_2$-receptors	Inhibition of excessive stomach acids, stomach ulcer	Dog / cat: 0.5 mg/kg, PO, IM, IV, SID–BID	Careful in patients with liver and renal insufficiency, can have negative ionotropic effects	Fall in blood pressure, vomiting with rapid IV application; serum ALT concentration is increased with high doses
Felbamate antiepileptic	Inhibition of NMDA receptors and potentiates GABA receptors	Epilepsy	Dog: 15–60 mg/kg, PO, TID; serum concentration: 20–100 mg/l	Liver insufficiency. Increases phenobarbitol concentration	Bone marrow and liver toxicity
Fentanyl opioid	Opioid receptor antagonist	Analgesia, sedation	Dog: 1–3 µg/kg, IV (effects last 15–20 min); 2–5 µg/kg/h, IV, continual infusion, after 2 h reduced to half with fentanyl patches: 2–4 µg/kg/h	Potentiates other sedatives, analgesics and anaesthetics; do not use with monoamine oxidase inhibitors	Respiratory depression, bradycardia
Fluconazole antifungal	Fungiostatic triazole derivative; increases cell membrane permeability and purine uptake	Systemic fungal diseases: *Candida, Cryptococcus, Histoplasma, Blastomyces*	Dog: 2.5–5 mg/kg, PO, SID for 8 to 12 weeks Cat: 2.5–10 mg/kg, PO, BID	Liver and renal insufficiency, pregnancy	Vomiting, diarrhoea, anorexia, increased liver values, thrombocytopaenia
Fluvoxamine antidepressant	Potentiates the effects of serotonin (inhibits re-uptake of serotonin)	Separation anxiety	Dog: 1 mg/kg, PO, SID Cat: 0.25–1 mg/kg, PO, BID	Hypersensitivity to fluvoxamine, epileptic seizures, diabetes mellitus. Monoamine oxidase inhibitors	Not known in dogs. In humans: nervousness, sleeplessness, inappetence, nausea, vomiting, diarrhoea

A5

A5

Active substance	Activity	Indication	Dosage	Contraindication/ interactions	Side effects
Fluoxetine antidepressant	Potentiates the effects of serotonin (inhibits re-uptake of serotonin)	Separation anxiety	Dog: 1 mg/kg, PO, SID Cat: 0.5–1 mg/kg, PO, BID	Hypersensitivity to fluoxetine, epileptic seizures, diabetes mellitus. Monoamine oxidase inhibitors	Not known in dogs. In humans: nervousness, sleeplessness, dizziness, tiredness, inappetence, nausea, vomiting, diarrhoea
Furosemide diuretic	Loop diuretic	Brain oedema: potentiates the effects of mannitol > 15 min	Dog/cat: 2–4 mg/kg, IV, SC, then 1–2 mg/kg, IV, SC, TID–QID	Dehydration	Dehydration, hyponatraemia, rarely hypokalaemia
Gentamycin antibiotic	Bactericidal, aminoglycoside, against gram-negative bacteria	Sepsis, peritonitis, otitis externa	Dog/cat: 2–4 mg/kg, IM, SC, IV slowly, max. 5 days	Renal insufficiency, myasthenia gravis	Nephrotoxic, ototoxic, neuromuscular blockade
Glycopyrrolate anticholinergic	Inhibition of acetylcholine at the postganglionic muscarinic receptors	Bradycardia	Dog/cat: 0.005–0.01 mg/kg, IV, IM, SC as needed	Glaucoma, tachycardia, tachyarrhythmia, hyperthyroidism, paralytic ileus. Parasympathomimetics	Initial bradycardia then tachycardia; reduced salivation and bronchial secretions; intestinal atony
Heparin anticoagulant	Low doses inhibit the conversion of prothrombin to thrombin; higher doses inactivate thrombin and block the conversion of fibrinogen to fibrin	Disseminated intravascular coagulation (DIC) Thromboembolism	Dog/cat: 75 IU/kg, SC, TID Dog/cat: 200 IU/kg, IV, SC, then 50 IU/kg, SC, TID–QID	Thrombocytopaenia, uncontrolled bleeding; do not give intramuscularly	Haemorrhage, thrombocytopaenia, hypersensitivity
Hydromorphone opioid	Opioid receptor agonist	Analgesia, sedation, premedication	Dog/cat: 0.1–0.4 mg/kg, IV, IM, SC, q 2–4 h	Liver failure, increased ICP. Potentiates the effects of other sedatives, analgesics and anaesthetics; do not give with monoamine oxidase inhibitors	Respiratory depression, hypotension, bradycardia
Imipramine antidepressant	Blocks amino acid pump and so increases serotonin and norepinephrine concentrations; central and peripheral anticholinergic activity	Cataplexy Separation anxiety Urinary incontinence	Dog: 0.5–1 mg/kg, PO, TID Dog: 2.2–4.4 mg/kg, PO, SID–BID Dog: 5–15 mg/dog, PO, SID–BID Cat: 2.5–5 mg/cat, PO, BID	Monoamine oxidase inhibitors	Sedation, hyperexcitation, bone marrow suppression, vomiting, diarrhoea
Itraconazole antifungal	Fungiostatic triazole derivative; increases cell membrane permeability and purine uptake	Systemic fungal diseases: *Aspergillus, Blastomyces, Candida, Cryptococcus, Histoplasma*	Dog/cat: 5 mg/kg, PO, SID–BID	Liver and renal insufficiency, pregnancy	Vomiting, diarrhoea, anorexia, increased liver values, thrombocytopaenia
Ketamine disassociative anaesthetic	Blocks GABA, serotonin, norepinephrine and dopamine receptors in CNS	Analgesia, anaesthesia	Dog: 3–10 mg/kg, IV, IM Cat: 10–30 mg/kg, IM or 2–4 mg/kg, IV	Head injuries, epileptic seizures, intracranial space-occupying lesions, myelography	Dyspnoea, vomiting, muscle tremors, seizures, hypertonus, opisthitonus, cardiac arrest
Ketoconazole antifungal	Fungiostatic triazole derivative; increases cell membrane permeability and purine uptake	Fungal diseases: *Aspergillus, Blastomyces, Candida, Cryptococcus, Histoplasma, Microsporum, Trichophyton*	Dog/cat: 5–10 (20) mg/kg, PO, BID	Liver insufficiency, thrombocytopaenia, pregnancy	Vomiting, diarrhoea, anorexia, increased liver values, thrombocytopaenia

Active substance	Activity	Indication	Dosage	Contraindication/ interactions	Side effects
Ketoprofen NSAID	Cyclic oxygenase inhibitor	Analgesia, anti-inflammatory, antipyretic	Dog/cat: 0.2 mg/kg, PO, IV, SID	Liver and renal insufficiency, GI haemorrhaging and ulcers. Do not combine with steroids	Vomiting, GI haemorrhage and ulcers
Lactulose laxative	Reduces ammonium concentration in blood; osmotic laxative	Hepatoencephalopathy	Dog: 5–30 ml/dog, PO, TID Cat: 2.5–1 ml/cat, PO, TID	Diabetes mellitus	Flatulence, diarrhoea; seizures (overdosage)
L-carnitine amino acid	Essential for metabolism of long-chain fatty acids	Chronic carnitine deficiency, hepatic lipidosis	Dog/cat: 50–100 mg/kg, PO, BID		Nausea, vomiting, diarrhoea
Levothyroxine thyroid hormone	Increases protein synthesis, gluconeogenesis, oxygen utilisation, cardiac frequency and output	Hypothyroidism	Dog: 20 µg/kg, PO, BID Cat: 10–20 µg/kg, PO, SID; fine dosage adjustment after 4 to 8 weeks	Myocardial ischemia, thyrotoxicosis, severe adrenal insufficiency	Nervousness and excitability, tachycardia, polyphagia, PU/PD
Lidocaine local anaesthetic	Blocks sodium channels in depolarised cell membrane	Ventricular tachyarrhythmias Local anaesthesia (EEG)	Dog: 2–4 ml/kg, IV as bolus, afterwards 50–80 µg/kg/min Dog: 2–4 ml/kg, SC	Additive effect with procainamide results in increased toxicity	Tremors and spasms with too rapid injection of bolus; apathy, bradycardia as sign of accumulative effect
Lomustine cytostatic	Inhibition of DNA and RNA synthesis	Neoplasia in CNS	Dog: 50–80 mg/m^2, PO, every 5 to 8 weeks	Anaemia, bone marrow insufficiency, infection, renal insufficiency, pregnancy. Increased risk of bone marrow suppression with chloramphenicol, colchicine and flucytosine; increased risk of infection with azathioprine, cyclophosphamide and corticosteroids	Anorexia, vomiting, diarrhoea, alopecia, anaemia, thrombocytopaenia, leukopaenia, hepatotoxicity, lung infiltration or fibrosis
Mannitol diuretic	Osmotic diuretic	Brain oedema	Dog/cat: 0.5–2 g/kg, IV over 20 min, q 4 h	Dehydration, intracranial haemorrhage, lung oedema	Electrolyte abnormalities
Medetomidine α2-adrenergic agonist	Stimulates α_2-adrenergic receptors	Sedation, premedication, analgesia	Dog/cat: 2–10 µg/kg, IV	Cardiovascular disease, shock, pregnancy. Effects potentiated by opioids	Bradycardia, AV block, vomiting
Meloxicam NSAID	Cyclic oxygenase inhibitor	Analgesia, anti-inflammatory, antipyretic	Dog: 0.2 mg/kg, PO, IV, SID	Liver and renal insufficiency, GI haemorrhaging and ulcers. Do not combine with steroids	Vomiting, GI haemorrhage and ulcers
Methadone opioid	Opioid receptor agonist	Strong analgesia, sedation	Dog/cat: 0.1–0.5 mg/kg, IV, IM, q 2–3 h	Potentiates effects of other sedatives, analgesics and anaesthetics	Mydriasis; overdosage leads to ataxia, disorientation
Methotrexate chemotherapeutic	Competitive inhibition of folic acid reductase in S phase of mitosis	Chemotherapy protocol	Dog: 2.5 mg/m^2, PO, SID or 5 mg/m^2, PO, twice/week Cat: 5 mg/m^2, PO, 2–3 ×/week	Liver and renal insufficiency, severe bone marrow suppression. Protein-binding drugs (salicylate, sulphonamide, phenytoin, phenylbutazone, tetracyclines, chloramphenicol)	Nausea, vomiting, diarrhoea, bone marrow suppression, hepatotoxicity, renal tubular necrosis, alopecia, depigmentation

A5

A5

Active substance	Activity	Indication	Dosage	Contraindication / interactions	Side effects
Methylprednisolone succinate corticosteroid	Phospholipase A_2 inhibition	CNS trauma within 8 h, spinal cord infarct, preoperative (spinal and cranial surgery)	Dog/cat: 30 mg/kg, IV as bolus; 15 mg/kg, IV after 2 and 6 h; then 2.5 mg/kg continual infusion for 24–48 h; or 30 mg/kg, IV as bolus; then 5.4 mg/kg continual infusion for 24–48 h	Sepsis; systemic fungal infection; viral, bacterial and protozoal infections; GI ulceration; liver and renal insufficiency; corneal ulceration	PU/PD, polyphagia, fluid retention, vomiting/diarrhoea, GI ulceration
Methysergide Synthetic ergot alkaloid – 5-HT receptor antagonist	Serotonin antagonist	Muscle hypertonia, migraine	Dog: 0.33 mg/kg, PO	Cardiac insufficiency, liver and renal insufficiency, pregnancy	Nausea, vomiting, dizziness, nervousness
Metoclopramide prokinetic drug, antiemetic	Sensibilises smooth muscles for acetylcholine in upper GI tract; central antagonism in the dopamine receptor domain	Nausea, vomiting, stimulates stomach emptying	Dog/cat: 0.2–0.5 mg/kg, IV, SC, PO, QID	GI haemorrhage, foreign bodies in stomach or duodenum, pancreatitis. Phenothiazine, narcotics and sedatives strengthen the central effects of metoclopramide	Rarely behavioural disturbances, nausea, diarrhoea
Metronidazole antibiotic	Bactericidal, antibacterial and antiprotozoal, broad spectrum especially against anaerobes	Tetanus, bacterial meningoencephalitis, hepatoencephalopathy	Dog: 25–30mg/kg, IV, PO, BID Cat: 10–25 mg/kg, IV, PO, BID	Hepatopathies. Barbiturates increase the metronidazole metabolism	GI disturbances, liver damage with high doses; ataxia, torticollis, nystagmus, tremor, epileptic seizures
Mexiletine antiarrhythmic	Inhibition of sodium channels	Myotonia Tachyarrhythmia	Dog: 8.3 mg/kg, PO TID Dog: 2–5 µg/kg/min, IV slowly, followed by 3–10 mg/kg, PO BID–TID	AV blocks, congestive heart disease, liver insufficiency. Cimitidine increases mexiletine concentration	Nausea, vomiting, dizziness
Midazolam benzodiazepine	GABA agonist, serotonin antagonist, reduced release of acetylcholine in CNS	Sedation, epileptic seizures	Dog/cat: 0.2–5 mg/kg, IV, IM as needed	Liver and renal insufficiency. Narcotics increases sedative effects of midazolam	Paradoxical behaviour (excitement, snuffling), respiratory depression
Misoprostol Prostaglandin E_1	Inhibits stomach acid and pepsin secretion; increases production of gastric mucous and bicarbonate	Inhibition of excess acid production in stomach; stomach and intestinal ulceration	Dog/cat: 1–5 µg/kg, PO, TID	Pregnancy (increased uterine contractions)	Vomiting, diarrhoea, abdominal pain, flatulence, uterus contractions
Morphine opioid	Opioid receptor agonist	Analgesia	Dog/cat: 0.2–0.6 mg/kg, IV, IM, SC, q 2–4 h	Renal failure, adrenal insufficiency, increased ICP. Potentiates effects of other sedatives, analgesics and anaesthetics; do not use with monoamine oxidase inhibitors	Respiratory depression, mydriasis; overdosage leads to ataxia, disorientation
Naloxone opioid antagonist	Competitive opioid antagonist	Opioid side-effects, overdosage	Dog/cat: 0.01–0.05 mg/kg, IV, IM	Also antagonises following opioid agonists/ antagonists: butorphenol, pentazocine, nalbupin	Not known
Naproxen NSAID	Cyclic oxygenase inhibitor	Analgesia, anti-inflammatory, antipyretic	Dog/cat: 2–5 mg/kg, PO, q 48 h	Heart, liver or renal diseases. Urine alkalisation agents, furosemide, corticosteroids, other NSAIDs	GI ulceration

Active substance	Activity	Indication	Dosage	Contraindication/ interactions	Side effects
Neostigmine parasympathomimetic	Acetylcholine esterase inhibitor	Myasthenia gravis	Dog/cat: 0.05 mg/kg IM, QID	Peritonitis, mechanical GI and urinary tract obstruction, pregnancy. Atropine antagonist	Diarrhoea, vomiting
Nizergoline peripheral vasodilator	Adrenolytic; inhibits thrombocyte aggregation; passes blood-brain barrier	Brain hypoxia	Dog/cat: 0.25 mg/kg PO	Haemorrhages, bradycardia, hypotension. Sympathomimetics	Dizziness, nausea, hypotension
Oestrogen steroidal hormone	Increases external urethral sphincter tone	Incontinence after castration	Dog: 0.1–1 mg/day, PO, for 3 to 5 days, then 1 mg/week		Oestrous, bone marrow toxicity
Omiprazole protects stomach	Blocks proton pumps	Inhibition of excessive stomach acid production, GI ulceration	Dog/cat: 0.5–1 mg/kg, PO, SID	Liver insufficiency	Rarely in human medicine: nausea, vomiting, diarrhoea, flatulence, proteinuria, bladder inflammation
Oxazepam benzodiazepine	GABA agonist, serotonin antagonist, reduced release of acetylcholine in CNS	Separation anxiety, appetite stimulant	Dog/cat: 0.2–1 mg/kg, PO, SID–BID	Careful with liver insufficiency. Potentiates effects of other sedatives and analgesics	Sedation, ataxia
Oxymorphone opioid	Agonist	Analgesia, sedation, premedication	Dog/cat: 0.03–0.1 mg/kg, IM, IV, SC, q 3–4 h	Liver failure, increased ICP. Potentiates effects of other sedatives, analgesics and anaesthetics; do not give with monoamine oxidase inhibitors	Respiratory depression, hypotension, bradycardia
Paroxetine Antidepressant; selective serotonin reuptake inhibitor	Inhibits serotonin uptake	Dominant behavioural attributes, anxiety, house soiling problems	Dog: 1 mg/kg, PO, SID Cat: 0.5–1 mg/kg, PO, SID	Monoamine oxidase inhibitors; careful using combinations with other antidepressants	Sedation, hyperexcitation, nausea, diarrhoea, urine and faeces retention
Penicillamine chelator	With cysteine, stable water-soluble complex; antirheumatic	Metal intoxication	Dog/cat: 20–30 mg/kg PO, TID–QID for 1 to 2 weeks	Pregnancy. Cyclophosphamide, azathioprine, phenylbutazone	Nausea, vomiting
Pentobarbital anaesthetic, barbiturate	Increased GABA activity; inhibition of acetylcholine, glutamate and norepinephrine in CNS	Status epilepticus when no response with phenobarbital	Dog/cat: 5–15 mg/kg, IV until sedation occurs; then according to effect 0.2–1 mg/kg for 24–36 h	Increased risk of liver and renal failure; careful with hypovolaemia and respiratory dysfunction	Respiratory depression, reduced blood pressure
Pethidine (meperidine) opioid	Opioid agonist	Analgesia, sedation, premedication	Dog/cat: 3–10 mg/kg, IM, IV, SC as needed	Liver failure; increased ICP. Potentiates effects of other sedatives, analgesics and anaesthetics; do not give with monoamine oxidase inhibitors	Hypotension, bradycardia, cardiovascular collapse with too rapid IV injection
Phenobarbital antiepileptic, barbiturate	Increased GABA activity; inhibition of glutamate activity	Epileptic seizure Status epilepticus Long-term oral therapy	Dog/cat: 2–5 mg/kg, IV Dog/cat: 5–10 mg/kg, IV; max. dose/day: 25 mg/kg Dog/cat: 2–5 mg/kg, PO, BID	Due to its induction of microsomal enzymes in the liver, influence on drugs degraded in this manner: steroids, phenytoin, phenylbutazone, oestrogens	Apathy for 2 to 3 weeks, PU/PD, polyphagia, induction of microsomal enzyme activity in liver; rare: bone marrow suppression, superficial necrolytic dermatitis; lymphadenopathy and cutaneous eruptions in cats

A5

A5

Active substance	Activity	Indication	Dosage	Contraindication / interactions	Side effects
Phenoxybenzamine sympatholytic	Blocks α-adrenergic receptors	Reduction of tone in internal urethral sphincter	Dog / cat: 0.25–0.5 mg/kg, PO, BID–TID	Careful in patients with glaucoma, diabetes mellitus and heart disease. Antagonism with α-sympathomimetics	Hypotension, tachycardia, weakness, dizziness, vomiting
Phenyl-propranolamine sympathomimetic	Stimulates α- and β-adrenergic receptors by causing a release of norepinephrine	Hypotonia of the urethral sphincter	Dog / cat: 1–1.5 mg/kg, PO, BID–TID	Hypertonia, cardiovascular disease, glaucoma, hyperthyroidism, diabetes mellitus. Not with other sympathomimetics, indomethacin, aspirin, tricyclic antidepressants	Increased excitability, nervousness, sleeplessness, hypertonia
Phenytoin antiepileptic	Causes sodium efflux from nerve cells leading to hyperpolarisation of nerve cell membrane	Epilepsy	Dog: 15–40 mg/kg, PO, TID serum concentration: 10–20 μg/ml	Liver insufficiency, pregnancy. Effects increased by allopurinol, cimetidine, chloramphenicol, diazepam, phenylbutone, sulphonamides and valproic acid; effects reduced by barbiturates, diazoxide, antacids, calcium, nitrofurantoin, pyridoxine and cytostatic drugs.	Anorexia, vomiting, ataxia, sedation, increased serum ALAT, hepatocellular hypertrophy and necrosis, hepatic lipidosis
Potassium bromide (KBr) antiepileptic	Substitution of bromide for chloride ions leading to an increase in the nerve membrane polarisation	Long-term oral antiepileptic therapy	Dog / cat: 20–40 mg/kg, PO, BID as loading dose; 40–60 mg/kg, PO, BID for 3 to 5 days: KBr concentration: 1–3 mg/ml	Renal failure	Depression, tiredness, ataxia, increased appetite, rarely erythema, pruritis, pancreatitis, asthma in cats
Potassium chloride		Hypokalaemia, myopathy	Cat: 0.5 mmol/kg/h, IV	Cardiac insufficiency, heart arrhythmias	Bradycardia
Potassium gluconate		Hypokalaemia, myopathy	Cat: recommended dose: 5–8 mmol/day PO; maintenance: 2–4 mmol/day PO depending on serum potassium concentration	Cardiac insufficiency, heart arrhythmias	Bradycardia
Pralidoxime chloride oxime; cholinesterase reactivator	Reactivates cholinesterase	Organophosphate intoxication	Dog / cat: 10–15 mg/kg, IV, IM, SC, BID–TID	Not in cabamate intoxication. Acetylcholinesterase inhibitors	Rapid intravenous injection can cause tachycardia, spasticity of the musculature and laryngeal spasm
Prednisolone Prednisone corticosteroid	Inhibition of phospholipase A_2, 12–36 h	Anti-inflammatory Brain and spinal cord swelling Immunosuppression Hypoglycaemia (insulinoma)	Dog / cat: 0.5–1 mg/kg, PO, SC, SID Dog / cat: 1–2 mg/kg, PO, SC, SID Dog / cat: 2–4 mg/kg, PO, SID Dog / cat: 0.25–0.5 mg/kg, PO, BID	Sepsis; systemic fungal infections; not prolonged treatment with viral, bacterial or protozoal infections; GI ulceration; liver and renal insufficiency	PU / PD, polyphagy, vomiting / diarrhoea, GI ulceration

Active substance	Activity	Indication	Dosage	Contraindication/ interactions	Side effects
Primidone (active metabolites: phenylethylmalone amide and phenobarbital) antiepileptic	Increases GABA activity and inhibits glutamate activity	Epilepsy	Dog/cat: 5–20 mg/kg, PO, BID–TID serum concentration: 15–40 µg/ml	Hepatopathies; be careful in cats. Careful when giving other drugs which are degraded by the microsomal enzyme system in the liver (steroids, phenytoin, phenylbutazone, oestrogens)	Apathy for 2 to 3 weeks; PU/PD, polyphagia, induction of the microsomal enzyme activity in the liver
Procainamide antiarrhythmic	Anticholinergic	Myotonia Tachyarrhythmia	Dog/cat: 40–50 mg/kg, PO, BID–TID Dog: 20–40 µg/kg/min, in continuous infusion; 10–25 mg/kg, PO, TID–QID	Myasthenia gravis; careful in congestive cardiac insufficiency and renal insufficiency	Anorexia, vomiting, diarrhoea, weakness, hypotension, negative ionotropism
Propofol intravenous anaesthetic	Short-acting hypnotic; effects not fully elucidated	Short-term sedation, induction of anaesthesia, status epilepticus	Dog/cat: 2–7 mg/kg, IV to effect; 0.1–0.6 mg/kg/min, IV	Careful in patients with shock and sensitive to cardiovascular and respiratory depression. Increased vasodilation and negative inotropic effects with acepromazine and opioids	Hypotension, respiratory depression to apnoea
Propranolol sympatholytic	Blocks $\beta_{1,2}$-receptors	Hypertrophic cardiomyopathy, hyperthyroidism in cats Tachyarrhythmia Atonic bladder	Cat: 2.5–5 mg/kg, PO, TID Dog/cat: 0.25–1 mg/kg, IV slowly Dog: 0.5–2 mg/kg, PO, BID–TID (max. 10 mg/dog)	Bradycardia, AV block, congestive cardiac insufficiency, hypoglycaemia	Bradycardia, AV block, weakness, bronchospasm, hypoglycaemia
Pyridostigmine parasympathomimetic	Long-acting acetylcholine-esterase inhibitor	Myasthenia gravis	Dog/cat: 0.2–2 mg/kg, PO, BID–TID	Atropine antagonist	Diarrhoea, vomiting
Pyrimethamine chemotherapeutic	Folic acid antagonist	Toxoplasmosis	Dog/cat: 0.5–1 mg/kg, PO, SID for 2 days, then 0.25 mg/kg for 2 weeks with sulfadiazine (30 mg/kg, PO, BID)	During pregnancy give folic acid substitution	Anorexia, vomiting, depression, anaemia, thrombocytopaenia, leukopaenia
Rantidine H_2-antagonist	Blocks H_2-receptors	Inhibition of excessive stomach acid secretion, stomach ulcer	Dog/cat: preventative: 0.5 mg/kg, diluted PO, IV, BID; chronic ulcer: 2 mg/kg, PO, IV, BID		With rapid IV, drop in blood pressure and vomiting; increased ALT concentration
Selegiline monoamine oxidase B inhibitor	Inhibition of monoamine oxidase B, reduces dopamine metabolism	Behavioural disturbances, cognitive dysfunctions in the dog, central Cushing's disease	Dog: 0.5–1 mg/kg, PO, SID Cat: 1 mg/kg, PO, SID	Opioids	Vomiting, diarrhoea, salivation, anorexia, nervousness, apathy, tremor, pruritis
Somatostatin (ocreotide – synthetic hormone)	Inhibition of insulin synthesis and secretion in β-cells	Insulinoma	Dog: 10–40 µg/dog, SC, BID–TID	Diabetes mellitus	Not known
Sucralfate antiulcer drug	Sucralfate + stomach acid complex binds with protein-containing exudates in ulcer	GI ulceration, reflux oesophagitis	Dog: 0.5–1 mg/dog, PO, TID Cat: 0.25–0.5 mg/cat, PO, BID–TID	Inhibits resorption of tetracyclines, digoxin and phenytoin	Constipation

A5

A5

Active substance	Activity	Indication	Dosage	Contraindication/ interactions	Side effects
Tetanus antitoxin equine antitetanus serum, human antitetanus immunoglobulin	Neutralisation of tetanus toxin	Tetanus	Dog/cat: 25–110 IU/kg, SC, IV (before IV application give 0.1 ml intradermal)		Anaphylactic shock with IV application
Thiamine (vitamin B1)	coenzyme of aerobic glycolysis	Thiamine deficiency	Dog/cat: 100–250 mg, SC, SID–BID	May increase activity of neuromuscular blockers	Induces anaphylaxis
Thiopental barbiturate	Increases GABA activity; inhibition of acetylcholine, glutamate and norepinephrine in CNS; ultra short effect	Induction of anaesthesia	Dog/cat: 10–20 mg/kg, IV according to effect	Use in greyhounds, shock, hypovolaemia	Respiratory depression (apnoea), sensitization of myocardium to catecholamines; phlebitis with extravascular injection; "top-up" dosing leads to accumulation
Trimethoprim/ sulphadiazine chemotherapeutic	Bacteristatic, antibacterial and antiprotozoal, broad spectrum	Bacterial meningoencephalitis, neosporosis, toxoplasmosis	Dog/cat: 15–30 mg/kg, PO, BID	Careful in Doberman. Careful with concomitant use of salicylates, phenylbutazone and narcotics (increased blood concentration of sulphonamides)	Keratoconjunctivitis sicca, transient weakness, renal damage due to crystalluria and haemolysis (especially in young animals), liver damage
Valproic acid antiepileptic	GABA transferase inhibition	Epilepsy	Dog: 75–200 mg/kg, PO, TID	Liver insufficiency, thrombocytopaenia, dysfunction of thrombocyte adhesion. Valproic acid increases the concentrations of phenobarbital and primidone if they are being used concurrently	Nausea, vomiting, diarrhoea, increased liver enzymes, sedation, behavioural disturbances, ataxia, thrombocytopaenia, dysfunction of thrombocyte adhesion, anaemia, leukopaenia, alopecia
Verapamil antiarrhythmic	Blocks calcium channels	Supraventricular tachyarrhythmia	Dog: 0.5 mg/kg, IV over 2 min, repeat every 15 to 30 min; max. dose 0.15–0.2 mg/kg	Congestive cardiac insufficiency, high grade AV block. Additive effects with β-blockers; increases serum digoxin concentration; increased effects with cimetidine	Hypotension, negative ionotropic effect, bradycardia
Vincristine chemotherapeutic	Inhibits mitosis by binding to tubulin	Chemotherapy protocol (lymphoma)	Dog/cat: 0.5–0.75 mg/m^2, IV, every 7 to 14 days	Careful with liver insufficiency, leukopaenia, neuromuscular disease. Neurotoxicity potentiated with asparaginase	Bone marrow suppression, polyneuropathy, perivascular necrosis
Vitamin E	antioxidant	Vitamin E deficiency, myopathy, degenerative myelopathy	Dog: 500–2000 IU, PO, SID		
Yohimbine α_2-adrenergic blocker	Central and peripheral antagonist effect to xylazine	Xylazine antagonist	Dog/cat: 0.1mg/kg, IV	Renal insufficiency	Excitability, muscle tremors, salivation, tachypnoea, hyperaemia of the mucosa

Abbreviations

IM = intramuscular; IV = intravenous; PO = per os; SC = subcutaneous; SID = every 24 hours; BID = every 12 hours; TID = every 8 hours; QID = every 6 hours; min = minute; h = hour; GI = gastrointestinal; NSAID = non-steroidal anti-inflammatory drug

Reference list

ETTINGER, S. J., FELDMAN, E. C. (2000): Textbook of Veterinary Internal Medicine. 5th Edition. W.B. Saunders Company.

JAGGY, A. (1979): Neurologische Notfälle beim Kleintier. Ferdinand Enke Verlag, Stuttgart.

Klinik für kleine Haustiere (1995): Pharmakotherapie-Büchlein, Universität Bern.

OLIVER, J. E., LORENZ, M. D., KORNEGAY, J. N. (1997): Handbook of Veterinary Neurology, 3rd Edition, W.B. Saunders, Philadelphia.

PLUMB, D. C. (1999): Veterinary Drug Handbook. 3rd Edition, Iowa State University Press./Ames.

Appendix 6:
Epidemiological overview of the neurological diseases seen in dogs between 1989 and 2000 at the Small Animal Clinic in Bern, Switzerland

Gaby Flühmann

A6

Introduction

The Institute of Animal Neurology at the University of Bern has a long tradition as a referral clinic for dogs and cats with neurological diseases. In addition, the entire clinic's patient data has been completely electronically recorded since 1985. In 2003, these data bases were systematically summarized and evaluated epidemiologically. This descriptive epidemiological study of the neurological diseases of dogs referred to us between 1989 and 2000 provided important information about our patients. In 2000, 14% of the dogs and cats referred to the Small Animal Clinic at the University of Bern were presented at the Institute for Animal Neurology.

Earlier studies that were carried out over a long time period focused either on the breed distribution (breed predisposition) or a particular disease (case series) (LING et al., 1998; BARONE et al., 2002; HARKIN et al., 2002). Some examples of such published studies include the risk factors associated with diabetes mellitus in dogs completed by analyzing case histories between 1970 and 1999 (GUPTILL et al., 2003), the risk factors for acquired myasthenia gravis in 1154 dogs between 1991 and 1995 (SHELTON et al., 1997), and the reasons for the euthanasia of 927 army dogs (MOORE et al., 2001). Another retrospective epidemiological study of diagnoses with respect to gender, age, and breed was undertaken in Sweden in 1996 (EGENVALL et al., 2000). In general, such extensive studies are very valuable due to the large number of data sets and the significance of their results.

The aim of the present study was to bring together information about case histories from different data bases and use it to do a frequency analysis of the neurological diseases with respect to age, gender, breed, and geographic distribution in the period between 1989 and 2000. This study is to our knowledge the most extensive descriptive epidemiological study of neurological disease undertaken in the field of veterinary medicine.

Materials and methods

Case histories

In 1985, the Institute for Animal Neurology began to store their patient data electronically in the DOS-based system, REFLEX (Borland Software Cooperation, Scotts Valley, California, USA). The REFLEX data base contained all the patient data including the neurohistopathological diagnosis. Six years later, the system was changed and two new data bases were set up using ACCESS for Windows (Microsoft Corporation, Redmond, USA). Since then for organizational reasons, these two separate data bases have been maintained. The veterinarians of the Institute for Animal Neurology, mainly residents of the European College of Veterinary Neurology (ECVN), had the task of maintaining a data base with the signalment, diagnostic results, and diagnoses of their patients. The second data base is managed by the neuropathologists and contains all the general pathology information as well as neurohistopathological results and diagnoses. Every patient, to presentation in our department, is given an individual number to ensure that the patient can be followed in both data bases.

The starting point for this study was, therefore, three data bases with, in part, different variables and contents. In order to undertake the study, a new data base (ACCESS for Windows) was set up to consolidate all the data sets for the time period in question. At the beginning of the study, the three data bases were analyzed so that the different structures could be understood and that the mutual variables could be found. The time period chosen was between January 1989 and December 2000, as in the first years of its existence the REFLEX data base had severe gaps in its information.

A total of 4497 dogs each with an individual patient number were included in the study. Additionally, the Swiss Cynological Society offered us an insight into their information about the different dog breed populations and their birth rates, so that we could use them to compare the breed frequencies of the neurological patients in our data sets.

Variables

The variables were redesigned for this study. In the original data bases, the information about the neurological localization, diagnostic workup, and diagnoses were filed in one or more text fields. In the new data base, non-overlapping, list-dependent text fields for each variable were defined. The existing information contained in the old free-text fields was verified, categorized, and fed into the respective fields in the new data base.

Localization

The information concerning the neurological localization was subdivided into: cerebrum; brain stem; cerebellum; peripheral vestibular; spinal segments C1–C5, C6–T2, T3–L3, L4–S3; cauda equina; peripheral nervous system (PNS); multifocal; and other (VANDEVELDE et al., 2001). The multifocal localization included more than one localization in the nervous system at the same point of time. Patients that could not have a localization ascribed to them were grouped together under "other". The classification "no localization" was given to dogs whose clinical examination and diagnostic workup were found to be normal.

A list with all the possible breeds was setup for the breed classification. The age classification was divided according to the stage of life: young dog (< 1 year), juvenile (1–2 years), adult (3–5 years), old (6–9 years), and geriatric (> 10 years). Three diagnosis fields were set up: "tentative diagnosis", "clinical diagnosis", and "neurohistopathological diagnosis". A key list with diagnoses was developed and used in the diagnosis fields. This diagnosis code consisted of a serial number, a code for the localization, and a code for the classification according to VITAMIN D.

VITAMIN D

The acronym VITAMIN D is used by clinicians for making the categorization of the etiology of diseases easier. The letters stand for **V** = vascular, **I** = inflammatory, **T** = traumatic, **A** = anomaly, **M** = metabolic / toxic, **I** = idiopathic, **N** = neoplastic, and **D** = degenerative (VANDEVELDE et al., 2001). All the diagnoses in the combined data base used in this study were classified according to the VITAMIN D system.

Diagnoses

The patients in this study were referral cases from private veterinarians. Every dog was given a clinical, a tentative diagnosis, or no diagnosis in addition to a neuro histopathological diagnosis, independent of its survival. A clinical diagnosis was made when a disease could be confirmed using a neurological examination or additional diagnostic methods such as radiography, MRI, electro-diagnostics, EEG, and / or CSF investigation. All those cases in which only a neurological investigation was undertaken or no abnormalities were found in the diagnostic workup, but were still suspected as having a neurological disease were classified as having a tentative diagnosis. All of the neuro histopathological investigations were undertaken by the Institute for Animal Neurology. Cases subjected to a neuro histopathological investigation were either directly referred by the private veterinarian or had been given a tentative or clinical diagnosis by the Institute for Animal Neurology.

Additional variables

Additional variables were set up in the data base that were not used in the present study. These included the electrodiagnostic results, laboratory results, muscle and nerve biopsies, CSF analysis, and EEG results. The list of the variables for the CSF investigation were divided into a normal and an abnormal group according to the reference values for normal CSF, a negative Pandy's test, and 8 white blood cells /ml (VANDEVELDE et al., 2001).

On principle, no information was entered into any fields in the research data base if the data in the original data base was missing.

Examples of specific diseases

In order to show the value of a well-arranged data base, the most frequent diagnosis (intervertebral disc disease) and the diagnosis of the most frequent localization (idiopathic epilepsy) have been chosen for further analysis and discussion.

A6

Intervertebral disc disease

The clinical diagnosis of vertebral disc disease was based on radiography, CSF investigation, myelography, and/or MRI. The neurohistopathological investigations were either done on a biopsy taken during an operation or post mortem.

Idiopathic epilepsy (IE)

The clinical diagnosis of IE was made by exclusion following a normal neurological examination, a normal EEG and/or a normal MRI, and normal CSF results. As a consequence, the neurohistopathological investigation was also defined as being normal, i.e. no abnormal pathological changes were found.

A6 Graphics and statistics

The graphics and figures were generated using Microsoft PowerPoint for windows (Microsoft Corporation, Redmond, USA). The descriptive statistics, frequency distribution, and cross-classified tables were calculated using NCSS 2001 for Windows (www.ncss.com). The X^2 test was used to calculate the significant differences of the data in the cross-classified table.

Geographic analysis

Each individual patient with a valid Swiss address (postal code and/or town) was shown as an event on a geographic map and evaluated using the software MapInfo version 4 (www.mapinfo.com).

Results

Diagnosis distribution

During the 12-year time frame of this study, 4497 dogs (average of 375/year) with neurological problems or a neurohistopathological diagnosis were registered in the data base. A neurohistopathological diagnosis was achieved in 1159 dogs (25.8%), although only 148 dogs (12.8%) had been directly sent in to have a neurohistopathological examination. At the small animal clinic, a clinical diagnosis was ascertained in 729 of these dogs (62.9%) and a tentative diagnosis in 282 (24.3%) before the neurohistopathological examination was undertaken. Within the whole group of probands, 1431 dogs (31.8%) had only a clinical diagnosis and 1491 dogs (33.2%) only a tentative diagnosis. For 416 dogs (9.3%), there was neither a clinical, a tentative, nor a neurohistopathological diagnosis available.

No pathological changes could be found in 48 (4.1%) of the neurohistopathological cases and these patients were considered to be normal.

Breed distribution

A total of 187 different breeds with neurological diseases were presented. The most commonly affected breeds included mixed-breed dogs (577; 12.8%), German Shepherd (466; 10.4%), Dachshund (389; 8.7%), and Labrador Retriever (235; 5.2%). Data for comparing the breed distribution of all the dogs in Switzerland were not available; however, the breed population for certain breeds in Switzerland could be calculated for the period 1989–2000 and compared with our neurological patients. For example, 2.7% of the German Shepherd population (17280), 2.8% of Labrador Retrievers (8488), and 7.0% of Dachshunds (5527) were referred as neurological patients to the Small Animal Clinic in Bern.

Age and sex distribution

The age distribution ranged from 2 days to 17 years, with a mean value of 5 years. Only 12% of the patients were younger than 1 year, 15% were between 1–3 years, 27% between 4–6 years, 32% between 7–9 years, and 14% were over 10 years old.

Of those dogs with known gender, 2,599 were male (86.7% intact, 13.3% castrated) and 1,858 female (57.2% intact, 42.8% spayed).

Frequency of the diagnoses

Every diagnosis which occurred in more than 2% of either the clinical, tentative, or neurohistopathological diagnosis groups is shown in Table 1. Intervertebral disc disease was the most common diagnosis in all three diagnosis groups.

The clinical diagnosis of a behavioral problem was only made in 25 dogs (0.6% of the 4497 cases). In these cases, an organic disease could be eliminated. In another 35 dogs (0.8%), there was a tentative diagnosis of a behavioral problem. A neurohistopathological investigation was undertaken in one animal in each of these two groups and in both cases found to be normal.

Table 1: Frequencies of the tentative, clinical, and neurohistopathological diagnoses. All diagnoses with an incidence of more than 2% are listed

	Clinical diagnosis Number (%)	Tentative diagnosis Number (%)	Neurohistopathological diagnosis Number (%)
Intervertebral disc disease	741 (34.3)	191 (10.8)	558 (48.1)
Idiopathic epilepsy	271 (12.6)	101 (5.7)	0
Space-occupying lesions	0	187 (10.6)	0
Degenerative lumbosacral stenosis	193 (8.9)	125 (7.1)	64 (5.5)
Fracture / luxation	153 (7.1)	94 (5.3)	51 (4.4)
Infarct	0	158 (8.9)	18 (1.6)
Non-neurological	111 (5.1)	91 (5.1)	0
Normal	87 (4)	0	48 (4.1)
Distemper	18 (0.8)	33 (1.9)	39 (3.4)
Metabolic encephalopathy	61 (2.8)	82 (4.6)	31 (2.7)
Inflammation of the middle ear	85 (3.9)	19 (1.1.)	0
Avulsion / neuropraxia of the brachial plexus	59 (2.7)	10 (0.6)	7 (0.6)
Congenital vestibular syndrome	48 (2.2)	5 (0.3)	0
Steroid-responsive meningitis	44 (2.0)	20 (1.1)	7 (0.6)
Degenerative myelopathy	28 (1.3)	62 (3.5)	11 (1.0)
Intoxication	17 (0.8)	60 (3.4)	11 (1.0)
Metastatic meningoencephalitis	0	35 (2.0)	20 (1.7)
Behavioural problems	25 (1.2)	35 (2.0)	0
Others < 2%	219 (10.1)	465 (26.2)	294 (25.4)
Total	2160 (100)	1773 (100)	1159 (100)

A6

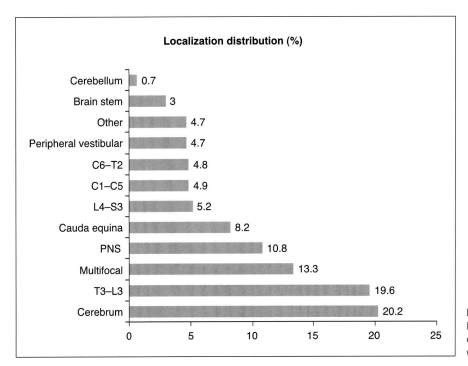

Fig. 1
Localization distribution (n = 4487; 10 dogs were considered to be healthy and so no localization was given for these patients).

A6

Distribution of disease localization

The most frequent localization was the cerebrum (20.2%), followed by T3–L3 (19.6%). Indeed, the other spinal localizations (C1–C6, C6–T2, and L4–S3) were far less commonly affected (Fig. 1). A multifocal localization was found in 13.3% of the dogs. The least affected region was the cerebellum with 0.7%. In ten dogs, no neurological or other problem could be diagnosed, which is why they were not given any localization. In 4.65% of the dogs, the clinical symptoms were not found to be neurological in origin and so they were given the localization "other".

VITAMIN D distribution

The degenerative diseases were the most common of all the VITAMIN D categories (38.0%). With regard to the other categories, there was a remarkable drop in the percentage registered to each one: inflammatory / infectious (14.0%) and idiopathic disease (13.0%) (Fig. 2). The cross-classified table of the localization and VITAMIN D categories showed that 441 (48.7%) of the diseases with a cerebral localization had an idiopathic etiology (Table 2). Almost a third of the diseases in the brain stem were classified as inflammatory / infectious and another third as neoplastic. In 12 dogs (57.1%) with a cerebellar localization, the problem had a neoplastic origin. The multifocal localization was classified as being inflammatory / infectious in 182 dogs (43.8%). In comparison, 639 cases (76.1%) with localization in the region T3–L3 had a degenerative disease. In general, if the localization was in the

spinal cord or cauda equina, the most common cause was a degenerative disease. An inflammatory / infectious disease was found in 105 dogs (56.8%) with a peripheral vestibular localization.

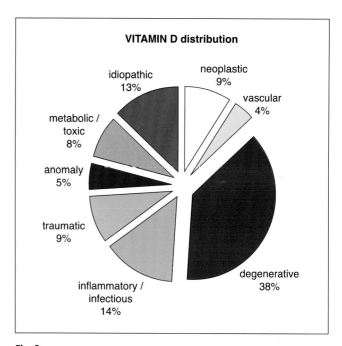

Fig. 2
Distribution of the neurological diagnoses according to VITAMIN D (n = 3727; the distribution could not be given for the remaining 770 dogs).

Table 2: Analysis between neurological localisation and VITAMIN D disease mechanism in a total of 3370 referred dogs

Localisation	Vascular	Inflammatory/ infectious	Traumatic	Anomaly	Metabolic	Idiopathic	Neoplastic	Degenerative	Total
Cerebrum	8	62	13	30	167	441	97	4	822
Brain stem	19	30	18	2	7	0	32	0	108
Cerebellum	0	2	0	2	0	0	12	5	21
Multifocal	3	182	40	19	39	0	58	75	416
C1–C5	9	7	33	33	0	0	22	97	201
C6–T2	17	6	13	25	0	0	19	122	202
T3–L3	48	16	72	22	0	0	43	639	840
L4–S3	50	12	23	4	0	0	14	107	210
Cauda equina	0	20	12	4	0	0	5	315	356
PNS	3	65	11	0	72	36	39	43	369
Peripheral vestibular	0	105	5	52	3	19	1	0	185
Total	157	507	340	193	288	496	342	1407	3730

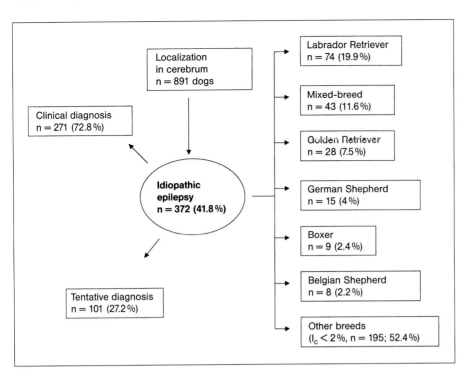

Fig. 3
Division of the tentative and clinical diagnoses as well as the breed and sex distribution of the dogs with idiopathic epilepsy.

Intervertebral disc disease

Intervertebral disc disease was the most common diagnosis with 946 cases (21.0%). Of these cases, 558 (59.0%) were confirmed neurohistopathologically. The thoracolumbar localization was most frequent, occurring in 596 dogs (63.0%). With respect to the other spinal segments, 84 cases (8.9%) occurred in the section L3–S3 and 199 (21.0%) in the cervical region (C1–T2). There was an almost equal distribution between C1–C5 (91; 9.6%) and C6–T2 (108; 11.4%). The remaining cases (67; 7.1%) had a multifocal localization.

Information with respect to the breed could be gleaned from 941 (99.5%) of the dogs. The Dachshund was overrepresented (320; 34.0%), followed by mixed-breed dogs (100; 10.6%), German Shepherds (64; 6.8%), and Pekinese (54; 5.7%).

The age distribution could be calculated from 926 (97.9%) of the dogs. The highest incidence of disc disease occurred between the ages of 6 and 9 years (422; 45.6%), followed by dogs between 3 and 5 years (308; 33.3%).

No sex predisposition could be determined: 520 dogs (55.9%) were male (453 intact; 67 castrated) and 410 (44.1%) were female (229 intact; 181 spayed). There were no significant sex differences in the occurrence of disc disease in comparison to the total number of dogs in the study (4456).

Idiopathic epilepsy

The cerebrum (906 cases; 20.2%) was the most common localization in our patients. A diagnosis of IE was made in 372 (41.1%) of these dogs. The frequency distribution of the tentative diagnosis, clinical diagnosis, breed, and age are shown in Fig. 3. The proportion of male dogs was significantly larger (249; 67.7%) than females (119; 32.3%). A significant difference (X^2 test; $p<0.001$) could also be found between the intact (207; 83.1%) and the castrated males (42; 16.9%). No significant differences were found between the intact females (49.6%) and the spayed ones (50.4%).

Geographic distribution

The majority of owners in the patient pool were from the canton of Bern. Communities with a higher number of canine patients were mainly distributed (1) throughout the region around Bern and (2) in regions with higher human population densities (Lake Geneva in the southwest, Zurich and Basel in the north). A considerably lower number of referrals were sent from regions with lower population densities, such as the Alpine regions.

A6

Discussion

To our knowledge, this is the most comprehensive data base on veterinary patients with neurological disease and an exactly defined diagnosis which has been statistically analyzed and classified. The main aim of the study was a descriptive epidemiological overview of individual neurological diseases as well as the representation of breed-specific, age-specific, sex-specific, and geographical distribution.

Data and evaluation of a data base

In compliance with the defined inclusion criteria, 4497 dogs between 1989 and 2000 were included in the study. The advantage of such a comprehensive study is the accumulated value of the analyzed patient information. As all the dogs had been examined by specialist veterinarians, a correct localization and diagnosis could be achieved. We are well aware that some data and information went missing; however, we consider this as being of little significance in comparison to the enormous yield of the rest of the data.

The available data reflect a selection of diseases seen "in the field", as all the patients were referred to the clinic by private veterinarians. This means that the diagnoses reached in these patients depended on the knowledge and therapeutic possibilities of the private veterinarians. Particularly in the past few years, small animal medicine has developed enormously and it is becoming more and more specialized. As a consequence, the analyzed values are not statistically significant and most probably the distribution of the different neurological problems will have other results in the future. In addition, other neurological diseases may become more important and new diseases could be discovered – both of which will change the distribution of the diagnoses and their composition.

We would have liked to compare our data with those of affected dogs from throughout Switzerland, but this information was not available. As our analysis therefore tends to reflect trends, it would be very interesting to undertake a similar epidemiological evaluation on a regular basis. Such a scheme can only be carried out when the complete patient data remains constant and is saved in a categorized format.

We suggest that in future the value of such patient data bases should be improved; all the input variables should be exactly defined, free-text fields should be avoided where possible, and all the patient information should be put in the same data base. It would also be sensible to make reference tables for each of the variables to prevent clerical errors, which make information retrieval difficult and make any statistical analyses questionable. In this study, these problems were eliminated by manual screening, which proved to be very time consuming.

Distribution of the individual diagnoses

The frequency analysis of the different diseases revealed many tentative diagnoses (37.4%). This relatively high number could have arisen due to lost information if after the complete workup of the disease the final diagnoses were no longer registered in the data base. In addition, in some cases, the owner may not have wanted, for various reasons, to provide further information that would have led to a clinical diagnosis. Neurohistopathological investigations were done on 26% of all the dogs included in the study. Only 148 dogs were actually sent directly by private veterinarians to the neuropathology unit for necropsy. There may have been many reasons for this: the veterinarians did not know enough to send in brain or spinal cord specimens for investigation or the owner did not wish to have a post-mortem investigation. Certainly, an increased number of submissions would widen the diagnosis spectrum and future epidemiological studies would better reflect the general population.

Breed distribution

It is amazing that the most common breed presented between 1989 and 2000 was the mixed-breed dog (577 = 12.8%). The breed-specific statistics provided by the Swiss Cynological Society for the past ten years show a tendency for the birth rate of the pure breed dogs to fall. This could have been the reason for the increased proportion of mixed-breed dogs. Alternatively, it could be speculated that diseases in the nervous system occur more commonly in these animals. We consider, however, the latter to be less probable.

During the study period, there was a large population of German Shepherds (17280) and Labrador Retrievers (8488) in Switzerland. Our data base included 2.7% and 2.8% of these populations, respectively. We assume that the relatively large number of these dogs in the study come from these breeding populations. Interestingly, 7% of all Swiss Dachshunds occurred in our data files. In comparison with the other two breeds, it can be presumed that the Dachshund is more commonly affected by neurological disease, for example, intervertebral disc disease.

Age distribution

The analysis of age distribution showed that 32% of the dogs were between 6–9 years and 27% between 3–5 years old. These results may be an indication that during the study period a population of older dogs was predominant, or possibly even due to the result of the reduced birth rate within the pure breeds.

It could also be that older dogs tend to develop neurological diseases more frequently than younger ones. It could also be speculated that the owners of geriatric dogs or those of dogs which are younger than 3 years, are less likely to decide on further clarification of a disease situation. In addition, there are certain diseases, such as intervertebral disc disease or IE, which occur more commonly in middle-aged dogs (DELA-HUNTA, 1983; HOERLEIN, 1987; OLIVER, et al., 1997; VANDER-VELDE et al., 2001). This situation would have increased the proportion of these animals in the respective age categories.

police or sport dogs. This type of work causes constant stress to the joints, including the intervertebral discs.

Information about the age of the dogs with intervertebral disc disease was available for 926 dogs (97.9%). In contrast to the age predisposition described in the literature (OLIVER et al., 1997), in our study problems predominantly arose between the ages of 6–9 years (45.0%) and 3–5 years (33.0%). If it is taken for granted that the clinical symptoms get worse with time, it could be that the dogs were only presented in an advanced stage of the disease.

The most common neurological disease: intervertebral disc disease

A total of 946 dogs with intervertebral disc disease were included in this study. Interestingly, only a clinical diagnosis was available in 21.4% of these dogs. If it is assumed that a myelographic investigation is only made when there is an indication for surgery, then this would mean that the prognosis for the disc problem was too poor in these dogs and that the owner had decided to have their pet euthanised. A tentative diagnosis without neurohistopathological investigation was made in 176 (18.6%) cases. Based on the literature on the surgical indications for intervertebral disc disease (OLIVER et al., 1997), it can be assumed that the clinical symptoms were not sufficient to indicate surgery and that the dog was treated conservatively. According to the experience at the Institute of Animal Neurology, only a few owners are willing to have further investigations performed if the prognosis is good.

The thoracolumbar region was significantly overrepresented (596; 63.0%) within the total number of cases of intervertebral disc disease (946). This percentage reflects that reported in the literature (OLIVER et al., 1997). The localization L3–S3 was diagnosed in 84 dogs (8.9%) and 199 dogs (21.0%) had a cervical localization (C1–T2). Both these results are higher than that found in the literature (HOERLEIN, 1987; OLIVER et al., 1997). The distribution for the localizations C1–C5 (91; 9.6%) and C6–T2 (108; 11.4%) were almost the same. However, the caudal cervical localization was somewhat more common, which is also different to that described in the literature (HOERLEIN, 1987; OLIVER et al., 1997).

The Dachshund was significantly more commonly affected (320; 34.8%) than other breeds. This can be an indication that of all the chondrodystrophic breeds, the Dachshund has the greatest predisposition for intervertebral disc disease. German Shepherds also show a remarkably high frequency of disc disease (6.8%). Disc herniation in the cauda equina is summarized under the diagnosis "degenerative lumbosacral stenosis". As a result, the incidence of protrusions could be higher than that reported. This high incidence in the German Shepherd is presumably the result of the breed being intensively used as

The most frequent disease associated with the most common localization: idiopathic epilepsy

If the combined localizations in the spinal cord are ignored, then the cerebrum was the most common localization in our probands. The significantly most common diagnosis was IE (41.0%). The breed analysis of the affected dogs was identical with that described in the literature: Labrador Retrievers (20.0%) and Golden Retrievers (7.5%) (OLIVER et al., 1997; KATHMANN et al., 1999; VANDEVELDE et al., 2001). There was also a remarkably high incidence of IE in mixed-breed dogs (12.0%). It is possible that these dogs were related to others affected with IE. If the high proportion of mixed-breed dogs is considered on the one hand with respect to the total number of dogs and on the other hand with respect to the proportion affected with IE, it may be speculated that there is a predisposition for neurological disease in mixed-breed dogs.

The highest incidence of IE occurred between the ages of 3–5 years (40.0%) and 1–2 years (30.0%). In the literature, it is described that first seizures often occur between 6 months and 5 years of age (OLIVER et al., 1997), and that there is an increased incidence between 1–3 years (HEYNOLD et al., 1997; JAGGY and BERNADINI, 1998). By comparison, in our data base, the highest incidence occurred in patients between 3–5 years of age. If one considers that the age reported reflects when the patient was presented in our clinic and not when the symptoms first appeared, this means that the dogs were either in an advanced stage of the disease or that the age when their disease first occurred was truly higher than that reported previously. Only 17 cases (4.6%) were presented before 1 year of age. It is possible that these dogs were the progeny of epileptic dogs – a very early juvenile occurrence of seizures has been described in such animals (GERARD and CORNACK, 1991; KATHMANN et al., 1999). The over-representation of male dogs in comparison to females has already been published (VAN DER VELDEN 1968; BIEFELT et al. 1971; FORRESTER, 1989).

A6

Transmissible spongiform encephalopathy (TSE)

Until now there has been no definitive proof that dogs can be affected by TSE. The diagnostic test, however, has been established and is used in our laboratory. A case of canine TSE would have, therefore, been diagnosed during the neuro histopathological investigation.

Geographic distribution

The density allocation of the patients' origins is comparable to the Swiss human population and is also affected by the distance to our clinic. As a consequence, the largest referral area was in the region around Bern. In any case, the importance of

the Institute of Animal Neurology as a referral clinic for neurological patients is enforced by the multifocal nature of its catchment area.

Conclusions

This study was aimed at showing how a data base can be structured and the possible uses of such collated patient information. Such studies are trend analyses and demonstrate the importance of data bases for retrospective studies. Other analyses should be undertaken using this data base to discover the regional distribution of certain neurological diseases and frequency analyses within the general canine population in Switzerland.

Literature and further reading

BARONE, G., ZIEMER, L.S., SHOFER, F.S., STEINBERG, S.A. (2002): Risk factors associated with development of seizures after use of iohexol for myelography in dogs: 182 cases (1998). Journal of the American Veterinary Medical Association 10, 1499–502.

BERGHAUS, R.D., O'BRIEN, D.P., THORNE, J.G., BUENING, GM. (2002): Incidence of canine dysautonomia in Missouri, USA, between January 1996 and December 2000. Preventive Veterinary Medicine 4, 291–300.

BIEFELT, S.W., REDMAN, H.C., BROADHURST, J.J. (1971): Sire and sexrelated differences in rates of epileptiform seizures in a purebred beagle dog colony. American Journal of Veterinary Research 32, 2039–2048.

BUSH, W.W., BARR, C.S., DARRIN, E.W., SHOFER, F.S., VITE, C.H., STEINBERG, S.A. (2002): Results of cerebrospinal fluid analysis, neurologic examination findings, and age at the onset of seizures as predictors for results of magnetic resonance imaging of the brain in dogs examined because of seizures: 115 cases (1992–2000). Journal of the American Veterinary Medical Association 6, 781–4.

CASE, L.C., LING, G.V., RUBY, A.L., JOHNSON, D.L., FRANTI, C.E., STEVENS, F. (1993): Urolithiasis in Dalmations: 275 cases (1981–1990). Journal of American Veterinary Medical Association 1, 96–100.

DE LAHUNTA, A. (1983): Veterinary Neuroanatomy and Clinical Neurology-2nd edition, W.B. Saunders Company, Philadelphia, USA.

EGENVALL, A., BONNETT, B.N., OLSON, P., HEDHAMMAR, A. (2000): Gender, age and breed pattern of diagnosis for veterinary care in insured dogs in Sweden during 1996. Veterinary Records 19, 551–7.

FALCO, M.J., BARKER, J., WALLEACE, M.E. (1974): The genetics of epilepsy in the British Alsatian. Journal of Small Animal Practice 15, 685–692.

FLÜHMANN, G., DOHERR, M., JAGGY, A. (2003): Descriptive epidemiology of neurological diseases in canine hospital admissions between 1989 and 2000. Vet. med. Dissertation.

FORRESTER, S.D. (1989): Current concepts in the management of canine epilepsy. Compendium on Continuing Education for the Practising Veterinarian 11, 811–820.

GANDINI, G., CIZINAUSKAS, S., LANG, J., FATZER, R., JAGGY, A. (2003): Fibrocartilaginous embolism in 75 dogs: clinical findings and factors influencing the recovery rate. Journal of Small Animal Practice 2, 76–80.

GERARD, V.A., CORNACK, C.N. (1991): Identifying the cause of an early onset of seizures in puppies with epileptic parents, Journal of Veterinary Internal Medicine 11, 1060–1061.

GLOOR, P., FARIELLO, R.G. (1988): Generalized epilepsy: Some of its cellular mechanisms differ from those of focal epilepsy. Trends Neuroscience 11, 63–68.

GUPTILL, L., GICKMAN, L., GLICKMAN, N. (2003): Time trends and risk factors for diabetes mellitus in dogs: analysis of veterinary medical data base records (1970–1999). Veterinary Journal 3, 240–7.

HARKIN, K.R., ANDREWS, G.A., NIETFELD, J.C. (2002): Dysautonomia in dogs: 65 cases (1993–2000). Journal of American Veterinary Medical Association 5, 633–9.

HEYNOLD, Y., FAISSLER, D., STEFFEN, F., JAGGY, A. (1997): Clinical, epidemiological and treatment results of idiopathic epilepsy in 54 Labrador Retrievers: a long term study, Journal of Small Animal Practice 38, 7–14.

HOERLEIN, B.F.: Intervertebral disk disease. In OLIVER J.E., HOERLEIN B.F., MAYHEW, I.G. (1987): Veterinary Neurology, W.B. Saunders Company, Philadelphia, USA.

A6

HOLLIDAY, T.A. Epilepsy in animals. In FREY, H-H., JANZ, D. (1985): Handbook of Experimental Pharmacology, Springer-Verlag, 55–76.

HOLLIDAY, T.A (1980): Seizure disorders. Veterinary Clinics of North America 10: 3–29.

HOLLIDAY, T.A., Cunningham J.G., Gutnick M.J. (1971): Comparative clinical and electroencephalographic studies of canine epilepsy. Epilepsia 11, 281–292.

JAGGY, A., BERNARDINI, M. (1998): Idiopathic epilepsy in 125 dogs: a long term study. Clinical and electroencephalographic findings. Journal of Small Animal Practice 39, 23–29.

KATHMANN, I., JAGGY, A., GAILLARD, C. (1999): Clinical and genetic investigations of idiopathic epilepsy in the Bernese mountain dog, Journal of Small Animal Practice 40: 319–325.

LING, G.V., RUBY, A.L., JOHNSON, D.L., THURMOND, M., FRANTI, C.E. (1998): Renal calculi in dogs and cats: prevalence, mineral type, breed, age, and gender interrelationships (1981–1993). Journal of Veterinary Internal Medicine 1, 11–21.

MOORE, G.E., BURKMAN, K.D., CARTER, M.N., PETERSON, M.R. (2001): Causes of death or reasons for euthanasia in military working dogs: 927 cases (1993–1996). Journal of American Veterinary Medical Association 2, 209–14.

OLBY, N., LEVINE, J., HARRIS, T., MUNANA, K., SKEEN, T, SHARP, N. (2003): Long-term functional outcome of dogs with severe injuries of the thoracolumbar spinal cord: 87 cases (1996–2001). Journal of American Veterinary Medical Association 11, 1502–3.

OLIVER, J.E., LORENZ, M.D., KORNEGAY, J.N. (1997): Handbook of Veterinary Neurology-3rd edition, W.B. Saunders Company, Philadelphia, USA.

OLIVER, J.E.: Seizure disorders and narcolepsy. In OLIVER, J.E., HOERLEIN, B.F., MAYHEW, I.G. (1987): Veterinary Neurology, W.B. Saunders Company, Philadelphia, 285–302.

OLIVER, J.E. (1978): Protocol for the diagnosis of seizure disorders in companion animals. Journal of American Veterinary Medical Association 172, 822–824.

SHELTON, G.D., SCHULE, A., KASS, P.H. (1997): Risk factors for acquired myasthenia gravis in dogs: 1,154 cases (1991–1995). Journal of American Veterinary Medical Association 11, 1428–31.

SRENK, P., JAGGY, A., GAILLARD, C., HORIN, P. (1994): Genetische Grundlagen der idiopathischen Epilepsie beim Golden Retriever. Tierärztliche Praxis 22, 574–8.

VAN DER VELDEN, A. (1968): Fits in Tervueren shepherd dogs: A presumed hereditary trait. Journal of Small Animal Practice 9, 63–70.

VANDEVELDE, M., FANKHAUSER, R. (1987): Einführung in die veterinärmedizinische Neurologie. Paul Parey Verlag, Hamburg und Berlin.

VANDEVELDE, M., JAGGY, A., LANG, J. (2001): Veterinärmedizinische Neurologie. Paul Parey Verlag, Berlin und Wien.

WALLACE, M.E. Keeshonds (1975): A genetic study of epilepsy and EEG readings. Journal of Small Animal Practice 16, 1–10.

A6

Subject Index

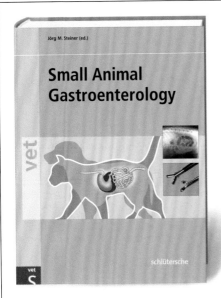

Jörg M. Steiner (ed.)

Small Animal Gastroenterology

2008. 384 pages, 281 illustrations,
8 ½ × 11"
ISBN 978-3-89993-027-6
€ 129,–

Gastrointestinal disorders are common in canine and feline patients and diagnosis and treatment require up-to-date knowledge of this expanding field. This book is designed to be both a pracitcal companion for veterinarians in general practice and a concise, yet comprehensive, resource for veterinary students, interns, and residents.

The book is structured into different sections. The first section covers diagnostic tools and provides a rational approach to common clinical problems. In the second section, diseases affecting each portion of the gastrointestinal tract are discussed in detail.

"The book is practical and is therefore eminently suitable for undergraduates and qualified veterinary surgeons alike. It is highly readable, and for those with more inquiring minds wanting to know about the 'scientific evidence', there are fairly extensive reference lists at the end of each chapter. Overall, I would highly recommend that this gastroenterology text is slotted swiftly between 'farming' and 'horses' on veterinary practice shelves."

The Veterinary Record

Contents

Diagnosis of Gastrointestinal Disorders
- Diagnostic Tools
- Clinical Evaluation of Dogs and Cats with Specific Clinical Signs

Diseases of the Gastrointestinal Tract
- Esophagus
- Stomach
- Small Intestine
- Large Intestine
- Liver
- Exocrine Pancreas
- Diseases that affect more than one Organ of the Gastrointestinal Tract

The authors

Jörg M. Steiner, Dr. med. vet., PhD, DACVIM, DECVIM-CA, Associate Professor of Small Animal Internal Medicine and Director of GI Laboratory, Texas A&M, University, USA

schlütersche

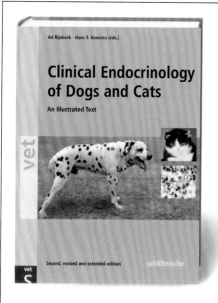

Ad Rijnberk · Hans S. Kooistra (eds.)

**Clinical Endocrinology
of Dogs and Cats**

An Illustrated Text
Second, revised and extended edition

2010. 352 pages, 446 coloured photographs,
radiographs and drawings, 20 tables
8 ½ × 11"
ISBN 978-3-89993-058-0
€ 119,–

The authors describe all the important endocrine diseases in the dog and cat. The case-oriented and organ-centered structure of the book as well as its numerous illustrations facilitate the use of the information in clinical practice. The second edition has been thoroughly revised and extended.

The chapters deal with separate endocrine glands, beginning with a brief review of the morphology and physiology of the gland, complete with drawings depicting the functional principles. This is followed by descriptions of the disorders of the gland with up-to-date information on diagnosis and treatment. Numerous photographs from clinical cases illustrate the presenting symptoms and the results of treatment. These pictures will be found to aid the reader in learning to recognize the endocrine diseases.

The clearly arranged diagnostic and therapeutic protocols in addition to flow diagrams on the most important clinical problems help simplify the attainment of a rapid and firm diagnosis.
This reference book is the definitive guide to endocrine problems in small animal practice.

Contents

- Fundamentals of Endocrinology
- Hypothalamo-Pituarity System
- Thyroids
- Adrenals
- Endocrine Pancreas
- Gonadal Development and Disorders in Sexual Differentiation
- Testes, Ovaries
- Calciotropic Hormones

- Parathyroids
- Bone Metabolism
- Tissue Hormones and Humoral Manifestation of Cancer
- Obesity
- Protocoles for Function Tests
- Treatment Protocoles
- Algorithms

The authors

Prof. Ad Rijnberk and Dr. Hans Kooistra are associated with the Department of Clinical Sciences of Companion Animals at Utrecht University, The Netherlands, and are internationally acknowledged in the field of clinical endocrinology of dogs and cats. They have prepared the book with the close cooperation and contribution of experts in the fields of biochemistry, diagnostic imaging, endocrinology, genetics, pathobiology, and reproduction.

schlütersche

CD-ROM to book

The enclosed CD-ROM contains video sequences demonstrating the neurological examination and use of visual diagnostics.

Part 1 "Clinical investigation" shows and explains the individual steps of the examination: (1) Mental status, behaviour, posture; (2) Gait; (3) Cranial nerves; (4) Postural and placement reactions; (5) Spinal reflexes; and (6) Sensation.

Part 2 "Clinical cases" provides demonstration material of neurological diseases affecting various localizations.

Instructions for use

Normally, the CD-ROM will start automatically when inserted (Autostart). If the Autostart is deactivated, then you can open the software application by doing a double click on **"start"**.

System requirements

CD-ROM drive
Pentium III 800 MHz
129 MB (RAM)
Windows 2000/Me/XP
AGP Interface is recommended
20 MB free hard disk space